Problem-based
Feline Medicine

For Elsevier:

Commissioning Editor: Joyce Rodenhuis
Development Editor: Rita Demetriou-Swanwick
Project Manager: Anne Dickie
Design Direction: Andy Chapman

Problem-based Feline Medicine

Edited by

Jacquie Rand BVSc (Hons), DVSc (Guelph),

Dip ACVIM (Int. Med.)

Professor of Companion Animal Health
Director, Centre for Companion Animal Health
School of Veterinary Science
The University of Queensland
Australia

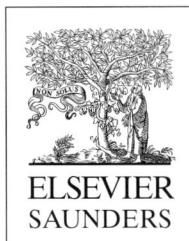

ELSEVIER
SAUNDERS

Edinburgh London New York Oxford Philadelphia St Louis Sydney Toronto 2006

ELSEVIER
SAUNDERS

© 2006, Elsevier Limited. All rights reserved.

First published 2006
Reprinted 2007 (three times), 2008

ISBN 978 0 7020 2488 7

British Library Cataloguing in Publication Data
A catalogue record for this book is available from the British Library

Library of Congress Cataloging in Publication Data
A catalog record for this book is available from the Library of Congress

Printed in China

Contents

Contributors

Abrams-Ogg, A – Department of Clinical Studies, Ontario Veterinary College, University of Guelph, Guelph, Ontario, Canada

Arrington, K.A. – Beltway Emergency Animal Hospital, Glenn Dale, MD, USA

Bagley, R.S – Associate Professor, Department of Veterinary Clinical Sciences, College of Veterinary Medicine, Washington State University, Pullman, WA, USA

Barber P.† – **Formerly** Lecturer, Department of Veterinary Clinical Studies, University of Edinburgh Hospital for Small Animals, Roslin, Midlothian, UK

Bartges, J.W. – Professor of Medicine and Nutrition, and The Acree Endowed Chair of Small Animal Research, College of Veterinary Medicine, University of Tennessee, Knoxville, Tennessee, USA.

Bernays, M. – Staff Veterinary Ophthalmologist, Animal Eye Services, MacGregor, Queensland, Australia

Boothe, D.M. – Anatomy, Physiology and Pharmacology, College of Veterinary Medicine, Auburn University, Auburn, Alabama, USA

Braz-Ruivo, L.A.H. – Beltway Emergency Animal Hospital, Glenn Dale, MD, USA

Breathnach, R.M.S – School of Agriculture, Food Science and Veterinary Medicine, University College Dublin, Belfield, Dublin, Ireland

Burton, G. – Animal Allergy and Dermatology Service, Springwood, Queensland, Australia

Campbell, F. – Veterinary Medical Teaching Hospital, University of California, Davis CA, USA

Cuddon, P.A. – Neurological Center for Animals, Lakewood, CO, USA

Dowers, K.L. – Department of Clinical Sciences, College of Veterinary Medicine & Biomedical Sciences, Colorado State University, Fort Collins, CO, USA

Filippich, L.J. – School of Veterinary Science, University of Queensland, Brisbane, Queensland, Australia

Gunn-Moore, D. – Senior Lecturer, Head of Feline Clinic, University of Edinburgh Hospital for Small Animals, Easter Bush Veterinary Centre, Roslin, Midlothian, UK

Jergens, A.E. – Associate Professor, CVMBS-VTH Veterinary Clinical Sciences, Iowa State University, Ames IA, USA

Johnstone, I.P. – Adjunct Associate Professor, Veterinary Teaching Hospital, School of Veterinary Science, University of Queensland, Brisbane, Queensland, Australia

Jones, B.R. – Professor of Small Animal Clinical Studies and Dean, School of Agriculture, Food Science and Veterinary Medicine, University College Dublin, Belfield, Dublin, Ireland

King, T. – Veterinary Specialist Services, Underwood, Queensland, Australia

Lappin, M.R. – Professor, CVMBS-VTH, Clinical Sciences, Colorado State University, Fort Collins, CO, USA

Levy, J. – Department of Small Animal Clinical Sciences, College of Veterinary Medicine, University of Florida, Gainesville, FL, USA

Litster, A.L. – School of Veterinary Science, University of Queensland, Brisbane, Queensland, Australia

Maddison, J.E. – Royal Veterinary College, North Mymms, Hatfield Hertfordshire, UK

Mason, R.A. – Oceanview Veterinary Specialists Nikken Wellness Consultant, Healthy Achievements International, Mill Creek, WA, USA

McCarthy, G.M. – School of Agriculture, Food Science and Veterinary Medicine, University College Dublin, Belfield, Dublin, Ireland

Menrath, V.H. – Adjunct Associate Professor, Creek Road Cat Clinic Pty Ltd, Mount Gravatt, Queensland, Australia

Miller, J.B. – Professor, Department of Companion Animals, Atlantic Veterinary College, University of Prince Edward Island, Charlottetown PE, Canada.

Parent, J. M. – Professor, Department of Veterinary Clinical Studies, Ontario Veterinary College, University of Guelph, Guelph, Ontario, Canada

Quesnel A.D.[†] – Formerly Professeure agrégée, Département de sciences cliniques, Université de Montréal, Faculté de médecine vétérinaire, Quebec, Canada

Rand, J.S. – School of Veterinary Science, University of Queensland, Brisbane, Queensland, Australia

Seksel, K. – Sydney Animal Behaviour Service, Seaforth, New South Wales, Australia

Shipstone, M. – Dermatology for Animals, Stafford Heights, Queensland, Australia

Smith, R.I.E. – Veterinary Ophthalmologist, Animal Eye Services, MacGregor, Queensland, Australia

Straw, R.C. – Director, Animal Cancer Care and Brisbane Veterinary Specialist Centre, Albany Creek, Queensland, Australia

Thomson, M. – Animal Cancer Care, School of Veterinary Science, The University of Queensland, Brisbane, Queensland, Australia

Wilson, G.J. – Animal Dental & Oral Care, Wellington Pt, Queensland, Australia

Zoran, D. – Small Animal Medicine and Surgery, CVM, Texas A & M University, College Station, TX, USA

† **Deceased**.

Preface

Problem-based feline medicine was inspired by teaching students in the clinic, and from consulting to veterinarians in practice. It was apparent that the way veterinary medicine was traditionally taught often caused problems when the students were in the clinic. Many times they did very well in written examinations, but could not utilize the material taught to make a diagnosis in the clinic. Traditional disease-based text books, divided into sections based on aetiology, assumed the clinician knew whether the disease was viral or bacterial, fungal or metabolic. Clients usually do not say "my cat has feline leukaemia and what is the most appropriate treatment". They say "my cat is losing weight and is not as active as normal". The dilemma for students is, which page of a text-book do I to turn to? Making a diagnosis is the most important part of being a veterinarian, because without a diagnosis, determining appropriate treatment is problematic.

My hope is that this book will support students and veterinarians in practice, and assist them in turning to the "right page" for the information they need to make a diagnosis. A challenge in writing a book like this, is the duplication of material, and differences between authors when writing about the same disease in different chapters. I think this contributes to the richness of information in the book, and reflects that life it is not black and white, and there are different opinions based on different experiences.

One difficulty students had using the acronym DAMNPIT, was that in formulating a list of likely diseases causing the problem, they often omitted obvious diseases. When they first listed the organs or body systems that could cause the signs, and then used DAMNPIT, it increased their score rate. Sometimes the organ system is not evident when the signs are not organ-specific, and to help them walk through the thought processes, they were first encouraged to answer the question "What mechanisms can be responsible for these signs?" Hence the first section in the summary table and introduction answers the questions: "What mechanism/s causes this problem?" (MECHANISM?), "Which organs or body systems cause this problem?" (WHERE?), "What diseases/s cause this problem?" (WHAT?)

The format for each chapter is the same. The chapter title is based on a presenting sign. A summary page lists the answers to "MECHANISM?", "WHERE?", and "WHAT?" This is followed by a quick reference guide to the diseases that should be considered as potential rule-outs. They are starred with 0-3 stars to indicate how important the disease is as a cause of the problem. Some diseases are common but rarely cause the sign (problem), and they did not get

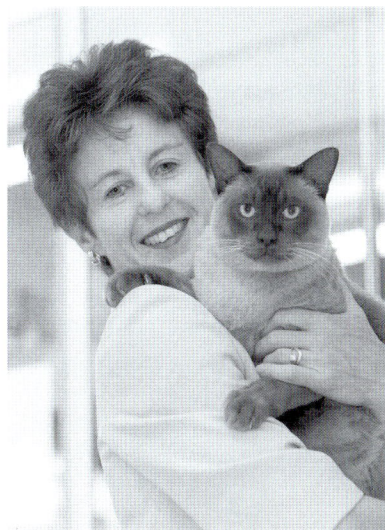

xi

a frequency star. Next is the introduction, which in more detail describes "MECHANISM?", "WHERE?", and "WHAT?". This is followed by the diseases, roughly listed in order of likelihood of causing the sign. Therefore, diseases with 3 stars are listed before those with no stars, that are rare causes of the signs. Some suggested reading lists are included if the reader wants to delve further. Although Veterinary Information Network (VIN) is not referenced specifically for most chapters, the reader is encouraged to utilize VIN to check new developments, particularly in diagnostic tests and treatment.

Strive for excellence and enjoy. Remember, making a diagnosis is one of the most important things you do as a veterinarian.

If you have suggestions for the next edition of the book, I would love to hear them (contact me by email: *j.rand@uq.edu.au*).

Jacquie

This book is dedicated to those who shaped my life:

To my dad who taught me that "if a job is worth doing, it is worth doing well", and that "a job is not done until it is finished".

To my mum who has always been a cheerful supporter in all the twists and turns in my life.

To the students who inspired, taught and challenged me.

To my husband Tom, my rock, my safe and welcoming harbor, and my sanctuary in stormy seas.

To my daughter Lisette, who reminded me when it was time to play, and the importance of having a balanced life.

Thank you all and bless you

Acknowledgments

There are many people I would like to thank who have helped turn my vision of a problem-based text into a reality. Firstly, the contributing authors, who helped make this text happen when it became apparent that it was expanding into too big a vision for one person to accomplish. Secondly, to Annette Litster who proof read many chapters, and joined as a contributing author late in the project, responding cheerfully to urgent requests to write and subedit the gastrointestinal tract section. Thirdly, to the many staff and students who helped with formatting the manuscript and editing, including Heidi Farrow, Joanne Chapel, Philippa Williams, Sarah Gestier and Desley Badrick.

I would like to acknowledge the invaluable resource of the Veterinary Information Network (VIN), which greatly assisted in my commitment to include the most recent material and practical information. Although sometimes the information sourced from VIN is not referenced in the text, I would especially like to acknowledge the usefulness and great support that this database provides to veterinarians in practice and academia.

I would also like to acknowledge the veterinary class of '95 at the University of Queensland, who inspired me to embark on this project, and all the students, before and after, who reinforced the belief that this format would help veterinarians in practice.

In the early mornings, Merlin our Burmese cat provided me with company and inspiration while I worked on the manuscript, by sitting on the keyboard, on pages I was reading, or on my lap purring.

Lastly, but most importantly, this book would not have been possible without the support and love of my husband Tom and daughter Lisette.

1. How to make a problem-based diagnosis

Jacquie Rand

- Competence at making a diagnosis is the most important part of being a veterinarian. Therefore, it is the most important skill learnt in veterinary education. High-level surgery skills and in-depth knowledge of drugs may be useless if the wrong diagnosis is made.
- Making a diagnosis involves problem-solving. If clinical signs are treated without first making a diagnosis, it is likely that corticosteroids, antibiotics and euthanasia will be over-prescribed.

There are two ways to make a diagnosis. Firstly there is the **"expert method"**. This is the way many veterinarians make a diagnosis, and it involves pattern recognition.

The disadvantages of the "expert method" are that it requires a lot of experience to be accurate, and there is a greater chance of being wrong, especially for the less-experienced practitioner, because the same signs may occur for many diseases. For example, diarrhea may be caused by many diseases including intestinal parasites, food intolerance, intussusception, lymphoma and inflammatory bowel disease. The appropriate treatment varies depending on the diagnosis.

The second method of making a diagnosis is by using a **problem-based approach**. This leads to fewer mistakes and facilitates better veterinary practice.

KEY ELEMENTS FOR MAKING A PROBLEM-BASED DIAGNOSIS

To make a problem-based diagnosis, the signs exhibited are separated out into individual problems, and each problem is considered separately.

The individual steps in making a problem-based diagnosis are as follows.

1. Obtain detailed data from a complete history and physical examination.

Take an exact and detailed history. It is critical that questions are asked to cover a detailed history in all areas of the pet's health, not just for the problem presented. To get the correct information it may be necessary to ask the same question in different ways.

Complete a thorough physical examination.

The history and physical examination are the most critical parts of making a diagnosis.

Diagnostic tests may not overcome deficiencies in the history and physical examination. For example, if hematology and biochemistry analyses were performed but a chest radiograph was not taken because increased frequency of coughing was missed in the history, or dyspnea was missed on the physical examination, a primary lung tumor may be missed despite performing many other tests to determine the cause of lethargy.

- Normal physical examination findings need to be appreciated before abnormal findings can be identified. Veterinary students are encouraged to take every opportunity to practice physical examinations so the range of normal is recognized.

2. **List the problems identified** based on the history and physical examination.

It is important to only **list the problem at the level that it is understood.** For example, if the cat has an abdominal mass, the problem is initially listed as an abdominal mass and not a neoplasm, because it may be caused by a number of other conditions including reactive lymphadenomegaly, feces, abscess, etc.

Characterize each problem listed based on duration, character and severity.

Characterize each problem by the 3 Cs:
- Chronicity (duration)
- Character
- Concern (severity/frequency/size).
  - For example, the problem "sneezing and nasal discharge" may be characterized as 2 months duration (chronicity), purulent (character), occurring approximately six times/day (i.e. moderate severity).

Select the problem/s to consider first. Choose those that are most likely to provide a diagnosis.

Choose problems for consideration first that are:
- **Severe or frequent problems.** Problems that are infrequent or mild may not lead to the main definitive diagnosis as quickly, or may be independent problems.
- **Represent the problem the owner was concerned about.**
- **Problems that are most specific for an organ or body system.** Avoid using non-specific problems such as lethargy or anorexia. These problems indicate severity of the problem, but are not organ-specific and can be caused by almost any disease in the body. They are not useful diagnostically because they require a wide range of diagnostic tests to be performed in an attempt to detect an organ-specific abnormality.

3. **List the differential diagnoses** (likely diseases) for each problem. To formulate a list of differentials, it helps to ask two questions, "WHERE?" and "WHAT?".

To answer **"WHERE?"**, ask yourself which organs or body systems can cause the problem?

If possible, try to first categorize the answer to "WHERE?" into sub-headings. For example, for seizures, the problem could have extra-cranial or intra-cranial causes. Similarly, for vomiting, there could be extra-gastrointestinal or gastrointestinal causes; and for jaundice, the sub-headings pre-hepatic, hepatic, and post-hepatic are appropriate.

"WHERE?" for an abdominal mass includes liver, GIT, spleen, urinary tract, omentum, reproductive tract, etc. "WHERE?" for alopecia is skin; "WHERE?" for PU/PD is kidney, which is the end organ influencing water intake and urine output. It is usually better to simplify the answer in this way, rather than listing all the organs that can cause polyuria/polydipsia, although this can also be done, e.g. kidney, liver, brain, kidney, adrenal, bladder, etc.

To answer "WHERE?", you may have to answer the question what is the **"MECHANISM?"** that results in this problem, and use your knowledge of pathophysiologic principles to answer "WHERE"?
- For example, abdominal effusion can be due to:
  - Decreased oncotic pressure as a consequence of hypoalbuminemia resulting from liver, GIT or kidney dysfunction.
  - Increased hydrostatic pressure resulting from cardiac disease or vascular obstruction.
  - Increased permeability of blood vessel walls.
  - Lymphatic obstruction involving abdominal lymphatics.

If the answer to "WHERE?" is more than one organ system, then **diagnostic tests are usually required to localize the problem.** For example, for an abdominal mass, results of diagnostic tests such as a serum biochemistry profile (showing increased liver enzymes), radiography (indicating hepatomegaly), and/or ultrasound (revealing a mass in area of liver), may be required to answer the question WHERE? (liver).

Once the organ systems involved have been identified, you can move on to answering the question **"WHAT?"**. That is, for each organ or body system identified as potentially being involved, what diseases are potential causes of the problem?

- **To assist in listing the diseases that can cause the problem, it helps to use an acronym such as DAMNPIT to aid the memory.**

D :	*	degenerative
A :	*	anomaly (congenital)
	*	accident (e.g. volvulus, intussusception)
M :	*	metabolic (e.g. electrolyte, hormonal)
	*	mechanical (e.g. foreign body, urolith)
N :	*	neoplastic
	*	nutritional

P : * physical (e.g. heat, cold, water, fire)
      * psychological
      * pharmacological (drug effect)

I : * infectious (viral, bacterial, mycoplasma, rickettsial, protozoal, fungal, parasitic)
      * immune
      * iatrogenic (caused by you)
      * idiopathic (unknown)
      * infarct

T : * trauma
      * toxic/adverse drug

For example, the answer to "WHAT?" diseases could cause polyuria/polydipsia in a 10-year-old male castrated domestic shorthair cat that has a history of losing weight for 2 months, a good appetite until the last couple of days, frequently urinating in the litter box, and drinking 1 liter/day include:

D :   Chronic renal failure

A :

M :   Diabetes mellitus
               Diabetes insipidus
               Hyperthyroidism
               Hyperadrenocorticism
               Hepatic failure
               Hypercalcemia
               Acromegaly
               Hypoadrenocorticism
               Hypercalcemia

N :   Renal neoplasia
               Lymphoma and
                  pseudohyperparathyroidism
               Polycythemia vera

P :

I : Infectious   Pyelonephritis
                      Cystic endometrial hyperplasia/
                         pyometra
      Immune   Glomerulonephritis/renal
                         amyloidosis

T :   Vitamin D toxicity
               Drugs such as
                 corticosteroids

After listing the diseases, rank the diseases as likely, possible or unlikely based on cross-matching the patient's data with the characteristics of the disease.

To rank diseases as likely, possible, or unlikely, **cross-match** the patient's signalment (breed, age, gender), clinical signs, and physical examination findings **with the known characteristics of the disease including** typical signalment, signs and physical examination findings of the disease and frequency of disease (how common it is).

● For the differential diagnosis "diabetes mellitus", consider whether the typical signalment, history and physical examination findings of this disease fit the patients findings. An example of the thought processes are the following: Diabetes mellitus is a **very likely** cause of the problem because it occurs in older cats, male cats are more often affected, and the patient has all the expected signs, including signs of chronic disease, polydipsia and polyuria, weight loss and a good appetite until recently. The high volume of water drunk by this cat can occur with diabetes mellitus.

● For the differential diagnosis, "chronic renal failure" an example of the thought processes is: Chronic renal failure is a **possible** cause of the problem because the expected signs include evidence of a chronic disease, with weight loss and recent inappetence. However, cats with renal failure that have marked polydipsia often have a more picky appetite once weight loss is apparent, and the volume of water drunk is usually less.

● For the differential diagnosis "hepatic failure", an example of the thought processes is: Hepatic failure is an **unlikely** cause of this cat's problem because although this cat has some of the clinical signs expected with hepatic failure, it does not have all of the typical signs. The signs of this patient that fit include: chronic disease with lethargy, inappetence and weight loss. Polydipsia can occasionally occur if there is liver failure. However, cats with hepatic failure sufficient to cause weight loss and affect renal concentrating mechanisms are usually inappetent and jaundiced. In addition, hepatic failure is a rare cause of polydipsia in cats.

● It helps to know **1–5 lines of information for each disease on your list of differential diagnoses. You should know more about the common diseases than uncommon diseases**. Learn the typical signalment, clinical signs, physical examination findings, and frequency of diseases that occur in your area.

4. Formulate a **diagnostic plan** to prove or disprove each possible disease. **Choose the initial diagnostic tests based on**:

- Prioritizing, ruling in or out the most likely diseases
- Choose tests initially that are least invasive, and to some extent easiest and/or cheapest to perform
- Choose the tests that have the best combination of specificity and sensitivity.

Remember that each negative or normal test result makes the list shorter.

For example, for the problem "liver mass" that was identified based on ultrasound, radiology and biochemistry profile, the following is an example of a diagnostic plan.

- Following ultrasound identification of the mass, fine-needle biopsy and cytological examination will be performed, with culture requested if no neoplastic cells are obvious. Although the sensitivity and specificity are not as high as with a wedge biopsy or laparotomy, it is balanced by the less-invasive nature, ease and cost. These diagnostic decisions need to be made in conjunction with the owner.
- If a definitive diagnosis is not possible from the results of the fine-needle biopsy, the next diagnostic tests that could be considered would be a needle biopsy suitable for histological examination, or laparotomy and wedge biopsy. The decision will require balanced consideration of many factors including input from the owner regarding cost, invasiveness, etc.

5. **Formulate a rational treatment plan** based on the diagnoses identified.

- Treatment may either be specific for a disease process, such as antibiotics and drainage of an abscess, or be non-specific, for example, IV fluids for dehydration. Initial treatment plans will often be formulated in parallel with diagnostic plans, because some problems such as dehydration or cyanosis need addressing early.

6. As diagnostic data are received and the response to initial therapy is observed, it is important to update the **problem list, differential diagnoses, diagnostic plan and treatment plan.**

Summary of the steps in making a problem-based diagnosis

1. Obtain data from a detailed history and physical examination.
2. List the problems identified based on the history and physical examination.
3. List the differential diagnoses for the major and most organ-specific problems.

   Use your answers to "WHERE?" and "WHAT?" to formulate a logical list of differential diagnoses. Cross-match the patient and disease characteristics to identify the most likely diseases.
4. Formulate a diagnostic plan to rule-in or rule-out the likely differential diagnoses.
5. Formulate a treatment plan.
6. Update points 2–5 as diagnostic data become available and the response to therapy is observed.

USING THE BOOK

This book is set out to facilitate making a problem-based diagnosis. At the start of each chapter there is a summary of the answers to the questions 'Mechanism?', 'Where?', and 'What?' for each problem. A quick reference summary lists the diseases that can be associated with that problem. Stars after each disease denote the importance of the disease as a cause of the problem.

PART 1

Cat with upper respiratory tract signs

2. The cat with acute sneezing or nasal discharge

Jacquie Rand

KEY SIGNS

- Serous, mucoid, purulent or bloody nasal discharge less than 2 weeks' duration.
- Acute sneezing or snuffling.

MECHANISM?

- Signs of acute sneezing or nasal discharge usually result from viral, chlamydophilial or mycoplasmal infection.

WHERE?

- Nose (nasal cavity, paranasal sinuses).

WHAT?

- Most cats (80%) with acute onset of sneezing or nasal discharge have calicivirus or herpesvirus.

QUICK REFERENCE SUMMARY

Diseases causing acute sneezing or nasal discharge

MECHANICAL

- Foreign body (p 15)

Acute onset of sneezing and rubbing face, progressing to chronic discharge, often unilateral, no systemic signs.

NEOPLASIA

- Bleeding ulcer on external nares (p 16)

Acute sneezing and bleeding may occur with a bleeding ulcer on the external nares, particularly the nasal septum. Usually caused by squamous cell carcinoma (SCC), but occurs occasionally with eosinophilic granuloma or associated with acute calicivirus infection. Signs are often episodic with squamous cell carcinoma.

- Intranasal tumors (p 17)

Occasionally present with acute sneezing, ± nasal discharge and bleeding.

INFECTIOUS

Bacterial:

- *Bordetella bronchiseptica* (p 14)

Pyrexia, sneezing, nasal discharge, mandibular lymphadenopathy, coughing and dyspnea.

Viral:

- **Feline rhinotracheitis virus (herpesvirus-1)*** (p 7)**

Paroxysms of sneezing, severe serous to mucopurulent oculonasal discharge, usually bilateral severe conjunctivitis with tearing, photophobia and chemosis, ± corneal lesions.

- **Feline calicivirus*** (p 11)**

Fever, mild upper respiratory tract signs, oral ulcers.

Chlamydophila, Mycoplasma:

- **Chlamydophila felis (Chlamydophila felis)**(p 13)**

Mainly conjunctivitis, initially unilateral, later bilateral and often chronic.

- *Mycoplasma* (p 14)

Mainly conjunctivitis, usually without systemic illness; often occurs as secondary infection in viral upper respiratory tract disease.

Fungal:

- *Cryptococcus* (p 16)

Usually chronic signs, but occasionally acute onset of sneezing and nasal discharge.

Immune:

- Allergic (p 17)

Serous or mucoid ocular and/or nasal discharge, without systemic signs. Signs may be seasonal in occurrence.

INTRODUCTION

MECHANISM?

Signs of acute sneezing or nasal discharge indicate inflammation of the nasal cavity, which in cats is almost always the result of infection, usually viral or associated with chlamydophilia or mycoplasma.

WHERE?

Nose (nasal cavity, paranasal sinuses).

WHAT?

Most cats (80%) with acute onset of sneezing or nasal discharge have calicivirus or herpesvirus.

DISEASES CAUSING ACUTE SNEEZING OR NASAL DISCHARGE

FELINE RHINOTRACHEITIS VIRUS (FELINE HERPESVIRUS-1), "RHINO" OR "SNUFFLES"***

> ### Classical signs
>
> - Acute onset of sneezing, pyrexia, depression.
> - Marked discharge from eyes and nose, initially serous but progressing to mucopurulent.
> - Severe conjunctivitis with chemosis and photophobia.
> - Corneal keratitis or ulcers in some cats.
> - Generally less than 10–14 days duration.

For more details of ocular changes see page 1212 (The Cat With Ocular Discharge or Changed Conjunctival Appearance) and page 1237 (The Cat With Abnormalities Confined to the Cornea).

Pathogenesis

Herpesvirus causes an **acute infection of the upper respiratory tract**, conjunctiva and cornea.

Virus multiplication is **temperature restricted**, and most lesions occur on cooler mucosal-epithelial surfaces, e.g. nasopharynx, conjunctiva, turbinates.

Necrosis of epithelium occurs within 24–48 h of viral contact.

Signs occur **2 to 6 days after infection.**

Secondary bacterial infection of lesions usually occurs, producing purulent ocular-nasal discharges.

Osteolysis of the turbinate bones may occur.

Virus may cause **corneal necrosis** resulting in keratitis, ulceration, and occasionally corneal rupture and loss of the eye.

Concurrent infections with calicivirus, *Chlamydophila*, *Mycoplasma* or *Bordetella bronchiseptica* are common, and may alter the clinical signs.

Clinical signs

Earliest sign is paroxysms of sneezing.

Severe conjunctivitis occurs, with tearing, photophobia and chemosis.

Severe ocular and nasal discharges occur which are initially serous, but progress rapidly to mucopurulent. Discharge is typically more marked than with calicivirus.

Later, discharge and crusting of nares and conjunctiva may produce nasal obstruction and sealing of the eyelids.

Anorexia, depression and pyrexia are common; dehydration may occur.

Tracheal and bronchial inflammation may result in coughing and dyspnea, and occasionally bacterial pneumonia occurs in kittens.

Very rarely, ulceration on the nose or tongue occurs, but this is much more frequent with calicivirus infection.

Corneal involvement resulting in keratitis may occur 1–2 weeks later. Keratitis is visible as corneal cloudiness (edema and inflammation), and punctate or branching ulcers, which may coalesce to large ulcers.

Corneal perforation and secondary bacterial infection may result in destruction of the eye; this occurs more often in young kittens (ophthalmia neonatorium).

Herpesvirus keratitis often occurs in the absence of signs of active upper respiratory tract infection.

Infection of the pregnant queen may lead to fetal absorption, **abortion,** or kittens either born infected or developing signs shortly after birth.

Signs in newborn kittens include continuous crying, nasal discharge, sneezing and dyspnea.

Signs are worse in:
- **Young kittens** once maternal antibody levels decrease.
- **Conditions of crowding**, e.g. animal shelters, breeding colonies and pet shops.
- **Stress factors** or other **intercurrent disease**, e.g. FIV, FeLV, renal failure.

Signs of rhinotracheitis usually resolve in 2 weeks, but purulent rhinitis and sinusitis may persist longer.

Superficial ulcerative dermatitis occasionally occurs on the face, trunk and footpads. The lesions are usually more severe on the face and occur on the nasal planum or haired skin. They consist of vesicles, ulcers and crusts, and may be pruritic. Upper respiratory tract signs may or may not be present, and signs appear to occur in situations of reactivation of latent infection.

Stomatitis may be associated with latent herpesvirus infection, and may or may not occur with dermatitis.

Diagnosis

A definitive diagnosis is usually not made, and a presumptive diagnosis is based on clinical signs.

The following diagnostic tests are offered by some laboratories: **fluorescent antibody** staining of **conjunctival** or **nasal mucosal scrapings or biopsy**, antibody titers (measured initially and after convalescence), virus isolation or polymerase chain reaction (PCR).
- These are **infrequently performed** for individual cats with signs of upper respiratory tract disease, because the result rarely changes the treatment.
- Obtaining a definitive diagnosis is more useful if a cattery problem persists despite vaccination.
- Diagnostic tests are indicated to confirm herpesvirus infection if corneal ulceration is poorly responsive to treatment, but false-negative results are common.

Histopathological examination of the skin lesions indicates ulcerative dermatitis with epithelial cell necrosis and eosinophilic inflammation. Epidermal cells may contain basophilic intranuclear inclusion bodies. PCR indicates the presence of herpesvirus in skin samples.

Differential diagnoses

Calicivirus usually has milder upper respiratory signs; oral ulcers are classical; **no** keratitis or corneal ulceration; occasionally viral pneumonia occurs.

Chlamydophila generally has milder signs, although young kittens can have severe conjunctivitis and ocular-nasal discharge; typically conjunctivitis lasts longer (weeks) with Chlamydophila.

Cryptococcosis or nasal tumors may occasionally present with an acute onset of sneezing; however, signs do not resolve, but become chronic and progressive.

Concurrent FeLV or FIV should be suspected in cats with very severe, prolonged signs, or in adult vaccinated cats with severe signs, and in cats with recurrent upper respiratory disease.

See page 1213 for more details of differential diagnoses in The Cat With Ocular Discharge or Changed Conjunctival Appearance.

Treatment

Minimize hospital contamination. Cats should be treated as outpatients, unless dehydrated or requiring oxygen.

Use **broad-spectrum antibiotics** if nasal discharge is mucopurulent, indicating secondary bacterial infection.
- Antibiotics also help prevent chronic rhinitis.
- Amoxicillin, cephalosporin, doxycycline or trimethaprim-sulfadiazine are indicated.
- Doxycycline is useful if concurrent infections of *Chlamydophila*, *Mycoplasma* or *Bordetella* are suspected.

Correct dehydration and maintain optimum hydration using subcutaneous or intravenous fluids.
- Dehydration is common, because cats will not eat or drink, and marked fluid loss may occur from the ocular-nasal discharge and salivation.

Improve airflow through the respiratory tract.
- **Clean crusted discharge** from the nose three times daily.
- Use a protective agent such as vaseline on the nose to prevent excoriation.
- Use a **vaporizer or nebulizer** to provide airway humidification, or have the owners put the cat in a steamy bathroom.

- Nasal decongestants (intranasal or oral) are generally not well tolerated by cats, but can be tried.
  - **Intranasal decongestants** (e.g. pediatric preparations of phenylephrine, neosynephrine or oxymethazoline, 1 drop in one nostril) may be useful, but do not use longer than a couple of days.
  - **Oral decongestants,** e.g. ephedrine or pseudoephedrine (e.g. Sudafed) can be tried, but are unpalatable to cats, and may induce severe salivation.

Treat eyes with topical therapy. For more treatment details see page 1214 (The Cat With Ocular Discharge or Changed Conjunctival Appearance) and page 1239 (The Cat With Abnormalities Confined to the Cornea).
- Clean discharges from eyes three times daily.
- **Antibiotic eye ointment** (**without steroids**), e.g. tetracycline or tobramycin. Avoid use of bacitracin-neomycin-polymyxin ointment because of reports of acute death associated with its use.
- **Antiviral eye drops** or ointment should be used if **herpetic keratitis** is present; they may also help conjunctivitis.
  - **Idoxuridine** q 4–5 h (Dendrid, Herplex, IDU, Stoxil), **vidarabine** q 5 h (Vira-A), **trifluorothymidine** q 2–4 h for 3 weeks (Viroptic). Viroptic was the most effective of the viricidal agents in vitro, but it is expensive, and may be very irritating to the eye.

Acyclovir (100–200 mg/cat q 8–12 h, per os; Zovirax) may be useful in resistant ulcers. If using this drug monitor white and red cell counts for evidence of bone marrow suppression. The efficacy is controversial in FHV-1 infection because the enzyme involved in conversion to the active form has low activity in cats compared to humans, and the drug is 100 times less active.

L-lysine (500 mg/cat q 24 h, per os) is recommended, and may help to reduce signs and viral shedding. It competes with arginine which is essential for viral replication.

Interferon (30 IU α-interferon) orally and topically (30 u/ml in artificial tears q 6 h) daily until lesions have resolved and then taper.

Support nutrition
- **Appetite stimulants.** Use diazepam (Valium; 0.1–0.2 mg/kg, IV) and immediately place food in front of cat, or oxazepam (Serax; 2–2.5 mg/cat, PO q 12 h) or cyproheptadiene (Periactin, 1–2 mg/cat PO q 12 h) just before feeding.
- Multivitamins (A, B and C) but especially **thiamine** and vitamin A.
- **Tempt to eat** with strong smelling foods, e.g. fried chicken or sardines. Warming food to body temperature increases palatability.
- Handfeed or force feed initially.
- **Tube feed via** a naso-osophageal, esphageal or gastrostomy tube if the cat is still depressed and anorexic after 3 days.

Warmth enhances recovery because the virus is temperature sensitive (e.g. use incubator or heating pad).

Prognosis

Mortality is usually low, although may be higher (up to 30%) in young kittens.

Persistent or recurrent **chronic bacterial rhinitis and sinusitis** occurs in some cats as a result of nasal epithelium damage and osteolysis.
- Chronic rhinitis is evident as recurrent sneezing, and mucopurulent nasal discharge, which responds temporarily to antibiotics.

Scarring and **occlusion of the lacrimal ducts** may produce chronic wetting of the face from tears.

Rarely, chronic keratitis, poorly healing corneal ulcers, conjunctival adhesions (symblephron), and keratoconjunctivitis sicca occur.

Herpesvirus **ulcerative facial dermatitis or stomatitis** syndrome appears to occur in some cats in situations associated with reactivation of latent infection.

Carrier state is common (up to 80% of recovered cats), and may last years.
- Virus is shed **intermittently**, often following stress; shedding may or may not be associated with mild clinical signs.
- Glucocorticoid administration or environmental stress such as from overcrowding or relocation may predispose to reactivation of infection.

Transmission

Herpesvirus is highly contagious with rapid spread in catteries, veterinary hospitals and multicat households.

- Infection rates may reach 100% in unvaccinated cats and kittens.
- Young kittens (5–8 weeks of age) are most susceptible.
- Occasionally kittens are born with infection.

Most infections occur via direct close contact with infected cats.

- **Fomites** are also important in spread, especially unwashed hands, food, bowels and contaminated cages.
- **Airborne transmission** occurs over short distances (approximately 1.2 m (4 feet)). Virus is present in the droplets formed by sneezing.
- **Virus is shed in secretions** (ocular, nasal and oral) for 1–3 weeks after infection.

Spread in boarding catteries, shelters and veterinary hospitals is facilitated by **the high frequency of carrier cats** in the population that shed virus at times of stress or glucocorticoid treatment and may show no signs of infection.

Vertical transmission occasionally occurs from a carrier queen, resulting in kittens born with disease.

- More usually, carrier **queens shed virus 4–6 weeks after queening**, infecting kittens at the time maternal immunity is waning.

Feline herpesvirus is relatively **fragile**, and is stabile for less than 24 h outside the host.

- The virus is **susceptible to most disinfectants**.

Prevention

Vaccination

Parenteral and intranasal vaccines are available in combination with feline calicivirus vaccine.

Combinations with feline parvovirus, chlamydophila, rabies and/or feline leukemia vaccines are also available.

- **Parenteral** vaccines for subcutaneous administration are available as modified live or inactivated vaccines.
  - Administer twice with a 3–4-week interval between doses.
  - If the kitten is less than 8 weeks old at the first dose, give a third dose 3–4 weeks after the second dose.
  - If a cattery problem occurs, vaccinate litters as early as 4 weeks of age, and repeat every 3–4 weeks until 14 weeks of age.
- **Intranasal** vaccine is a modified live vaccine, which produces rapid immunity (1–4 days). Some cats have transient mild sneezing and naso-ocular discharge after vaccination.
  - Vaccinate with a single dose. If less than 10 weeks of age at the first dose, give second dose 3–4 weeks later.
  - If a cattery problem occurs, divide the dose amongst the litter and give at 2 weeks of age, and follow with a parenteral vaccination every 4 weeks until 14 weeks of age.
- The **combination of intranasal and subcutaneous vaccination** reduced the incidence of upper respiratory tract disease (31% of cats developed signs) in a shelter compared with subcutaneous vaccination alone (51% of cats developed signs), and was cost-effective.

The frequency of **booster vaccinations is controversial.** Annual boosters are typically recommended, particularly because occurrence of upper respiratory tract signs is common in vaccinated cats, especially when exposed to stress. However, measurement of serum titers suggests that humoral immunity lasts for 48 months or more. Serological titers are not equivalent to protection from challenge, although the predictive value for resistance to challenge for a positive serum antibody titer was 70% for herpesvirus and 92% for calicivirus. Additional boosters are recommended before a heavy challenge, e.g. boarding in a cattery.

Live parenteral vaccine can produce signs of upper respiratory tract disease if aerosolized or spilt on the cat's hair, so take care with administration.

Maternal antibodies can block the effect of the vaccine.

- Antibody levels vary between kittens, and **may last 5–6 weeks with herpesvirus (7–8 weeks with calicivirus)**.

Vaccinating queens 1–4 weeks before partum increases colostrum-derived maternal immunity.

- DO NOT USE WITH **LIVE** PANLEUKOPENIA VACCINE in pregnant queens.

Localized viral infection can occur in vaccinated cats, and may produce mild ocular and nasal discharge, and viral shedding.

Disease control in the cattery or shelter

Vaccinate kittens early, and vaccinate all cats regularly to maintain immunity.

Isolate sick cats, and pregnant and nursing queens from the main cattery.

Vaccinate and **isolate** incoming cats for 3 weeks.
- Avoid introducing cats that are likely carriers, i.e. from catteries with known infection problems.

Carrier queens shed virus and infect nursing kittens, therefore, remove queens that repeatedly have infected litters, or wean kittens early.

Avoid overcrowding and other causes of stress.

Clean and disinfect cages daily and **bowels** with **sodium hypochlorite** (0.175%, i.e. 1:32 dilution of household bleach) added to detergent.

FELINE CALICIVIRUS (FCV)***

> **Classical signs**
>
> - Lethargy, anorexia, fever.
> - Oral ulcers of less than 1 week duration.
> - Mild upper respiratory tract signs (sneezing, discharges).

See other reference on page 1137 for details (The Fading Kitten and Neonate).

Pathogenesis

Calicivirus replicates in epithelial cells of the upper respiratory tract, conjunctiva, tongue and in pneumocytes of the lung alveoli.

Multiple antigenic subtypes occur with differing pathogenicity.
- Most isolates cause low mortality.
- Some very pathogenic isolates cause severe pneumonia and significant mortality.
- Other isolates cause "limping kitten syndrome".
- FCV-Ari isolate produces high mortality.

Clinical signs

Clinical signs vary from mild to severe, depending on viral subtype and immune status of the cat.

- Signs are often milder than feline herpesvirus infection.

Early signs are often non-specific, and typical of a sick cat, i.e. **lethargy, anorexia and pyrexia.**

Nasal and ocular discharge is often only **mild and serous** or mucoid, or may be absent.

Sneezing is less prominent than in herpesvirus and is not paroxysmal.

Oral ulcers are characteristic and present in 70% of cats.
- Oral ulcers may occur either as small ulcers (2–5 mm in diameter) or as a large ulcer.
- Typically ulcers are located on the **anterior or lateral margin of the tongue.** Less frequently they occur at the angle of the jaws, on the hard palate, nasal philtrum or lips.
- Footpad ulcers occur occasionally, hence the name "paw and mouth disease".

Salivation may be profuse in the first few days after ulcers form.

Conjunctiva are generally only **mildly hyperemic,** and are not chemotic, as occurs with herpesvirus or chlamydophila.

Viral pneumonia occurs occasionally with certain strains, and may produce significant mortality. Death is often sudden and preceded by labored respiration.

Rarely, vomiting and diarrhea occur as a result of enteritis.

"**Limping kitten syndrome**" occurs occasionally with some strains of virus.
- Acute viral arthritis results in reluctance to move, and acute swelling and pain on palpation of the joints.

A **rare variant strain (FCV-Ari)** reported from California, USA, produces a **high fever, facial and paw edema** (50% of cats), ocular and nasal discharge, conjunctivitis and ulcerative stomatitis (50% of cats), **hemorrhage from the nose, GIT**, etc. (30–40% of cats), **icterus** (20% of cats) and **rapid death. Mortality is high** (30–50%).
- Swelling of the feet and face is a combination of edema and hemorrhage, which is thought to result from vasculitis. Hemostatic abnormalities have

been attributed to vasculitis and disseminated intravascular coagulation (DIC).

- Some cats also had pneumonia, pleural effusion, pancreatitis and abdominal effusion.

Diagnosis

Presumptive diagnosis of calicivirus infection is **based on clinical signs**

A definitive diagnosis is usually not made except where there is an ongoing cattery problem, and is based on demonstrating a **rising antibody titer, or on PCR or viral isolation**. These tests are available through some laboratories.

Identification of **FCV-Ari** is based on the clinical syndrome, pathology and **culture of virus from blood, nasal or ocular discharge, spleen or lungs**. Thrombocytopenia and prolonged PT and aPTT may be evident in some cats.

Differential diagnosis

Herpesvirus generally has more pronounced ocular-nasal discharge and paroxysms of sneezing. Corneal lesions in herpesvirus infection are usually diagnostic, and mouth ulcers rarely occur.

Mycoplasma often occurs as a secondary infection in viral upper respiratory tract disease, rather than a primary disease, and is not associated with mouth ulcers.

Chlamydia generally has mild upper respiratory tract signs, but no mouth ulcers; conjunctivitis often persists longer and is more severe than with calicivirus.

Caustic stomatitis generally does not cause fever. Ocular-nasal discharge is usually absent, or if present, is a mild, serous discharge.

Concurrent infection with herpesvirus, mycoplasma or *Bordetella* may confuse the clinical picture.

Acetaminophen (paracetamol) toxicity produces similar facial and paw swelling in an acutely ill cat as does FCV-Ari, but cats are not febrile.

Other acute infectious illnesses may appear similar to FCV-Ari, for example *Yersinia pestis* (feline plague), *Salmonella* spp. (song-bird fever), *Francisella*

tularensis (tularemia), all may be difficult to differentiate pre-mortem if the illness progresses rapidly to death.

Pancreatitis does not usually produce such a high fever as FCV-Ari.

Treatment

Treatment for calicivirus infection including the hemorrhagic form involves **supportive therapy** (see treatment of herpesvirus for details, page 8).

- Maintain good hydration.
- Humidify airways using a vaporizer or nebulizer.
- Use broad-spectrum antibiotics for secondary infections.
- Clean discharges from face.
- Provide oxygen if dyspneic.
- Analgesics (e.g. buprenorphine) may help make the cat more comfortable if there is severe ulceration.

No specific therapy is available, and no antiviral drug is effective.

Prognosis

Signs generally resolve within 5–7 days.

Rarely, mortality is high with strains causing severe viral pneumonia or vasculitis (FCV-Ari), and kittens may die suddenly.

Chronic gingivitis and stomatitis occurs in some carriers.

Persistent mild conjunctivitis or ulcerative keratitis may be a problem.

Transmission

Calicivirus is highly contagious, with nearly 100% morbidity in susceptible cats.

Infection spreads rapidly when multiple cats are housed together.

- Young unvaccinated kittens 2–6 months of age are most susceptible.

Incubation period is 2–4 days. First signs generally occur 3 days after exposure, but this varies with dose and virulence of virus.

Transmission is primarily **via direct contact with infected cats**.

- **Fomite** transmission occurs, e.g. food and water bowls, cages, human hands, shoes and clothing.
- Virus can survive several days, and in some situations up to 8–10 days, on contaminated objects.

Virus is shed in secretions from the mouth and nose of sick cats.

The carrier state is common, and may last years. Carrier cats provide a source of infection, and shed virus **continuously,** mainly from the tonsils.

Virus is resistant to lipotrophic disinfectants, and **sodium hypochlorite** (1:32 dilution of household bleach) is efficacious.

Prevention

Vaccines are available **combined with feline herpesvirus** vaccine (see herpesvirus (page 10) for administration details).

Vaccination decreases severity and duration of signs.
- Vaccination may **not afford 100% protection** if challenged by a subtype that is different from the vaccine strain.

Cattery control involves vaccination, isolation of incoming cats and good hygiene (see herpesvirus, page 11).

CHLAMYDOPHILA FELIS (CHLAMYDOPHILA FELIS PSITTACI)**

> ### Classical signs
>
> - Conjunctivitis, initially acute but progressing to chronic inflammation.
> - Sneezing and nasal discharge is usually mild and often becomes chronic.

See other reference on page 1215 for details (The Cat With Ocular Discharge or Changed Conjunctival Appearance).

Pathogenesis

Chlamydophilosis causes approximately 20% of upper respiratory tract disease in cats, but is a frequent cause of conjunctivitis.

Infection may occur concurrently with herpes or calicivirus infection.

Clinical signs

Conjunctivitis is often initially unilateral, but progresses to bilateral involvement.
- Conjunctiva are **hyperemic**, which is usually mild but can be severe, and are occasionally edematous and chemotic.
- Ocular discharge is initially seromucous, but rapidly becomes mucopurulent.

Sneezing and nasal discharge result from ocular discharge draining through the nasolacrimal duct.

Pneumonia occasionally occurs in kittens.

Chlamydophila may cause abortion and infertility, although this is controversial and poorly documented in cats.

Diagnosis

Visualization of inclusion bodies in epithelial cells obtained from conjunctival scraping (Diff-Quick stain) is diagnostic.
- Inclusion bodies are visible as groups or clusters of organisms in the cytoplasm (in the same plane as the nucleus).
- Inclusions are most often visible in the first 2 weeks of infection, and numbers decrease with chronicity.

Antibody-based detection in conjunctival scrapings using **ELISA or latex agglutination** is available. False positives occur with both tests if many bacteria are present.
- Use a dry swab, and roll well to get sufficient tissue for the test.

PCR is becoming more commonly available from diagnostic laboratories, and is the technique now used predominantly for studies involving chlamydophila.

Differential diagnosis

Herpesvirus generally produces more severe ocular-nasal discharge and systemic signs. If ulcerative keratitis is present, it is usually diagnostic for herpesvirus.

Calicivirus typically causes oral ulcers, which are not present with chlamydophila.

Mycoplasma may not be clinically distinguishable from chlamydophila.

Treatment

Use **tetracycline ophthalmic** ointment. Continue for **10 days after clinical remission** (usually 2–4 weeks of treatment 3–4 times daily). Avoid use of bacitracin-neomycin-polymyxin ointment because of reports of acute death associated with its use.

Oral doxycycline therapy may also be required in **resistant cases**. It is excreted in tears, and is also effective as a sole agent. Treat for 21 days, although up to 6–8 weeks treatment may be required in refractory cases.

Oral azithromycin (Zithromax, Pfizer, 5 mg/kg q 24 h PO for 14 days) is an alternative treatment to tetracycline.

Some chronic cases may require long-term systemic therapy.

Prognosis

Chlamydophilosis frequently **progresses to chronic signs**, with conjunctival thickening and prominent conjunctival lymphoid follicles.

Untreated cats frequently relapse after apparent recovery.

Transmission

Transmission is by direct contact with an infected cat.

MYCOPLASMA

Classical signs

- Conjunctivitis with purulent ocular discharge; unilateral progressing to bilateral.

See main reference on page 1218 for details (The Cat With Ocular Discharge or Changed Conjunctival Appearance).

Pathogenesis

Causal agents are *Mycoplasma felis* and *M. gatae*.

Mycoplama more often plays a secondary role to herpesvirus or calicivirus infections.

Clinical signs

Conjunctivitis is initially unilateral, progressing to bilateral involvement.
- Conjunctiva may be normal, hyperemic or edematous.
- In severe infections, conjunctiva may be covered in a gray pseudomembrane (diptheritic membrane).

Nasal discharge is mild, and results from ocular discharge draining into the nose.

Diagnosis

Diagnosis is based on visualization of clusters of **coccoid or coccobacillary organisms** in the periphery of epithelium cells from stained (e.g. Diff-Quik stain) conjunctival scrapings.

Isolation of the organism can be done in most laboratories from clean conjunctival swabs. Remove ocular discharges with sterile normal saline solution prior to taking the sample, to reduce contamination from secondary bacterial infections.

Differential diagnosis

Chlamydophila has similar clinical signs, but is more common.

Treatment

Chloramphenicol or doxycycline ophthalmic ointment (6 mm (1/4 inch) strip q 6 h).

BORDETELLA

Classical signs

- Pyrexia.
- Sneezing and nasal discharge.
- Mandibular lymphadenopathy.
- Coughing.
- Dyspnea, cyanosis, pneumonia.

Pathogenesis

Bordetella bronchiseptica may act as a primary pathogen, or play a secondary role to herpesvirus or calicivirus infection.

Infection appears **widespread in the feline population**. *B. bronchiseptica* may be a normal commensal in the respiratory tract of cats, because it can be isolated from many healthy cats. It can be isolated from as many as 20% of cats in rescue catteries. The lowest rates of isolation are from one- and two-cat households.

Overgrowth of the organism may produce upper respiratory tract inflammation or pneumonia.

Severe cases with **bronchopneumonia** have occurred in situations of **overcrowding** and other stress factors.

The incidence in cats is reported to be higher in households where signs were present in dogs.

In most cats, **signs resolve after approximately 10 days**. Occasionally, coughing persists longer.

Clinical signs

Signs are most likely to occur in cats from **multi-cat environments, especially rescue or shelter catteries**, where calicivirus and herpesvirus are also a problem.

Typically there is an **acute onset of pyrexia, and sneezing and nasal discharge**.

Mandibular lymphadenopathy may be palpable.

Coughing may be spontaneous, or only evident on tracheal pressure. Generally, coughing is not as pronounced as in dogs.

Dyspnea, cyanosis, crackles and wheezes may be auscultated over lung fields in some cats. Death from **pneumonia** may occur, especially in young kittens less than 8 weeks old.

Diagnosis

Bacteria can be isolated from the nasal discharge, oropharyngeal secretions, tonsillar swabs, or a transtracheal wash.

- Samples should be transported in **special medium** (e.g. charcoal Amies transport medium), and need special media for culture.
- Although *B. bronchiseptica* is a normal commensal in many cats, in cats with disease from the organism, **large numbers of organisms** are often isolated.

Differential diagnosis

Herpesvirus and calicivirus can have similar signs, and mixed infections are common, making definitive diagnosis impossible based solely on signs.

Treatment

Use **appropriate antibiotics** based on susceptibility data and the ability to reach therapeutic concentrations in respiratory secretions such as oxytetracycline, doxycycline or enrofloxacin. Beware of sudden retinal degeneration if using enrofloxacin.

Montelukast (Singulaire, 0.25–1 mg/kg SID) is a leukotriene receptor blocker. Although the cat has insufficient leukotriene receptors for cysteinyl leukotrienes to cause bronchoconstriction, anecdotal evidence suggests that montelukast may **reduce sneezing and nasal discharge** associated with *Bordetella*. This effect may be mediated through blockage of leukotriene-mediated attraction of inflammatory cells such as eosinophils and neutrophils, and their subsequent release of inflammatory cytokines and other chemicals.

Prevention

An **intranasal modified live vaccine** is available which does not prevent or eliminate infection with *Bordetella*, but usually prevents severe overgrowth and clinical signs. It is most useful in catteries or shelters with culture-proven outbreaks of disease. It is effective in 3–5 days.

The rate of adverse signs (e.g. sneezing) associated with *Bordetella* vaccination probably exceeds the frequency of disease caused by the organism in cats living in one- or two-cat households.

Improve cattery/shelter conditions to decrease overcrowding if the organism appears to be causing recurrent problems.

FOREIGN BODY

Classical signs

- Acute onset of sneezing and face rubbing, progressing to chronic signs.
- Unilateral discharge.
- Gagging.

See main reference on page 28 for details (The Cat With Chronic Nasal Disease).

Grass or seeds may occasionally enter the nose of cats. Other foreign bodies such as gun pellets are less common.

Clinical signs

Typically there is an **acute onset of sneezing and distress**, and rubbing at the face.

Signs may progress to chronic gagging, or sneezing and discharge.

A unilateral serosanguinous discharge is typically present.

Diagnosis

Visualize foreign body using an otoscope, fiberoptic scope, or with a dental mirror in the nasopharynx. Use a spay hook to retract the soft palate for better visualization.

Flushing the nose using a naso-esophageal feeding catheter may remove parts or all of the whole foreign body for diagnosis.

CRYPTOCOCCOSIS

Classical signs

- Chronic nasal discharge and sneezing, progressing in severity.
- Soft tissue swelling over the nasal bones (Roman nose), or polyp-like mass in nasal cavity.
- Facial distortion.

See main reference on page 25 for details (The Cat With Signs of Chronic Nasal Disease).

Clinical signs

Occasionally, the initial signs of cryptococcosis are **acute in onset.**

Upper respiratory tract signs are most common, and include **sneezing, snuffling and chronic nasal discharge**.

Nasal discharge may be unilateral or bilateral, and serous, mucopurulent or hemorrhagic.

Distortion and swelling over the bridge of nose, or a **polyp-like mass** projecting from the nasal cavity are present in 70% of cats with the respiratory form.

Depression, **anorexia** or inappetence and **weight loss** are often present with nasal or CNS involvement.

Submandibular lymph nodes are often **enlarged**.

Diagnosis

Diagnosis is based on **cytological identification of the organism** in nasal discharge, exudate from skin lesions, lymph node aspirate, cerebrospinal fluid (CSF), or ocular aspirate. *Cryptococcus* appears as **yeast-like organisms** (5–15 μm) surrounded by a **wide, clear capsule.**

Serology to detect cryptococcal capsular antigen in blood, CSF, or urine is **sensitive and specific**.

Tissue biopsy of the granulomatous mass or skin lesion, and histological identification of the organism may be required if cytology is negative.

Fungal isolation with **culture** is rarely required for diagnosis, but is **useful for sensitivity testing**.

BLEEDING ULCER ON EXTERNAL NARES

Classical signs

- Bleeding ulcer on external nares.
- ± Sneezing.

See main reference on page 27 for details (The Cat With Signs of Chronic Nasal Disease).

Clinical signs

Acute sneezing and/or discharge may occasionally occur associated with a bleeding ulcer on the external nares, particularly the nasal septum. It is usually associated with **squamous cell carcinoma** (SCC), but occasionally with **eosinophilic granuloma** or with **acute calicivirus infection**.

Diagnosis

Cytological examination of an **impression smear,** or **biopsy and histological** examination of the lesion is usually diagnostic for squamous cell carcinoma of the external nares.

Eosinophilic granuloma requires biopsy for diagnosis.

Acute calicivirus infection is diagnosed based on clinical signs, and in some cases PCR.

INTRANASAL TUMORS

Classical signs

- Chronic nasal discharge and sneezing, progressing in severity.
- Facial distortion.

See main reference on page 23 for details (The Cat With Signs of Chronic Nasal Disease).

Clinical signs

Acute sneezing and/or discharge may occasionally occur associated with an **intranasal tumor**. Suspect this disease when signs do not resolve over 2–3 weeks, and instead progress with worsening discharge, and often nasal distortion.

Intranasal tumors are associated with **chronic sneezing and snuffling**, which **progressively worsen** with time and a **purulent or bloody nasal discharge, which may temporarily respond to antibiotics.** The discharge may initially be unilateral and progress to bilateral involvement.

Snoring, snorting, inspiratory stridor, stertor or dyspnea may result from **nasal obstruction.**

Facial distortion, e.g. elevation of bridge of nose (Roman nose) or facial swelling may occur.

Diagnosis

Intranasal tumors usually require an **invasive approach** for diagnosis. Cytological examination of the discharge or atraumatic nasal flush usually reveals evidence of inflammation (neutrophils and bacteria) but no tumor.

- **Radiography** demonstrates increased opacity of the nasal cavity and often **destruction of the turbinates, nasal septum, lateral bone and loss of teeth** adjacent to the lesion. Radiographic changes are often unilateral or asymmetrical.
- A **traumatic flush using a stiff catheter** and syringe (e.g. cut-off dog urinary catheter) yields better results than an atraumatic flush.
- A **biopsy** is often required to obtain tissue for a histological diagnosis. Tissue may be obtained using biopsy **forceps** through the external nares or via a **rhinotomy.**

ALLERGIC RHINITIS

Classical signs

- Acute or chronic serous or mucoid nasal discharge, often seasonal.

Clinical signs

Allergic rhinitis appears to be a rare and poorly documented condition in cats.

It presents as serous or mucoid ocular and/or nasal discharge without systemic signs, and may be seasonal in occurrence.

It has been reported associated with allergy to **Japanese cedar** (*Cryptomeria japonica*).

Diagnosis

Diagnosis is based on **exclusion of all other causes** of nasal discharge, and biopsy results indicating rhinitis with no evidence of underlying pathogens. A mixed neutrophilic and eosinophilic rhinitis has been reported.

Most cases with similar signs are the result of viral upper respiratory disease, often with chronic bacterial rhinitis cases.

Treatment

A combination of antihistamine and steroid may work well in some cats. For example, trimeprazine tartrate (5 mg) and prednisolone (2 mg) in Temaril-P (1/4 to 1/2 tablet PO q 12–24 h).

RECOMMENDED READING

Binns SH, Dawson S, Speakman AJ, et al. A study of feline upper respiratory tract disease with reference to prevalence and risk factors for infection with feline calicivirus and feline herpesvirus. J Feline Med Surg 2000; 2(3): 123–133.

Gaskell R, Dawson S. Feline respiratory disease. In: Greene CE (ed.) Infectious Diseases of the Dog and Cat, 2nd edn. Philadelphia, PA: WB Saunders Co., 1998, pp 97–106.

Jacobs GJ, Medleau L, Calvert C, et al. Cryptococcal infection in cats: factors influencing treatment outcome, and results of sequential serum antigen titers in 35 cats. J Vet Int Med 1997; 11: 1–4.

Kate F, Hurley KF, Pesavento PA, et al. An outbreak of virulent systemic feline calicivirus disease. J Am Vet Med Assoc 2004; 224(2): 241–249.

Lappin MR. Sneezing and nasal discharge; viral diseases. In: Lappin MR (ed.) Feline Internal Medicine Secrets, 1st edn. Philadelphia, PA: Hanley and Belfus, 2001, pp 8–11.

Ramsey DT. Feline chlamydophila felis and calicivirus infections. Vet Clin North Am Small Anim Pract 2000; 30(5): 1015–1028.

Stein JE. Sneezing and nasal discharge; bacterial diseases. In: Lappin MR (ed.) Feline Internal Medicine Secrets, 1st edn. Philadelphia, PA: Hanley and Belfus, 2001, pp 4–8.

Stein JE, Lappin MR. Bacterial culture results in cats with upper or lower respiratory disease. J Vet Int Med 2001; 15: 320.

Sykes JE. Feline upper respiratory tract pathogens: herpesvirus-1 and calicivirus. Compend Contin Educ Pract Vet 2001; 23(2): 166–175.

Sykes JE, Allen JL, Studdert VP, et al. Detection of feline calicivirus, feline herpesvirus 1 and *Chlamydophila felis psittaci* mucosal swabs by multiplex RT-PCR/PCR. Vet Microbiol 2001; 81(2): 95–108.

3. The cat with signs of chronic nasal disease. (chronic > 3 weeks duration)

Jacquie Rand

KEY SIGNS

- Chronic mucoid, purulent and/or bloody nasal discharge.
- Chronic sneezing or snuffling.
- Stertorous respiration, snoring, dyspnea or mouth breathing.
- Facial distortion or nasopharyngeal distortion.
- Gagging.

MECHANISM?

- Signs of chronic disease result from chronic inflammation or obstruction of the nasal structures or its junction with the pharynx.

WHERE?

- External nares, nasal cavity, frontal sinuses and nasopharynx

WHAT?

- Most cats with signs of chronic nasal disease have secondary bacterial infection following herpes or calicivirus infection; less common causes are *Cryptococcus* and neoplasia.

QUICK REFERENCE SUMMARY

Diseases causing signs of chronic nasal disease

ANOMALY

- **Congenital anomaly of the nose or hard palate**(p 27)

Breed-related obstruction of the external nares (e.g. Persian cats) causes chronic snuffling and stertorous respiration.

Cleft palate, and congenital anomalies of the nasal cavity cause signs in young kittens which depend on the type and severity of the anomaly, e.g. nasal discharge and inability to suckle associated with a cleft palate.

MECHANICAL

- Foreign body (p 28)

Acute onset of sneezing and rubbing face or gagging, followed by chronic unilateral nasal discharge and sneezing, or gagging. Often associated with a blade of grass, a grass seed or awn.

continued

continued

NEOPLASTIC

- **Neoplasia**(p 23)**
Chronic mucopurulent or hemorrhagic nasal discharge, often unilateral initially, but progressing to bilateral; sneezing, stertorous respiration ± facial distortion.

- Nasopharyngeal polyp (p 30)
Chronic snuffling, stertorous respiration and dyspnea from nasal obstruction; retching or gagging with eating, ± mucopurulent nasal discharge.

INFLAMMATION

- **Secondary rhinitis associated with dental disease* (p 27)**
Mild, chronic mucopurulent or hemorrhagic discharge and sneezing.

- Nasopharyngeal stenosis (p 30)
Chronic snuffling, partial nasal obstruction, retching or gagging with eating.

INFECTIOUS

Bacterial:

- **Secondary bacterial rhinitis*** (p 21)**
Occurs secondary to viral upper respiratory tract disease. Signs include chronic mucopurulent or hemorrhagic nasal discharge, sneezing, stertorous respiration, occasionally nasal distortion.

Fungal:

- ***Cryptococcus*** (p 25)**
Chronic mucopurulent or hemorrhagic nasal discharge, sneezing, stertorous respiration, distortion over bridge of nose (Roman nose), polyp-like mass in nasal opening.

- Other fungi
Aspergillus, *Penicillium*, *Sporothrix* or other fungi are very rare causes of chronic nasal disease.

Chlamydophila felis and *Mycoplasma*:

- *Chlamydophila felis (Chlamydophila felis psittaci)* and *mycoplasma* (p 29)
Chronic ocular and nasal discharge, chronic conjunctivitis and sneezing.

Immune:

- Allergic rhinitis (p 31)
Acute or chronic serous or mucoid nasal discharge, which is often seasonal.

Trauma:

- Oronasal fistula or nasal fractures following trauma (p 29)
Chronic snuffling, sneezing and nasal discharge associated with cleft palate, oronasal fistula or obstructed nasal cavity.

INTRODUCTION

MECHANISM?

Chronic nasal disease should be suspected when a cat has any of the **following signs for more than 3 weeks**.
- **Chronic sneezing** or snuffling.
- **Nasal discharge which may be mucoid, purulent or bloody**.
- **Signs of nasal** obstruction, such as stertorous respiration (snoring), stridor (high-pitched whistling indicating obstruction), dyspnea or mouth breathing.
- **Gagging**.
- **Facial distortion**.
- **Nasopharyngeal distortion** or bulging of the soft palate into the oral cavity.

The nasal mucosa responds to chronic disease by increased mucoid discharge.
- A **purulent discharge** occurs with infection or necrosis.
- **Blood** may be present if there is severe **inflammation or erosion**.
  - **Bleeding without other signs of nasal disease**, such as a purulent nasal discharge, may indicate a **systemic bleeding problem**, rather than nasal disease.

Facial distortion occurs with **neoplasia or chronic infection**.
- Fungal (usually *Cryptococcus*) more often causes nasal distortion than chronic bacterial infection.

Gagging occurs when there is **nasopharyngeal stimulation** from a mass lesion, a **foreign body**, or caudal nasal discharge.

Ciliated columnar epithelium lining of the nasal cavity **undergoes squamous metaplasia after herpesvirus** infection.
- This decreases mucociliary clearance and predisposes to secondary bacterial infection.

WHERE?

Signs of chronic nasal disease result from problems in any of the following sites:
- **External nares, nasal cavity, frontal sinuses and nasopharynx**.

Careful **history taking** and **physical examination** help localize the lesion.

Examination of the oropharynex under anesthesia and **radiography** aid localization and diagnosis.

WHAT?

The most common cause of chronic nasal disease is **secondary bacterial infection following herpes or calicivirus infection**
- Less common causes are *Cryptococcus* and neoplasia.
- **Foreign bodies are generally rare** causes of chronic nasal signs in cats.
  - **Grass in the nasopharyngnx** is more common, and causes **gagging**.

Diagnosis is based on history and physical examination findings, radiography, *Cryptococcus* titer, and cytological or histopathological examination of tissue samples.

DISEASES CAUSING SIGNS OF CHRONIC NASAL DISCHARGE

SECONDARY BACTERIAL RHINITIS***

Classical signs

- Chronic sneezing and snuffling following acute upper respiratory tract signs.
- Chronic mucopurulent nasal discharge.
- Stertorous respiration.
- Occasionally, nasal distortion.

Pathogenesis

Secondary bacterial infection of the nasal cavity and sinuses following feline herpesvirus or calicivirus infection is one of the most common causes of chronic sneezing and nasal discharge in cats.

Feline herpesvirus (feline rhinotracheitis virus) predisposes to **persistent** or **recurring** bacterial infection of the nose and sinuses.

Herpesvirus **causes structural changes in the nose and sinuses**.

These changes decrease mucociliary clearance from the nose, and cause nasal and sinus obstruction.

- Structural changes include necrosis of the nasal epithelium, **squamous metaplasia,** osteolysis of the turbinates, and mucosal gland hypertrophy.
- The result is decreased density of cilia and increased viscosity of mucus. This **decreases mucociliary clearance** from the nose and sinuses.
- Persistent **thickening of the lining tissues of the nasal cavity** and **sinuses** leads to nasal and sinus obstruction, predisposing to chronic sinusitis.
- The normal opening between the nasal cavity and frontal sinuses is small in cats, and is relatively easily obstructed.

Organisms most frequently isolated are those that comprise the normal flora of the nose (e.g. *Staphylococcus*, *Streptococcus*, *Pseudomonas*).

Cats with feline immunodeficiency virus (FIV) or feline leukemia virus (FeLV) may be more susceptible.

Clinical signs

Chronic sneezing, snuffling and mucopurulent nasal discharge is often present for months or years.

Stertorous respiration, (snoring) or stridor (whistling), may be audible from the nasal area.

Occasionally, nasal distortion is present when signs have been present for years.

Diagnosis

History of chronic snuffling following acute upper respiratory tract infection.

Radiographic findings
- Usually there is **loss of lucency in the nasal cavity** (fluid density) and often in the frontal sinuses.
- Radiographic changes are usually **bilaterally symmetrical**.
- **Osteolysis of the turbinates** and/or nasal septum may be evident.

Cytology or histology reveals many neutrophils with intra- and extracellular bacteria, and no evidence of *Cryptococcus neoformans* or neoplastic cells.
- **Beware of similar cytologic findings with neoplasia,** and sometimes cryptococcosis. Often neoplasia is misdiagnosed as bacterial infection, because of the presence of neutrophils and bacteria.
- To exclude neoplasia, material must be collected via a **traumatic flush** using a stiff polypropylene catheter attached to a syringe, or via a **biopsy** using a pinch biopsy technique through the nares, or a core biopsy via a trephine, or surgical biopsy via rhinotomy.
- Cytological examination of the **nasal discharge or atraumatic nasal flush is inadequate to exclude neoplasia** as a cause of the secondary bacterial infection.
- Surgical **rhinotomy** and biopsy may be necessary to exclude neoplasia when the history and radiographic findings are equivocal.

Negative *Cryptococcus* titer.

Check FeLV and FIV status.

Differential diagnosis

Neoplasia produces similar signs, but duration of signs is usually less than 6 months, and cats are often older than 10 years of age. **Radiographic lesions are often unilateral or asymmetric**, whereas chronic rhinitis tends to be bilaterally symmetrical.

Cryptococcosis produces similar signs, although 70% of cats with nasal involvement have distortion over the bridge of the nose, or a polyp-like mass visible in the nasal cavity.
- **Only rarely do cats with chronic bacterial infection have nasal distortion**, and this is usually only after signs have been evident for years.
- Diagnosis of cryptococcosis is based on finding evidence of the organism on cytology, histology or serology.

Treatment

Treatment requires prolonged antibiotic therapy for 1–4 months. Many cats cannot be cured, and nasal discharge and sneezing persist, requiring repeated therapy when signs are exacerbated. Different combinations of therapy work better in individual cats.
- Use **broad-spectrum antibiotics**, or base choice on culture and sensitivity. Because of the large number of normal flora in the nasal cavity, culture, and therefore sensitivity results, are hard to interpret. The best antibiotics to use are broad spectrum with efficacy against anaerobes, and that penetrate bone and cartilage.

– Commonly used antibiotics include doxycycline, cephalexin, amoxicillin-clavulanic acid, clindamycin, enrofloxacin and azithromycin. Amoxicillin-clavulanic acid, metronidazole, clindamycin and azithromycin are good first choices.

– Doxycycline and metronidazole may be advantageous because they have an **immunomodulating effect** which may help **reduce inflammation.**

– Azithromycin is attractive because of the alternate day dosing, and in cattery and breeder situations the pharmacokinetics allow twice weekly dosing (q 72 h).

- One regime that is effective in many cats is **enrofloxacin** (Baytril; 2.5 mg/kg q 12 h for 30 days) together with **azithromycin** (Zithromax; 20 mg QD for 30–45 days).

– Fluroquinolones, particularly enrofloxacin may be associated with **retinal degeneration and blindness**, especially at high doses, and many ophthalmologists avoid using these drugs.

- Cats with *Pseudomonas* cultured from the sinuses may respond to a long course of carbenicillin.

- If signs return rapidly after stopping antibiotics, long-term antibiotics administered once daily at half the total daily dose may help control signs in some cats. However, resistance to antibacterial action commonly occurs, and a better strategy is a longer course of antibiotics based on culture and sensitivity using dosages suitable for osteomyelitis, followed by a course of antibiotics when signs relapse.

- **Intranasally administered antibiotics** such as gentomicin ophthalmic drops sprayed into each nostril twice daily for 30 days may help, if the cat will tolerate them.

- **Acetylcysteine** (Mucomyst) helps to liquefy nasal secretions when used with nebulization, but may be expensive for long-term use.

- In some cats, **intermittent flushing of the nasal cavity** under anesthesia (with tracheal intubation) can be useful in controlling clinical signs.

- Occasionally, cats will tolerate local instillation of **saline drops** in the nasal cavity. This stimulates a sneeze response and encourages evacuation of mucus.

- Individual cats may show improvement with antihistamines especially second-generation **antihistamines** such as loratidine (Claritin; 2.5 mg/day) because of their anti-inflammatory effects as well as their ability to dry up excessive mucus.

- Leukotriene antagonists like **zafirlukast** (Accolade; 0.5–1.0 mg/kg PO q 12–24 h) or **montelukast** (Singulaire, 0.25–1.0 mg/kg SID) help by reducing pain and inflammation, and may be effective in some cats.

If signs persist despite antibiotics, **surgical removal of chronically inflamed tissue** via a rhinotomy is sometimes successful.

- Surgery is generally **more successful for chronic sinusitis** with radiographic evidence of fluid in the sinuses, than for chronic rhinitis. Opening the foramen between the sinus and nasal passages facilitates drainage of the sinus.

- **Surgery involves turbinectomy and/or ablation of the frontal sinuses.** For frontal sinus ablation, the sinuses are curetted out, the periosteum removed, and the cavity filled with subcutaneous abdominal fat or methylmethacrylic.

Interferon alone or with ATZ (zidovudine) or PMEA (phosphonomethoxyethyl adenine) may help in FeLV- and FIV-infected cats to stimulate immunity and improve signs.

Prognosis

Most cats have a good quality of life, although signs often persist and must be controlled with antibiotics.

Prevention

Regular vaccination to prevent feline calicivirus and herpesvirus infection is recommended, because most chronic bacterial rhinitis occurs secondary to upper respiratory viral infection.

NEOPLASIA**

Classical signs

- Progressively worsening chronic sneezing and snuffling.
- Purulent or blood-tinged nasal discharge, which may temporarily respond to antibiotics.
- Epiphora, ± signs of retrobulbar pressure, e.g. exophthalmos.
- Nasal obstruction, and occasionally facial distortion.

Pathogenesis

Neoplasia may involve primarily the external nares, the nasal cavity or the paranasal sinuses.

- Neoplasia typically causes purulent nasal discharge, bleeding, sneezing and/or obstruction.

Neoplasia involving **primarily the external nares** is most commonly **squamous cell carcinoma**. Less frequently fibrosarcoma or fibroma are involved.

- **Squamous cell carcinoma** usually occurs in older cats with a non-pigmented nose, that live in a sunny climate and are outside during the day.

Neoplasia primarily involving **the nasal cavity or the frontal sinuses** is most commonly **adenocarcinoma and lymphoma**.

- Less common tumors are undifferentiated carcinoma or sarcoma, olfactory neuroblastoma, fibrosarcoma, chondrosarcoma, chondroma, osteosarcoma and squamous cell carcinoma.

Neoplasia usually occurs in **older cats** (> 8–10 years).

Most occur in the **caudal third of the nasal passage**.

Clinical signs

Squamous cell carcinoma involving the **external nares** may cause **sneezing** and a **bloody nasal discharge**.

- Lesions causing signs of nasal disease many consist of a bleeding ulcer on the nasal septum, or an **advanced erosive lesion on the external nares**.
  - Signs may be present for **months or years.**

Intranasal tumors are associated with the following signs:

- **Chronic sneezing and snuffling**, which **progressively worsen** with time.
- **Purulent or bloody nasal discharge, which may temporarily respond to antibiotics**.
  - The discharge may initially be unilateral and progress to bilateral involvement.
- **Snoring, snorting, inspiratory stridor, stertor or dyspnea from nasal obstruction**.
- Facial distortion, e.g. elevation of bridge of nose (Roman nose) or facial swelling.
- Epiphora (associated with obstruction of the lacrimal duct), or a bloody ocular discharge.
- Signs of **retrobulbar pressure** may be present, e.g. exophthalmos and ocular deviation.

- Occasionally, central nervous system signs occur, e.g. seizures, circling, ataxia, behavioral change.
  - Signs may be present for days, or in rare cases, for as long as 2 years. Usually, signs are present for less than 6 months prior to diagnosis.

Diagnosis

Cytological examination of an **impression smear,** or **biopsy and histological** examination of the lesion is usually diagnostic for squamous cell carcinoma of the **external nares**.

Intranasal tumors require a more **invasive approach**. Cytological examination of the discharge or atraumatic nasal flush usually reveals evidence of inflammation (neutrophils and bacteria) but no tumor.

- **Radiography** demonstrates increased opacity of the nasal cavity and often **destruction of the turbinates, nasal septum, lateral bone and loss of teeth** adjacent to the lesion. Radiographic changes are often unilateral or asymmetrical.
- A **traumatic flush using a stiff catheter** and syringe (e.g. cut-off dog urinary catheter) yields better results than an atraumatic flush.
- A **biopsy** is often required to obtain tissue for a histological diagnosis. Tissue may be obtained using biopsy **forceps** through the external nares or via a **rhinotomy**.

Differential diagnosis

Cryptococcosis can produce very similar signs to intranasal tumors. However, 70% of cats with cryptococcosis have either **distortion of the bridge of the nose** or a **polyp-like mass** visible projecting from the nasal cavity.

- Most have a positive *Cryptococcus* titer.
- Cats with cryptococcosis tend to be younger than cats with neoplasia.
- **Chronic bacterial infection** of the nasal cavity secondary to viral upper respiratory disease may produce similar signs. However, signs are typically present for longer, and only very rarely is there nasal distortion.

Treatment

Treatment of squamous cell carcinoma involving the external nares depends on the extent of local invasion.

- **Radiotherapy, cryotherapy, intralesional chemotherapy, or resection of the nasal planum** are indicated depending on the lesion.
- If ulcerated and erosive, radical resection of the nasal planum yields best results.

Lymphoma is best treated with radiotherapy and/or **chemotherapy**.

Other tumors of the nasal cavity have a guarded to poor prognosis. At the time of diagnosis, there is usually **extensive local invasion**, and the **recurrence rate after radiotherapy and/or surgery is high**.

Prognosis

Squamous cell carcinoma of the external nares can have a good prognosis if the lesion is small, or if radical resection of the nasal planum totally removes the tumor. Local recurrence may occur, but the tumor is slow to metastasize.

Lymphoma has a guarded prognosis, but may respond to chemotherapy or radiotherapy.

Other **intranasal tumors** have a **very poor prognosis**, especially if destruction of the turbinates is evident radiographically.

CRYPTOCOCCOSIS*–**

Classical signs

- Chronic nasal discharge and sneezing, progressing in severity.
- Soft-tissue swelling over the nasal bones (Roman nose), or polyp-like mass in nasal cavity.

Pathogenesis

Cryptococcus neoformans most commonly produces granulomatous lesions in the nasal cavity or paranasal sinuses.

Disease is caused by *Cryptococcus neoformans neoformans* or *Cryptococcus neoformans gattii*.

Cryptococcus neoformans neoformans **is shed in pigeon feces**; high concentrations of organisms are found in soil contaminated by pigeon droppings, and in the debris of pigeon roosts.

Cryptococcus neoformans gattii **is found in the developing flower of Red River gums** and forest red gums; high concentrations of organisms are found in the bark and the accumulated debris surrounding the base of the tree.

- These trees have been widely exported around the world from Australia.

Organisms are **viable for at least 2 years**, if protected from direct sunlight and drying.

Nasal infection occurs via inhalation of airborne organisms or contamination of the wound with organisms.

- There are **no reports** of **transmission between animals or people**; infection is from the environment.
- Cell-mediated immunity may be compromised in infected animals; there are some reports of a higher incidence of FIV infection in cats with *Cryptococcus*.
- **Cats are more susceptible** than dogs or humans.
- Any age of cat can be infected, but the **average age is 5 years** (younger than cats with neoplasia).
- Following inhalation, the organism deposits in the **upper respiratory tract producing nasal granulomas**, or deposits in the alveoli producing pulmonary granulomas, which are usually subclinical.
- The organism **may disseminate through the cribriform plate** or via the blood to the central nervous system (CNS).
- If CNS signs develop, cats may or may not have concurrent signs of respiratory infection.

In cats with cryptococcosis, **50–80% have respiratory disease** involving mainly the nasal cavity, and **10–40% have cutaneous or subcutaneous lesions**. **Central nervous system** (CNS) involvement and **ocular disease** are less common.

Clinical signs

Upper respiratory tract signs are most common, and include **sneezing, snuffling and chronic nasal discharge**.

- Nasal discharge may be unilateral or bilateral, and serous, mucopurulent or hemorrhagic.

Distortion and swelling over the bridge of the nose, or a **polyp-like mass** projecting from the nasal cavity are present in 70% of cats with the respiratory form.

Depression, **anorexia** or inappetence and **weight loss** are often present with nasal or CNS involvement.

Submandibular lymph nodes are often **enlarged**.

Skin lesions consist of **papules or nodules** varying from 0.1–1 cm in diameter.
- Lesions may ulcerate and exude serous fluid, or remain as intact nodules.
- Skin lesions may be single or multiple, and occur alone, or with involvement of other organs.

Central nervous system signs result from inflammation of the brain and meninges or a mass lesion (granuloma).
- Signs reported are referable to the **cerebrum** (seizures, circling, ataxia, behavioral change, head pressing, blindness), or **brainstem** (head tilt, nystagmus, facial paralysis, paresis, ataxia, circling).
- Occasionally, signs are referable to the spinal cord.

Ocular signs include epiphora, dilated unresponsive pupils, blindness and anterior uveitis.

Occasionally, other organs are involved, e.g. bone, kidney.

Diagnosis

Diagnosis is based on **cytological identification of the organism** in nasal discharge, exudate from skin lesions, lymph node aspirate, cerebrospinal fluid (CSF) or ocular aspirate.
- Stain sample with **new methylene blue**, Indian ink or Diff-Quick.
- *Cryptococcus* appears as **yeast-like organisms** (5–15 μm) surrounded by a **wide, clear capsule.**
- Organism **buds from a narrow base**, in contrast to *Blastomyces* which has broad-based budding and thinner capsule.

Serology to detect cryptococcal capsular antigen in blood, CSF, or urine is **sensitive and specific**.

Tissue biopsy of the granulomatous mass or skin lesion, and histological identification of the organism may be required if cytology is negative.

Fungal isolation with **culture** is rarely required for diagnosis, but is **useful for sensitivity testing**.

Radiographs often reveal **turbinate lysis and opacity** of the nasal cavity (soft-tissue density). Sinus involvement is common.

Differential diagnosis

Neoplasia may have similar signs. The presence of a polyp-like mass in the nose, or swelling over the bridge of the nose suggest cryptococcosis rather than neoplasia. Cats with neoplasia are on average older than cats with cryptococcosis.

Chronic bacterial infection of the nasal cavity secondary to viral upper respiratory disease has similar signs. However, it is only rarely associated with nasal distortion.

Treatment

Best success occurs using a **multi-drug regime** comprising of **amphotericin** (fungicidal) plus **5-fluorocytosine** (flucytosine), combined with or followed by **fluconazole** or **itraconazole** (fungistatic).
- **Amphotericin B is very nephrotoxic**, so use diuresis to protect the kidneys. Liposomal or lipid-encapsulated amphotericin B are safer than regular amphotericin B but are expensive.
  - Amphotericin B can be given IV (see standard texts) or SC (0.5–0.8 mg/kg) in 400 ml of 0.45% saline containing 2.5% dextrose. Administer subcutaneously two or three times a week for 1–3 months, until a total cumulative dose of 12–26 mg/kg is reached. Monitor serum creatinine, urea (more sensitive, but influenced by many non-renal factors) and urine specific gravity and sediment for casts. If azotemia develops, discontinue amphotericin until it resolves and reduce dose (Malik et al. 1996).

Sensitivity to amphotericin toxicity varies considerably between cats, and some cats develop acute renal failure with relatively small doses. It is imperative that serum urea concentration and urine are checked prior to each dose. The client should be instructed to return immediately if the cat becomes lethargic, inappetent or is vomiting.

Combine with 5-fluorocytosine 50 mg/kg q 8 h PO.

Either during or after the course of amphotericin is completed, **use an imadizole/triazole** to mop up infection (fungistatic):
- **Ketaconazole is cheapest**, but has most side effects (anorexia, vomiting, hepatic disease) and is perhaps least potent (10 mg/kg PO q 12–24 h).
- **Itraconazole** may work better than ketaconazole, and has fewer side effects (5 mg/kg PO q 12–24 h).

- **Fluconazole** is better for CNS infection, but is expensive (2.5–10 mg/kg PO q 12 h).

Approximately **3 weeks of treatment are required before there is an improvement in clinical signs**.

A decreasing serum *Cryptococcus* titer is predictive of recovery, but depending on the laboratory, it may be expensive to get the actual titer measured.

Clinical signs return if treatment is stopped too early. Ideally, **treat until titer is negative, which may be longer than 1 year.** However, some healthy cats remain antibody positive. If the cat is clinically healthy and the titer drops 16–32-fold, it is unlikely to relapse.

Alternatively treat for 4 weeks after resolution of all signs, with a minimum treatment period of 8 weeks. Relapses are more common with these shorter treatment periods.

Prognosis

Prognosis is variable. A falling titer in response to therapy suggests optimistic prognosis for cure. Prognosis is guarded if there is CNS involvement.

CONGENITAL ANOMALY OF THE NOSE OR HARD PALATE**

Classical signs

- Chronic snuffling and stertorous respiration.
- Dyspnea or mouth breathing.
- Narrow external nares.

Pathogenesis

Congenital stenosis of the external nares is common in some breeds, e.g. **Persians, Himalayans**.
- The combined effects of stenosis of the external nares and reduced nasal air space cause respiratory obstruction.
- Partial obstruction results in **increased respiratory effort and stertorous respiration**.
- **With stress** (e.g. visit to veterinarian or cat show), stridor becomes more pronounced, and **cats may become severely dyspneic and mouth breath**.

Clinical signs

Typically, there is **chronic snuffling and stertorous respiration** from the nasal region. Signs may be evident most or all of the time if the stenosis is severe.

Dyspnea or mouth breathing occurs with **stress**.

Narrow external nares are visible on physical examination.

Diagnosis

The diagnosis is usually based on clinical signs (nasal stridor) and physical examination (stenotic nares).

Differential diagnosis

The features of stenotic nares (signs since the cat was a young adult, cranial nasal stertor and narrow external nares) make most other diseases unlikely.

Treatment

Treatment involves surgical removal of the wing of the nostril.

Prognosis

Prognosis is good with surgery, provided there is not concurrent marked narrowing of the nasal cavity.

SECONDARY RHINITIS ASSOCIATED WITH DENTAL DISEASE*

Classical signs

- Chronic sneezing.
- Chronic unilateral or bilateral mucopurulent nasal discharge, which may be bloody.
- Oronasal fistula.

Pathogenesis

An **oronasal fistula** may result in **low-grade chronic rhinitis**, because **food and fluids enter the nose** from the mouth.

An oronasal fistula usually results from **advanced periodontal disease** of the **canine teeth**, with or without loss of the tooth.

- Often, the tooth is still present, and a **deep periodontal pocket** extends into the nasal cavity or maxillary sinus.
- Occasionally, a **periapical abscess from a dental fracture** or **caries** results in rhinitis.
- Iatrogenic oronasal fistula may result from poor dental extraction technique.

Clinical signs

Chronic sneezing, and mucopurulent nasal discharge, which may be blood-tinged.

Presence of an **oronasal fistula** associated with tooth loss or advanced periodontal disease, or a tooth fracture suggesting a periapical abscess.
- Examination under deep sedation or general anesthesia is often required for diagnosis.

Diagnosis

Diagnosis is based on signs of chronic nasal disease and the presence of an oronasal fistula.

Rarely, a periapical abscess is the cause. This is visible on radiograph.

Differential diagnosis

Visualization of the oronasal fistula is diagnostic.
- Very rarely another disease process is also present, and is responsible for the signs of chronic nasal disease, e.g. oronasal fistula with concurrent neoplasia or chronic bacterial infection secondary to viral upper respiratory tract disease.
- **Radiograph the nose prior to surgery**. Evidence of turbinate lysis suggests tumor, cryptococcosis or chronic bacterial rhinitis secondary to herpesvirus.
- Failure to respond to surgery suggests another disease process.

Treatment

Seal oronasal fistula surgically using a mucoperiosteal pedicle flap.

Prognosis

Prognosis is excellent, if the fistula is successfully closed, but some fistulas may be difficult to close.

FOREIGN BODY

> ### Classical signs
>
> - Acute onset of sneezing and rubbing face, progressing to chronic signs.
> - Unilateral discharge.
> - Gagging.

Pathogenesis

Most foreign bodies are of **plant origin**, and are either **grass, grass seeds or awns**.

Shotgun or airgun pellets, wood or bone are less frequent.

Clinical signs

Signs depend on where the foreign body lodges. Foreign bodies lodging in the nasal cavity cause sneezing and nasal discharge. Blades of grass tend to lodge in the nasopharynx and produce gagging.

Typically, there is a sudden onset of:
- **Sneezing**, which initially is **marked and paroxysmal**, and then becomes chronic.
- **Rubbing or pawing** at the nose.
- **Unilateral nasal discharge**, which is initially **serous or blood-tinged**, but progresses to **mucopurulent** and may be bloody.
- **Gagging** occurs when the foreign body lodges in the nasopharynx, or discharge drains into the pharynx from a foreign body in the posterior nasal cavity.

Diagnosis

Diagnosis is **based on visualizing** the foreign body using:
- An **otoscope or rhinoscope** for foreign bodies in the anterior nasal cavity.
- A **dental mirror** (warmed and sprayed with defogging agent) for foreign bodies in the caudal nasal cavity and nasopharynx. Pull the soft palate rostrally to improve the view.
- A **nasal flush** may remove all or parts of the foreign body for diagnosis.
- **Rhinotomy,** when all else fails.

Radiographs are rarely diagnostic, except for gun pellets.

Differential diagnosis

Chronic bacterial rhinitis secondary to viral upper respiratory infection may produce **similar laboratory findings** with neutrophils and bacteria, and no neoplastic or fungal elements. However, the **discharge** is typically **bilateral**, whereas with a foreign body it is typically unilateral.

Neoplasia and cryptococcosis may have similar signs, and the discharge is initially often unilateral. Positive diagnosis can be difficult with neoplasia and foreign bodies, and may require a rhinotomy.

Treatment

Treatment involves **removing the foreign body** by flushing, or grasping with forceps via the nares, nasopharynx or rhinotomy.

Prognosis

The prognosis is excellent if the foreign body can be entirely removed.

ORONASAL FISTULA OR NASAL FRACTURES FOLLOWING TRAUMA

> **Classical signs**
> - Chronic snuffling, sneezing and nasal discharge.
> - Cleft hard palate (lateral or midline).

Pathogenesis

Cats that have been **hit by a car**, or have **jumped out of a high-rise building** often have **splitting of the hard palate along the symphyses**.

Signs of chronic nasal discharge and sneezing result when food and water enter the nasal cavity.

Spontaneous healing of the cleft often occurs within 2–3 weeks.

If the hard palate is shattered into several pieces, **necrosis of a fragment** may occur, forming an **oronasal fistula**.

Clinical signs

Typically there is chronic snuffling, sneezing and nasal discharge in a cat that sustained facial injuries in a fall or car accident.

Examination reveals a **split hard palate** either **centrally along the palatine symphysis, or laterally adjacent to the teeth** along the maxillary symphysis.

Signs often resolve spontaneously with spontaneous healing of the cleft.

Diagnosis

Diagnosis is based on a history of trauma, signs of nasal disease and visual evidence of the cleft.

Differential diagnosis

Congenital cleft palate may look similar, but usually signs are present from a few weeks of age, rather than a recent onset following trauma.

Oronasal fistula associated with dental disease may produce similar signs; evidence of advanced periodontal disease and lack of history or evidence of facial trauma should allow differentiation.

Treatment

If spontaneous resolution does not occur in 2–3 weeks, surgical repair is necessary.

Prognosis

Good.

CHLAMYDOPHILA FELIS (CHLAMYDOPHILA FELIS PSITTACI) AND MYCOPLASMA

> **Classical signs**
> - Chronic ocular-nasal discharge.
> - Chronic conjunctivitis.
> - Chronic sneezing.

See main references on page 13 for details (The Cat With Acute Sneezing or Nasal Discharge) and Page 1215 (The Cat With Ocular Discharge or Changed Conjunctival Appearance).

Clinical signs

Chlamydophilia and mycoplasma infection may result in **chronic mucopurulent ocular and nasal discharge**.

Typically there is **chronic conjunctivitis. Follicular hyperplasia of lymphoid tissue** in the conjunctiva and nictitating membrane is often visible as multiple, small white nodules.

Chronic sneezing may occur.

Diagnosis

A **presumptive diagnosis** is often made based on signs. A **definitive diagnosis** is based on identification of the organism.
- Examine a stained (e.g. Diff-Quick) preparation of a conjunctival scraping or smear obtained with a dry cotton bud. *Chlamydophila felis* infection is associated with **inclusion bodies** in epithelial cells but they are difficult to identify in chronic disease. Mycoplasma is seen as clusters of coccoid or coccobacillary organisms in the periphery of epithelium cells.

Antibody-based detection in conjunctival scrapings using ELISA or latex agglutination may be useful for *Chlamydophila felis*, but false positives occur with both tests if many bacteria are present.

Polymerase chain reaction (PCR) and **IFA techniques** for detection of the organisms are also available from some laboratories.

NASOPHARYNGEAL STENOSIS

Classical signs
- Stertorous respiration from nasal area, ± dyspnea.
- No nasal discharge.

See main reference on page 38 for details (The Cat With Stridor).

Clinical signs

Chronic snuffling is typically present for 3 months to 2 years.

Stertorous respiration (snoring) or stridor (whistling noise) may be evident, and results from partial nasal obstruction. **Dyspnea** may occur, particularly when the cat is stressed.

Retching or gagging may occur on eating.

No or minimal nasal discharge is present.

Diagnosis

With the cat under general anesthesia, visualize the stenosis with a dental mirror. Pull the soft palate rostrally for an improved view.
- Stenosis is visible as a **pin-point opening in the nasopharynx.** The normal opening is approximately 5 mm in diameter.

Radiographs are generally normal.

NASOPHARYNGEAL POLYP

Classical signs
- Stertorous respiration from nasal area, or dyspnea.
- ± Nasal discharge.

See main reference on page 37 for details (The Cat With Stridor).

Clinical signs

Stertorous respiration is audible from the nasal area. If the obstruction is severe, there may be dyspnea, and open mouth breathing may occur with stress.

There may be **no nasal discharge,** or a mucopurulent discharge may be evident.

Discharge from ear and **signs of otitis media** may also be present.

Diagnosis

With the cat under general anesthesia, **visualize the polyp directly or with a dental mirror**. Pull the soft palate rostrally for an improved view. The rostral soft palate may bulge down into the oral cavity with pressure from the polyp.

Radiography reveals a rounded density in the nasopharynx, just caudal to the hard palate.

ALLERGIC RHINITIS

> **Classical signs**
>
> - Acute or chronic serous or mucoid nasal discharge, often seasonal.

Clinical signs

Allergic rhinitis appears to be a rare and poorly documented condition in cats.

It presents as serous or mucoid ocular and/or nasal discharge, with no systemic signs and is typically seasonal in occurrence.

It has been reported associated with allergy to **Japanese cedar** (*Cryptomeria japonica*).

Diagnosis

Diagnosis is based on **exclusion of all other causes** of nasal discharge and biopsy results indicating rhinitis with no evidence of underlying pathogens. A mixed neutrophilic and eosinophilic rhinitis has been reported.

Most cases with similar signs are the result of viral upper respiratory disease often with chronic bacterial rhinitis cases.

Treatment

A combination of antihistamine and steroid may work well in some cats. For example, Temaril-P (1/4 to 1/2 tablet PO q 12–24 h).

RECOMMENDED READING

Disorders of the nasal cavity In: Nelson RW, Couto CG (eds) Small Animal Internal Medicine, 2nd edition. St Louis, Mosby, 1998, pp 225–237.

Gaskell R, Dawson S. Feline respiratory disease. In: Greene CE (ed) Infectious Diseases of the Dog and Cat, 2nd edition. Philadelphia, WB Saunders Co., 1998, pp 97–106.

Jacobs GJ, Medleau L, Calvert C, et al. Cryptococcal infection in cats: factors influencing treatment outcome, and results of sequential serum antigen titers in 35 cats. J Vet Int Med 1997; 11: 1–4.

Lappin MR. Sneezing and nasal discharge; viral diseases. In: Lappin MR (ed) Feline Internal Medicine Secrets, 1st edition, Hanley and Belfus, Philadelphia, 2001, pp 8–11.

Malik R, Craig AJ, Wigney DI, et al. Combination chemotherapy of canine and feline cryptococcosis using subcutaneous administered amphotericin B. Aust Vet J 1996; 73: 124–128.

O'Brien RT, Evans SM, Wortman JA, Hendrick MJ. Radiographic findings in cats with intranasal neoplasia or chronic rhinitis: 29 cases (1982–1988). J Am Vet Med Assoc 1996; 208: 385–389.

Stein JE. Sneezing and nasal discharge; bacterial diseases. In: Lappin MR (ed) Feline Internal Medicine Secrets, 1st edition. Hanley and Belfus, Philadelphia, 2001, pp 4–8.

Stein JE, Lappin MR. Bacterial culture results in cats with upper or lower respiratory disease. J Vet Int Med 2001; 15: 320.

4. The cat with stridor or stertor

Jacquie Rand and Robert Allen Mason

> ### KEY SIGNS
> - Stridor.
> - Snuffling.
> - Snoring.

MECHANISM?

- Stridor is a harsh, high-pitched respiratory sound and stertor is a snoring sound created by upper airway obstructive diseases, such as laryngeal obstruction. Airflow through a narrowed upper airway has increased resistance and becomes more turbulent.
- With dynamic obstructions, such as laryngeal paralysis and tracheal collapse, the airflow limitation occurs mainly during inspiration. Fixed obstructions, such as foreign objects and mass lesions, affect airflow during both inspiration and expiration.

WHERE?

- Stridor or stertor arise from luminal narrowing in the upper airways, generally involving the pharynx, soft palate, laryngeal structures and the upper trachea. Nasal stridor may also be encountered.

WHAT?

- Most cats with respiratory stridor have nasal disease. Persians and Himalayans frequently have respiratory stridor from stenotic nares. Chronic bacterial rhinitis following viral upper respiratory tract infection, neoplasia or *Cryptococcus* infections are the most common acquired causes of stridor.

NASAL STRIDOR

QUICK REFERENCE SUMMARY

Diseases causing stridor or stertor

ANOMALY

- **Stenosis of the external nares** ** (p 35)
Breed-related obstruction of the external nares (e.g. Persian cats) causes chronic snuffling and stertorous respiration.

MECHANICAL

- Foreign body (grass, grass seed, awn) (p 40)

Acute onset of sneezing and rubbing face or gagging followed by chronic unilateral nasal discharge and sneezing. Occasionally stridor.

NEOPLASTIC

- **Neoplasia** (p 36)**

Chronic mucopurulent or hemorrhagic nasal discharge, often initially unilateral progressing to bilateral, sneezing, stertorous respiration ± facial distortion.

- Nasopharyngeal polyp (p 37)

Chronic snuffling, stertorous respiration and dyspnea from nasal obstruction, retching or gagging with eating ± mucropurulent nasal discharge.

INFLAMMATION

- Nasopharyngeal stenosis (p 38)

Chronic snuffling, partial nasal obstruction, retching or gagging with eating.

INFECTIOUS

Bacterial:

- **Secondary bacterial rhinitis*** (p 35)**

Typically there is a history of signs of chronic bacterial rhinitis occurring following acute viral upper respiratory tract disease. Signs include chronic mucopurulent or hemorrhagic nasal discharge, sneezing, stertorous respiration and occasionally nasal distortion.

Fungal:

- **Cryptococcosis and other fungi** (p 36)**

Cryptococcosis typically results in chronic mucopurulent or hemorrhagic nasal discharge, sneezing, stertorous respiration and distortion over bridge of nose (Roman nose), or a polyp-like mass in the nasal opening. Occasionally there are signs of a nasopharyngeal mass only. Other fungi such as *Aspergillus, Penicillium, Sporothrix* and some other fungi are very rare causes of chronic nasal disease.

Chlamydophila and *Mycoplasma spp*:

- *Chlamydophila* and *Mycoplasma* spp (p 38)

Chronic ocular and nasal discharge, and chronic conjunctivitis. Sneezing and occasionally stridor.

Trauma:

- Oronasal fistula or nasal fractures following trauma (p 39)

Chronic snuffling, sneezing, stridor or stertor and nasal discharge associated with cleft palate or obstructed nasal cavity.

continued

continued

STRIDOR FROM PHARYNGEAL, LARYNGEAL OR TRACHEAL AREA

Degenerative:

● Laryngeal paralysis (p 43)

Generally neurogenic paresis/paralysis of the abductor muscles of the arytenoid cartilages of the larynx. Often idiopathic, although traumatic causes are reported. Inspiratory dyspnea with stertor (snoring sounds) or stridor (whistling obstructive sounds) is the hallmark of laryngeal paralysis. Changes in voice and character of purring are often reported by owner.

● Tracheobronchial collapse (p 44)

Harsh, "honking" cough caused by degeneration of the cartilage support of the large airway walls. If upper cervical trachea is involved, stridor may be present. Rare in cats.

Anomaly:

● **Congenital anomalies of the upper respiratory tract* (p 39)**

Dyspnea usually indicates fixed obstruction (inspiratory and expiratory) because of the stenotic nature of most defects. Inspiratory dyspnea, stertor and stridor occur with the brachycephalic syndrome.

Mechanical:

● Airway foreign bodies (p 40)

Harsh, productive cough and acute dyspnea occur with foreign objects that have been inhaled, regurgitated or aspirated into the nasopharynx, trachea or bronchi. Stridor is noted when the foreign body is lodged in the larynx or trachea. Nasal foreign bodies create a form of stridor that has a more whistling character than laryngeal stridor. Sneezing and nasal discharge are common with nasal foreign bodies.

Neoplastic:

● Airway tumors (p 41)

Signs depend on the site of the tumor. Nasal tumors causing obstruction may produce stridor and open-mouth breathing. Pharyngeal tumors causing obstruction may result in dysphagia, stridor, stertor and voice changes. Tracheal tumors result in a fixed obstruction, and inspiratory and expiratory dyspnea, stridor and commonly a cough.

Inflammation:

● Laryngeal edema (p 42)

Usually occur secondary to an allergic reaction, following alphaxalone/alphdolone anesthesia or laryngeal trauma. Signs include inspiratory dyspnea and stertorous breathing or stridor.

● Laryngeal stenosis (p 42)

Common in cats after laryngeal trauma or surgery. Results in dyspnea and stridor on inspiration.

● Laryngeal eosinophilic granuloma (p 45)

Occurs weeks or months after signs of viral upper respiratory tract infection. Signs include stridor from the laryngeal region and swollen, edematous arytenoid cartilages of larynx.

INTRODUCTION

MECHANISM?

Airflow through a narrowed upper airway has increased resistance and becomes more turbulent. This resistance is a function of the diminished luminal diameter of the tube, **the resistance increasing to the fourth power of the radius**.

With **dynamic obstructions, dyspnea occurs during inspiration**, because the negative intraluminal airway pressure creates a vacuum, pulling the walls inwardly. Any weakened area of the airway wall will tend to move into the lumen, decrease the luminal diameter, and create an obstruction.

Fixed obstructions cause both inspiratory or expiratory stridor, although inspiratory noises are more prominent.

Stertor are snoring sounds. Stridor is a harsh, high-pitched whistling respiratory sound created by upper airway obstructive diseases, such as the inspiratory sound of acute laryngeal obstruction.

WHERE?

Stridor or stertor arise from luminal narrowing in the **upper airways**, generally involving the pharynx, soft palate, laryngeal structures and the upper trachea. Nasal stridor or stertor may also be encountered.

WHAT?

With dynamic obstructions, the airflow limitation occurs mainly during inspiration. Dynamic obstructions include **laryngeal paralysis, tracheal collapse and epiglottic entrapment**.

Fixed obstructions, such as **foreign objects and mass lesions**, affect airflow during both inspiration and expiration, although inspiratory noises are generally more prominent.

DISEASES CAUSING NASAL STRIDOR

SECONDARY BACTERIAL RHINITIS***

Classical signs

- Chronic sneezing and snuffling.
- Chronic mucopurulent nasal discharge.
- Stertorous respiration or stridor.
- Occasionally, nasal distortion.

See main reference on page 21 for details (The Cat With Signs of Chronic Nasal Disease).

Clinical signs

Chronic secondary bacterial rhinitis occurs in some cats following viral upper respiratory tract disease.

Typically there is a history of chronic sneezing and snuffling following acute upper respiratory tract signs.

Chronic mucopurulent nasal discharge.

Stertorous respiration (snoring) or stridor (high pitched whistling respiration).

Occasionally, nasal distortion.

Diagnosis

Diagnosis is based on a history of chronic signs of long duration (>6 months), especially if the history includes acute upper respiratory tract signs preceding the chronic problem. Diagnosis is based on exclusion of neoplasia and cryptococcosis.

STENOSIS OF THE EXTERNAL NARES**

Classical signs

- Chronic snuffling and stertorous respiration or stridor.
- Dyspnea or mouth breathing.
- Narrow external nares.

Pathogenesis

Congenital stenosis of the external nares is common in some breeds, e.g. Persians, Himalayans.

The combined effects of stenosis of the external nares and reduced nasal air space cause respiratory obstruction.

Partial obstruction results in increased respiratory effort and stertorous respiration or stridor.

With stress (e.g. visit to veterinarian or cat show), stridor becomes more pronounced, and cats may become severely dyspneic and mouth breath.

Clinical signs

Chronic snuffling and stertorous respiration or stridor.

Dyspnea or mouth breathing.

Narrow external nares in a brachycephalic cat.

Diagnosis

Based on clinical signs and physical examination.

Treatment

Surgical removal of the wing of the nostril.

NEOPLASIA **

> ### Classical signs
>
> - Progressively worsening chronic sneezing and snuffling.
> - Purulent or blood-tinged nasal discharge, which may temporarily respond to antibiotics.
> - Nasal obstruction and epiphora.
> - Occasionally facial distortion ± signs of retrobulbar pressure, e.g. exophthalmos.

See main reference on page 23 for details (The Cat With Signs of Chronic Nasal Disease).

Clinical signs

Chronic sneezing and snuffling, which progressively worsen with time.

Purulent or bloody nasal discharge, which **may temporarily respond to antibiotics**.

The discharge may **initially be unilateral** and **progress to bilateral involvement**.

Snoring, snorting, inspiratory stridor, stertor or dyspnea from nasal obstruction are common.

Facial distortion, e.g. elevation of bridge of nose (Roman nose) or facial swelling may be evident.

Epiphora (associated with obstruction of the lacrimal duct), or a bloody ocular discharge may occur.

Signs of **retrobulbar pressure** may be present, e.g. exophthalmos and ocular deviation.

Occasionally, central nervous system signs, e.g. seizures, circling, ataxia, behavioral change occur.

Nasal signs may be present for days, or in rare cases, for as long as 2 years. Usually, signs are present for less than 6 months prior to diagnosis.

Diagnosis

Radiography demonstrates increased opacity of the nasal cavity and often destruction of the turbinates, nasal septum, lateral bone and loss of teeth adjacent to the lesion. Radiographic changes are often unilateral or asymmetrical.

Cytological examination of the discharge or atraumatic nasal flush usually reveals evidence of inflammation (neutrophils and bacteria) but no tumor.

A traumatic flush using a stiff catheter and syringe (e.g. cut-off dog urinary catheter) yields better results than an atraumatic flush.

A biopsy is often required to obtain tissue for a histological diagnosis. Tissue may be obtained using biopsy forceps through the external nares or via a rhinotomy.

CRYPTOCOCCOSIS AND OTHER FUNGI**

> ### Classical signs
>
> - Chronic nasal discharge, stridor and sneezing, progressing in severity.
> - Soft tissue swelling over the nasal bones (Roman nose), or polyp-like mass in nasal cavity.

See main reference on page 25 for details (The Cat With Signs of Chronic Nasal Disease).

Clinical signs

Sneezing, snuffling, stridor or stertor and chronic nasal discharge are most common with cryptococcosis.

Nasal discharge may be unilateral or bilateral, and serous, mucopurulent or hemorrhagic.

Distortion and swelling over the bridge of nose, or a **polyp-like mass projecting from the nasal cavity** are present in 70% of cats with the respiratory form of cryptococcosis.

Depression, anorexia or inappetence and weight loss are often present with nasal or CNS involvement.

Mandibular lymph nodes are often enlarged.

Vestibular disease has been reported associated with cryptococcal infection.

Aspergillus, Penicillium, Sporothrix and some other fungi are very rare causes of chronic nasal disease.

Diagnosis

Cytological identification of the organism in nasal discharge, exudate from skin lesions, lymph node aspirate, cerebrospinal fluid (CSF), or ocular aspirate is diagnostic. Note that very occasionally small numbers of organisms may be cultured from the nasal exudate of normal cats.

Serology to detect cryptococcal capsular antigen in blood, CSF, or urine is **sensitive and specific**.

Tissue biopsy of the granulomatous mass or skin lesion, and histological identification of the organism may be required if cytology is negative.

PCR (polymerase chain reaction) assays are now available to detect cryptococcal antigens in biopsy material.

Fungal isolation with **culture** is rarely required for diagnosis, but is **useful for sensitivity testing**.

Radiographs often reveal **turbinate lysis and opacity** of the nasal cavity (soft tissue density). Sinus involvement is common.

NASOPHARYNGEAL POLYP

Classical signs

- Nasal discharge and congestion.
- Inspiratory dyspnea and stridor.

Classical signs—Cont'd

- Chronic non-responsive otitis, head tilt and Horner's syndrome.

Clinical signs

Nasopharyngeal polyps are thought to **occur secondary to chronic upper respiratory tract inflammation** as they consist of inflammatory tissue covered by epithelium. They are thought to **arise from the Eustachian tube** or **bulla**.

They are a **relatively common cause of stridor and dyspnea**, and typically occur in young cats (average age 1½ years old), and most begin to exhibit signs before they are 1 year of age. Abyssinians may be predisposed.

Chronic mucopurulent nasal discharge and congestion is common, but may be absent.

Inspiratory noises, usually stridor, but sometimes stertor, along with dyspnea and open-mouth breathing have been reported.

Signs of ear disease, including chronic discharge, head tilt and possibly Horner's syndrome on the affected side, may be present.

Diagnosis

Radiographs or CT may show a soft tissue **mass lesion in the nasopharynx**

Rhinoscopy and otoscopy are valuable in visualizing the mass and obtaining biopsy material. The polyp may be visualized directly or with a dental mirror. The rostral soft palate may bulge down into the oral cavity with pressure from the polyp. Pull the soft palate rostrally for an improved view.

Differential diagnosis

Tracheitis from feline rhinotracheitis virus is generally associated with other upper respiratory signs.

Laryngeal paralysis or edema, **tracheal foreign body**, and **tracheobronchial neoplasm** can be differentiated endoscopically.

Nasopharyngeal stenosis may have similar signs, and caudal rhinoscopy is required to distinguish this from polyp formation.

Treatment

Surgical therapy to remove the polyp is required. Concurrent bulla osteotomy may be needed to remove the entire source of the polyp and prevent recurrence. Generally, removal is via the mouth. The soft palate is retracted and the base of the polyp grasped with forceps. Gentle traction should be applied until the polyp detaches. Alternatively, the stalk may be cut. Bleeding may be profuse, but more often is minimal.

NASOPHARYNGEAL STENOSIS

Classical signs

- Stertorous respiration from nasal area.
- Dyspnea.
- No or minimal nasal discharge.

Pathogenesis

Rare condition thought to arise secondary to chronic nasal inflammation or trauma.

A strong membrane forms across the nasopharynx. It may completely occlude the nasopharyngeal opening, or more often it reduces the opening to pin-point size.

Clinical signs

Chronic snuffling of 3 months to 2 years duration is reported.

Any age of cat from < 1 year to 10 years may be affected.

Stertorous respiration (snoring) or stridor (whistling noise) occurs from partial nasal obstruction.

Dyspnea, or open-mouth breathing may occur.

Retching or gagging may be evident on eating.

No or minimal nasal discharge.

Diagnosis

With the cat under general anesthesia, visualize the stenosis with a dental mirror. Pull the soft palate rostrally for an improved view.

Stenosis is visible as a pin-point opening in the nasopharynx (normal opening is approximately 5 mm).

Radiographs are generally normal.

Diagnosis

Diagnosis is based on the history, signs and visual evidence of the stenosis.

Treatment

Treatment involves surgical removal of the stenosis.

Prognosis

Prognosis is good with surgery

CHLAMYDOPHILIA AND MYCOPLASMA

Classical signs

- Chronic ocular-nasal discharge.
- Chronic conjunctivitis.
- Acute or chronic sneezing.
- Stertor and stridor.

See main references on page 13 for details (The Cat With Acute Sneezing or Nasal Discharge) and pages 1215, 1218 (The Cat With Ocular Discharge or Changed Conjunctival Appearance).

Clinical signs

Chlamydophila felis and *Mycoplasma* spp. infection may result in initial acute signs of upper respiratory tract infection progressing to chronic conjunctivitis, chronic mucopurulent ocular and nasal discharge.

Sneezing and occasionally stridor or stertor may occur.

Follicular hyperplasia of lymphoid tissue in the conjunctiva and nictitating membrane is often visible as **multiple, small white nodules** in *Chlamydophila* infection.

Diagnosis

A **presumptive diagnosis** is often made based on signs. A **definitive diagnosis** is based on identification of the organism.

Examine a stained (e.g. Diff-Quick) preparation of a conjunctival scraping or smear obtained with a dry cotton bud. *Chlamydophila felis* infection is associated with **inclusion bodies** in epithelial cells but they are difficult to identify in chronic disease. Mycoplasma is seen as clusters of coccoid or coccobacillary organisms in the periphery of epithelium cells.

Antibody-based detection in conjunctival scrapings using ELISA or latex agglutination may be useful for *Chlamydophila felis*, but false positives occur with both tests if many bacteria are present.

Polymerase chain reaction (PCR) and IFA techniques for detection of the organisms are also available from some laboratories.

ORONASAL FISTULA OR NASAL FRACTURES FOLLOWING TRAUMA

Classical signs

- Chronic snuffling, sneezing, stridor or stertor and nasal discharge .
- Cleft hard palate (lateral or midline).

See main reference on page 29 for details (The Cat With Signs of Chronic Nasal Disease).

Clinical signs

Typically there is chronic snuffling, sneezing, **stridor or stertor,** and nasal discharge in a cat that sustained facial injuries in a fall or car accident.

Examination may reveal a **split hard palate** either **centrally along the platine symphysis, or laterally adjacent to the teeth** along the maxillary symphysis.

Signs often resolve spontaneously with spontaneous healing of the cleft or nasal fracture.

Diagnosis

Diagnosis is based on a history of trauma, signs of nasal disease, visual evidence of the cleft and radiography.

FOREIGN BODY (GRASS, GRASS SEED, AWN)

Classical signs

- Acute onset of sneezing and rubbing face, progressing to chronic signs.
- Unilateral discharge.
- Gagging.

See main reference on page 28 for details (The Cat With Signs of Chronic Nasal Disease).

Grass or seeds may occasionally enter the nose of cats. Other foreign bodies such as gun pellets are less common.

Clinical signs

Typically there is an **acute onset of sneezing and distress**, and rubbing at the face.

Signs may progress to chronic gagging, or sneezing and discharge.

A unilateral serosanguineous discharge is typically present.

Diagnosis

Visualize foreign body using an otoscope, fiber-optic scope, or with a dental mirror in the nasopharynx. Use a spay hook to retract the soft palate for better visualization.

Flushing the nose using a naso-esophageal feeding catheter may remove parts or all of the whole foreign body for diagnosis.

THE CAT WITH PHARYNGEAL, LARYNGEAL OR TRACHEAL STRIDOR OR STERTOR

CONGENITAL ANOMALIES OF THE UPPER RESPIRATORY TRACT*

Classical signs

- Usually inspiratory and expiratory dyspnea.
- Inspiratory dyspnea with both stridor and stertor occurs with the brachycephalic syndrome.

Pathogenesis

Congenital anatomic anomalies characteristic of **brachycephalic breeds (Persians, Himalayans)**, are related to the flat face and short neck. Stenotic nares is the most commonly evident anomaly.

Brachycephalic syndrome includes stenotic nares, elongated soft palate, eversion of the lateral laryngeal ventricles, laryngeal collapse and hypoplastic trachea.

Clinical signs

Stenotic nares, hypoplastic trachea, etc., create a non-dynamic, fixed obstruction leading to inspiratory and expiratory dyspnea.

Dynamic obstructions occur with an elongated soft palate and create **inspiratory dyspnea with stertor**.

Stridor is present with laryngeal collapse or lateral ventricular eversion.

Collapse, exercise intolerance, dyspnea or dysphagia may also be reported.

Oronasal reflux, especially with fluids, occurs with a cleft palate.

Diagnosis

Diagnosis is based mostly on **clinical signs of stertor and stridor in a brachycephalic** cat. Nasal stenosis can be assessed visually. **Pharyngoscopy and laryngoscopy** are required to diagnose and stage the severity of **palatal** and **laryngeal involvement**.

Lateral cervical and thoracic radiographs are needed to assess tracheal hypoplasia.

Differential diagnosis

Upper airway foreign bodies and **masses** may mimic brachycephalic syndrome in a brachycephalic breed, although careful history-taking will usually differentiate them based on time of onset. Laryngeal edema may occur due to causes other than congenital malformation.

Treatment

If possible, **surgically correct** the defect, if the signs are severe. This includes wedge resection of the nares,

palatal resection, and resection of the everted lateral ventricles.

Prognosis

The prognosis is excellent for nasal, palatal and laryngeal defects with surgical intervention, if indicated. **Tracheal hypoplasia is currently not treatable**. **Prevention or treatment of obesity** is a major prognostic factor, as lean cats tolerate this much better than obese cats.

Prevention

Prevention is via selected breeding programs. Not using severely affected cats for breeding will help to reduce the prevalence.

AIRWAY FOREIGN BODIES

> **Classical signs**
>
> - Sneezing and stridor (nasal foreign bodies).
> - Coughing and stridor (pharyngeal and tracheobronchial foreign bodies).

Clinical signs

Grass is one of the most common foreign bodies. The blade of grass becomes adherent to the roof of the pharynx and extends into the nasopharyngeal region.

Cuterebra larvae may bury in the **retropharyngeal tissue or in the pharyngeal soft palate**. A clue to diagnosis is evidence of a hole in the mucosa or a mass lesion.

Bone fragments and sewing needles may become embedded in the pharnx. **Cotton, string and fishing line** may get caught around the base of the tongue. **Grass seeds** may cause nasal foreign bodies.

Acute onset of sneezing and nasal discharge are common signs of nasal foreign bodies. The cat may be in sudden and severe distress attempting to dislodge the foreign body. Pawing at the face and mouth is commonly observed.

Signs of **fixed obstruction** occur with nasal and tracheobronchial foreign bodies because airflow is limited during inspiration and expiration due to constant partial obstruction of the airway. This may result in increased breathing sounds, and often stridor and dyspnea during inspiration and expiration.

Typically **nasal foreign bodies have sneezing, stridor and pawing or rubbing of the face**, while **pharyngeal and tracheobronchial foreign bodies present with coughing, stridor, gagging or retching,** pawing at the mouth, salivation and dyspnea. Typically the signs are frequent, marked and have a sudden onset.

Diagnosis

Some nasal and most tracheal foreign bodies may be seen radiographically.

Rhinoscopy and tracheobronchoscopy can be both diagnostic and therapeutic. Rigid tracheoscopy allows for larger retrieval instruments to be utilized than with flexible endoscopy.

Differential diagnosis

Nasopharyngeal polyps may cause similar signs of nasal obstruction and sneezing, but tend to have a more chronic course.

Tracheal or bronchial neoplasia may have similar signs, but again are more chronic in nature and can be distinguished bronchoscopically.

Treatment

Removal of the foreign body, either surgically or endoscopically, is often curative. Nasal foreign bodies may be endoscopically retrieved or hydropulsed, but occasionally require surgical rhinotomy.

AIRWAY TUMORS

Classical signs

- Nasal obstruction: stridor, open-mouth breathing.
- Pharyngeal obstruction: dysphagia, stridor, stertor and voice changes.
- Tracheal tumors: fixed obstruction, inspiratory and expiratory dyspnea and stridor. Cough is common.

See reference on page 23 for details (The Cat With Signs of Chronic Nasal Disease).

Pathogenesis

Nasal tumors are most commonly squamous cell carcinoma (SCC) of the nasal planum, solid nasal carcinomas and nasal lymphoma.

SCCs of the tonsil are common pharyngeal masses, along with **benign nasopharyngeal polyps**.

Tracheal tumors consist of lymphoma, SCC, leiomyosarcoma and osteochondral tumors from the tracheal rings. Adenocarcinomas have increased prevalence in the Siamese.

Lymphosarcoma and squamous cell carcinomas are the most frequent tumor types involving the larynx.

Clinical signs

Nasal obstruction produces stridor, open-mouth breathing, unilateral nasal discharge and coughing from post-nasal drip. Anosmia may lead to inappetence.

Pharyngeal masses produce dysphagia, stridor, stertorous dyspnea and voice changes. **Fetid halitosis** is also reported.

Tracheal tumors cause fixed obstruction, leading to **both** inspiratory and expiratory dyspnea with stridor, which is often louder on inspiration. A harsh, dry cough is common.

Diagnosis

Diagnosis is made via rhinoscopy, pharyngoscopy or tracheoscopy with biopsy. It is possible to image soft tissue masses radiographically, but endoscopy is still advised for biopsy. Other imaging modalities (CT and MRI) provide excellent images and aid in surgical and radiotherapy planning.

Differential diagnosis

Inhaled and penetrating foreign bodies may produce similar signs, but usually have a history of acute onset. Benign or parasitic **granulomas** of the airways may mimic neoplastic masses but can be differentiated on biopsy.

Treatment

Solid nasal tumors often respond well to external beam radiotherapy, with survival times of 20–27 months. Rhinotomy with turbinatectomy has been reported to be successful.

Often, there is extensive local invasion by the neoplasm, and the recurrence rate after radiotherapy with or without surgery is high.

Nasal lymphoma responds well to standard chemotherapy for lymphoma, with remission times of 16 months reported. See page 676 for therapy.

Pharyngeal and tracheal masses and nasopharyngeal polyps (see page 37) are best addressed with surgical resection.

Laryngeal tumors are difficult to resect and generally carry a poor prognosis.

LARYNGEAL EDEMA

Classical signs

- Inspiratory dyspnea.
- Stertorous breathing, stridor.

Pathogenesis

Usually occurs **secondary to an allergic reaction** (type I hypersensitivity) from an **insect sting**, or following **vaccination**.

Acute laryngeal edema occurs in some cats associated with the intravenous anesthetic agent **alfaxalone/alphdolone (Saffan,** Scherng-Plough) which is available in Europe and other countries. The oil-based preparation causes histamine release.

Edema may be the result of **laryngeal trauma**, either blunt trauma to the throat, penetrating trauma (cat-bite wound), or from the **ingestion of sharp objects** or **caustic materials** (phenols, alkalis, acids) or **plants** (poinsettias, philodendrons, dieffenbachia).

Clinical signs

Inspiratory dyspnea, which may be associated with severe respiratory distress and cyanosis.

Stertor occurs, which is worsened with excitement or exercise.

Diagnosis

Acute onset of inspiratory dyspnea.

Laryngoscopic inspection under heavy sedation or light anesthesia with a rigid laryngoscope and blade reveals erythema and edema of the laryngeal mucosa.

Differential diagnosis

Laryngeal paralysis, laryngeal mass lesion or foreign bodies may have similar signs, but are differentiated on history and visualization of the larynx.

Treatment

Corticosteroids are indicated.
- Dexamethasone (0.1–0.25 mg/kg IV or IM), or prednisolone sodium succinate (10–30 mg/kg IV) are good parenteral choices.

Antihistamines may be useful, but histamine release has generally already occurred at the time of presentation.

Intubation or tracheostomy may be indicated in severe situations.

Prognosis

Generally good, but severe obstruction, if untreated, can be fatal. Laryngeal edema can also be a harbinger of systemic anaphylaxis.

Prevention

Avoidance of insect stings, access to poisonous plants and caustic agents such as dishwashing powder and cleaning agents.

Use of the new formulation of alfaxalone (Alsaxon-CD, Turox, Australia), which is water-based.

LARYNGEAL STENOSIS

Classical signs

- Dyspnea and stridor on inspiration.
- Common in cats after laryngeal trauma or surgery.

Pathogenesis

The cat appears to be more prone to fibrosis and stricture formation of the upper airway than is the dog. **Trauma from external penetrating wounds, aspirated foreign bodies**, or from **caustic chemical damage**, or **post-operative scarring** can **lead to excessive scar formation and stricture**.

The narrowed lumen creates the airway resistance and stridor. A **web of fibrosis** may **form across the larynx** and is especially dangerous.

Clinical signs

Laryngeal stenosis causes a dynamic airflow limitation, resulting in **inspiratory stridor and dyspnea**.

Stridor is worse with excitement or exercise.

Occasional stertor is evident.

Voice changes (absent or whisper-like meow), or harsh purring sounds may be reported.

Diagnosis

Diagnosis is based on clinical signs and history of prior laryngeal damage or surgery.

Laryngoscopic inspection under heavy sedation or light anesthesia with a rigid laryngoscope and blade reveals the stricture.

Low-dose ketamine (4–6 mg/kg IV), ketamine/diazepam (3–5 mg/kg/0.1–0.2 mg/kg IV) or propofol (4–6 mg/kg IV) allows visual inspection.

Differential diagnosis

Other causes of fixed upper respiratory tract obstruction are considerations, but can usually be differentiated visually or on biopsy. They include the following:
- **Oropharyngeal neoplasia** (SCC, oral melanoma, nasopharyngeal polyp).
- **Laryngeal or tracheal neoplasia** (intraluminal adenocarcinoma, extraluminal masses) or foreign bodies.

Treatment

Surgical intervention is generally required.
- Surgical resection of the stricture, if possible, is indicated. Laryngeal tie-back surgery (**arytenoid**

lateralization) may be required (see Laryngeal paralysis section).

In emergency respiratory distress, temporary tracheostomy may be required below the stricture, although this too can lead to future stricture formation.

Prognosis

Depends upon the nature and location of the stricture.

Prevention

At the time of laryngeal trauma or surgery, corticosteroids may help diminish scar formation.

LARYNGEAL PARALYSIS

Classical signs
- Inspiratory dyspnea and increased airway noise.
- Stertorous breathing (*snoring*).
- Stridor (high-pitched whistling = obstructive).
- Voice changes, absence of purring.

Pathogenesis

Exact pathomechanism is unclear in cats because of the small numbers reported.

It may be congenital, although most cases appear in **middle-aged to older cats**.

Peripheral neuropathies of recurrent laryngeal nerves can cause laryngeal paralysis. In dogs they have been associated with endocrinopathies (hypothyroidism – but this is rare in cats), myasthenia gravis, immune-mediated or paraneoplastic peripheral neuropathies, but this association has not been documented in cats.

Trauma, either to the recurrent laryngeal nerve (head, cervical or thoracic trauma) or to the structure of the larynx itself, can impair the laryngeal function. **Temporary or permanent damage** to the recurrent laryngeal nerve may occur following **cervical surgery, for example following thyroidectomy**.

Neoplasia, affecting either the innervation of the larynx (i.e., thyroid adenocarcinoma) or affecting the laryngeal structures directly (i.e., squamous cell carcinoma) can create laryngeal paralysis.

Parasitic involvement of the larynx and lead poisoning are very rare associations.

Percutaneous ultrasound-guided radiofrequency heat ablation and ethanol injections for treatment of hyperthyroidism in cats are both recent procedures, and laryngeal paralysis was a reported side effect of both.

Clinical signs

Inspiratory dyspnea, tachypnea.

Stridor, worse with excitement or exercise.

Occasional stertor.

Voice changes (absent or whisper-like meow), harsh purring sounds.

Dysphagia and weight loss.

Diagnosis

Diagnosis is based on clinical signs of laryngeal stridor and inspiratory dyspnea.

Laryngoscopic inspection under heavy sedation or light anesthesia with a rigid laryngoscope and blade reveals **absent or paradoxical motion** of the arytenoid cartilages. Normally they should abduct on inspiration. If they close on inspiration, it is paradoxical motion.

One retrospective study of 16 cases revealed 12 to be bilateral, and four to be unilateral.

Erythema and swelling of the arytenoid mucosa ("kissing lesions") may be evident from the repetitive trauma at the contact surfaces.

Low-dose ketamine (4–6 mg/kg IV), ketamine/diazepam (3–5 mg/kg/0.1–0.2 mg/kg IV) or propofol (4–6 mg/kg IV) allows visual inspection without diminishing laryngeal function.

Differential diagnosis

Other causes of dynamic or fixed upper respiratory tract obstruction are distinguished on laryngoscopic inspection.

Dynamic causes of upper respiratory tract obstruction are:
- **Brachycephalic airway syndrome** (elongated soft palate, lateral ventricle eversion).
- **Cervical tracheal collapse**.
- Pyogranulomatous or lymphoplasmacytic **laryngitis**.

Other causes of fixed upper respiratory tract obstruction include:
- **Oropharyngeal neoplasia** (SCC, oral melanoma, nasopharyngeal polyp).
- **Tracheal neoplasia** (intraluminal adenocarcinoma, extraluminal masses).
- **Tracheal foreign bodies**.

Treatment

Correction of the underlying cause of the neuropathy is rarely possible.

Surgical intervention is generally required for bilateral disease.
- Laryngeal tie-back surgery (**arytenoid lateralization**) is recommended by most surgeons, although other techniques are described. Success is directly correlated with skill of the operator.

In emergency respiratory distress, temporary tracheostomy may be required.

Prognosis

Generally good to excellent long-term prognosis with successful surgery.

Prevention

None known.

TRACHEOBRONCHIAL COLLAPSE

Classical signs
- Harsh, honking cough.
- Stridor on inspiration if cervical segment involved.
- Very rare in cats.

Clinical signs

Tracheobronchial collapse is **very rare in cats** and generally occurs **secondary to trauma or to com-**

pression caused by an **extraluminal mass**. It has been reported associated with proximal tracheal obstructions from a trachael granuloma or polyp.

The **cough is often harsh, non-productive and paroxysmal**, ending in a gagging episode which may appear to be productive.

Cervical trachea collapse produces inspiratory dyspnea, while intrathoracic tracheal or bronchial collapse will lead to mostly expiratory dyspnea. Stridor is occasionally reported.

Diagnosis

Radiographs may show attenuation of the tracheal or bronchial lumina. Fluoroscopy may be more sensitive for dynamic collapse.

Tracheobronchoscopy is valuable in both diagnosing and grading the severity of the collapse.

Differential diagnosis

Tracheitis from feline rhinotracheitis virus is generally associated with other upper respiratory signs.

Laryngeal paralysis or **edema, tracheal foreign body** and **tracheobronchial neoplasm** can be differentiated endoscopically.

Small airway disease (feline asthma/bronchitis complex) can worsen upper airway collapse, but generally diagnosis is based on the radiographic peribronchiolar pattern and airway inflammation on lung wash cytology.

Treatment

Medical treatment is indicated for a short and minimally attenuated collapsing segment, and consists primarily of antitussive therapy (**butorphanol** 1 mg/cat PO q 6–12 h as needed).

Surgical therapy may be indicated with severe collapse due to trauma. This generally requires referral to a specialist with experience in airway surgery. Extraluminal spiral ring prostheses made from a 3 ml syringe case were successful in reducing signs in two cats.

Weight loss and avoidance of neck collars can be very beneficial in affected cats.

LARYNGEAL EOSINOPHILIC GRANULOMA

Classical signs

- Stridor from laryngeal region.
- Swollen, edematous arytenoid cartilages of larynx.

Clinical signs

Syndrome often occurs **weeks or months** after signs of **viral upper respiratory tract infection.**

Stridor from laryngeal region is evident.

The larynx appears edematous and swollen.

With stress, cats become dyspneic and may mouth breathe.

Diagnosis

Visual appearance and biopsy are diagnostic. Biopsy reveals an eosinophilic granuloma.

Differential diagnosis

Invasive squamous cell carcinoma may have a similar appearance but can be differentiated on biopsy.

Other inflammatory infiltrations of the larynx, for example with lymphocyte, may appear similar, but are differentiated on biopsy.

Treatment

Oral steroids such as **prednisolone** 2 mg/kg bid PO for 10 days, then taper dose.

If oral medication cannot be given, methylprednisolone acetate (2–4 mg/kg 7 days for 2–6 treatments), can be used.

Occasionally, refractory cases need chlorambucil (0.1–0.2 mg/kg q 24 h initially PO, IM, then q 48 h).

RECOMMENDED READING

Little CJL. Nasopharyngeal polyps. In: August J (ed) Consultations in Feline Internal Medicine. W.B Saunders, Philadelphia, 1997, pp 310–316.

McKiernan BC. Respiratory diseases. In: Kirk R (ed) Current Veterinary Therapy. W.B Saunders, Philadelphia, 1983, pp 191–261.

McKiernan C. Sneezing and nasal discharge. In: Ettinger S, Feldman E. (eds) Textbook of Veterinary Internal Medicine. W.B Saunders, Philadephia, 2000, pp 194–197.

Schachter S, Norris CR. Laryngeal paralysis in cats: 16 cases (1990–1999). J Am Vet Med Assoc 2000; 216(7): 1100–1103.

Sherding R. The Cat: Diseases and Clinical Management. W.B Saunders, New York, 1994.

PART 2

Cat with lower respiratory tract or cardiac signs

5. The dyspneic or tachypneic cat

Robert Allen Mason and Jacquie Rand

KEY SIGNS

Dyspnea
- Anxious, uncomfortable breathing.
- Increased respiratory effort.
- Respiratory distress.

Tachypnea
- Rapid breathing, not necessarily labored.

MECHANISM?

- Dyspnea can be caused by several mechanisms:
    obstruction to airflow.
    weakness of ventilatory muscles.
    pleural space disease, inhibiting expansion of the lungs.
    diminished oxygen-carrying capacity of the blood.

WHERE?

- Upper respiratory tract (nasal cavity, paranasal sinuses, pharynx, larynx, trachea).
- Lower respiratory tree (bronchial tree, small airways).
- Lung parenchyma, pleural space, chest wall and ventilatory muscles.

WHAT?

- Acute severe dyspnea in cats is often caused by an acute asthma attack, trauma or decompensating congestive heart failure.

QUICK REFERENCE SUMMARY

Diseases causing a dyspneic or tachypneic cat

DEGENERATIVE

● **Cardiomyopathy** (p 54)

Dilated cardiomyopathy (DCM), hypertrophic (HCM), intermediate (ICM) or restrictive (RCM) often present as acute dyspnea. Abnormal heart sounds are often audible as mumurs, gallops and arrhythmias. Advential lung sounds, such as crackles may be audible with pulmonary edema. Occasionally, marked pleural effusion is present and heart and lung sounds are muffled ventrally. Coughing is an uncommon presenting sign in the cat.

● Tracheobronchial collapse (p 69)

Very rare in cats. Degeneration of the cartilage support of the large airway walls results in tracheo-bronchial collapse. Cervical collapse causes inspiratory dyspnea, while intrathoracic collapse causes expiratory dyspnea. Harsh honking cough and stridor may be evident.

● Laryngeal paralysis (p 67)

Idiopathic laryngeal paralysis is reported in cats. Iatrogenic paralysis may occur after cervical surgery or trauma. Inspiratory dyspnea, stridor and stertor are common signs.

ANOMALIES

● Congenital heart defects (p 67)

Atrioventricular valve dysplasia, septal defects, aortic and pulmonic stenosis (rare) and patent ductus arteriosus all lead to pressure and/or volume overload on the heart and potentially result in congestive heart failure. Dyspnea, open-mouth breathing, cyanosis, exaggerated chest excursions with minimal airflow all may occur. Abnormal heart sounds are common.

● Congenital anomalies of the upper respiratory tract (p 68)

Stenotic nares, elongated soft palate, hypoplastic trachea (i.e., brachycephalic syndrome) create variable upper airway resistance. Stertor and inspiratory dyspnea are common signs.

● **Acquired or congenital diaphragmatic defects*** (p 57)

Abdominal contents lie within the pleural or pericardial cavities, creating variable degrees of dyspnea. Signs include increased chest excursions with decreased airflow, muffled heart and lung sounds, and reluctance to lie in lateral recumbency. Palpation of the abdomen has an empty feel.

MECHANICAL

● Grass awns, foreign bodies (p 65)

Foreign bodies may be inhaled into the nasal cavity, upper respiratory tract or lower airways. The character of the dyspnea is dependent on location.

● **Pleural effusion** (p 54)

Dyspnea characterized by excessive chest excursions with poor airflow, orthopnea, muffled heart and lung sounds. Signs of chronic illness may be present such as weight loss.

METABOLIC

● Myopathy/neuropathy (p 61)

Hypokalemia, myasthenia gravis, polyradiculoneuritis (rare in cats), botulism, polymyositis and other causes of weakness of the respiratory muscles cause poor ventilatory muscle excursions.

● **Anemia/hypoxemia* (p 57)**

Reduced oxygen-carrying capacity of the blood results from anemia (blood loss, hemolysis, myelodysplastic disease) or altered hemoglobin (methoxyhemoglobinemia from acetaminophen toxicity, carboxyhemoglobinemia from CO toxicity). Tachypnea, pallor, cyanosis or brick-red mucous membranes may be seen.

● **Pulmonary thromboembolism***

Secondary to hypercoagulable states, blood flow stasis, vascular injuries and heartworm disease. Creates significant ventilation/perfusion mismatch, with sudden onset of severe dyspnea and tachypnea. Cyanosis and collapse may occur. Lung parenchyma may appear normal radiographically.

● **Aortic thromboembolism* (p 58)**

Acute single-limb paresis or, with "saddle" thrombus, bilateral hindlimb paralysis. The affected limb is cold, painful and the foot pads are cyanotic. Signs of congestive heart failure may be severe, with marked worsening of dyspnea.

NEOPLASTIC

● **Pleural/mediastinal masses***

Signs relate to the space-occupying nature of the mass. Dyspnea with muffled heart and lung sounds or pleural effusion. Heart sounds are typically asymmetric because of displacement of the heart by the mass. Compression of the chest wall may reveal decreased compliance.

● Airway tumors

Nasal, laryngeal and cervical tracheal masses create stertor, stridor and inspiratory dyspnea. Thoracic tracheal and bronchial masses create expiratory dyspnea. Coughing may occur with tracheal masses.

● Pulmonary neoplasia

Dyspnea may be subtle. Systemic signs such as weight loss and possibly coughing may be evident. Inappetence, weight loss, fetid breath and reluctance to play may also be noted.

● Cardiac tumors

Extremely rare in cats. Space-occupying effect in chest or signs of congestive heart failure from obstruction of blood flow may produce dyspnea.

INFLAMMATORY

INFECTIOUS

● **Acute and chronic infectious upper respiratory tract disease****

Sneezing, acute or chronic oculonasal discharge, and sometimes conjunctivitis are present. Inspiratory dyspnea occurs if there is marked nasal obstruction. Nasal distortion may be present with cryptococcosis, neoplasia or rarely with secondary bacterial rhinitis.

Bacterial:

● **Pyothorax****

Dyspnea characterized by excessive chest excursions with poor airflow, orthopnea, muffled heart and lung sounds. Signs of chronic illness may be present such as weight loss. Signs of sepsis such as hypothermia and hypoglycemia are occasionally present. Often signs of chronic illness such as weight loss and inappetence were evident before presentation for dyspnea.

continued

continued

   ● Pneumonia
   Uncommon in cats. Fever, fetid halitosis, crackles and wheezes heard over lung fields.

Parasitic:

   ● Parasites
   Heartworm (*Dirafilaris immitus*), lung worm (*Aleurostrongylus abstrusus, Capillaria aerophilia*), lung flukes (*Paragonomus kellicoti*), and migrating nematodes (*Toxocara cati*) are potential lung pathogens. Coughing may be seen. Inappetence, weight loss and poor hair coat may be evident. Vomiting is reported in feline heartworm disease along with dyspnea. Acute marked respiratory distress and sudden death may also occur with heartworm.

Immune:

   ● **Feline asthma/bronchitis complex)*****
   Acute dyspnea occurs with s*tatus asthmaticus.* Cats are air-starved, and present with frantic, open-mouth breathing, increased expiratory effort, and with possible wheezing and coughing.

   ● Laryngeal edema (p 64)
   Laryngeal edema may follow a hypersensitivity reaction. Inspiratory dyspnea, stridor and stertor are common signs.

   ● Acute systemic anaphylaxis (p 68)
   Clinical signs include acute dyspnea, collapse, pale mucus membranes and other signs of hypotensive shock. There may be a history of exposure to a foreign antigen, usually protein. Anaphylaxis may occur on the first exposure to the inciting antigen.

Idiopathic:

   ● Pulmonary fibrosis (p 69)
   Pulmonary fibrosis causes both inspiratory and expiratory dyspnea. It is a very rare condition and may be associated with feline asthma/bronchitis complex. A syndrome consistent with usual interstitial pneumonia in human beings has been reported in cats.

   ● Fibrosing pleuritis (p 70)
   Restrictive fibrosing pleuritis cause both inspiratory and expiratory dyspnea. It is a rare sequel of pyothorax and other chronic pleural effusions, especially chylothorax. Heart and lung sounds are muffled ventrally.

Trauma:

   ● **Upper airway/chest wall trauma*****
   Character of the dyspnea corresponds to the area of injury. Marked inspiratory dyspnea, stridor and subcutaneous emphysema may be evident with laryngeal or trachea trauma. Chest wall trauma may result in dyspnea, cyanosis, abnormal or decreased lung sounds and evidence of shock.

INTRODUCTION

MECHANISM?

Dyspnea is the distressful feeling associated with difficult or labored breathing. In animals, the term dyspnea is often applied to labored breathing that appears to be uncomfortable.

Tachypnea is rapid breathing (not necessarily labored).

Hyperpnea is deep breathing.

Hyperventilation refers to increased air entering the pulmonary alveoli, brought about by prolonged, rapid and deep breathing.

Panting, however, refers to swift and shallow breathing, with a rapid respiratory frequency and a small tidal volume.

Respiratory causes of dypsnea include upper and lower airway obstruction.

Upper airway obstructions may be fixed or dynamic. Airflow through a narrowed upper airway has increased resistance and becomes more turbulent. This resistance is a function of the diminished luminal diameter of the tube, **the resistance increasing to the fourth power of the radius**.

- **Fixed obstructions** affect both **inspiration** and **expiration.**
- **With dynamic obstructions, dyspnea occurs during inspiration**, because the negative intraluminal airway pressure creates a vacuum, pulling the walls inwardly. Any weakened area of the airway wall will tend to move into the lumen, decrease the luminal diameter, and create an obstruction.

Lower airway obstructions may be **obstructive** or **restrictive.**

- **Obstructions** include intraluminal masses and foreign bodies, bronchoconstriction, extraluminal compression by masses or left atrial enlargement, and rarely tracheobronchial collapse.
- **Restrictive obstructions** include pleural space disease (pneumothorax, hydrothorax, pleural masses) and primary pulmonary disease (pulmonary fibrosis, pneumonia) that restrict expansion of the lung.

Non-respiratory causes of dyspnea are varied and include:

- Weakness of ventilatory, muscles or diseases which restrict thoracic expansion (myopathies, neuropathies, neuromuscular disease, obesity and organomegaly).
- Pulmonary vascular disease (pulmonary hypertension, pulmonary thromboembolism, shock).
- Diminished oxygen-carrying capacity (methemoglobinemia, anemia).
- Cardiac disease (congestive heart failure, cyanotic heart disease with right-to-left shunting).
- Miscellaneous (pain, fever, anxiety, hyperthermia).

WHERE?

Upper respiratory tract (nasal cavity, paranasal sinuses, pharynx, larynx, trachea). With upper respiratory tract obstructions, stertor and stridor may be evident. Stertor is a snoring sound. Stridor is a harsh, high-pitched whistling respiratory sound created by upper airway obstructive diseases. Stridor arises from luminal narrowing in the upper airways, generally involving the pharynx, soft palate, laryngeal structures and the upper trachea. Nasal stridor may also be encountered.

Lower respiratory tree (bronchial tree, small airways).

Lung parenchyma, pleural space, chest wall and ventilatory muscles. Pleural space disease often has dyspnea with excessive chest wall excursions accompanied by minimal nasal airflow.

Oxygen delivery system (blood vessels, RBCs, heart).

What?

Acute severe dyspnea in cats is often caused by an acute asthmatic attack, decompensating congestive heart failure or trauma.

The dyspneic cat is extremely fragile, and needs to be handled very gently and with minimal restraint. Cats with open-mouth breathing and cyanosis have very little respiratory reserve left, and the slightest additional stress may be lethal.

In most cases, we need to resist the temptation to make a definitive diagnosis until our patient is more stable. These cats are focusing on their next breath, and are not in the least concerned with our welfare and well-being.

These cats often require much less restraint than a well cat. If there is the slightest resistance to restraint – **STOP RESTRAINING THEM** – and proceed with supportive care in as least a stressful manner as possible.

DISEASES CAUSING DYSPNEA OR TACHYPNEA

UPPER AIRWAY/CHEST WALL TRAUMA***

Classical signs

- Inspiratory dyspnea (in upper airway trauma).
- +/– Subcutaneous emphysema.
- +/– Paradoxical chest wall motion with flail chest.
- Evidence of superficial trauma.

Clinical signs

The character of the dyspnea corresponds to the area of injury and whether the upper or lower respiratory tract is involved.

Blunt (car injury, horse kick or fall) or penetrating (bite or firearm wound) trauma to the larynx or trachea, may cause inspiratory dyspnea.

Air leakage from a wound to the upper or lower respiratory tract may lead to **subcutaneous emphysema and pneumomediastinum**. Crepitus is evident on palpation with subcutaneous emphysema.

Dyspnea, cyanosis, abnormal or decreased lung sounds occur with severe pulmonary contusions, and signs of shock may be evident.

Paradoxical chest wall motion of a flail chest segment can occur, that is, inward motion during inspiration.

Traumatic hemothorax may produce increased chest wall motion with poor air movement.

Other signs of superficial trauma and shredded nails are usually evident with automobile trauma.

Pyrexia often occurs within 24 hours of cat-bite wounds.

Diagnosis

Diagnosis is based on the history and physical exam findings.

Radiographic assessment of the severity of lung trauma may be misleading in the early stages. Often there is a lag time of 12–18 hours from the time of blunt trauma of the chest wall to appearance of interstitial fluid densities in the lung. This is analogous to deep bruising on the skin and muscle after trauma – it takes time for the bruise to fully develop.

Complete focal lung consolidation with severe contusion may be evident radiographically after chest wall trauma.

Differential diagnosis

Upper airway neoplasia or foreign body in some situations may present similarity to trauma, but can be differentiated on diagnostic findings such as radiography or endoscopy.

Pleural space disease, pneumonia and pulmonary neoplasia can be differentiated based on history, physical exam and diagnostic findings.

Treatment

Treatment involves supportive care, wound cleaning and microbial therapy. Surgical repair of upper respiratory tract trauma may be required.

Flail chest is defined as a segment of the rib cage with proximal and distal fractures, resulting in an unstable segment of the chest wall.
- **Temporary stabilization** may be provided with techniques using Bachaus towel clamps, wooden tongue depressors, etc.
- Rapid definitive surgical correction of the flail chest is not as important as **stabilizing the patient** from the severe trauma, and treating the severe pulmonary contusion with oxygen supplementation, antibiotics, analgesics, bronchodilators, etc.

Tube thoracostomy and intermittent or continuous drainage of the pleural space is indicated when significant pneumothorax requires that air be removed more than three times within 24 h.

Positive-pressure ventilation must be used with extreme caution due to the fragility of the traumatized lung and susceptibility to additional barotrauma.

FELINE ASTHMA/BRONCHITIS COMPLEX***

Classical signs

- Expiratory dyspnea with wheezing.
- Cough is a prominent sign.
- *Status asthmaticus* – severe acute respiratory distress.
- Cyanosis, open-mouth breathing.

See main reference on page 92 for details (The Coughing Cat).

Clinical signs

Signs can occur at any age, although average is 2–8 years.

Signs may be episodic (with asthma) or chronic (with bronchitis).

There may or may not be a history of coughing for weeks or months preceding an episode of mild to severe, life-threatening respiratory distress from bronchoconstriction. Cats may present severely air-starved, with cyanosis, open-mouth breathing and a significant expiratory push.

Diagnosis

Adventitial lung sounds such as wheezing and crackles are very common.

Thoracic radiographs may be normal or have the following changes:

- **Hyperlucency, hyperinflation**, and flattening of the diaphragm due to air trapping may be seen with asthma.
- Diffuse prominent peribronchiolar pattern is the hallmark of chronic bronchitis.
- Right heart enlargement may be present.

Lung wash for cytology and culture.

- Transtracheal wash may be perfomed in the awake cat.
- Bronchoscopy for bronchoalveolar lavage (BAL) or unguided catheter BAL are performed in the anesthetized cat and are preferred by most clinicains over a transtracheal wash.

Cytology reveals highly cellular samples with **intact non-degenerative neutrophils** as the primary cells.

- Eosinophils are not a reliable marker of inflammation in the cat due to the increased prevalence (up to 24%) in normal airways.

Pulmonary function testing for increased airway resistance includes spirometry, whole-body plethysmography, and tidal breathing flow–volume loops (TBFVL). These are rarely available outside of teaching institutions.

Differential diagnosis

Main differential for *status asthmaticus* is acute congestive heart failure of cardiomyopathy.

Other respiratory diseases, such as parasitic pneumonia, aspiration pneumonia, bronchopulmonary neoplasia and pleural space diseases may present with dyspnea.

Treatment

- The cornerstone of therapy for cats with *status asthmaticus* is to minimize handling until signs abate, and administer oxygen, bronchodilators and glucocorticoids.
- **Oxygen supplementation** is required during respiratory distress and an oxygen chamber or tent seems to be best tolerated by air-starved patients. Oxygen hoods made with an Elizabethan collar and cellophane, or oxygen delivery via a nasal canula have proven useful in some cats, but may stress other cats and exacerbate signs.
- **Minimal handling** and restraint of acutely dyspneic patients is essential.
- For severe signs (dyspnea, open mouth breathing +/- cyanosis) which are a life-threatening emergency, it is important not to stress the cat as this may precipitate death. Administer **oxygen** via oxygen cage or nasal canula, **methylprednisolone** sodium succinate (100 mg/cat IV) or **dexamethasone**

(2 mg/kg IV) and **terbutaline** (0.01 mg/kg IV) q30 minutes for up to 4 h until a response is observed.

- Once stabilized cats are discharged with **fluticasone (Flovent®)** 220 mcg q 12 h and **albuterol** (*Proventil, Ventolin*) q 6 h as needed
- See page 94 The Coughing Cat for details of acute and chronic therapy

CARDIOMYOPATHY**

Classical signs

- Dyspnea – mild to acute and severe with cyanosis.
- Abnormal heart sounds (murmurs, gallops, arrhythmias).
- +/– Signs of pleural effusion or pulmonary edema.

See main reference on page 128 for details (The Cat With Abnormal Heart Sounds and/or an Enlarged Heart).

Clinical signs

Dyspnea varies from **mild** and associated with reduced activity levels and reluctance to play, to **acute, fulminant air-starvation** with open-mouth breathing and cyanosis.

Abnormal heart sounds (murmurs, gallops, arrhythmias) may be present, or may be difficult to assess in the distressed patient.

Pleural effusion is occasionally present especially with DCM, and results in increased chest excursions with little airflow (can be detected by listening close to the muzzle during breathing) and muffled ventral sounds.

Pulmonary edema is more common especially with hypertrophic and restrictive/intermediate cardiomyopathies, and results in increased adventitial lung sounds such as crackles.

Diagnosis

Definitive diagnosis is based on ultrasonographic characterization of the type and severity of the cardiomyopathy present.

Differential diagnosis

Acute marked dyspnea is most often associated with status asthmaticus and is differentiated from cardiogenic dyspnea on signs, expiratory push, wheezing, prior history of coughing and radiographic findings.

Treatment

Oxygen therapy (O_2 chamber or tents).

Furosemide (1–2 mg/kg IV or IM).

Provide **sedation** if the cat is frantic (morphine 0.1 mg/kg IM prn, or butorphanol 0.2–0.4 mg/kg IM q 4–6 h as needed).

If there are signs of pleural effusion, **emergency thoracocentesis** in cats with severe respiratory distress may be life saving.

- A butterfly set on a 60 ml syringe is introduced at the 5th–7th intercostal space (ICS) on the right, just above the costochondral junction. Remove as much fluid as possible, or until breathing improves.

Definitive therapy is based on ultrasonographic characterization of the type and severity of the cardiomyopathy present. See page 130 for treatment details (The Cat With Abnormal Heart Sounds and/or an Enlarged Heart).

PLEURAL EFFUSION**

Classical signs

- Muffled heart and/or lung sounds ventrally.
- Dyspnea characterized by excessive chest excursions with poor airflow.
- Orthopnea (positional dyspnea).

See main reference on page 71 for details (The Cat With Hydrothorax).

Clinical signs

Marked chest wall excursions and minimal airflow.

Orthopnea (worsening dyspnea in lateral recumbency) and reluctance to lie in lateral recumbency.

Muffled heart and lung sounds ventrally, dull chest percussion.

Depending on the etiology of the effusion, signs of chronic illness may be present such as weight loss. Inappetence or anorexia and pyrexia may be present with pyothorax.

Diagnosis

With mild to moderate clinical signs, thoracic radiography may be diagnostic. Signs are evident when fluid exceeds 50 ml/kg.

With severely affected cats in respiratory distress, radiography should be delayed until after thoracocentesis.
- CATS WITH PLEURAL EFFUSIONS DIE IN RADIOLOGY!

Fluid analysis is essential to determine etiology.

Differential diagnosis

Hemothorax, transudation from increased hydrostatic pressure (cardiac disease) or decreased oncotic pressure (protein-losing enteropathies, nephropathies or hepatic disease), lymphatic obstruction (thoracic neoplasia), chylothorax and pyothorax are all forms of hydrothorax that need to be differentiated.

Treatment

Thoracocentesis is part of the universal therapy for all forms of pleural effusion.

Definitive therapy is based upon the underlying cause.

PYOTHORAX**

Classical signs
- Dyspnea related to pleural effusion.
- Signs of chronic disease (weight loss, inappetence).
- +/– Fever.
- Turbid, flocculent and other fetid-smelling pleural fluid.

See main reference on page 75 for details (The Cat With Hydrothorax).

Clinical signs

Pyothorax is more common in intact males and is likely associated with fight wounds.

Dull or muffled heart and lung sounds are audible ventrally.

Marked chest wall excursions with minimal airflow are evident, and dyspnea is worsened by lateral recumbency (orthopnea).

The cat typically has a sick, septic, thin, unkempt appearance and may be febrile.

Diagnosis

A thick, fetid, septic, suppurative exudate is obtained on thoracocentesis. Cytology and Gram stains reveal many degenerate neutrophils, some with intracellular bacteria. Culture and sensitivity should be performed, but may show no growth of organisms.

ACUTE AND CHRONIC INFECTIOUS UPPER RESPIRATORY TRACT DISEASE**

Classical signs
- Acute or chronic nasal discharge (bilateral, copious, mucopurulent).
- Open-mouth breathing.
- Coughing.
- Ocular discharge.
- +/– Nasal distortion.

See main reference on page 19 for details (The Cat With Signs of Chronic Nasal Disease) and page 5 (The Cat With Acute Sneezing or Nasal Discharge).

Clinical signs

Upper respiratory tract disease may cause inspiratory dyspnea as a result of nasal obstruction.

Signs may be acute and associated with calici or herpes virus infection or chronic associated with cryptococcosis, neoplasia or chronic secondary bacterial rhinitis following calici or herpes viral infection.

When dyspnea is present, **nasal discharge** is usually bilateral, often mucopurulent and copious.

Open-mouth breathing may occur especially with stress.

Coughing may be present if *Bordetella bronchiseptica* or herpes virus are involved.

Ocular discharge, conjunctivitis and chemosis occur with acute upper respiratory tract infection with calici or herpes virus and *Chlamydophila felis*.

Stertorus respiration (snoring) may be evident.

Nasal distortion may occur with cryptococcosis, neoplasia or rarely with chronic secondary bacterial rhinitis.

Diagnosis

Signalment, clinical signs and history are often suggestive of the etiology. In acute upper respiratory tract infection, multiple cats in the home are often affected.

Radiographic findings:
- Usually there is loss of lucency in the nasal cavity resulting from fluid (fluid density). In chronic nasal diseases causing dyspnea, there is often osteolysis of the nasal turbinates. Lysis tends to be asymmetrical with neoplasia and is more often symmetrical with cryptococcosis and chronic bacterial rhinitis secondary to viral disease.

Culture or PCR is now available for calicivirus, herpesvirus and *Chlamydophila felis*. Bacterial culture may be useful to identify bacteria in secondary bacterial rhinitis so the most appropriate antibacterial therapy can be selected, e.g. *Pasteurella* spp.

Cats with cryptococcosis frequently have nasal distortion over the bridge of the nose or a polyp-like mass visible in the nasal cavity. Diagnosis is based on cytology, histology or a positive serology titer.

Neoplasia is most reliably diagnosed on histology, although a cytological sample may be diagnostic.

PLEURAL/MEDIASTINAL MASSES*

Classical signs

- Muffled heart and lung sounds ventrally or asymmetrical sounds.
- Dyspnea characterized by excessive chest excursions with poor airflow.
- Orthopnea (positional dyspnea).

Clinical signs

Mediastinal masses are often thymomas, thymic lymphoma, or mediastinal lymphoma. Occasionally, ectopic thyroid adenocarcinoma may create a space-occupying mass of the mediastinum. Pleural masses include mesotheliomas, osteosarcoma or chondrosarcoma of the ribs or sternabrae.

Signs are related to the space-occupying nature of the mass, or to obstruction of lymphatic drainage, leading to pleural effusion.

Orthopnea (dyspnea worsened by lateral recumbency), tachypnea, minimal airflow with increased chest excursions, muffled heart and lung sounds, or **asymmetrical sounds if the heart is displaced laterally**.

Extraluminal compression of the trachea can cause dyspnea and cough.

Compression of the anterior chest wall may reveal decreased compliance.

Diagnosis

Thoracic radiography may reveal the mass lesion or the secondary pleural effusion.

Thoracic ultrasound can be extremely useful.
- Small mediastinal masses surrounded by aerated lung may not be visible from a paracostal approach, and may require a thoracic inlet window.
- Transesophageal ultrasonography is excellent for demonstrating mediastinal masses, but requires specialized equipment and general anesthesia.

Analysis of the thoracocentesis fluid may be diagnostic on the rare occasions that the neoplasm has exfoliated into the fluid. Pleural effusions associated with tumors are usually modified transudates, but may be transudates, exudates or chylous. Surgical or ultrasound-guided biopsy of the mass is usually required for a definitive diagnosis.

Mediastinal lymphoma occasionally has hypercalcemia as a paraneoplastic syndrome.

Differential diagnosis

Other causes of pleural effusion need to be differentiated. Chylothorax is more commonly idiopathic and associated with lymphatic lymphangiectasia, although cardiac disease and trauma need to be excluded. History, signs (evidence of murmurs, gallops and arrhythmias), radiography and ultrasound help to differentiate these causes from thoracic neoplasia.

Treatment

Lymphoma of the thymus or mediastinal lymph nodes is best handled with standard chemotherapy protocols for lymphoma (see page 676).

Surgical excision is the treatment of choice for thymoma, and may be curative.

Mesothelioma is an infiltrative disease that cannot be readily resected, and there are few reports in the literature of effective chemotherapy. Local infusion of carboplatin may be helpful with or without intravenous doxirubicin. Prognosis is grave.

ANEMIA/HYPOXEMIA*

Classical signs

- Dyspnea, tachypnea and tachycardia.
- Pallor from anemia, cyanosis with methemoglobinemia.

Clinical signs

Signs may be acute or chronic in onset depending on the underlying disease process.

Pale mucous membranes, tachycardia and **tachypnea** occur with anemia.

Cyanosis occurs with methemoglobinemia.

Cherry red mucous membranes occur with carboxyhemoglobinemia from carbon monoxide (CO) toxicity.

Diagnosis

Diagnosis of anemia is based on finding a decreased hematocrit on CBC.
- PCV < 10% may be associated with dyspnea, especially if the cat is stressed.
- Evidence of blood loss or poor RBC production may be evident.

- Bone marrow biopsy may be indicated if there is evidence of anemia of longer than 4–6 days duration without a regenerative response.
- Measurement of carboxyhemoglobin concentration is required for diagnosis of CO toxicity. Routine STAT assays are available in human hospitals.

ACQUIRED OR CONGENITAL DIAPHRAGMATIC DEFECTS*

Classical signs

- May or may not have clinical signs.
- Muffled heart and/or lung sounds.
- Occasionally dyspnea, cyanosis.
- Vague gastrointestinal signs, gaunt abdomen on palpation.

Clinical signs

Diaphragmatic hernia may occur as a **congenital defect** allowing abdominal organs to move into the thoracic space or pericardium, or may follow **trauma, especially a motor-car accident or fall from a building.**

With congenital hernias, signs may be evident as a kitten or there may be no signs until later in life, depending on the severity of the hernia.

With aquired hernias, signs may or may not be evident immediately following trauma, and worsen or improve as adhesions form to limit movement of viscera. In some cats, signs are only present with activity or stress.

Typically there are muffled heart and lung sounds, and occasionally borborygmus is audible in the chest.

The **severity of dyspnea** is variable from mild, to acute and severe. Sudden worsening of signs may occur when more abdominal viscera move into the chest.

Tachypnea, orthopnea (worsened dyspnea in lateral recumbency) and cyanosis may occur depending on the volume of abdominal organs in the thorax.

On palpation, the abdomen has a gaunt or empty feel. **Other ventral midline defects** such as umbilical hernias, *pectus excavatum,* etc., may be present with congenital hernias.

Intermittent vomiting and inappetence are the most common gastrointestinal signs.

Diagnosis

Thoracic radiographs demonstrate bowel loops, or space-occupying soft tissue densities within the pleural or pericardial space. Globose cardiomegaly is evident with peritoneopericardial diaphragmatic hernia.

Other imaging modalities such as ultrasonography, positive contrast upper GI series, pneumoperitoneography or contrast injected into the abdomen (celiogram) may be useful for diagnosis.

Differential diagnosis

Pleural space disease (effusions, pneumothorax, mass lesions), pericardial effusion and cardiomyopathy may have similar signalment and signs to traumatic diaphragmatic hernia, but can usually be differentiated on radiography and ultrasonography.

Treatment

Treatment consists of **surgical repair** after stabilizing the patient. If dyspnea is the major clinical sign, stabilization may not be possible until the pericardial or pleural cavities are evacuated. Oxygen therapy is of little value in a patient with severe pleural occupation.

AORTIC THROMBOEMBOLISM*

Classical signs

- Acute single or bilateral limb paresis or paralysis, most often involving hindlimbs.
- Signs of congestive heart failure – cyanosis, respiratory distress, pleural effusion.
- Heart murmurs, arrhythmias and gallops.

See main reference on page 915 for details (The Weak and Ataxic Cat or Paralyzed Cat).

Clinical signs

Cardiomyopathy in cats is sometimes associated with thrombus formation in the left atrium. The thrombus may be dislodged, and most commonly obstructs the aorta at its trifurcation (saddle thrombus).

Typically, there is **acute onset of single limb paresis or paralysis**, which most often involves the **hindlimbs**. Signs may be bilateral with a "saddle thrombus" at the aortic trifurcation.

On physical examination the **limb is cool and pulseless, with cyanotic foot pads or nail beds**. The gastrocnemius muscle is firm and painful on palpation.

Signs of congestive heart failure including cyanosis, respiratory distress, or evidence of pleural effusion may be present. **Dyspnea and tachypnea** may be acutely exacerbated. Heart murmurs, arrhythmias and gallops are often evident.

Diagnosis

Diagnosis is based on the clinical signs and confirmed by evidence of lack of blood flow in the distal limb measured by a Doppler flow meter.

Thoracic radiography and ultrasonography demonstrate underlying heart disease, often with significant chamber enlargement, especially of the left atrium.

Contrast arteriography of the affected limb is the "gold standard", but not frequently used in clinical cases.

PULMONARY THROMBOEMBOLISM*

Classical signs

- Sudden onset of severe dyspnea with normal lung parenchyma radiographically.
- Peracute dyspnea, orthopnea, tachypnea.
- Cyanosis, collapse.
- Cough, with or without hemoptysis.

Pathogenesis

Pulmonary thromboembolism involves **embolic showering** of the pulmonary arterial tree, causing obstruction of blood flow to that portion of the lung.

Thrombi may be produced locally (i.e., feline heartworm disease), or may embolize from distant locations. Thrombi may originate in the right atrium (**cardiomyopathy, advanced tricuspid valvular disease**), caudal vena cava, femoral veins, mesenteric venous system or jugular veins.

Hypercoagulable states such as **protein-losing nephropathies** (i.e., glomerulonephritis, renal amyloidosis, hypertension) or **enteropathies** (i.e., IBD, lymphangiectasia), stasis of blood flow, **exposure of vascular subendothelial tissue** (i.e., vasculitis, right atrial dilation, post-stenotic "jet lesions", trauma and indwelling jugular catheters) all predispose to thrombus formation.

Pulmonary arterial obstruction causes ventilation/perfusion (V/Q) mismatch, resulting in **hypoxemia and dyspnea**.
- Increased pulmonary arterial pressure may induce cor pulmonale, or right-sided heart failure.

Feline heartworm disease frequently presents as severe peracute pulmonary inflammation, edema and pulmonary thromboembolism resulting in acute respiratory failure and death.

Clinical signs

Severity of signs is proportional to the degree of arterial obstruction.

Acute onset of severe dyspnea and tachypnea is typical. Cyanosis or collapse may also occur. Massive disease may result in sudden death.

Orthopnea (positional dyspnea), especially in lateral recumbency, and reluctance to lie in lateral recumbency, may be an early sign.

Coughing may be evident, and ranges from mild to severe, and may involve hemoptysis.

Signs of right-sided heart failure may occur, such as tachycardia, jugular venous distension and split second heart sounds.

Often presenting signs relating to the primary condition are also evident, i.e., weight loss and diarrhea with protein-losing enteropathy.

Diagnosis

Thoracic radiographs may be totally normal, and in the presence of severe dyspnea, increase the index of suspicion of pulmonary thromboembolism.
- Enlarged or truncated pulmonary arteries may be seen.

When lesions are evident radiographically, lung patterns range from focal areas of hyperlucency to alveolar infiltration, and mild to moderate pleural effusion.

Pulmonary arterial angiography is the "gold standard" for evaluation of pulmonary thromboembolism (PTE) in people. This requires catheterization of the right heart and injection of contrast material into the pulmonary arterial tree. Areas of obstruction or decreased blood flow may be detected.

Scintigraphic ventilation/perfusion studies utilize both aerosolized and injected radioisotopes to identify areas of V/Q mismatch. Special facilities and expertise are required, which are generally unavailable outside of teaching institutions.

Echocardiography may reveal right atrial enlargement with thrombus formation, pulmonary arterial dilation, right ventricular enlargement, pulmonary hypertension on Doppler studies of the tricuspid and pulmonic valves, or evidence of heartworm in the right heart or pulmonary arteries.

Tall P waves on ECG may indicate right atrial enlargement, and right axis shift supports right ventricular enlargement consistent with cor pulmonale.

Differential diagnosis

Severe dyspnea and cyanosis with normal thoracic radiographs may accompany upper airway obstruction or feline asthma.

Treatment

Oxygen therapy during the respiratory crisis is **important**, but limited in efficacy if the blood delivery to the lung is compromised.

The **primary disease condition**, if identified, should be addressed as a priority.

Thrombolytic therapy is controversial. The use of tissue plasminogen activator (TPA) has been advocated, but requires local delivery into the pulmonary arterial circulation. This requires cardiac catheterization under fluoroscopy. There are inherent risks involved with the procedure, and the risk of inducing a bleeding diathesis.

Anti-thrombotic therapy using heparin has been advocated to prevent further thrombin formation. Various protocols ranging from low (100 IU/kg SQ q 8 hours) to moderate doses (300 IU/kg SQ q 8 h) have been published, with no clear advantages of any one protocol.

Coumadin is a more potent anti-thrombotic agent in the cat. Having an oral liquid suspension compounded makes the titration of the dosage much more reliable in the cat. Doses of 0.1 mg/kg PO q 24 h are a recommended starting point. Monitoring the prothrombin time (PT) and the INR (international normalization ratio), with a treatment endpoint of an INR of 2.0–3.0, may help to prevent overdosage, although trials in cats are lacking.

Fluid therapy must be used judiciously, due to the predisposition of right-sided heart failure.

Prognosis

Prognosis is directly proportionate to the severity of the lesion, as well as to the underlying cause. Resolvable causes (i.e., trauma or catheter-induced) have a better long-term prognosis that do patients with irreversible causes (i.e., renal amyloidosis).

Prevention

Treat underlying risk factors early in the disease course, for example, protein-losing nephropathies and enteropathies.

Acetylsalicylic acid or heparin theoretically may help prevent further thrombus formation, although there are no studies demonstrating efficacy in cats.

AIRWAY TUMORS

> ### Classical signs
>
> - Nasal obstruction produces stridor and open-mouth breathing.
> - Pharyngeal obstruction results in dysphagia, stertor and voice changes.
> - Tracheal tumors produce fixed obstruction with inspiratory and expiratory dyspnea, and often coughing.

See main reference on pages 41 and 24 for details (The Cat With Stridor, and The Cat With Signs of Chronic Nasal Disease).

Clinical signs

Nasal tumors are most commonly squamous cell carcinoma of the nasal planum, solid nasal carcinomas and nasal lymphoma.

Nasal obstruction produces stridor, stertor or open-mouth breathing, uni- or bilateral nasal discharge and coughing from post-nasal drip. Anosmia may lead to inappetance.

Squamous cell carcinomas of the tonsil are common pharyngeal masses, along with benign nasopharyngeal polyps.

Pharyngeal masses produce dysphagia, stertorous dyspnea and voice changes. Fetid halitosis is also reported.

Tracheal tumors consist of lymphoma, squamous cell carcinoma, leiomyosarcoma and osteochondral tumors from the tracheal rings. Adenocarcinomas have increased prevalence in Siamese cats.

Tracheal tumors cause fixed obstruction, leading to **both** inspiratory and expiratory dyspnea. A harsh, dry cough is common.

Diagnosis

Diagnosis is by rhinoscopy, pharyngoscopy or tracheoscopy with biopsy. It is possible to image soft tissue masses radiographically, but endoscopy is still advised for biopsy.

Differential diagnosis

Inhaled and penetrating foreign bodies, and benign or parasitic granulomas of the airways may mimic neoplastic masses. Foreign bodies result in acute onset of signs and often distress, compared to chronic signs in neoplasia and granulomas. Visualization and biopsy will differentiate these diseases.

Treatment

Solid nasal tumors respond well to external beam radiotherapy, with survival times of 20–27 months. Rhinotomy with turbinatectomy has been reported to be successful.

• Often, there is extensive local invasion by the neoplasm, and the recurrence rate after radiotherapy and/or surgery is high.

Nasal lymphoma responds well to **standard chemotherapy** for lymphoma, with remission times of 16 months reported.

Pharyngeal and tracheal masses and nasopharyngeal polyps are best treated with surgical resection.

PARASITIC DISEASE

> ### Classical signs
>
> • Coughing.
> • Reduced physical activity and reluctance to play.
> • Mild to severe dyspnea.
> • Weight loss, poor coat, inappetance.
> • Sudden marked respiratory distress (feline heartworm).

See main reference on page 104 for details (The Coughing Cat).

Clinical signs

Heartworm (*Dirafilaria immitis*), lungworm (*Aelurostrongylus abstrusus*, *Capillaria aerophilia*), lung flukes (*Paragonomus kellicoti*), migrating nematodes (*Toxocara cati*) and toxoplasmosis all may cause respiratory signs.

Coughing may be present and is typically harsh, productive and paroxysmal.

Mild to marked dyspnea and reduced activity may be observed, depending on the severity of the lung disease.

Weight loss, poor coat and ill-thrift may be evident.

Vomiting is a common sign with feline heartworm disease. Sudden death or sudden extreme respiratory distress and generalized respiratory failure occur in approximately 30% of symptomatic cats with heartworm disease.

Diagnosis

Feline heartworm disease is suggested by a positive heartworm antibody test, radiographic changes of dilated and blunted pulmonary arteries and evidence of heartworms on ultrasound. Occasionally peripheral basophilia is evident (see Feline heartworm page 104, The Coughing Cat).

Lungworm infection with *Capillaria aerophilia* is diagnosed by finding eggs in the stools or lung wash, and with *Aelurostrongylus abstrussus,* by finding larvae in the lung wash or fecal Baermann.

Lung flukes (*Paragonimus kellicotti*) produce operculated eggs in the stool.

Toxoplasmosis rarely produces clinical disease in cats. Mixed fluffy interstitial and alveolar patterns are typically evident on radiographs. Tachyzoites may be recovered in the lung wash.

Differential diagnosis

Other forms of pneumonia, including bacterial, viral, fungal, inflammatory and neoplasia, need to be considered if no larvae or ova are found in the stool or lungwash.

Treatment

Feline heartworm disease therapy is usually symptomatic, as adulticide therapy is associated with a high mortality rate (see Feline heartworm disease, page 105, The Coughing Cat).

Lungworm – *Capillaria aerophilia* and *Aelurostrongylus abstrussus* – **fenbendazole** (50 mg/kg PO q 24 h for 3 days) or *ivermectin* (400 µg/kg PO, SQ).

Lung flukes – *Paragonimus kellicotti*, fenbendazole (50 mg/kg PO q 24 h for 3 days), or **praziquantel** (25 mg/kg PO q 8 h for 2 days).

Toxoplasmosis – **clindamycin**, 12.5 mg/kg PO q 12 h, potentiated sulfa (trimethoprim or ormetoprim) or azithromycin.

MYOPATHY/NEUROPATHY

> ### Classical signs
>
> • Dyspnea characterized by weakened chest excursions.
> • Weakened gait, ventroflexion of the head.
> • Regurgitation may lead to aspiration pneumonia.

See main reference on page 941 for details (The Cat With Generalized Weakness).

Clinical signs

Dyspnea associated with myopathy or neuropathy is related to weakness of the intercostal and diaphragmatic muscle, causing diminished ventilation.

Signs related to the underlying disease will be evident, for example:

- **Hyperthyroid myopathy** is usually seen in older cats. Signs include ravenous appetite, restlessness, weight loss, poor haircoat, generalized muscle wasting and weakness.
- **Hypokalemic myopathy** occurs in older cats usually secondary to renal insufficiency, or in Burmese cats less than 1 year of age. Ventroflexion of the head, a stiff stilted gait, inability or reluctance to walk or jump are common signs. Sensitivity to palpation of the larger muscle groups may be evident.
- **Hypocalcemic myopathy** results in episodic generalized weakness, tetany or tremors. It occurs most commonly after thyroidectomy, but occasionally occurs with hypoparathyroidism, chronic renal failure, pancreatitis, eclampsia or phosphate-containing enemas.
- **Hyperadrenocorticism** results in poorly controlled diabetes mellitus, unkempt haircoat, pot-bellied appearance and generalized muscle weakness.
- **Myasthenia gravis** occurs typically in adult cats or Siamese < 1 year of age and presents as generalized muscle weakness and stiff stilted gait exacerbated with exercise. Severe dyspnea may be evident if aspiration pneumonia is present.
- **Polymyositis** produces generalized pain on palpation of muscle groups, and a stiff stilted gait.
- **Botulism toxicity** results in flaccid paralysis of skeletal or respiratory muscles.
- **Polyradiculoneuritis** produces an ascending flaccid paralysis of skeletal and respiratory muscles.
- **Tick paralysis** from *Demacentor* spp. and *Ixodes* spp. ticks, produces a rapidly progressive skeletal and respiratory paralysis.

Diagnosis

Serum electrolytes (i.e., potassium and calcium) should be measured to rule out hypokalemia and hypocalcemia.

Endocrine testing involves measurement of total T4 and free-T4 (hyperthyroidism), blood and urine glucose, fructosamine concentration (diabetes mellitus), or ACTH stimulation testing (hyperadrenocorticism) if clinical signs are consistent.

Acetylcholine receptor antibodies assay is used for myasthenia gravis.

Measurement of muscle enzymes (creatine phosphokinase activity) and muscle biopsy are necessary for diagnosis of myositis.

PNEUMONIA

Classical signs

- Cough.
- Inspiratory/expiratory dyspnea.
- Fever.
- Occasional nasal discharge.

Pathogenesis

Pneumonia may be primary or secondary and associated with bacterial, mycoplasmal, *Chlamydophila felis*, fungal or viral agents.

Primary bacterial pathogens include *Bordetella bronchiseptica* and *Pasteurella multocida*, which are common flora of the oropharynx, and can colonize the lower respiratory tree.

Secondary bacterial infection is possible with many opportunist organisms including streptococci, *Bordetella bronchiseptica*, *Pseudomonas* spp., *Nocardia* spp. and *Actinomyces* spp.

Pneumonia may occur following lung damage from various sources, or associated with diseases that reduce immunocompetence such as:

- Aspiration as a result of esophageal dysmotility, or during recovery from general anesthesia, etc.
- Metabolic disease including uremic pneumonitis, hyperadrenocorticism and diabetes mellitus.
- Trauma (blunt, penetrating or surgical trauma).
- Immunosuppression from drugs, neoplasia, or retroviral infection.
- Pre-existing infection.

Mycoplasma pneumonia is rare, but may be a sequel of severe URT infection.

Chlamydiosis can result in pneumonitis in kittens.

Protozoal (toxoplasmosis) and parasitic (capillariasis, aelurostrongylosis, *Paragonimus kellicotti*) pneumonia may occur.

Primary fungal pneumonia is mainly restricted to *Cryptococcus neoformans*. Infection can occur as a sequel to fungal rhinosinusitis, or as primary pneumonia.

Viral interstitial pneumonia with feline calici virus has been reported.

Less common fungal pneumonias include blastomycosis, histoplasmosis, aspergillosis and candidiasis.

Clinical signs

A **deep productive cough** may be heard, although coughing is not as common as in dogs.

Fetid breath halitosis.

Fever is common, although a subnormal body temperature can occur if the cat is septic.

Inspiratory and expiratory dyspnea may be evident, often with open-mouth breathing.

Adventitial breath sounds, including crackles, wheezes, snaps and pops may be audible. Breath sounds may be absent over areas of lobar consolidation.

Lethargy and anorexia are typically present, and weight loss and ill thrift may be evident if the pneumonia is more chronic.

Infectious pneumonia is uncommon in cats. A recent study of 39 cats with infectious pneumonia showed that a substantial proportion had no clinical signs that were referable to the respiratory tract (36% of cats), they lacked clinical signs of systemic illness (41%), and had unremarkable findings on hematology (22%) and thoracic radiography (23%).

Diagnosis

Thoracic radiography findings include focal or generalized alveolar densities with air bronchograms, or focal areas of complete consolidation.
- A ventral distribution of lesions may signal aspiration as the cause of pneumonia.
- A miliary interstitial pattern is seen with blastomycosis.

- **Hilar lymphadenopathy** supports **fungal or mycobacterial** pneumonia, although infiltrative **lymphosarcoma** may mimic this.

Hematology may reveal neutrophilia with or without a left shift and toxic neutrophils (Doehle bodies, etc.).
- Low-grade non-responsive anemia and monocytosis may support chronicity.

Hypoxemia (PaO_2 < 80 mmHg on room air or SPO_2 < 90%) may be present, with trends monitored by arterial blood gas or pulse oximetry.
- **Note:** the oxygen saturation curve **drops steeply** with SPO_2 values <90%.

Samples for cytology and culture can be obtained using percutaneous lung aspiration, transtracheal wash, unguided bronchioalveolar lavage or bronchoscopic lavage. Cultures for aerobic and anaerobic bacteria should be performed and a fungal culture is indicated if infection is possible within the geographical region. Results of cultures must be evaluated in light of other data including the concentration of bacteria, cytological findings, etc.
- Bacterial pneumonia is characterized bysuppurative inflammation involving degenerative neutrophils with intracellular bacteria.
- Fungal and mycobacterial diseases have pyogranulomatous inflammation, with characteristic organisms seen on routine or special stains.

Cryptococcal titers may aid in the diagnosis.

Differential diagnosis

Chronic small airway disease (feline asthma/ bronchitis), pulmonary infiltrate with eosinophils (PIE) and lymphomatoid granulomatosis may share many similar historical, clinical and radiographic signs and need to be differentiated on clinical and histopathologic findings.

Pulmonary neoplasia, either primary (squamous cell carcinoma, bronchogenic carcinoma), or metastatic disease, is differentiated on histopathology.

Treatment

Bacterial pneumonia requires antimicrobial therapy.
- The parenteral route is used in debilitated or septic patients, and oral therapy in outpatients.
- Antibiotic selection is best based upon specific culture and sensitivity testing.

- Initial empirical choices can be based upon Gram stain of the cytology sample.
  - Gram negative rods – amikacin, fluoro-quinolones, trimethoprim-sulfa, chloramphenicol.
  - Gram positive cocci – beta-lactams, trimetho-prim-sulfa, chloramphenicol.
  - *Bordetella* – amikacin, tetracycline, chloramphenicol.
  - Anaerobes – beta-lactams, second-generation cephalosporins, clindamycin.

Fungal pneumonia requires antifungal therapy.
- **Itraconazole** at 5–10 mg/kg PO daily is the drug of choice, with 50–60% response rates quoted in cats.
- **Amphotericin B** (0.25 mg/kg IV q 2 days), alone or in combination with itraconazole.
- If CNS signs are present with cryptococcosis, **fluconazole** (2.5–5.0 mg/kg PO daily) is the drug of choice to cross the blood–brain barrier (see Cryptococcosis, page 27 in The Cat With Signs of Chronic Nasal Disease).

Viral pneumonia treatment is mostly supportive. There is no clear evidence to suggest antiviral therapy is of benefit. Low-dose oral **alpha interferon** (30 IU PO daily) may possibly be beneficial, although reports are anectdotal.

Supportive care is vital. Airway and systemic hydration are essential for mucociliary clearance.
- Intravenous crystalloids need to be used judiciously if there is increased vascular permeability in the lung.
- Nebulization with saline may be helpful.
- **Physical therapy**, such as positional changes, coupage of the chest wall (percussion with a cupped hand) and enforced mild exercise, all enhance the clearance of debris from the lung.
- **Oxygen enrichment** via nasal O_2 catheter, oxygen tent or cage may be essential in critical cases.
- Bronchodilator therapy remains controversial in the treatment of pneumonia.

Prognosis

Prognosis depends on the agent and the severity of the infection.

Bacterial pneumonia has a fair to good prognosis if there are no other debilitating factors, but prognosis is worse in patients with pre-existing illness (neoplasia, multiple trauma, multiple organ failure), or patients on immunosuppressive therapy for immune-mediated disease or organ transplantation.

Prognosis for **cryptococcal pneumonia** is generally fair to good provided the cat is not debilitated on presentation, and therapy is continued sufficiently long enough for antibody titers to fall to zero.

Prevention

Avoid the source of infectious agents, such as bird droppings and other risk factors, for example, aspiration after anesthesia.

LARYNGEAL EDEMA

> ### Classical signs
>
> - **Inspiratory dyspnea.**
> - **Stertorous breathing.**

See main reference page 42 (The Cat With Stridor).

Clinical signs

Inspiratory dyspnea which may be associated with severe respiratory distress.

Stertor occurs, which is worsened with excitement or exercise.

Diagnosis

Acute onset of inspiratory dyspnea.

Laryngoscopic inspection under heavy sedation or light anesthesia with a rigid laryngoscope and blade reveals erythema and edema of the laryngeal mucosa.

Differential diagnosis

Laryngeal paralysis, laryngeal mass lesion or foreign bodies.

GRASS AWNS, FOREIGN BODIES

Classical signs

- Sneezing (nasal foreign bodies), coughing (tracheobronchial foreign bodies).
- Inspiratory/expiratory dyspnea, depending on location.
- Nasal discharge.

Pathogenesis

Foreign bodies are usually **inhaled or regurgitated** and rarely penetrate through the skin. Barbed grass awns or seeds or blades of grass favor one-way migration (i.e., difficult to expel backwards).

Inhaled foreign bodies tend to lodge in the nasal cavity in cats.

- As cats rarely mouth-breathe, inhaled tracheal foreign bodies occur much less commonly than in dogs.

Penetrating foreign bodies can lodge in the nasal cavity, such as pellets or a tooth broken from an opponent during a cat fight.

Nasopharyngeal foreign bodies may lodge above the soft palate after vomiting. Food, hairballs and blades of grass are more common than grass seeds in this area.

Tracheobronchial foreign bodies are often the **result of aspiration** of regurgitated ingesta.

Clinical signs

Nasal foreign bodies create intense sneezing, pawing or rubbing the nose along the ground, and nasal discharge (often unilateral) with stridorous (*whistling*) nasal breathing.

Nasopharyngeal foreign bodies cause gagging, dysphagia and reverse sneezing. Coughing may occur secondary to post-nasal drip (aspiration of caudal nasal discharge). Stertorous breathing (*snoring*) may occur.

Tracheobronchial foreign bodies cause **coughing** and **signs of fixed obstruction** (i.e., both inspiratory and expiratory dyspnea).

- The coughing is often harsh and productive, and may be elicited with tracheal palpation.

Diagnosis

Nasal and nasopharyngeal foreign bodies often result in little change on radiographs other than a unilateral fluid density. Rhinoscopy is often both diagnostic and therapeutic, if the foreign body can be retrieved.

Tracheal foreign bodies may be seen radiographically. Rigid tracheoscopy allows for larger retrieval instruments to be utilized than with flexible endoscopy.

Bronchial foreign bodies may cause complete lobar atelectasis or abscessation radiographically. **Right caudal and accessory lobes** are most **often affected** with **inhalation foreign bodies**. **Right middle lobe** is affected commonly with **aspiration of vomitus**.

Differential diagnosis

Other nasal diseases, such as infectious (especially fungal), nasal cuterebriasis or neoplastic disease, tend to have a more insidious onset. Upper respiratory tract viral infection, especially calicivirus, causes acute paroxysms of sneezing, which in the early stages could appear similar to a nasal foreign body.

Nasopharyngeal polyps tend to have a more insidious onset.

Tracheal or bronchial neoplasia have a more insidious onset.

Treatment

Effective treatment involves removal of the foreign body and most can be removed endoscopically. Nasal foreign bodies may be endoscopically retrieved or hydropulsed. Occasionally, rhinotomy is required, especially for foreign bodies that have migrated into the frontal sinuses.

If a lung lobe is abscessed with a bronchial foreign body, lobectomy may be required.

Prognosis

Prognosis is excellent with removal of the foreign body.

Prevention

Appropriate hairball prophylaxis with combing and oral lubricant/laxatives reduces the likelihood or vomiting and aspiration of vomitus or the hairball.

Avoidance of grass fields during seed time.

PULMONARY NEOPLASIA

Classical signs

- Non-productive cough, with or without hemoptysis.
- Reduced activity.
- Tachypnea and dyspnea – subtle to marked, especially if pleural effusion is evident.
- Fetid halitosis.
- Mass lesion radiographically.
- Anorexia, weight loss, muscle wasting.

Pathogenesis

Pulmonary neoplasia may be **primary** or result from **secondary** metastases from distant neoplasms.

Primary tumors include **bronchogenic carcinoma, pulmonary adenocarcinoma** and **squamous cell carcinomas**.

Secondary metastatic tumors include a wide variety of carcinomas (i.e., mammary adenocarcinomas) and sarcomas (i.e., osteosarcoma), and local metastases from primary lung tumors.

Pleural malignancy may cause dyspnea, either by the space-occupying nature of the mass, or from secondary pleural effusion.

Clinical signs

Reduced activity with reluctance to play or run may be observed.

Inappetance or anorexia and weight loss are often present.

Fetid halitosis may be noticed on physical exam or by the owner.

A non-productive cough, with or without hemoptysis is sometimes present. Dyspnea (inspiratory and expiratory) and respiratory distress may be evident in the later stages, or if pleural effusion develops.

Pleural effusion results in muffled heart and lung sounds ventrally and worsening of dyspnea in lateral recumbency.

Very rarely, lameness occurs from peripheral appendicular bone lesions of hypertrophic osteopathy.

Diagnosis

Chest radiographs demonstrate a solid tissue mass(es) or nodular interstitial pattern.

- Sensitivity is limited to masses > 10 mm diameter, and multiple views are important to maximize diagnosis. Hilar lymphadenopathy may be present.

Other imaging modalities, such as CT or MRI are useful if available.

Biopsy of mass(es) is required for definitive diagnosis, as well as for distinguishing the origin of tumor.

- Biopsy options include percutaneous needle aspiration or core biopsy, bronchoscopy, or unguided bronchioalveolar lavage, or transbronchial lung biopsy.
- Ultrasound is often a poor tool to guide percutaneous biopsy needles, unless the entire lung lobe has become consolidated, as the sonic beam is reflected by any aerated lung tissue.
- Triangulating the landmarks based on two orthogonal radiographic views is extremely effective for percutaneous biopsy.
- Transbronchial cytology (TTW or BAL) is often disappointing, due to the interstitial nature of the lesion.
- Transbronchial lung biopsy is a promising technique for obtaining samples for histopathology, but is only available at some institutions.

Surgical biopsy may be performed via thoracotomy, generally during lobectomy.

- Local lymph nodes should be aspirated or biopsied for staging.

Thoracocentesis and cytology of pleural fluid is occasionally diagnostic if neoplastic cells have exfoliated.

Differential diagnosis

Infectious disease, especially fungal and parasitic granulomas, foreign body reactions, inflammatory granulomatous lesions, and lung lobe torsions may mimic neoplastic disease clinically and radiographically.

Treatment

Surgical resection is the treatment of choice for solitary primary neoplasms. Cure or long-term remission is possible with wide surgical margins. If non-resectible, excision of nodules may palliate clinical signs temporarily.

Chemotherapy and radiation have been attempted in generalized pulmonary neoplasms, with disappointing results. Metastases from distant tumors carry a grave prognosis, although pulmonary lymphoma may attain remission with chemotherapy.

General supportive care and nutrition are important.

Prognosis

Fair to excellent with surgically resectible **primary pulmonary neoplasms** without metastasis.

Grave with metastatic disease or malignant pleural effusions.

CONGENITAL HEART DEFECTS

Classical signs

- Reluctance to play or run.
- Anxious, uncomfortable breathing.
- Dyspnea – if present varies from mild to severe.
- Abnormal heart sounds (murmurs, gallops, arrhythmias).
- Signs of pleural effusion – increased chest excursions with little airflow.

Clinical signs

Atrioventricular valve dysplasia, septal defects, aortic and pulmonic stenosis (rare) and patent ductus arteriosus all lead to pressure and/or volume overload on the heart, and potentially result in congestive heart failure.

Heart murmurs at various locations (left apex for mitral valve dysplasia, right apex for ventricular septal defect), and intensities (continuous murmur of patent ductus arteriosis) occur depending on the type of congenital heart defect.

The **cat may be reluctant to play or run**, and if present, **dyspnea** varies from mild to severe. Open-mouth breathing or cyanosis may occur with severe defects.

Signs of pleural effusion include increased chest excursions with little airflow.

Treatment

Corrective surgery for patent ductus arteriosis and pulmonic stenosis (rare in cats) is available in specialist centers.

Most other problems require medical management depending on the presenting signs (see page 140, The Cat With Abnormal Heart Sounds and/or an Enlarged Heart).

LARYNGEAL PARALYSIS

Classical signs

- Inspiratory dyspnea and increased airway noise.
- Stertorous breathing (*snoring*).
- Stridor (high-pitched *whistling* = *obstructive*).
- Voice changes, absence of purring.

See main reference page 43 (The Cat With Stridor).

Clinical signs

Inspiratory dyspnea.

Stridor which is worse with excitement or exercise.

Occasional stertorous breathing or snoring.

Voice changes such as an absent or whisper-like meow, or harsh purring sounds.

Diagnosis

Diagnosis is based on signs of laryngeal stridor, inspiratory dyspnea and visualization of the larynx.

Laryngoscopic inspection under heavy sedation or light anesthesia with a rigid laryngoscope and blade reveals absent or **paradoxical motion** of the arytenoid cartilages. Normally they should abduct on inspiration. If they close on inspiration, it is paradoxical motion.

Erythema and swelling ("kissing lesions") of the arytenoid mucosa may be evident as a result of repetitive focal impact of the touching surfaces of the corniculate processes.

Low-dose ketamine (4–6 mg/kg IV), ketamine/diazepam (3–5 mg/kg/0.1–0.2 mg/kg IV) or propofol (4–6 mg/kg IV) allows visual inspection without diminishing laryngeal function.

Differential diagnosis

Other causes of dynamic or fixed upper respiratory tract obstruction are distinguished on laryngoscopic inspection (see Chapter 4, The Cat With Stridor).

Dynamic causes of upper respiratory tract obstruction are:

- Brachycephalic airway syndrome. This results in an elongated soft palate causing partial laryngeal obstruction and entrapment of the epiglottis, and lateral ventricle eversion causing ballooning of the mucosa of the lateral ventricles into the lumen.
- Cervical tracheal collapse.
- Pyogranulomatous or lymphoplasmacytic laryngitis results in a roughened, proliferative mucosa of the arytenoids and epiglottis.

Fixed causes of upper respiratory tract obstruction are:

- Oropharyngeal neoplasia (squamous cell carcinoma, oral melanoma, nasopharyngeal polyp).
- Tracheal neoplasia (intraluminal adenocarcinoma, extraluminal masses).
- Tracheal foreign bodies.

CONGENITAL ANOMALIES OF THE UPPER RESPIRATORY TRACT

> **Classical signs**
>
> - Dyspnea, usually fixed obstruction (inspiratory and expiratory) due to stenotic nature of most defects.
> - Inspiratory dyspnea and stertor occur with the brachycephalic syndrome.

See main reference on page 39 for details (The Cat With Stridor).

Clinical signs

Stenotic nares, hypoplastic trachea, etc., potentially create a non-dynamic, fixed obstruction leading to inspiratory and expiratory dyspnea, although inspiratory dyspnea may be more prominent with stenotic nares and hypoplastic trachea, if there is a dynamic component to the obstruction.

Dynamic obstructions such as occur with elongated soft palate create **inspiratory dyspnea with stertor**.

Oronasal reflux, especially with fluids, occurs with cleft palate.

With stress, nasal obstruction may result in mouth breathing.

Treatment

Treatment involves surgical correction of the defect, if possible.

ACUTE SYSTEMIC ANAPHYLAXIS

> **Classical signs**
>
> - Acute dyspnea
> - Hypotensive shock
> - Collapse
> - Pale mucous membranes

See main reference on page 566 for details (The Cat With Polycythemia).

Clinical Signs

- Pulmonary signs such as **severe acute dyspnea** predominate, because the lung is the **"shock organ" in cats.**
- Signs of **hypotensive shock,** such as pallor and collapse, accompany the pulmonary signs.
- **The onset of clinical signs occurs in seconds to minutes after exposure** to the inciting antigen.
- Occasionally, **cutaneous swelling** may be noted around the face and paws.

Diagnosis

- Diagnosis is made by a **combination of appropriate history and characteristic clinical signs.**
- **No laboratory tests are currently available to make a definitive diagnosis** of acute systemic anaphylaxis.

CARDIAC TUMORS

> **Classical signs**
>
> - Dyspnea and trachypnea.

Clinical signs

Cardiac tumors are extremely rare in cats.

Dyspnea may occur from obstruction of blood flow to or from the heart (i.e., aortic body chemodectomas), or because the tumor acts as a space-occupying mass compressing the mainstem airways at the hilus.

Malignant pleural or pericardial effusion may occur, creating dyspnea and weakness or lethargy.

Diagnosis

Diagnosis is based or finding a mass lesion on the heart base when imaged with radiography or ultrasonography.

TRACHEOBRONCHIAL COLLAPSE

> **Classical signs**
> - Harsh, honking cough.
> - Stridor on inspiration if cervical segment involved.
> - Very rare in cats.

See main reference on page 44 for details (The Cat With Stridor).

Clinical signs

Tracheobronchial collapse is **very rare in cats** and generally occurs **secondary to trauma or to compression** caused by an **extraluminal mass**. It has been reported associated with proximal tracheal obstructions from a trachael granuloma or polyp.

The **cough is often harsh, non-productive and paroxysmal**, ending in a gagging episode which may appear to be productive.

Cervical trachea collapse produces inspiratory dyspnea, while intrathoracic tracheal or bronchial collapse will lead to mostly expiratory dyspnea. Stridor is occasionally reported.

Diagnosis

Radiographs may show attenuation of the tracheal or bronchial lumina. Fluoroscopy may be more sensitive for dynamic collapse.

Tracheobronchoscopy is valuable in both diagnosing and grading the severity of the collapse.

PULMONARY FIBROSIS

> **Classical signs**
> - Dyspnea.
> - Rare in cats.

Clinical signs

Chronic progressive dyspnea associated with restrictive pulmonary disease and tachypnea.

Occasionally cats will cough, especially if a secondary bacterial infection occurs.

Very rare in cats, and may be associated with chronic small airway disease (feline asthma/bronchitis complex) or chemotherapy.

A recent paper cited an emerging syndrome of spontaneous feline idiopathic pulmonary fibrosis. In this study, chronic respiratory disease with pathology consistent with usual interstitial pneumonia (UIP) spontaneously developed in domestic short- and longhair cats and Persians.
- Duration of respiratory signs ranged from years (6/22 cats) to acute death (3/22 cats). Cough (12/16), dyspnea (16/19) and increased respiratory rate (19/19 cats) were present. Crackles, wheezes, and harsh or loud lung sounds were auscultated in some cats.

Diagnosis

Marked interstitial pattern is visible on radiographs.

Bronchioalveolar fluid may contain a predominance of lymphocytes or non-lytic neutrophils, eosinophils and macrophages. Culture sample to rule out secondary bacterial infection.

Diffuse interstitial fibrosis is evident on histopathology of a lung biopsy.

Treatment

Bronchdilators orally such as sustained release theophylline (TheoDur or Slo-bid Gyrocaps 25 mg/kg q

24 h in the evening) or inhaled via a face mask (albuterol).

Steroids at anti-inflammatory doses are usually the cornerstone of therapy (prednisone 1 mg/kg q 12 h for 7 days then 1 mg/kg q 24 h, then reducing to the minimum effective dose over 2–4 months).

Antibiotics are indicated when signs worsen and do not respond to steroids. If there are many neutrophils in the BAL fluid, a preliminary course of antibiotics may be indicated before steroids are used, to see if there is any improvement in signs. Be careful about combined use of enrofloxacin and theophylline, as enrofloxacin has the potential to inhibit liver metabolism of theophylline and increase plasma concentrations.

FIBROSING PLEURITIS

Classical signs

- Dyspnea.
- Muffled heart and lung sounds ventrally.

Pathogenesis

Fibrosing pleuritis is a rare sequence of pyothorax and other chronic pleural effusions, especially chyothorax.

Chronic pleuritis results in restrictive fibrosis of the pleura, which prevents the lungs expanding.

Because of the restricted expansion of the lungs during inspiration, negative pressure is increased in the pleural space, resulting in rapid reaccumulation of fluid.

Clinical signs

Dyspnea occurs which is inspiratory and expiratory.

Muffled lung and heart sounds are audible ventrally as a result of the pleural effusion.

There is rapid return of hydrothorax, even after the pyothorax has been successfully treated.

Diagnosis

Radiography may reveal distorted poorly expanded rounded lung lobes.

Diagnosis is frequently only made at surgery.

Treatment

Stripping of the fibrotic pleura from the lungs followed by glucocorticoid therapy has been attempted, but is rarely successful.

Prognosis

Prognosis is generally poor.

RECOMMENDED READING

Mason RA. Dyspnea, tachypnea and panting. In: Tilley LP, Smith FWK (eds) The 5 minute veterinary consult, 2nd edition. Baltimore, Lippincott Williams & Wilkins, 2000, pp 68–69.
Turnwald GH. Dyspnea and tachypnea. In: Ettinger SJ (ed) Textbook of Veterinary Internal Medicine, 4th edition. Philadelphia, Saunders, 1995, pp 61–64.
Ware W. Dyspnea: diagnosis and management. In: August JR (ed) Consultations in feline internal medicine. Philadelphia, Saunders, 1991, pp 147–169.
Williams K, Malarkey D, Cohn L, Patrick D, Dye J, Toews G. Identification of spontaneous feline idiopathic pulmonary fibrosis: morphology and ultrastructural evidence for a type II pneumocyte defect. Chest 2004; 125(6): 2278–2288.

6. The cat with hydrothorax

Robert Allen Mason

> **KEY SIGNS**
>
> - Dyspnea worsened in lateral recumbency.
> - Dull heart and lung sounds ventrally.
> - Fluid aspirated from chest (chyle, blood, transudate, modified transudate, exudates).

MECHANISM?

- Accumulation of fluid (blood, transudate, modified transudate, exudate, chylous) in the pleural cavity.
- There is a delicate balance of the normal fluid dynamics between the slight transudation across the parietal pleura and the slight absorption across the visceral pleura.
- Factors which facilitate pleural effusion include decreased oncotic or increased hydrostatic pressure within blood vessels, increased vessel wall permeability, and lymphatic obstruction.
- Excessive fluid in pleural cavity (chlye, blood, transudate, modified transudate, exudate).
- Pleural effusion encroaches on the space generally occupied by the lungs, and creates hydraulic pressure opposing expansion of the lungs.

WHERE?

- Pleural space is the cavity between the **visceral** and the **parietal pleura**. Generally, this space contains a few milliliters of fluid to act as a lubricant.

WHAT?

- Chylothorax – secondary to congestive heart failure, mediastinal neoplasia, lymphangiectasia, or trauma.
- Hemothorax – secondary to trauma, coagulopathy, or neoplasia.
  Pyothorax – from penetrating chest wound, ruptured lung abscess, or systemic bacteremia.
- Transudation – secondary to hypoalbuminemia from hepatic failure, protein-losing enteropathy, or protein-losing nephropathy. May also occur from increased hydrostatic pressure from congestive heart failure or lymphaticovenous obstruction from a neoplastic or granulomatous disease of the chest.
- Modified transudates result either from causes of chronic transudates or occur early in diseases, which cause exudates such as vasculitis secondary to feline infectious peritonitis, uremia, neoplasia or pancreatitis.

QUICK REFERENCE SUMMARY

Diseases causing hydrothorax

DEGENERATIVE

- **Congestive heart failure (cardiomyopathy)* (p 83)**

Pleural effusion may result from right-sided or biventricular failure, most commonly associated with cardiomyopathies. Cardiac tamponade from pericardial effusion may cause pleural effusion. Abnormal heart sounds (gallops, murmurs, arrhythmias) are commonly noted. Cardiomegaly, pulmonary venous congestion and pulmonary edema may be seen radiographically. Effusion fluid is commonly a modified transudate or chylous effusion. Rarely, heartworm disease has been associated with pleural effusion of a clear transudate.

ANOMALY

- **Chylothorax** (p 77)**

Milky white, lipid-rich lymphatic fluid accumulates in the pleural space secondary to thoracic duct hypertension. Idiopathic chylothorax is the most common form. Less commonly chylothorax is associated with cardiomyopathy, or mediastinal neoplasia. Affected cats are often chronically ill for several months prior to the onset of dyspneic signs of pleural space disease.

MECHANICAL

- Pleural/mediastinal masses (p 84)

Malignancies like thymoma or thymic lymphoma may cause obstruction of the lymphatic drainage of the pleural cavity, leading to hydrothorax and dyspnea. Mass lesions may be observed radiographically, especially after thoracocentesis. Dyspnea rarely may not improve significantly after drainage. Transudate or exudate found on fluid analysis.

- Hemothorax (p 87)

Trauma or bleeding diatheses from congenital coagulopathies (hemophilia, Chediak–Higashi) or acquired coagulopathies (rodenticide toxicity) may create hemothorax. Fluid is pink to frankly red in color, but often defibrinated and does not clot. Evidence of blunt or penetrating chest trauma is common. There may be other signs of coagulopathy (scleral hemorrhages, hematoma formation, epistaxis, etc.).

METABOLIC

- Hypoproteinemia (p 88)

Protein-losing enteropathy, **protein-losing nephropathy**, and **hepatic failure** are common causes of low serum protein, specifically hypoalbuminemia, which may result in decreased oncotic pressure and transudation. This fluid is clear to lightly straw-colored. Signs include dyspnea, weight loss, especially loss of muscle mass +/− icterus.

NEOPLASTIC

- Airway / Pulmonary neoplasia (p 87)

Tracheal adenocarcinomas (i.e., Siamese), primary pulmonary masses (pulmonary adenocarcinoma) or secondary metastatic disease from distant neoplasms may create effusions. Fluid is often modified transudate and is often grossly opaque. It is more common in middle-aged to older cats.

INFECTIOUS

● Pneumonia (p 84)

Moist, productive cough, fever, halitosis may be seen. Parapneumonic pleural effusions are commonly sterile inflammatory exudates, often grossly serous or hemorrhagic rather than purulent. They often resolve with treatment of the lung disease.

● **Feline infectious peritonitis (FIP)* (p 81)**

Vasculitis caused by the immune response to feline coronavirus causes exudation of a protein-rich fibrinous fluid into various body cavities including the pleura. Systemic illness is common.

● **Pyothorax*** (p 75)**

There is an accumulation of grossly obvious purulent exudate in the pleural cavity. Turbid, flocculent, often fetid-smelling fluid with cells that are primarily degenerative neutrophils. Dyspnea, signs of chronic disease (weight loss, ill-thrift), and fever are common signs.

INTRODUCTION

MECHANISM?

Pleural space is the cavity between the **visceral pleura** (covering the lungs and the pericardium) and the **parietal pleura** (covering the internal thoracic wall, diaphragm and mediastinum).

Generally, this space contains a few milliliters of fluid to act as a lubricant for motion of the lungs and the heart. This fluid is very close to the composition of serum.

Visceral and parietal pleurae have distinctly separate vascular supplies and lymphatics. The parietal pleural lymphatics have **stomata** – gaps that exist to remove particulate matter from the pleural space. Absorption through these stomata may be facilitated by motion of the chest wall during breathing. Obstruction of the stomata may decrease absorption of exudative effusions.

Normal fluid dynamics of the pleura balance between opposing **hydrostatic** and **oncotic pressures** across the pleurae. There is a delicate balance between the slight transudation across the parietal pleura and the slight absorption across the visceral pleura, that maintains a steady ratio of production to drainage of fluid through the pleural space.

Disease conditions that disrupt this balance can lead to pleural effusion by changing;

● oncotic pressure.
● systemic or pulmonary vascular pressure.
● lymphatic hydrostatic pressure, compliance or permeability.
● vascular permeability.

Hydrothorax is the accumulation of fluid in the pleural cavity, which may consist of blood, transudate, modified transudate, exudate or chylous fluid

Various fluid types that may accumulate include:

● **Hemorrhage** consists of frank blood, and may be caused by neoplasia, coagulation defects or trauma. The hematocrit of the fluid is often much lower than the peripheral blood, and it rarely clots after removal.

● **Transudates** are low protein (< 15 g/L), low cellularity (< 1.0×10^9/L) fluids that leak out of the vascular space secondary to lymphatic or venous occlusion from congestive heart failure, mediastinal mass obstruction or infiltration of the pleura.

● **Modified transudates or exudates** are more cellular (1.0–7.0×10^9/L and 5.0–20×10^9/L, respectively), and higher protein (25–50 g/L and 30–80 g/L, respectively) fluids.

  – **Modified transudates** are associated either with **diseases that cause chronic transudates**, or occur **early in diseases that produce exudates**. Over time, chronic transudates produce pleural irritation that results in increased cell numbers and slightly increased protein in the fluid, which is then classified as a modified transudate. Modified transudates also occur early in diseases that produce exudates from leaking blood vessels such as neoplasia, and vasculitis associated with feline infectious peritonitis, uremia, pancreatitis or neoplasia.

- **Pyothorax** is pus in the chest cavity from bacterial infection. Protein is high (30–70 g/L) and nucleated cell counts are high ($5–300 \times 10^9$/L).
- **Chylothorax** is a lipid-rich tissue fluid from obstruction or trauma to the thoracic duct. Protein content ranges from 25–60 g/L and cell counts from $1.0–20 \times 10^9$/L.

The fluid from these various forms of pleural effusion encroaches on the space generally occupied by the lungs, and creates hydraulic pressure that opposes the expansion of the lungs. Fluid volumes greater than 50 ml/kg result in dyspnea.

WHERE?

Hydrothorax is the result of conditions that affect the pleural space, especially conditions affecting the blood vessels or lymphatics of the pleura.

Blood vessel problems that contribute to hydrothorax include:

- Increased hydrostatic pressure from congestive heart disease or vascular obstruction.
- Decreased oncotic pressure from hypoalbuminemia secondary to liver disease, kidney or gastrointestinal protein loss.
- Increased vascular permeability from inflammation (vasculitis).
- Vascular rupture and hemorrhage (trauma, neoplasia).

Lymphatic diseases that contribute to hydrothorax include:

- Obstruction from congestive heart disease, lymphangiectasia or neoplasia.
- Rupture from trauma.

WHAT?

The following conditions are most commonly associated with the different forms of hydrothorax in cats:

- **Hemothorax** usually results from trauma or coagulopathy.
- **Transudation** results from either **increased hydrostatic pressure** (mediastinal mass, lymphatic infiltration or obstruction, and cardiac disease) or from

decreased oncotic pressure as a result of hypoalbuminemia (protein-losing enteropathy, protein-losing nephropathy or hepatic failure).

- **Chylothorax** is usually idiopathic and associated with lymphangiectasia, or may occur in association with congestive heart failure, mediastinal neoplasia or thoracic duct rupture.
- **Pyothorax** is most often associated with mixed bacterial infections presumed from a penetrating wound or foreign body.
- **Thoracic exudates** are most commonly associated with feline infectious peritonitis, but may also occur with neoplasia, pancreatitis and uremia.
- **The most common forms of hydrothorax** in the cat are pyothorax, neoplastic effusions, transudation from cardiac disease and chylothorax.

DIAGNOSIS

For cats with **mild to moderate clinical signs**, thoracic radiography may be diagnostic. Pleural fissure lines, separation of the lung borders from the thoracic wall, loss of cardiac detail, blunting of the costophrenic angles (lateral and VD views), widening of the mediastinum (DV view) can all indicate the presence of fluid in the pleural space.

With **severely affected cats** in respiratory distress, **radiography should be delayed** until after thoracocentesis (**cats with pleural effusions die in radiology!**).

An algorithm for the approach to the dyspneic cat follows;

- **A** – Airway – establish a patent airway.
- **B** – Breathing – be certain the patient is ventilating.
- **C** – Centesis – if the dyspnea has not resolved with steps A and B, then evaluating for the presence of pleural space disease via thoracocentesis is not only diagnostic, but therapeutic for both hydrothorax and pneumothorax. A negative tap would suggest the presence of a mass lesion or primary parenchymal disease such as *status asthmaticus*.

Thoracocentesis

- In the acute, emergency setting, a butterfly set may be rapidly introduced to alleviate life-threatening accumulations.
- In chronic or more stable cases, a polypropylene or Silastic IV catheter on an IV extension set with a three-way stopcock attached to a 20–60 ml syringe

works very well. Local anesthetic blockade may or may not be required, depending on the level of respiratory distress.

- **Technique**
  - Have the patient sitting, standing or in sternal recumbency.
  - Clip and aseptically prepare the 4th–7th intercostal space – above and below the costochondral junction.
  - Infiltrate around the 7th intercostals space just above the costochondral junction with local anesthetic field block (optional if peracute and in severe distress), using 2% lidocaine or 2% mepivicaine. Block the skin, muscles and parietal pleura, as this is the most painful area.
  - **Use 25 gauge needles and INJECT SLOWLY!**
  - Place the catheter at the 7th intercostal space just above the costochondral junction. With a syringe on the catheter, aspirate using minimal negative pressure.
  - Direct the catheter ventrally for fluid removal. If drainage is inadequate use a butterfly needle and aspirate the intercostal junction from the 4th–6th intercostals or place a chest drain.
- **Fluid analysis** should be performed to determine the etiology of the hydrothorax.
  - Cytologic, clinicopathologic, and bacteriologic analysis will help determine the etiology. Common assessments include **physical parameters** such as color, transparency, specific gravity (SG), total protein (TP), and total nucleated cell counts (TNCC) and some **biochemical parameters** such as triglyceride, cholesterol, glucose and certain enzyme levels, such as lactate dehydrogenase (LDH).
  - Hemothorax is characterized by frank blood. Erythrophagocytosis which is usually defibrinated may be evident cytologically, and generally has a hematocrit lower than peripheral blood.
  - Transudates are clear and colorless with a specific gravity (SG) $\leq$ 1.013, total protein (TP) < 2.5 g/L and low cellularity (total nucleated cell count [TNCC] < 1.5×10^9/L).
  - Modified transudates are typically straw-colored to pink-white. Total protein is between 2.5 and 4.0 g/L, and TNCC between 1.0 and 7.0×10^9/L. Modified transudates result from transudates modified from chronicity, prolonged increased

hydrostatic pressure (i.e., heart failure), or occur in acute inflammatory disease prior to exudation.
  - Exudates vary from white to red, turbid to opaque, are high protein (> 3.0 g/L), and highly cellular (TNCC > 7.0×10^9/L. They are associated with inflammatory or neoplastic disease.
- **Thoracic radiography** should be performed after thoracocentesis to help to assess the success of pleural drainage and to facilitate imaging of mediastinal masses, pulmonary lesions or cardiac changes that may have contributed to the effusion. These changes may have been previously masked by the presence of the effusion.

Other imaging may be required depending on the character of the effusion (i.e., cardiac ultrasound if transudate, lymphangiography if chylous effusion, etc.).

DISEASES CAUSING HYDROTHORAX

PYOTHORAX***

> **Classical signs**
>
> - Dyspnea with exaggerated chest excursions/poor airflow.
> - Muffled heart and/or lung sounds ventrally.
> - Orthopnea (positional dyspnea – reluctance to lay in lateral recumbency).
> - Signs of chronic disease (weight loss, ill-thrift), and fever are common.
> - Grossly purulent exudate in the pleural cavity.
> - History of fight wounds several weeks previous to presentation.

Pathogenesis

Septic bacterial infection of the pleural cavity results in purulent exudation.

Multiple routes of infection, include:
- Hematogeneous with systemic sepsis spread via vasculature or lymphatics.
- **Extension from an adjacent infected structure**, including parapneumonic spread from lung infection or abscess, or from esophageal rupture, or mediastinitis.

- **Penetrating wound** as a result of a fight, a foreign body or thoracic surgery.

Fibrinous exudation and cellular infiltration occurring in response to bacterial infection results in obstruction of the parietal pleural stomata, which further reduces drainage of the exudation.

Clinical signs of systemic illness result from the chronic sepsis. Eventually respiratory signs become evident as fluid reaches critical volume (estimated in cats to be 50 ml/kg).

Clinical signs

Pyothorax is more common in **intact males**, and there is a **history of fight wounds** several weeks prior to presentation.

Heart and lung sounds are dull ventrally. Breathing sounds are harsh dorsally in standing or sternal recumbency. Chest wall percussion may be dull ventrally.

Dyspnea is characterized by marked chest wall excursions with minimal airflow. Orthopnea, or positional dyspnea is common. Dyspnea is worsened in lateral recumbency and cats often are **reluctant to lie in lateral recumbency**.

Signs of chronic disease are often evident. The cat may appear sick, septic, thin and unkempt.

Fever or, in the latter stages, hypothermia may be present.

There may be caudal displacement of the liver due to pleural fluid pressure on the diaphragm.

Diagnosis

Typically there is a vague history of being unwell for weeks, with inappetance, weight loss and recent onset of dyspnea.

Thoracic radiographs show significant pleural effusion with pleural fissure lines and loss of the cardiac silhouette. Effusions are usually bilateral, although not always.

Thoracocentesis may be both diagnostic and therapeutic in pleural space disease.

- Thoracocentesis should be **performed in all acutely dyspneic animals**, especially trauma patients, **prior to radiography.** These patients are extremely fragile, and even the minimal restraint involved in radiography may be excessive, and they may die during the procedure!
- A negative tap for air or fluid suggests solid pleural space disease (mass or herniated viscus), primary pulmonary (i.e., contusion in the trauma patient) or cardiac disease. If the tap is positive, remember that small animals may accommodate up to 50 ml/kg free fluid in the chest prior to becoming dyspneic.
- Be certain to remove as much fluid as possible, do not stop after you have a diagnostic sample.

Cytology

Cytology and Gram stain are important in identification of the pathogen, as culture is often negative.

Pyothorax is characterized by a thick, fetid, septic suppurative exudate. Cytology reveals a high protein fluid (TP > 30 g/L), highly cellular (TNCC > 7.0 × 10^9/L) with mostly degenerative neutrophils, often with intracellular bacteria. Macrophages and reactive mesothelial cells are common.

- Bacterial infection is characterized by suppurative inflammation involving degenerative neutrophils with intracellular bacteria.
- Fungal and mycobacterial diseases have pyogranulomatous inflammation, with characteristic organisms seen on routine or special stains.

Bacteriology

Bacterial culture for aerobic and anaerobic bacteria is important, but negative cultures are not surprising, as many bacteria have been killed or had their growth inhibited by the lysozymes present in the exudate. Gram staining is an excellent way to document the initial categories of bacteria present, as well as following the response to therapy.

Hematology

Blood smear may reveal neutrophilia with or without a left shift and toxic neutrophils (Doehle bodies, etc.).

A low-grade non-responsive anemia and monocytosis may support chronicity.

Differential diagnosis

All causes of pleural effusion show similar signs of dyspnea and dull chest sounds. Most other causes, however, do not show the same severe systemic signs, other than some forms of pleural or pulmonary neoplasia.

Treatment

Thoracostomy (T) tube placement and chest drainage is the cornerstone of therapy.

- Tubes may be placed surgically or via a trocar. Placement along the ventral thoracic floor helps maximize complete drainage.
- **Continuous underwater sealed suction** with 20 cmH$_2$O of vacuum appears to be superior to intermittent drainage, but requires 24-hour direct supervision. Disposable, self-contained collection units are easily adaptable to cats. These are commercially available one-piece plastic chambers that adapt to a suction line on one end, and to the thoracostomy tube on the other. The effusion is collected and volume measured in the calibrated chamber.
- Occasionally bilateral T-tubes are required for complete drainage. Average duration of tube use is 3–5 days with continuous suction. Intermittent suction generally requires longer duration of therapy. Tubes are usually removed once less than 2 ml/kg of fluid is drained.
- Controversy exists as to the benefit of pleural lavage. There has been no convincing evidence showing any advantage to lavage, and the risk of contamination is high.

Systemic support with **IV fluid hydration** and antibiotic therapy is very important. Most patients are hypovolemic on presentation, and the initial fluid losses via the T-tube can be tremendous. Fluid requirements must include **volume replacement, maintenance, and ongoing losses** through the T-tube. Keeping the patient well-hydrated helps to promote the "dialysis membrane" effect of the pleura, effectively "washing" the pleural space and draining the excess fluid through the T-tube. Serum potassium and phosphorus levels should be monitred and supplemented, when indicated.

Antibiotics

Antibiotic selection is best based upon specific culture and sensitivity testing. Initial empirical choices can be based on the Gram stain of the cytology sample.

- **Gram-positive rods** – fluoroquinolones, chloramphenicol, clindamycin.
- **Gram-positive cocci** – beta-lactams, chloramphenicol.
- **Note**: aminoglycosides require oxygen-rich environments to be effective, and trimethoprim-sulfa drugs may be inactivated in purulent debris. For these reasons, these medications are not indicated in pyothoraces.

Beta lactams such as **ampicillin** at 20–40 mg/kg IV initially q 4 hours for 48 hours, then PO q 6–8 hours are sufficient for the majority of community-acquired infections.

Clindamycin is effective against *Bacteriodes fragilis*, found in approximately 15% of cases, and is dosed at 25 mg/cat PO q 12 hours.

Recommendation for length of antibiotic therapy varies from 4 to 12 weeks.

Prognosis

Prompt, aggressive and complete drainage of the abscess cavity in the pleural space is essential for successful therapy. The use of T-tube(s) with continuous suction has increased the treatment success rate of this disease tremendously.

Prognosis also varies with the presence or absence of underlying risk factors, such as pre-existing immunosuppressive disease with retroviral infection or systemic neoplasia.

With aggressive therapy, lack of significant risk factors, and long-term therapy with appropriate antibiotics, prognosis is very good to excellent.

Prevention

Neuter intact males. Prevent roaming and fighting.

CHYLOTHORAX**

Classical signs

- Muffled heart and/or lung sounds ventrally.
- Exaggerated chest excursions with poor airflow.
- Orthopnea (positional dyspnea with reluctance to lie in lateral recumbency).

Pathogenesis

Chyle is the lymphatic fluid being transported from the abdominal organs to the prehepatic circulation. It contains lipid-rich products such as chylomicrons, and grossly it is pink to milky white. Protein content may vary, and measurement may be interfered with by the presence of the lipids. Cells are primarily small lymphocytes, and the count (TNCC) is $< 10 \times 10^9$/L.

The **thoracic duct** is the cranial continuation of the **cysterna chyli**, the major lymphatic structure draining the abdominal organs. The **thoracic duct passes through the diaphragm at the aortic hilus** and proceeds cranially in the mediastinum dorsal to the thoracic aorta and ventral to the azygous vein. It terminates cranially at the lymphaticovenous junction **at the thoracic inlet, either into left jugular, subclavian, or brachiocephalic veins**. Here the lymphatic fluid from the entire body, except the right side of the face, the right pectoral limb, and the right thoracic wall, which drain into the right lymphatic duct, re-enters the venous circulation.

The rate of lymph flow through the thoracic duct in cats has been estimated **at 2 ml/kg/hour**, increasing up to 10-fold after a high-fat meal. Rapid accumulation of several hundreds of milliliters of fluid can occur with obstruction of or leakage from lymphatic drainage.

Chylous effusion in cats is most often idiopathic. The most commonly known causes are associated with increased lymphatic hypertension from congestive heart failure or obstructive neoplasia (see sections under Cardiomyopathy or Mediastinal masses in this chapter).

Increased systemic venous pressure associated with dilated cardiomyopathy and rarely heartworm diseases may result in lymphatic hypertension and, occasionally chlyothorax.

Mediastinal neoplasia, especially lymphosarcoma and thymoma are most common neoplasias associated with chylothorax.

Occasionally thrombus formation associated with an indwelling jugular catheter results in chylothorax.

Idiopathic chylous **effusions** are associated with thoracic duct disease.
- Thoracic duct lymphangiectasia, demonstrated via contrast lymphangiography, is the most common finding in primary chylothorax in cats. There is controversy whether this finding represents a cause and effect of lymphatic hypertension.
- Thoracic trauma is a less common cause of thoracic duct rupture, although this has been documented.
- Chronic chylothorax is irritating to the pleura and may cause fibrosing pleuritis and pericarditis.
- New evidence suggests this secondary fibrosing pericarditis may lead to increased right-sided pressures and decreased lymphaticovenous drainage, resulting in diminished drainage of the thorax, and persistence of the chylothorax.

Clinical signs

Chylothorax generally occurs in **middle-aged cats**, possibly more common in purebreds.

Vague signs of depression and lethargy, often for greater than 1 month, are common.

Tachypnea, dyspnea and the ventilation pattern typical for pleural space disease are present. This involves increased chest wall excursion, often with the head and neck extended, but very little airflow present. Dyspnea may be reported as acute in onset. Dyspnea is often worsened in lateral recumbency and cats are reluctant to lie in lateral recumbency.

Heart sounds are muffled but become more apparent after the chest tap and are generally normal.

Abnormal heart sounds such as murmurs, gallops or arrhythmias may be present if the chylous effusion is associated with congestive heart disease, but are generally absent in idiopathic chylous effusion.

Coughing may be present from pleural irritation.

Diagnosis

Clinically there are signs of pleural effusion and muffled heart sounds.

Thoracocentesis should be performed prior to radiography in the severely dyspneic patients, both as an emergency treatment and a diagnostic procedure.
- The typical effusion is grossly chylous with milky-white to pink fluid. Cell count is usually $<1 \times 1^9$/L and is largely lymphocytes, unless the effusion is chronic in which case large numbers of neutrophils and macrophages may be present.

- Cholesterol and triglyceride levels of the serum and the effusion may be measured and compared to definitively diagnose true chylous effusion, but these findings rarely change the prognosis or the management. True chylothorax has higher triglyceride and lower cholesterol levels than serum.
- So-called pseudochylous effusions have the same gross appearance but with higher cholesterol and lower triglyceride concentrations than serum. Pseudochylous effusion has been discussed in the veterinary literature for years, but there is little evidence that this exists as a clinical entity in cats.

Thoracic radiography should be performed after thoracocentesis.
- If cardiac or pulmonary vessel abnormalities are evident radiographically, this indicates the pleural effusion may be secondary to congestive heart failure.
- Chronic chylothorax may result in fibrosing pleuritis evidenced by rounded or collapsed lung lobes on radiography.
- Contrast lymphangiography may be performed if no underlying cardiac disease or neoplasia is detected.
  - A mesenteric lymphatic vessel is cannulated via celiotomy, and iodinated contrast media are injected. Thoracic duct lymphangiectasia is the most common finding with primary chylothorax in cats. Radiographically, dilated, tortuous lymphatics are found in the cranial mediastinum of affected cats. This procedure adds significant time under anesthesia, and may be technically difficult to perform without intraoperative radiography or fluoroscopy capabilities. There is current debate whether this finding of lymphangiectasia is the cause or an effect of thoracic lymphatic hypertension.

Echocardiography is the definitive modality for ruling out cardiomyopathy, pericardial effusion, or other causes of congestive heart failure.

If the cat is only mildly dyspneic, ultrasound should be performed before the pleural fluid is drained as the fluid aids in the detection of a mediastinal mass. Severely dyspneic cats should have some fluid drained first, as the stress of ultrasound can be fatal.

Differential diagnosis

Other forms of pleural effusion may have similar clinical signs but the appearance of the fluid is different.

Chylous effusions may occur as part of **congestive heart failure**. If cardiac abnormalities are detected, than a complete cardiac diagnostic evaluation should be performed (see Cardiomyopathy section in this chapter).

Treatment

Emergency thoracocentesis should be performed immediately in cats with severe respiratory distress.
- A 23 G butterfly infusion set on a 60 ml syringe is introduced at the 5th–7th intercostal space (ICS) on the right, just above the costochondral junction. Remove as much fluid as possible, or until breathing improves. This can usually be performed without sedation or local anesthetic block with the cat standing or in sternal recumbancy. Drainage at multiple locations below the costochondral junction between the 4th and 6th intercostal space is sometimes more effective.
- Placement of a chest drain is recommended for all patients except those that are very debilitated.
- Fluid should be aspirated 1–2 times/day and the tube removed once less than 1–2 ml/kg daily is obtained.
- Intermittent thoracocentesis may be required until definitive therapy has been effective.

Definitive therapy if congestive heart failure is diagnosed is based upon ultrasonographic characterization of the type and severity of the cardiomyopathy present (see page 128 The Cat With Abnormal Heart Sounds and/or an Enlarged Heart).

Removal of the jugular catheter and drainage of the chlye usually results in resolution of the chylothorax in those cases associated with an indwelling jugular catheter.

For idiopathic primary chylothorax, both medical and surgical management have been advocated.

Medical management
- **This is based around decreasing the lymphatic flow through the thoracic duct**. **Restricting dietary fats** is the cornerstone of medical management. Parenteral intravenous feeding is used in humans, but is not a practical long-term solution in cats. Low-fat-reducing diets, commercial or homemade, help reduce chyle flow, but must be formulated to meet the nutritional needs of the patient. MCT oil (medium chain triglycerides) is a way to

supply calories from fats that are absorbed directly into the portal circulation and bypass the thoracic duct lymphatics. Whether this truly decreases thoracic duct flow has come under question in the dog, and information is still lacking in cats. MCT oil is generally reserved for extremely cachectic cats. It tastes terrible, and may worsen inappetance.

- **Nutriceutical "fat binders" such as Chitin/Chitosan** may be beneficial to decrease the fat-induced chlye flow.
- **Rutin**, another oral nutriceutical therapy, has shown mixed results in idiopathic chylothorax.
- Rutin is a bioflavanoid and a derivative of vitamin C. It stimulates macrophage uptake of protein and processing of inflammatory cells, thus improving the absorption of the remaining fluid. Dose is 50 mg/kg tin, which can be mixed up with food.
- Octreotide (Sandostatin, Novartis) a synthetic somatostatin is being trialled in cats as a SQ injection tid, but its efficacy is currently unknown.
- Medical management together with intermittent thoracocentesis may be used during the treatment for the underlying disease (cardiac therapy, cancer treatments, etc.).

Surgical management.

- Surgery should only be considered for patients who do not respond to medical management within 6–10 days. Success following surgery is disappointingly low. Surgery is best performed by a specialist with experience in thoracic duct ligation.
  - **Ligation of the thoracic duct** is the definitive therapy for idiopathic chylothorax. Surgical approaches and techniques are described in standard surgical texts. Some surgeons prefer to give cream orally prior to surgery so that the thoracic duct is filled with white chyle at the time of surgery, for easier identification. Others prefer to perform a mesenteric lymphatic dye study similar to what is described for lymphangiography, but using new methylene blue dye rather than radiographic contrast material. This dye is visible at the time of surgery to ease identification.
  - A postoperative contrast lymphangiogram may be performed through the same mesenteric lymphatic catheter to assess the success of the ligation. A thoracostomy tube is placed postoperatively

and removed once the fluid production through the tube falls below 1 ml/kg daily.
  - There is current debate whether this procedure is useful in idiopathic lymphangiectasia, or whether the lymphatic hypertension continues despite ligation.
  - **Pleuroperitoneal drainage**, either with passive drains with diaphragmatic mesh implants, or active sump drains between the pleural and peritoneal cavities have been described, but there is a lack of data on the outcomes of these procedures in cats. Blockage of the drain is a problem.
  - Some surgeons report success with pericardectomy, as a means to decrease the underlying lymphatic hypertension. Recent studies combining pericardectomy with thoracic duct ligation have resulted in 80% success in a group of ten cats with chylothorax.

Prognosis

The success of medical management has been documented at 20% or less. The author's clinical experience has been somewhat below that figure. Traumatic injuries to the thoracic duct may have a slightly better response rate to medical management. Successful treatment of the underlying disease process usually results in resolution of the chylothorax for taurine-responsive dilated cardiomyopathy and neoplasia. The poor success rate in idiopathic chylothorax likely relates to persistence of the underlying pathophysiology.

Prognosis for success of surgical ligation varies from 25–53%, and likely varies directly with the skill and experience of the surgeon. Continued effusion occurred in 30% of cats after thoracic duct ligation in one study. Proponents of the primary lymphatic hypertension theory feel that surgical ligation does not change the underlying pathophysiology. New data regarding the success rate of pericardectomy are very promising, with one report of an 80% remission rate in ten cats.

Chyle is a very irritating fluid to the pleura. Chylofibrosis and restrictive pleuritis may follow as a complication even after successful surgical ligation. If the fibrosis is severe, the lungs may fail to expand even after thoracocentesis. Pleural stripping has been described, but is not commonly performed in cats, so the success rate is unknown.

Prevention

Taurine supplementation of commercial cat foods in North America has dramatically decreased the incidence of dilated cardiomyopathy in cats. Other causes of cardiomyopathies remain unclear at this time.

FELINE INFECTIOUS PERITONITIS (FIP)*

Classical signs

- Muffled heart and/or lung sounds ventrally.
- Exaggerated chest excursions with poor airflow.
- Orthopnea (positional dyspnea with reluctance to lie in lateral recumbency).
- Anorexia, weight loss, depression, dehydration and fever are common early signs.

See main reference on page 372, for details (The Pyrexic Cat).

Pathogenesis

Feline infectious peritonitis (**FIP**) is caused by a strain of feline coronavirus called feline infectious peritonitis virus (FIPV).

- **This virus specifically infects the mononuclear phagocytic cells** of the spleen, liver and lymph nodes. Replication of the virus occurs primarily in these cells and creates a systemic viremic state within 1 week of experimental exposure.
- **Virus and virus-infected circulating monocytes deposit** in the endothelial lining of venules. Immune complex interaction to the viral antigen creates an intense vasculitis with complement-mediated damage to the vessel walls.
- The "holes" created in the vessels result in the **exudation of the fibrin-rich characteristic "FIP fluid".**

Three forms of FIP exist. The **effusive or "wet" form** is of most significance in creating pleural effusion. It is the damage caused by the humoral immune system, rather than viral cytotoxicity per se, that is the major pathogenic mechanism in the formation of the effusion.

The large body cavities such as the chest and abdomen are most prone to fluid accumulation.

Clinical signs

No real age, sex or breed predisposition. **Kittens 6–12 months old** and **purebred queens up to 5 years** of age are over-represented. Another peak is reported in aged cats. Cats from **multi-cat environments** are as greatest risk.

Anorexia, weight loss, depression, fever or hypothermia (terminally), and dehydration may all occur, but none are specific to FIP.

The effusive form is more rapid and fulminant than the non-effusive form.

Progressive accumulation of ascites and pleural effusion in an inappetant, lethargic and pyrexic cat is characteristic of effusive FIP. **Dyspnea occurs in about 1/3 of cats** and results from the pleural restriction of the pleural effusion as well as the compromised diaphragmatic excursions secondary to the ascites.

Typically the wet form progresses to **death within 5–7 weeks** of onset of clinical signs. This progression may be shortened to a few days in young kittens.

Diagnosis

Clinical signs of pleural and abdominal effusion with normal heart sounds in an inappetant, lethargic and often pyrexic cat are highly suggestive of FIP.

Serology
- **Up to 10–40% of healthy cats have positive coronavirus titers**. A positive titer means exposure to a feline coronavirus, but not necessarily FIPV.
- High titers in the presence of typical signs of FIP in a cat from a one- or two-cat household may suggest FIP, however, methodology is not standard between labs. Some healthy cats, especially pure-bred or from multi-cat households, have very high titers.
- **PCR (polymerase chain reaction)** may be more accurate at detecting viral antigens. One study, however, showed 8/9 cats suspected with FIP (87.5%) were positive, but 51/84 cats (61%) were positive in non-suspects.
- **A 7B FIP ELISA** test is available which detects antibody to the 7B protein, which is specific to some coronavirus strains causing FIP. Specificity and sensitivity data have not been published. Anecdotal evidence suggests this is not sensitive for FIP.

Thoracocentesis or abdominocentesis and examination of the fluid are very valuable.

The high protein (50–120 g/L) and fibrin content of the fluid makes it thick, viscous and straw-colored. Cell count is moderate (10×10^9/L), and consists predominantly of non-degenerative neutrophils.

Electrophoretic separation of the proteins within the fluid may be helpful.
- Fluid with gamma globulins > 32% has a high positive predictive value for FIP.
- Fluids with protein comprised of > 48% albumin had a very high negative predictive value for ruling out FIP.
- **Histopathology** of liver, kidney or other abdominal tissue with inflammation is diagnostic.

Differential diagnosis

There are few other differential diagnoses for hydrothorax with a clear or straw-colored, highly proteinaceous fluid. Other forms of pleural effusion with an exudative fluid are usually turbid, such as pyothorax.
- **Pyothorax** may have systemic clinical signs and effusion fluid that resembles FIP. FIP fluid has high protein content (50–120 g/L) with low to moderate cellularity (10×10^9/L), and predominantly non-degenerative neutrophils, while pyothorax fluid has moderately high protein levels (30–70 g/L), and extremely high nucleated cell counts (5–300×10^9/L), which are mostly degenerative septic neutrophils. Electrophoresis and bacterial culture of the fluid may help separate these entities. FIP fluid has high gamma globulin and is sterile, where pyothorax fluid has a balanced albumin/globulin ratio, and is a septic exudate, based on Gram stain or culture results.

Pericardial effusion may present with ascites and pleural effusion.

Treatment

Emergency thoracocentesis should be performed in cats with severe respiratory distress (see section on Pleural effusions, this chapter).

Medical management
- **Management strategies for FIP** take advantage of the different immunopathogenic mechanisms of the

effusive (humoral, beta cell mediated) and granulomatous (cell-mediated, T-cell response) forms of the disease, but generally have a very poor outcome in almost all cases. For a more thorough discussion, see page 458, The Cat With Abdominal Distention or Abdominal Fluid.
- For effusive FIP, several strategies have been advocated, including:
  - **Corticosteroids**: prednisone 2–4 mg/kg/day PO.
  - **Cytotoxic drugs**: cyclophosphamide 2.2 mg/kg/day PO 4 days each week, or 50 mg/m² PO q 48 hours, or melphalan 2 mg/m² PO q 48 h, or chlorambucil 1.5 mg/m² PO q 24 hours.
  - **Antiviral drugs**: ribavirin 5 mg/kg IV q 24 h. Ribavirin is very toxic to cats, mainly myelosuppressive. It has not been shown to substantially improve the longevity, although a slight increase in survival time (10 days) with fewer clinical signs has been documented. Ribavirin can be combined with interferon therapy. Low-dose oral human interferon-alpha (Roferon) 30 IU/day PO has been advocated.
  - **NB: in high risk, systemically ill cats, omitting the cytotoxic and antiviral agents is recommended.**

Ancillary treatment consists of using the serotonin antagonist **cyproheptadine** (1–2 mg PO q 12 hours) for appetite stimulation. Antibiotics have been used, especially with neutropenia and fever, but with no data to support efficacy. Amphotericin B has been shown to have in vitro antiviral effects against FIP, but its nephrotoxicity limits its use in cats.

Prognosis

Long-term prognosis for effusive FIP is extremely poor. Average survival from onset of clinical signs is 5–7 weeks, although some stronger "healthier" individuals may have a more insidious disease course, and may survive for 6–8 months.

Prevention

Management strategies
- One study showed kittens raised in catteries with all other cats or isolated from other cats except queens had 30–50% positive titers for FIPV, and 1–2% death rate from clinical FIP. However, kittens raised in a cattery, that were weaned and

separated from queens at 4–6 weeks of age had 0% positive titer, 0% died of FIP.

- The recommendation from this study was to **wean early and separate kittens from the queen** before the maternal antibodies are lost.

Vaccination

- **A heat-sensitive modified-live intranasal vaccine** was tested for efficacy. In this study, of 550 cats arriving at shelter, half were vaccinated and 2/254 developed clinical FIP, where 8/246 unvaccinated controls developed FIP. However, an experimental study using a different challenge strain to the vaccine strain found no protection and antibody-dependent enhancement occurred resulting in accelerated disease.

CONGESTIVE HEART FAILURE (CARDIOMYOPATHY)

Classical signs

- Muffled heart and/or lung sounds ventrally.
- Exaggerated chest excursions/poor airflow.
- Orthopnea (positional dyspnea – reluctance to lay in lateral recumbency).
- Dyspnea ranging from mild to acute and severe with cyanosis.
- Abnormal heart sounds (murmurs, gallops, arrhythmias).

See main reference on page 128 for details (The Cat With Abnormal Heart Sounds and/or an Enlarged Heart).

Pathogenesis

Mechanism of pleural effusion in cats with congestive heart failure is currently unknown, but there are two leading theories:

- **Left-sided failure** results in pulmonary venous and capillary hypertension, which leads to reflex pulmonary vasoconstriction. The resultant pulmonary hypertension leads to **right-sided heart failure** and pleural effusion. Evidence against this theory is that other signs attributed to right heart failure (right heart enlargement, hepatic venous distention, etc.) are rarely found in cats with congestive heart failure and pleural effusion.
- The **visceral pleural veins in cats drain into the pulmonary veins** (as seen in humans), and pulmonary venous hypertension leads to pleural effusion. This is suspected, but not proved, in cats.

Pleural fluid tends to be a **modified transudate or chylous** in nature with congestive heart failure.

Cardiomyopathies such as hypertrophic, dilated or intermediate forms are most often associated with pleural effusions. Dilated cardiomyopathy is more often associated with pleural effusion than the other forms of cardiomyopathy, but it is now a rare disease following taurine supplementation of commercial pet food.

Rarely heartworm disease has been associated with pleural effusion.

Clinical signs

Dyspnea varies from **mild and associated with reduced activity levels and reluctance to play**, to acute, fulminant air-starvation with open-mouth breathing and cyanosis.

Abnormal heart sounds (murmurs, gallops, arrhythmias) may be present, or may be difficult to assess in the distressed patient.

Signs of pleural effusion include increased **chest excursions with little airflow** (can be detected by listening close to muzzle during breathing).

The cat may present with signs of aorto-iliac thromboembolism, such as paresis of one or more limb, nail bed cyanosis, cool anesthetic limb, firm cramping of the gastrocnemius muscle, vocalization and tachypinea or dyspnea.

Orthopnea (worsened dyspnea in lateral recumbancy) or reluctance of the patient to lay in lateral recumbency may be reported.

Muffled heart and lung sounds are audible ventrally, with harsh breathing sounds dorsally in the standing or sternal recumbency positions. Dull percussion of the chest wall is evident ventrally.

The liver may be displaced caudally due to fluid pressure exerted on the diaphragm.

Diagnosis

Typically there are **clinical signs of pleural effusion** together with abnormal heart sounds.

Thoracocentesis is indicated in the dyspneic patient with clinical signs of effusion.

- Thoracocentesis should be performed in all acutely dyspneic animals, **prior to radiography.** These patients are extremely fragile, and even the minimal restraint involved in radiography may be excessive, and they may die during the procedure.
- **A transudate, modified transudate, or chylous effusion** are the most common fluid types in heart disease.
- **Heart sounds are often more apparent** after the chest tap, and murmurs, gallops or dysrhythmias may be heard. Be certain to remove as much fluid as possible, do not stop after you have a diagnostic sample.
- A negative tap for fluid suggests pulmonary edema rather than effusion from cardiac disease.

Thoracic radiography
- This is best performed in the acutely dyspneic patient **after** thoracocentesis and stabilization.
- Findings may include enlarged cardiac outline, pulmonary venous distention, and patchy alveolar infiltrates indicating pulmonary edema.

Echocardiography
- This is the definitive modality for diagnosis of cardiomyopathy, as well as the primary tool for categorization of the type and severity of disease. Various forms of cardiomyopathy include hypertrophic (HCM), dilated (DCM), restrictive (RCM) and intermediate (ICM). Therapeutic strategies and prognosis rely heavily on the echocardiographic information. Thoracocentesis should be performed prior to echocardiography in the severely dyspneic patient, otherwise death may occur during the procedure.
- **Electrocardiography** is important if an arrhythmia is detected during physical exam or ultrasound exam.

Differential diagnosis

Other forms of pleural effusion are not associated with abnormal heart sounds (murmurs, gallops, arrhythmias).

Pericardial effusion may create pleural effusion, an enlarged heart shadow on radiographs and possibly an abnormal ECG pattern. *Electrical alternans* on ECG tends to signal pericardial effusion, especially if the pleural effusion has been drained. Ultrasound is definitive in distinguishing cardiomyopathy from pericardial effusion.

Treatment

Emergency thoracocentesis can be **life saving** in cats with severe respiratory distress.
- A 23 G butterfly set on a 60 ml syringe is introduced at the 5th–7th intercostal space (ICS) on the right, just above the costochondral junction. Remove as much fluid as possible, or until breathing improves. Thoracocentesis can usually be performed without sedation or local anesthetic block

Oxygen therapy should be administered using an O_2 chamber, masks or tents.

Furosemide (1–2 mg/kg IV or IM) should be administered without stressing the patient.

Use sedation if the cat is frantic (morphine 0.1 mg/kg IM prn, or butorphanol 0.2–0.4 mg/kg IM q 4–6 h as needed).

Nitroglycerin 2% cream – 1/8 to 1/4 inch applied to the skin of the medial pinna q 4–6 hours for 24 hours.

Take a "hands off" approach until stable, as the **slightest stress can cause lethal decompensation** in these fragile cases.

Definitive therapy is based upon ultrasonographic characterization of the type and severity of the cardiomyopathy present, but this is not performed until the patient is stable.

Prognosis

The prognosis is related to the clinical and echocardiographic severity. Severe left atrial enlargement predisposes to aorto-iliac thromboembolism, which worsens the prognosis.

Prevention

Taurine supplementation of commercial cat foods in North America has dramatically decreased the incidence of dilated cardiomyopathy in cats. Causes for the other cardiomyopathies remain unclear at this time.

PLEURAL/MEDIASTINAL MASSES

Classical signs

- Muffled heart and lung sounds ventrally.
- Dyspnea characterized by excessive chest excursions with poor airflow.
- Orthopnea (positional dyspnea with reluctance to lie in lateral recumbency).

See main reference on page 56 for details (The Dyspneic or Tachypneic Cat).

Clinical signs

Mediastinal masses are often **thymomas, thymic lymphoma** or **mediastinal lymphoma**. Occasionally, ectopic thyroid adenocarcinoma may create a space-occupying mass of the mediastinum. **Pleural masses** include mesotheliomas, osteosarcoma or chondrosarcoma of the ribs or sternabrae.

Signs are related to the space-occupying nature of the mass, or to obstruction of lymphatic drainage and secondary pleural effusion.

Signs include increased **dyspnea in lateral recumbency** (i.e., orthopnea), tachypnea, minimal airflow with increased chest excursions, **muffled heart and lung sounds** or **asymmetrical sounds if the heart is displaced laterally.**

Extraluminal compression of the trachea can cause dyspnea and cough.

Compression of the anterior thorax may reveal decreased compliance.

Diagnosis

Thoracic radiography may reveal the mass lesion or the secondary pleural effusion.
- Separation of the "cupolae" (anterior tips of the cranial lobes) on ventrodorsal projection, representing widening of the anterior mediastinum, may be a sensitive indicator of a subtle mass lesion.

Thoracic ultrasound can be extremely useful.
- Small mediastinal masses surrounded by aerated lung may not be visible from a paracostal approach, and may require a **thoracic inlet window**.

- **Transesophageal ultrasonography** is excellent for demonstrating mediastinal masses, but requires specialized equipment and general anesthesia.
- Surgical or ultrasound-guided biopsy of the mass may be required for a definitive diagnosis.

Thoracocentesis and analysis of the fluid may be diagnostic if the neoplasm has exfoliated into the fluid. This is, however, a rare occurrence. Typically the fluid is a modified transudate, although occasionally it is an exudate.

Mediastinal lymphoma may have **hypercalcemia** as a paraneoplastic syndrome, but this is **rare** in the cat.

Tissue biopsy and histopathology are required for definitive diagnosis.

Differential diagnosis

Other causes of pleural effusion that typically cause a modified transudate are cardiac disease and other airway neoplasias. Radiography and ultrasound can usually differentiate these.

Treatment

Lymphoma of the thymus or mediastinal lymph nodes is best handled with standard chemotherapy protocols for lymphoma (see page 676).

Surgical excision is the treatment of choice for **thymoma**, and may be curative.

Mesothelioma is an infiltrative disease that cannot be readily resected, and there are few reports in the literature of effective chemotherapy. Local infusion of carboplatin may be helpful with or without the addition of doxirubicin intravenously. Prognosis is grave.

PNEUMONIA

Classical signs

- Moist, productive cough, with adventitial lung sounds.
- Fever.
- Fetid halitosis.
- **Parapneumonic pleural effusion** can create dyspnea and decreased ventilation, possibly with exaggerated chest excursions/poor airflow.

continued

Classical signs—Cont'd

- Muffled heart and/or lung sounds ventrally.
- Orthopnea (positional dyspnea with reluctance to lie in lateral recumbency).

See main reference on page 62 for details (The Dyspneic or Tachypneic Cat).

Clinical signs

Infectious pneumonia is rare in cats.

A deep productive cough may be present, which generally is infrequent unless the pneumonia is secondary to bronchitis (see page 104, The Coughing Cat).

Inspiratory and expiratory dyspnea, often with open-mouth breathing is present when pneumonia is severe and associated with a parapneumonia pleural effusion.

Adventitial breath sounds, including crackles, wheezes, snaps and pops are audible.

Heart sounds may be muffled and lung sounds poorly audible ventrally, although the effusion volume is usually small.

Systemic signs include lethargy, anorexia, weight loss, fever and ill thrift.

Halitosis may be noted.

Deep chest excursion and diminished oral airflow occurs when parapneumonic pleural effusion is present.

Geographical location and other signs might suggest the etiology of the pneumonia, including bacterial, fungal, viral and *Chlamydophila felis* pneumonitis.

Diagnosis

Thoracic radiography reveals alveolar densities (focal or generalized) and possible areas of complete consolidation. There is subtle radiographic evidence (e.g. pleural fissure lines) of a **small-volume pleural effusion.**
- Hilar lymphadenopathy supports fungal or mycobacterial pneumonia.

On hematology neutrophilia is common, with or without a left shift or signs of toxicity.
- Low-grade, non-responsive anemia and monocytosis may support chronicity.

- **On thoracocentesis** there is a **small volume of effusion** which is commonly a **sterile inflammatory exudate**, and is often grossly serous or hemorrhagic rather than purulent.

Cytology and culture samples from percutaneous lung aspiration, transtracheal wash or bronchoscopic lavage may be diagnostic. Fungal, aerobic and anaerobic bacterial cultures are generally submitted.

Cryptococcal titers may aid in the diagnosis.

Differential diagnosis

Other causes of pleural effusion, such as pyothorax, congestive heart failure, chylothorax, FIP and mediastinal masses may mimic the parapneumonic effusion of some pneumonias. Typically, pneumonic patients are more severely dyspneic than would be attributed to the subtle effusion, because of the associated compromise of the lung parenchyma in pneumonia, which is not usually found in other causes of effusion.

Each of the infectious pneumonias can have overlapping features.

Treatment

Bacterial pneumonia
- Appropriate antimicrobial therapy is the mainstay of therapy. The parenteral route is used if the patient is debilitated or septic. The oral route can be used with outpatients. Antibiotic selection is best based upon specific culture and sensitivity testing.
- Pending culture results, some therapeutic decisions may be based upon Gram stain results.
  - **Gram-positive cocci** – ampicillin, amoxicillin, amoxicillin-clavulanic acid, trimethoprim-sulfa, cephalosporins.
  - **Gram-negative rods** – chloramphenicol, trimethoprim-sulfa, fluoroquinolones.
  - **Bordetella** – tetracycline, doxycyline, chloramphenicol, fluoroquinolones.
  - **Suspected anaerobes** – clindamycin, amoxicillin-clavulanic acid, metronidazole.

Fungal pneumonia
- Systemic **itraconazole** given at 5–10 mg/kg PO daily is the drug of choice. If there are CNS signs with cryptococcosis, use **fluconazole** (2.5–5.0 mg/kg PO daily) as it crosses the blood–brain barrier.

Viral pneumonia mostly involves supportive treatment.

Supportive care includes airway and systemic hydration, which are essential for mucociliary clearance. Intravenous crystalloids should be used judiciously. Nebulization with saline may be helpful. Physical therapy including coupage, positional drainage, position changes, etc., and oxygen enrichment are indicated. **Bronchodilator therapy** with beta agonists such as terbutaline (0.625–1.25 mg PO q 12 hours) or methylxanthines such as sustained-release theophylline (*Theo-Dur* 25 mg/kg PO q 24 hours) may be helpful.

Thoracocentesis is rarely required for treatment, as the parapneumonic pleural effusion generally resolves with appropriate therapy for the pneumonia.

AIRWAY/PULMONARY NEOPLASIA

Classical signs

- Muffled heart and/or lung sounds ventrally.
- Exaggerated chest excursions with poor airflow.
- Orthopnea (positional dyspnea with reluctance to lie in lateral recumbency).
- Non-productive cough, with or without hemoptysis.
- Mass lesion seen radiographically.
- Anorexia, weight loss, muscle wasting.

See main reference on page 66 for details (The Dyspneic or Tachypneic Cat).

Clinical signs

Tracheal adenocarcinomas (i.e., Siamese), primary pulmonary masses (pulmonary adenocarcinoma) or secondary metastatic disease from distant neoplasms may create effusions. It is more common in middle-aged to older cats.

A non-productive cough may be present, with or without hemoptysis. Dyspnea (inspiratory and expiratory) and reluctance to lie in lateral recumbency, or respiratory distress is present if pleural effusion is of large volume.

Very rarely, lameness occurs from peripheral appendicular bone lesions of hypertrophic osteopathy.

Systemic signs such as anorexia and weight loss (cancer cachexia) are often present.

Dull chest sounds and dyspnea result from pleural effusion.

Diagnosis

Diagnosis is usually made by radiography followed by biopsy via endoscopy, thorocolony or is ultrasound-guided.

Pleural effusion fluid is often a modified transudate and is often grossly opaque.

Differential diagnosis

Other causes of pleural effusion such as congestive heart failure and mediastinal masses may produce a similar type of effusion but are differentiated on radiography, ultrasound and biopsy.

Treatment

Surgical resection via partial or total lobectomy is the treatment of choice for solitary primary neoplasms. Cure or long-term remission is possible with wide surgical margins. If non-resectible, excision of nodules may palliate clinical signs temporarily.

Chemotherapy and radiation have been attempted in generalized pulmonary neoplasms, with disappointing results. Metastases from distant tumors carry a grave prognosis, although pulmonary lymphoma may attain remission with chemotherapy.

HEMOTHORAX

Classical signs

- Muffled heart and lung sounds ventrally.
- Dyspnea characterized by excessive chest excursions with poor airflow.
- Orthopnea.
- Pallor, possibly other sites of bleeding (epistaxis, hyphema, etc.).

See main reference on page 493 for details (The Bleeding Cat).

Clinical signs

Hemorrhagic effusions generally result from either **trauma or coagulopathy**. History and physical exam findings are vital in the separation of these causes.

Signs related to pleural effusion and anemia include dyspnea, orthopnea (positional dyspnea), tachypnea, minimal airflow with increased chest excursions and muffled heart and lung sounds ventrally.

Weakness, hemic heart murmur, watery thready femoral pulse, pale mucous membranes all support possible blood loss.

Trauma may have **signs of external trauma** such as skin abrasions, rib fractures, penetrating thoracic wounds, etc., present.

Coagulopathies may involve other bleeding sites such as abdominal effusion (hemoabdomen), epistaxis, hyphema and hematoma formation. Common coagulopathies include rodenticide toxicity, factor VIIIC deficiency (hemophilia A), and factor XII deficiency (although this rarely causes clinical bleeding).

Diagnosis

Thoracic radiography reveals signs of pleural effusion, indistinguishable from other causes. Alveolar densities may be also present, indicating intrapulmonary hemorrhage.

Thoracocentesis
- Analysis of the fluid reveals obvious bloody fluid, often with a packed cell volume (PCV) lower than peripheral blood, except in cases of severe peracute frank hemorrhage where the PCV is similar to peripheral blood. The blood is generally defibrinated with no platelets observed cytologically, but, in acute bleeding situations, frank clotting blood with platelets may be present.

Coagulation testing.
- Coagulation tests help rule in and categorize types of coagulation disorders.
- In-clinic tests include activated clotting time (ACT, generally normal considered to be less than 65 seconds in the cat) to test the intrinsic cascade, blood smear for platelet numbers (should be 11–25 per high-power field), and buccal mucosal bleeding time (BMBT, normal considered to be 1–3 minutes) for platelet function (i.e., Von Willebrand's disease).

- Send-out lab tests include prothrombin time (PT – extrinsic system), partial tissue thromboplastin time (PTT – intrinsic system), and PIVKA test for rodenticide toxicity. Factor analysis for deficiencies of factors II, VII and X may be requested.
- Common coagulopathies include rodenticide exposure and genetic bleeding diatheses.

Differential diagnosis

Differential diagnoses include any cause of pleural effusion with bleeding into the pleural fluid, such as bleeding neoplasms, some chylothoraces (the fluid is less bloody and more "tomato soup-like"), as well as iatrogenic bleeding from previous thoracocenteses.

Treatment

Thoracostomy tube placement is generally contraindicated, especially in coagulopathies as it may trigger further bleeding.

Gentle handling and supportive care are indicated in trauma patients, as well as tending to other injuries.

Whole blood transfusion may be lifesaving in severe thrombocytopenia or coagulopathy. Depending on the breed (i.e., Persians) and the geographic location, cats with type B blood may be common. Cross-matching must be performed to avoid catastrophic transfusion reactions.

Results of coagulation tests may help with therapeutic decisions.
- **Vitamin K1** may be used for rodenticide toxicity.
- **Fresh frozen plasma transfusions** may be used for coagulation factor deficiency, etc.

HYPOPROTEINEMIA

Classical signs
- Muffled heart and lung sounds ventrally.
- Dyspnea characterized by excessive chest excursions with poor airflow.
- Orthopnea (positional dyspnea).
- Muscle wasting, weight loss, ascites, limb edema.

See main reference on pages 358 and 760 for details (The Thin, Inappetant Cat and The Cat With Signs of Chronic Small Bowel Diarrhea).

Clinical signs

Protein-losing enteropathy, **protein-losing nephropathy** and **hepatic failure** are common causes of low serum protein, specifically hypoalbuminemia, which may result in decreased oncotic pressure and transudation.

Signs are related to pleural effusion, ascites and muscle loss.

Orthopnea, tachypnea, minimal airflow with increased chest excursions, muffled heart and lung sounds may be present if the pleural effusion volume is > 50 ml/kg.

Weight loss with prominent muscle wasting is common. Distention of the abdomen from weakness of abdominal muscles, as well as presence of ascites may be present. Hair coat is typically poor quality.

Appetite may be ravenous in protein-losing enteropathy, and diarrhea and weight loss are evident.

Rarely, signs of hepatic encephalopathy including ptyalism, dementia, somnolence and pica occur with liver failure.

Icterus may be present.

Diagnosis

Thoracic radiography demonstrates signs of pleural effusion, indistinguishable from other causes.
- Thoracocentesis reveals a clear and colorless fluid, which is a pure transudate with a specific gravity (SG) < 1.013, low total protein (TP) < 2.5 g/L, and low cellularity (TNCC < 1.5×10^9/L).

Hypoalbuminemia (< 15 g/L) is a persistent finding.
- Protein-losing enteropathy (PLE) has panhypoproteinemia as the hallmark (hypoalbuminemia, globulin < 20 g/L) (see page 760, The Cat With Signs of Chronic Small Bowel Diarrhea).
- Protein-losing nephropathy (PLN) is characterized by proteinuria, urine protein:creatinine ratio > 2, hypoalbuminemia, possible hypertension and hypercholesterolemia (nephrotic syndrome) (see page 358, The Thin, Inappetent Cat).
- Hepatic failure may be characterized by low urea, hypoalbuminemia, low to elevated cholesterol, possible hypoglycemia, normal to low liver enzyme levels, elevated serum bilirubin levels may be present (see page 421, The Yellow Cat or Cat With Elevated Liver Enzymes).

Differential diagnosis

Once hypoalbuminemia has been established and the pleural effusion has been characterized as a pure transudate, a general biochemistry panel will help to distinguish the major causes of hypoproteinemia.

Treatment

Thoracostomy tube placement is generally not indicated.

Treatment for the underlying disorders will be covered in the chapters for those conditions. If serum albumin can be increased above 15–20 g/L with treatment of the underlying disease, the hydrothorax and ascites will resolve providing there is not underlying hypertension or vasculitis.

RECOMMENDED READING

Bauer T, Woodfield JA. Mediastinal, pleural, and extrapleural diseases. In: Ettinger SJ (ed) Textbook of Veterinary Internal Medicine, 4th edition. Philadelphia, Saunders, 1995, pp 817–822.

Lehmkuhl LB, Smith FWK. Pleural effusion. In: Tilley LP, Smith FWK (eds) The 5 Minute Veterinary Consult, 2nd edition. Baltimore, Lippincott, Williams & Wilkins, 2000, pp 1084–1085.

Padrid PA. Pulmonary diagnostics. In: August JR (ed) Consultations in Feline Internal Medicine 3. Philadelphia, Saunders, 1997, pp 292–302.

7. The coughing cat

Robert Allen Mason and Jacquie Rand

KEY SIGNS

- Cough ranging from soft to harsh or honking.
- Gagging, which may appear as vomiting or regurgitation.

MECHANISM?

- Coughing is a reflex that produces **rapid expulsion of air** in response to mechanical or chemical irritation of the pharynx, larynx, trachea, bronchi and small airways, to free the airway of foreign material.

WHERE?

- Coughing occurs in response to irritation of the upper respiratory tract (nasal cavity, pharynx, larynx, trachea), lower respiratory tract (bronchial tree, small airways), lung parenchyma or the pleural space.

WHAT?

- **Coughing is usually a sign of small airway disease in cats.** Unlike dogs, coughing is rarely associated with congestive heart failure (CHF).

QUICK REFERENCE SUMMARY
Diseases causing a coughing cat

DEGENERATIVE

- Cardiomyopathy (Dilated cardiomyopathy (DCM), hypertrophic (HCM), intermediate (ICM) or restrictive (RCM)) (p 107)

Although dyspnea is common with congestive heart failure and pulmonary edema, coughing is an uncommon presenting sign in the cat.

- Trachebronchial collapse (p 102)

Harsh "honking" cough caused by degeneration of the cartilage support of the large airway walls. Rare in cats.

MECHANICAL

- Grass awns/foreign bodies (p 98)

Sudden onset of a harsh, productive cough and acute dyspnea from foreign objects that have been inhaled, regurgitated or aspirated into the nasopharynx, trachea or bronchi.

- Inhalation of noxious agents (p 99)

Inhalation of gas, smoke, fumes, dust particles or hair can stimulate an aggressive cough reaction.

NEOPLASTIC

- Airway/pulmonary neoplasia (p 97)

Tracheal masses and primary or metastatic pulmonary masses in middle-aged to older cats may cause coughing ranging from soft to harsh and productive. Weight loss and ill-thrift are also seen.

- Pleural/mediastinal masses (p 107)

These masses cause pleural effusion or extraluminal compression of the trachea resulting in dyspnea, orthopnea, tachypnea and rarely cough. Heart and lung sounds are muffled from pleural effusion.

INFECTIOUS

Bacterial:

- Pneumonia (p 103)

Lethargy, inappetence, tachypnea, fever and halitosis are typical signs. Moist, productive cough and dyspnea may be present. Causes may include bacterial, fungal, viral, protozoal (toxoplasmosis) and chlamydophila felis pneumonitis.

- **Bordetella* (p 98)**

Acute onset of pyrexia, sneezing and nasal discharge. Coughing may be spontaneous or only evident on tracheal pressure. Signs resolve in 1–2 weeks.

Parasitic:

- Parasitic pneumonia (p 106)

A variable degree of coughing occurs. Peripheral eosinophilia or parasitic larva/ova may be present in the stool or lungwash. Lungworm (*Aleurostrongylus abstrusus, Capillaria aerophilia*), lung flukes (*Paragonumus kellicoti*) and migrating nematodes (*Toxacara cati*) are potential causes.

- **Heartworm disease* (p 104)**

Coughing, dyspnea and vomiting may occur together. Acute respiratory failure and death may occur from acute pulmonary inflammation and edema. Generally limited to cats from heartworm endemic areas.

Immune:

- **Feline asthma/bronchitis complex*** (p 92)**

An inhalant allergic response leads to bronchitis and bronchospasm. Coughing is the most common clinical sign, along with expiratory dyspnea and wheezing.

- **Pulmonary infiltrates with eosinophils (PIE)/Eosinophilic bronchopneumopathy* (p 96)**

Coughing varies from mild to severe. Crackles or wheezes, or areas of diminished lung sounds are heard on auscultation. Cats may have peripheral eosinophilia on CBC. Thoracic radiographs often show an interstitial pattern, although patchy alveolar or nodular densities may occur.

- Laryngitis (p 101)

Laryngeal edema from allergic reactions and idiopathic laryngeal paralysis have been reported in the cat. They may lead to aspiration of food, water or saliva and create significant harsh coughing. Stridor, dysphonia and inspiratory dyspnea are reported.

INTRODUCTION

MECHANISM?

Coughing is a reflex rapid expulsion of air in response to mechanical or chemical irritation of the pharynx, larynx, trachea, bronchi and small airways, to free the airway of foreign material.

Afferent impulses from epithelial receptors reach the cough center in the medulla via the vagus nerve. A complex series of events transpires from this point, namely:

- Air is inspired to 2–3 times the tidal volume.
- There is closure of the epiglottis and vocal folds.
- Contraction of the diaphragm, intercostal and external abdominal muscles occurs against the closed glottis, which increases intrapleural pressure (Valsalva maneuver) and decreases the luminal diameter of the small airways.
- Sudden opening of the glottis occurs with rapid expulsion of air from the small airway at speeds of 75–100 miles per hour.
- Explosive release carries the offending particulate matter clear of the lower airways.

In **acute conditions** (aspiration, inhalation of noxious fumes, etc.) this cough reflex is a **protective mechanism**. In the **chronic state**, however, it **becomes a debilitating problem.** Chronic airway irritation decreases the threshold of the cough receptor, which brings about more coughing and more mucosal damage and irritation.

WHERE?

Cough receptors are found along the entire airway, but are **especially dense at the larynx and the carina**. All receptors are innervated by the parasympathetic system.

In cats, receptors have been found as far distally as the alveoli.

WHAT?

The most common cause of acute coughing in the cat is foreign body aspiration, often associated with hairballs trapped in the oropharynx.

Aspiration of food or fluid can be more serious, creating aspiration pneumonia.

Chronic coughing in cats is often caused by feline asthma/bronchitis complex.

Unlike dogs, coughing is rarely associated with congestive heart failure (CHF).

DISEASES CAUSING COUGHING

FELINE ASTHMA/BRONCHITIS COMPLEX***

> **Classical signs**
>
> - Cough is a prominent sign.
> - Expiratory dyspnea with wheezing.
> - *Status asthmaticus* –severe acute respiratory distress.
> - Cyanosis, open-mouth breathing, wheezing.

Pathogenesis

Exposure of the respiratory epithelium to an inhaled antigen results in multiple inflammatory responses that create airway obstruction, namely:

- Edema.
- Cellular infiltration into airway walls.
- Epithelial hypertrophy or metaplasia with erosion or ulceration.
- Excessive mucus production.
- Decreased mucus clearance.
- Inflammatory exudation within the lumen.
- Hyperreactivity of the airway smooth muscle causing bronchoconstriction fibrosis.
- Emphysema.

Coughing results from enhanced airway sensitivity.

Wheezing is generated by air forced through narrowed airways, caused by mucosal thickening (epithelial hypertrophy, infiltration and edema) and bronchoconstriction.

Crackles result from excessive airway mucus.

The systemic inflammatory reaction, increased work of breathing and airflow limitation all create **systemic lethargy**.

There are **multiple inflammatory mediators** involved in the airways of cats:

- **Serotonin**
  - Serotonin is released from feline mast cell granules during exposure to an allergen.
  - Serotonin antagonists are useful in decreasing associated signs.
  - Mast cell stabilizing agents may play a role in decreasing the severity and frequency of attacks.
- **Histamine**
  - It has been demonstrated that histamine does not play a role in feline asthma.
  - Stimulation of the H3 receptors in the feline airway causes relaxation of the airway smooth muscle, the exact opposite effect seen in humans.
  - This work might suggest that antihistamines are contraindicated in feline asthma.
- **Leukotrienes**
  - Cats have far fewer leukotriene (LT) receptors in the airways than do people, but enough are present to make a significant contribution to the inflammatory cascade.
  - Leukotrienes are released from eosinophils, and via the lipoxygenase cascade, are converted to various forms of leukotrienes, all with variable inflammatory effects.
  - Because cats have poor glutathione pathways, the inflammatory leukotrienes LTC4 and LTD4 are not produced in significant amounts, but the pathway is directed toward LTB4 production.
  - LTB4 is a known chemotactic agent for eosinophils.
  - Recent evidence questions the role of leukotriene in asthmatic cats.
  - Mast cells have recently been incriminated in having a more profound role is asthmatic pathogenesis in humans than previously thought. Research is on-going in cats.

Clinical signs

Signs can occur at any age, although the **average is 2–8 years.**

Typically there is a **history of coughing for weeks or months.** The cough may be mild to severe and intermittent or continuous. It may be productive and stimulated with *coupage of the chest wall.*

Dyspnea may range from mild, to severe life-threatening respiratory distress from bronchoconstriction.

Signs may be episodic (with asthma) or chronic (with bronchitis).

There may be a **history of exposure to the offending allergen**, including dusty litter, perfumes, carpet cleaners, smoke from fireplaces, cigarette smoke and insulation materials.

Cats may present severely air-starved, with **cyanosis, open-mouth breathing**, and a significant abdominal expiratory push.

Diagnosis

Many cats with asthma may have eosinophilia on hematology.

On auscultation, typical lung sounds are wheezes and crackles, which may be worse on expiration.
- Severely affected cats may have diminished air sounds from emphysema.

Thoracic radiographs may be normal or abnormal.
- Asthma is characterized by hyperlucency, hyperinflation and flattening of the diaphragm from air trapping.
- Chronic bronchitis typically has a diffuse, prominent peribronchiolar pattern, with or without patchy alveolar infiltrates (especially the right middle lobe from atelectasis). Right heart enlargement may be present.
- A **lung wash for cytology and culture** can be obtained via transtracheal wash in the awake cat, or using a catheter or bronchoscope to lavage the bronchi and alveoli in the anesthetized cat, which is the method preferred by most clinicians. Culture for mycoplasma should be requested, because mycoplasmal infection may cause chronic coughing.
- **Cytological examination** typically reveals highly cellular samples with intact non-degenerative neutrophils as the primary cells. Eosinophils are not a reliable marker because of the increased prevalence (up to 24%) in the airways of normal cats. Neutrophilic or mixed inflammatory cellular patterns are common.
- There is on-going research looking for other biochemical markers of asthma leukotriene levels, IgA, IgG and IgE titers, etc., but none is yet clinically available as a test.

- Pulmonary function testing includes spirometry, whole-body plethysmography and tidal breathing flow–volume loops (TBFVL). Increased airway resistance with aerosol challenge, and decreased resistance with bronchodilator therapy are diagnostic of asthma. This testing is rarely available outside of teaching or research institutions.
- Asthma is differentiated from bronchitis on the basis of a positive response to an inhaled bronchodilator with asthma.

Differential diagnosis

Main differential for *status asthmaticus* is **acute congestive heart failure**, usually due to cardiomyopathy, although cats with heart failure rarely cough.

Other respiratory diseases, such as upper airway obstruction (laryngeal paralysis), pulmonary disease (pneumonia, neoplasia), and pleural space disease may also cause chronic coughing.

Treatment

Status asthmaticus – **oxygen** supplementation is required during respiratory distress. An O_2 chamber or tent is best tolerated by air-starved patients. Use injectible **terbutaline** (0.01 mg/kg SQ), and **dexamethasone** (0.25–0.5 mg/kg IV or IM), and in severe cases, **epinephrine** (0.5 ml 1:10 000) SQ as a bronchodilator. Minimal handling and restraint of acutely dyspneic patients is essential.

Asthma
- As this is a bronchoconstrictive disorder, it responds more briskly to bronchodilators.
- Bronchodilators seem to have a synergistic effect when used with steroids, or when two classes of bronchodilator are combined.

Bronchitis
- As this is an inflammatory disease, anti-inflammatories, and perhaps leukotriene inhibitors and mast cell stabilizing agents are more indicated for long-term therapy.

Bronchodilators
Bronchodilators are an important part of therapy for asthmatic cats, and can be administered orally, parentally or by inhalation.

- **Terbutaline** 0.01 mg/kg SQ will usually result in bronchodilation within 10–15 mins; for longer term therapy it can be administered orally (0.1 mg/kg PO q 12 h (1/4 – 1/2 × 2.5 mg tablet) or inhaled (*Brethine*). In a crisis, it can be given IV (0.01 mg/kg IV q 30 min for up to 4 h) until a response is observed, or by inhalation.
- **Inhalant bronchodilators (beta$_2$-adrenergic agonists such as terbutaline (*Brethine*), albuterol [also known as salbutamol] (*Proventil, Ventolin*)** may be used in a crisis situation (q 30 min repeated for 2–4 h) with an effect seen in 5–10 min. This route is more effective than IM, SC, or oral administration. They are administered using a spacer chamber attached to the metered dose inhaler at one end and a face mask at the other end. *Aerokat®* (www.aerokat.com) mask and spacer chamber is made specifically for cats, or ones made for infants such as the *Pocket Chamber®* combined with the smallest *Panda Mask®* (Ferraris Medical Inc) can be used to deliver drug inhalant therapy. Empty toilet paper rolls or paper coffee cups have also been used successfully as spacing chambers in cats. Two "puffs" or metered doses of the bronchodilator is used to fill the spacer chamber, and the mask is gently placed over the cat's mouth and nose while the cat breathes 10–15 times (approx 30–45 secs). There are several anecdotal reports of success, leading to weaning off systemic drug dosages or decreasing severity and frequency of attacks. Albuterol is reported to be rapid acting, and may be used in an emergency situation, or for chronic therapy q 12 h as needed (prn). **Salmeterol** [Serevent] has a slower onset and a 12 hour duration, and can be used for chronic therapy. Adverse effects of beta$_2$-adrenergic agonists are musculoskeletal twitchiness, excitability, insomnia, and anorexia, but are very rare in cats, suggesting these drugs have a high safety margin in cats.
- **Sustained release theophylline** 25 mg/kg PO q 24 h or 10 mg/kg PO q 12 h. Consistent pharmacokinetics have only been demonstrated with a few products (*Theo-Dur®* (Key Pharmaceuticals), *Slo-Bid Gyrocaps®* (Rhone-Poulene Rorer Labs), and *Theocap ER®* and *Theochron ER®* (Inwood Laboratories or Forest Laboratories), and the first two are unavailable in the US. *Theochron ER®* tablets can only be broken along the scored line into half, and *Theocap ER®* capsules can be opened

and divided into smaller doses by a compounding pharmacy. Beta$_2$-adrenergic agonists are more effective than the xanthine derivatives (theophylline) in producing bronchodilation.

Glucocorticoids
- **Prednisone** 1 mg/kg PO q 12 h for 5 days, then 1 mg/kg PO q 24 h and slowly weaned to a minimum effective dosage over 2 to 4 months. For seasonal allergy, prednisone may be weaned entirely until the following year. Alternatively, the cat may require chronic low dose therapy, 2.5–5.0 mg PO q 48 h. Some cats respond poorly to oral prednisone, and may respond better to **dexamethasone** 0.25 mg/kg PO q 12 h for 5 days, then wean slowly or switch to oral prednisone. Other cats require parenteral dosing with 20 mg **methylprednisolone acetate** IM q 3-6 weeks. However, this potentially has greater side effects, including inducing diabetes mellitus, than alternate day prednisone therapy. In a crisis, methylprednisolone sodium succinate (100 mg/cat IV) or dexamethasone (0.5–2 mg/kg IV or IM) can be given.
- **Inhaled steroids** scuh as fluticasone (**Flovent®**) are beneficial in cats that tolerate face mask inhalers. Topical therapy has less systemic side effects, which may be important in diabetic cats and cats predisposed to diabetes. In general, inhaled steroids are preferred because of their reduced side-effects, but they are more expensive. Fluticasone may take 5–10 days to work, so oral steroids should be administered concurrently for 5–10 days, depending on the severity of signs.

Oxygen supplementation is required during respiratory distress and an oxygen chamber or tent seems to be best tolerated by air-starved patients. Oxygen hoods made with an Elizabethan collar and cellophane have proven very useful in cats.

Minimal handling and restraint of acutely dyspneic patients is essential.

Serotonin antagonists
- **Cyproheptadine** (Periactin®) – 2–4 mg/cat PO q 12–24 h. This drug blocks serotonin, the major inflammatory mediator from feline mast cells in airway disease.

Leukotriene receptor blockers
- **Zafirlukast** (Accolade®) 0.5–1.0 mg/kg PO q 12–24 h. This drug is not useful in acute attacks, but can be used to stabilize long-term patients. Use may allow for a decrease of steroid dosages (beneficial in diabetic patients). It may decrease eosinophil chemotaxis. This drug should be considered in cases of severe eosinophilic inflammation, or cases refractory to standard therapy. Liver damage has been infrequently reported in cats.
- **Montelukast** (Singulaire®, 0.25–1.0 mg/kg SID) is a leukotriene blocker that has been used in cats for maintenance therapy but by itself is rarely effective. Although the cat has insufficient leukotriene receptors for cysteinyl leukotrienes to cause bronchoconstriction, anecdotal evidence suggests that montelukast may reduce bronchial inflammation and coughing. This effect may be mediated through blockage of leukotriene-mediated attraction of inflammatory cells such as eosinophils and neutrophils and their subsequent release of inflammatory cytokines and other chemicals. Montelukast may allow for the dose of steroids to be reduced or for cyroheptadine to replace the steroids.

Other agents
- **Mast cell stabilizers**
  - **Cromolyn** is an inhalant that stabilizes mast cell degranulation. It may be helpful for long-term control, and to diminish maintenance doses of steroids. Use 1 metered dose (800 mcg) q 12–24 h.
  - **Amitryptiline** is a systemic mast cell stabilizer. There is no information on its use in cats for airway disease, but it has been used for urine marking and psychogenic dermatoses at 1.1–2.2 mg/kg PO q 12 h.
- Antitussives
  - Debate exists whether the cough of bronchitis should be suppressed, as it is a protective mechanism of the airway.
  - **Butorphanol (Torbutrol)** can be dosed at 0.05–0.6 mg/kg PO q 6–12 h, prn to control cough. "Pulse antitussive therapy" may be helpful. This involves treating for 2–3 days to break the cycle of the harmful effects of the cough, then stopping for 2–3 days to allow improved airway clearance. Administration must be judged on a case-by-case basis.

Therapeutic protocol recommended by Dr Phil Padrid:

- For mild signs (cough only): fluticasone 110 mcg q 12 h and albuterol prn
- For moderate signs (cough and tires easily, and sleep disruption for client): prednisolone 1 mg/kg PO q 12 h for 5 days, and on an ongoing basis, fluticasone (**Flovent®**) 220 mcg q 12 h and albuterol prn;
- For marked signs (cough and dyspnea at rest with diminished quality of life): prednisolone 1 mg/kg PO q 12 h for 5 days, q 24 h for 5 days, q 48 h for 5 days, and on an ongoing basis, fluticasone 220 mcg q 12 h and albuterol prn;
- For severe signs (dyspnea, open mouth breathing +/− cyanosis) which are a life-threatening emergency, it is important not stress the cat as this may precipitate death. Administer oxygen via oxygen cage or nasal canula, methylprednisolone sodium succinate (100 mg/cat IV) or dexamethasone (2 mg/kg IV) and terbutaline (0.01 mg/kg IV) q 30 minutes for up to 4 h until a response is observed. Once stabilized, cats can be discharged with fluticasone 220 mcg q 12 h and albuterol q 6 h as needed.

Prognosis

Patients in *status asthmaticus* are extremely fragile, and may decompensate and die without rapid therapy administered with minimal handling.

Chronic cases, or once *status asthmaticus* resolves, have a fair to good prognosis with prolonged therapy.

Cure is rare, but with long-term therapy, management is frequently quite successful.

Prevention

Identification and removal of the offending antigen is highly desirable, but often difficult.

Clean the furnace or air-conditioning air ducts, shampoo carpets (avoiding perfumed cleansers), remove scented candles or potpourri, avoid using hair spray or aerosol cleaners near the patient, switch to **dust-free and unscented cat litter**, and quit smoking.

High-quality home air-filtration systems have been shown to help human asthmatics, and it is logical that cats would also benefit. HEPA filters (class III and above) decrease inhaled particles significantly.

Recently, there appears to be epidemologic evidence of decreased risk of asthma in male cats neutered before 5.5 months of age.

PULMONARY INFILTRATES WITH EOSINOPHILS (PIE) (EOSINOPHILIC BRONCHOPNEUMOPATHY)*

> **Classical signs**
>
> - Coughing – mild to severe.
> - Crackles, wheezes or diminished lung sounds.
> - Possible peripheral eosinophilia on CBC.

Pathogenesis

Interstitial or alveolar infiltration of pulmonary parenchyma with **eosinophils**. The infiltrate may form space-occupying eosinophilic granulomas measuring up to 20 cm diameter. Varies from mild, self-limiting disease, to severe and life-threatening.

Antigenic source, such as migrating parasites (*Toxocara* spp.) or heartworms may be found. Eosinophil-derived cytokines (leukotrienes, major basic protein, etc.) can damage the offending parasite or the host tissue, depending on the circumstances or severity.

In most cases, the inciting allergen is not identified.

Clinical signs

Mild to severe coughing for weeks to months prior to presentation is common.

Signs of systemic illness such as weight loss, anorexia and depression, may be present.

Adventitial lung sounds such as crackles or wheezes, or areas of diminished lung sounds may be present on thoracic auscultation.

Coughing may be elicited on tracheal palpation or coupage of the chest.

Diagnosis

Peripheral eosinophilia is present on CBC in 50–75% of patients.

Thoracic radiography
- **Interstitial or alveolar patterns** with air bronchograms, ranging from mild to severe.
- Nodular interstitial densities may mimic neoplastic masses. Dilated and truncated pulmonary arteries indicate potential heartworm disease or pulmonary hypertension. Hilar lymphadenopathy may be present.

Cytology
- Method of sample acquisition is dependent upon the predominant radiographic pattern.
- **Peribronchiolar or alveolar infiltrates** may produce excellent samples via **airway wash** (transtracheal or bronchoscopic lavage).
- **Interstitial densities** exfoliate poorly into the airways, and are better sampled via **percutaneous lung aspirates**.
- Cytology reveals a heavy infiltration of non-neoplastic eosinophils. Samples should be evaluated for the presence of antigens (parasites, fungal agents). Some neoplasms may be chemotactic to eosinophils.

Allied testing includes heartworm antigen or antibody testing, fecal floatation and Baermann exams for parasite ova and larvae, fungal culture (*Cryptococcus* spp.) from lung fluid, and fungal serology.

Differential diagnosis

Pulmonary neoplasia may mimic the nodular infiltrates radiographically. Cytology or lung biopsy is required for differentiation.

Congestive heart failure may also have alveolar infiltrates, but usually other clinical signs (tachyarrhythmias, murmurs, gallop rhythms) or radiographic signs of heart disease such as cardiomegaly, pulmonary venous congestion, pleural effusion are present.

Treatment

Treatment of the underlying disease is preferable, where possible (i.e., parasiticide therapy with fenbendazole for lungworm, praziquantel for lung flukes, etc.). Changing to a dust free cat litter and eliminating passive smoke from the environment may help.

Glucocorticoids – prednisone 1–2 mg/kg PO q 12 h for 5–7 days. Repeat thoracic radiographs, and if there is improvement noted, slowly taper the dosage over several months. Serial radiographs are useful for long-term monitoring. Many cases require long-term therapy for months to years, at the minimum effective dosage.

Cytotoxic drugs – if large mass lesions are present (eosinophilic granulomatosis), more aggressive immunosuppression may be required. **Cyclophosphamide** (50 mg/m^2 PO q 48 h) has been used in conjunction with prednisone. **Azathioprine should be avoided in cats due to toxicity**.

Prognosis

Eosinophilic inflammation can be very damaging to the host tissues.

If identification and elimination of the offending allergen is possible, the prognosis is excellent. If no allergen can be identified, the prognosis for cure is poor, but good to excellent control may be achieved with long-term therapy.

Eosinophilic granulomatosis carries a **poor long-term prognosis**, although remission of weeks to months is possible.

Prevention

Parasite prevention programs.
- Heartworm prophylaxis in endemic areas.
- Routine anthelmintic treatments with pyrantel pamoate or fenbendazole for nematodes such as *Toxocara cati* and *Aelurostrongylus* spp.
- Limit exposure to intermediate hosts (i.e., crayfish for *Paragonimus kellicotti*).

Limit exposure to inhalant allergens. Clean the furnace or air-conditioning air ducts, steam-clean carpets (avoiding perfumed cleansers), remove scented candles or potpourri, avoid using hair spray or aerosol cleaners near the patient, switch to dust-free and unscented cat litter (clumping litters may be especially dusty), and reduce exposure to cigarette smoke (quit or smoke outside), high-efficiency in-home air filtration systems may reduce antigenic load.

Avoid exposure to cats with respiratory tract infections, as PIE patients may be more prone to serious respiratory infections, especially if receiving immunosuppressive therapy.

BORDETELLA*

> ### Classical signs
>
> - Pyrexia.
> - Sneezing and nasal discharge.
> - Mandibular lymphadenopathy.
> - Coughing.
> - Dyspnea, cyanosis, pneumonia.

See main reference on page 14 for details (The Cat With Acute Sneezing or Nasal Discharge).

Clinical signs

Signs are most likely to occur in **cats from multi-cat environments, especially rescue or shelter catteries** where calicivirus and herpesvirus are also a problem.

Typically there is an acute onset of pyrexia, sneezing and nasal discharge.

Mandibular lymphadenopathy may be palpable.

Coughing may be spontaneous, or only evident on tracheal pressure; generally, coughing is not as pronounced as in dogs.

Dyspnea, cyanosis, crackles and wheezes may be auscultated over lung fields in some cats. Death from pneumonia may occur, especially in young kittens less than 8 weeks old.

Treatment

Oxytetracycline, doxycycline or enrofloxacin.

Montelukast (Singulaire, 0.25–1 mg/kg SID) is a leukotriene receptor blocker. Although the cat has insufficient leukotriene receptors for cysteinyl leukotrienes to cause bronchoconstriction, anecdotal evidence suggests that montelukast may reduce sneezing and nasal discharge associated with *Bordetella*. This effect may be mediated through blockage of leukotriene-mediated attraction of inflammatory cells such as eosinophils and neutrophils and their subsequent release of inflammatory cytokines and other chemicals.

GRASS AWNS/FOREIGN BODIES

> ### Classical signs
>
> - Sneezing with nasal foreign bodies, and coughing with pharyngeal and tracheobronchial foreign bodies.
> - Inspiratory/expiratory dyspnea, depending on location.

Pathogenesis

Foreign bodies may be inhaled directly into the rostral nasal cavity or tracheobronchial tree, or may be regurgitated into the caudal nasopharynx. Common solid foreign bodies include grass, seeds, hairballs, twigs and occasionally stones, while particulate foreign bodies include coal dust (UK) and metal dust from road grime (Australia).

Occasionally, penetrating foreign bodies, such as projectiles (pellets) or a broken tooth from an opponent during a cat fight, can lodge in the nasal cavity or airway.

Tracheobronchial foreign bodies may be caused by aspiration of vomited or regurgitated ingesta.

Clinical signs

Acute onset of sneezing and nasal discharge are common signs of nasal foreign bodies, although coughing may be the predominant sign with post-nasal drainage into the pharynx. These cats may be in sudden and severe distress attempting to dislodge the foreign body. Pawing at the face and mouth is commonly observed.

Coughing and signs of **fixed obstruction** – meaning there is airflow limitation during both inspiratory and expiratory due to constant partial obstruction of the airway – may be seen with tracheobronchial foreign bodies. The coughing is often harsh, and may be elicited with tracheal palpation.

Diagnosis

Tracheal foreign bodies may be seen radiographically. Tracheobronchoscopy can be both diagnostic and therapeutic. Rigid tracheoscopy allows for larger retrieval instruments to be utilized than with a flexible endoscopy.

Bronchial foreign bodies may cause complete lobar atelectasis or abscessation radiographically. The right caudal and accessory lobes are most often affected with inhalation foreign bodies. The right middle lobe is affected commonly with aspiration of vomitus.

Differential diagnosis

Nasopharyngeal polyps may cause similar signs of nasal obstruction and sneezing, but tend to have a more chronic course.

Tracheal or bronchial neoplasia may have similar signs, but again are more chronic in nature and can be distinguished bronchoscopically.

Treatment

Removal of the foreign body, either surgically or endoscopically, is often curative. Nasal foreign bodies may be endoscopically retrieved or hydropulsed, but occasionally require surgical rhinotomy.

Bronchial foreign bodies, especially with lung lobe abscesses, require lung lobectomy.

Prognosis

Excellent with removal of the foreign body.

Prevention

Hairball prophylaxis.

Avoidance of grass fields during seed time.

INHALATION OF NOXIOUS AGENTS

Classical signs

- Acute onset of severe coughing.
- Evidence of inhalation of gas, smoke, fumes, dust particles or hair.

Pathogenesis

Poor ventilation, engine exhaust, smoke from fires or cigarettes, all can stimulate an aggressive cough reaction.

Fires may cause thermal damage to the upper airway. Burning plastics release toxic fumes causing direct chemical damage to lungs.

Carbon monoxide exposure results in carboxyhemoglobin formation, lowering the oxygen-carrying capacity of hemoglobin, and worsening the hypoxemia.

Airways irritated by underlying disease such as bronchitis, may be hyperresponsive to cigarette smoke or household fumes.

Clinical signs

Patients rescued from fires smell of smoke, have burned hair or vibrissae, may be coughing, and are often expectorating soot-tinged sputum.

Cherry-red mucus membranes indicate carboxyhemoglobinemia, and cyanosis indicates hypoxemia.

Stridor and inspiratory dyspnea suggest **laryngeal edema**.

Crackles indicate increased airway fluid.

Wheezes indicate diminished airway diameter via bronchoconstriction, congestion, mucus accumulation, and airway edema.

Diagnosis

Presumptive diagnosis is based upon evidence of recent exposure to noxious agent and acute onset of coughing.

Thoracic radiography.
- May vary from peribronchiolar to patchy interstitial lung pattern, with possible lobar consolidation.
- Infiltrates are generalized, although the caudodorsal fields may be more affected.
- These changes may lag several hours behind clinical signs.

Pulse oximetry may indirectly assess oxygenation through **SPO$_2$** (hemoglobulin saturation).

Blood gases.
- **Arterial oxygen (PaO$_2$)** represents dissolved oxygen content not bound to hemoglobin.
- PaO$_2$ < 60 mmHg indicates severe hypoxemia, ofetn associated with cyanosis.

- PaO$_2$ may be misleading in CO toxicity due to extreme carboxyhemoglobinemia and very low O$_2$-carrying capacity.
- A profound mixed acidosis may be present.

Measuring **carboxyhemoglobin** levels are needed to diagnose carbon monoxide toxicity. Routine STAT assays are available in human hospitals.

Treatment

Emergency treatment focuses on assessing three critical areas – **ABC – airway, breathing, circulation**.

A – airway
- If the upper airway is burned or edematous, establishing a patent airway may require laryngeal suctioning, tracheal intubation, or transtracheal catheterization, or tracheostomy.

B – breathing
- **Oxygen is the single most important drug to use**. Carbon monoxide is displaced from the carboxyhemoglobin complex 8–10 times faster on 100% O$_2$ than on room air. Continue 100% O$_2$ until carboxyhemoglobin < 10% on follow-up samples.
- Bronchodilators – **terbutaline** (0.01 mg/kg SQ) can be repeated every 4 hours.

C – circulation
- **Crystalloid** administration supports the blood pressure and cardiovascular status, promotes diuresis of absorbed toxins, but must be used judiciously and monitored carefully for iatrogenic pulmonary edema. **Colloids** (fresh frozen plasma, synthetic starch products, synthetic blood substitutes) may be beneficial.

The prophylactic use of **antibiotics** is controversial. Antibiotics reduce the normal flora, and may predispose to a more serious nosocomial infection. If infection is suspected, antibiotic selection should be based on culture results of lung wash fluid.

Prognosis

The prognosis is directly related to the extent of the injuries, both to the airways and non-respiratory damage (i.e., skin burns, other organ damage, etc.). Signs may progressively worsen over the initial 24–48 hours.

Prevention

Ensure proper ventilation for heaters and wood stoves, avoid exposure to aerosol chemicals, and reduce exposure to cigarette smoke (quit smoking or smoke outdoors).

AIRWAY/PULMONARY NEOPLASIA

> ### Classical signs
>
> - Dyspnea, other inspiratory and expiratory
> - Coughing, ranging from harsh and dry to soft and productive.

Pathogenesis

Upper respiratory tract masses may produce a cough from post-nasal drip.

Pulmonary or airway masses cause coughing by stimulation of cough receptors within the airway lumina, or from extraluminal compression and distortion of the airway.

Upper airway neoplasms include:
- Nasopharyngeal polyps, oropharyngeal squamous cell carcinoma, tracheal adenocarcinoma (Siamese), nasal adenocarcinoma.

Pulmonary neoplasms include:
- Primary pulmonary neoplasia.
  - Bronchogenic carcinoma, pulmonary adenocarcinoma, and squamous cell carcinomas.
- Secondary metastases from distant neoplasms, including a variety of carcinomas (i.e., mammary adenocarcinomas) and sarcomas (i.e., osteosarcoma), as well as local metastases from primary lung tumors.

Pleural malignancy may cause coughing.

Clinical signs

Tracheal tumors create **fixed obstruction**, leading to inspiratory and expiratory dyspnea, and a harsh, dry cough. Hemoptysis may be present.

Bronchial tumors may be associated with a softer, productive cough, fetid halitosis and hemoptysis.

Very rarely, lameness from hypertrophic osteopathy occurs.

Diagnosis

Radiographs.
- **Cervical radiographs** may show soft tissue masses of the throat and trachea.
- **Thoracic radiographs** showing solid tissue masses or nodular interstitial pattern are highly supportive of neoplasia. Multiple orthogonal views (left and right lateral projections, as well as both dorsoventral and ventrodorsal views) are important to assess potential mass lesions. Hilar lymphadenopathy may be present.

Other imaging modalities, such as CT or MRI may be employed.

Histological examination of the mass(es) is required for definitive diagnosis, as well as for distinguishing the origin of the tumor. Biopsy options include percutaneous fine-needle (20–22 gauge) aspiration, percutaneous core biopsy with 14–18 gauge *TruCut*®-style needle, bronchoscopy for cytology via BAL or bronchial brushings, or transbronchial lung biopsy.
- Ultrasound is a poor tool to guide percutaneous biopsy needles, unless the entire lung lobe has become consolidated, as the sonic beam is reflected by any aerated lung tissue. Triangulating the landmarks based on two right-angled radiographic views is extremely effective. However, pulmonary tumors in cats often have a thin rim of neoplastic tissue surrounding a large necrotic mass, which makes it very difficult to get diagnositic tissue using needle biospy techniques.
- **Transbronchial cytology** (TTW or BAL) is often disappointing, because of the interstitial nature of the lesion, as neoplastic diseases rarely cross into the airway lumen. Transbronchial lung biopsy is a promising technique.
- **Surgical biopsy** during open thoracotomy is an option, generally during lobectomy. Local lymph nodes should be biopsied for staging of the tumor. There is evidence that any mass in the lung large enough to biopsy requires thoracotomy and surgical excision, because even benign inflammatory diseases (i.e., eosinophilic granulomatosus) respond poorly to medical management, and that eventually, thoracotomy is required.

Thoracocentesis and cytology of pleural fluid may be diagnostic.

Differential diagnosis

Inhaled and penetrating foreign bodies, benign or parasitic granulomas of the airways, and lung lobe torsions, abscesses and pulmonary infiltrates with eosinophils (PIE) may mimic neoplastic masses. Biopsy is often required to differentiate.

Treatment

Tracheal (adenocarcinoma) and some bronchial tumors (bronchogenic carcinoma) may be surgically resectible.

Surgical resection is the treatment of choice for solitary pulmonary neoplasms. Cure or long-term remission is possible with wide surgical margins, generally meaning complete lung lobectomy. If non-resectible, excision of nodules may palliate clinical signs.

Chemotherapy and radiation have been disappointing in generalized pulmonary neoplasms. Metastases from distant tumors carry a grave prognosis, although pulmonary lymphoma may attain remission with chemotherapy.

General supportive care and nutrition are important.

Prognosis

Prognosis is fair to excellent with surgically resectible primary pulmonary neoplasms that have not metastasized at the time of surgery.

Prognosis is grave with metastatic disease or malignant pleural effusions.

Prevention

None known.

LARYNGITIS

Classical signs
- Dysphonia (voice changes) and stridor.
- Harsh gagging cough.
- Inspiratory dyspnea.

Pathogenesis

Laryngeal edema may occur secondary to laryngeal trauma (bite wounds, endotracheal intubation, near-strangulation from neck collars), excessive vocalization (senility, sexual behavior), or other laryngeal disease (laryngeal paralysis).

Laryngeal trauma may directly inflame the larynx, or may cause nerve damage, secondary laryngeal paralysis and subsequent mucosal edema from abnormal arytenoid cartilage motion.

Aspiration of lavage solutions from dental prophylaxis or endodontics may be caustic to the laryngeal mucosa, creating significant edema.

Laryngeal edema may occur as part of a **type I hypersensitivity** reaction to insect stings or vaccination.

Inflammatory diseases like eosinophilic laryngeal granuloma can cause edema (see The Cat With Stridor, page 45).

Coughing may occur from irritation of the laryngeal cough receptors, or from aspiration of food, water or saliva due to laryngeal paresis.

Clinical signs

The cough is usually non-productive, but is typically harsh and may stimulate a gag reflex and expectoration of pharyngeal contents.

Inspiratory dyspnea and stridor, which is worse with excitement or exercise, may be evident.

Dysphonia or voice change, often a whisper-like or hoarse sound, is frequently observed in cats.

Diagnosis

Laryngoscopy requires deep sedation or anesthesia and a rigid laryngoscope and blade, and often reveals erythema and edema of the laryngeal mucosa.

Samples of abnormal tissue may be taken for cytology and histology. Culture of the larynx is of questionable value.

If biopsies are taken, this may worsen edema. Postoperative steroids may decrease iatrogenic edema. Occasionally, temporary tracheostomy may be required after biopsy.

Differential diagnosis

Laryngeal mass lesion or foreign bodies are differentiated visually and by biopsy. Other causes of upper airway obstruction such as tracheal collapse, are differentiated with laryngotracheobronchoscopy.

Treatment

Anti-inflammatories, especially glucocorticoids, are used to diminish the local inflammation.
- **Dexamethasone** (0.1–0.25 mg/kg IV or IM), or prednisone (0.5–1.0 mg/kg PO q 12–24 h).
- Little is known about the application of **NSAIDs** in laryngeal edema.

Antibiotics are only indicated if there is evidence of bacterial infection.

Antitussives may be indicated when the cough has become protracted and debilitating, and lower respiratory disease has been ruled out.
- **Butorphanol** (0.2 mg/kg SQ q 6 h or 1 mg/cat PO q 6–8 hours prn) may be effective.

Prognosis

Fair to excellent.

Prevention

Use of break-away neck collars on outdoor cats may significantly decrease strangulation injury to the larynx and the laryngeal nerves.

Avoidance of insect stings is helpful.

Neutering tom cats helps to prevent both fighting and mating behaviors such as excessive vocalization.

TRACHEOBRONCHIAL COLLAPSE

Classical signs

- Harsh, honking cough.
- Dynamic airflow limitation on inspiration if cervical segment, and expiratory if intrathoracic segment involved.
- Very rare in cats.

Clinical signs

The cough is often harsh, non-productive and paroxysmal, ending in a gagging episode which may appear to be productive.

Cervical trachea collapse produces inspiratory dyspnea, while intrathoracic tracheal or bronchial collapse will lead to mostly expiratory dyspnea.

Generally occurs **secondary to trauma** or to compression caused by an **extraluminal mass.**

Diagnosis

Radiographs may show attenuation of the tracheal or bronchial lumina. Fluoroscopy may be more sensitive for dynamic collapse.

Tracheobronchoscopy is valuable in both diagnosing and grading the severity of the collapse.

Differential diagnosis

Tracheitis from feline rhinotracheitis virus is generally associated with other upper respiratory tract signs.

Laryngeal paralysis or edema, tracheal foreign body and tracheobronchial neoplasm can be differentiated endoscopically.

Small airway disease (feline asthma/bronchitis complex) can worsen upper airway collapse, but generally diagnosis is based on radiographic peribronchiolar pattern and airway inflammation on lung wash cytology.

Treatment

Medical treatment is indicated if the collapsing segment is short and minimally attenuated, and consists primarily of antitussive therapy (**butorphanol** 1 mg/cat PO q 6–12 h prn).

Surgical therapy may be indicated with severe collapse due to trauma. This generally requires referral to a specialist with experience in airway surgery.

Weight loss and avoidance of neck collars can be very beneficial in affected cats.

PNEUMONIA

Classical signs

- Moist, productive cough.
- Fever or hypothermia may be present.
- Fetid halitosis.
- Adventitial lung sounds are common.

See main reference on page 64 for details (The Dyspneic or Tachypneic Cat).

Clinical signs

Deep productive cough, may be soft and ineffective.

Inspiratory and expiratory dyspnea, often with open-mouth breathing.

Adventitial breath sounds, including crackles, wheezes, snaps and pops.

History of signs consistent with bacterial, fungal, viral, mycoplasmal and *Chlamydophila felis* pneumonitis.

Constitutional signs include lethargy, anorexia, weight loss, fever and ill thrift.

Diagnosis

Thoracic radiography shows alveolar densities (focal or generalized) and possible areas of complete consolidation. Hilar lymphadenopathy supports fungal or mycobacterial pneumonia.

Hematology often shows neutrophilia with or without a left shift or signs of toxicity. Low-grade, non-responsive anemia and monocytosis may support chronicity.

Cytology and culture of lung samples may be obtained via percutaneous lung aspiration, transtracheal wash, or bronchoscopic lavage. Fungal, aerobic and anaerobic bacterial cultures are generally submitted.

Serology may aid in the diagnosis of cryptococcal pneumonia.

Differential diagnosis

Chronic small airway disease (feline asthma/bronchitis), PIE and lymphomatoid granulomatosis, and pulmonary neoplasia, either primary or metastatic disease, may mimic pneumonia.

  Small airway disease tends to have peribronchiolar infiltrates compared to the alveolar pattern of pneumonia. Also, although asthmatic cats may be severely dyspneic, systemic signs of fever, or neutrophilic leukocytosis are rare.

  PIE, granulomas or neoplasms tend to have a nodular or interstitial density on radiographs, but biopsy results are required to distinguish these diseases.

Each of the infectious pneumonias can have overlapping features.

Treatment

Bacterial pneumonia – antimicrobial therapy, parenteral if debilitated or septic, and oral if cat is an outpatient. Antibiotic selection best based upon specific culture and sensitivity testing.

Fungal pneumonia – systemic **itraconazole** at 5–10 mg/kg PO daily is the drug of choice. If there are CNS signs with cryptococcosis, **fluconazole** (2.5–5.0 mg/kg PO daily) crosses the blood–brain barrier.

Viral pneumonia – mostly supportive.

Supportive care is essential. Adequate airway and systemic hydration are essential for mucociliary clearance. Intravenous crystalloids are important for systemic hydration, but should be used judiciously to avoide over-hydration. Nebulization with saline may be helpful. Physical therapy, oxygen enrichment and bronchodilator therapy may be helpful.

Prognosis

Prognosis depends on the etiological agent and the severity of the infection.

Bacterial pneumonia has a fair to good prognosis, but the prognosis is worse in patients with pre-existing illnesses or patients on immunosuppressive therapy.

The prognosis for **aspiration pneumonia** depends on the degree of tissue damage.

Cryptococcal pneumonia generally has a fair to good prognosis, although it is poor if CNS signs are present.

Prevention

Avoid the source of infectious agents (i.e., aspergillus from bird droppings) and risk factors (i.e., aspiration).

FELINE HEARTWORM DISEASE

Classical signs

- Cough.
- Acute-onset dyspnea.
- Vomiting together with respiratory signs.

Pathogenesis

Dirofilaira immitis **larvae (L3) infect the cat** following a bite from an infected mosquito.

Larvae molt and migrate to the pulmonary arteries, **arriving as immature heartworms (L5) approximately 100 days** or more after **initial infection**.

Cats typically have **fewer adult worms than dogs**. Less than six adults is usual and often only one or two worms are present. Adult worms live shorter lifespans in cats compared to dogs, typically 18 months to 3 years.

The **prevalence** of heartworm infection in cats is **approximately 5–10% of the infection rate in dogs** in the same location, although the ratio may be higher in some areas. A recent report from Florida showed 5% of necropsied cats were positive for the parasite, and 17% of tested cats were seropositive. In a similar study in Georgia, *D. immitis* were found in four of 184 cats (2.1%).

Indoor cats are as likely to be infected as outdoor cats.

In some studies, male cats had a higher incidence of infection and had a higher worm burden.

Cats infected with heartworm may be **asymptomatic, have chronic coughing, acute respiratory distress or die suddenly**.

Clinical signs are most likely to occur at the time of arrival of the immature heartworms in the lungs or with death of adult worms.

Initial arrival of the immature worms results in a marked inflammatory response, and signs similar to the feline asthma/bronchitis complex may occur. With maturation to the adult worm, signs may improve or resolve.

Death of adult heartworms may produce acute severe pulmonary inflammation with edema, and an acute respiratory distress syndrome characterized by generalized respiratory failure.

Clinical signs

Harsh and productive coughing is the most common sign.

Dyspnea may be **acute and life threatening**. Acute dyspnea is associated with pulmonary thromboembolism, or **acute pulmonary inflammation and edema** associated with worm death. Acute respiratory distress syndrome (ARDS) and generalized respiratory failure are not uncommon.

Acute death is reported in approximately 30–45% of cats presenting with clinical signs of heartworm disease.

Vomiting is often reported and when it occurs together with respiratory signs, it is suggestive of chronic feline heartworm disease.

A gallop rhythm is sometimes audible.

Neurological signs such as blindness and vestibular signs may be associated with aberrant migration of **L4 larvae** to the brain.

A report describes two cases of **cutaneous nodular lesions** associated with *D. immitis* adult parasites in domestic short-haired cats living in an endemic area in northern Italy.

Diagnosis

Mild non-regenerative anemia, peripheral basophilia, eosinophilia and hyperglobulinemia are sometimes evident.

Heartworm testing.
- **Antigen tests** (ELISA test) are **highly specific, but only moderately sensitive.** False negatives occur with low numbers (< 5) worms, and as most cats have only one or two worms, the test is positive in less than 50% of infected cats.
- **Antibody tests** are more sensitive, but less specific for active infection than antigen testing, as they may remain positive for 18 months after infection has resolved.
- A higher sensitivity and specificity is obtained if both the antigen and antibody tests are performed and the results considered together.
- **Microfilarial tests are unreliable** in the cat because the concentration of microfilaria is very low and microfilaremia is transient, lasting only 1–2 months.

Thoracic radiographs may show **dilated and blunted pulmonary arteries**, which are most prominent in the caudal pulmonary arteries, particularly the right side. The dilation may not be evident beyond the cardiac shadow.

- **Lung changes vary** from **patchy pulmonary infiltrates** to **severe alveolar densities** suggestive of lung lobe atelectasis or consolidating pneumonia. Occasionally pleural effusion is present.

Cardiac ultrasound may show hollow linear densities (worms) in the **right chambers** and **pulmonary artery**, as well as pulmonary arterial dilation.
- Cardiac ultrasound has similir sensitivity to antigen tests. False negatives occur because worms may reside in the extremities of the pulmonary arteries where they cannot be detected with the ultrasound. Occasionally, false-positive results may occur from linear densities detected where the main pulmonary artery branches.

Differential diagnosis

Other causes of chronic coughing or acute respiratory distress should be considered as differentials.
- **Lungworm and lung flukes** are diagnosed with fecal Baermann exams.
- **Feline asthma** is not associated with vomiting, and basophilia is uncommon.
- **Cardiomyopathy** is diagnosed with echocardiography.
- **Hydrothorax** is diagnosed radiographically and classified based on examination of the fluid.
- **Other forms of pneumonia**, (bacterial, viral, fungal, inflammatory), and **neoplastic disease** may appear similar, and are differentiated by lack of evidence of feline heartworm on serology, radiology and ultrasound. Radiography, serology and cytological or histological examination of tissue may provide a definitive diagnosis.

Treatment

Asymptomatic cats do not require treatment and spontaneous resolution of infection may occur as worms live only about 1.5–2 years in cats.

Symptomatic cats.
- Stabilize with oxygen therapy, **prednisone** (1–2 mg/kg PO q 12–24 h for 10–14 days, then slowly wean down), **bronchodilator therapy** (Theophylline, **TheoDur®** 25 mg/kg PO q 24 h) and if needed **antiemetics**.

- **Adulticide therapy is not recommended** as there is a **high risk (25–30%) of mortality**, mostly from pulmonary thromboembolism within the first 5 days. The death rate following treatment is at least as high as the death rate in untreated cats.
- **Manual removal of worms by a specialist** is associated with a lower mortality rate than killing the worms with parasiticides. This technique is only recommended in symptomatic cats with worms visible in the right heart and main pulmonary arteries on ultrasound. Shock-like signs and death may occur if the worms are damaged during extraction.

Prevention

The currently available drugs licensed for **prevention of heartworm** in cats are **ivermectin** (24 µg/kg once monthly) and **selamectin** (*Revolution*®, Pfizer Animal Health, 6 mg/kg once every 30 days). **Milbemycine oxime** (*Interceptor*®, Novartis Animal Health, 500 µg/kg once monthly) is effective but not licensed for use in cats.

Imidacloprid and **moxidectin** (*Feline Advantage Heart*®, Bayer Health Care) topical solution as monthly treatment for prevention of heartworm infection in cats.

As indoor cats are as likely to be infected as outdoor cats, restricting the cat to indoors is not effective prevention.

PARASITIC PNEUMONIA

> ### Classical signs
>
> - Variable cough.
> - +/− Eosinophilia.
> - +/− Larva/ova in stool.

Clinical signs

Etiological agents include heartworm disease, lungworm (*Capillaria aerophilia* or *Aelurostrongylus obstrussus*), lung flukes (*Paragonimus kellicotti*), migrating nematodes and toxoplasmosis.

Coughing may be present, and is typically harsh and productive.

Dyspnea and exercise intolerance, evidenced as lethargy, physical inactivity, reluctance to play or weakness, may occur.

Weight loss, poor coat and ill-thrift may be evident.

Vomiting sometimes occurs with feline heartworm disease.

Diagnosis

Feline heartworm disease – peripheral basophilia, positive heartworm antibody testing, dilated and blunted pulmonary arteries and patchy pulmonary infiltrates on radiographs, and evidence of heartworms on ultrasound (see page 105 for details).

Lungworm infection with *Capillaria aerophilia* is diagnosed by finding eggs in the stools or lung wash, and with *Aelurostrongylus abstrussus* by finding larvae in the lung wash or fecal Baermann.

Lung flukes (*Paragonimus kellicotti*) produce operculated eggs in the stool.

Toxoplasmosis rarely produces clinical disease in cats. Mixed fluffy interstitial and alveolar patterns are typically evident on radiographs. Tachyzoites may occasionally be recovered on lung wash.

Differential diagnosis

Other forms of pneumonia, namely bacterial, viral, fungal, inflammatory and neoplasia need to be considered if no larvae or ova are found in the stool or lung wash.

Treatment

Feline heartworm disease, see page 105 for main reference.

Lungworm – *Capillaria aerophilia* and *Aelurostrongylus abstrussus* – **fenbendazole** (50 mg/kg PO q 24 h for 3 days) or **ivermectin** (400 µg/kg PO, SQ).

Lung flukes – *Paragonimus kellicotti*, **fenbendazole** (50 mg/kg PO q 24 h for 3 days), or **praziquantel** (25 mg/kg PO q 8 h for 2 days).

Toxoplasmosis – **clindamycin** (12.5 mg/kg PO q 12 h), potentiated sulfa (trimethoprim or ormetoprim), or azithromycin (7–15 mg/kg PO q 12 h).

Migrating nematodes – *Toxocara* spp., **pyrantel pamoate** (20 mg/kg PO, repeat 7–10 days).

CARDIOMYOPATHY (DILATED CARDIOMYOPATHY (DCM), HYPERTROPHIC (HCM), INTERMEDIATE (ICM) OR RESTRICTIVE (RCM))

Classical signs

- Dyspnea.
- Gallop rhythm, murmur or arrhythmia.
- Coughing is an uncommon presenting sign in the cat.

See main reference on page 54 for details (The Dyspneic of Tachypneic Cat).

Clinical signs

Coughing is very uncommon in cats, even in advanced congestive failure.

Dyspnea is common with CHF and pulmonary edema, and signs vary from mild exercise intolerance (lethargy, weakness, reluctance to move or play) to severe, open-mouth breathing with cyanosis.

Abnormal heart sounds (murmurs, gallops, arrhythmias) are often present.

Treatment

Oxygen therapy (O_2 chamber or tents work well), **furosemide** (1–2 mg/kg IV or IM), sedation if frantic (**morphine** 0.1 mg/kg IM prn, or **butorphanol** 0.2–0.4 mg/kg IM q 4–6 h prn), and emergency thoracocentesis if hydrothorax is present. See page 84 for treatment details.

PLEURAL/MEDIASTINAL MASSES

Classical signs

- Dyspnea, orthopnea, tachypnea or rarely, coughing.
- Muffled heart and lung sounds from pleural effusion.

See main reference on page 85 for details (The Cat With Hydrothorax).

Clinical signs

Mediastinal lymphoma, thymomas, and mesothelioma cause pleural effusion or extraluminal compression to the trachea.

Extraluminal compression of the trachea can cause **dyspnea and coughing**.

Other signs that may be present include orthopnea (recumbent dyspnea), tachypnea, minimal airflow with increased chest excursions, or muffled heart and lung sounds from a mass or effusion.

Treatment

Lymphoma is best handled with standard chemotherapy protocols. See page 676 for details.

Surgical excision is the treatment of choice for **thymoma**, and may be curative.

Mesothelioma is an infiltrative disease that cannot be readily resected. Although there are few reports in the literature of effective chemotherapy, local infusion of **carboplatin** may be helpful. Prognosis is grave with or without doxirubicin intravenously.

RECOMMENDED READING

Atkins CE, DeFrancesco TC, Coats JR, Sidley JA, Keene BW. Heartworm disease in cats: 50 cases (1985–1997). JAVMA 2000; 217(3): 355–358.

Court EA, Litster A, Menrath V, Gunew M. Forty five cases of feline heartworm disease. Australian Veterinary Practitioner 2000; 30(1): 11.

Dye JA, McKiernan BC, Rozanski EA, et al. Bronchopulmonary disease in the cat: historical, physical, radiographic, clinicopathologic, and pulmonary functional evaluation of 24 affected and 15 healthy cats. J Vet Int Med 1996; 10: 385–400.

Ettinger SJ. Coughing. In: Ettinger SJ (ed) Textbook of Veterinary Internal Medicine, 5th edition. Philadelphia, Saunders, 2000, pages 162–166.

Ettinger SJ. Dirofilariasis in dogs and cats. In: Ettinger SJ (ed) Textbook of Veterinary Internal Medicine, 5th edition. Philadelphia, Saunders, 2000, pages 937–963.

Noone KE. Asthma, bronchitis – cats. In: Tilley LP, Smith FWK (eds) The 5 Minute Veterinary Consult, 2nd edition. Baltimore, Lippincott Williams & Wilkins, 2000, pages 464–465.

Padrid PA. Feline asthma. In: Bonagura J (ed) Current Veterinary Therapy XIII. Philadelphia, Saunders, 1999, pages 805–810.

Padrid PA. Feline asthma – diagnosis and treatment. *Vet Clin Nth Am: SA pract* 2000; 30(6): 1279–1293.

8. The cyanotic cat

Grainne Muire McCarthy

KEY SIGNS

Bluish discoloration of the skin and/or mucous membranes.

MECHANISM?

- Cyanosis is **bluish discoloration of the skin and/or mucous membranes** due to **reduced oxygen saturation of hemoglobin** in the blood causing hypoxia. Hypoxia producing cyanosis results either from **central** (cardiac or respiratory) or **peripheral causes.**

WHERE?

- Central hypoxia results from **cardiac or respiratory disease,** including disease of the upper or lower respiratory tract, pleural cavity, thoracic wall or diaphragm.
- Peripheral hypoxia may be generalized and associated with generalized vasoconstriction, or is localized and the result of **arterial or venous obstruction.**
- Occasionally abnormal hemoglobin with decreased oxygen carrying capacity is the cause of the cyanosis.

WHAT?

- The **commonest causes of cyanosis** are central causes and include bronchial and pulmonary disease, pleural effusions, cardiac disease, mediastinal neoplasia, diaphragmatic hernia and poisoning with acetaminophen.
  Peripheral cyanosis is usually the result of arterial thromboembolism.

QUICK REFERENCE SUMMARY

Diseases causing a cyanotic cat

CENTRAL HYPOXIA

WHERE? – CARDIAC HYPOXIA

ANOMALY

- Congential heart anomaly (p 113)
  Tetralogy of Fallot, reversed shunting (R–L), patent ductus arteriosus, tricuspid valve atresia, Eisenmenger's syndrome, endocardial cushion defect, and transposition of the great arteries can all cause cyanosis. Cats with congenital cyanotic heart conditions are usually stunted and cyanotic, and frequently present with a history of lethargy and syncope. Abnormal heart sounds may be audible.

continued

continued

NEOPLASTIC

● Heart base tumors (p 113)

Muffled heart and lung sounds, pleural effusion and ascites.

INFECTIOUS (PARASITIC)

● **Dirofilariasis** (p 112)

Most cats are asymptomatic, others may have non-specific signs of cough, lethargy, anorexia. Sudden death may occur.

IDIOPATHIC

● **Cardiomyopathy*** (p 112)

Dyspnea and tachypnea and cats with arterial thromboembolism may present with posterior paresis.

WHERE? – RESPIRATORY HYPOXIA

ANOMALY

● Diaphragmatic hernia (p 115)

Usually occurs following trauma, but may be congenital. Clinical signs of dyspnea and tachypnea may be present early in life or may not occur for years. Vomiting, regurgitation or inappetence may also occur.

MECHANICAL

● Airway obstruction (p 117)

Acute onset of inspiratory dyspnea and cough occur with foreign bodies lodged in airways. Coughing and wheezing occur when the obstruction is due to bronchoconstriction.

● **Pleural effusion/pneumothorax*** (p 114)

Multiple causes of pleural effusion, both cardiac and non-cardiac, result in dyspnea and tachypnea. Inappetence, weight loss and pyrexia may occur depending on the cause.

● Pulmonary thromboembolism associated with heartworm disease (p 116)

Sudden onset of coughing, dyspnea, pulmonary crackles on ausculation and occasionally hemoptysis. Vomiting may also occur.

NEOPLASTIC

● **Cranial mediastinal lymphosarcoma** (p 115)

Dyspnea, tachypnea, regurgitation and reduced compressibility of the cranial thorax may be evident. Inappetence and weight loss may also occur.

INFLAMMATION (INFECTIOUS)

● Bacterial/viral/fungal/parasitic/protozoal/mycoplasmal

Pneumonia; depression, fever, tachypnea, cough and dyspnea. The cat may also show signs of upper respiratory tract disease.

INFECTIOUS (IMMUNE)

● **Feline bronchopulmonary disease/feline bronchitis complex/feline asthma** (p 114)

Typically, there is wheezing and coughing which may progress to severe dyspnea, open-mouthed breathing and cyanosis.

TRAUMA

● **Diaphragmatic hernia* (p 115)**
Dyspnea and tachypnea may occur acutely or months or years following blunt trauma. Vomiting, regurgitation, inappetence and weight loss may also occur.

● Central nervous system damage to the respiratory center (p 118)
Persistent or episodic weakness, Cheyne–Stokes respiration and cyanosis.

TOXIC

● Drug overdosage (p 117)
Excessive administration of barbiturates, narcotics, opiates, tranquilizers or anesthetic agents may lead to decreased respiratory effort, loss of consciousness and cyanosis. During anesthesia, reduced bleeding at surgical sites and indicators of a deep plane of anesthesia are present.

PERIPHERAL HYPOXIA
WHERE? – GENERALIZED
MECHANICAL

● **Vasoconstriction* (p 118)**
Peripheral hypoxia occurs due to vasoconstriction as a consequence of hypovolemic, cardiogenic or septic shock or due to hypothermia. Clinical signs, physical findings and history point to one of these causes. There may be evidence of shock, trauma, dehydration, pyrexia, blood loss or reduced urinary output. Signs of cardiac failure include dyspnea, cardiac murmur, gallop rhythm, slow capillary refill time, pale/cyanotic mucous membranes and pulse deficits. Frequent or severe vomiting, diarrhea or diuresis may indicate fluid loss.

LOCALIZED
MECHANICAL

● **Arterial thromboembolism** (p 120)**
Ninety percent lodge at the distal aortic bifurcation causing bilateral hindlimb pain and paresis, weak or absent femoral pulses, cold, cyanotic footpads and lack of spontaneous movement of the muscles of the hindlimbs. Other areas embolized less commonly are the thoracic aorta, renal, mesenteric, coronary, cerebral and branchial arteries which cause acute, severe and variable clinical signs.

● Venous obstruction (p 121)
Clinical signs relate to the area drained by the obstructed vein, mainly edema and vasodilatation distal to the site of obstruction. Cranial vena caval obstruction results in edema of the neck, ventral head, cranial thorax and forelimbs.

ABNORMAL HEMOGLOBIN WITH DECREASED OXYGEN-CARRYING CAPACITY
WHERE? – HEMOGLOBIN IN RED BLOOD CELLS
WHAT?

TOXICITY

● Paracetamol/acetaminophen toxicity (p 121)
Acute onset and rapid progression of salivation, vomiting and depression. Cyanosis develops within 4–12 hours of ingestion. Subcutaneous edema of the face may be evident, which may be accompanied by lacrimation and puritis. Hematuria, hemolysis and Heinz bodies occur associated with methemoglobin formation.

INTRODUCTION

MECHANISM?

Cyanosis is bluish discoloration of the skin and/or mucous membranes due to reduced oxygen saturation of hemoglobin in the blood causing hypoxia. Cyanosis most commonly results from **decreased oxygen saturation of normal hemoglobin.** Only rarely it results from abnormal hemoglobin with decreased oxygen-carrying capacity. Hypoxia producing cyanosis results either from **central (cardiac or respiratory) or peripheral causes**.

WHERE?

Hypoxia (i.e. decreased oxygen saturation of normal hemoglobin).

Central hypoxia results from congenital **cardiac** anomalies such as tetralogy of Fallot and pulmonary arterial hypertension secondary to a large PDA, VSD, ASD or truncus arteriosus, **respiratory** diseases including tracheal and laryngeal neoplasia (rare), pleural effusions, pulmonary edema, pneumonia, thoracic wall lesions and rupture of the diaphragm.

Peripheral hypoxia is either **generalized** as a result of generalized vasoconstriction due to hypothermia, heart failure or shock or **localized** as a result of **arterial or venous obstruction.** Acute arterial obstruction may result from thromboembolism or thrombosis occurring with cardiomyopathy, bacterial endocarditis, hypercoagulable conditions and cold agglutinin disease. Venous obstruction occurs as a result of thrombophlebitis and restrictive devices such as a rubber band around the limb.

Abnormal hemoglobin with decreased oxygen-carrying capacity.

WHAT?

In the cat, the commonest causes of cyanosis include bronchial and pulmonary disease, pleural effusions, cardiac disease, mediastinal neoplasia, diaphragmatic hernias and poisoning with acetaminophen. Peripheral cyanosis is usually the result of arterial thromboembolism.

CARDIAC HYPOXIA

CARDIOMYOPATHY***

> **Classical signs**
> - Dyspnea and tachypnea.
> - Lethargy.
> - Anorexia/vomiting.
> - Posterior paresis.
> - Abnormal heart sounds.

See main reference on page 128 for details (The Cat With Abnormal Heart Sounds and/or an Enlarged Heart).

Clinical signs

Dyspnea and tachypnea, or in severe cases open-mouthed breathing, occur because of pleural effusion and/or pulmonary edema.

Lethargy, anorexia and occasional vomiting may be present.

Occasionally, acute onset of posterior paresis occurs with painful hardening of the quadriceps and gastrocnemius groups of muscles, cyanosis of the nail beds and cold extremities associated with aortic thromboembolism.

Diagnosis

Thoracic radiography may show cardiac enlargement, pleural effusion and pulmonary edema.

Echocardiography may show left ventricular hypertrophy and left atrial enlargement in hypertrophic cardiomyopathy or left atrial and ventricular dilation with reduced contractility in dilated cardiomyopathy.

DIROFILARIASIS**

> **Classical signs**
> - Most cats are asymptomatic.
> - Cough, lethargy, anorexia, vomiting, dyspnea and syncope.
> - Acute dyspnea and sudden death.

See main reference on page 104 for details (The Coughing Cat).

Clinical signs

Many cats are **asymptomatic.**

Sudden death occurs in 30–40% of cats with clinical signs from dirofilaria.

Most cats are presented with non-specific signs such as lethargy, anorexia, vomiting, coughing, dyspnea and syncope.

Acute dyspnea may result from acute thromboembolism.

Right-sided heart failure is rare.

Diagnosis

Thoracic radiography may show prominent blunted or tortuous caudal lobar arteries and right heart enlargement.

Laboratory tests reveal eosinophilia and a non-regenerative anemia in 33% of cases. **Adult antigen tests** detect only about 25% of infected cats because of low worm numbers. **Tests for circulating antibody** to heartworm are more sensitive, but there are problems with false positives and negatives. Antibodies may persist for up to 18 months after worms have died, so a positive test does not necessarily indicate current infection.

Echocardiography may reveal worms in the pulmonary artery, right heart or vena cava.

Non-selective angiography may show linear filling defects associated with the presence of worms.

CONGENITAL HEART ANOMALY

Classical signs

- Stunting.
- Cyanosis.
- Signs of congestive heart failure.
- Abnormal heart sounds.

See main reference on page 140 for details (The Cat With Abnormal Heart Sounds and/or an Enlarged Heart).

Pathogenesis

Congenital cardiac anomalies causing cyanosis result from **defects in the partitions of the heart or** great vessels and an obstruction to pulmonary blood flow.

This leads to **right-to-left shunting** and results in mixing of unsaturated and saturated blood which is then ejected into the systemic circulation.

Tetralogy of Fallot, reversed shunting (R–L), patent ductus arteriosus, tricuspid valve atresia, Eisenmenger's syndrome, endocardial cushion defect and transposition of the great arteries can all cause cyanosis.

Clinical signs

Cyanosis in a young cat or kitten frequently is suggestive of a congenital heart anomaly.

They may present with lethargy, exercise intolerance, syncope and tachypnea.

Signs of **congestive heart failure** or **abnormal heart sounds** may be present.

Diagnosis

Dorsoventral thoracic radiographs may show **enlargement of the right atrium** at the 8–11 o'clock position, right ventricular enlargement at the 5–9 o'clock position or post-stenotic dilation of the pulmonary artery at the 1–2 o'clock position.

Lateral thoracic radiographs may show rounding of the cranial border of the heart with **increased sternal contact** and elevation of the trachea in the cranial thorax. On both views the **pulmonary vessels may be underperfused**.

Echocardiography is useful for visualizing the abnormal cardiac and vascular shunts. Doppler studies will help to identify the presence and direction of shunts.

Hematological examination may indicate a **polycythemia with a PCV often in excess of 75%.**

HEART BASE TUMORS

Classical signs

- Muffled heart sounds.
- Right heart failure.
- Pale mucous membranes.
- Weak arterial pulses.

See main reference on page 137 for details.

Clinical signs

Heart base tumors **are rare in cats.**

Heart sounds are often muffled **associated with a pericardial/pleural effusion.**

Weakness, dyspnea and tachypnea are often present.

Ascites is commonly present due to cardiac tamponade.

Edema of the head, neck and forelegs occurs if the tumor presses on the cranial vena cava.

Weight loss may be present.

Diagnosis

Thoracic radiography may show a rounded cardiac silhouette and pleural effusion.

Pericardiocentesis, cytological analysis and contrast pericardiography may help diagnose a heart base tumor.

Echocardiography may enable visualization of the tumor and enable ultrasound-guided fine-needle aspirate biopsy of the tumor for histologic analysis.

RESPIRATORY HYPOXIA

PLEURAL EFFUSION/PNEUMOTHORAX***

> **Classical signs**
> - Dyspnea.
> - Tachypnea.

See main reference on page 54 for details (The Dyspneic or Tachypneic Cat).

Clinical signs

Progressively worsening dyspnea frequently occurs with thoracic fluid accumulation.

Acute dyspnea may occur with **traumatic pneumothorax** and **tension pneumothorax**.

Muffled lung sounds occur due to the presence of thoracic fluid.

Lung sounds may be inaudible with a pneumothorax.

If due to a cranial mediastinal mass it may result in a non-compressible cranial thorax.

Diagnosis

Thoracic radiograph may show the presence of fluid, air or a mediastinal or other space-occupying mass.

Thoracocentesis may yield fluid which can be classified as transudate, exudate, chylous or hemorrhagic effusion.

Thoracocentesis may yield air indicative of a pneumothorax.

FELINE BRONCHOPULMONARY DISEASE/FELINE BRONCHITIS COMPLEX/FELINE ASTHMA**

> **Classical signs**
> - Cough.
> - Wheeze.
> - Severe dyspnea, open-mouthed breathing and cyanosis.

See main reference on page 92 for details (The Coughing Cat).

Clinical signs

Coughing of variable severity is frequently seen as a result of bronchoconstriction.

Dyspnea and tachypnea will appear if there is severe bronchconstriction or marked cellular infiltration into the lung parenchyma.

Dyspnea may be inspiratory or there may be **end-expiratory grunting** due to difficulty in expelling air from the cat's hyperinflated lungs.

Acute exacerbations may cause severe dyspnea, orthopnea, open-mouth breathing and cyanosis, which may be life-threatening.

Diagnosis

The **clinical findings** are very supportive of a diagnosis as there are few other clearly recognized causes of **coughing and dyspnea** in the cat.

Wheezing and crackling with moist gurgling sounds can be heard on auscultation.

Thoracic radiographs may show a bronchial or a mixed bronchial/interstitial or alveolar pulmonary pattern throughout the entire lung field.

In the **acute phase** there may be **hyperinflation** of the lungs and **flattening of the diaphragm.** Occasionally collapse of the right middle lung lobe may be seen.

Bronchoalveolar lavage fluid usually shows an inflammatory response which is usually eosinophilic but may be neutrophilic in nature.

Differential diagnosis

Lungworm and lung fluke infestation are diagnosed with fecal Baermann exams.

Heartworm disease is often associated with vomiting, and sometimes basophilia. On radiographs, **dilated and blunted pulmonary arteries,** which are most prominent in the caudal pulmonary arteries, particularly the right side, may be seen. **Lung changes vary** from **patchy pulmonary infiltrates** to **severe alveolar densities,** and sometimes are difficult to differentiate from those of feline bronchopulmonary disease/ asthma.

Treatment

Acute respiratory distress requires a **rapid-acting corticosteroid** such as methylprednisolone sodium succinate given intravenously at a dose of 30–50 mg/kg, oxygen and **terbutaline** at a dose of 0.01 mg/kg IM or SQ q 4 h.

Long-term management involves eliminating potential allergens and intermittent anti-inflammatory and bronchodilator therapy.

CRANIAL MEDIASTINAL LYMPHOSARCOMA**

Classical signs

- Dyspnea.
- Tachypnea.
- Regurgitation.
- Pleural effusion.
- Non-compressible cranial thorax.

See main reference on page 56 for details (The Dyspneic or Tachypneic Cat) and page 676 for details of treatment.

Clinical signs

Dyspnea and tachypnea are often associated with a pleural effusion.

Regurgitation may occur due to compression of the esophagus by the mass.

Cyanosis may result from compression of the mediastinal vessels.

Reduced compressibility of the cranial mediastinal thorax may be evident because of a space-occupying mass.

Diagnosis

Thoracic radiography shows a space-occupying lesion causing widening of the cranial mediastinum. A pleural effusion is frequently present.

Cytologic evaluation of pleural fluid is useful as it often contains **lymphoblastic cells.**

Fine-needle aspiration of the mass under ultrasound guidance will yield a sample for histopathologic examination.

Test cat for FeLV as approximately 60% of cats with mediastinal lymphosarcoma are FeLV-positive in USA. This may be lower in countries where FeLV is rare.

Test for FIV as this virus is also associated with increased rates of lymphosarcoma.

DIAPHRAGMATIC HERNIA (CONGENITAL ANOMALY OR TRAUMATIC)*

Classical signs

- Dyspnea.
- Tachypnea.

See main reference on page 58 for details (The Dyspneic or Tachypneic Cat).

Clinical signs

Acute tachypnea/dyspnea may develop **after a blunt traumatic event.** There may be signs of shock and other injuries related to an event such as a road traffic accident.

Acute exacerbations of chronic diaphragmatic hernia may occur following the development of a **pleural effusion or dilation of a herniated stomach.**

In **chronic cases**, signs may be restricted to **exercise intolerance**, or **signs of gastrointestinal upset** may occur, weeks or months after the trauma.

Entrapment of viscera following traumatic diaphragmatic hernia may lead to **pleural effusion**. Even partial herniation of liver may result in significant effusion.

Congenital peritoneo-pericardial hernias also occur causing similar clinical signs.

Diagnosis

Clinical findings of **muffled lung sounds, displacement of cardiac apex, gut sounds audible in thorax and reduced volume of abdominal contents are suggestive**.

Thoracic radiography may show loss of diaphragmatic line, abdominal contents in the thorax or pleural effusion.

Thoracic ultrasound can identify the presence of abnormal contents in the thorax and loss of continuity of the diaphragmatic line.

PULMONARY THROMBOEMBOLISM ASSOCIATED WITH HEARTWORM DISEASE

Classical signs

- Severe dyspnea.
- Tachypnea.
- Cyanosis.

See main reference on page 104 for details (The Coughing Cat).

Clinical signs

Acute dyspnea is associated with **pulmonary thromboembolism** or **acute pulmonary inflammation and edema** associated with worm death. **Acute respiratory distress syndrome** (ARDS) and generalized respiratory failure is not uncommon.

Cats usually have an **acute onset of severe dyspnea, tachypnea and cyanosis**, and may mouth breathe.

Dyspnea may be **worsened in lateral recumbency** (orthopnea) and the cat is reluctant to lie in this position.

There may be splitting of the second heart sound, resulting in a **gallop rhythm**, due to acute pulmonary arterial hypertension.

Diagnosis

Thoracic radiographs may show evidence of **parenchymal lung disease, right-sided cardiomegaly, or enlargement of the caudal lobar arteries or may be normal**.

Ultrasound examination may reveal heartworm as **hollow linear densities** in the main pulmonary artery or right atrium, as well as pulmonary arterial dilation.

Definitive diagnosis of the thromboembolism requires angiography or **pulmonary scintigraphy**.

Blood chemistries may indicate the presence of a hypercoagulable condition.

Heartworm tests may be positive.

PNEUMONIA

Classical signs

- Fever.
- Tachypnea.
- Cough.
- Dyspnea.
- Inappetance.

See main reference on page 62 for details (The Dyspneic or Tachypneic Cat).

Clinical signs

Cats are usually **inappetent, dull, febrile and lethargic** and may have a productive cough or fetid halitosis with bacterial pneumonia.

Tachypnea and dyspnea may be evident, and **open-mouth breathing** may occur with stress.

Aspiration pneumonia after oral dosing with liquid paraffin or mineral oil, or associated with megaesophagus may also result in **coughing**.

Viral pneumonia with feline calicivirus causes a non-productive cough.

Diagnosis

Crackles and wheezes may be heard on **pulmonary auscultation** especially in the **ventral lung fields**.

Thoracic radiographs show a **patchy interstitial or alveolar pattern, and possibly lung lobe consolidation in the cranioventral lung fields**. There may be evidence of **megaesophagus** present.

Tracheal and bronchoalveolar lavage cytology may reveal a neutrophilic inflammatory response with many degenerate neutrophils. Alternately, the presence of eosinophils may indicate an allergic, parasitic or neoplastic etiology.

Microbial culture of cytospun lavage fluid deposit may reveal a primary pathogen (bacterial, fungal, parasitic or myoplasma).

Bronchoscopy may show inflammatory exudate in the airways.

Routine hematologic examination may reveal a left shift in bacterial pneumonia.

Check FeLV and FIV status in cats with chronic pneumonia as they may be immunosuppressed.

AIRWAY OBSTRUCTION

Classical signs

- Inspiratory dyspnea.
- Cough.
- Stridor.
- Cyanosis.

See main reference on page 65 for detail. (The Dyspneic or Tachypneic Cat (Foreign bodies)) and page 92 (The Coughing Cat (Feline asthma/bronchitis complex)).

Clinical signs

Acute-onset inspiratory dyspnea and stridor occur shortly after inhalation of a foreign body. **Tracheal foreign bodies** are more common in cats than dogs.

Coughing is likely with bronchial foreign bodies and the right middle lobe most likely to be involved.

Tracheobronchial compression caused by **space-occupying** lesions (most often lymphoma or thymoma) usually lead to coughing and dyspnea.

Airway obstruction caused by **bronchoconstriction** associated with feline asthma or bronchitis complex leads to severe dyspnea, wheezing and coughing.

Diagnosis

Thoracic radiography may reveal foreign bodies, tumors or other structures compressing or obstructing the airways.

Bronchoscopy may reveal structures compressing the airway or a foreign body or other material in the airways.

DRUG OVERDOSAGE

Classical signs

- Decreased respiratory effort.
- Absence of voluntary respiration.
- Loss of consciousness.
- Cyanosis.
- Reduced bleeding from surgical site.

Clinical signs

Respiratory depression or even failure can result from **excessive administration of barbiturates, narcotics, opiates, tranquillizers or anesthetic agents.**

This leads to **loss of consciousness and cyanosis** due to hypoxemia.

If it occurs during a surgical procedure, there may be **reduced bleeding** from the surgical site and the color of the **blood darkens**. **Loss of blink reflex** indicates a deep plane of anesthesia and is associated with increased respiratory depression.

Diagnosis

Diagnosis is based on **clinical signs** together with **anesthetic records** indicating drug overdose, or a **history of access** to sedative, narcotic or anesthetic drugs.

CENTRAL NERVOUS SYSTEM DAMAGE TO THE RESPIRATORY CENTER

Classical signs

- Persistent or episodic weakness.
- Cheyne–Stokes respiration.
- Cyanosis.

Clinical signs

Central respiratory depression as a result of CNS infection, increased intracranial pressure or head injury leads to slow, gasping respirations (Cheyne–Stokes respiration).

The cat may be unconscious and cyanotic.

Other evidence of trauma, or neurologic deficits may be present.

Diagnosis

Neurological examination demonstrates neurologic deficits consistent with a medullary lesion together with a typical respiratory pattern.

PERIPHERAL HYPOXIA – GENERALIZED

VASOCONSTRICTION*

Classical signs

- Generalized cyanosis.
- Signs of hypovolemic, cardiogenic, or septic shock or hypothermia.

Pathogenesis

Peripheral hypoxia occurs due to vasoconstriction as a consequence of **hypovolemic, cardiogenic or septic shock or due to hypothermia.** This leads to inadequate capillary perfusion and oxygen delivery to peripheral tissues becomes impaired, which may lead to generalized peripheral cyanosis.

Hypovolemia occurs when blood volume is diminished by **whole blood loss or by extracellular fluid losses.** Compensatory mechanisms include splenic and venous constriction to translocate blood from the venous capacitance vessels to the central arterial circulation; arteriolar constriction to maintain diastolic blood pressure and increasing heart rate to increase cardiac output. When severe, hypovolemic shock ensues resulting in generalized peripheral hypoxia.

Cardiogenic shock occurs with any condition that **interferes with forward outflow from the heart** to such an extent that adequate tissue perfusion is not achieved. Examples include acute or chronic heart failure, cardiomyopathy, intracardiac thrombosis, pericardial tamponade, heartworm disease and severe arrhythmias.

When an animal's blood has become **infected by bacteria, viruses, rickettsia, fungi or protozoa it is considered septic**. Some of these organisms produce **toxins** which are directly **vasoactive** or release vasoactive substances. When the infection is affecting the animal to the extent that tissue perfusion is compromised, **septic shock** has ensued.

Hypothermia results when heat loss exceeds heat production. Decreasing body temperature decreases the partial pressure of oxygen, increases solubility and shifts the oxygen–hemoglobin dissociation curve to the left. These changes impede oxygen unloading at the tissue level. Thermoregulatory vasoconstriction further decreases oxygen delivery.

Clinical signs

Generalized cyanosis together with **signs of severe hypovolemia**, **severe cardiac disease, hypothermia or sepsis,** which suggest vasoconstriction is leading to inadequate capillary perfusion and impaired oxygen delivery to peripheral tissues.

Signs of cardiac failure include dyspnoea, cardiac murmur, gallop rhythm, slow capillary refill time, pale/cyanotic mucous membranes and pulse deficits.

Evidence of shock, trauma, pyrexia, blood loss or reduced urinary output may indicate cause of peripheral vasoconstriction.

History of frequent or **severe vomiting, diarrhea or diuresis** are suggestive of marked fluid loss leading to **hypovolemia.**

Fluid accumulations in the thoracic or abdominal cavities or in intracellular spaces suggest cardiac disease, sepsis, bleeding or severe hypoalbuminemia is the cause of the vasoconstriction and cyanosis.

Acute weakness, bradycardia and cyanosis, with or without a history of polyuria/polydipsia or GIT signs, in a young to middle-aged dog is suggestive of **hypoadrenocorticism** (Addisons disease).

Diagnosis

Diagnosis is based on clinical signs and physical findings which suggest that hypovolemia, severe cardiac disease, sepsis or hypothermia are causing marked vasoconstriction and generalized peripheral cyanosis.

Cardiovascular examination, including echocardiography are important in assessing cardiac function.

Complete blood profile may indicate sepsis or hypovolemia.

Thoracic and abdominal radiographs may show cardiomegaly, fluid accumulations, evidence of hypovolemia, evidence of trauma or masses such as abscesses.

Treatment

For cardiogenic shock, treatment is directed at restoring organ perfusion to provide adequate tissue oxygenation, i.e. supporting arterial blood pressure, forward cardiac output and vascular volume. Diuresis, vasodilation, calcium channel- or beta-blocking drugs, anti-arrhythmics, oxygen and thoracocentesis may be required in hypertrophic cardiomyopathy. Continuous monitoring of cardiac, pulmonary and renal status is essential. Supportive therapy includes cage rest where necessary, weight reduction, avoidance of pregnancy and general reduction in cardiac workload. See page 130 (The Cat With Abnormal Heart Sounds and/or an Enlarged Heart) for treatment.

For shock, treatment depends on the cause. For hypovolemia administer intravenous fluids, and if indicated, a blood transfusion and control any continuing blood loss. For septic shock, fluid therapy and intravenous broad-spectrum antibiotic therapy is indicated. For anaphylactic shock, in addition to fluid therapy, epinephrine is of proven efficacy. Careful monitoring of acid–base balance, urine output, heart rate, pulse quality, capillary refill time, mucous membrane color and mental state are important. The reader is advised to consult a specialist source for an in-depth review of shock therapy.

Rewarming is required for hypothermia. When the **body temperature is less than 32 degrees** Centigrade (90 degrees Fahrenheit) **active central rewarming is required.** This includes the use **of warmed (to 35 degrees Centigrade/95 degrees Fahrenheit) IV fluids, flushing stomach, rectum and open body cavity with warmed isotonic fluids**, and providing warmed, humidified air. If body temperature is between **32 and 36 degrees Centigrade** (90 and 96 degrees Fahrenheit) **active surface rewarming** can be carried out using hot water bottles, heat pads, radiant heaters and hair dryers. At body temperatures above 36 degrees Centigrade (96 degrees Fahrenheit) passive rewarming by covering the cat with blankets is sufficient.

Prognosis

With **hypovolemia** recovery rates can be high, providing adequate correction of fluid deficits can be achieved.

Cardiogenic shock is usually associated with advanced heart disease and so recovery rates are less.

Mortality rates in **septic shock** are high.

The systemic consequences of mild to moderate **hypothermia** are minimal but those of severe prolonged hypothermia are serious and fraught with many complications including cardiac arrhythmias, electrolyte disturbances, coagulopathies, blood glucose upset and cold diuresis.

PERIPHERAL HYPOXIA – LOCALIZED

ARTERIAL THROMBOEMBOLISM**

> **Classical signs**
>
> - Acute onset of posterior paresis/paralysis.
> - Cyanosis of footpads and cold extremities.
> - Marked pain and swollen, turgid hind limb muscles.
> - Weak or absent femoral pulses.

See main reference on page 915 for details (The Weak and Ataxic or Paralyzed Cat).

Pathogenesis

Arterial thromboembolism is a relatively common and serious **sequela to feline cardiomyopathy**. **Thrombi form in the left atrium** due to a combination of factors including sluggish blood flow, endothelial damage and increased blood coagulability. The blood flow through the atria of cats with cardiomyopathy is normal to slow. Slow blood flow enables red cells and other blood factors to clump together and platelet aggregability in cats with cardiomyopathy is reported to be increased.

Once a thrombus is formed it may remain in the atrium and cause no symptoms. It may become an **embolus and travel to the distal aorta** and extend down the external iliac arteries forming a **"saddle thromboembolus"** obstructing blood flow to the hindlimbs. Ninety percent of cats with arterial thromboembolism are thus affected.

It is thought that the embolus releases **serotonin and thromboxane A$_2$**, which are powerful **vasoconstrictors.** This results in very poor collateral blood flow beyond the embolus, leading to tissue hypoxia and muscular ischemia.

Other emboli may obstruct the **femoral, brachial, renal, mesenteric, coronary or cerebral** arteries causing a wide variety of clinical signs.

Clinical signs

Many cats are in heart failure and therefore are **tachypneic and dyspneic,** and may have a heart murmur or a gallop rhythm.

Typically there is an **acute onset of posterior paresis/paralysis.**

Weakness or absence of one or both **femoral pulses** is evident.

There is **early severe pain** in **hindlimb muscles** which are **swollen and turgid**. The pain subsides as sensory nervous input is lost over several hours.

Pallor and cyanosis of footpads and **coldness of extremities** are evident.

Later over days to weeks, depending of the degree of arterial obstruction, neurological deficits begin to resolve.

Other organs may be affected depending on deposition of emboli.

Diagnosis

Diagnosis is based primarily on **clinical findings**.

Lack of blood flow to hindlimbs can be confirmed using a **Doppler arterial blood pressure** monitor.

Echocardiography is valuable to identify cardiomyopathy.

Biochemical profiles may help to identify other organ involvement.

Differential diagnosis

Other causes of posterior paresis/paralysis such as road traffic accidents and trauma should be considered.

Treatment

Treatment is mostly palliative, such as cage rest and consider the administration of drugs such as aspirin, heparin or arteriolar dilators. **Heparin** is given to prevent new thrombus formation at an initial dose of 220 U/kg IV followed by a maintenance dose of 70–200 U/kg SC every 6 hours. The dose should be tailored to increase the activated thromboplastin time to at least 1.5 times baseline.

Surgical intervention to remove the embolus and balloon embolectomy may lead to reperfusion syndrome and most cats will be in heart failure, so are poor anesthetic risks.

Thrombolytic therapy using **tissue plasminogen activator** reduces time to reperfusion and ambulation, however 50% of treated cats died during clinical trials.

Pain treatment in the early stages of the disease using oxymorphone (0.05–0.15 mg/kg IM or IV every 6 hours) and butorphanol (0.02–0.4 mg/kg every 4 hours IM or SC) is essential.

Acetylpromazine (0.05–0.1 mg/kg IV) may be useful as an anxiolytic.

Treatment of the heart failure must also be undertaken.

VENOUS OBSTRUCTION

Classical signs

- Localized cyanosis and edema referable to site of obstruction.
- Edema of neck, ventral head, cranial thorax and forelimbs (vena cava obstruction).

Pathogenesis

Localized peripheral hypoxia resulting from venous obstruction is usually the result of thrombosis, phlebitis or venous obstruction from external compression.
- **Thrombosis** is typically caused by blunt trauma and perforating injury, such as venepuncture or prolonged venous catheterization.
- **Phlebitis** may result from tissue inflammation extending to the veins, or originate from a venous intimal lesion.
- Venous obstruction may be caused by **compression** by **abscesses, hematomas, tumors or enlarged lymph nodes.**

Clinical signs

Clinical signs **depend on the anatomic location** and the extent of the obstructive process, the collateral vessel reserve and the capacity of the draining lymphatics.

Large lesions may result in **edema and cyanosis** in the area, which is usually short-lived because of large collateral circulation.

If all veins draining an area are obstructed, edema, cyanosis and **necrosis** may occur.

Cranial vena caval obstruction results in edema of the neck, ventral head, cranial thorax and forelimbs.

Diagnosis

Diagnosis is based on historical and clinical findings.

Treatment

Thrombosis is usually self-limiting once catheters are removed. Broad-spectrum antibiotic cover may be necessary for septic lesions.

Surgical management is by drainage of abscesses and hematomas, and debulking of tumors where indicated.

Treat the underlying cause of **lymphadenopathy** using antibiotics, chemotherapy or surgical excision where appropriate.

Prognosis

Prognosis depends on the primary disease process.

ABNORMAL HEMOGLOBIN WITH DECREASED OXYGEN-CARRYING CAPACITY

ACETAMINOPHEN (USA)/PARACETAMOL (EUROPE, AUSTRALIA) TOXICITY

Classical signs

- Salivation, vomiting and depression and cyanosis.
- Subcutaneous edema of face and extremities.
- Lacrimation and facial pruritis.
- Hematuria and hemolysis.

Pathogenesis

Feline hemoglobin is particularly **susceptible to oxidative damage**, and therefore to the formation of **methemoglobin** and **Heinz bodies** in erythrocytes.

Most species biotransform acetaminophen by hepatic conjugation with glucuronic acid and excrete it in the urine.

However, **cats have limited ability to conjugate drugs as glucuronides** and so they **excrete** the majority of acetaminophen as a **sulfate conjugate**.

This pathway is saturated at relatively low drug concentrations leading to early oxidative toxicity in the cat.

Hepatocellular injury associated with acute acetaminophen toxicity in other species is not seen in cats because cats develop oxidative toxicity at much lower doses than those required for hepatotoxicity in other species.

Accumulation of oxidative metabolites produces methemoglobin, which reduces oxygenation of blood.

Methemoglobinemia leads to the **denaturing of hemoglobin and Heinz bodies** are formed from the **precipitation of this denatured haemoglobin** within the red blood cells.

Heinz bodies lead to **increased osmotic fragility** of red blood cells causing **hemolysis and anaemia**.

The **feline toxic dose of acetaminophen is 50–100 mg/kg**, and the average size of a regular tablet is 325 mg (USA) or 250 mg (Europe).

Clinical signs

Salivation, vomiting and depression progress rapidly and **cyanosis** develops **within 4–12 hours** of ingestion.

Hematuria and hemolysis appear when blood levels of **methemoglobin reach 20%.**

Subcutaneous edema of face and extremities may happen and be accompanied by **lacrimation and pruritis**.

Death may occur.

Jaundice is seen 2–7 days post-exposure if the cat survives.

Diagnosis

Diagnosis is based on the history of exposure and clinical signs.

Finding the pills in stomach contents is confirmatory.

Frequent laboratory findings include; **methemoglobinemia, depletion of erythrocyte-reduced glutathione, Heinz bodies and a decreased packed cell volume.**

Elevated hepatic enzyme levels and total and direct bilirubin levels are evidence of hepatic necrosis.

Differential diagnosis

Other causes of methemoglobinemia include, **benzocaine** (used as a laryngeal local anesthetic spray to facilitate intubation), **DL methionine** (used as a urinary acidifier), **phenacetin** (used as an analgesic in humans) and **phenazopyridine** (used as a urinary analgesic drug).

Methylene blue, a drug previously used to treat cats with methemoglobinemia may actually cause Heinz body formation and hemolytic anemia.

Familial methemoglobin reductase deficiency has been reported in a family of domestic shorthair cats and is thought to have an autosomal recessive form of inheritance.

Treatment

Induce emesis and administer **activated charcoal** if the cat is treated **within the first 4 hours post-ingestion.**

N-acetylcysteine will provide the cysteine moiety required for the increased **synthesis of gluthathione** and may increase the concentration of **free serum sulfate**. A dose of 140 mg/kg IV should be followed by 70 mg/kg IV every 6 hours for a total of seven treatments.

Ascorbic acid provides a reserve system for the **nonenzymatic reduction of methemoglobin back to hemoglobin** and can be given at a dose of 30 mg/kg IV four times a day.

Blood transfusion may provide a lifesaving fraction of **functional hemoglobin** until the methemoglobin can be reduced.

Cimetidine, which works differently to acetylcysteine and ascorbic acid in the metabolism of acetaminophen, has been used in an attempt to **reduce hepatotoxicity**. The suggested dose rate is 15 mg/kg IV every 8 hours or 100 mg/kg orally every 8 hours.

Prognosis

The time between ingestion and initiation of therapy is of primary importance and the dosage of acetaminophen ingested is the other important consideration. The sooner the animal is treated the better the outcome. **Most cats treated within the first 24 hours will survive**.

RECOMMENDED READING

Aronson LR, Drobatz K. Acetaminophen toxicosis in 17 cats. J Vet Emerg Crit Care 1996: 6: 65–69.

Dunn J. Cyanosis. In: Textbook of Small Animal Medicine. W.B. Saunders, London, 1999, pp 118–122.

Ettinger S, Feldman E. Cyanosis. In: Textbook of Veterinary Internal Medicine, Volume 1, Sixth Edition, 2005, W.B. Saunders, London, pp 219–222.

Osweiler GD. In: Toxicology. The National Veterinary Medical Series. Williams and Wilkins, Philadelphia, 1996.

PART 3

Cat with signs of heart disease

9. The cat with abnormal heart sounds and/or an enlarged heart

Luis A H Braz-Ruivo and Kathy A Arrington

KEY SIGNS

- Heart murmur.
- Gallop rhythm.
- Muffled, displaced or absent heart sounds.

MECHANISM?

- Murmurs are abnormal heart sounds caused by turbulent blood flow due to valvular stenosis or insufficiency.
- Innocent or functional murmurs may be present in the absence of morphologic heart disease.
- Gallop rhythms are caused by extra heart sounds and are due to abnormalities in myocardial relaxation.
- Displaced, absent, or muffled heart sounds are caused by intrathoracic masses, effusions or structural changes.
- Cardiac enlargement is the result of alterations of blood flow causing volume overload, myocardial hypertrophy or due to primary myopathic processes.

WHERE?

- Heart.
- Mediastinum.

- Diaphragm.
- Thoracic skeleton.

WHAT?

- Most cats with heart murmurs **are not symptomatic** for heart disease.
- The most common form of acquired heart disease in cats is **hypertrophic cardiomyopathy.**
- Some cats with cardiac enlargement have normal physical exam findings.

QUICK REFERENCE SUMMARY

Diseases causing abnormal heart sounds and/or an enlarged heart

DEGENERATIVE

- Valvular endocardiosis (p 155)

A murmur localized to the left sternal apex is heard. It is a rare disease of old cats. Some cats may present with congestive heart failure.

ANOMALY

- **Ventricular septal defect* (p 140)**

A congenital systolic murmur is heard which is loudest over the right sternal border. Most cats are asymptomatic.

- Patent ductus arteriosus (p 142)

A congenital continuous murmur loudest over the left cranial thorax is heard. A palpable thrill is usually present. It is more common in Siamese and Persian cats.

- Tetralogy of Fallot (p 149)

A systolic murmur is heard over the left cranial thorax (pulmonic area). A split second heart sound may also be found. Cyanosis is usually present.

- Atrial septal defect (p 144)

A breed predilection in Persian cats is reported. A systolic murmur over the left cranial thorax is heard.

- Mitral valve dysplasia/stenosis (p 145)

This is the most commonly encountered congenital valvular malformation and is associated with a systolic and/or diastolic murmur over the left cardiac apex.

- Aortic stenosis (p 146)

Aortic stenosis is associated with a systolic murmur over the left aortic area. There is an increased incidence in Siamese cats.

- Pulmonic stenosis (p 148)

Pulmonic stenosis is associated with a systolic murmur over the pulmonic area and is usually seen with other defects.

- Tricuspid dysplasia

Tricuspid dysplasia is associated with a low-frequency systolic murmur over the right thorax.

continued

continued

● Peritoneal–pericardial diaphragmatic hernia (p 153)

A murmur may or may not be heard. The cardiac silhouette is extremely enlarged on thoracic radiographs. Many cats are asymptomatic, but some cats present for gastrointestinal signs or respiratory distress.

METABOLIC

● Hypertensive heart disease*** (p 133)

A systolic murmur, tachycardia and/or gallop rhythm may be heard. Hypertension in cats is most commonly secondary to chronic renal failure or hyperthyroidism. Essential or idiopathic hypertension is less common.

● Hyperthyroid heart disease*** (p 131)

A systolic murmur, tachycardia and/or gallop rhythm may be heard. Hyperthyroid heart disease is associated with other clinical signs of hyperthyroidism including weight loss, restlessness, palpable thyroid nodule, low frequency of gastrointestinal signs and is seen in older cats.

● High cardiac output state* (p 138)

A murmur, gallop rhythm or tachycardia may be heard on auscultation. It can be caused by anemia secondary to other disease states or hyperthyroidism. The heart size may be variable depending on the disease or the chronicity of the anemia.

NEOPLASTIC

● Neoplasia** (p 137)

Displaced or muffled heart sounds can be caused by neoplasia from a mass or effusion. Lymphoma is the most common neoplasia seen in cats and occasionally infiltrates the myocardium.

INFECTIOUS

● Infectious

Infectious diseases can rarely cause secondary cardiomyopathies in cats. Most cats die unexpectedly and/or are systemically ill. Etiologies suspected are viral (feline infectious peritonitis), secondary bacterial or parasitic (toxoplasmosis). Bacterial (pyothorax, myocarditis, pericarditis) and viral (myocarditis, pericarditis) infections can cause displaced or muffled heart sounds and/or arrhythmias (p 157).

● Heartworm disease* (p 139)

Dirofilaria immitis (heartworm disease) in cats is less common than in dogs. Cardiac signs are variable and may include signs of right heart failure, gallop rhythm or murmurs. Coughing, vomiting or sudden death may also occur. Heartworm disease in cats is more common in male cats, outdoor cats, and occurrence depends on geographical location.

IDIOPATHIC

● Hypertrophic cardiomyopathy*** (p 128)

A systolic murmur varying in location, arrhythmia and/or gallop rhythm may be heard. It is the most common form of heart disease in cats and occurs usually in male and middle-aged cats. It can also be seen in young (less than 1 year of age) cats and older cats. It may be genetically transmitted in some pure-breed cats. The heart may or may not be enlarged on radiographs.

- ● **Restrictive and unclassified cardiomyopathies** (p 135)**
  A systolic heart murmur, gallop rhythm and/or arrhythmia may be heard. Abnormal heart sounds are not always heard on auscultation. The heart is usually enlarged.

- ● Dilated cardiomyopathy (p 151)
  A systolic murmur, gallop rhythm and/or arrhythmia may be heard. The heart shows generalized enlargement. Dilated cardiomyopathy can occur in cats eating taurine-deficient diets.

- ● **Chylous effusion* (p 139)**
  Displaced or muffled heart sounds may be heard. Etiologies are trauma, infection, cardiomyopathy, neoplasia and idiopathic. In most cases, the cause is idiopathic.

TRAUMATIC

- ● Diaphragmatic hernia (p 154)
  Displaced and/or muffled heart sounds may be heard. Dyspnea may or may not occur.

INTRODUCTION

MECHANISM?

Abnormal heart sounds are defined as follows:

Systolic murmurs are **common** and are caused by turbulent blood flow secondary to a valvular stenosis or insufficiency. **Systolic murmurs** are the most common and account for >95% of murmurs.

Diastolic and continuous murmurs are rare.

Continuous murmurs occur during diastole and systole and most commonly occur from a patent ductus arteriosus.

In thin cats, murmurs may be caused by mechanical compression of the chest during auscultation.

Gallop rhythms are extra heart **sounds** due to abnormalities in relaxation. The gallop rhythm is classified as either S_4 or S_3 but it is difficult to distinguish between these in cats.

Arrhythmias are disturbances in **rate** and **rhythm** and are noted by an irregular rhythm.

Tachycardia is defined as a heart rate greater than **220 bpm.**

Loud heart sounds are usually normal in thin cats and during tachycardia.

Displaced heart sounds and **muffled** heart sounds are most commonly caused by masses within the thorax (neoplasia) and/or effusions (cardiomyopathy, neoplasia or infection) or rarely structural changes (hernias or pectus excavatum).

Cardiac enlargement most commonly results from cardiomyopathy secondary to hypertrophy.

WHERE?

Abnormal heart sounds and/or cardiac enlargement result from problems in any of the following sites:

Heart, mediastinum, diaphragm, thoracic skeleton, lungs.

WHAT?

The most **common** cause of cardiac disease is **hypertrophic cardiomyopathy**. It is usually **acquired** and **idiopathic.**

Congenital heart disease is **rare** and a **murmur** is **usually** heard at a young age.

The most **common** congenital defect in cats is ventral septal defect followed by mitral valve dysplasia.

Most cats with **heart murmurs** are **asymptomatic.**

Abnormal heart sounds in **asymptomatic** cats **always** warrants a **cardiovascular** work-up.

Cats with **abnormal heart sounds** may or may not have cardiac enlargement.

Lack of **cardiac enlargement** on radiographs in cats with **abnormal heart sounds** does not exclude heart disease.

Diagnosis is based on history, physical examination, radiography, electrocardiography and echocardiography.

Normal echocardiographic values for the **interventricular septum and left ventricular posterior wall** in diastole are up to 5 mm in thickness. The dimension between 5–6 mm represents questionable hypertrophy.

Normal echocardiographic values of the **left atrium** are up to 13 mm or a left atrium to aorta ratio less than 1.5.

Normal **left ventricular dimension** in diastole is up to 17 mm. Increased dimensions are consistent with left ventricular eccentric hypertrophy (dilation).

Fractional shortening (percent change between the left ventricular diastolic and systolic dimensions) ranges from 35–55%.

The above values can be obtained from the two-dimensional image or the M mode.

Cardiomegaly on radiographs is an indicator of heart disease although a **normal-size heart does not rule out heart disease.** Cardiac enlargement on radiographs can be determined by conventional methods or the vertebral heart scale.

The vertebral heart scale (VHS) compares cardiac dimensions to the length of the thoracic vertebrae, which is an indicator of body size.

The VHS method is as follows: The long axis and short axis dimensions of the heart are transposed onto the vertebral column and recorded as the corresponding number of vertebrae as measured caudally from the cranial edge of T4. These values are added to obtain the vertebral heart size (VHS).

The depth of the thorax is measured from the dorsocaudal border of the seventh sternebra to the closest edge of the vertebral column.

Normal cats' VHS are: mean VHS in lateral radiographs, 7.5 v (upper limit 8.0 v), mean cardiac short axis in lateral radiographs, 3.2 v (upper limit 3.5; mean cardiac short axis in VD or DV radiographs, 3.4 v (upper limit 4 v); The cardiac long axis in the lateral view approximates the length of three sternebrae, measured from S2 to S4.

Conventional methods of evaluating heart size in cats are on the lateral view with the normal heart width approximately 2–2.5 intercostal spaces. On the ventrodorsal view or dorsoventral view, the maximum width of the normal heart occupies up to 50% of the width of the chest cavity at the same level.

DISEASES CAUSING ABNORMAL HEART SOUNDS AND/OR AN ENLARGED HEART

HYPERTROPHIC CARDIOMYOPATHY***

Classical signs

- Heart murmur (in some cases it may not be present).
- Gallop rhythm.
- Arrhythmia.
- Dyspnea.
- Collapse.
- Lameness, paralysis or paresis from systemic thromboembolism.

Pathogenesis

Hypertrophic cardiomyopathy is defined as the presence of left ventricular hypertrophy in the absence of systemic disease causing secondary hypertrophy. Hypertrophy may be generalized or focal.

Focal hypertrophy **may be recognized in the** interventricular septum, **left ventricular free wall** or papillary muscles.

Any combination of hypertrophic changes is possible.

Hypertrophic cardiomyopathy (HCM) is recognized to be **genetically determined** in selected families of cats: Persian, Maine Coon, American Shorthair and possibly in Ragdolls. Transmission is suspected to be **autosomal dominant.**

The cause for hypertrophy is probably related to **genetic alteration** of the β-myosin heavy chain.

An association with increased levels of **growth hormone** concentration has also been found.

Echocardiographically there are two distinct varieties, a **non-obstructive** form and an **obstructive** form.

The **non-obstructive** form results primarily in **diastolic dysfunction** due to delayed or decreased **myocardial relaxation.**

The **obstructive form** is caused by **anterior motion of the mitral valve** during systole, which obstructs the left ventricular outflow tract. This results in **decreased cardiac output** at faster heart rates, in addition to abnormal diastolic function.

The outflow obstruction may contribute to the presence of ventricular concentric hypertrophy.

Histologically there is myocardial fiber disarray and diffuse myocardial fibrosis. HCM is usually limited to the left ventricle but in some cases, concurrent right ventricular hypertrophy is present.

The development of **left ventricular hypertrophy** is associated with altered intracellular calcium regulatory mechanisms. This results in the development of **relaxation abnormalities** during diastole.

The **chronic diastolic** dysfunction ultimately results in **left atrial dilatation**, elevation of **left atrial pressures** and finally **congestive heart failure**.

Clinical signs

Hypertrophic cardiomyopathy most commonly occurs in **middle-aged male cats**.

A heart murmur is usually present, but in some cases may not be present. When present, the murmur is systolic and varies in location and intensity.

A gallop rhythm is commonly heard. It is identified when more than two heart sounds are present on auscultation. The extra sound is classified as S_3 or S_4.

The fast heart rate in cats makes it often impossible to distinguish between a S_3 and S_4 sound.

Arrhythmias are occasionally heard as premature heart beats with pulse deficits. Ventricular arrhythmias are most common.

Dyspnea is seen in symptomatic cases together with an increased respiratory rate (greater than 30 breaths/min) at rest or with open-mouth breathing in extreme cases.

Collapse may result from impaired cardiac output associated with either ventricular tachycardia or the obstructive form of hypertrophic cardiomyopathy.

Sudden onset of lameness, paralysis or paresis may occur and is usually the result of systemic thromboembolism.

Most cats with aortic saddle thrombosis present for acute onset of hindlimb paralysis, hypothermia, pain, absent femoral pulses, cool extremities and cyanosis of the nail bed. In some cases a history of episodic lameness is given.

Diagnosis

Clinically, cats with hypertrophic cardiomyopathy present with a history of a heart murmur, arrhythmia, collapse or respiratory distress. Radiographic and electrocardiographic findings may support the diagnosis, but echocardiography is required for a definitive diagnosis.

Radiographic findings

The cardiac image varies from normal to obvious left ventricular and atrial enlargement.

Enlargement of the pulmonary veins may be seen, representing venous congestion.

Areas of focal alveolar densities representing pulmonary edema may be found. In some cases, pleural effusion may be present.

Electrocardiographic findings

Tachycardia (HR > 220 bpm), **left anterior fascicular block** (evidenced as left axis deviation with a mean electrical axis (MEA) from 0 to –60 degrees, a QRS in lead I and aVL with a QR pattern, and large S waves in leads II, III, aVF), **tall R waves on lead II** (>0.9 mV), and notched QRS in any lead may be seen.

Ventricular arrhythmias are more common than supraventricular arrhythmias.

Atrial fibrillation is rare but if present is always associated with extreme dilatation of the left and/or right atria.

Echocardiographic findings

Left ventricular hypertrophy (diastolic dimension of the interventricular septum and/or LV posterior wall greater than 6 mm), which may be global or focal (see Pathogenesis), and left atrial enlargement (dimension greater than 13 mm) can be seen.

- Elongated mitral valve leaflets with systolic anterior motion (anterior displacement into the left ventricular outflow of the anterior mitral valve leaflet) causing secondary left ventricular outflow obstruction as determined by Doppler study (velocity of blood flow >2.0 m/s) is seen in the obstructive form.

Differential diagnosis

Congenital heart disease
- A murmur is usually present from birth. Most congenital murmurs do not change in loudness with alterations of the heart rate. Congenital murmurs are usually relatively loud.

Dilated cardiomyopathy.
- Murmurs are usually very soft, and in many cases may not be present. A gallop rhythm is usually present.

Restrictive cardiomyopathy.
- It is difficult to differentiate from hypertrophic cardiomyopathy on auscultation; many cases have a gallop rhythm.

Intra-thoracic masses.
- A murmur may not be present unless there is compression of the heart by the mass or concurrent unrelated heart disease. Most commonly, dyspnea and lethargy are seen.

Feline asthma or chronic bronchitis.
- Unless cardiac disease is also present, most cats do not have a murmur. Cough and increased respiratory rate are common. Symptoms in the cat with feline asthma may be episodic and seasonal.

Chylous effusion.
- A murmur may not be present. In most cases, cardiac disease is not present. The most common clinical signs are dyspnea, increased respiratory rate and lethargy.

Neurological disease causing collapse or hindlimb paralysis

Cardiac signs are usually absent, however a full cardiac work-up may be warranted to rule out the presence of silent heart disease. Neurological disease usually is not associated with alterations of peripheral systemic perfusion.

Treatment

The treatment recommended depends on the severity of signs and the presence of left ventricular outflow tract (LVOT) obstruction.

Treatment of the asymptomatic cat.
- **Hypertrophic non-obstructive cardiomyopathy (HCM)** – Wall dimensions larger than 6 mm and normal Doppler LV outflow study ($LVOT_{max}$ less than 1.8 m/s).
  - **Normal** left atrial size – no therapy.
  - **Increased** left atrial size (>13 mm or LA/Ao > 1.5).
    - **Beta-blocker**
      Atenolol 12.5 mg/cat PO q 12–24 h.
    OR
    - **Calcium channel blockers:**
      Diltiazem 7.5–15 mg PO q 8 h **OR**
      Diltiazem slow release – 60 mg PO daily.
- **Hypertrophic obstructive cardiomyopathy (HOCM)** with presence of systolic anterior motion of the mitral valve and LV outflow obstruction ($LVOT_{max}$ <3.5 m/s).
  - **Normal** left atrial size – no therapy.
  - **Increased** left atrial size – beta-blocker as above.
- **Hypertrophic obstructive cardiomyopathy** (presence of systolic anterior motion of the mitral valve and LV outflow obstruction -$LVOT_{max}$ >3.5 m/s).
  - **Normal or increased** left atrial size – beta-blocker as above.

Treatment of the symptomatic cat with congestive heart failure (**acute management**).
Criteria to start therapy:
- Respiratory distress (open-mouth breathing or very abnormal respiratory pattern).
- Pulmonary congestion (moderate to severe) on radiographs and/or pleural effusion.
- Hypothermia.
  - Oxygen.
  - Diuretics
    - Furosemide 1–2 mg/kg IV or IM q 6–12 h until respiration rate and pattern are normalized.
    - Furosemide constant rate infusion (if normal renal values at presentation) 0.5–1 mg/kg/hr until congestion is resolved but not for longer than 24 hours.
  - Nitroglycerin ointment (2%) 1/4 of an inch (6 mm) q 8 h until resolution of the congestion.
  - Angiotensin-converting enzyme inhibitor.
    - Enalapril 0.25–0.5 mg/kg q 24 h **OR**
    - Benazepril 0.25–0.5 mg/kg q 24 h.
  - Thoracocentesis if there is evidence of moderate to severe pleural effusion on radiographs.

– Aspirate from the right thorax to avoid puncturing the enlarged auricles.
– Hypertrophic non-obstructive cardiomyopathy – use calcium channel blocker OR beta-blockers as above.
– Hypertrophic obstructive cardiomyopathy – use beta-blockers as above.

Symptomatic cat with congestive heart failure (**chronic management**).

Criteria to start therapy:

● Maintenance therapy after initial therapy to control signs of acute onset of congestive heart failure.
● Any patient found to have early evidence of congestive heart failure (usually on radiographs) but without symptoms, that will require acute intervention if untreated.

Hypertrophic non-obstructive cardiomyopathy – use calcium channel blocker or beta-blocker as above.

Hypertrophic obstructive cardiomyopathy – use beta-blocker as above.

Diuretics:

● Furosemide 1–2 mg/kg IV or IM q 6–12 h until respiration rate and pattern are normalized.
● Furosemide constant rate infusion (if normal renal values at presentation) 0.5–1 mg/kg/hr and congestion is resolved but not for longer than 24 hours.
● **Hydrochlorothiazide** 1–2 mg/kg PO q 12 h **OR/AND**
● **Spironolactone** 2–4 mg/kg PO q 12 h.

Angiotensin-converting enzyme inhibitor:

● **Enalapril** 0.25–0.5 mg/kg q 24 h **OR**
● **Benazepril** 0.25–0.5 mg/kg q 24 h.

Diuretics should be used cautiously in cats. Overzealous therapy for 1–2 days may rapidly result in severe fluid and electrolyte imbalances and **metabolic alkalosis**.

Judicious concurrent administration of **low-sodium solutions** (NaCl concentration $\leq 0.45\%$) with potassium supplementation may be required in some cases that are clinically dehydrated after diuretic therapy.

The volume of fluid administered varies with the degree of dehydration present, but in severe cases rates up to twice maintenance can be infused. While infusing fluids in a cardiac patient, special attention to respiratory function is recommended.

Potassium supplementation should be based on serum levels. Patients with normal potassium (3.5–5.5 mmol/L

[Meq/L]) should receive solutions with 20 mmol/L [Meq/L] added.

In cases of hypokalemia refer to standard guidelines of therapy. Do not exceed rates of potassium 0.5 mmol/L (Meq)/kg/h.

Chronic diuretic administration is **not required in some cases**. **Multiple diuretic therapy** can be used for refractory cases but monitor renal function and hydration carefully.

Renal function and electrolytes should be monitored in all cats on diuretics and angiotensin-converting enzyme inhibitor therapy.

Some cats develop **anorexia or poor appetite** while taking Diltiazem slow-release preparations.

Prognosis

Hypertrophic cardiomyopathy and hypertrophic obstructive cardiomyopathy ultimately result in congestive heart failure and/or aortic saddle thromboembolism. Sudden death occurs in some cases, usually in younger cats less than 3 years old.

Median survival time for cats without congestive heart failure is 732 days (over 33% alive after 5 years).

Median survival for cats with congestive heart failure is 92 days.

Median survival time for cats with thromboembolism is 61 days.

Heart rate less than 200 beats per minute at initial presentation is associated with longer survival (1830 days vs 152 days).

HYPERTHYROID HEART DISEASE***

Classical signs

● Weight loss.
● Polyphagia.
● Heart murmur.
● Tachycardia.

See main reference page 304 (The Cat With Weight Loss and a Good Appetite).

Clinical signs

Cats are usually older than 8 years of age (mean age is 13 years old) with no breed or sex predilection.

Typically there is progressive **weight loss** with a good appetite.

A heart murmur **is heard in some cases, and a gallop rhythm may be noticed.**

Tachycardia **is persistent even at rest. Many cats have heart rates above 240 bpm.**

Arrhythmias are present in more advanced cases.

A hyperkinetic peripheral pulse, **usually the femoral pulse, is very easy to palpate.**

Loud heart sounds and a strong precordial impulse are **typically present, which is the result of increased sympathetic tone and decreased fat deposits over the chest.**

Increased respiratory rate or panting is particularly seen in cats in a crisis (thyroid storm). This may be mistaken for respiratory distress when it is only hyperventilation.

Respiratory distress may occur secondary to heart failure when pulmonary edema and/or pleural effusion are present.

Cats are often difficult to handle and owners report a change in behavior (irritability and restlessness).

Polyuria, polydipsia and vomiting are seen in approximately 50% of the cases.

Palpable thyroid nodules are common.

Diagnosis

An **increased serum total thyroxine** (T_4) is usually diagnostic. The upper range of normal is 51 nmol/L (4.0 µg/dl).

A single random serum T_4 level is usually diagnostic.

If a random serum T_4 level does not confirm the disease in a highly suspected case, repeat serum T_4 or free T_4 in 1–2 weeks or perform a T_3 suppression test.

Radiographic findings

Heart size varies from normal to severe dilation of all chambers.

Pleural effusion and/or pulmonary edema may be present in severe cases.

Electrocardiographic findings

Sinus tachycardia (Heart rate > 220 bpm) is common. Increased R wave amplitude (>0.9 mV), supraventricular premature beats and ventricular arrhythmias are commonly found.

Echocardiographic findings

Heart chambers may be of normal size but in many cases, **some degree of ventricular concentric hypertrophy is present.** Interventricular septum and LV free wall measurements in diastole are greater than 6 mm.

The "typical" hyperthyroid heart shows mild to moderate increase in wall thickness (see above), upper range of normal ventricular chamber size (LV diastolic dimension 16–17 mm) and increased contractility (fractional shortening higher than 55%) reflecting hyperdynamic cardiac function.

Variable degrees of left atrial dilation are present.

In some cases (usually advanced cases), a dilated form of cardiomyopathy may be seen. It is difficult to differentiate from restrictive or dilated cardiomyopathy.

Systemic blood pressure

Hypertension is commonly found. Systolic arterial blood pressure, measured by Doppler technique, consistently **above 180 mmHg is diagnostic.**

Treatment

Antithyroid drugs (**Methimazole, Carbimazole**), **radioactive iodine** and **thyroidectomy** are treatment choices for hyperthyroidism (for further details refer to page 305).

Tachycardia and **hypertension** should be treated with beta-blocking drugs. This class of drugs controls the cardiovascular effects of hyperthyroidism and improves clinical signs.

Beta-blockers do not decrease serum thyroid hormones. Beta-blockade therapy is discontinued upon normalization of serum thyroid hormones and resolution of cardiovascular signs.
- **Propranolol** 0.5–1.0 mg/kg PO q 8 h **OR**
- **Atenolol** 12.5 mg/cat PO q 12 h.

If **congestive heart failure is present** refer to the section on hypertrophic cardiomyopathy for therapeutic options (page 128).

HYPERTENSIVE HEART DISEASE***

> ### Classical signs
>
> - **Heart murmur.**
> - **Gallop rhythm.**
> - **Tachycardia.**
> - **Blindness due to retinal hemorrhage or detachment.**
> - **Hyphema.**

Pathogenesis

Hypertension is defined as systemic arterial pressure **higher than 180/100 mmHg** (systolic/ diastolic).

Hypertension is most commonly **secondary** to an underlying etiology.
- The two most common causes in cats are **hyperthyroidism** and **chronic renal failure** (CRF).
- The **mechanism for development of hypertension** in **hyperthyroidism** is the increased number and sensitivity of **adrenergic receptors** coupled with an **increase in cardiac output.**
- The **mechanism for development of hypertension in CRF** is renal hypertension with retention of salt and activation of the renin-angiotensin aldosterone system.
- **The hypertension of hyperthyroidism is reversible** upon control of the thyroid state while the hypertension secondary to CRF requires continued therapy and monitoring.
- **There is no correlation between the degree of renal disease and the severity of hypertension**.
- **Essential hypertension** is an exclusion diagnosis when diagnostic tests failed to identify **a specific cause**.

Chronic untreated hypertension has several long-term adverse effects.

The increase in systemic vascular resistance results in increased afterload and **development of left ventricular hypertrophy.**

Chronic elevation of arterial pressure results in dysregulation of endothelial homeostasis leading to hypertensive vasculopathy.

- The vascular beds **most sensitive to chronic hypertension** are the ocular, renal, cerebrovascular and cardiac vessels.

Clinical signs

Signs directly related to the systemic hypertension **are not common**.

Ocular changes (retinal hemorrhages, hyphema, arterial tortuosity and retinal detachments) are the **most common** clinical signs seen in hypertensive cats.
- Most cats initially present for **blindness** secondary to retinal detachment and hemorrhages.
- Retinal examinations should be done in all cats diagnosed with systemic hypertension.
- Retinal examination is a good way to evaluate the organ damage resulting from systemic hypertension.

Weight loss, polyuria and polydipsia seen in hypertensive cats are secondary to the underlying disease (CRF or hyperthyroidism) and are not directly referable to the hypertension.

Seizures and syncope are **rare** neurological abnormalities seen in hyertensive cats.
- They are the results of cerebrovascular accidents from the hypertension.

Diagnosis

Retinal vascular changes with evidence of retinal hemorrhage and detached retinas **are commonly seen in hypertensive cats** on ocular examination.
- Indirect and direct ophthalmoscopy should be done on all hypertensive cats.
- Cats are **often presented blind** with **dilated non-responsive pupils**. Aged cats with a sudden onset of blindness should be evaluated for hypertension.
- Common findings are retinal hemorrhages, hyphema, retinal edema and partial or complete retinal detachments.

Elevated systemic arterial pressure (higher than 180 mmHg systolic pressure) is seen.

Hyperthyroidism or **chronic renal disease** are common underlying etiologies.
- Hyperthyroidism is diagnosed with an increased total thyroxine greater than 51 mmol/L (4 µg/dl) and

consistent clinical signs (weight loss, ravenous appetite, palpable thyroid nodules, polyuria, polydipsia).

- Chronic renal disease is diagnosed with an increased urea of greater than 11.6 mmol/L (32.5 mg/dl), increased creatinine greater than 163 µmol/L (1.84 mg/dl) with a decreased urine specific gravity less than 1.035.

Radiographic findings

Heart size varies from normal to marked generalized cardiomegaly.

Enlarged aortic arch is seen in chronic cases.

Undulation of the caudal aorta is suggestive of hypertension.

Electrocardiographic findings

Tachycardia with a heart rate greater than 220 bpm is usually present with hyperthyroidism.

Electrocardiogram is usually normal but evidence of left ventricular hypertrophy (R wave > 9 mm on lead II) may be seen.

Echocardiographic findings

Mild to moderate **left ventricular hypertrophy** may be seen. Left atrial size is usually normal.

Transmitral inflow velocity Doppler profile may show evidence of impaired relaxation (small E and tall A wave).

Enlarged aortic arch equal or greater than 11 mm is seen in chronic cases.

For findings in hyperthyroidism see page 132 (Hyperthyroid heart disease).

Differential diagnosis

Cats with either hypertension or cardiomyopathy commonly have murmurs.

- However, cats with hypertension **most commonly present with ocular signs.**
- **Most** hypertensive cats have polyuria, polydipsia or weight loss consistent with chronic renal disease or hyperthyroidism.

- **Cats with cardiomyopathy** usually do not have weight loss but may show dyspnea secondary to congestive heart failure.

Cats with **coagulopathy, optic neuritis, systemic infectious disease and neoplasia** may have similar ocular signs (retinal hemorrhages, hyphema and detached retinas) as hypertensive cats.

Documentation of hypertension is needed to **help differentiate** these diseases from hypertensive cats. Cerebrovascular accidents in cats with hypertension are **rare.**

Cats with cerebrovascular accidents are **usually secondary** to an underlying neurological disease.

Treatment

Beta-blockers – refer to page 306 on hyperthyroidism.

Amlodipine is the **drug of choice if the etiology is CRF or unknown**. The dose is 0.625 mg (cat < 5 kg) to 1.25 mg (cat ≥ 5 kg) orally once a day for hypertension caused by diseases other than hyperthyroidism.

ACE inhibitors (Enalapril or Benazepril) can be used as adjuvant therapy.
- ACE inhibitors can be used carefully in cases with concurrent chronic renal failure. Close follow-up of renal function is mandatory.
- If serum creatinine is higher than 265 µmol/L (3.0 mg/dl) at baseline, ACE inhibitors should not be used.
- Start at 0.25–0.5 mg/kg once a day for Benazepril OR Enalapril.
- Obtain baseline renal values and recheck at 5 and 10 days after starting medications.

In refractory cases, multiple drug therapy may be required (amlodipine, beta-blockers, diuretics, ACE inhibitors).

Low-salt diets may be used in refractory cases.

The **goal of therapy** is to decrease systolic blood pressure to **140–160 mmHg**.
- Drugs should be titrated to effect.

Prognosis

Hypertension caused by **hyperthyroidism is usually reversible** with normalization of the serum thyroid levels.

Hypertension caused by **other diseases requires long-term life-long management**.

RESTRICTIVE AND UNCLASSIFIED CARDIOMYOPATHIES**

> **Classical signs**
>
> - Heart murmur (in some cases may not be present).
> - Gallop rhythm.
> - Arrhythmia.
> - Dyspnea.
> - Hypothermia.
> - Collapse.
> - Lameness, paralysis or paresis from systemic thromboembolism.

Pathogenesis

Endocardial, **subendocardial and myocardial fibrosis** are the primary **pathologic characteristics** of **restrictive** cardiomyopathy. Myocardial fibrosis is also present in **intermediate/unclassified** cardiomyopathy. Geometrically the left ventricle may be normal or misshapen.

Histopathologically, **myocardial infarction** is reported to be a **feature of intermediate/ unclassified** cardiomyopathy, but it can also be seen in cases with restrictive cardiomyopathy.

Adhesions of papillary muscle and chordae tendinae may interfere with normal ventricular blood flow during systole, causing mid-ventricular obstruction. Mononuclear infiltration of the myocardium suggests an **inflammatory** process, resulting in endomyocarditis.

Left atrial (echocardiographic dimension > 13 mm), **biatrial** and right **ventricular** enlargement (maximal internal diameter > 7 mm) are often found. **Intracardiac thrombi** are frequently observed. **Infiltrative myocardial** disease may be present.

Hemodynamically this disease is **characterized by pure diastolic dysfunction** due to abnormally low compliance of the ventricular chambers. **Systolic function** is usually preserved or just slightly decreased.

Abnormal chamber compliance results in inadequate ventricular filling. The non-compliant ventricle rapidly reaches end-diastolic filling pressure typically during the first half of the diastolic phase.

Chronic **diastolic** dysfunction leads to the progressive development of **increased left atrial** size and secondary increase in left **atrial pressures** resulting in **pulmonary venous** congestion, **pulmonary edema** and in advanced cases **pulmonary artery hypertension**.

Chronic **pulmonary artery hypertension** will result in **right-sided** congestive heart failure.

Classification of these forms of cardiomyopathies is poorly defined.

Clinically it is difficult to distinguish between restrictive and unclassified forms of cardiomyopathy.

Clinical signs

There is no age or sex predilection.

Burmese cats seem to have a higher incidence of restrictive cardiomyopathy.

Heart murmur is often present but in some cases may not be present. When present, a systolic murmur varies in location and intensity with variations in heart rate.

Gallop rhythm is commonly heard. It is identified when more than two heart sounds are present on auscultation.

Arrhythmias are frequently heard as premature heart beats with pulse deficits. Ventricular arrhythmias are most common.

Dyspnea is seen in symptomatic cats with an increased respiratory rate (greater than 30 breaths/min) at rest or with open-mouth breathing in extreme cases.

In symptomatic cats, hypothermia is common.

Collapse may result from impaired cardiac output (ventricular tachycardia).

Lameness, paralysis or paresis is usually the result of systemic thromboembolism. Aortic saddle thrombosis resulting in hindlimb paralysis may be seen. In some cases, embolism may only cause lameness.

Most cats with aortic saddle thrombosis present for acute onset of hindlimb paralysis, pain, absent femoral pulses, cool extremities and cyanosis of the nail bed. In some cases a history of episodic lameness is given.

Diagnosis

Usually a history of **heart murmur, arrhythmia, collapse or respiratory distress** is present. Some cats may not have an audible murmur but a gallop rhythm is commonly heard.

Diagnosis is based on supportive radiographic, electrocardiographic and especially echocardiographic findings.

Radiographic findings

Severe **left atrial** or **biatrial** enlargement.

Enlarged pulmonary veins can be seen.

Pulmonary edema with or without **pleural effusion** may be present.

Electrocardiographic findings

Ventricular arrhythmias are more **common** than with other types of feline myocardial disease.

Atrial fibrillation is more common than with HCM; and if present is usually associated with **extreme dilatation of the left** and/or right atria.

Tachycardia (heart rate above 220), ventricular conduction disturbances (notched QRS), tall R waves on lead II (>0.9 mV) may be seen.

Echocardiographic findings

Severe left atrial or biatrial enlargement is commonly found. Left atrial to aortic ratio is usually >2.0.

Left ventricular size may be normal to mildly dilated (LV end-diastolic dimension up to or above 16 mm).

Systolic function is normal or mildly decreased (normal FS is between 35–55%)

Right ventricular dilatation may be seen (RV end-diastolic dimension > 7 mm)

Hyperechoic endocardium and/or myocardium are frequently observed.

Focal areas of myocardial hypertrophy bordering areas of **myocardial thinning** are seen which probably represent myocardial **infarction**.

The **mitral inflow profile** is recorded at the tips of the mitral valve from the four-chamber left parasternal view. It commonly shows increased early inflow velocity (E wave > 1.1 m/s) and normal or decreased atrial flow component.

Thrombi (homogeneous mass) in the left atrium and/or ventricle may be found.

Differential diagnoses

Congenital heart disease.
- A murmur is usually present from birth. Most congenital murmurs do not change in loudness with alterations of the heart rate. Congenital murmurs are usually relatively loud.

Dilated cardiomyopathy.
- Murmurs are usually very soft, and in many cases may not be present. A gallop rhythm is usually present.

Hypertrophic cardiomyopathy.
- It is difficult to differentiate on auscultation from restrictive or intermediate/unclassified cardiomyopathy. A gallop rhythm may be more common in restrictive or intermediate/unclassified cardiomyopathies.

Intrathoracic masses.
- A murmur may not be present unless there is compression of the heart by the mass or concurrent unrelated heart disease. Most commonly, dyspnea and lethargy are seen.

Feline asthma or chronic bronchitis.
- Unless cardiac disease is also present, most cats do not have a murmur. Cough and increased respiratory rate are common. Symptoms may be seasonal.

Chylous effusion.
- A murmur may not be present. In most cases, cardiac disease is not present. The most common clinical sign is dyspnea, increased respiratory rate and lethargy.

Neurological disease causing collapse or hindlimb paralysis.
- Cardiac signs are usually absent, however a full cardiac work-up may be warranted to rule out the presence of silent heart disease. Neurological disease usually is not associated with alterations of peripheral systemic perfusion.

Treatment

Asymptomatic cat.
- Angiotensin-converting enzyme inhibitors

- **Enalapril** 0.5 mg/kg PO q 24 h **OR**
- **Benazepril** 0.5 mg/kg PO q 24 h.

Symptomatic cat with congestive heart failure (acute management). Criteria to start therapy:
- Respiratory distress (open-mouth breathing or very abnormal respiratory pattern).
- Pulmonary congestion (moderate to severe) on radiographs and/or pleural effusion.
- Hypothermia.
- **Oxygen.**
- Diuretics.*
  - **Furosemide** 1–2 mg/kg IV or IM q 8–12 h until respiratory rate and pattern are normalized.
  - Furosemide constant rate infusion (if normal renal values at presentation) 0.5–1 mg/kg/hr until congestion is resolved but not for longer than 24 hours.
- Venodilator.
  - **Nitroglycerin** ointment (2%) 1/4 of an inch (6 mm) q 8 h.
- **Thoracocentesis (right thorax** to avoid puncturing of the enlarged auricles) if there is evidence of moderate to severe pleural effusion on radiographs.
- Angiotensin-converting enzyme inhibitor.
  - **Enalapril** 0.25–0.5 mg/kg PO q 24 h **OR**
  - **Benazepril** 0.25–0.5 mg/kg PO q 24 h.

Symptomatic cat with congestive heart failure (chronic management). Criteria to start therapy:
- Maintenance therapy after initial therapy to control signs of acute congestive heart failure.
- Any patient found to have early evidence of congestive heart failure (usually on radiographs) but without symptoms, that will require acute intervention if untreated.
- Diuretics*
  - **Furosemide** 0.5–1.0 mg/kg PO q 12–24 h **OR**
  - **Hydrochlorothiazide** 1–2 mg/kg PO q 12 h **OR/AND**
  - **Spironolactone** 2–4 mg/kg PO q 12 h.
- Angiotensin-converting enzyme inhibitor
  - **Enalapril** 0.25–0.5 mg/kg PO q 24 h **OR**
  - **Benazepril** 0.25–0.5 mg/kg PO q 24 h.
- Arrhythmia control
  - **Sotalol** 15–30 mg/cat PO q 8 h **OR**
  - **Propranolol** 0.5–1.0 mg/kg PO q 8 h **OR**
  - **Atenolol** 12.5 mg/cat PO q 12–24 h **OR**
  - **Diltiazem** 15 mg/cat PO q 8 h.
- Associated intracardiac thrombus or systemic thromboembolism.

- Anti-thrombotic therapy:
  - **Heparin** and **Warfarin** therapy are controversial and should be utilized under the guidance of an experienced clinician.
  - **Low-molecular-weight heparins** have been recently suggested. This class of heparins does not require continued monitoring of coagulation parameters.
  - **Enoxaparin** (Lovenox ®) 1 mg/kg SQ q 24 h.
  - **Aspirin** 80 mg PO q 48–72 h is recommended by some clinicians but its efficacy has not been established. A lower dose (5 mg/cat PO q 24 h) has also been recommended, because of concerns of that prostacyclin production is inhibited at the higher dose.

Thrombolytic therapy is contraindicated if an intracardiac thrombus is present, and controversial in aortic saddle thrombus (see page 916, The Weak and Ataxic or Paralyzed Cat).

Prognosis

Almost **all cats after** development of congestive heart failure **have a poor prognosis.**

It is unknown if early therapy **of asymptomatic cats results in delay of onset of clinical signs.**

NEOPLASIA**

> **Classical signs**
>
> - Anorexia.
> - Weight loss.

Clinical signs

Cats commonly present with anorexia and secondary weight loss.

A cranial mediastinal mass may cause a **non-compliant chest wall during compressive palpation**.

The presence of intrathoracic or pericardial masses may cause **effusions** which will result in **muffled heart sounds** or displaced lung and/or heart sounds.

If a mass compresses the heart, a new murmur can result.

Some cats with pericardial effusion secondary to neoplasia present for the evaluation of **ascites**.

Diagnosis

Radiographic findings

Soft tissue density seen within the cranial mediastinum.

Elevated trachea.

Pleural effusion.

Electrocardiographic findings

Normal.

Echocardiographic findings

Normal cardiac function unless concurrent heart disease is present.

A cardiac mass may be seen (rare).

Ultrasound of the cranial mediastinum may reveal a mass.

Pleural effusion may be seen.

HIGH CARDIAC OUTPUT HEART DISEASE*

Classical signs

- Heart murmur.
- Gallop rhythm.
- Tachycardia.

Pathogenesis

High cardiac output heart disease in cats is secondary to hyperthyroidism or chronic anemia.

High cardiac output heart disease is uncommon.

Etiologies of chronic anemia are infectious (feline leukemia virus, feline immunodeficiency virus), neoplastic (lymphoma, thymoma), and metabolic diseases (chronic renal failure). Refer to page 526, (The Anemic Cat) for a more detailed description of anemia.

In chronic anemia, increased cardiac output results from decreased blood viscosity and systemic arteriolar tone augmenting stroke volume.

Anemia causes high cardiac output, which increases cardiac work and results in congestive heart failure when a co-existing cardiac disease or a hyperkinetic state is present.

In chronic anemia, the heart rate may be normal or only mildly increased.

For hyperthyroid heart disease refer to page 131.

Clinical signs

A systolic blowing murmur louder at the heart base is usually present.

A gallop rhythm may be present.

Sinus tachycardia is usually present, with heart rates above 220 bpm.

Displaced and/or muffled heart sounds are heard secondary to intrathoracic masses displacing the heart. In some cases, this finding may be due to the presence of pleural effusion.

Other systemic signs:
- Pale mucus membranes, prolonged capillary refill time, petechiae, anorexia, ravenous appetite, weight loss and palpable thyroid glands bilaterally.

Diagnosis

Anemia is present if the hematocrit is less than 0.24 L/L (PCV = 24%).

Secondary cardiac changes are not usually present unless a chronic anemia with a hematocrit less than 0.15 L/L (PCV ≤ 15%) is present.

Hyperthyroidism is considered present if total thyroxine is increased and there are consistent clinical signs. Refer to page 304 (The Cat With Weight Loss and a Good Appetite).

Radiographic findings

Heart size ranges from normal to severe enlargement.

Pulmonary edema may be present in rare cases.

Electrocardiographic findings

Tachycardia (>220 bpm) and increased R wave amplitude in lead II (>0.9 mV).

Echocardiographic findings

In **anemia,** a normal to moderate increase in left ventricular dimension (LVIDd > 18 mm) with hyperkinetic (FS > 55%) cardiac function is found. Left atrial size is usually normal to mildly increased.

In rare cases, findings similar to dilated cardiomyopathy are present.

Refer to page 132 for echocardiographic findings in hyperthyroidism.

Differential diagnosis

Cardiomyopathy.

Hyperthyroidism.

Treatment

Treatment should be directed towards the underlying disease.

Refer to page 305 (The Cat With Weight Loss and a Good Appetite) for hyperthyroidism and page 526 (The Anemic Cat) for anemia.

If congestive heart failure is present, with concurrent myocardial failure refer to section on dilated cardiomyopathy, page 151.

If congestive heart failure is present without myocardial failure refer to section on hypertrophic cardiomyopathy, page 128.

Prognosis

Varies depending on disease process.

CHYLOUS EFFUSION*

Classical signs

- Dyspnea/tachypnea.
- Anorexia.
- Lethargy.

See main reference page 77 (The Cat With Hydrothorax).

Clinical signs

Chylous effusion in cats is often of **unknown cause**. The **most common causes are right heart failure** from cardiomyopathy or heartworm or mediastinal neoplasia associated with lymphoma or thymoma. Chylothorax may occur secondary to a thrombus associated with an indwelling **jugular catheter**.

Dyspnea and tachypnea are common presenting clinical signs. Commonly an abdominal respiratory component is seen.

The presence of chest fluid results in muffled heart sounds and absent lung sounds in the ventral thorax.

Cats develop **poor appetite** when a large amount of fluid is present (> ~150 ml).

Cats with symptoms may show **open-mouth breathing and/or cyanosis** after mild to moderate exercise.

Diagnosis

Thoracocentesis findings

Aspiration of the chest fluid commonly yields a milky white fluid (can be slightly pink). This fluid may feel greasy.

Determination of fluid triglyceride level with a paired serum triglyceride sample (obtained at the same time) always reveals a **higher triglyceride level** in the chest fluid.

Cytological evaluation usually reveals a homogeneous population of **mature lymphocytes** and **neutrophils**.

Bacterial culture is negative.

Radiographic findings

Marked pleural effusion.

Elevated trachea.

Obscured cardiac silhouette.

Collapsed lung lobes.

Electrocardiographic findings

Normal.

Abnormalities may be seen if there is concurrent heart disease.

Echocardiographic findings

Many cats have a normal echocardiogram.

In some cases, chylous effusion may be secondary to severe heart disease of any etiology.

HEARTWORM DISEASE*

Classical signs

- Respiratory distress.
- Coughing.
- Vomiting.
- Sudden death.

Clinical signs

Many cats are asymptomatic.

Sudden death is seen in some cases.

Vomiting, lethargy, anorexia and syncope are seen in symptomatic cases.

Respiratory signs such as **cough or dyspnea** are common.

Respiratory signs may be quite **similar to feline chronic bronchitis or asthma.**

Some cats can present for evaluation of pneumothorax/chylothorax.

Occasionally aberrant larval migration results in neurological signs such as seizures, collapse, blindness and vestibular signs.

See main reference page 104 (The Coughing Cat).

Diagnosis

Radiographic findings

Enlarged and tortuous caudal pulmonary arteries are visible on both projections of the chest, but especially the DV/VD views.

Diffuse pulmonary infiltrates characterized by a mixed interstitial and peribronchial pattern.

Electrocardiographic findings

The ECG is generally not useful in diagnosis of feline heartworm disease.

Sinus tachycardia (HR > 220 bpm)

Right heart enlargement in advanced cases. The MEA is usually beyond +180 degrees clockwise.

Echocardiographic findings

Main pulmonary artery may be normal or enlarged.

Linear parallel densities may present in the main pulmonary artery or the main branches.

Dilatation of the right ventricle is seen in advanced cases; RV internal dimension in diastole > 6 mm.

Echocardiography has high specificity for the diagnosis of feline heartworm disease, but sensitivity is highly dependent on the experience of the ultrasonographer.

Cardiac catheterization findings

Non-selective angiography may show:
- Linear filling defects within the pulmonary arterial tree.
- Dilated and tortuous pulmonary arteries.
- Dilated right ventricle.

Blood examination and serologic findings

Microfilaremia is rare in cats and transient (possibly about 1 month). If present, the number of microfilaria is small.

Serologic testing should include both an **antibody and antigen test.**

A positive antibody test is consistent with exposure with or without current infestation. It is a useful screening test and cats with a positive test should be followed up with antigen test.

A **positive antigen test** may be consistent with current infestation. The sensitivity of the current antigen tests is considerably less than the antibody test.

Combining results from serum Ab and Ag tests achieves higher sensitivities than using serum Ab and Ag test results alone.

Negative serologic findings do not absolutely rule out heartworm infestation. If clinical signs are compatible, repeat Ab and Ag testing by a different method, **evaluate chest radiographs and consider echocardiographic examination**.

Treatment

Adulticide treatment is not usually recommended in cats because of severe side effects. Infestation is small (1–2 worms) and their lifespan is short (average 2 years).

Surgical removal of the worms through a jugular approach can be attempted in severe cases.

Medical treatment is mainly symptomatic.

VENTRICULAR SEPTAL DEFECT*

> ### Classical signs
> - **Systolic murmur** loudest over the right sternal border.

Pathogenesis

The shunting of blood depends on the size of the defect and the relative resistance of the systemic and pulmonary circulations.

- **Normally, shunting occurs from the left to the right**, unless right heart pressures rise above systemic pressures causing reversal of shunting of blood flow.

In most cases, the defect is present in the **perimembranous area of the interventricular septum**, immediately below the aortic valve annulus.
- The right ventricular location of the defect is commonly situated below the septal leaflet of the tricuspid valve, but can also be located in other areas of the perimembranous septum.
- Primary muscular defects of the septum are rare.

With small defects, the amount of blood being shunted is small and unlikely to create volume overload of the pulmonary circulation and the left heart.
- However, with large defects different degrees of volume overload can be expected, depending on the shunt fraction.
- In some cases chronic volume overload may lead to the development of **left-sided congestive heart failure.**
- In rare instances, chronic volume overload of the pulmonary circulation may result in increased pulmonary vascular resistance with significant elevation of right ventricular systolic pressures that may result in **reversal of the direction of shunting (Eisenmenger's syndrome).**
- Large defects can result in abnormal morphology of the aortic valve annulus leading to aortic valve prolapse and variable degrees of aortic insufficiency.

Clinical signs

No sex or breed predilection is reported and it is seen usually in cats less than 1 year old.

Systolic murmur is heard over the right sternal border **(the louder the murmur the smaller the VSD).**

In many cases, a **thrill** is felt over the right sternal border.

Most cases are **asymptomatic.**

Tachypnea and/or dyspnea may be a clinical complaint.

The **femoral pulses** are normal.

Bounding pulses occur in cases with significant aortic insufficiency (usually with large VSDs).

Diagnosis

Congenital systolic ejection murmur is heard over the right sternal border in a young cat.

VSD is the most **common cause** of a congenital murmur in the cat.

Radiographic findings

Pulmonary over-circulation demonstrated by a prominent and enlarged vasculature of the lungs.

Left atrium and ventricular dilation with variable degrees of right ventricular enlargement can be seen.

Echocardiographic findings

Most defects are not visualized except for large ones.

Demonstration of shunting and direction of blood flow across the interventricular septum is possible using Doppler technique.

Left atrial and ventricular dilation may be present.

High-velocity flow across the pulmonic valve may be found (relative stenosis due to high volume if large shunting fraction is present). Usually maximal blood flow velocity obtained with continuous flow Doppler is higher than 1.8 m/s.

In severe cases, right ventricular dilation is observed.

If shunting from right to left, an injection of saline from a peripheral systemic vein will demonstrate "bubbles" traveling from the right ventricle to the left ventricle and/or aorta.

In large defects, aortic insufficiency is commonly found.

Cardiac catheterization

Left ventricular injection with angiographic contrast shows shunting of blood from the left ventricle to right ventricle.

If direction of shunting is right to left, a right ventricular injection of contrast shows shunting to the left ventricle.

Increase in oxygen saturation equal to or above 5% from the right atrium to the right ventricle is diagnostic for a left to right ventricular septal defect.

Differential diagnosis

Cardiomyopathy is uncommon in young cats. **Cardiomyopathy murmurs are usually not as loud**. Cardiomyopathy murmurs may sound different with serial auscultations.

In pulmonic or aortic stenosis, the murmur is usually **louder on the left cranial thorax** and its character is harsher than a VSD murmur.

In tricuspid valve dysplasia, the murmur is usually lower frequency and a thrill is uncommon.

In tetralogy of Fallot, peripheral cyanosis may be present; the murmur is similar to the murmur of pulmonic stenosis.

Treatment

Treatment is not required in most cases.

Pulmonary arterial banding should be considered in cases where severe volume overload of the left heart is evident.

If signs of congestive heart failure are present refer to hypertrophic cardiomyopathy section for treatment detail (page 130).

Prognosis

The prognosis is good in most cases, unless congestive heart failure is present at the time of presentation.

Most cats have a normal lifespan.

PATENT DUCTUS ARTERIOSUS

Classical signs

- Continuous murmur **is heard loudest over the left cranial thorax.**
- Palpable thrill, which may be present bilaterally.
- Bounding arterial pulses.
- Strong precordial impulse.
- Signs of left-sided heart failure may be present (respiratory distress, tachypnea, crackles).

Pathogenesis

The ductus arteriosus should normally close within the first 72 hours of life. **Failure of the ductus arteriosus** to close will maintain a **patent ductus** and allow for shunting between the aorta and pulmonary artery and is called a patent ductus arteriosus (PDA).

The **most common** direction of shunting is **left to right** (aorta to pulmonary artery).

The amount of blood being shunted is **proportional to the size of the ductus**.

Volume overload of the pulmonary circulation and the left heart may be present and ultimately lead to the development of congestive heart failure.

Chronic overload of the left atrium and ventricle results in progressive dilatation of these chambers, and increased left ventricular filling pressures.

Ventricular dilatation causes changes in geometry of the left ventricle and results in functional mitral regurgitation.

Typically, systolic **arterial pressures are increased** due to the increased stroke volume and **diastolic pressures are lower** than normal explaining the bounding pulse.

In some cases, it is believed that **chronic volume overload of the pulmonary circulation** results in vascular changes, which **increase pulmonary vascular resistance.**

If **pulmonary vascular resistance is elevated** above systemic vascular resistance, the direction of **shunting of blood is right to left** (pulmonary artery to aorta) resulting in **lower arterial oxygen content** and an **increase in red blood cell numbers (polycythemia).**

Systemic hypoxemia results in signs of dyspnea, panting and decreased energy, which may be followed by collapse.

Right to left shunting is uncommon.

Clinical signs

No breed or sex predilection is seen. Cats at presentation are usually less than 1 year of age.

No symptoms are present in 1/3 of the cases at initial presentation.

Cats are usually presented for **abnormal respiration** (29%), **lethargy** (24%) and **stunted growth** (14%).

A continuous murmur is located over the heart base in 71% of the cases. The other 29% have systolic murmurs only.

Bounding arterial pulses are commonly found.

A strong precordial impulse is commonly found and results from the cardiomegaly.

Arrhythmias can be found in severe cases.

Faint diastolic murmur or no murmur is present in right to left PDAs.

Polycythemia with PCV exceeding 65% may be found in right to left PDA.

Concurrent cardiac defects are found in 29% of the cases.

Diagnosis

Left to right shunt:
- Congenital **continuous murmur** is heard with bounding arterial pulses.

Radiographic findings

Left atrial and ventricular enlargement can be seen.

Large pulmonary vessels suggesting over-circulation can be seen.

Enlarged main pulmonary artery and aortic arch can be seen.

Pulmonary edema may be present in complicated cases.

Electrocardiography

Left ventricular hypertrophy (R wave in lead II > 0.9 mV) is common.

Left atrial enlargement (P wave > 40 ms) can be seen.

Tachycardia can be seen.

Arrhythmias are uncommon.

Echocardiographic findings

Left heart enlargement (LVIDd > 18 mm), hyperkinetic left ventricular function (FS > 55%), enlarged main pulmonary artery (MPA > 10 mm) and aortic arch are seen.

Doppler shows **persistent flow of blood within the main pulmonary artery** through all phases of the cardiac cycle.

Mitral regurgitation may be present.

A small amount of aortic insufficiency may be seen.

Diagnosis

Right to left shunt.
- These cases are rare.
- There is a history of a loud murmur that resolved or is only diastolic now.
- A loud second heart sound, which may be split, may be heard.
- Lethargy, dyspnea and/or collapse are common.

Radiographic findings

Generalized cardiomegaly with a large main pulmonary artery is seen.

Pulmonary over-circulation is not seen with a right to left shunt.

Electrocardiographic findings

Right heart enlargement pattern (right axis deviation) is seen.

Echocardiographic findings

Right ventricular hypertrophy is seen (RVIDd > 6 mm and RVFWd > 3 mm).

Left heart enlargement (LVIDd > 18mm) may also be present.

Doppler flow across PDA from right to left or bi-directional flow can be seen.

Differential diagnosis

Aorticopulmonary window can only be differentiated by echocardiographic study; continuous blood flow with shunting between the aorta and MPA is seen at the level of the aortic root.

Truncus arteriosus can be differentiated by echocardiography; a common large outlet for the left and right ventricles is seen.

Pulmonary arteriovenous fistula will produce similar hemodynamic abnormalities as a left to right PDA but the flow within the main pulmonary artery is normal.

Treatment

Surgery is curative for left to right PDA. The success rate of surgery is 85% when performed by an experienced surgeon.

- Surgery should be accomplished as soon as the patient is a good anesthetic risk.
- If heart failure is present, a period of stabilization prior to surgery is required.
- See treatment for HCM (page 130) for therapy of heart failure.
- **Surgery is contraindicated** in right to left shunts. Treatment is mainly palliative.
- If clinical signs of lethargy, tachypnea and/or collapse are present and if the **packed cell volume is above 60–65%** periodic phlebotomy is indicated. Phlebotomy decreases blood viscosity and improves peripheral perfusion. The presence of clinical signs alone is an indication for phlebotomy.
- If there are signs of right-side heart failure, diuretics will be necessary.
- Rest is recommended.

Prognosis

Left to right PDA.
- Prognosis is good for long-term survival after surgical correction.
- Even in animals presented in heart failure, successful correction of the PDA results in resolution of signs. A normal life expectancy is seen in most of these cases.
- Right to left PDA.
  - **Prognosis is poor for long-term survival**, however many cats can still live for several years with minimal symptoms.

ATRIAL SEPTAL DEFECT

Classical signs

- Soft **systolic murmur** is heard over the left heart base and may radiate to the apex.
- **Dyspnea.**
- **Collapse.**

Pathogenesis

Left to right shunting occurs through the atrial septal defect.

In the absence of significant **mitral regurgitation,** the **shunt fraction** is small and animals may not have any symptoms. With increased amounts of mitral regurgita-

tion, the shunt fraction increases and if significant, **volume overload** of the right and left heart is present.

Mitral regurgitation may occur secondary to left heart volume overload or congenital abnormalities of the formation of the valve.

Kittens with severe disease develop left-sided **congestive heart failure** by 6 weeks of age.

Clinical signs

Signs depend on the degree of **shunt fraction.**

Most cats are **asymptomatic.**

At the left heart base, a soft **systolic ejection murmur** is heard. It is often also heard on the right side of the chest.

Signs of **increased respiratory rate, dyspnea or collapse** may be seen while playing.

Stunted growth is seen in severe cases.

Some cases present with **ascites**, suggesting right-side heart failure.

Diagnosis

Congenital murmur is found over the left heart base. The murmur is systolic and usually soft.

Radiographic findings

Pulmonary over-circulation demonstrated by a prominent and enlarged vasculature of the lungs.

Areas of focal alveolar densities representing **pulmonary edema** may be found.

Generalized cardiomegaly.

Electrocardiographic findings

Sinus tachycardia (HR > 220 bpm) if heart failure is present

Evidence of left ventricular hypertrophy with a tall R wave in lead II (> 0.9 mV)

In cases where the defect may interrupt or deviate the His bundle, notching and prolongation of the QRS may be seen.

Echocardiographic findings

Echocardiographic evidence of an atrial septal defect is seen as **echo drop out** at the regions of the interatrial septum.

It is important to note that due to the thickness of the septum in a normal heart, many times there is the illusion of an echo drop out. Multiple views must be obtained to reach a diagnosis.

Doppler confirmation of left-to-right shunting is documented across the atrial septal defect.

Doppler study may show variable degrees of mitral regurgitation.

Relative pulmonic stenosis (blood flow velocity > 2.0 m/s) secondary to increased volume of blood may be seen with significant shunt fractions.

In severe cases, biatrial and bi-ventricular enlargement can be seen.

Cardiac catheterization

A catheter can be passed across the interatrial septum into the left atria and ventricle.

An increase greater than 5% in oxygen saturation at the level of the right atrium when compared with blood from the caudal vena cava is indicative of an atrial septal defect with left-to-right shunting.

Angiographic contrast study from the left atria will show shunting of blood into the right heart with opacification of the right atria and ventricle.

Differential diagnosis

Cardiomyopathy is uncommon in young cats. Cardiomyopathy murmurs are usually not as loud. Cardiomyopathy murmurs may sound different with serial auscultations.

Ventricular septal defects usually have a louder murmur on the right sternal border and the character is harsher.

Mitral valve dysplasia occurs with a murmur louder at the apex, in some cases a diastolic murmur may be present if there is significant mitral stenosis.

Pulmonic or aortic stenosis present with louder and harsher murmurs than atrial septal defects.

Treatment

Many cases are asymptomatic and there is no need for therapy.

Definitive therapy requires surgical repair, which is very difficult to accomplish in veterinary medicine.

If the patient is in congestive heart failure, refer to hypertrophic cardiomyopathy section (page 130) for treatment details.

Prognosis

Prognosis is good in most cases, but it depends on the degree of shunt fraction, which is dependent on the degree of mitral regurgitation present.

Many cats have a normal lifespan.

MITRAL VALVE DYSPLASIA/STENOSIS

> ### Classical signs
> - Systolic and/or diastolic murmur is heard over the left apex.
> - Dyspnea.
> - Thromboembolic disease

Pathogenesis

Congenital mitral valve malformation will result in poor coaptation of its leaflets and secondary regurgitation.

In some cases, the mitral valve is thick and misshapen with restricted motility during diastole, causing impaired blood flow from the left atrium to the left ventricle.

In some cases, more than two leaflets may be present. Most commonly, the anterior leaflet may be subdivided and it is called a cleft mitral valve.

Clinical signs

A heart murmur is heard loudest over the left heart apex and is present from a young age.

Dyspnea or respiratory distress occur if congestive heart failure is present.

Signs of **increased respiratory rate, dyspnea or collapse** may be seen while playing.

Lameness, paralysis or paresis may result from systemic thromboembolism.

Atrial arrhythmias may be present if there is severe left atrial enlargement. Atrial premature contractions, paroxysmal atrial tachycardia or atrial fibrillation can be seen.

Diagnosis

Radiographic findings

Marked left atrium enlargement is seen, as demonstrated by elevation of the carina and bulging of the caudal atrial wall on the lateral view. A valentine-shaped heart may be seen on the V/D view.

Pulmonary venous congestion defined by a larger pulmonary vein than the accompanying artery, with or without **pulmonary edema** may be present.

Left ventricular enlargement is seen with the cardiac silhouette larger than two intercostal spaces on the lateral view, secondary to severe mitral valve regurgitation.

Electrocardiographic findings

Left ventricular hypertrophy demonstrated by a **tall R wave in lead II** (> 0.9 mV).

Sinus tachycardia (HR > 220 bpm) if heart failure is present.

Some cases may have **atrial premature contractions** or paroxysmal atrial tachycardia. If **atrial fibrillation** is present, there is invariably severe left atrial enlargement.

Echocardiographic findings

A thick and misshapen mitral valve is seen which may have poor motility during diastole.

Systolic anterior motion of the mitral valve may be seen (anterior displacement into the left ventricular outflow of the anterior mitral valve leaflet causing outflow obstruction).

Variable degrees of mitral regurgitation are found on Doppler study.

Determination of the mitral valve inflow velocity profile is essential to determine the presence and degree of mitral stenosis.
- The early diastolic wave (E wave) of mitral inflow shows delayed deceleration of blood flow in mid-diastole, and there is fusion with the atrial diastolic wave (A wave). This results in an M-shaped mitral inflow profile or in severe cases a rectangular shape.

Secondary **left atrial enlargement** occurs with the left atrial to aortic ratio usually > 2.0. Left atrial enlargement is either secondary to restriction of filling of the left ventricle by a stenotic valve or because of severe regurgitation.

In cases with **severe mitral regurgitation,** secondary **left ventricular enlargement** (LV end-diastolic dimension >17 mm) is usually seen.

Severe mitral regurgitation and stenosis do not necessarily have to co-exist in the same patient.

Differential diagnosis

Cardiomyopathy is uncommon in young cats. Cardiomyopathy murmurs are usually not as loud. Cardiomyopathy murmurs may sound different with serial auscultations.

Pulmonic or aortic stenosis is present with louder and harsher murmurs than mitral valve dysplasia/ stenosis.

Atrial septal defects usually have soft murmur present at the left heart base.

Differential diagnosis solely based on physical exam may be difficult.

Treatment

Many cases are asymptomatic and there is no need for therapy.

If the patient is in congestive heart failure, refer to the hypertrophic cardiomyopathy section (page 130) for treatment details.

Prognosis

Prognosis is good in most cases. Cats with marked mitral regurgitation may only develop symptoms of congestive heart failure between 5–10 years of age.

Patients with severe regurgitation may present in congestive heart failure within the first year of life.

Prognosis is worse with the presence of co-existent thromboembolic disease.

AORTIC STENOSIS

> **Classical signs**
> - Systolic murmur is heard over the left heart base or over the cranial aspect of the sternum.

Pathogenesis

With congenital valvular malformation of the aortic valve, there is **thickening of the valve leaflets and** poor motility during systole, resulting in fixed obstruction of outflow of blood. In some cases, supravalvular or subvalvular stenosis may be found.

Secondary left ventricular hypertrophy may develop. The degree of hypertrophy is directly dependent on the severity of the stenosis. Valvular gradients above 100 mmHg are classified as severe.

Clinical signs

A systolic murmur is heard over the left heart base or over the cranial aspect of the sternum.

Most cats are asymptomatic. Most common symptoms in severe cases are exercise intolerance and syncope.

If severe, in the first 1–2 years of life, cats may die suddenly or develop congestive heart failure.

Diagnosis

Radiographic findings

There is widening of the cranial mediastinum as a result of **post-stenotic dilation of the aortic arch**. This is evident on both views (dorsoventral view and lateral view).

Left ventricular enlargement with elongation of the left heart occurs secondary to hypertrophy.

If congestive heart failure is present, pulmonary venous distention (pulmonary vein larger than accompanying pulmonary artery) and evidence of pulmonary edema may be seen (focal areas of marked interstitial or alveolar densities).

Electrocardiographic findings

The electrocardiogram may be normal or have evidence of left ventricular hypertrophy with a tall R wave in lead II (> 0.9 mV).

Left axis deviation and/or left fascicular anterior block may be present.

Ventricular arrhythmias may be present, but are not common.

Echocardiographic findings

Left ventricular hypertrophy is seen (diastolic dimension of the interventricular septum and/or LV posterior wall greater than 6 mm).

If valvular stenosis is present, the valve appears thick and has restricted opening.

A subvalvular or supravalvular fibrous ridge may be identified.

In some cases, left atrial enlargement may be present.

Doppler study of the left ventricular outflow reveals **increased velocity of blood flow (> 2.0 m/s)**.

Cardiac catheterization findings

Cardiac catheterization is not routinely done, since the introduction of echocardiography.

Injection of contrast in the left ventricle will show:
- Left ventricular hypertrophy.
- Narrow left ventricular outflow.
- Filling defect at the aortic valve level (due to a thickened valve).
- Post-stenotic dilatation of the aortic arch.
- Subvalvular or supravalvular filling defects may be seen.

Differential diagnosis

Hypertrophic obstructive cardiomyopathy (HOCM) differs from aortic stenosis in the location and pathophysiology of the stenosis. With HOCM the stenosis is dynamic (changes with heart rate) while in aortic stenosis the obstruction to blood flow is fixed.

Treatment

In mild and moderate cases (Doppler-derived pressure gradient less than 100 mmHg and asymptomatic), there is no benefit from medical therapy.

In cases complicated with ventricular arrhythmias and/or left ventricular concentric hypertrophy, beta-blockers may reduce the likelihood of sudden death and/or collapse. Refer to section in hypertrophic cardiomyopathy (page 130).

If congestive heart failure is present, refer to hypertrophic cardiomyopathy section (page 130).

Caution with the use of angiotensin-converting enzyme inhibitors, which may increase the pressure gradient across the stenosis.

No surgical therapy is currently being offered for treatment of this disease.

Prognosis

Prognosis is dependent on severity of the stenosis and the presence of congestive heart failure with or without collapse.

Some cats may have a normal lifespan.

Severely affected cats die within the first 1–2 years of life.

Cats with aortic stenosis are at an increased risk of developing bacterial valvular endocarditis.

PULMONIC STENOSIS

> **Classical signs**
>
> • Systolic murmur is heard over the left heart base over the pulmonic area.

Pathogenesis

With congenital valvular malformation of the pulmonic valve, there is **thickening of the valve leaflets and poor motility during systole,** resulting in fixed obstruction of outflow of blood. In some cases, supravalvular or subvalvular stenosis may be found.

The increased resistance to blood flow across the pulmonary valve stenosis results in elevation of right ventricular systolic pressure. Secondary right ventricular hypertrophy and dilation may develop, along with arrhythmias.

Dilation and hypertrophy of the right ventricle may result in secondary tricuspid insufficiency.

Signs of right-sided congestive heart failure may develop.

Pulmonic stenosis is often seen with other cardiac defects such as tetralogy of Fallot, septal defects and tricuspid dysplasia.

It is a rare congenital defect in cats.

Clinical signs

Many cats are asymptomatic and present for evaluation of a heart murmur.

The age of presentation varies from the **first few months of life until middle age**.

Cats with symptoms may show dyspnea or open-mouth breathing after mild to moderate exercise.

The murmur is best heard at the **left heart base**. It is an ejection systolic murmur, which varies in intensity during systole because of the crescendo and decrescendo character.

Characterization of the ejection murmur may be difficult in a cat because of the fast heart rate.

Diagnosis

Radiographic findings

Normal cardiac size or right ventricular enlargement is found.

Dilated main pulmonary artery (post-stenotic dilatation) is seen as a bulge in the left cranio-lateral part of the cardiac silhouette in the ventro-dorsal view or dorso-ventral view.

Under-perfused pulmonary circulation is seen as hypovascular lung fields characterized by hyperinflated lungs and a decreased peripheral pulmonary vasculature.

Electrocardiographic findings

Tachycardia is frequently seen with a heart rate greater than 220 bpm.

Right axis deviation is seen between −60 and −180 degrees in the frontal plane.

Deep S waves are seen on leads II, aVF and III.

Echocardiographic findings

Pulmonary valve stenosis is present. Pulmonary artery hypoplasia and a dysplastic pulmonic valve may be evident.

Doppler study across the pulmonary valve will determine the degree of stenosis. Velocities of blood flow obtained by continuous wave Doppler above 2.0 m/s are diagnostic of stenosis.

Cardiac catheterization findings

Selective angiography of the right ventricle will show:
• Right ventricular hypertrophy.
• Pulmonary valve stenosis and post-stenotic dilatation of the main pulmonary artery.

Differential diagnosis

Tetralogy of Fallot.

- The murmur of pulmonic stenosis may be similar to the murmur heard in tetralogy of Fallot.
- Cyanosis or brick-red mucus membranes are not seen with pulmonic stenosis.

Cardiomyopathies.
- The murmur is usually not as loud and may vary in intensity.

Treatment

Use **furosemide** if congestive heart failure is present and treat arrhythmias (see page 160 The Cat With Tachycardia, Bradycardia or an Irregular Rhythm).

Surgical options are available but rarely performed.
- Blalock–Taussig shunt can be recommended (artificial shunt from the left subclavian artery to the pulmonary artery). This increases blood flow through the pulmonary circulation.
- Other modified techniques have been described. Consult with an experienced surgeon.

Catheter balloon valvuloplasty can be very successful in reducing the gradient across the stenotic valve. The catheter is positioned through the valve and the balloon inflated to dilate the stenosis.

Prognosis

Most cats reach middle age and some even have a normal lifespan.

Long-term prognosis depends on the severity of obstruction to blood flow.

TETRALOGY OF FALLOT

Classical signs

- Systolic murmur over the cranial ventral thorax.
- Cyanosis or brick-red mucus membranes may be present.
- Signs of increased respiratory rate (with open-mouth breathing), dyspnea or collapse may be seen while playing.
- Many cats are asymptomatic on presentation.

Pathogenesis

Tetralogy of Fallot implies four separate anatomic abnormalities:
- Large ventricular septal defect (VSD).
- Pulmonic valvular stenosis.
- Overriding aorta (dextroposition of the aorta) results from the cranial displacement of the aorta relative to the interventricular septum. This leads to the abnormal alignment of the aorta and the left ventricular outflow tract. A portion of the aorta is positioned over the right ventricular outflow tract.
- Right ventricular hypertrophy.

These abnormalities have a common morphogenetic cause and **result from anterior deviation of the interventricular septum** during development.

It is a rare congenital disease in the cat and is inherited as a **simple autosomal recessive** trait.

The increased resistance to blood flow across the pulmonary valve stenosis results in elevation of right ventricular systolic pressures above left ventricular systolic pressures. These hemodynamic alterations cause the shunting of blood through the large ventricular septal defect.

The cranial displacement of the aortic root allows for direct ejection of blood from the right ventricle into the aorta.

The degree of shunting is relative to the amount of pulmonary stenosis and dextroposition of the aorta. In some patients, minimal shunting occurs at rest, and symptoms are only present during exercise.

Chronic hypoxia results in polycythemia (PCV > 65%).

Clinical signs

Many cats are asymptomatic at rest and present for evaluation of a heart murmur.

The age of presentation varies from the **first few months of life until middle age**.

Cats with symptoms may show open-mouth breathing and/or cyanosis after mild to moderate exercise. In some cats, syncope is seen.

The **mucus membranes may be pink or cyanotic** depending on the degree of the polycythemia and shunting.

The murmur is usually due to the pulmonic stenosis and best heard at the **left heart base**. It is an ejecti on systolic murmur, which varies in intensity during systole because of the crescendo and decrescendo character.

Characterization of the ejection murmur may be difficult in a cat because of the fast heart rate.

Diagnosis

Radiographic findings

Normal cardiac size or right ventricular enlargement is found.

Dilated main pulmonary artery (post-stenotic dilatation) is seen as a bulge in the left cranio-lateral part of the cardiac silhouette in the ventro-dorsal view or dorso-ventral view.

Under-perfused pulmonary circulation is seen as hypovascular lung fields characterized by hyperinflated lungs and a decreased peripheral pulmonary vasculature.

Electrocardiographic findings

Tachycardia is frequently seen with a heart rate greater than 220 bpm.

Right axis deviation is seen between −60 and −180 degrees in the frontal plane.

Deep S waves are seen on leads II, aVF and III.

Echocardiographic findings

A large **perimembranous ventral septal defect** is seen below an overriding aorta.

Pulmonary valve stenosis is present. Most cases have pulmonary artery hypoplasia and a dysplastic pulmonic valve.

Doppler study of the flow across the VSD will determine the direction of shunting of blood. Most frequently, there is right to left shunting.

Doppler study across the pulmonary valve will determine the degree of stenosis. Velocities of blood flow obtained by continuous wave Doppler above 2.0 m/s are diagnostic of stenosis. Usually the degree of stenosis is severe (Vmax > 5.0 m/s).

Saline contrast studies may be helpful in identifying the direction of shunting.

Cardiac catheterization findings

Selective angiography of the right ventricle will show:
- Right ventricular hypertrophy.
- Large VSD.
- Pulmonary valve stenosis and post-stenotic dilatation of the main pulmonary artery.
- Overriding aorta.

Cardiac catheterization demonstrates equalization of right ventricular and left ventricular pressures.

Pulmonary artery pressures are normal.

Differential diagnosis

Pulmonary stenosis.
- Cyanosis or brick-red mucus membranes are not seen with pulmonic stenosis.
- The murmur of pulmonic stenosis may be similar to the murmur heard in tetralogy of Fallot.

Right to left PDA.
- In many cases, no murmur is heard although cyanosis and exercise intolerance are usually present.
- Cyanosis of the right-to-left PDA is usually peripheral and localized to the caudal portion of the body.

Cardiomyopathies.
- Cyanosis is only present in cases of severe pulmonary edema.
- The murmur is usually not as loud and may vary in intensity.

Treatment

Medical therapy consists of periodic phlebotomy to control clinical signs.
- Blood of volume removed = [BW (kg) × 0.08] × 1000 ml/kg × Actual Hct.–Desired Hct./ − Actual Hct.
- Repeat PCV in 2 hours. The goal is to decrease PCV to ~60%. CAUTION–removing too much red cell mass may render the patient symptomatic at rest.

Avoid heavy playing and keep confined within the household.

Use **beta-blockers** if the **heart rate** is greater than 200 bpm at rest.
- Propranolol – 0.5–1 mg/kg q 8 h **OR**
- Atenolol 6.25–12.5 mg/cat q 12 h.

Surgical options are available but rarely performed.

- Blalock–Taussig shunt can be recommended (artificial shunt from the left subclavian artery to the pulmonary artery). This increases blood flow through the pulmonary circulation.
- Other modified techniques have been described. Consult with an experienced surgeon.

Prognosis

Most cats can reach middle age and some even have a normal lifespan.

Long-term prognosis depends on the severity of blood flow.

DILATED CARDIOMYOPATHY

Classical signs

- Heart murmur (in some cases may not be present).
- Gallop rhythm.
- Arrhythmia.
- Dyspnea.
- Hypothermia.
- Collapse.
- Lameness, paralysis or paresis from systemic thromboembolism.

Pathogenesis

This disease **in most cats is due to a deficiency in taurine concentration**. Taurine supplementation in commercially available diets has reduced significantly its incidence.

Any cat fed a non-commercial diet should have taurine supplementation. Cats fed home-made vegetarian diets are at high risk of taurine deficiency. However, not all cats experimentally fed a taurine-deficient diet have developed dilated cardiomyopathy.

Dilated cardiomyopathy (DCM) is not always the result of taurine deficiency. Currently most of the cases are idiopathic.

Retinal degeneration changes consistent with taurine deficiency are present in 33% of cats.

Other potential causes for DCM include a late expression of chronic myocarditis, genetic abnormalities, and in some cats, the cause is unknown.

In cats fed commercially available feline diets, DCM is a **rare form of cardiomyopathy**.

All cardiac chambers are dilated. Atrophy of papillary muscles is present.

Myocardial sections on post-mortem show patchy white areas. Microscopically there is myocyte atrophy with interstitial fibrosis.

The hemodynamic hallmark is severe systolic dysfunction.

Clinical signs

There is no age or sex predilection.

Usually cats with dilated cardiomyopathy have a history of being fed a non-commercial diet, or dog food.

A heart murmur is often present, but in some cases may not be. When present, a systolic murmur varies in location and intensity with variations in heart rate.

Gallop rhythm is commonly heard. It is identified when more than two heart sounds are present on auscultation.

Arrhythmias can be heard as premature heart beats with pulse deficits.

Dyspnea is seen in symptomatic cats with an increased respiratory rate (greater than 30 breaths/ min) at rest or with open-mouth breathing in extreme cases. Pleural effusion may be present and result in muffled heart sounds.

In symptomatic cats, hypothermia is common.

Collapse may result from impaired cardiac output (ventricular tachycardia)

Lameness, paralysis or paresis are usually the result of systemic thromboembolism.

Most cats with aortic saddle thrombosis present for acute onset of hindlimb paralysis, pain, absent femoral pulses, cool extremities and cyanosis of the nail bed. In some cases a history of episodic lameness is given.

Ascites is found in a small minority of cases.

Diagnosis

Radiographic findings

Severe generalized cardiomegaly and enlarged pulmonary veins are seen. Pulmonary edema with or without pleural effusion may be present. Pleural effusion is more common in dilated cardiomyopathy than in other forms of cardiomyopathy. The fluid may be a transudate, modified transudate or chylous.

Electrocardiographic findings

Ventricular arrhythmias are present in about 50% of cases.

Tachycardia, ventricular conduction disturbances (notched QRS), or tall R waves on lead II (> 0.9 mV) are **commonly** found.

Atrial fibrillation is more common than in HCM and is usually associated with **extreme dilatation** of the left and/or right atria.

Echocardiographic findings

The echocardiographic findings reveal **severe biventricular dilatation with severe biatrial enlargement**. The left atrial to aortic ratio is usually >2.0.

Left ventricular systolic function is markedly diminished (fractional shortening is less then 20–25% in most cases). Normal FS is between 35–55%.

Left ventricular internal dimensions in diastole is usually larger than 20 mm. Intracardiac thrombi may be found. Normal LV end-diastolic dimension is up to 17 mm.

In **taurine-deficient cats**, improvement in chamber size and contractility is seen 6–8 weeks after starting supplementation.

Laboratory findings

Plasma **taurine levels** (heparinized sample) are less than 30 nmol/ml in most cats. Plasma levels of 40–60 nmol/ml may be consistent with taurine deficiency.

Cats with congestive heart failure may show **azotemia** due to decreased renal perfusion.

Treatment

Treatment of the asymptomatic cat:
- Angiotensin-converting enzyme inhibitors
  - **Enalapril** 0.25–0.5 mg/kg PO q 24 h **OR**
  - **Benazepril** 0.25–0.5 mg/kg PO q 24 h.
- Nutraceuticals
  - **Taurine** PO 250–500 mg q 12 h.

Treatment of the symptomatic cat with congestive heart failure (**acute management**).
Criteria to start therapy:
- Respiratory distress (open-mouth breathing or very abnormal respiratory pattern).
- Pulmonary congestion (moderate to severe) on radiographs and/or pleural effusion.
- Hypothermia.
- Oxygen.
- Diuretics.
  - **Furosemide** 1–2 mg/kg IV or IM q 8–12 h until respiratory rate and pattern are normalized.
  - Furosemide constant rate infusion (if normal renal values at presentation) 0.5–1 mg/kg/hr until congestion is resolved but not for longer than 24 hours.
- Venodilator.
  - **Nitroglycerin** ointment (2%) 1/4 of an inch (6 mm) q 8 h.
- Inotropic support.
  - **Dobutamine** continuous rate infusion, IV 1–3 μg/kg/min (watch for vomiting or seizures). **OR**
  - **Pimobendan** 0.25 mg/kg PO q 12 h (only if able to pill without causing distress)
- **Thoracocentesis (right thorax** to avoid puncturing of the enlarged auricles) if there is evidence of moderate to severe pleural effusion on radiographs.
- **Angiotensin-converting enzyme inhibitor** (see above).
- **Taurine** supplement (see above).
- **Thermoregulatory support** (heating blanket).
  - Fluid therapy should be done cautiously until stable cardiac function is established.

Symptomatic cat with congestive heart failure (**chronic management**).
Criteria to start therapy:
- Maintenance therapy after initial treatment for acute congestive heart failure.
- Any patient found to have early evidence of congestive heart failure (usually on radiographs) but without symptoms, that will require acute intervention if untreated.
  - Diuretics
  - **Furosemide** 0.5–1.0 mg/kg PO q 12–24 h **OR**
  - **Hydrochlorothiazide** 1–2 mg/kg PO q 12 h **OR/AND**
  - **Spironolactone** 2–4 mg/kg PO q 12 h.
- Angiotensin-converting enzyme inhibitor (see above)
- Taurine supplement (see above)

Inotropic Support
- Digoxin 0.016 mg/cat PO q 24–48 h (monitor for anorexia and gastrointestinal signs). **OR**
  - For monitoring, obtain a serum sample 8 hours after giving digoxin dose. Do not store the serum in plastic tubes, since digoxin binds to plastic. Therapeutic serum concentrations range from 1.3–3.2 nmol/L (1.0–2.5 ng/ml). The authors prefer not to exceed levels higher than 1.9 nmol/L (1.5 ng/ml). The side effects usually are GI signs and anorexia.
- **Pimobendan** 0.25 mg/kg PO q 12 h.
- Arrhythmia control.
  - Improvement is usually seen with supportive treatment.
  - Caution should be exercised if beta-blockers or calcium channel blockers are used, due to the negative inotropic effects of these drugs.
  - For ventricular or supraventricular arrhythmias:
  - **Procainamide SR** 10–20 mg/kg PO q 8 h.
  - Associated intracardiac thrombus or systemic thromboembolism.
- Anti-thrombotic therapy:
  - **Heparin** and **Warfarin** therapy are controversial and should be utilized under the guidance of an experienced clinician.
  - **Low-molecular-weight heparins** have been recently suggested. This class of heparins does not require continued monitoring of coagulation parameters.
  - **Enoxaparin** (Lovenox ®) 1 mg/kg SQ q 24 h.
  - **Aspirin** 80 mg PO q 48–72 h is recommended by some clinicians but its efficacy has not been established. A lower dose (5 mg/cat PO q 24 h) has also been recommended, because of concerns that prostacyclin production is inhibited at the higher dose.

Thrombolytic therapy is contraindicated if an intracardiac thrombus is present, and controversial in aortic saddle thrombus.

Prognosis

Prognosis is good if the etiology is taurine deficiency.

Most cases currently seen are not due to taurine deficiency and the prognosis is poor.

Prevention

Cats should be maintained on a diet designed for the feline patient, which has adequate amounts of taurine.

PERITONEAL–PERICARDIAL DIAPHRAGMATIC HERNIA (PPDH)

Classical signs

- Vomiting.
- Diarrhea.
- Weight loss.
- Dyspnea.

Pathogenesis

Persistent communication occurs between the **pericardial and peritoneal cavities** because of abnormal fusion of the septum transversum with the pleuroperitoneal folds during development.

The hernia is of variable size.

The most likely organs to be herniated are the **liver and gallbladder, small intestine, spleen, stomach**.

Clinical signs

Signs are mostly related to the gastrointestinal system and include vomiting, diarrhea and weight loss.

Most cases are asymptomatic and it is an incidental finding. An increased incidence in Persian cats is suspected.

Physical exam is often normal. In some cases, the heart sounds may be muffled.

In symptomatic patients, respiratory signs can be present, particularly under stressful conditions.

Diagnosis

Radiographic findings

Extreme enlargement of the "cardiac" silhouette.

Dorsal displacement of the trachea.

Silhouetting of the caudal border of the heart with the diaphragm.

Heterogeneous densities of the "cardiac" silhouette due to varied contents of the pericardial cavity.

Abdominal radiographs may show an absent or smaller than normal liver.

Electrocardiographic findings

Some patients have a normal ECG.

The expected QRS complexes in a cat with a severely enlarged heart diagnosed by radiography are not present in patients with peritoneopericardial diaphragmatic hernia.

The mean electrical axis may be shifted (depending on the abnormal deviation of the heart by the viscera).

Echocardiographic findings

The cardiac exam is commonly normal.

In cases where primary cardiac disease is present, it is difficult to obtain a true evaluation of the heart due to compression by nearby organs.

Abnormal blood flow patterns may be caused by compression forces of the viscera against the heart.

The liver and other organs can be visualized in direct contact with the heart.

Cardiac catheterization findings

Non-selective angiography demonstrates that the pericardial sac is filled with other organs.

Differential diagnosis

Pericardial effusion is usually associated with clinical signs of cardiac or infectious disease. Radiographically the cardiac silhouette lacks heterogeneous densities.

Dilated cardiomyopathy is usually associated with signs indicative of heart disease. Radiographically the heart never develops the degree of enlargement seen with PPDH.

In a diaphragmatic hernia the heart, size is normal and displaced. There is loss of distinct diaphragmatic borders. A history of trauma is common.

Treatment

If the patient is asymptomatic and the diagnosis is incidental, then surgery is not necessary.

Surgical correction should be reserved for cases with symptoms attributed to this condition.
- Post-operative care may be complicated in some cases. Consult with an experienced surgeon.

Prognosis

Asymptomatic patients have a good prognosis in general.

Surgically corrected patients have an excellent prognosis.

DIAPHRAGMATIC HERNIA

> ### Classical signs
> - Dyspnea/tachypnea.

See main reference page 57 (The Dyspneic or Tachypneic Cat).

Clinical signs

Trauma associated with a **motor vehicle accident** or a **fall from several stories** is the most common cause, although it can occasionally occur as a **congenital problem**.

Tachypnea and **dyspnea** are often evident, and may begin at the time of trauma or a few hours later. In some cats, the respiratory signs improve after a few days and are most evident only after physical activity.

Typically there is a **vague history of gastrointestinal signs** including vomiting, inappetance and weight loss, usually beginning some time after a motor vehicle accident or fall.

Physical examination may be normal. Often the **heart sounds are muffled** on one or both sides of the chest. There may be an impression of an **"empty" abdomen** on abdominal palpation because of organ displacement.

Diagnosis

Radiographic findings

Abdominal viscera are identified within the thorax. Stomach and small intestine can be easily identified as gas-filled or fluid-filled structures.

Displacement of abdominal and thoracic structures is found due to shifting of the organs through the diaphragmatic surface.

Partial or complete **loss of the thoracic–diaphragmatic surface** outline is seen.

In some cases, pleural effusion is detected.

Electrocardiographic findings

Mean electrical axis may be shifted due to the altered position of the heart in the chest.

A typical mean electrical axis shift cannot be expected, due to the variable position of the heart in each individual case.

Echocardiographic findings

A normal echocardiogram is found, unless concurrent heart disease is present.

The abdominal viscera may displace the heart making it difficult to obtain standard imaging planes.

Abdominal organs are visualized **within the chest cavity**.

VALVULAR ENDOCARDIOSIS

Classical signs

- Systolic murmur.
- Gallop.
- Dyspnea or tachypnea if symptomatic.

Pathogenesis

This is a **rare disorder** in cats.

Degeneration of the collagen matrix of the valve occurs resulting in laxity of the chord apparatus and prolapse of the valve.

There is **thickening of the valve leaflets**.

Clinical signs

Systolic murmur located over the apex of the heart.

Gallop rhythm may be present.

Tachypnea or dyspnea may be present in cases with concurrent congestive heart failure.

Diagnosis

Radiographic findings

Marked left atrial enlargement.

Left ventricular enlargement.

Dorsal displacement of the trachea.

Pulmonary edema.

Dilatation of the pulmonary veins relative to the pulmonary arteries.

Pleural effusion may be present (rare).

Electrocardiographic findings

Sinus tachycardia if heart failure is present.

Left ventricular enlargement (R wave > 0.9 mV on lead II).

Left anterior fascicular block (LAFB) may signify left ventricular enlargement. In LAFB the QRS duration is normal, there is marked left axis deviation (between −60 and −90 degrees), small Q wave and tall R wave in leads I and aVL, deep S waves in lead II, III and aVF.

Arrhythmias are uncommon.

Echocardiographic findings

Thick and prolapsing mitral valve.

Marked mitral regurgitation.
- Marked left atrial enlargement
- Variable degrees of left ventricular enlargement occur depending on the degree of valvular insufficiency.
- **Hyperkinetic left ventricle** (contraction is exuberant, stronger than normal) with a fractional shortening often greater than 55%.

Differential diagnosis

Any type of cardiomyopathy.
- Cardiomyopathy cases have in general **normal valvular morphology**.
- In cardiomyopathy patients, the degree of valvular insufficiency is usually less than with endocardiosis.

Treatment

If not in congestive heart failure:
- Treatment is not required and probably will not change the outcome.
- If severe left atrial enlargement is present (left atrial to aortic ratio >2), consider beta-blocker therapy (refer to HCM section for doses, page 130).

If in congestive heart failure (respiratory distress with open-mouth breathing or very abnormal respiratory pattern, pulmonary congestion on radiographs with or without pleural effusion and hypothermia) refer to section on HCM for therapy (page 130).

Prognosis

The prognosis is variable and depends on the severity of the mitral regurgitation and degree of cardiac enlargement present.

If congestive heart failure is present, life expectancy is around 1–2 years.

RECOMMENDED READING

Ettinger SJ, Feldman EC. Textbook of Veterinary Internal Medicine. Philadelphia, PA, WB Saunders Co., 2005.

Fox PR. Textbook of Canine and Feline Cardiology: Principles of Clinical Practice. Philadelphia, WB Saunders, 1999.

Kittleson MD, Kienle RD. Small Animal Cardiovascular Medicine. St. Louis, MO, Mosby, 1998.

Tilley LP. Essentials of Canine and Feline Electrocardiography, 3rd edition. Interpretation and Treatment. Malvern, PA, Lea and Febiger, 1992.

Tilley LP, Smith FWK (eds) The Five Minute Veterinary Consult, 3rd Edition. Baltimore, Lippincott, Williams & Wilkins, 2004.

10. The cat with tachycardia, bradycardia or an irregular rhythm

Luis A H Braz-Ruivo, Kathy A Arrington and Fiona Campbell

KEY SIGNS

- Tachycardia.
- Bradycardia.
- Irregular heart sounds or pulse.

MECHANISM?

- Arrhythmias are caused by two basic abnormalities: disorders of impulse formation and disorders of impulse conduction.
- Alterations of impulse formation are usually the result of diseased myocardial cells.
- Alterations of electrical impulse conduction occur secondary to primary diseases of the conduction system.

WHERE?

- Arrhythmias can occur wherever there is excitable cardiac tissue in the heart.

WHAT?

- Most cats with a cardiac arrhythmia are asymptomatic.
- The most common arrhythmia is ventricular premature contractions (VPCs).

QUICK REFERENCE SUMMARY

Diseases causing tachycardia, bradycardia or an irregular rhythm

TACHYARRHYTHMIAS

ANOMALY

- Ventricular pre-excitation

This is a rare cardiac arrhythmia resulting from the presence of a congenital bundle of muscle across the atrioventricular annulus – allowing bypass of the electrical impulse to the ventricles.

It can occur at any age; in many cases, it is an incidental finding. The most common symptom is syncope or lethargy during the periods of supraventricular tachycardia.

continued

continued

METABOLIC

- **Tachyarrhythmias (sinus tachycardia, supraventricular/atrial tachycardia, ventricular premature beats and ventricular tachycardia)*** (p 160)**

Tachyarrhythmias can result from hyperthyroidism, acidosis and uremia or be drug-induced.

Cats tolerate tachycardia better than other species. Syncope, lethargy and weakness are the most common signs in addition to the sign of the underlying disease.

- **Ventricular arrhythmias (ventricular premature beats, ventricular tachycardia)*** (p 164)**

Ventricular arrhythmias may result from hyperthyroidism, acidosis, uremia or be drug-induced. In addition to the signs related to the underlying disease, cats may present with lethargy, weakness, anorexia and syncope.

- **Atrial arrhythmias (supraventricular/atrial tachycardia, atrial fibrillation) (p 161)**

Atrial arrhythmias may be seen in hyperthyroidism. In addition to the signs related to the underlying disease, cats may present with lethargy, weakness and syncope.

NEOPLASTIC

- **Ventricular arrhythmias (ventricular premature beats, ventricular tachycardia) (p 164)**

Ventricular arrhythmias may be seen in primary or metastatic cardiac disease. Most patients do not show clinical signs from the arrhythmia. Most of the clinical signs are related to the underlying disease.

INFECTIOUS

- **Ventricular arrhythmias (ventricular premature beats, ventricular tachycardia) (p 164)**

Ventricular arrhythmias may be seen with bacterial infections (endocarditis, myocarditis) and viral infections (myopericarditis). Fever, lethargy, anorexia and a new heart murmur are the most common clinical signs.

IDIOPATHIC

- **Ventricular arrhythmias (ventricular premature beats, ventricular tachycardia)*** (p 164)**

Ventricular arrhythmias are most commonly seen in cases of feline cardiomyopathies. The majority of the cases do not have symptoms related to the arrhythmia. Periods of ventricular tachycardia (rates above 300 bpm) may cause lethargy or syncope.

- **Atrial fibrillation* (p 162)**

Atrial fibrillation can be seen in end-stage cardiomyopathies when severe left atrial enlargement is present. Clinical signs include worsening of heart failure, weakness or syncope. Signs related to systemic thromboembolism (paresis/paralysis of hindlimbs) may be present.

- **Supraventricular arrhythmias (supraventricular/atrial tachycardia, atrial fibrillation)** (p 161)**

Atrial tachycardias, atrial premature beats and other forms of supraventricular tachycardias can occur in cats with cardiomyopathies. The majority of the cases do not have symptoms related to the arrhythmia. Periods of supraventricular tachycardia (rates above 300 bpm) may cause lethargy or syncope.

TRAUMATIC

● Ventricular arrhythmias (ventricular premature beats, ventricular tachycardia) (p 164)
Ventricular arrhythmias can be seen in cases following severe trauma to the chest. These are usually secondary to traumatic myocarditis. The majority of the cases do not have symptoms related to the arrhythmia. Periods of tachycardia (rates above 300 bpm) may cause lethargy or syncope

BRADYARRHYTHMIAS

DEGENERATIVE

● Atrioventricular block (p 169)
Several degrees of atrioventricular block are due to His bundle degeneration, vacuolization and fibrosis.
   Bradyarrhythmias cause clinical signs of lethargy, weakness and syncope. Depending on the degree of the bradyarrhythmia, many cats may not show clinical signs and usually are an incidental finding.

METABOLIC

● Sinus bradycardia (p 168)
Sinus bradycardia can result from hyperkalemia, hypokalemia, hypoglycemia, acidosis and hypothermia or be drug-induced. In addition to the signs related to the underlying disease, cats may present with lethargy, weakness, anorexia and syncope. Heart rate is <120 beats/min.

● Atrial standstill (p 168)
Atrial standstill can result from hyperkalemia primarily associated with urethral obstruction or from long-standing cardiac disease, most commonly dilated cardiomyopathy. In addition to the signs related to the underlying disease, cats may present with lethargy, weakness, anorexia and syncope.

TOXIC

● **AV block** (p 169)**
AV block can be drug-induced with digitalis, beta-blockers and calcium-channel blockers. In addition to the signs related to the underlying disease, cats may present with lethargy, weakness, anorexia and syncope.

INTRODUCTION

MECHANISMS?

The normal electrical impulse is generated in the **SA node** and spreads through the atria via the Bachmann bundles, continues down through the **AV node**, **His bundle**, **bundle branches** and **Purkinje fibers** and finally reaches the **ventricles**.

Arrhythmias are caused by two basic abnormalities, disorders of **impulse formation** and disorders of **impulse conduction**.

Alterations of **electrical impulse formation** occur secondary to **instability of the resting membrane potential** and are usually the result of **diseased myocardial cells**.
● If the electrical impulse forms **earlier** than expected, a **premature beat** is generated. If the electrical impulse forms **later** than expected, a **pause** in the cardiac rhythm is seen.

Alterations of **electrical impulse conduction** occur secondary to **primary diseases of the conduction system.** These either result in **block of conduction** of the electrical wave, or alterations that facilitate the **perpetuation of the electrical wave** in a circuit (re-entry).

Abnormal conduction of the electrical impulse can be either **blocked,** choose an **alternative pattern of conduction** (aberrantly conducted) or **re-enter** previously excited tissue (re-entry).

An arrhythmia should always be suspected whenever an **irregularity in cardiac rhythm** or **arterial pulse** is detected.

WHERE?

Arrhythmias can occur wherever there is **excitable** cardiac tissue in the heart.

Arrhythmias that originate in the **atria, interatrial septum, or above the AV node** are termed **supraventricular**.

Arrhythmias that originate in the ventricles or anywhere below the bifurcation of the His bundle are termed ventricular.

WHAT?

The most common arrhythmia is ventricular premature contractions (VPCs).

Cats with cardiac arrhythmias are generally suspected of having myocardial disease, even if radiographic and echocardiographic findings are within normal limits.

Cardiomyopathies are the most common form of cardiac disease associated with arrhythmias.

The diagnosis of atrial fibrillation in a cat is almost invariably associated with the presence of severe left atrial enlargement.

Most cats with a cardiac arrhythmia are asymptomatic.

Ventricular arrhythmias in young cats with severe left ventricular hypertrophy may be associated with a high risk of sudden death.

TREATMENT

Most cats do not require specific therapy with anti-arrhythmics unless they are symptomatic.

Class I anti-arrhythmics block the sodium channels and result in decreased excitability of the diseased cells. The most common examples are procainamide and lidocaine (high risk of toxicity).

Class II anti-arrhythmics are beta-blockers. This group antagonizes the action of cathecolamines and is most useful when increased sympathetic tone is present. Most common examples include propranolol (non-selective) and atenolol (beta-1 selective). They are contraindicated for cats with symptomatic respiratory disease.

Class III anti-arrhythmics block the potassium channels. This group hyperpolarizes the cells making it more difficult to reach threshold, and they prolong the refractory period. The most common used drug is sotalol. Sotalol, besides class III properties, also has class II properties.

Class IV anti-arrhythmics block the calcium channels. These drugs inhibit transmembrane calcium transport and the most pronounced effects are at the sinoatrial and atrioventricular nodes. The most common example is diltiazem.

DISEASES CAUSING TACHYCARDIA OR AN IRREGULAR RHYTHM

SINUS TACHYCARDIA***

> **Classical signs**
>
> - Heart rate greater than 220 beats per minute.
> - Strong precordial impulse.
> - Loud S1 heart sound.

Pathogenesis

This **arrhythmia** originates from the **sinoatrial node**, the normal pacemaker of the heart.

It results from **increased sympathetic tone**. The **causes of increased sympathetic tone** include stress, fever, pain, metabolic disease (hyperthyroidism), hypovolemia, thromboembolic disease, shock and anemia.

Clinical signs

In the majority of patients, clinical signs are related to the underlying disease.

Clinical signs related to a fast heart rate (> 280 bpm) include restlessness, tachypnea, open-mouth breathing, poor pulse quality and delayed capillary refill time.

Diagnosis

The diagnosis is based on physical examination and an electrocardiogram (Figure 10.1).

The **heart rate** is above **220 bpm**.

The **cardiac rhythm** is regular.

There is a **P wave for every QRS complex** with a constant P-R interval.

The morphology of the **P wave is normal**.

The **QRS complex morphology is normal**.

The **changes in the heart rate occur gradually** (i.e. gradual acceleration or deceleration of the heart rate).

Differential diagnosis

Supraventricular tachycardias including atrial tachycardia, AV nodal re-entrant tachycardia, atrial flutter with 2:1 conduction need to be differentiated from sinus tachycardia. Supraventricular tachycardia may look identical to sinus tachycardia on the ECG. Excessive heart rate (greater than 250 bpm) is more likely to be supraventricular tachycardia. Supraventricular tachycardia may have abnormal P wave morphology or lack P waves compared to sinus tachycardia where P waves are normal.

Treatment

Before initiating treatment, **determine the underlying etiology,** and treat appropriately.

If associated with **low systemic blood pressure** and the **cause is not** hypovolemia, shock or blood loss, and systolic myocardial function is preserved, consider **heart rate control** with:

- Propranolol at 0.5–1 mg/kg PO q 8–12 hours.
- Atenolol at 6.25–12.5 mg/cat PO q 12 hours.
- Sotalol at 10–20 mg/cat PO q 12 hours.
- Diltiazem at 7.5–15 mg/cat PO q 8 hours.

Prognosis

The **prognosis** depends on the underlying **etiology**.

Most cases have a favorable outcome.

SUPRAVENTRICULAR/ATRIAL TACHYCARDIA**

> **Classical signs**
>
> - Fast and regular heart rate above 220 bpm.
> - Strong precordial impulse.
> - Loud S1 heart sound.
> - Weakness/collapse.

Pathogenesis

The arrhythmia originates from anywhere above and including the atrioventricular node.

Supraventricular/atrial tachycardias most commonly result from primary myocardial disease.

These arrhythmias are most commonly seen in association with hypertrophic or restrictive cardiomyopathies.

Clinical signs

In the majority of patients, clinical **signs are related to** the underlying disease such as **cardiomyopathy** rather

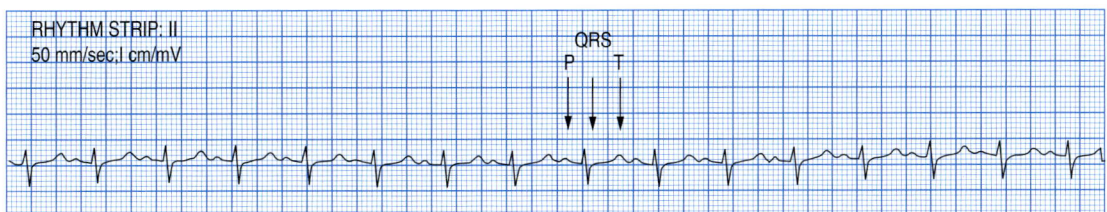

Figure 10.1. Sinus tachycardia at 225 bpm.

than the tachycardia, and include a heart mumur, dyspnea, weakness, collapse and lameness, paralysis or paresis from systemic thromboembolism.

Clinical signs related to a fast heart rate (> 280 bpm) include restlessness, tachypnea, open-mouth breathing, poor pulse quality and delayed capillary refill time.

Diagnosis

The diagnosis is based on physical examination and an electrocardiogram.

The **heart rate** is above **220 bpm**.

The **cardiac rhythm** is **regular.**

The **QRS complex** morphology is **normal.**

There is a P wave for every QRS complex, but the **P wave morphology may or may not** be **different** from normal sinus beats.

P waves may be "buried" in the S–T segment.

The **arrhythmia** may be **sustained** or **occur in paroxysms**.

The **changes** in the **heart rate are abrupt**. The **arrhythmia may terminate spontaneously** with a sudden decrease in heart rate.

The **QRS complex** may be slightly **aberrant** in the beginning of the paroxysm of tachycardia.

The QRS complex may alter its configuration (electrical alternans) in the first few seconds of the run of tachycardia.

Differential diagnosis

Sinus tachycardia may look identical to supraventricular tachycardia sinus on the ECG. Excessive heart rate (greater than 250 bpm) is more likely to be supraventricular tachycardia. Supraventricular tachycardia may have abnormal P wave morphology or lack P waves compared to sinus tachycardia where P waves are normal.

Motion or electrical artifact can usually be resolved by improved ECG recording technique: repositioning the electrodes, moistening the skin with alcohol, positioning the cat on a non-metal table isolated from other electrical devices.

Treatment

If the patient is **symptomatic** (hypotension, cardiogenic shock, collapse) for the arrhythmia, then treatment is required. The following drugs can be used in succession and are written in order of preference if the previous drug is not effective.

- **Diltiazem** at 0.1–0.3 mg/kg IV slow bolus over 3–5 minutes. The dose can be repeated in 5–10 minutes if sustained SVT. After IV bolus an intravenous constant rate infusion can be started at 5–20 µg/kg/min. Diltiazem is compatible with any type of IV fluids.
- **Esmolol** at 250–500 µg/kg IV bolus given slowly over 1 minute. The bolus can be followed with a constant rate infusion at 50–200 µg/kg/min. Esmolol is compatible with 5% dextrose.
- **Propranolol** at 20 µg/kg IV slow bolus over 5 minutes. Propranolol can be given up to a total dose of 100 µg/kg in repeated boluses.

If the patient is **not symptomatic** for the arrhythmia:
- Atenolol at 6.25–12.5 mg/cat PO every 12 hours.
- Diltiazem at 7.5–15 mg/cat PO every 8 hours.
- Propranolol at 2.5–5 mg/cat PO every 8–12 hours.
- Sotalol at 10–20 mg/cat PO every 12 hours.

Prognosis

The **prognosis** depends on the underlying **etiology**.

In general, the presence of this arrhythmia suggests advanced underlying cardiac disease.

In cases where the etiology is due to the existence of a by-pass tract, the cat may have a good prognosis, providing there is good control of the tachycardia.

ATRIAL FIBRILLATION*

Classical signs

- Fast and irregularly irregular variable heart rate.
- Strong precordial impulse.
- Loud and variable S1 heart sound.
- Weakness/collapse (rare).

Pathogenesis

This arrhythmia results from rapid disorganized atrial activity "bombarding" the AV node.

The heart rate may be normal or increased.

Its presence is usually associated with severe left atrial enlargement.

Clinical signs

In the majority of patients, clinical signs are related to the underlying cardiac disease.

Clinical signs related to a fast heart rate (> 280 bpm) include restlessness, tachypnea, open-mouth breathing, poor pulse quality and delayed capillary refill time.

The onset of atrial fibrillation may be marked by decompensation of the heart disease with pulmonary congestion.

Diagnosis

The heart rate may be normal or increased (Figure 10.2).

There are no visible P waves in any lead.

Small fluctuations on the baseline (f waves) may be seen and are not related to the QRS complex.

The ventricular rate is irregularly irregular, and the QRS complex has a normal configuration.

Differential diagnosis

Atrial flutter with variable conduction: With atrial fibrillation the baseline may have some deflections which appear similar to P waves, but these can be distinguished from true P waves because they do not occur in every lead. With atrial flutter, P waves can be identified in all leads with a regular P–P interval.

Frequent paroxysmal supraventricular tachycardia: Usually paroxysmal supraventricular tachycardia is sustained for several beats. These beats have a regular R–R interval compared to atrial fibrillation where the R–R interval is always irregular.

Treatment

The goal is to obtain a **heart rate** below **180 beats per minute** in the exam room. The **heart rate** should be **determined by ECG rhythm strip**. Several recheck visits, usually weekly, may be needed for adjustment of medication to reach the target heart rate.

For cats with underlying dilated cardiomyopathy:
- Digoxin at 1/4 of 0.125 mg tablet/cat PO every 24–48 hours. Cats should be monitored carefully for signs of toxicity, and medication stopped if anorexia or vomiting develop.

For cats with preserved myocardial systolic function:
- Atenolol at 12.5 mg/cat PO every 12 hours.
- Diltiazem at 7.5–15 mg/cat PO every 8 hours.
- Propranolol at 2.5–5 mg/cat PO every 8–12 hours.
- Sotalol at 10–20 mg/cat PO every 12 hours.

Prognosis

In general, this arrhythmia is associated with **end-stage cardiac disease** and with **severe left atrial enlargement**. It may predispose to the development of thromboembolic disease.

The **prognosis** for long-term survival is **poor.**

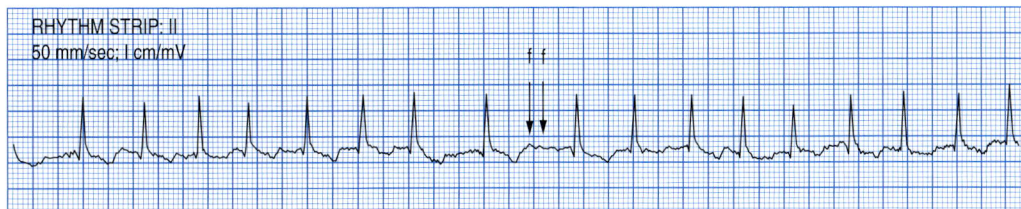

Figure 10.2. Atrial fibrillation. Note fibrillatory "f" waves.

VENTRICULAR TACHYCARDIA***

Classical signs

- Fast and regular heart rate above 220 beats per minute.
- Strong precordial impulse.
- Loud S1 heart sound.
- Weakness/collapse (rare).

Pathogenesis

The arrhythmia originates from the ventricles.

Ventricular tachycardias most commonly result from primary cardiac disease.

Most often, it is the result of myocardial fibrosis associated with a cardiomyopathy.

Sustained ventricular tachycardia may be caused by myocardial infarction.

Other causes of ventricular tachycardia include metabolic acidosis and drug-induced (digitalis).

Clinical signs

In the majority of patients, clinical signs are related to the underlying disease.

Some patients do not show clinical signs from the tachycardia.

Clinical signs related to a fast heart rate (> 280 bpm) include restlessness, tachypnea, open-mouth breathing, poor pulse quality and delayed capillary refill time.

Diagnosis

The heat rate is above 220 bpm (Figure 10.3).

There is no association between P waves and the QRS complex (P waves may be seen anywhere in the cardiac cycle).

The QRS morphology is aberrant.

This arrhythmia is usually regular, but some degree of variability of the cardiac rhythm may be present.

This arrhythmia may be sustained or occur in paroxysms.

Changes in heart rate are abrupt.

Differential diagnosis

Supraventricular tachycardia (supraventricular tachycardia with aberrant ventricular conduction, or atrial flutter without variable conduction but with aberrant ventricular conduction) may appear similar to ventricular tachycardia on the ECG. Supraventricular tachycardia may have P waves preceding the QRS complex.

Motion or electrical artifact can usually be resolved by improved ECG recording technique: repositioning the electrodes, moistening the skin with alcohol, positioning the cat on a non-metal table isolated from other electrical devices.

Treatment

If the patient is **symptomatic** (hypotension, cardiogenic shock, collapse), or sustained **heart rate** greater than **220 bpm**, then immediate therapy is recommended.

Correct any metabolic, electrolyte or acid–base abnormalities.

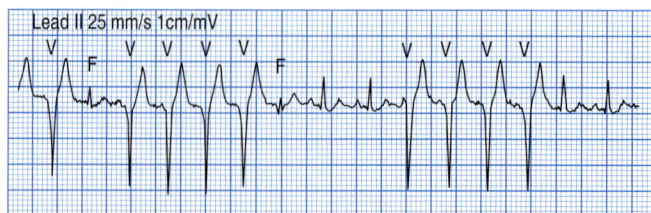

Figure 10.3. Ventricular tachycardia. "V" marks VPCs. Fusion beats are marked "F".

- The authors use **procainamide** at 5–10 mg/kg slow IV bolus. This bolus can be repeated once if necessary.
- **Esmolol** at 250–500 µg/kg IV bolus given slowly over 1 minute. The bolus can be followed with a constant rate infusion at 50–200 µg/kg/min. Esmolol is compatible with 5% dextrose.
- **Propranolol** at 20 µg/kg slow IV bolus. Repeat boluses can be given up to a total maximum dose of 100 µg/kg.

DO NOT USE LIDOCAINE IN CATS. Severe neurotoxicity can occur.

If patient is **not symptomatic** for the arrhythmia:
- Atenolol 6.25–12.5 mg/cat PO every 12 hours.
- Propranolol at 2.5–5 mg/kg PO every 8 hours.
- Sotalol 10–20 mg/cat PO every 12 hours.
- Procainamide 10–20 mg/kg PO every 8–12 hours.

Prognosis

Most cats with sustained ventricular tachycardia have severe myocardial damage and are at high risk of sudden death.

The prognosis is fair.

PREMATURE BEATS

The following are definitions of electrocardiographic findings necessary to understand the distinguishing features between supraventricular and ventricular premature beats:

- A **fusion beat** occurs when the ventricles are **activated** by **two different wave** fronts, resulting in **abnormal/aberrant appearance** of the QRS complex.
- An **interpolated beat** is when a ventricular beat occurs between **two normal beats** without **disturbing** the cardiac rhythm.
- The **re-setting** or **non-resetting** of the **sinoatrial node** refers to the **influence** of the **premature beat** on the **basic sinus rhythm**.
- If the rhythm is **disturbed** by the **premature beat** then the rhythm is **reset**. **Resetting** of the basic rhythm is also referred to as **non-compensatory pause**.

SUPRAVENTRICULAR PREMATURE BEATS (SVPBS)***

Classical signs

- Pulse deficits.
- Interruptions of rhythm regularity.

Pathogenesis

Premature beats result from two mechanisms, alterations in impulse formation and alterations in impulse conduction.

Alterations of impulse formation depend on the intrinsic automaticity of diseased cardiac cells.
- Diseased myocardial cells outside the specialized conduction system can acquire automaticity because of changes in the resting membrane potential.

Alterations of impulse conduction result from re-entry and by-pass tracts.
- **Re-entry**, is a self-sustaining electrical circuit that **repeatedly depolarizes** surrounding tissue.
- **By-pass tracts** alter the normal pathway of conduction by providing an **alternative pathway around the AV node.**

Clinical signs

Most patients show no evidence of clinical signs.

In some cases panting, restlessness and anxiety may be seen.

Diagnosis

The heart rate is normal and the cardiac rhythm is irregular because of the premature beats (Figure 10.4).

The ectopic P wave is premature, the configuration may be different from normal sinus beats.

The **morphology** of the **QRS complex** is **similar** to a normal sinus beat.

The **QRS complex** is usually **narrow, but in very premature beats it may be wider (longer duration) than normal.**

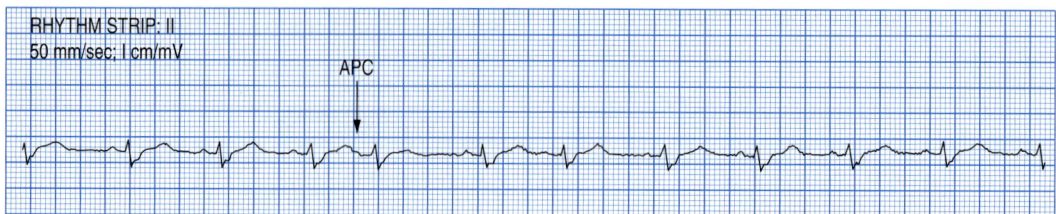

RHYTHM STRIP: II
50 mm/sec; I cm/mV

APC

Figure 10.4. Atrial premature contraction (APC).

There is **association** between **P waves** and the **QRS complex**.

Supraventricular premature beats cause **re-setting** of the **sinoatrial node**.

Supraventricular tachycardia is always **regular**.

Differential diagnosis

Marked respiratory sinus arrhythmia is rare in cats but may mimic the presence of premature beats. **Sinus arrhythmia is rare** in cats and only occurs at slow heart rates. Increasing the heart rate above 180 bpm by excitement or atropine (0.04 mg/kg parenterally) will abolish sinus arrhythmia.

Motion or electrical artifact may mimic premature beats. Premature beats can be distinguished from motion artifact because they occur simultaneously in all leads.

Ventricular premature beats without a wide QRS complex may be erroneously classified as supraventricular premature beats. Supraventricular premature beats will usually reset the sinus rate.

Treatment

Isolated premature beats do not require therapy unless they present with other more severe arrhythmias.

If there is suggestion of hemodynamic compromise therapy may be considered:
- Atenolol at 6.25–12.5 mg/cat PO every 12 hours.
- Diltiazem at 7.5–15 mg/cat PO every 8 hours.
- Propranolol at 0.5–1 mg/kg PO every 8–12 hours.
- Sotalol at 10–20 mg/cat PO every 12 hours.

Prognosis

The prognosis depends on the underlying cardiac disease, but in general, this class of arrhythmias is not likely to severely compromise the patient's outcome.

If the arrhythmia is frequent and is a result of **severe left atrial enlargement**, these beats may reflect atrial electrical instability and **precede the development of atrial fibrillation.**

VENTRICULAR PREMATURE BEATS (VPBS)***

Classical signs

- Pulse deficits.
- Interruptions of rhythm regularity.

Pathogenesis

Premature beats result from two mechanisms, alterations in impulse formation and alterations in impulse conduction.

Alterations of impulse formation depend on the intrinsic automaticity of diseased cardiac cells.
- Diseased myocardial cells outside the specialized conduction system can acquire automaticity because of changes in the resting membrane potential.

Alterations of impulse conduction result from re-entry and by-pass tracts.
- **Re-entry**, is a self-sustaining electrical circuit that **repeatedly depolarizes** surrounding tissue.
- **By-pass tracts** alter the normal pathway of conduction by providing an **alternative pathway around the AV node.**

Clinical signs

Most patients show no evidence of clinical signs.

In some cases with frequent VPBS panting, restlessness and anxiety may be seen.

Diagnosis

The heart rate is normal and the cardiac rhythm is irregular because of the premature beats (Figure 10.5).

The **morphology** of the QRS complex is **abnormal/aberrant** when compared with the normal sinus beat.

The **QRS complex** is **wider** than normal and has a **bizarre appearance**.

VPBs may occur as a **fusion beat**.

VPBs may occur as an **interpolated beat**.

There is **no association** between the P waves and the QRS complex.

VPBs do **not re-set** the sinoatrial node.

Differential diagnosis

Marked respiratory sinus arrhythmia is rare in cats but may mimic the presence of premature beats. **Sinus arrhythmia is rare** in cats and only occurs at slow heart rates. Increasing the heart rate above 180 bpm by excitement or atropine (0.04 mg/kg parenterally) will abolish sinus arrhythmia.

Motion or electrical artifact may mimic premature beats. Premature beats can be distinguished from motion artifact because they occur simultaneously in all leads.

Supraventricular premature beats with aberrant ventricular conduction may be erroneously classified as ventricular premature beats. Supraven-tricular premature beats will usually reset the sinus rate.

Treatment

Isolated premature beats do not require therapy unless present with other more severe arrhythmias.

If there is a large number of ventricular premature beats where the **premature QRS falls within the preceding T wave** (R on T phenomenon), therapy should be considered.

If there is suggestion of hemodynamic compromise therapy may be considered:
- Atenolol at 6.25–12.5 mg/cat PO every 12 hours.
- Propranolol at 0.5–1 mg/kg PO every 8–12 hours.
- Procainamide at 10–20 mg/kg PO every 8–12 hours.
- Sotalol at 10–20 mg/cat PO every 12 hours.

Prognosis

The prognosis depends on the underlying disease.

In most cases isolated premature beats are not life threatening.

When R on T phenomenon is present, patients may be predisposed to the development of ventricular tachycardia and/or sudden death.

If VPBs are due to **primary heart disease,** this likely reflects an advanced stage and may be associated with a **less-favorable prognosis**.

If due to causes **other than primary heart disease**, the **prognosis** is dependent on the **underlying disease**.

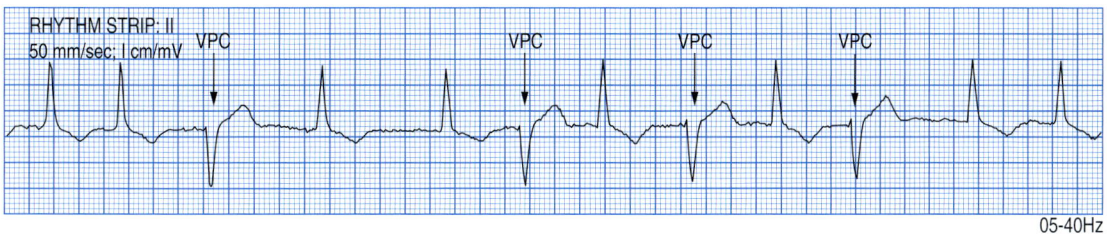

RHYTHM STRIP: II
50 mm/sec; 1 cm/mV
VPC   VPC   VPC   VPC
05-40Hz

Figure 10.5. Ventricular premature contractions.

DISEASES CAUSING BRADYCARDIA

SINUS BRADYCARDIA*

Classical signs

- Heart rate less than 120 beats per minute.
- Pulse is regular.
- Weakness.
- Collapse.

Pathogenesis

This arrhythmia originates from the sino-atrial node, the normal pacemaker of the heart. It is usually indicative of **severe underlying cardiac disease** or secondary to **extracardiac** disease.

Extracardiac causes most commonly associated with this arrhythmia are:
- Respiratory disease.
- Intracranial disease.
- Electrolyte disturbances (hyper or hypokalemia).
- Metabolic disturbances (acidosis, hypoglycemia).
- Hypothermia and hypoxia.
- Overdose of beta-blockers or calcium channel blockers, anesthetic agent or digitalis.

Clinical signs

If the heart rate is less than 100 beats per minute, weakness, collapse and lethargy may be seen.

In the majority of patients, clinical signs are related to the underlying disease.

Diagnosis

The heart rate is lower then 120 bpm.

There is a P wave for every QRS complex.

The QRS complex morphology is normal.

The atropine response test is normal (give 0.04 mg/kg IV while recording rhythm strip, if no response in 2 minutes repeat dose).

Differential diagnosis

Sinus bradycardia may be diagnosed as a junctional escape rhythm in cases where P waves are isoelectric.

Recording several leads, especially chest leads, will facilitate identification of P waves.

Treatment

Treat the underlying disease.

The response to atropine administration should be determined to assess normal sinus node function.

Prognosis

The prognosis depends on the underlying disease.

ATRIAL STANDSTILL*

Classical signs

- Weakness.
- Collapse.
- Lethargy.

Pathogenesis

The arrhythmia can result from atrial cardiomyopathy.

The arrhythmia can occur in **long-standing cardiac disease**, more commonly seen in the **dilated form**.

The arrhythmia can result from **hyperkalemia,** primarily because of feline urethral obstruction syndrome.

A serum potassium greater than 8.5 mEq/L (mmol/L) results in disappearance of P waves and results in atrial standstill.

Clinical signs

Signs may be related to the underlying disease.

Weakness, lethargy and collapse are most commonly seen.

Diagnosis

The heart rate is slower than 120 bpm (Figure 10.6).

There are no P waves in any lead.

The ventricular rhythm is regular.

The QRS complex morphology may be normal or increased in duration and bizarre in morphology.

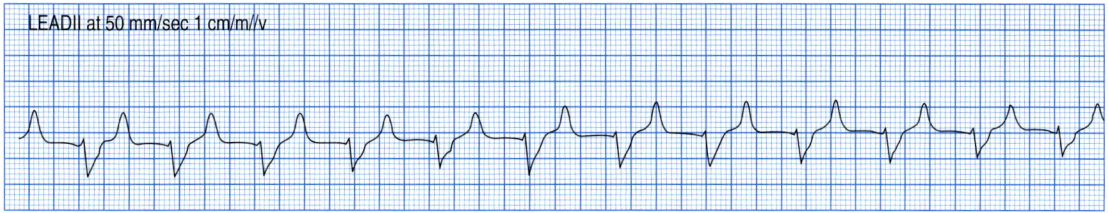

Figure 10.6. Atrial standstill with right bundle branch block. Note lack of P waves.

P waves should not be present in any lead.

In hyperkalemia T waves are tall and peaked.

Differential diagnosis

Sinus bradycardia with isoelectric P waves can mimic atrial standstill.

Recording several leads, especially chest leads, will facilitate identification of P waves.

Treatment

Treat the **underlying disease.** If patient is **symptomatic** for the slow heart rate, a pacemaker is indicated.

Pacemaker lead should be implanted on the epicardium.

Prognosis

Normal atrial activity will not be restored unless the cause is **hyperkalemia**.

After a successful pacemaker implantation, the prognosis is fair because the underlying atrial myopathy is likely to progress to congestive heart failure or thromboembolic disease.

SECOND DEGREE ATRIO-VENTRICULAR BLOCK**

Classical signs

- Weakness.
- Lethargy.
- Collapse.

Pathogenesis

The arrhythmia results from intermittent block of the atrial electrical wave through the AV node. There are two different types:

Mobitz type I
- This type of second-degree AV block is usually the result of **enhanced parasympathetic** tone and is **not associated** with **conduction system disease**.
- The **block** is usually **located above** the **His bundle bifurcation.**
- It is found in some patients with cardiomyopathy and in some cases may be drug induced (digitalis, beta-blockers, calcium channel blockers).

Mobitz type II
- This type of second-degree AV block is the result of **primary conduction system disease**, either due to degeneration of the His bundle, infiltrative cardiac disease or cardiomyopathy.
- The site of **block** is **located** at or **below** the **His bundle.**

Clinical signs

Mobitz type I
- This type of AV block is usually not associated with clinical signs.

Mobitz type II
- Most cases are asymptomatic, when symptoms are present the most common are:
  - Weakness.
  - Lethargy.
  - Collapse.

Diagnosis

Second degree AV block Mobitz type I (Figure 10.7).
- The basic rhythm is a **sinus** rhythm.

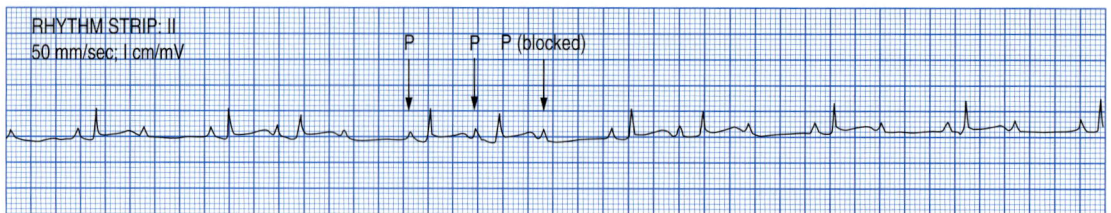

Figure 10.7. Second-degree AV block Mobitz type 1. Note progressive lengthening of the P–R interval.

- The **heart rate** may be **normal** or **lower** than normal.
- There is **progressive prolongation** of the **P–R interval**.
- The P–R interval prolongation is seen at progressively decreasing increments.
- There is progressive shortening of the R–R interval.
- One or more of the P waves are blocked.
- The P–R interval of the beat immediately after a blocked P wave is shorter than the beat immediately before the blocked beat.

Second-degree AV block Mobitz type II.
- The basic rhythm is a **sinus** rhythm.
- The **P–R interval** and the **R–R interval** are **constant**.
- There is unexpected failure of a P wave to conduct to the ventricle.
- The **ventricular rate** is **slower** than the **atrial rate**.
- The **degree of block,** i.e. the relative number of P waves and QRS complex is **variable**.
- The **QRS complex** morphology may be **abnormal**.

Differential diagnosis

When the atrial and ventricular rates are multiples of each other and variable in rate, **third-degree AV block** may mimic second-degree AV block Mobitz type II. Usually the QRS complexes are wide and bizarre with third-degree AV block, but look normal with second-degree AV block.

Artifact mimicking a blocked P wave. Premature beats can be distinguished from motion artifact because they occur simultaneously in all leads.

Treatment

Second-degree AV block Mobitz type I:
- Usually **does not** require **therapy**.

- The response to atropine should be determined. With normal AV nodal function, blocked P waves should disappear and the rhythm becomes regular.

Second-degree AV block Mobitz type II:
- The **treatment** depends on the **severity** of the **block**.
- If the ventricular rate is adequate and the patient does not have symptoms that are explained by the cardiac rhythm, then treat the underlying disease.
- If the patient is **symptomatic** for the bradyarrhythmia:
  - Medical therapy can be tried:
  - Theophylline 20 mg/kg PO every 24 h.
  - Propantheline bromide 7.5 mg/cat PO every 8–12 h.
  - Terbutaline 0.625 mg/cat PO every 8–12 h.
  - Responses to medical therapy are variable and usually temporary, and a **pacemaker** is usually indicated.

Prognosis

Second-degree AV block Mobitz type I:
- The prognosis is good.

Second degree AV block Mobitz type II:
- If the patient is **asymptomatic** and there is no progression of the severity of the AV block, then the prognosis is **favorable**.
- This **form** of AV block may **progress** to **third-degree AV block**.
- Restoration of normal AV conduction is not expected.

THIRD-DEGREE AV BLOCK

Classical signs

- Weakness.
- Lethargy.
- Collapse.

Pathogenesis

This arrhythmia results from **complete block** of the atrial electrical wave through the AV node.

The site of **block** is **at** or **below** the **bundle of His**.

The most common etiologies are:
- Cardiomyopathy.
- Degeneration, fibrosis or infiltration of the conduction system.

Clinical signs

In some cases, no clinical signs are present.

If there are clinical signs these are due to a combination of the underlying disease and the degree of bradycardia.

Usually the heart rate is below 100 beats per minute and the signs are:
- Weakness.
- Lethargy.
- Collapse.

Diagnosis

In third-degree AV block there is **complete dissociation** between the **atrial rhythm** and the **ventricular rhythm** (Figure 10.8).

The **P–P interval** and **R–R interval** are usually **constant**.

The atrial rate is higher than the ventricular rate.

The **P wave** configuration is **normal**.

The QRS complex morphology is normal if the escape focus responsible for ventricular activation is located above the bifurcation of the His bundle.

The **QRS complex** morphology is more **commonly abnormal** and is wide and bizarre.

Differential diagnosis

Advanced second-degree AV block may mimic intermittent third-degree AV block.

Treatment

Many cats are **asymptomatic** with this arrhythmia; therefore treatment is not indicated for these patients.

If **symptoms** of collapse or weakness are present medical therapy can be tried:
- Theophylline 20 mg/kg PO every 24 h.
- Propantheline bromide 7.5 mg/cat PO every 8–12 h.
- Terbutaline 0.625 mg/cat PO every 8–12 h.

Responses to medical therapy are variable and usually temporary and **a pacemaker** is indicated.

Prognosis

The prognosis is poor for restoration of normal AV conduction.

Successful pacemaker implant is associated with a good prognosis if severe morphologic cardiac disease is not present.
- **Epicardial leads are recommended.** The authors do not recommend the use of transvenous pacemaker leads in cats. Transvenous pacemaker leads are commonly associated with post-operative complications, resulting in severe pleural effusion due to thrombosis of the cranial vena cava.

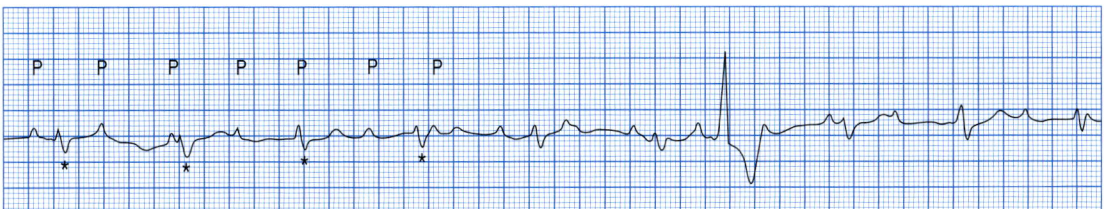

Figure 10.8. Third-degree AV block. Note the lack of relationship between P waves and QRS complexes marked with asterisk.

RECOMMENDED READING

Ettinger, J and Feldman, C. Textbook of Veterinary Internal Medicine. Philadelphia, PA W.B. Saunders., 2004.

Fox P, Sisson D, Moise NS. Textbook of Canine and Feline Cardiology: Principles and Clinical Practice. Philadelphia, PA, WB Saunders Co., 1999.

Kittleson MD, Kienle RD. Small Animal Cardiovascular Medicine. St Louis, MO, Mosby, 1998.

Tilley LP. Essentials of Canine and Feline Electrocardiograph: Interpretation and Treatment. Philadelphia, PA, Lea & Febiger, 1992.

Tilley LP. ECG for the Small Animal Practitioner. Jackson, WY, Teton NewMedia, 1999.

PART 4

Cat with urinary tract signs

11. The cat straining to urinate

Lucio John Filippich

> **KEY SIGNS**
> - Straining to urinate.
> - Excessive time spent in the litter box.
> - Urination in inappropriate places.

MECHANISM?

- Straining in cats during micturition is due to **increased urethral outflow resistance and/or lower urinary tract inflammation or pain**.
- Hematuria associated with difficult or painful urination indicates lower urinary tract bleeding.
- Cats straining to urinate may also **spend excessive time in the litter box** or have **inappropriate urination** which needs to be differentiated from constipation, and behavioral causes of inappropriate urination.

WHERE?

- Lower urinary tract (urinary bladder, urethra and prostate gland).

WHAT?

- Although several lower urinary tract diseases can cause cats to strain, most are idiopathic, followed by urolithiasis and bacterial cystitis/urethritis.

QUICK REFERENCE SUMMARY

Diseases causing straining to urinate

MECHANICAL

● Hypercontractile bladder* (p 190)

Occurs when detrusor muscle contractions are triggered at low volumes and pressure, resulting in urinary bladder storage dysfunction. It may be due to reduced bladder capacity, excessive sensory input or neurologic disorders. Clinical signs include incontinence and pollakiuria associated with a relatively empty urinary bladder.

● Urethral stricture (p 191)

Dysuria associated with urine dribbling and an over-distended urinary bladder.

METABOLIC

● Urolithiasis** (p 184)

Mainly seen in middle-aged cats showing persistent or recurring cystitis and hematuria. The formation of small uroliths can lead to urethral obstruction, especially in male cats. Most frequent uroliths are calcium oxalate and struvite.

NEOPLASTIC

● Neoplasia* (p 191)

Tumors of the lower urinary tract are rare, often malignant and mainly seen in cats over 8 years of age. Dysuria and intermittent or persistent hematuria may occur depending on the type and location of the neoplasm.

INFLAMMATORY

● Infectious cystitis/urethritis* (p 187)

Infectious agents, usually bacterial, may cause inflammation of the urinary tract. Most bacterial infections are secondary to other causes of lower urinary tract disease or the use of indwelling urinary catheters. Clinical signs include dysuria, pollakiuria with or without hematuria. The urinary bladder is usually empty.

IDIOPATHIC

● Obstructed lower urinary tract disease (LUTD)** (p 179)

Urethral plugs are formed causing mechanical urethral obstruction that can lead to bladder distention, post-renal renal failure and death. Occurs mainly in male cats under 5 years of age. Acute onset of dysuria, pollakiuria and stranguria. Abdominal palpation reveals a non-expressible, firm, often painful, over-distended urinary bladder. Signs of uremia include depression, vomiting, dehydration, hypothermia, bradycardia and general muscle weakness.

● Non-obstructed lower urinary tract disease (LUTD)/feline idiopathic cystitis*** (p 176)

Hemorrhagic cystitis of unknown etiology mainly seen in cats 2–6 years of age. History of recurring bouts of dysuria, pollakiuria and hematuria. Abdominal palpation reveals a small contracted, painful urinary bladder. The urine usually contains frank blood and the duration of the hematuria varies.

TRAUMA

- **Urethral trauma* (p 189)**
  May result from pelvic fractures, surgery and catheterization especially when associated with urethral obstruction. Urethral rupture may result in subcutaneous accumulation of urine in the perineal region leading to swelling, discoloration and necrosis of the skin.

TOXIC

- Cyclophosphamide toxicity (p 191)
  The use of cyclophosphamide as a therapeutic agent can lead to hematuria and dysuria.

INTRODUCTION

MECHANISM?

Straining in cats during micturition is due to increased urethral outflow resistance and/or lower urinary tract inflammation or pain.

Straining cat exhibits clinical signs such as **dysuria** (difficult or painful urination), **stranguria** (slow and painful urination with a narrow or dribbling urine stream), **pollakiuria** (abnormally frequent urination) with or without hematuria.

Hematuria associated with dysuria indicates lower urinary tract bleeding.

Owners may complain of **inappropriate urination** or **excessive time spent in the litter box**, so these need to be differentiated from behavioral causes of inappropriate urination and constipation.

Urinary bladder **innervation is primarily autonomic. The storage phase is controlled by sympathetic innervation**.
- During the **filling phase, sympathetic autonomic activity (hypogastric nerve)** dominates and causes the body of the **bladder to relax (β-adrenergic stimulation)** and the **internal sphincter** to **contract (α-adrenergic stimulation)**.
- There is also an α-receptor-mediated inhibition of parasympathetic ganglion transmission.

Pudendal nerves (somatic innervation) stimulate contraction of the external urethal sphincter (and anal sphincter).

Bladder emptying is under parasympathetic control.

Stretch receptors in the detrusor muscle are gradually stretched during bladder fill. **Afferent pelvic nerve fibers (parasympathetic) detect changes in the amount of stretch** during filling and when the threshold of bladder capacity is reached, they **discharge impulses to the sacral spinal cord**.
- These impulses are relayed through the spinoreticular pathways to the **pons** (pontine mesencephalic reticular activating system) in the brain stem where a detrusor response is integrated.
- Efferent motor impulses descend the spinal cord via the reticulospinal pathway to the sacral parasympathetic nucleus, and then on to the **detrusor muscle via the pelvic nerve**.

Each muscle fiber in the detrusor muscle does not receive direct innervation; rather **"pacemaker" fibers** scattered through the detrusor are depolarized with subsequent **spread** of excitation to adjoining muscle fibers through **"tight junctions"**. Tight junctions are areas of fusion of the outer components of the cell membrane.

The resulting wave of excitation causes **contraction of the detrusor, which pulls the neck of the bladder open like a funnel and squeezes out the urine**.

Simultaneously with detrusor muscle contraction, **inhibitory interneurons** are activated in the sacral spinal cord, which synapse on **pudendal motor neurons**. The **pudendal neurons are inhibited, resulting in relaxation of the external urethral sphincter.**

Once the bladder is empty, pelvic nerve activity ceases and the hypogastric and pudendal nerves are no longer inhibited. Detrusor muscle relaxation and urethral sphincters contraction returns and the filling phase begins again.

A **thin mucus layer of glycosaminoglycans** (GAGs) which help **prevent transepithelial movement of urinary substances** covers the urinary bladder mucosa. Defects in surface GAGs may allow urinary substances (protons, potassium ions or hyperosmolar fluid) to penetrate the bladder mucosa initiating sensory nerve stimulation, mast cell activation and/or induce an immune-mediated or neurogenic inflammatory response.

Excitation of sensory afferent neurons (c-fibers) and **release of neuropeptides** and/or **activation of mast cells** in proximity to neuropeptide-containing sensory neurons may **lead to inflammation, pain and tissue injury.**

Mast cell activation results in secretion of biologically active substances (histamine) that may be responsible for the inflammation, pain and smooth muscle contraction seen in bladder disease.

WHERE?

Lower urinary tract (urinary bladder, urethra and prostate gland).

WHAT?

Incidence is about 0.5–0.8% of hospital admissions. Although several lower urinary tract diseases can cause cats to strain, **most are idiopathic**, followed by **urolithiasis and bacterial cystitis/urethritis.**

DISEASES CAUSING SIGNS OF STRAINING

NON-OBSTRUCTED IDIOPATHIC LUTD (IDIOPATHIC CYSTITIS, INTERSTITIAL CYSTITIS)***

Classical signs

- Frequently seen trying to urinate (pollakiuria).
- Spends more time in litter box.
- Strains with little or no urine passed (stranguria/dysuria).
- Blood tinged urine ± blood clots (hematuria).
- Cat may cry out during urination.
- Cat may urinate in inappropriate places.

Pathogenesis

Non-obstructed idiopathic LUTD, also known as **idiopathic or interstitial cystitis,** commonly **presents as hemorrhagic cystitis.** It is the most common cause of signs of lower urinary tract disease in cats, and accounts for 60–70% of cases.

The syndrome is **self-limiting, but recurring**.

Although the etiology is unknown, uropathogens, and inflammation triggered by neurogenic mechanisms or urinary constituents have been postulated.

Stress may play a precipitating role in some cases.

Cats were significantly more likely to be **male, overweight and pedigree.** Several **stress factors** were found to be involved including **living with another cat with which there was conflict.**

Signs and pathophysiology appear analogous to **interstitial cystitis in human beings.**

Feline idiopathic or interstitial cystitis has been associated with local abnormalities in the bladder, and abnormalities in the endocrine system, the central nervous system, and the efferent and afferent neurons.

Bladder abnormalities include decreased urine glucosaminoglycan (GAG) excretion, submucosal petechial hemorrhage (glomerulations) visible when the bladder is distended with water at low or high pressure, increased mast cells in the bladder wall, and increased bladder permeability.

Increased concentrations of the neurotransmitter P and its receptor are present in the bladder wall which may increase the inflammatory response.

Increased sympathetic outflow from the brain is present, and this may result in increased inflammatory response in the bladder and increased permeability.
- Stress and pain increase the sympathetic outflow from the brain, and stress appears to precipitate signs in susceptible cats.

Cats with interstitial cystitis have **reduced cortisol concentrations after stimulation with ACTH,** and have smaller adrenal glands with smaller zona fasciculata and reticularis than healthy cats. These findings suggest cats with interstitial cystitis have primary adrenal insufficiency. Reduced adrenal cortical reserve may result in increased sympathetic nervous system output. Replacement therapy is not effective and not indicated.

Cats with interstitial cystitis are more likely to have **gastrointestinal signs and behavior abnormalities,** suggesting **multiple organ abnormalities.** Recent data suggest interstitial cystitis represents a neuroendocrine disorder rather than a primary bladder disorder.

Clinical signs

More common in female cats in some countries, for example Australia, although equal sex distribution is reported in other countries (USA).

Mainly occurs in **cats 2–6 years of age.**

Typical history is of **recurring bouts of hematuria lasting a few hours to several days** associated with frequent urination and straining. The cat urinating in inappropriate places is also often reported.

Abdominal palpation reveals a **small contracted urinary bladder,** which is often painful on palpation.

The **urine usually contains frank blood** and the duration of the hematuria may vary from a few hours to many days. Blood clots may be seen occasionally in the voided urine.

Diagnosis

Diagnosis of non-obstructed idiopathic LUTD or idiopathic cystitis **is one of exclusion.** It is based on the presence of signs of lower urinary tract disease, and exclusion of other causes of signs using urine culture, and imaging techniques such as plain radiographs, contrast radiography and ultrasonography.

History and physical examination can exclude urethral obstruction. External abdominal palpation reveals a small, often firm, urinary bladder that may go into spasm on palpation. In contrast, with urethral obstruction, the bladder is large on palpation.

Urinalysis.
- A voided sample is sufficient to confirm hematuria but a **cystocentesis sample is required for urinalysis and culture.** If the bladder is empty at presentation, the cat will need to be admitted and bladder fill monitored (see page 188, Infectious Cystitis).

- Urinalysis is more suggestive of a bleeding disorder **(hematuria; >5 RBC/hpf, <5 WBC/hpf)** than an inflammatory disease (pyuria > 5 WBC/hpf).
  - Erythrocytes in urine may be at various stages of degeneration, suggesting chronic bleeding.
  - **Pyuria (>5 WBC/hpf) is not a feature of this disease.**
- Urine is bacteriologically sterile.
- Crystalluria is usually absent, and when present, the crystals (struvite) are of normal size and number.

Radiography or ultrasonography.
- Survey abdominal radiographs are usually normal.
- Contrast radiographs may reveal **bladder wall thickening and mucosal irregularities**.
- **Ultrasonographic** finding **may be normal** or reveal hyperechoic material presumed to be crystalline in nature, blood clots and **mural irregularities or thickenings**.
- Imaging can be used to exclude urolithiasis and neoplasia.

Cystoscopic examination may show increased mucosal vascularity, superficial urothelial desquamation and **submucosal hemorrhage.**

Bladder wall biopsy via cystoscopy is increasingly being used in practice and may show epithelial hyperplasia, mucosal necrosis, muscular degeneration, edema, fibrosis, and perivascular accumulation of lymphocytes and hemorrhage.

Differential diagnosis

Cystitis/urethritis typically occurs in middle-aged or older cats and is characterized by pyuria and bacteriuria.

Urolithiasis occurs in middle-aged or older cats, and imaging reveals a urolith.

Hypercontractile bladder is usually not associated with hematuria, despite signs of straining and pollakiuria.

Neoplasia occurs in older cats and ultrasound or contrast radiography reveals a mass.

Behavioral causes of inappropriate urination are generally **not associated with hematuria, dysuria and stranguria.**

TREATMENT

Goals of therapy are to relieve the discomfort and pain associated with cystitis and to reduce the frequency of recurrence.

Signs are self-limiting despite therapy. Remission usually occurs within 7 days.

Several treatments, such as antimicrobials, glucocorticoids, progestagens (megestrol acetate), intravesicular administration of DMSO (10–20 ml of 10% solution instilled in bladder for 10 minutes under general anesthesia), anticholinergic agents, diuretics (furosemide), elimination diets, pentosan polysulfate and the surgical placement of a copper ring in to the bladder have been advocated, but their efficacy is questionable.

Antispasmodic drugs can provide symptomatic relief from straining. Flavoxate (50 mg BID), propantheline bromide (7.5 mg/cat sid PO), or phenoxybenzamine (2.5–10 mg PO q 8–12 h).

Pain relief via opiates (including a fentyl patch, butorphanol elixir) are indicated for cats that are frequently straining to urinate.

Anti-inflammatory drugs such as piroxicam (0.3 mg/kg PO sid) may decrease straining and pollakiuria.

Megestrol acetate 5 mg sid PO for 5 days has been reported by one author (Norsworthy) to be the most effective drug for relieving dysuria.

Hydrodistension of the urinary bladder (80 cm of water for 10–15 minutes) may give relief of signs in some cats and prevent reoccurence.

Cosequin (pentosan polysulfate (Elmiron) 8 mg/kg PO q 12 h) is a **glycosaminoglycan (GAG)** which is used in humans with interstitial cystitis to promote urothelial GAG formation. It can be mixed in the food and given indefinitely to reduce recurrence. However, GAG replacers have not been proven to be more effective than placebo in cats with interstitial cystitis.

Feed exclusively a specially formulated non-calcinogenic **diet that is used to minimize struvite crystal formation** and **maintain a low urine pH (<6.5)** and **specific gravity (<1.030)**. Such diets have been shown to be effective. However, struvite crystalluria does not appear to be a significant factor in non-obstructed LUTD, and the benefit of these diets may be from the reduction in urine SG.

Canned food has been shown to reduce the incidence of feline lower urinary tract disease compared to dry food, probably because of the lower urine SG produced. **Constancy of diet may help as dietary change can precipitate signs.**

Aim for a **low urine specific gravity (eg. 1.020),** by adding water or a meat-flavored liquid to the food. Urine should look like water and have no odor. If feeding dry food, add 1 cup of water to 1 cup of dry food and allow it to soak for at least 5 minutes.

Amitryptyline (2.5–5 mg/cat orally at night) may be useful in some cats to reduce signs of irritative voiding but not hematuria. It is a tricyclic antidepressant which prevents mast cell degranulation and has anti-inflammatory, analgesic, anticholinergic and alpha adrenergic blocking effects. A significant reduction in the frequency of recurrence may occur with prolonged use, without improvement in urinalysis or cystoscopy findings. Adverse reactions reported in cats include sedation, weight gain, unkempt haircoat, urine retention, thrombocytopenia and neutropenia.

Reduction of stress and environmental change may help to prevent recurrence. In susceptible cats, episodes can be triggered by environmental change (e.g. changes in food, house, animals or people in the house).

- Use of the synthetic **feline facial pheromone** (Feliway, Ceva Animal Health), which reduces anxiety in cats may be beneficial in some situations. In cats with interstitial cystitis, there was a trend to show fewer days with clinical signs of cystitis in cats where the environment was treated with the pheromone.

Ensure that there are sufficient litter boxes and they are cleaned frequently.

If signs do not resolve within 7 days, the cat should be re-evaluated for other diseases causing these signs.

Prognosis

Prognosis for recurrence is guarded because the etiology is unknown and treatment is largely supportive in nature.

Recurrence of signs within 6–12 months occurs in a high percentage of cats.

OBSTRUCTED IDIOPATHIC LUTD**

Classical signs

- Straining with little or no urine passed (stranguria/dysuria).
- Frequently seen trying to urinate (pollakiuria).
- Cat may cry out during urination.

Pathogenesis

Historically, diets or components of diets, such as magnesium and phosphate, have been implicated in the pathogenesis of some forms of idiopathic LUTD in cats.

Although the etiology is unknown, **urethral plugs** are formed causing mechanical urethral obstruction that can lead to bladder distention, post-renal renal failure and death.

- It occurs **mainly in male cats** possibly because their **urethra is longer, narrower** and less distensible.
- The **urethral plugs are composed of colloidal matrix** into which are embedded crystals, usually struvite crystals (magnesium ammonium phosphate).
  - The ratio of matrix to crystalline material varies with **some urethral plugs (about 5%) lacking crystalline material** and are known as non-crystalline matrix plugs.
  - Other **crystals that occur less commonly** include ammonium acid urate, and **calcium phosphate** and calcium oxalate.
  - Some urethral plugs may also contain erythrocytes.
  - The exact chemical composition and **origin of the matrix are unknown** although Tamm-Horsfall protein of renal origin has been implicated.
- The factors(s) involved in the formation of urethral plugs are unknown and may be different for the different plugs.
- Since minerals other than struvite may be found in some urethral plugs, suggesting matrix per se may play an important primary role in the formation of some plugs.

- Acid–base status of the urine is important in crystal formation, with alkaline urine favoring struvite formation and acid urine favoring oxalate formation.
- The role of viruses is controversial.

Occasionally urethral obstruction is from a urolith, rather than a plug. Calcium oxalate urate and cystine uroliths are more common causes of urethal obstruction than struvite uroliths. The mechanism for urolith formation is different from plug formation, and is covered on page 184 in Urolithiasis.

Urethral obstruction **can result** in **post-renal renal failure** (obstructive nephropathy).

- The severity of the renal failure depends on the degree and duration of the obstruction.
- **Post-renal renal failure can be biochemically detected by 24 hours after complete obstruction,** and by **48 hours** clinical and metabolic changes can become **life threatening.**
- Post-renal renal failure is invariably reversible with appropriate treatment.

Bladder over-distention may result in ischemia, edema, hemorrhage and **loss of epithelium**. The **urethra, proximal to the obstruction, will have similar injuries** with desquamation of epithelium, edema and infiltration of neutrophils around blood vessels, lamina propria and muscle layers.

Post-obstructive diuresis may occur following relief of the obstruction and last for several days.

- The diuresis is possibly due to the clearance of accumulated metabolites and a temporary loss of concentrating ability by the renal tubules.
- Dehydration and possibly hypokalemia can occur during this polyuric phase.

Clinical signs

Almost always seen in **male cats under 5 years of age**.

History of **excessive licking around the perineal area and the penis** is often seen extruded from the prepuce.

Acute onset of dysuria.

The cat may cry out during urination.

Close inspection of the penis may show a **whitish, chalky material blocking the urethral orifice** and the tip of the penis traumatized due to excessive licking.

Abdominal palpation reveals a **non-expressible, firm, often painful, over-distended bladder**. Cats **obstructed for over 48 hours may show little or no signs of pain** on abdominal palpation and in such cases, the **bladder may rupture** if handled other than with extreme care and gentleness.

Cats with partial obstruction may be able to maintain a small bladder size and not develop renal failure. Such cats show stranguria (painful urination with a narrower urine stream).

Signs of uremia indicate complete obstruction for at least 48 hours.

- **Depression, anorexia**, vomiting, dehydration and **hypothermia**.
- **Hyperkalemia can cause bradycardia**, ventricular arrhythmia and general muscle weakness.
- Metabolic acidosis may exacerbate the effects of hyperkalemia on the myocardium.
- Shock.

Diagnosis

History and physical examination.

- **Acute onset of dysuria in a male cat**.
- A **distended, firm** and often painful urinary **bladder** on abdominal palpation.
- Whitish, chalky material seen blocking the urethral orifice or around the prepucal/perineal area.

Urinalysis.

- Varying degrees of **hematuria** depending on the duration of the obstruction.
- Pyuria is variable.
- **Crystalluria is often seen** and on many occasions large crystals are found in the urine. The significance of these large crystals is unclear.
- Urinary pH and specific gravity values, at presentation, are variable, but pH is usually acidic and **specific gravity generally approaches 1.020 with prolonged obstruction**.
- Glucosuria is variable.

Radiography. Urethral plugs are often not visible on plain radiographs.

Electrocardiography.

- Hyperkalemia (>6.0 mmol (mEq)/L). ECG changes are often evident when K > 7 mmol(mEq)/L.
  - Bradycardia.
  - Absence of a P wave.
  - Widened QRS interval.
  - Spiked T wave.

Blood tests.

- Changes in blood values (urea, creatinine, potassium, phosphorus, pH) depend on the severity of the renal failure.
- Serum values are usually normal in cats with lower urinary tract disease unless there is outflow obstruction or rupture.
  - **Post-renal azotemia (increased urea, creatinine), hyperphosphatemia, hyperkalemia** become evident by **24 hours**. Hypocalcemia is variable. Mild hyperglycemia may be present.
- The absence of clinical signs of hyperkalemia (bradycardia) does not eliminate the possibility of severe hyperkalemia.

Differential diagnosis

Urolithiasis occurs more often in middle-aged or older cats.

Functional urethral obstruction is often associated with other neurologic signs (see The incontinent cat).

Urethral trauma usually has a history and hindquarter lesions which are suggestive.

Stricture is usually preceded by a history of catheterization or trauma.

Neoplasia.

TREATMENT

Depends on the severity of the clinical signs at presentation.

If the cat is not showing clinical signs of renal failure or has not been obstructed for more than **24–36 hours, relieving the urethral obstruction** and giving a **balanced electrolyte solution**, subcutaneously or intravenously at 70 ml/kg is usually sufficient.

If the cat is showing **signs of renal failure**, or has been **obstructed for more than 36–48 hours, correcting the fluid and electrolyte imbalance takes priority over restoring urethral patency**.

- Cats in post-renal renal failure must first be stabilized before diagnostic tests, other than blood and urine sampling, are undertaken.

- Consider **cystocentesis** for **temporary relief of bladder distention**.
- Give **dextrose saline solution** IV (0.9% NaCl with 5% dextrose – add 100 ml of 50% dextrose per liter of fluids) to rehydrate the patient over 4–6 hours and reduce hyperkalemia, metabolic acidosis and azotemia.
- Cats in renal failure are frequently **hypothermic** and **should be warmed** to normal body temperature.

Remove the obstruction.
- **Immobilization.**
- **Sedation during catheterization will help minimize further urethral trauma and urethral or bladder rupture.**
- Urethral trauma from catheterization can lead to inflammation with edema of the periurethral tissue and subsequent functional urethral obstruction.
- Inappropriate force or the cat struggling during catheterization may result in urethral or bladder rupture.
- The degree of sedation required will depend on the cat's clinical condition and temperament.
- An opiate (pethidine (meperidine)) 1 mg/kg SC; butorphanol (0.05–0.4 mg/kg IV, SC; buprenorphine 0.005–0.01 mg/kg IV, SC) and acepromazine (0.02–0.05 mg/kg IV, SC) or an opiate and diazepam (0.25 mg/kg SC, IV) can be used.
- Premedicate with atropine sulfate (0.03 mg/kg) subcutaneously or intravenously combined in the same syringe as the opiate. **Intravenous ultra short-acting barbiturates** (sodium thiamylal or thiopentone (thiopental)), propofol, alfaxalone and **inhalant anesthetics** (isoflurane) can be used. Depressed cats can be masked down with isoflurane and oxygen. Beware of intubating the cat before it has reached a suitable plane of anesthesia, as intubation may cause reflex bradycardia or cardiac arrest. Spray the larynx with lignocaine (lidocaine) prior to attempting intubation.
- Succinylcholine is contra-indicated as it increases serum potassium levels.
- Catheterization of the bladder in cats with severe renal failure may be possible by using physical restraint only.
- **Catheterization.**
  - The method employed and the instrumentation used to remove the obstruction must ensure that no further urethral or bladder trauma occurs.

- Exteriorize the penis from the prepuce and extend it caudally so as to straighten the natural curvature of the cat's penis. Clean with warm water.
- As aseptically as possible, fill a **3.5 French, open-ended urinary catheter (olive tip urethral catheters, Jorgensen Laboratories) with lubricating gel (xylocaine jelly at room temperature)** and gently pass the catheter into the urethra, until it comes in contact with the obstructing material, which is **usually at the level of the bulbo-urethral gland** where the urethra narrows and becomes the penile portion.
- **Instill 0.25 ml of lubricating gel** through the catheter into the urethra and remove the catheter. **After 3 minutes,** the jelly usually has lubricated and broken up the obstructing mass, allowing it to be spontaneously extruded like toothpaste by the high urethral pressure cranial to the obstruction. **If the material re-obstructs, repeat the procedure several times using 0.15 ml** of gel, until urine appears. This technique ensures that all the obstructing material in the urethra has been removed and little if any has been pushed into the bladder. If spontaneous resolution of the obstruction does not occur, **apply gentle pressure to the bladder.** Great care should be exercised when applying pressure to the urinary bladder, as it can lead to bladder rupture.
- Retropulsion with a saline flush is commonly used in practice, but is more likely to lead to re-obstruction, because obstruding material is pushed into the bladder.
- If **local anesthetic agents** are combined in the lubricating gel to anesthetize the urethral mucosa, they **should be used sparingly to avoid local and systemic toxic** effects that are more likely to occur in the presence of damaged urothelium.
- **Recatheterize** with a **long, soft, flexible Teflon urinary catheter (3.5–4 French),** secured in place with sutures, to empty the bladder completely.
- Once the bladder has been catheterized, urine is allowed to drip freely. **Avoid removing urine by negative pressure** (syringe) **or by applying external pressure** on the urinary bladder as this can unnecessarily traumatize the bladder mucosa.
- **If the urine is visibly clear: Instill 5–10 ml of sodium acetate/acetic acid** buffer solution

(**Wallpoles buffer solution**) into the **bladder** to **dissolve any struvite crystals**. If the catheterization was achieved with minimal trauma, an indwelling catheter is not required.

- **If hematuria is present: Wallpoles buffer solution should not be used.**
- **Instill 100 mg of ampicillin in 20 ml of normal saline** into the bladder. Give parenteral antimicrobials that are not nephrotoxic, such as amoxicillin/clavulanate, enrofloxacin. Leave the urinary catheter in situ for as shorter a time as possible. Indwelling catheters can induce further damage to the urothelium by disrupting its glycosaminoglycan coating and thus promote microbial adherence and urinary tract infection. **Remove the indwelling catheter once hematuria is no longer visible.**

- **An indwelling catheter is required if**:
  - Obstructing material was expelled into the urinary bladder.
  - Severe urethral trauma occurred associated with removal of the plug. Significant trauma occurs if excessive force or repeated catheterization attempts are necessary to unblock the urethra.
  - A large amount of potentially obstructing debris is present in the bladder, which may be determined during bladder empting, by palpation of the empty bladder, or by radiography/ultrasonography.
  - Urine stream after relief of the obstruction is narrower than normal.
  - The urinary bladder does not contract normally after emptying, indicating atony.
  - Re-obstruction occurs, especially within 24 hours.
  - Measurement of urine flow rate is required during intensive care of critically ill cats.
  - In these situations, the advantages of maintaining urethral patency and decompression of a chronically distended, devitalized bladder outweighs the disadvantages of ascending bacterial infection and ongoing damage to the urethral mucosa.
  - Silicone elastomer catheters (Wysong urethral catheter) are preferred as they are soft, pliable, less irritant to the urethral mucosa and curl up inside the bladder without kinking as the bladder empties, thus avoiding bladder wall irritation.

- A closed urine drainage system is often impractical in the cat. However, it should be used if indwelling catheters are to be left in for more than 3–4 days. A closed drainage system involves connecting the urinary catheter, via extension tubing, to a sterile, empty fluid bag below the cat.
- Indwelling catheters should be used for as short a time as possible to minimize catheter-induced iatrogenic disease.
- Beginning the cat on phenoxybenzamine (2.5–10 mg PO q 8–2 h) may help to reduce re-obstruction or dysinergia once the catheter is removed.
- An Elizabethan collar and/or hobbles on the hind legs using self adhesive tape or elastoplast may be necessary to prevent the cat interfering with the urinary catheter.
- Most cats will not interfere with a properly placed or correctly selected indwelling urinary catheter. Interference usually indicates poor catheter placement or catheter-induced irritation.
- The use of antimicrobial therapy to prevent secondary urinary tract infection is controversial.
- To avoid developing resistant organisms, it is recommended that a broad-spectrum antimicrobial, such as amoxicillin be used only once infection occurs.
- Evidence that an infection is occurring includes the appearance of hematuria or increasing hematuria, bacteriuria and pyuria.
- Removal of the catheter at the first signs of urinary infection may obviate the need for antimicrobial therapy.
- Follow-up urine culture and susceptibility tests are essential to determine treatment success.
- Once the catheter is removed, the cat should be keep in hospital for a further 24 hours to ensure that it can urinate freely.

- **If the obstruction cannot be relieved**:
  - **General anesthesia** in an unanesthetized patient **may help to relieve urethral spasm,** and the intraluminal pressure present in the urinary bladder and urethra may facilitate the removal of the obstructing material.
  - The **use of acid buffer solutions** to dissolve the obstructing material **is ineffective** and time wasting, especially if the cat is in post-renal renal failure.

- **Decompress the bladder by cystocentesis** using a 23 G × 32 mm (1.25 in) needle attached to an extension tube, a 2-way valve and 50 ml syringe. Removal of approximately 30 ml of urine from the bladder **may trigger spontaneous micturition.** The bladder should not be manually palpated for the next 24 hours.
- Consider **cystotomy** with **placement of an indwelling catheter** (Foley catheter, 8 French; Stamey suprapubic catheter, 10 French) in the urinary bladder, and percutaneous prepubic urinary drainage or a perineal urethrostomy.
- **Perineal urethrostomy is only recommended as a last resort** because it does not prevent reoccurrence of non-obstructed disease and it can predispose to ascending urinary tract infection, urine scald dermatitis and urethral stricture.
- **Perineal urethrostomy is recommended** if frequent urethral obstruction occurs despite **adequate medical management or urethral lesions** exist that cause recurrent or persistent obstruction.

Prednisolone (2.5 mg/cat orally every 12 hours for 3–5 days) may reduce urethral inflammation but may predispose to urinary tract infection.

Functional urethral obstruction due to urethral irritation and inflammation resulting in urethral spasm can occur following mechanical obstruction. This is difficult to differentiate from mechanical urethral obstruction, however, failure to encounter obstructing material or a grating sensation during recatheterization, suggests function urethral obstruction.

Phenoxybenzamine (5 mg/cat orally daily for 3–5 days) may help reduce urethral outflow resistance.

Bladder atony may occur due to overdistention and can be corrected (see The Incontinent Cat).

Postobstructive diuresis.
- Following relief of the obstruction, a **marked diuresis may occur and last for 2–10 days**.
- Intravenous fluid therapy is required to maintain hydration and electrolyte balance. Initially a **dextrose saline solution** is used to hydrate the patient over **4–6 hours**, followed by a **balanced electrolyte solution (lactated Ringers solution)** to maintain hydration and correct electrolyte imbalance.

- Hypokalemia may occur with prolonged diuresis or the use of potassium-free fluids. **Potassium supplementation** can be given in intravenous fluids (0.5 mmol/kg/h) or orally (2–6 mmol/cat/day) until the cat starts eating.
- The gluconate form of potassium is preferred orally.
- Once the cat voluntarily eats and drinks, the fluid rate is decreased over 24 hours while hydration status is monitored.

Prevention.
- Feed exclusively a specially formulated non-calcinogenic diet to minimize struvite crystal formation and maintain a low urine pH (<6.5) and low specific gravity (<1.030, ideally 1.020). Meat- or fish-flavored liquid or water can be added to increase water intake.
  - Canned food produces a lower urine specific gravity than dry food, and decreases the frequency of recurrence in cats. If feeding dry food, add 1 cup of water per 1 cup of diet and allow to soak at least 5 minutes before feeding.

Prognosis

The prognosis depends on the duration of the obstruction, on the ease of obtaining and maintaining urethral patency, and correction of renal failure.

Prognosis is grave if:
- The duration of the **obstruction is more than 60 hours**.
- The **packed cell volume of centrifuged bloody urine is greater than 2%**.
- **Urinary specific gravity is below 1.020**.

The **recurrence rate is 35–50%,** mainly within 6 months after hospitalization. Recurrence appears to be **higher in cats under 4 years of age.**

Studies on the efficacy of specially formulated diets in naturally occurring idiopathic LUTD are limited but the results are encouraging. Such diets have been formulated to reduce magnesium and phosphate intake and promote a dilute, acid urine. However, the pH of these diets may predispose to oxalte uroliths in susceptible cats.

The **prognosis** following **urethrostomy is good** in that recurrence of urethral obstruction is unlikely, but **recurring episodes** of **non-obstructed cystitis** may occur. Post-surgically, urethral strictures and/or incontinence have been reported, but are uncommon following uncomplicated surgery. Urethrostomy may **predispose to ascending urinary tract infection.**

UROLITHIASIS**

> ### Classical signs
>
> - Blood-tinged urine (hematuria).
> - Frequently seen trying to urinate (pollakiuria).
> - Spends more time in litter box.
> - Straining to urinate (dysuria).
> - Cat may urinate in inappropriate places.

Pathogenesis

Urolithiasis in cats is uncommon and represents less than 5% of cats presented with hematuria and dysuria.

Urolithiasis is the formation of stones called uroliths (calculi) in the urinary tract.

Uroliths are made up of **crystalloid with very little organic matrix**, and although a particular chemical type usually predominates, the chemical composition of the urolith can be mixed.

- The main chemical composition of uroliths reported in cats, include **magnesium ammonium phosphate (struvite; 42%), calcium oxalate (46%),** purine (uric acid and urates; 6%), calcium phosphate (<1%) and cystine (<1%).
- Each chemical type should be considered a separate disease process.
- The incidence of struvite uroliths appears to be decreasing while calcium oxalate uroliths are increasing. This is thought to be due to the increased use of acidifying diets in cats.

Urolithiasis is not a single disease entity, but rather the end result of one or more physiological and/or pathological processors, interrelated with some **predisposing factor**(s), **such as urine pH and concentration,** excessive **excretion of endogenous crystalloid-forming substances** (uric acid, amino acid cystine), **excessive mineral** intake and **genetic factors**.

Unlike the dog, struvite uroliths in cats are **usually not associated with urinary tract infection**.

Hypercalcemia (primary hyperparathyroidism, pseudohyperparathyroidism, idiopathic, hypercalcemia and vitamin D intoxication) results in hypercalciuria, which has been **associated with calcium oxalate urolith formation.** However, most cats with calcium oxalate uroliths have normal serum mineral levels.

Congenital portovascular anomalies and renal tubular reabsorptive defects have been associated with purine (urate) uroliths. Urate uroliths consist of either ammonium biurate (which occur with porto/vascular anomalies), uric acid or sodium acid urates (occur with tubular defects). Predisposed cats fed a high purine diet (e.g. liver) and producing concentrated, acidic urine are at a greater risk of producing purine uroliths.

Cystinuria due to **proximal renal tubular dysfunction** can **predispose to cystine urolith formation**.

Uroliths, especially those in the bladder, **can cause lower urinary tract disease**.

The formation of **small uroliths** can lead to **urethral obstruction**, especially in male cats.

Clinical signs

Mainly seen in **middle-aged adult cats**.

There appears to be no sex or breed predisposition.

Most cystoliths are asymptomatic.

Persistent or recurring cystitis may occur and present as increased frequency of urination, straining to urinate or increased time spent in the litter box or urinating in inappropriate places.

Hematuria varies from microscopic hematuria (>5 RBC/hpf) to gross hematuria.

Urethral obstruction may occur occasionally, more commonly with calcium oxalate, urate or cystine uroliths than with struvite uroliths.

Diagnosis

Physical examination. Cystic uroliths are usually difficult to palpate (<10%) because most are flattened disc-shape and few in number.

Urinalysis.
- Most uroliths and crystals in a urine sample are calcium oxalate or struvite, although heavy crystal-

luria with amorphous urates and phosphates is occasionally seen.

- **Urine sediment containing struvite crystals** (three- to six-sided colorless **prisms**) **suggests that the urolith is struvite** in composition.
- **Urine sediment containing calcium oxalate dihydrate** (colorless **envelopes** with dipyramidal or octahedral form) or monohydrate crystals (small spindles or dumbbells) suggests that the urolith is calcium oxalate in composition.
- **Ammonium biurate crystals** (yellow-brown spherulites; thorn apples) are common in cats with portosystemic vascular anomalies, however urate uroliths are uncommon. Rarely urate uroliths also occur due to tubular disease (cat has no signs of liver disease and normal pre- and post-prandial bile acids). Urate crystals associated with tubular disease appear different from biurates, and are composed of uric acid or sodium acid urate.
- However, **crystal type in urine and urolith composition can be different**.
- Uroliths found in alkaline urine are likely to be struvite or calcium phosphate (amorphous or long thin prisms).
- **Urinary tract infections are usually absent (<2%).**
- Hypercalciuria may occur with calcium containing uroliths.

Radiography.
- Plain abdominal radiographs may detect radiodense uroliths in the kidneys, bladder or urethra.
  - **Radiodense uroliths contain calcium salts**, such as calcium oxalate.
  - Struvite uroliths may contain calcium and become slightly radiodense.
- **Double-contrast cystography** can be used to detect radiolucent uroliths. The technique involves instilling, via a urinary catheter, 1–2 ml of water-soluble iodinated contrast material (positive contrast) into the urinary bladder, followed by a slow infusion of carbon dioxide or nitrous oxide gas (negative contrast), sufficient to distend the bladder (approximately 30 ml). Fatal air embolism can occur in cats with hematuria when air is used.
- **Retrograde contrast urethrography.** The technique involves infusing, as a bolus, 5 ml of positive contrast material through an open-ended urinary **catheter positioned in the distal ure-**

thra. To minimize back leakage, digital pressure around the catheter and urethra can be applied or balloon-tipped catheters (4 or 5 French) can be used to occlude the urethra. Radiographs are taken **during the infusion of the last portion of the bolus dose.**

Ultrasonography.
- Abdominal ultrasonography can be used to **identify radiodense and radiolucent cystic uroliths**, as well as soft tissue masses.

Blood tests (biochemistry).
- Elevated serum urea and creatinine levels suggest renal involvement.
- Elevated liver enzymes and/or low urea levels suggest liver dysfunction. Typically cats with ammonium biurate uroliths associated with portosystemic shunts have reduced serum urea levels, increased serum uric acid and bile acid levels and hyperammonemia.
- Hypercalcemia may suggest a calcium-containing urolith.

Urolith analysis.
- **Urolith analysis** provides valuable information that can be used in therapy to prevent the recurrence of urolithiasis.
- Crystallographic, X-ray diffraction and infrared spectroscopy techniques are preferable to qualitative chemical analysis (Oxford Stone Analysis Kit). A proper **quantitative analysis gives all the mineral components of the urolith by percentage and by location (surface, middle and center). Prevention therapy is based on the mineral composition of the center of the urolith** as precipitation of the central mineral initiates urolith formation.

Differential diagnosis

Infectious cystitis/urethritis is differentiated on the presence of bacteriuria and a positive culture.

Idiopathic LUTD tends to occur in young adult cats.

Treatment

Uroliths can be removed by medical dissolution or surgical resection. The type and location of the urolith, the severity of the clinical signs, the anesthetic risk, concurrent diseases, the sex and age of the cat, and the owner's wishes will all influence which procedure is most appropriate.

- **Surgical removal**.
  - Cystotomy is performed via a ventral midline abdominal approach. An avascular area near the apex of the bladder is selected, stay sutures (3-0 silk) placed on either side of the intended incision line and the bladder is emptied by cystocentesis. A 2-cm incision is made into the bladder wall and the uroliths removed. Before closure of the bladder, a urinary catheter attached to a saline-filled syringe is used to flush out any uroliths in the bladder neck and urethra.
- **Medical dissolution**.
  - **Only nephroliths and cystoliths can be medically dissolved. Medical dissolution of uroliths in the ureters or urethra should not be attempted**.
  - **Calcium oxalate uroliths can not be medically dissolved**.
  - **Struvite uroliths can be medically dissolved**.
  - Mineral composition of the urolith should be determined before dissolution therapy is attempted. However, this is often not possible, and crystals in the urine sediment are used as a guide.
  - Dissolution diets are designed to produce an acidic, low-mineral, dilute urine environment in which cystic struvite uroliths dissolve over a period of 4–8 weeks. Nephroliths usually take longer to dissolve.
  - The **dissolution diet should be fed for at least 2–4 weeks after uroliths are no longer visible radiographically or on ultrasound**.
  - **Failure to dissolve the uroliths** may be due to poor owner compliance, the presence of urinary tract infection or the mineral composition of the urolith is not struvite.

Prevention

Long-term prevention strategies to prevent or minimize reoccurrence should be based on mineral composition of the urolith.

If infection is present, this must be treated and the urine (culture, urinalysis especially pH) monitored long term to ensure that the infection has been eliminated. **Urine**

pH should stay below 6.5 long term. Cats passing alkaline urine should be recultured.

Struvite urolithiasis.
- An acidifying, low-magnesium, low-phosphorus and low-calcium diet is recommended.
- Alternatively, urine acidifiers (ammonium chloride or DL methionine) to effect (approximately 1000 mg/cat/day) can be given orally at mealtime to ameliorate the postprandial alkaline tide. Acute toxicity with high doses cat occur, especially in kittens.
- Chronic metabolic acidemia due to long-term acidification can have adverse effects.

Calcium oxalate urolithiasis.
- A non-acidifying regular diet is recommended.
- Diets used to prevent struvite urolithiasis should not be used.
- If the diet does not maintain the **urine pH above 7.5, potassium citrate** (50–75 mg/kg orally 12 hourly) therapy may be used. Monitor total CO_2 to ensure alkalosis does not occur. Keep TCO_2 about 20 mmol(mEq)/L.
- **Vitamin B6** (2 mg/kg orally every 24–48 hours) may be useful.
- The cause of hypercalcemia, if present, should be determined and treated.
- **Thiazide diuretics** (chlorthiazide, 10 mg/kg orally 12 hourly) with potassium supplementation have been used in normocalcemic dogs with oxalate uroliths.

Urate urolithiasis.
- Avoid acidifying diets and diets high in purine precursors (e.g. liver).

Cystine urolithiasis.
- Acidifying diets should not be fed.

Prognosis

Recurrence rates of 19% and 37% have been reported.

Prognosis is guarded because in some cases recurrences occur despite the implementation of adequate preventative measures.

Unless preventative measures are implemented, urolithiasis will reoccur.

INFECTIOUS CYSTITIS/URETHRITIS*

Classical signs

- Frequently seen trying to urinate (pollakiuria).
- Straining with little urine passed (dysuria).
- Blood-tinged urine (hematuria).
- Cat may urinate in inappropriate places.

Pathogenesis

Inflammation of the feline urinary tract is rarely caused by an infectious agent.

About **5–10%** of cats with **lower urinary tract disease have urinary tract infections**, which may be primary or secondary.

The prevalence of urinary tract infections **increases with age**, being uncommon in young adult cats to middle age of either sex.

- Urinary tract infection accounts for **less than 2%** of cases of lower urinary tract disease in **cats from 1–10 years of age.**
- Of **cats older than 10 years of age** with signs of lower urinary tract disease, **46%** had a positive urine culture and a further **17%** had a positive culture associated with **urolithiasis.** Two thirds of cats with a positive culture not associated with urolithiasis had **chronic renal failure.**
- Of **cats with chronic renal failure, 30%** had one or more positive urine cultures over a period of 4–8 months which were all **E. coli.**

Most bacterial infections in cats are **secondary** to other causes of lower urinary tract disease, perineal urethrostomy, the use of indwelling urinary catheters or chronic renal failure.

Predisposing causes of urinary tract infection include:

- **Anatomical abnormalities** (ectopic ureter, patent urachus, perineal urethrostomy).
- **Urethral incompetence** (usually associated with perineal urethrostomy).
- Loss of mechanical washout of the bladder and urethra due to bladder atony, **urolithiasis**, painful hindquarters and debility.

- Damage to the bladder mucosal defense barrier due to **trauma** (catheterization, surgery, uroliths) or **neoplasia.**
- **Changes in urine composition** (alkaline pH, glucosuria).
- **Chronic renal failure.**

Infectious agents include:
- **Bacterial** cystitis/urethritis (cystourethritis).
  - Rare in cats and **most are aerobic infections**.
  - Common organisms cultured include **Escherichia coli**, **Staphlococcus** intermedius, **Streptococcus** spp., Proteus, Pasteurella, Klebsiella, Pseudomonas and Enterobacter. Occasionally Mycoplasma and Ureaplasma are reported and these organisms do not grow on routine culture media.
  - **Mycoplasma cultures should be considered if pyuria is present but no aerobic bacterial growth** occurs.
  - Recurrent ascending urinary tract infections occur in **immunosuppressed** cats (FeLV, FIV, diabetes mellitus), and are common in cats with urethral incompetence, which occurs most frequently following **perineal urethrostomy.**
- **Viral**
  - A **herpesvirus** has been isolated from cats with sterile lower urinary tract inflammation but its significance is unclear.
- **Fungal**
  - Infections are **rare** and due to **Candida** albicans or **Aspergillus** fumigatus.
  - Mainly reported in cats on long-term antibiotic therapy with impaired host defenses (perineal urethrostomy and urine stasis).
- **Parasitic**
  - Rarely reported but include **Capillaria feliscati** and **Encephalitozoon** cuniculi.
  - **Capillaria feliscati** has been reported in Australia and USA. It is a trichurid nematode that usually attaches superficially to the bladder mucosa and so most cats are asymptomatic. However, on rare occasions it may produce recurrent bouts of hematuria and dysuria.

Clinical signs

Dysuria, pollakiuria with or without hematuria.

Cats with **chronic renal failure may or may not have clinical signs, and pyuria and bacteriuria** may not be obvious on examination of the urinary sediment.

Cats with urinary tract infection are rarely systemically affected.

- **Clinical signs of fever**, lethargy, dehydration, anorexia, vomiting, polydipsia, polyuria, weight loss, anaemia are consistent with **renal involvement and indicate ascending pyelonephritis.**

Capillaria infestation is usually reported in cats over 8 months of age and produces minimal clinical signs, but recurring bouts of hematuria and dysuria have been observed.

Encephalitozoon infestation may lead to renal failure.

Diagnosis

Urinalysis.

- **If the urinary bladder is empty,** cats can be given **normal saline (70 ml/kg)** subcutaneously, and bladder fill monitored. Alternatively, **frusemide (1 mg/kg) intravenously** can be used. Animals with acute lower urinary tract infection are usually pollakiuric, so several attempts to collect urine may be necessary throughout the day.
- **Hematuria** (>5 RBC/hpf), **pyuria** (>5 WBC/hpf) and **proteinuria** (>3.5 g (35mg)/kg/day) or increased protein/creatinine ratio >1.0 (N.B protein and creatinine values must be converted to mg/dl and μmol/L, respectively to calculate the ratio) **indicate inflammation of the urinary tract.** If bacteria are also seen or cultured, then the inflammatory process is due to or complicated by bacteria. If bacteria are not seen under light microscopy, it does not mean that an infection is not present as they, **especially cocci, are not always readily visualized**.
- **White blood cell casts or granular casts indicate renal tubular** involvement as in pyelonephritis. White blood cell casts appear as **tubular structures** composed of white cells and Tamm–Horsfall mucoprotein. These may degenerate and form granular casts, which are indistinguishable from degenerated renal tubular epithelial casts.
- Blastospores (yeast) or hyphae (*Aspergillus* spp.) in urine indicate fungal infection.
- *Capillaria* ova (bipolar) or Encepalitozoon spores can be seen in the urine. Heavy infestations of *C. feliscati* may be associated with proteinuria.

Bacteriology.

- Quantitative bacterial cultures $\geq 10^3$/ml of urine obtained by cystocentesis indicate urinary tract infection.
- **Aerobic cultures** and antimicrobial susceptibility testing are **indicated in cats with pyuria (>5 WBC/hpf) or elevated urine pH (>6.5) whether or not bacteriuria is seen.**
- Fungal cultures are indicated if blastospores (yeast) or hyphae are seen in the urine.

Blood tests.

- Leucocytosis and elevated serum urea and creatinine levels indicate renal involvement in lower urinary tract disease.

Radiology.

- Plain and contrast radiography may help to identify some predisposing causes of urinary tract infections, as well as, determine the chronicity of the infection (thickened bladder wall, bladder fill capacity).

Differential diagnosis

Non-obstructed idiopathic LUTD. Some cats diagnosed as having bacterial cystitis/urethritis often represent with a recurrence of lower urinary tract disease with sterile urine during or after appropriate antimicrobial therapy. These cats have non-obstructed idiopathic LUTD with secondary bacterial infection and can only be identified by reoccurrence of signs associated with sterile urine.

Treatment

The principal objectives in the treatment of urinary tract infection are to eliminate the infectious agent, correct the predisposing cause, if possible, and prevent the recurrence of infection.

Eliminate the infectious agent.

- **For bacterial infections**.
  - Antimicrobial drugs, selected on the bases of bacterial sensitivity, should be used at appropriate doses for **14 days for acute urinary tract infection and for 28 days for chronic or recurrent urinary tract infection**.
  - Antimicrobial drugs often effective include **sulfa-trimethoprim, enrofloxacin and amoxicillin with clavulinic acid.**

- Nephrotoxic antimicrobials (aminoglycosides) should be avoided and when used, they should not be given for more than 7–10 days without carefully monitoring renal function, especially urinalysis for evidence of casts.
- **Response to therapy should be based on urinalysis and bacterial culture, rather than on clinical response to treatment**, as most cats will show a marked clinical improvement, despite unsuccessful eradication of the urinary tract infection.
- **Repeat urinalysis without culture should be done 7 days** after commencement of therapy to ensure that bacteriuria is no longer present.
- A urine sample for urinalysis should be examined on the **last day of antimicrobial therapy** for evidence of **pyuria** (>5 WBC/hpf). **Urinalysis and bacterial culture should be repeated 7 days after antimicrobial therapy has ceased and again at monthly intervals** until two consecutive urine samples are negative.
- Treatment for urinary tract infections associated with indwelling catheters may be delayed, if signs are absent, until the urinary catheter is removed, to avoid developing antimicrobial resistance.
- **For viral infections**.
  - Use lysine (250 mg/cat orally every 12 hours) or interferon alpha (30 U/cat orally daily).
- **For fungal infections**.
  - Ketoconazole and itraconazole have been suggested but their efficacy in the cat with urinary tract infection has not been determined.
- **For parasitic infestations**.
  - For Capillaria use fenbendazole (25 mg/kg orally every 12 hours for 3–10 days). Alternatively, methyridine 200 mg/kg orally once has been used.
  - No known effective treatment has been reported for Encephalitozoon in cats, but albendazole and the antibiotic fumagillin have been shown to have efficacy in humans and mice.

Correct predisposing cause, if possible.
- Anatomical abnormalities, such as ectopic ureter(s) should be surgically corrected.
- Urethral incompetence and loss of mechanical washout should be corrected, if possible.
- The continued use of indwelling catheters associated with secondary urinary tract infections should be reassessed.

Prevent the recurrence of infection.
- **Bacterial**.
  - If urinary tract infection recurs, determine if it is due to a relapse or reinfection. **Reoccurrence of infection with the same organism** (relapse) usually **indicates that the original treatment did not eliminate the infection**. Recurrence of infection with a different organism (reinfection) suggests that the original treatment was effective but predisposing factors have allowed a new infection to occur.
  - **Urinary acidifiers** can be used for long-term therapy to provide a less-favorable environment (pH < 6.5) in the urinary tract.
  - **Encourage the patient to urinate more frequently** by providing clean litter trays or ready access to outdoors, thus utilizing mechanical washout.
  - If urinary tract infection persists because predisposing causes cannot be corrected, **ampicillin, amoxicillin, sulfa-trimethoprim and methenamine can be used for long-term therapy**. Give half the daily dose late in the evening.

Prognosis

Prognosis depends on the causative agent, the use of appropriate drug therapy and the identification and correction of predisposing causes.

URETHRAL TRAUMA*

> ### Classical signs
>
> - History of trauma, especially following motor vehicle accidents, falling from high places and after forceful or excessive urethral catheterization.
> - Dysuria.
> - Perineal swelling.

Pathogenesis

Urethral trauma may result from **motor vehicle accidents** or abdominal trauma, especially those that result in pelvic fractures, perineal surgery via scalpel blade or **excessive handling of the urethra, and catheterization,** especially when associated with urethral obstruction.

Urethral rupture may result in **subcutaneous accumulation of urine in the perineal region** leading to swelling, discoloration and necrosis of the skin.

Clinical signs

Dysuria.

Stranguria.

Perineal swelling.

Red discoloration of the perineal skin.

Abdominal pain.

Signs of post-renal renal failure.

Diagnosis

History of trauma or catheterization.

Clinical signs of swelling, discoloration or necrosis in the perineal region.

Positive-contrast urethrography will demonstrate extravasation of contrast into the periurethral soft tissue. If the rupture is at the proximal end of the urethra, contrast agent may enter the abdomen.

HYPERCONTRACTILE BLADDER*

> ### Classical signs
> - Small urinary bladder.
> - Dribbling urine.
> - Pollakiuria.

Pathogenesis

Hypercontractility of the urinary bladder occurs when **detrusor muscle contractions are triggered at low volumes and pressure**, resulting in dysfunction of urinary bladder storage.

It may be due to reduced bladder capacity **(hypoplastic bladder, neoplasia),** excessive sensory input **(inflammation)** or neurologic disorders **(upper motor neuron lesions).**

Bladder hypercontractibility (idiopathic detrusor instability), not associated with any known cause, has been reported in one cat with FeLV that responded to anticholinergic therapy.

Clinical signs

Small amounts of urine are frequently voided while the urinary bladder is still small.

Dribbling urine (incontinence) associated with a small bladder.

Pollakiuria.

Palpation of the bladder often initiates the act of urination.

*Diagnosis

Diagnosis is based on **clinical signs,** especially that the cat frequently urinates or **dribbles urine when the bladder is quite small.**

Urodynamic procedures, such as cystometrography, demonstrate reduced threshold volumes and pressure, which indicate reduced bladder compliance or detrussor hypercontractility.

Urinalysis may reveal pyuria or neoplasia.

Radiography may help to determine the underlining cause, for example neoplasia and cystitis (thickened bladder wall).

FeLV test.

Differential diagnosis

Infectious cystitis/urethritis – hematuria, pyuria and bacteriuria are usually present.

Non-obstructed LUTD – hematuria is usually present.

Treatment

Management of storage dysfunction of the urinary bladder may include elimination of urinary tract inflammation, correction of neurologic disorders or pharmacologic manipulation to reduce detrusor muscle excitability.
- Always treat urinary tract infections first before attempting pharmacologic manipulation.
- **Parasympathetic inhibitors (anticholinergic agents),** such as **propantheline** (5–7.5 mg /cat orally every 72 hours or more frequently as required) and **oxybutynin** (0.5–1.25 mg/cat orally every 8–12 hours) may be used.

- **Tricyclic antidepressants, such as imipramine** (2.5–5 mg/cat orally every 12 hours) may improve urinary bladder compliance.

Clip the hair and clean around the perineal/abdominal area to minimize urine scolding.

NEOPLASIA*

Classical signs

- Hematuria.
- Distended bladder.
- Dysuria.

Pathogenesis

Tumors of the urinary bladder are rare and those of the ureters and urethra even rarer.

Most are **malignant epithelial tumors** such as **transitional cell carcinomas, squamous cell carcinomas and adenocarcinomas.**

Benign tumors occur very infrequently.

Clinical signs

Usually occurs in cats **over 8 years of age.**

Dysuria and intermittent or persistent hematuria may occur depending on the type and location of the neoplasm.

Soft tissue mass may be palpable in the bladder neck.

Secondary infection may occur.

History of unresponsiveness to treatment for cystitis.

Diagnosis

Urinalysis.
- Hematuria (RBC > 5 phf).
- Pyuria and bacteriuria occur due to secondary urinary tract infection.
- Sediment may show abnormal transitional cells.

Blood tests (hematology and biochemistry).
- Normal unless urinary tract obstruction has occurred.

- One cat with transitional cell carcinoma also had hypereosinophilia.

Abdominal palpation of a soft tissue mass in the bladder neck.

Ultrasonography or contrast radiography shows a soft tissue, space-occupying mass. Generally, a water-soluble iodinated contrast agent (5–10 ml/kg or enough to moderately distend the bladder) is used.

Biopsy via exploratory laparotomy or cystoscopy provides a definitive diagnosis.

Treatment

Surgical resection is rarely feasible due to the high percentage of tumors that are malignant, the frequently late presentation and location of the tumor.

URETHRAL STRICTURE

Classical signs

- Dribbling urine.
- Distended bladder.
- Dysuria.
- Stranguria.

See main reference on page 199 for details (The Incontinent Cat).

Clinical signs

Incontinence associated with a distended bladder (overflow incontinence) and dysuria.

Diagnosis

Radiography. Retrograde urethrography.

Urodynamic procedures. Urethral pressure profilometry may be used to identify focal urethral obstructions.

CYCLOPHOSPHAMIDE TOXICITY

Classical signs

- Hematuria.

Clinical signs

Hemorrhagic cystitis may occur during **cyclophos-phamide therapy** (< 5% of cases) in cats due to the action of acrolein on the mucosa resulting in mucosal edema, necrosis and ulceration.

Diagnosis

History of access to toxic material.

Urinalysis reveals a **sterile hematuria** (RBC >5 hpf).

RECOMMENDED READING

Barsanti JA, Finco DR, Brown SA. Diseases of the lower urinary tract. In: Sherding RG (ed) The Cat: Diseases and Clinical Management, 2nd edn, Churchill Liverstone, Melbourne, 1994, pp 1769–1823.

Cameron ME, Casey RA, Bradshaw JW, Waran NK, Gunn-Moore DA. A study of environmental and behavioural factors that may be associated with feline idiopathic cystitis. J Small Anim Pract 2004; 45(3): 144–147.

Kalkstein TS, Kruger JM, Osbourne CA. Feline idiopathic lower urinary tract disease. Parts I to IV. Compendium 21, 1999: 15, 148, 387, 497.

Norsworthy GD. Feline Urologic Syndrome; Urolithiasis The Feline Patient: Essentials of Diagnosis and Treatment, Williams and Wilkins, Baltimore 1998.

Osborne CA, Finco DR. Canine and Feline Nephrology and Urology. Williams and Wilkins, Baltimore, 1995.

Westropp JL, Buffington CA. Feline idiopathic cystitis: current understanding of pathophysiology and management. Vet Clin North Am Small Anim Pract 2004; 34(4):1043–1055.

Westropp JL, Welk KA, Buffington CA. Small adrenal glands in cats with feline interstitial cystitis. J Urol 2003; 170(6 Pt 1): 2494–2497.

12. The incontinent cat

Lucio John Filippich

KEY SIGNS

- Urinary incontinence.
- Urine soiling around the perineal area.
- Perineal dermatitis.

MECHANISM?

- The incontinent cat has lost voluntary control over urination and intermittently or continuously dribbles urine. Maintenance of urinary continence in the cat depends on normal lower urinary tract anatomy and function and an intact nervous system. Urinary incontinence results from abnormalities of either the filling or emptying processes.
- During the filling phase (sympathetic stimulation), the body of the bladder acts as a reservoir with flaccid walls that generate little pressure, while the outlet of the bladder is a high-resistance duct preventing the passage of urine.
- During the emptying phase (parasympathetic stimulation), the roles are reversed and the body of the bladder becomes a pump that expels urine under high pressure while the outlet of the bladder reflexly opens and becomes a low-resistance duct.
- The two phases are functionally independent and depend on the cerebral cortex for co-ordination and voluntary control.

WHERE?

- Lower urinary tract (lower ureter, urinary bladder, urethra).

WHAT?

- Urinary incontinence in cats is uncommon. In juvenile cats, it is more likely due to a congenital abnormality (ectopic ureter); in the adult cat it is more likely neurologic in origin. Secondary urinary tract infections are common.

QUICK REFERENCE SUMMARY

Diseases causing an incontinent cat

ANOMALY

- **Ectopic ureter(s)* (p 198)**

A congenital or acquired anomaly where one or both ureters fail to terminate normally into the urinary bladder. Mainly seen in young cats showing continuous or intermittent dribbling of urine with wetness and dermatitis around the perineal area. The urinary bladder, if palpable, is not distended.

- Patent urachus (p 201)

Kittens show urine leakage from the umbilicus because the urachus between the urinary bladder and the umbilicus remains functionally patent after birth.

- Spinal dysraphism (p 201)

Young cats, especially Manx cats. Overflow incontinence occurs because of malformation of the sacral spinal cord segments and disruption of nerve pathways responsible for micturition. Commonly seen with other hindquarter abnormalities.

- Colorocystic fistula (p 202)

The fistula between the urinary bladder and colon predisposes to urinary incontinence and urinary tract infection.

- Ectopic uterine horns (p 202)

Ectopic uterine horns terminate in the urinary bladder and result in persistent urinary incontinence and cystitis.

- Exstrophy (p 203)

Urine dribbling from defects in the ventral abdominal wall, urinary bladder and external genitalia.

MECHANICAL

- **Hypocontractile bladder (detrusor atony)*** (p 195)**

Results from detrusor dysfunction or occurs secondary to increased urethral outflow resistance. Overflow incontinence occurs and the bladder may or may not be easily expressed. Often associated with hindquarter abnormalities.

- **Urethral incompetence* (p 200)**

Intermittent leakage occurs without a distended badder, often while the cat is sleeping or relaxed. Results from trauma, dysraphism, urethral hypoplasia and possibly feline leukemia virus infection and desexing. More common in aged cats.

- **Urethral stricture* (p 199)**

May present as overflow incontinence and dysuria in a young cat (congenital), but more common secondary to trauma, inflammation or iatrogenic following traumatic catheterization of a blocked cat.

IDIOPATHIC

- Dysautonomia (p 203)

Overflow incontinence is associated with gastrointestinal and ocular signs due to an autonomic polyganglionopathy. Sudden onset of anorexia and depression occurs together with dilated unresponsive pupils, bradycardia, dry mucous membranes and GIT signs.

INTRODUCTION

MECHANISM?

The incontinent cat **intermittently or continuously dribbles urine** because it has **lost voluntary control over urination**.

Cats that urinate at inappropriate times or in inappropriate places need to be differentiated from incontinent cats through history taking and clinical examination.

Maintenance of urinary continence in the cat **depends on normal lower urinary tract anatomy** and an **intact sympathetic, parasympathetic** and **somatic nervous system**.
- Anatomical abnormalities can bypass (ectopic ureter) or negate (urethral hypoplasia) neuromuscular control mechanisms.

Continence during the filling stage is maintained via the following mechanisms: **sympathetic stimulation (hypogastric nerve) during the filling phase** causes the body of the bladder (detrusor muscle) to relax (β-receptors) and the bladder neck and urethral smooth muscles to contract (α-receptors).
- Additional urethral resistance is supplied by the **urethral striated muscle**, which reflexively contracts and is under voluntary control (pudendal nerve).

The emptying phase occurs as follows: **Parasympathetic stretch receptors in the detrusor muscle** detect bladder fill, and when the threshold of bladder capacity is reached, they discharge impulses via the sacral spinal cord to the pons in the brain stem, where a detrusor response is integrated.

Efferent motor impulses descend the spinal cord to the detrusor muscle via the **pelvic nerve causing detrusor muscle contraction**.
- Simultaneously, **inhibitory interneurons** are activated in the sacral spinal cord, which **synapse** on **pudendal motor neurons**, resulting in a **relaxation of the external urethral sphincter**.

Once the bladder is empty, parasympathetic activity ceases and the sympathetic and pudendal nerves are no longer inhibited.

Detrusor muscle relaxation and urethral sphincter contraction returns and the filling phase begins again.

Incontinence, pollakiuria or nocturia associated with an empty bladder reflect storage disorders (reduced bladder capacity, hyperactivity of the detrusor muscle, urethral incompetence).

In contrast, **urine retention with overflow**, or **incomplete voiding and a distended bladder indicate emptying disorders** (detrusor atony, urethral obstruction).

Following spontaneous bladder emptying there should be less than 0.5 ml of urine remaining in a normal cat.

WHERE?

Lower urinary tract (lower ureter, urinary bladder, urethra).

WHAT?

Urinary incontinence in cats is uncommon. In **juvenile cats**, it is more likely due to a congenital abnormality (**ectopic ureter**): in the **adult cat** it is more likely neurologic in origin. Secondary urinary tract infections are common.

DISEASES CAUSING SIGNS OF URINARY INCONTINENCE

HYPOCONTRACTILE BLADDER*** (DETRUSOR ATONIC/HYPOTONIC BLADDER)

Classical signs
- Dribbling urine.
- Distended urinary bladder.
- ± Hindquarter ataxia or paresis.
- ± Tail paralysis.

Pathogenesis

Hypocontractile bladder can occur due to detrusor dysfunction or secondary to prolonged bladder distention.

Detrusor dysfunction.
- **Lesions cranial to the sacral spinal cord** may disrupt sensory and motor pathways to the urinary bladder. This results is an upper motor neuron bladder:

– Detrusor function is lost resulting in a flaccid bladder.
– Urethral sphincter tone is maintained.
– Loss of inhibition may lead to increased pudendal nerve activity and thus, increased urethral outflow resistance.
– Over time, intrinsic spinal reflexes may re-establish detrusor activity but voiding is usually involuntary and incomplete.

● **Lesions involving the sacral spinal cord segments**, cauda equina (sacrum) or peripheral nerves supplying the bladder and urethra result in a lower motor neuron bladder.
– Loss of most sensory and all motor input to the detrusor muscle.
– Loss of urethral sphincter tone.
– The urinary bladder is areflexic and easily expressed.
– Overflow incontinence occurs when the bladder is distended or when intravesicular pressures exceed urethral pressure.

Prolonged bladder distention.

● Prolonged bladder distention leads to loss of tight muscular junctions in the bladder wall resulting in detrusor atony. Prolonged bladder distention results from reduced bladder emptying which may be from a number of causes:
– Mechanical (urethroliths, urethral plugs, strictures, bladder neck or urethral masses, inflammation).
– Functional (neurologic injury, urethral muscle spasm). When bladder fill pressures exceed urethral resistance, overflow of urine occurs.
– Associated with hindquarter disorders (pain) or forced recumbency.

Neurologic injury, resulting in **urethral hyperactivity/dyssynergia**, has been rarely documented in cats. It can occur with **sacral spinal cord and cauda equina injuries**, resulting in the urethral musculature failing to relax during detrusor contraction, thus maintaining a high outflow resistance.

Urethral muscle spasm may occur following **urethral or pelvic surgery** or secondary to **urethral inflammatory disease**.

Functional urethral obstruction and detrusor atony are **common sequels** to **mechanical urethral obstruction**.

Feline dysautonomia may result in urinary incontinence. There is an inability to contract the bladder and the bladder is easy to express manually. Urinary incontinence is one of the less common signs. Typically there is a sudden onset of depression and anorexia over 24–48 h, and a variety of signs reflecting autonomic dysfunction, such as pupillary dilation with loss of PLR, dry eyes and nose, regurgitation, prolapsed 3rd eyelids, bradycardia and constipation or fecal incontinence.

Clinical signs

A hypocontractile bladder presents as urinary incontinence associated with a **distended urinary bladder** and **inability to completely void urine**.

The cat may or may not voluntarily attempt to urinate.

The **bladder may or may not be easily expressed** manually.

With **suprasacral (cranial to sacrum) spinal cord lesions**, the **bladder is initially distended**, **firm** and **difficult to express**.
● Over time there is emergence of the sacral reflex, and some bladder contractile function may return, resulting in frequent, uninhibited, incomplete voiding of small volumes of urine.
● If outflow resistance is high at this time, detrusor-urethral dyssynergia occurs resulting in dysuria (difficult or painful urination) and interrupted urination.
● Other clinical signs associated with suprasacral spinal cord lesions may include proprioceptive deficits, paraparesis or tetraparesis and hyperreflexia.

With **sacral spinal cord and peripheral nerve lesions**, the urinary bladder is usually distended but flaccid, and outflow resistance is generally low, so the **urinary bladder is easily expressed**.
● The cat may attempt to urinate, but fail to produce an adequate stream of urine.
● Clinical signs may also include hindlimb paresis or paralysis, reduced anal tone and perineal reflexes, fecal incontinence and tail paralysis.

Incontinence associated with **increased urethral outflow resistance** is initially characterized by bladder distention and difficulty in manually expressing urine, a large residual urine volume following voiding, dysuria and an attenuated urine stream (paradoxic incontinence).

If the cat initiates voiding but the urine stream is rapidly interrupted, consider detruso–urethral dyssynergia.

Fecal incontinence and/or constipation may also be present.

Diagnosis

History may help to characterize the problem, differentiate it from inappropriate urination and identify the possible cause (trauma, prolonged recumbency).

Physical examination.
- Abdominal palpation reveals a distended bladder.
- If detrusor dysfunction is neurological in origin, other signs of neurological disease such as hindquarter paralysis are commonly seen.

Neurologic examination.
- Neurologic deficits in the limbs suggest a neurologic cause for the incontinence.
- Loss of anal tone, perineal sensation and tail function indicate a sacral spinal cord lesion.
- Ophthalmological signs (mydriasis) may suggest the incontinence is associated with dysautonomia.

Observe micturition.
- This should always be done.
- Assess the urine stream passed.
- Note change in bladder size and residual urine volume after voiding.

Detrusor dysfunction is suspected on the basis of the history, physical examination, and the exclusion of a mechanical obstruction to urine outflow.

Catheterize the urinary bladder to determine patency.
- If an obstruction is detected, survey and contrast radiographs are often necessary to further characterize the obstruction. If the obstruction is due to a urethrolith, survey abdominal radiographs are necessary to determine if other uroliths are present in the urinary tract (kidney, ureter and bladder).
- If an obstruction is not detected, retrograde urethrography and contrast cystography may be needed to exclude soft tissue masses in the bladder and urethra.

If mechanical obstruction is ruled out, subjectively evaluate urethral resistance by palpating the urinary bladder and applying constant, firm digital pressure on the urinary bladder. The degree of pressure applied should not cause undue discomfort or pain to the cat.

- If detrusor activity is initiated and the cat begins to urinate, observe if the urine stream is abruptly interrupted and voiding is incomplete (functional urethral obstruction).
- If detrusor activity is not initiated and the bladder is easily expressed, bladder atony is present.

Ultrasonography is often useful in bladder diseases (neoplasia, urolithiasis) but does not visualize most of the urethra.

Urodynamic procedures.
- These are not readily available in veterinary practice.
- Cystometry, urethral pressure profilometry, uroflowmetry and electromyography can provide useful objective information about detrussor and urethral function.
- Cystometrography showing large filling volumes, and lack of sustained contractile peaks indicate detrussor atony.
- Urethral pressure profilometry can identify urethral incompetence and urethral hypertonicity.

Urinalysis is useful in detecting the presence of inflammation and infection.

Blood tests including serum urea, creatinine and electrolyte concentrations can be done to detect renal failure.

Biopsy a soft tissue mass, if detected.

Treatment

Immediately correct any life-threatening conditions, such as postrenal renal failure, and fluid and electrolyte imbalance.

Correct the primary cause, if possible.

Always treat urinary tract infections first before attempting pharmacologic manipulation.

For **bladder atony.**
- To facilitate smooth muscle recovery, the **residual urine volume** needs to be **kept small** by frequent manual expression, intermittent catheterization or temporary indwelling urinary catheter placement.
- Use pharmacologic manipulation, such as **parasympathomimetics (bethanechol chloride**, a cholinergic agonist, 1.25–2.5 mg/cat orally every 8–12 hours) to increase detrusor contractility and an **alpha-adrenergic antagonist (phenoxybenzamine**, 0.25 mg/kg

orally every 12 hours) to minimize urethral resistance, if necessary. Parasympathomimetic drugs are most likely to be effective when some neurologic innervation is still present. Drug doses may be increased incrementally, if needed, every 4–5 days, but patients should be carefully monitored for potential side effects (lacrimation, salivation, abdominal cramps, vomiting, diarrhea).

For increased **urethral resistance or detrussor–urethral dyssynergia**.

- The direct-acting skeletal muscle relaxant, **dantrolene sodium** (0.5–2 mg/kg orally 12 hourly or 1 mg/kg IV) may be effective in reducing striated-muscle resistance.
- The alpha-adrenergic antagonist (phenoxybenzamine) may be effective in reducing smooth-muscle resistance.
- Benzodiazepines such as diazepam (valium 2–5 mg PO tid) may reduce striated-muscle resistance.

Laboratory investigation, including plasma urea, creatinine and electrolyte concentrations and urinalysis, should be done to determine the degree of post-renal azotemia and to identify if hematuria, pyuria and/or infection are present.

Prognosis

Prognosis in neurologic cases is guarded and generally depends on the chronicity and severity of the neurologic lesion, response to medical therapy and the ease of manually maintaining an empty urinary bladder.

ECTOPIC URETER(S)*

Classical signs

- Young cat.
- Continuous dribbling of urine.
- Wetness around the perineal area.
- Perineal dermatitis.

Pathogenesis

A **congenital anomaly** where **one or both ureters fail to terminate normally in the trigone of the urinary bladder**. Ectopic ureter occurs because the origin or migration of the metanephric ducts (which become the ureters) was abnormal.

Ectopic ureters **usually terminate in the urethra** and **less frequently** in the **vagina**.

Approximately **50% are unilateral**.

Because of the close relationship of the mesonephros and the metanephros and development of other urogenital organs, other anomalies such as cystic (bladder) hypoplasia, renal hypoplasia, hydronephrosis and megaureter may also occur.

Acquired ureteral ectopia may occur due to a vaginoureteral fistula developing as a sequel to cesarian and ovario-hysterectomy.

Clinical signs

Congenital ureteral ectopia has been infrequently reported in cats and there appears to be no breed or sex predisposition.

Usually reported in **cats less than 18 months of age**.

Signs depend on the site of termination of the ectopic ureter(s) and the presence of other congenital or acquired abnormalities.

Continuous or intermittent dribbling of urine is typical.

Cats with bilateral ectopic ureters may or **may not urinate normally**, depending on how much urine refluxes back into the bladder.

Incontinent cats with unilateral ureteral ectopia urinate normally.

Urine scalding may result in vaginal discharge, phimosis (contraction of the prepucial orifice), and perivulvar or periprepucial dermatitis.

Soiled hair may discolor.

The **urinary bladder** on abdominal palpation **is not distended** (in contrast to urine retention with overflow).

Abdominal palpation may reveal an abnormal kidney(s).

Secondary **bacterial urinary tract infections are common** and may result in intermittent bouts of hematuria, cystitis and/or ascending pyelonephritis. With bilateral ectopia, renal failure may occur.

Diagnosis

A history of urinary incontinence since birth or when acquired as a kitten indicates congenital ureteral ectopia. Onset of signs following recent abdominal surgery at any age would suggest acquired ureteral ectopia.

Clinical signs which are suggestive are:
- Urinary incontinence without urinary bladder distention.
- Incontinence despite normal urination (unilateral ectopic ureter).

Radiographic techniques such as excretory urography/pneumocystography and retrograde urethrography or vaginourethrography provide information on the site of ureteral termination, renal size and ureteral shape.
- One or both ureters fail to terminate normally in the urinary bladder.
- Other anomalies, such as cystic and renal hypoplasia, hydronephrosis and megaureter may be seen.

Vaginoscopy may reveal the ectopic ureteral orifice if the ureter enters the vagina.

Ultrasonography may help to demonstrate the abnormal termination of the urethra or vagina.

Biochemistry
- Serum urea and creatinine estimations can be used to evaluate renal function.
- Urea and creatinine are more likely to be elevated with bilateral ureteral ectopia, especially if chronic.
- Elevations indicate both kidneys are diseased from ascending pyelonephritis or an associated congenital renal anomaly.

Urinalysis and bacterial culture can identify the presence of secondary infection.

Differential diagnosis

Urinary retention with overflow (overflow incontinence) is differentiated from ectopic ureter by finding a distended bladder on palpation.

Treatment

Vesico-ureteral transplantation is the treatment of choice when the kidney function is normal and the ureter is not markedly abnormal.

Ureteronephrectomy may be considered when the affected kidney is diseased and the contralateral kidney is normal.

Renal infarction by ligation of the renal blood vessel may be considered in azotemic cats with unilateral ureteral ectopia.

Continued incontinence after surgery may be due to concomitant urethral incompetence or reduced bladder capacity due to disuse. If the latter, bladder capacity usually improves with time.

Secondary bacterial infections are not uncommon and antimicrobials based on culture and sensitivity tests should be administered.

Prognosis

Following surgical correction, prognosis is generally good with immediate cessation of urinary incontinence.

Cats with ectopic ureters that terminate in the vagina are more likely to be continent after surgery.

Reimplantation of dilated ureters into the bladder may result in increased vesicoureteral reflux that can predispose to ascending pyelonephritis.

URETHRAL STRICTURE*

Classical signs

- Dribbling urine.
- Distended bladder.
- Dysuria.

Pathogenesis

Congenital urethral strictures are occasionally seen in young cats.

Acquired strictures are more common and occur secondary to trauma, inflammation or iatrogenic causes following catheterization or surgery.

Clinical signs

Typical signs are incontinence associated with a distended bladder (overflow incontinence) and dysuria (difficulty urinating) with a narrow urine stream.

Diagnosis

Diagnosis is via **radiography** using retrograde urethrography.

Following catheterization of the urethera using an open-ended cat catheter, contrast is injected (1–2 ml) while the radiographs are taken. Avoid over-distending the urinary bladder.

Urodynamic procedures such as urethral pressure profilometry may be used to identify focal urethral obstructions.

Treatment

Treatment depends on location and size of the stricture.

Extrapelvic strictures may be managed by urethrostomy, whereas, intrapelvic strictures may require urethral resection and anastomosis.

URETHRAL INCOMPETENCE*

> ### Classical signs
> - Small urinary bladder.
> - Intermittent dribbling of urine.

Pathogenesis

Incontinence occurs because of reduced urethral outflow resistance during urine storage. This results from lost or **reduced urethral smooth or striated muscle tone.**

Reported causes of urethral incompetence include:
- **Pelvic and pudendal nerve damage** following trauma (**cystotomy, perineal urethrostomy**) and rarely neoplasia (acquired urethral incompetence).
- **Dysraphism** in Manx cats.
- **Urethral hypoplasia** has been reported in young female cats (congenital urethral incompetence).
- A relationship between incontinence and **feline leukemia virus** (FeLV) infection is suspected.
- **Reproductive hormone-responsive incontinence** has been reported in two female cats following ovariectomy and suspected in three neutered males.

Clinical signs

Normal or small urinary bladder.

Intermittent leakage of small volumes of urine, often while the cat is sleeping or relaxed.

If congenital in origin, other anomalies, such as vaginal aplasia and cystic hypoplasia are commonly present.

Many **FeLV-positive cats with urinary incontinence** may also have **anisocoria**, reproductive disorders, weight loss, vomiting and ptyalism suggesting a **multifocal autonomic dysfunction**. In cats with FeLV-associated incontinence, digital palpation of the urinary bladder often elicits a urine flow.

In cats with urethral incompetence due to neoplasia, abdominal palpation may reveal a mass at the bladder neck. Others signs, such as dysuria and hematuria are often present.

Secondary urinary tract infections are common.

Diagnosis

Diagnosis is based on history and clinical signs of leakage of small amounts of urine, often when sleeping, and a normal or small bladder.

Ophthalmological signs (anisocoria) may suggest the incontinence is associated with FeLV infection.

A positive FeLV test.

Retrograde contrast vaginourethrography in female cats with urethral hypoplasia shows marked urethral shortening and other anomalies, such as vaginal aplasia and cystic hypoplasia.

Cystography or retrograde urethrography may reveal a mass at the bladder neck. Biopsy is necessary for a definitive diagnosis.

Urodynamic procedures, including urethral pressure profilometry can be used to identify urethral incompetence.

Differential diagnosis

Hypercontractile bladder (urge incontinence) is characterized by frequent conscious urination and a small bladder.

Treatment

Bladder neck reconstructive surgery may be considered in cats with urethral hypoplasia.

Alpha-adrenergic agonists, such as **phenylpropanolamine** (1.5–2.2 mg/kg PO 8–12 h) and **ephedrine** (2–4 mg/cat PO 8–12 h) may be used to alleviate the incontinence. Once the incontinence is controlled, the dosage can be reduced and/or the frequency lengthened.

High doses of oral estrogen therapy were reportedly effective in two cats that developed urinary incontinence following ovariectomy. However, at such doses nymphomania and toxic bone marrow effects may occur.

Testosterone propionate (5–10 mg intramuscularly), given to three neutered male cats suspected of reproductive hormone-responsive incontinence, gave **variable success**.

Prognosis

Response to drug therapy in severely affected animals is often poor.

PATENT URACHUS

Classical signs

- Immature cat.
- Dribbling urine from the umbilicus.
- Omphalitis.
- Ventral dermatitis.

Pathogenesis

Patent (persistent) urachus occurs when the entire urachus between the urinary bladder and the umbilicus remains functionally patent after birth.

Clinical signs

Kittens show **urine leakage from the umbilicus**.

A patent urachus is often associated with omphalitis (inflammation of the umbilicus), **ventral dermatitis** and signs of urinary tract infection.

Diagnosis

Physical examination reveals urine leakage from the umbilical region.

Differential diagnosis

Exstrophy of the bladder. The bladder wall and abdominal wall are not fully formed and are joined, with leakage of urine to the exterior.

Treatment

Surgical correction and antimicrobial therapy for secondary infection.

Prognosis

Good.

SPINAL DYSRAPHISM

Classical signs

- Young cat.
- Dribbling urine.
- Distended urinary bladder.
- ± Hindquarter abnormalities.

Pathogenesis

Incomplete closure of the neural tube during early prenatal development leads to **malformation of the sacral spinal cord segments** and disruption of nerve pathways responsible for micturition, resulting in **loss of detrusor responsiveness and urethral sphincter control**.

Sacrocaudal dysgenesis in Manx cats is due to a semilethal, autosomal dominant gene.

Clinical signs

Signs occur in young cats (< 6 months of age).

Severity of the clinical signs vary and may include abnormalities of urination, defecation and hindlimb gait.

Typically there is urinary incontinence (dribbling urine) with a distended urinary bladder that is easily expressed.

Perivulvar or periprepucial dermatitis.

Secondary urinary tract infections are common.

Other signs commonly seen include **fecal incontinence**, constipation, **locomotor disturbances** of the **hindlimbs** (plantigrade stance, hopping gait) and abnormal hindquarter conformation.

Diagnosis

Diagnosis is based on age, breed and clinical signs.

Survey radiographs may confirm vertebral abnormalities of the caudal spine.

Contrast myelography may demonstrate the presence of meningoceles.

Urodynamic procedures.
- Cystometrography may show large filling volumes and lack of a sustained contractile peak, consistent with detrussor atony.
- Urethral pressure profilometry can identify urethral incompetence.

Differential diagnosis

Most other congenital abnormalities do not produce the classical combination of dribbling urine from the penis/vulva and distended easily expressible bladder in a young cat.

Treatment

Treatment depends on the severity of the clinical signs.

Therapy should be directed at minimizing or overcoming overflow incontinence by **manual bladder compression** (provided there is not excessive urethral sphincter tone) and appropriate **treatment of urinary tract infections.**

Prognosis

Poor in severe cases.

COLO-UROCYSTIC FISTULA

Classical signs
- Dribbling urine in young cat.

Clinical signs

Colorocystic fistula has been reported in a male domestic shorthaired kitten.

This anomaly may result from incomplete division of the cloaca during embryogenesis.

Signs were of persistent urine dribbling and cystitis in a young cat.

Diagnosis

The abnormality predisposes to **urinary incontinence and urinary tract infection**.

Diagnosis can be established by contrast urography.

Treatment

Treatment is surgical correction of the fistula while preserving the colonic and urinary bladder function.

ECTOPIC UTERINE HORNS

Classical signs
- Urinary incontinence.

Clinical signs

Ectopic uterine horns terminating into the urinary bladder have been reported in a young female domestic shorthaired cat showing signs of persistent urinary incontinence and cystitis.

Diagnosis

Diagnosis based on contrast cystography.

EXSTROPHY

Classical signs

- Urine dribbles from abdominal defect.

Clinical signs

Very rare disorder in cats characterized by ventral mid-line defects in the ventral abdominal wall, urinary bladder, intestines and external genitalia.

Easily differentiated from other causes of incontinence as urine dribbles from the abdominal defect.

Diagnosis

Diagnosis is based on clinical signs. Exstrophy should be differentiated from patent urachus.

FELINE DYSAUTONOMIA

Classical signs

- Dribbling urine.
- Distended bladder.
- Gastrointestinal and ocular signs.

Pathogenesis

Feline dysautonomia is an autonomic polyganglionopathy (Key–Gaskell syndrome).

Autonomic ganglia (sympathetic and parasympathetic) are affected resulting in detrusor atony and urethral sphincter incompetence.

Overflow incontinence occurs as a result.

Clinical signs

Mainly seen in young cats.

Affected cats may voluntarily pass a small amount of urine with difficulty.

Typically there is a large flaccid urinary bladder (detrusor atony), which is easily manually expressed.

Other clinical signs usually predominate, such as an acute onset over 24–48 h of depression and anorexia, gastrointestinal signs (dysphagia, regurgitation, vomiting, tenesmus, diarrhea, constipation), mydriasis, prolapsed third eyelids, dry mucous membranes and bradycardia.

Diagnosis

Diagnosis is based on clinical examination findings of a flaccid bladder associated with acute onset of depression and gastrointestinal and ocular signs.

Radiographic signs are of megesophagus and a distended urinary bladder.

Ophthalmological examination reveals reduced tear production, dilated poorly responsive pupils in a visual cat, and prolapsed third eyelids.

Urodynamic procedures include the following:
- Cystometry and urethral pressure profilometry may be used to objectively evaluate detrusor and urethral function.
- Cystometrograms can be used to show large filling volumes, and lack of a sustained contractile peak indicates detrussor atony.
- Urethral pressure profilometry can be used to identify urethral incompetence.

Treatment

Bethanecol is effective in inducing urination in some cases, although it should not be used in cats with slow resting heart rates, as profound bradycardia and cardiac arrhythmia may occur.

RECOMMENDED READING

Barsanti JA, Finco DR, Brown SA. Diseases of the lower urinary tract. In: Sherding RG (ed) The Cat Diseases and Clinical Management. Churchill Livingstone, Melbourne, 1994, pp 1769–1823.

Lane IF. Disorders of micturition. In: Osborne CA, Finco DR (eds) Canine and Feline Nephrology and Urology. Williams and Wilkins, Baltimore, 1995, pp 593–717.

Lane IF, Barsanti JA. Urinary incontinence. In: August JR (ed) Consultations in Feline Internal Medicine. WB Saunders Company, Sydney, 1994, pp 373–382.

13. The cat with discolored urine

Joseph William Bartges

KEY SIGNS

- Red, pink, orange, brown, black, white, blue or colorless urine.

MECHANISM?

- Urine color other than yellow including red, orange, white, blue, brown and black is abnormal.
  Red, brown or orange urine suggests blood, hemoglobin, myoglobin or bilirubin.
  Cloudy or white urine suggests pus, lipid or crystals.
  Pale yellow or colorless urine is associated with dilute urine and increased urine volume.
  Blue or green urine is uncommon, and is usually associated with excretion of drugs or toxins.

WHERE?

- Urogenital tract – urine is formed in the kidney and is usually yellow.
  Pigments that are filtered by the glomerulus may alter urine color.
  Blood cells may alter urine color if added to urine after formation.

WHAT?

- Red, pink, orange, brown or black urine***

QUICK REFERENCE SUMMARY

Diseases causing discolored urine

MECHANICAL

- **Urolithiasis causing hematuria*** (p 209)**
  *Occurs in 15–30% of cats with lower urinary tract disease; *struvite most common in young cats;
  *calcium oxalate is most common in middle-aged or older cats; *nephroliths are often composed
  of calcium oxalate.

NEOPLASIA

- **Neoplasia causing hematuria* (p 210)**
  *urinary tract neoplasia is rare in cats; *renal neoplasia is often associated with renomegaly;
  *hematuria may be the only clinical sign.

continued

continued

METABOLIC

● Coagulopathy or thrombocytopenia causing hematuria (p 212)

*coagulopathy and thrombocytopenia are rare in cats; *evidence of bleeding at other sites is often-present, although hematuria may be the only clinical sign; *coagulation testing should be performed in cats with undiagnosed hematuria.

● Bilirubinuria** (p 211)

*bilirubinuria is always abnormal in cats; *it may result from prehepatic, hepatic, or post-hepatic causes; *most common causes are hepatic disease.

● Hemoglobinuria (p 212)

*associated with hemolysis; *hemolytic anemia is uncommon in cats; *myoglobinuria; *results from muscle breakdown; *may occur secondary to polymyopathy, but uncommon.

INFECTIOUS

● Urinary tract infection causing hematuria** (p 209)

*bacterial UTI occurs in 1–2% of cats < 10 years of age, but may occur in >45% of cats > 10 years; * *E. coli* is the most common organism isolated from cats with bacterial UTI; *urine should be collected by cystocentesis to adequately assess bacterial UTI.

IDIOPATHIC

● Idiopathic lower urinary tract disease causing hematuria*** (p 208)

*Most common cause of lower urinary tract disease in cats less than 10 years. Clinical signs include hematuria, stranguria, pollakiuria, and inappropriate urination; *urethral obstruction may occur in male cats.

TRAUMA

● Trauma causing hematuria* (p 210)

*Trauma to any part of the urinary tract may result in hematuria; *evaluate for other signs of trauma; *if hematuria is secondary to trauma, assess integrity of urinary tract.

● Cloudy white or white urine** (p 206)

● Crystalluria*** (p 213)

*Commonly associated with urolithiasis, matrix-crystalline urethral plug formation in males; *struvite and calcium oxalate most common; *struvite and urate more common in kittens; *may or may not be pathologic.

● Pyuria** (p 214)

*Signifies inflammation, which is often but not always associated with bacterial UTI; *may result from lower or upper urinary tract diseases.

● Lipiduria (p 214)

*May be normal; * may be an indication of lipid metabolism disorders.

- **Pale yellow or colorless urine*** (p 207)**

- **Dilute urine*** (p 215)**

*Occurs with polyuric states; *most common causes of PU/PD are renal failure, diabetes mellitus, and hyperthyroidism; *other clinical signs may be present and relate to an underlying disorder.

- **Blue or green urine (p 207)**

*Drug discoloration; *occurs with some drugs or dyes especially methylene blue.

INTRODUCTION

MECHANISM?

Urine that is anything other than yellow is abnormal.
- **Normal urine** is typically transparent and yellow or amber on visual inspection.
- Two pigments, **urochrome** and **urobilin**, impart the yellow color.
- The intensity of the yellow color is in part related to the **volume of urine** collected and concentration of urine produced.
- Significant disease may exist when urine is normal in color.

Abnormal urine color is caused by the presence of several endogenous or exogenous pigments, and indicates a problem.
- **Pink, red, brown, orange or black** urine suggests the presence of **blood, hemoglobin, myoglobin or bilirubin.**
- **Cloudy or white urine** suggests the presence of **pus, lipid or crystals.**
- **Pale yellow or colorless** urine is associated with **decreased urine concentration** and **increased urine volume**.
- **Blue or green** urine is uncommon, and is usually associated with excretion of **drugs or toxins.**

Owners may observe discolored urine in the litter box or in areas of inappropriate urination.

Examination of urine sediment (for red blood cells) and plasma or serum color will aid diagnosis.

Whole blood, hemoglobin and myoglobin **all give a positive reaction on the blood test pad** on dipsticks.
- These can be distinguished as follows:

- **Blood (hematuria)** is present when centrifuged or settled urine is clear with a red sediment at the bottom of the tube, or there are > 10–20 red cells/HPF on microscopic examination of sediment.
- **Hemoglobin** is present if the urine remains pink after centrifugation or on settling, few red cells (< 10 RBC/HPF) are evident on microscopic examination of the sediment, and there is clinical and hematologic evidence of hemolytic anemia. Plasma has a reddish discoloration.
- **Myoglobin** is present if the urine remains pink after centrifugation or on settling, few red cells are evident on microscopic examination of the sediment, and there is clinical and biochemical evidence of muscle damage. Plasma is clear.

Clinical signs associated with discolored urine will aid in diagnosis.
- **Hematuria** (red or pink urine) indicates urinary tract disease (upper or lower) or bleeding disorders.
  - Signs that suggest the cause is **lower urinary tract disease** are stranguria, pollakiuria and dysuria (urine may be pink, red, brown, orange or cloudy in color).
  - Signs that suggest hematuria is from **upper urinary tract** disease include polyuria and polydipsia (urine is usually pale yellow or colorless, however, cloudy or red urine may occur).
  - A **bleeding disorder** is indicated by evidence of bleeding from other sites.
  - **Hemoglobin** in urine suggests **intravascular hemolysis.** Marked hemoglobinuria may occur in kittens with neonatal isoerythrolysis. Hemoglobinuria rarely occurs with *Hemobartonella* infection and immune-mediated anemia, which present mainly as extravascular hemolysis.

- Signs that suggest intravascular hemolysis and hemoglobinuria include acute illness, fever, pale mucous membranes, +/− jaundice, +/− splenomegaly, or acute lethargy and death in 1–3-day-old kittens.
  - Hemoglobinuria and bilirubinuria may be both present with intravascular hemolysis.
- **Myoglobinuria** (red or brown urine) suggests acute muscle damage. In cats this is most often associated with ischemic myopathy secondary to an aortic thrombosis, muscle injury from trauma or ischemia (e.g. entrapment in window), or snake bite (especially Australian tiger snake).
  - Muscle damage with leakage of myoglobin is suggested by signs of muscle pain, biochemical evidence of muscle damage (increased creatine kinase) and other historical and clinical signs of trauma, thrombosis or snakebite.
- **Bilirubinuria** (dark yellow urine) suggests marked erythrocyte breakdown (hemolytic anemia), hepatic disease or bile duct obstruction.
  - Bilirubinuria is most often associated with hepatic disease including cholangiohepatitis complex, hepatic lipidosis, neoplasia and feline infectious peritonitis.
  - Occasionally it occurs when *Hemobartonella*-associated hemolysis is severe enough to cause jaundice.
  - Clinical signs are varied depending on the cause of bilirubinuria. Serum and plasma are also jaundiced.
- Cats with hematuria from upper urinary tract disease or hemoglobinuria, myoglobinuria or bilirubinuria may be systemically ill.
- Mucus membranes may be pale or yellow if urine discoloration is associated with hyperbilirubinemia or hemolytic anemia.
- Some cats with abnormal urine may have no other clinical signs.

WHERE?

Discolored urine is produced in the urinary tract. It may result from urinary tract disease (most common), a systemic bleeding disorder, or from excretion of pigments from the plasma.

Careful history and physical examination may help to determine if the discoloration is clinically significant.

WHAT?

Hematuria is the **most common** cause of discolored urine. This is most often associated with idiopathic lower urinary tract disease and less frequently with urolithiasis.

DISEASES CAUSING DISCOLORED URINE

RED, PINK, ORANGE, BROWN OR BLACK URINE

Red, pink, orange, brown or black urine suggests the presence of hematuria (frank blood), hemoglobin, myoglobin or bilirubin. Red or pink urine is most commonly associated with hematuria.

Cats with discolored urine may or may not have signs of lower urinary tract disease (stranguria, pollakiuria, dysuria, urination in inappropriate places).

Systemic illness may or may not be present.

Mucous membranes may be pale or yellow if associated with hyperbilirubinemia or anemia.

Diagnosis is aided by examination of urine sediment for red and white blood cells, and plasma or serum color.

IDIOPATHIC LOWER URINARY TRACT DISEASE CAUSING HEMATURIA*** (IDIOPATHIC FELINE LOWER URINARY TRACT DISEASE, IDIOPATHIC CYSTITIS–URETHRITIS COMPLEX, FELINE UROLOGIC SYNDROME, INTERSTITIAL CYSTITIS)

> **Classical signs**
>
> - Stranguria, pollakiuria, inappropriate urination and hematuria are present.
> - Occurs most commonly in cats less than 10 years of age.

See main reference on page 176 for details on idiopathic lower urinary tract disease.

Clinical signs

Clinical signs are similar to other causes of lower urinary tract disease: **hematuria, pollakiuria, stranguria and urination in inappropriate places**.

Most commonly occurs in cats less than 10 years of age; **average age is 2–4 years.**

Occurs with even frequency in male and female cats.

May be associated with urethral plug formation and obstruction in male cats.

Diagnosis

Must be differentiated from other causes of lower urinary tract disease such as urolithiasis and bacterial urinary tract infection.

In cats less than 10 years of age, it occurs in 55–70% of cases of lower urinary tract disease; in cats greater than 10 years of age, it occurs in 5–10% of cases of lower urinary tract disease.

Diagnosis is made by excluding other causes of lower urinary tract disease.

Urinalysis reveals hematuria (>5 RBC/hpf) without a urinary tract infection; white blood cells are usually present at < 5–10/hpf and urine culture is negative.

Crystals may or may not be present on urine sediment examination.

Radiographs and ultrasonography of the lower urinary tract are usually normal; however, bladder wall thickening or intraluminal blood clots may be present.

Cystoscopy often reveals small mucosal hemorrhages called glomerulations, without identifying other diseases processes.

UROLITHIASIS CAUSING HEMATURIA***

Classical signs

- Stranguria, pollakiuria, inappropriate urination and/or urethral obstruction.
- Renal pain, hematuria, or uremia if uroliths present in upper urinary tract.

See main reference on page 184 for details on urolithiasis.

Clinical signs

If uroliths are located in the **lower urinary tract, stranguria, pollakiuria, inappropriate urination, hematuria** and/or urethral obstruction may occur.

If uroliths are located in the **upper urinary tract, renal pain, hematuria** or **uremia** (if bilateral) may be present.

Uremia is present with urethral obstruction or bilateral ureteral obstruction.

Clinical signs may also be absent with uroliths.

Diagnosis

Microscopic examination of urine sediment reveals RBCs.

Crystalluria may or may not be present. If present, they may aid in estimating mineral composition (see page 213 for description of crystal appearance).

Most common mineral composition includes struvite (magnesium ammonium phosphate hexahydrate) and calcium oxalate; urate (purine), cystine, calcium phosphate, and drug metabolites have also been observed to occur.

Struvite and calcium oxalate uroliths are usually radiodense; urate and cystine are usually radiolucent and require contrast radiography or ultrasonography to identify.

URINARY TRACT INFECTION CAUSING HEMATURIA**

Classical signs

- Hematuria, stranguria, pollakiuria, and/or inappropriate urination (urinary bladder infection).
- Urinary tract infection may occur secondary to another disease, and other clinical signs may be present.
- Asymptomatic or associated with fever, renal pain, or uremia (upper urinary tract infection).

See main reference on page 187 for details on urinary tract infections.

Clinical signs

Bacterial urinary tract **occurs in approximately 1–2% of cats less than 10 years of age** that have lower urinary tract disease, **40–50% of cats greater than 10 years of age** that have lower urinary tract disease, and in approximately **20% of cats with renal failure**.

Bacterial urinary tract infection is more common than other infectious agents and usually involves the lower urinary tract.

Less common infectious agents causing hematuria include feline infectious peritonitis (FIP).

Urinary bladder is most common site of urinary tract infection. Clinical signs include **hematuria, stranguria, pollakiuria and/or inappropriate urination**; however, some cats may be asymptomatic.

If the upper urinary tract is involved, fever, renal pain and/or uremic signs may be present.

Bacterial urinary tract infection may occur secondary to diseases that alter normal host defense mechanisms such as renal failure, diabetes mellitus, urolithiasis or neoplasia; therefore, additional clinical signs may relate to the underlying disease.

Diagnosis

Urinalysis may reveal pyuria (> 5 WBC/hpf), bacteriuria, hematuria (> 5 RBC/hpf), and/or proteinuria; however, a bacterial urinary tract infection may be present with an inactive urinary sediment on microscopic examination, especially in cats with concurrent disease(s).

An aerobic culture and sensitivity should be performed on a urine sample collected by cystocentesis.

- This allows identification of the organism as well as selection of the appropriate antimicrobial for treatment.
- Nitrite and leukocyte test pads present on some dipsticks are not reliable and should not be used.
- **Urine may be stained with Wright's stain or Gram stain to aid in identification** of bacteria and to assist in selecting an appropriate antibiotic until culture results are returned.

TRAUMA CAUSING HEMATURIA*

Classical signs

- Hematuria.
- History of trauma may be present.
- Evidence for other trauma-induced injury (such as broken bones, diaphragmatic hernia, dyspnea, etc.).

Clinical signs

Evidence for trauma such as broken bones, dyspnea, pneumothorax, shredded nails, lacerations, etc., are often present.

History of traumatic episode, such as being hit by a car or attacked by a dog is often present.

Shock may be present.

Hematuria is present if the urinary tract is injured due to trauma (hemorrhage may be from upper urinary tract, lower urinary tract or both).

Diagnosis

Hematuria (numerous RBCs) is found on urinalysis.

- **Hemorrhage may be from the lower urinary tract, the upper urinary tract or both.**
- It is important to determine if the urinary tract is intact. This may require an excretory urogram to evaluate the upper urinary tract and/or contrast urethrocystography to evaluate the lower urinary tract.
  - Unexplained azotemia or uroabdomen (abdominal fluid with composition of urine, i.e. creatinine concentration > plasma) is an indication for contrast radiography and possibly surgical intervention.

Evidence for other organ systems being traumatized aids diagnosis.

NEOPLASIA CAUSING HEMATURIA*

Classical signs

- Hematuria, pollakiuria, stranguria and/or inappropriate urination may be present.

Classical signs—Cont'd

- Hematuria may be only clinical sign if upper urinary tract involved.

See main reference on page 191 for details on bladder/urethral neoplasia and page 250 for details on renal neoplasia.

Clinical signs

If the neoplasm involves the lower urinary tract, clinical signs may include **hematuria, stranguria, pollakiuria and/or inappropriate urination.**

If the neoplasm involves the **upper urinary tract**, **hematuria** may be present; renomegaly may be palpated.

Diagnosis

Most common lower urinary tract neoplasms include **transitional cell carcinoma and lymphoma.**
- Neoplastic cells may be present on microscopic examination of urine sediment.
- A bladder or urethral mass may be detected by ultrasonography, contrast urethrocystography, urethrocystoscopy or cystotomy.
- Definitive diagnosis is made by fine-needle aspiration, biopsy or excision of mass.

Most common upper urinary tract neoplasms include **lymphoma and carcinoma.**
- **Renomegaly is usually present; lymphoma often involves both kidneys.**
- Neoplastic cells may be present on microscopic examination of urine sediment.
- Survey abdominal radiography may reveal renomegaly.
- Renal ultrasonography may reveal a discreet renal mass or **diffuse hyperechogenicity if lymphoma** is involved.
- Definitive diagnosis is made by fine-needle aspiration, biopsy or nephrectomy.

BILIRUBINURIA**

Classical signs

- Urine is dark yellow.
- Mucous membranes and skin are icteric.

See main reference on page 421 (The Yellow Cat or Cat With Elevated Liver Enzymes) for details on the icteric cat.

Clinical signs

Urine is dark yellow or brown from presence of bilirubin.

Cat may be weak and icteric.

Mucous membranes are pale if associated with hemolytic anemia.

Abdominal palpation may reveal hepatomegaly, hepatic masses or the liver may not be palpable.

Bilirubinuria may be associated with vomiting, anorexia, diarrhea and/or neurologic signs (seizure, hypersalivation, tremors).

Diagnosis

Bilirubinuria is diagnosed by a color change on the bilirubin pad on a urine dipstick.
- Bilirubinuria is always abnormal in a cat.
- **The bilirubin test pad may change color if the urine is heavily pigmented as with hematuria.**

Bilirubinuria may occur because of prehepatic, hepatic or posthepatic causes of excess bilirubin in the plasma.
- Bilirubinemia and bilirubinuria occur when the hepatic capacity to process bilirubin is overwhelmed by marked hemolysis. Hemolysis is associated with anemia that is usually regenerative, and most commonly caused by **Hemobartonellosis** or **immune-mediated** mechanisms.
- Bilirubinuria also occurs when the capacity of the liver to process bilirubin is reduced, causing bilirubinemia. There are many causes for **hepatic-related icterus**, but **hepatic lipidosis, cholangio-**

hepatitis complex, **feline infectious peritonitis** and **lymphosarcoma** are most common.
- ALT, GGT and/or alkaline phosphatase activities are abnormal.
- Liver function tests, such as provocative serum bile acid concentrations or blood ammonia concentrations, are abnormal.
- Abdominal radiography and ultrasonography may reveal focal or diffuse hepatomegaly with abnormal echotexture.
- Liver biopsy or fine-needle aspiration is necessary to confirm the underlying disease.

Bile duct obstruction (posthepatic cause of bilirubinemia and bilirubinuria) is associated with cholestatic icterus, and is most commonly associated with pancreatitis, pancreatic or duodenal neoplasia, or sludge bile syndrome.
- **Alkaline phosphatase activity is usually extremely elevated relative to other liver enzyme activities.**
- Enlarged bile duct may be observed by abdominal ultrasonography.

COAGULOPATHY OR THROMBOCYTOPENIA CAYSING HEMATURIA

Classical signs

- Hematuria may occur.
- Other evidence of hemorrhage is usually present.

See main reference on page 487 (The Bleeding Cat) for details on coagulopathies.

Clinical signs

Hematuria may be the only clinical sign, but hemorrhage may occur from other orifices or in body cavities; **petechiations may be present.**

There may be a history of exposure to an anticoagulant toxin.

Pale mucous membranes.

Diagnosis

Anemia due to blood loss is present.

- **Marked thrombocytopenia** is present if it is the cause of the bleeding disorder or if associated with **DIC.**
- Coagulation tests are prolonged if associated with rodenticide poisoning or clotting factor deficiency.

Hematuria is present; however, white blood cell counts are usually < 5–10/hpf.

HEMOGLOBINURIA

Classical signs

- Urine is red or pink.
- Mucous membranes may be pale if associated with anemia.

See main reference on page 532 for details (The Anemic Cat) on hemolytic anemia.

Clinical signs

Hemoglobinuria indicates severe intravascular hemolysis has occurred.

Urine is usually red or pink due to excretion of hemoglobin, which has exceeded the saturation limit of the carrier plasma protein (haptoglobin).

Pale mucous membranes may be present and the cat may be weak or may collapse due to anemia.
- Tachypnea and tachycardia may be present.

Other signs suggestive of intravascular hemolysis and hemoglobinuria include acute illness, fever, pale mucous membranes, +/– jaundice, +/– splenomegaly or acute lethargy.

Marked hemoglobinuria is **most common in kittens with neonatal isoerythrolysis**. Kittens are normal at birth but develop acute lethargy or death in the first 1–3 days of life. In adult cats, hemoglobinuria is very **rarely associated** with *Mycoplasma haemofilis* or **immune-mediated anemia**.

Diagnosis

Although **urine is red or pink, RBCs are not observed on microscopic examination** of urine sediment.

Hemoglobinuria may be differentiated from myoglobinuria by examination of **plasma or serum; plasma**

5

or serum is pink with hemoglobinuria but clear with myoglobinuria.

Anemia may be present.
- Plasma and serum are pink.
- May be Coombs positive if associated with immune-mediated hemolytic anemia.

MYOGLOBINURIA

Classical signs
- Urine is red or brown.
- Muscle weakness or pain present.

See main reference on page 950 (The Cat With Generalized Weakness) for details on snake bite, and page 915 (The Weak and Ataxic or Paralyzed Cat) for details on aortic thrombosis.

Clinical signs

Myoglobinuria is most **commonly associated with aortic thrombosis or snake bite.** Rarely, toxoplasmosis results in myoglobinuria or bilirubinuria in young cats.

Urine is red, brown, or black.

Muscle weakness or pain is present.

Vomiting, anorexia, or other polysystemic signs may be present.

Arrhythmia or heart murmur may be present if an aortic saddle thrombus is present secondary to underlying cardiomyopathy.

Diagnosis

Urine is red, brown or black.

No RBCs observed on microscopic examination of urine sediment.

Plasma and serum are normal in color.

Hyperkalemia and **metabolic acidosis** is often present if due to muscle injury.

There is evidence for other organ dysfunction if myoglobinuria is associated with toxoplasmosis, including dyspnea, anemia, vomiting, diarrhea, neurological signs or jaundice.

Evidence of cardiac disease is usually present with aortic-saddle thrombus.

Snake bite may be complicated by a coagulopathy and hemolysis, resulting in hemoglobinuria, hematuria, as well as myoglobinuria.

CLOUDY WHITE OR WHITE URINE

Cloudy or white urine suggests the presence of pus, lipid, or crystals.

Diagnosis is aided by microscopic examination of urine sediment for pyuria, crystalluria or lipiduria.

Consideration of the clinical signs aids diagnosis. Signs of lower urinary tract disease or systemic illness may or may not be present.

CRYSTALLURIA***

Classical signs
- White or cloudy urine.
- May or may not be associated with urolithiasis.

See main reference on page 184 (The Cat Straining to Urinate) for details on urolithiasis.

Clinical signs

Crystalluria may result in white or cloudy urine if the crystalluria is marked or the urine is concentrated.

Crystalluria may occur with or without urolithiasis, and uroliths may be present without crystalluria.
- Uroliths in the lower urinary tract may be associated with hematuria, stranguria, inappropriate urination, pollakiuria or urethral obstruction.
- Uroliths in the upper urinary tract may be associated with hematuria or renal pain.
- Uroliths may not be associated with clinical signs.

Diagnosis

Crystals are identified on microscopic examination of urine sediment.
- **Struvite** crystals are **typically "coffin-lid"-shaped or amorphous**, and occur in a neutral to alkaline pH.

- **Calcium oxalate** crystals are typically "**dumb-bell**"-**shaped** (**monohydrate**) or are "**square-shaped** with an '**X**' in the center" (dihydrate), and occur in an acidic pH.
- **Urate crystals** are typically **yellow or brown** and **amorphous**, and occur in an acidic pH.
- **Cystine crystals** are **six-sided**, and occur in an acidic pH.
- Other crystals include other minerals (calcium phosphate), normal metabolites (leucine, bilirubin, tyrosine) or drugs (iodinated contrast media, sulfa-containing antibiotics).

Crystals may be present as artifact.
- Crystals may form due to a change in pH or temperature after collection; **struvite crystals commonly form in healthy cats if the urine is allowed to cool to room temperature** or colder (as with refrigeration).
- Crystals may also occur if the urine sample is allowed to evaporate.
- For accurate interpretation, a complete urinalysis including microscopic examination of sediment should be done on a **freshly collected sample in order to avoid artifact.**

PYURIA**

> ### Classical signs
>
> - Cloudy white or white urine.
> - Stranguria, pollakiuria if inflammation involves lower urinary tract.
> - Fever, vomiting, renal pain if inflammation involves upper urinary tract.

See main reference on page 187 (The Cat Straining to Urinate) for details on bacterial cystitis and page 225 (The Cat With Inappropriate Urination) for pyelonephritis.

Clinical signs

Pyuria is indicative of inflammation.
- This is usually associated with an infectious process.
  - **Bacterial infection is most common**.
  - Funguria is rare and is usually associated with a decrease in the host defense mechanisms such as diabetes mellitus, urolithiasis, chronic antibiotic administration, feline leukemia virus or feline

immunodeficiency virus infection, or neoplasia (see page 228, The Cat With Inappropriate Urination).
- Occasionally pyuria occurs without an infection.

Inflammation of the lower urinary tract is usually associated with **stranguria, dysuria, pollakiuria and/or inappropriate urination**; however, clinical signs may be absent.

Inflammation of the kidneys/ureters may be associated with **systemic illness** (fever, vomiting, renal pain and/or anorexia).

Diagnosis

Urine is white or cloudy.

Microscopic examination of urine sediment reveals increased numbers of WBC (typically > 50–100/hpf).
- Normal urine contains < 3–5 WBC/hpf.
- The significance of cell counts should be considered in association with the urine specific gravity.

Nitrite and leukocyte test pads present on some urine dipsticks are **not reliable** and should not be used.

LIPIDURIA

> ### Classical signs
>
> - White urine.
> - Not usually associated with a systemic disease although may be associated with lipid metabolism abnormalities.

See main reference on page 425 (The Yellow Cat or Cat With Elevated Liver Enzymes) for details on hepatic lipidosis and page 569 (The Cat With Hyperlipidemia).

Clinical signs

Lipiduria may result in white urine.

Lipiduria is **not usually associated with clinical signs**; it appears to be normal in some cats particularly those that are **obese** and consuming **normal or increased amounts of dietary fat.**

It may be present with lipid metabolism disorders such as idiopathic hyperlipidemia, inherited hyperchylomicronemia and idiopathic feline hepatic lipidosis.

Diagnosis

Lipid droplets identified **on microscopic sediment examination**.

Lipid droplets may be stained using Sudan IV.

PALE YELLOW OR COLORLESS URINE

DILUTE URINE***

Classical signs

- Polyuria and polydipsia are usually present.
- Most common causes of polyuria in cats are renal failure, diabetes mellitus and hyperthyroidism.

See main reference on page 231 for details (The Cat With Polyuria and Polydipsia).

Clinical signs

Pale yellow or colorless urine implies increased urine volume; therefore, **polyuria and polydipsia** are usually present.

Polysystemic signs such as **vomiting, weight loss** and anorexia may be present with some diseases (renal failure and diabetes mellitus) and increased appetite may occur with hyperthyroidism and diabetes mellitus.

Diagnosis

Urine is pale yellow or colorless.

Urine specific gravity is isosthenuric (1.008–1.014) or hyposthenuric (< 1.008).

Pale yellow or colorless urine may be normal with consumption of a large quantity of water, consumption of a low-protein diet or administration of fluids or agents that induce diuresis.

Pale yellow or colorless urine should be considered abnormal if present with azotemia or dehydration.

BLUE OR GREEN URINE

DRUG DISCOLORATION

Classical signs

- Blue or green urine.
- History of administration of drugs especially methylene blue.

Clinical signs

A number of drugs and dyes cause blue or green urine but few are used in cats.

Blue or green urine occurs in cats following methylene blue use. In humans amitriptyline and riboflavin have been reported to cause blue or green urine.

Diagnosis

Careful questioning of the owner will usually identify the drug causing the urine discoloration.

RECOMMENDED READING

Bartges JW. Discolored urine. In: Ettinger SJ, Feldman EC (eds) Textbook of Small Animal Internal Medicine. Philadelphia, WB Saunders, 2000, pp 96–99.

Bartges JW. Diseases of the urinary bladder. In: Birchard S, Sherding R (eds) WB Saunders Manual of Small Animal Practice. Philadelphia, WB Saunders, 2000, pp 943–957.

Lulich JP, Osborne CA, Bartges JW, et al. Canine lower urinary tract disorders. In: Ettinger SJ, Feldman EC (eds) Textbook of Small Animal Internal Medicine. Philadelphia, WB Saunders, 2000, pp 1747–1781.

Osborne CA, Lulich JP, Kruger JM (eds) Feline lower urinary tract disorders. Vet Clin North Am Small Anim Pract 1996; 26.

Osborne CA, Lulich JP, Bartges JW (eds) The ROCKet science of canine urolithiasis. Vet Clin North Am Small Anim Pract 1999; 29.

14.   The cat with inappropriate urination

Joseph William Bartges

KEY SIGNS

- Urination in inappropriate places.

MECHANISM?

- Urination occurs outside the litter box in inappropriate places.
  Urine may or not be of normal consistency and composition.
  Inappropriate urination occurs as a result of lower urinary tract diseases (urgency, irritation), polyuric states (inability to retain large volume of urine), incontinence (uncontrolled urination), or behavioral problems.
  In addition to inappropriate urination, clinical signs are variable depending on the underlying disease, if present.

WHERE?

- Urogenital tract.

WHAT?

- Most cats with inappropriate urination have an underlying disease process.
  Many lower urinary tract diseases are associated with inappropriate urination.
  Inappropriate urination may also be associated with polyuric states or behavioral problems.

QUICK REFERENCE SUMMARY

Diseases causing inappropriate urination

DEGENERATIVE

- Hormonally responsive incontinence (p 227)
  Incontinence is uncommon in cats; cats unconsciously urinate especially when sleeping.

ANOMALY

- Congenital anatomic diseases of the bladder or urethra (p 226)
  Congenital bladder and urethral diseases are uncommon; usually stranguria, pollakiuria or complete inability to urinate is observed in addition to inappropriate urination.

continued

continued

• Incontinence (p 227)

Incontinence resulting from congenital disease is uncommon. Affected cats may continuously pass small drops of urine.

METABOLIC

• Polyuric states (p 224)

Any disease associated with increased urine volume may result in cats urinating inappropriately if they are not able to adequately retain urine and use the litter box. Examples include chronic renal failure, diuretic therapy, diabetes mellitus and hyperthyroidism.

• **Urolithiasis** (p 222)**

Signs of lower urinary tract disease including pollakiuria, stranguria and hematuria are usually present, although uroliths may be present without clinical signs; may cause urethral obstruction.

NEOPLASTIC

• Neoplasm involving urethra and/or urinary bladder (p 225)

Pollakiuria, stranguria and hematuria usually present; may be associated with recurrent bacterial urinary tract infections or urethral obstruction.

• Meningioma (p 227)

May be associated with proprioceptive deficits, alteration of spinal reflexes and alteration of mentation: however, only clinical sign may be urinary incontinence.

PSYCHOLOGICAL

• **Behavioral*** (p 219)**

Inappropriate urination without clinical, biochemical or radiological evidence for an underlying disease involving the urinary bladder or urethra; may be associated with other behavioral problems or develop as a consequence of lower urinary tract disease.

INFECTIOUS

• **Bacterial urinary tract infection** (p 225)**

Pollakiuria, dysuria and hematuria are usually present; bacterial urinary tract infections are uncommon in cats and usually occur secondarily to another disease.

• Fungal urinary tract infection (p 228)

Cat may be asymptomatic or show pollakiuria, stranguria, hematuria and inappropriate urination; often occurs secondary to an underlying disease or immunosuppressive process.

• Viral urinary tract infection (p 226)

May result in secondary bacterial or fungal urinary tract infection (FeLV, FIV), or hypothesized to be one of the causes of idiopathic lower urinary tract disease.

IDIOPATHIC

• **Non-obstructive idiopathic lower urinary tract disease**** (idiopathic cystitis, feline urologic syndrome, interstitial cystitis, idiopathic FLUTD)*** (p 222)**

Cats show pollakiuria, hematuria, stranguria and inappropriate urination without an identifiable cause.

IATROGENIC

- **Catheterization of the urinary bladder or urethra* (p 224)**
  History of catheterization for relief of urethral obstruction, bladder disease or for diagnostics.

TRAUMATIC

- **Trauma to urethra and/or urinary bladder*** (p 223)**
  History of trauma or physical examination findings of trauma (fractures, skin abrasions, uroabdomen, etc.). Cats may be able to urinate even when the urinary bladder is compromised.

INTRODUCTION

MECHANISM?

Inappropriate urination is **defined as cats urinating in inappropriate places** (typically outside of a litter box) or at inappropriate times.

Lower urinary tract disease is the most common cause of inappropriate urination, and signs such as pollakiuria, stranguria and/or hematuria, are usually present.

Inappropriate urination **may also occur with incontinence, polyuric states** and an inability to retain urine appropriately, or as a **behavioral problem.**
- Inappropriate urination may be a behavioral problem that is learned while the cat is suffering from another lower urinary tract disease, such as idiopathic lower urinary tract disease or urolithiasis.
- Cats are inherently fastidious creatures and do not normally soil where they live.
- Male cats may urinate outside of the litter box to mark their territory.
- **Female cats usually do not mark territory;** however, they may do so if they are, or become, the **dominant cat** in the household.

WHERE?

Brain, bladder and urethral sphincter (mucosa, muscle, nerves).
- If pollakiuria, stranguria and hematuria are present, it localizes the disease to the lower urinary tract.

WHAT?

Most commonly, inappropriate urination occurs with lower urinary tract disease.

- In **young cats, idiopathic lower urinary tract disease is the most common cause** of lower urinary tract disease occurring in 50–70% of cases.
  - **Urolithiasis** is the second most common cause occurring in 15–25% of cases.
  - Bacterial urinary tract infection, trauma, neoplasia and incontinence are uncommon in young cats.
- **In cats older than 10 years, bacterial urinary tract infection** is the most common cause of lower urinary tract disease, occurring in 35–50% of cases.
  - Urolithiasis occurs in 10–15% of cases.
  - Idiopathic disease, trauma, neoplasia and incontinence are uncommon causes.

Inappropriate urination, however, may occur without signs of lower urinary tract disease.
- It may occur with **incontinence.**
- It may occur with **polyuric states.**
- It may be **behavioral.**

Diagnosis is based on historical information, physical examination findings and results of laboratory and radiological evaluation.

DISEASES CAUSING INAPPROPRIATE URINATION

BEHAVIORAL***

Classical signs
- Behavioral elimination problems are the most common behavior complaints of owners.
- Cats may urinate outside of the box.
- Behavioral urination problems may include inappropriate urination or urine marking.
- Underlying medical problems may result in a behavioral component causing inappropriate urination.

Pathogenesis

House-soiling problems are the most common behavior complaints made by cat owners.

Urine house-soiling problems include inappropriate urination and urine marking.

- Inappropriate urination involves elimination of urine outside the litter box at locations unacceptable to the owner.
  - **Inappropriate urination usually occurs on horizontal surfaces** outside the litter box.
  - Any age, breed or gender cat may be affected.
  - Location of inappropriate urination is variable.
  - **Inappropriate urination** often **results from a problem with the litter box** including, unwillingness by the cat to use certain types of litter, infrequent cleaning, change in litter consistency or amount and a deterrent to using the litter box because of other cats in the household.
- **Urine marking involves the use of urine in the act of olfactory communication, which may occur independent of the act of urination.**
  - Urine spraying occurs **more frequently in males than in females**, and in **intact animals** compared with neutered animals.
  - Urine marking may act as a means for cats to communicate their presence so that other cats will avoid using the same space at the same time.
  - Urine marking may be indicative of a high level of arousal, **often associated with the presence of other cats inside or outside of the house.**
  - Urine marking **often involves surfaces other than horizontal ones (such as drapes, walls and furniture);** however, it may involve horizontal surfaces similar to inappropriate urination.
  - Urine marking is not usually associated with a medical condition.

Clinical signs

Inappropriate urination occurs when the cat urinates a normal amount of urine assuming a normal posture consciously outside of the litter box; inappropriate fecal elimination may also occur. Urinalysis may or may not be normal.

Urine marking involves passing small amounts of urine on surfaces other than horizontal to mark a territory that a cat inhabits or is passing through; urinalysis is normal.

Diagnosis

Underlying medical problems must be ruled-out for a diagnosis of a behavioral problem, although behavioral urination problems may occur in conjunction with or following an underlying medical condition.

A behavioral history should be performed once medical problems have been eliminated.

- The owner should be asked to keep a daily record of the number of eliminations in each litter box and the number of eliminations outside the litter box with the location noted.
- Information should also be obtained concerning the care of the litter box by the owner.
- It is beneficial to ask the owner to make a map of the interior of the home, with sites of elimination and litter boxes marked so patterns can be visually identified.
- If multiple cats are in the household or **if it is uncertain as to where a cat may be urinating** inappropriately, **fluorescein dye** (0.3 ml SQ, 0.5 ml PO, or six fluorescein strips in gel capsules given PO) may be administered; any urine that is found outside the litter box during the next 24 hours can be checked for fluorescence using a Wood's light.

Urine marking is typically characterized by a cat passing small amounts of urine in different places ("spraying").

- Owners may or may not observe this behavior.
- In a multi-cat household, more than one cat may exhibit this behavior.
- Although isolation of cats in a household may identify the individual, urine marking may cease when separated from housemates.
- Fluorescein dye as described before may also be used to identify offenders.

Differential diagnosis

Inappropriate urination may or not occur secondary to a medical disorder.

- Diseases associated with **polyuria**, such as **renal failure** and **diabetes mellitus**, may result in inappropriate urination, because the **cat finds the litter excessively wet.**
- Causes of **lower urinary tract disease**, such as **urolithiasis or idiopathic disease** (non-obstructive FLUTD or interstitial cystitis), result in inappropriate urination.

- **Incontinence** associated with a congenital or acquired anatomical problem may be interpreted as inappropriate urination.

Urine marking must be differentiated from inappropriate elimination.
- This can usually be accomplished on the basis of historical information and a good behavior history.
- **Underlying medical problems rarely result in urine marking.**

Treatment

The goal of treatment of inappropriate urination is to **enhance the appeal and accessibility of the litter box and to decrease the availability and appeal of alternate sites**.
- The litter box should contain a litter that is preferred by the cat and kept clean.
- A litter box may be used in the **area where inappropriate urination has occurred.**
  - Once the cat begins to use this litterbox, it may be moved slowly to a site more acceptable to the owner.
  - Deterrents such as an unacceptable substrate, e.g. plastic covers or odor may be used at the inappropriate site.
- **Positive reinforcement** when the cat uses the appropriate litter box is better than negative reinforcement when the cat inappropriately eliminates.
- Pharmacologic therapy is not usually necessary; **environmental therapy is much more effective** with behavioral inappropriate urination.
- Owners' compliance can be a problem, and owners should maintain records of the cat's elimination patterns; owners also need positive reinforcement.

Treatment of urine marking can be accomplished by environmental, behavior, surgical and pharmacological methods.
- Environmental treatment involves deterring the cat from urine marking.
  - Restrict the cat from areas where spraying occurs.
  - Block the indoor cat's view of outdoor cats.
  - Reduce the number of cats outside or inside the house.

  - Make the location where the cat marks aversive to the problem cat.
  - An **odor deterrent** such as citrus spray may be effective.
  - **Spray synthesized facial pheromone** (the F3 fraction) **at the site**(s).
- Behavior modification consists of positive interactions with the cat in **scheduled play or grooming times.**
  - **Avoid punishment** because it may increase the cat's fear and anxiety.
- Pharmacologic treatment of urine marking attempts to attenuate the cat's arousal and/or anxiety in response to social or environmental situations.
  - **Benzodiazepines** have been used for their anxiolytic property.
  - They may not only decrease anxiety and fear, but they produce mild sedation.
  - Dosage of diazepam is 1–4 mg/cat q 12–24 h PO.
  - Side effects include sedation, muscle relaxation, increased appetite and paradoxical excitation; hepatic necrosis has been reported to occur rarely in cats.
  - Other **benzodiazepines** have not been thoroughly evaluated in cats.
  - Alprazolam may be given at 0.125–0.25 mg PO q 12 h or 0.05–0.1 mg/kg PO q 8 h.
  - Dosage for clonazepam is 0.016 mg/kg PO q 6–24 h.
  - Clorazepate dosage is 0.55–2.2 mg/kg PO q 12–24 h.
  - Flurazepam has been used primarily as an appetite stimulant at 0.2–0.4 mg/kg PO as needed.
  - Triazolam may also be tried at 0.03 mg PO q 12 h.
  - **Azaperones have serotonergic and dopaminergic mechanisms.**
  - **Buspirone** has been shown to be efficacious for the treatment of urine marking.
  - Dosage is 5–7.5 mg PO q 12 h, or 2–10 mg PO q 12–24 h, or 0.5–1 mg/kg PO q 12–24 h.
  - The drug has no potential for abuse and does not cause sedation.
  - It may take 1–3 weeks to show an effect.
  - Side effects include idiosyncratic changes in social behavior and mild gastrointestinal side effects.

- **Tricyclic antidepressants are used commonly to treat behavioral disorders.**
- Amitriptyline is used most commonly although clomipramine has been used.
- Dosage for **amitriptyline** is 2.5–10 mg PO q 24 h or 0.5–1 mg/kg PO q 24 h, and for **clomipramine**, it is 1–5 mg PO q 12–24 h.
- Side effects include sedation and possible anticholinergic effects.
- **Selective serotonin reuptake inhibitors** act selectively on the serotonin neurotransmitter system.
- Fluoxetine and paroxetine have been used to treat urine marking.
- Dosage for **fluoxetine** is 0.5 mg/kg PO q 12 h or 1–2.5 mg PO q 24 h, and for **paroxetine**, 0.5 mg/kg PO q 24 h or 1.25–2.5 mg PO q 24 h.
- Fluoxetine may take 3–4 weeks before an effect is observed; paroxetine has a shorter half-life and is quicker acting.
- Side effects include vomiting, diarrhea, nausea, inappetence, sleep disturbances and irritability.
- Historically, progestational compounds have been used to treat urine marking; however, because severe side effects such as diabetes mellitus may occur, other pharmacotherapy should be used.
- **Surgical treatment** can affect the incidence of urine marking.
  - **Castrate intact males**.
  - Olfactory transaction has been used rarely and is reserved for cats that are refractory to all other forms of therapy.

Prognosis

Prognosis for behavioral inappropriate urination is good; however, owner compliance is necessary.

Prognosis for urine marking is good; however, cats that are refractory to treatment often become unacceptable as indoor pets and are put outdoors or are euthanized.

Prevention

Inappropriate urination may be prevented by treating underlying medical problems and by appropriate care of the litter box.

Urine marking may be prevented by **castrating cats when kittens**, by **minimizing stress in the environment**, and by **early treatment of the problem.**

NON-OBSTRUCTIVE IDIOPATHIC LOWER URINARY TRACT DISEASE*** (IDIOPATHIC CYSTITIS, FELINE UROLOGIC SYNDROME, INTERSTITIAL CYSTITIS, IDIOPATHIC FLUTD)

Classical signs

- Inappropriate urination, hematuria, stranguria and pollakiuria.
- Signs are usually transient lasting between 3 and 7 days.

See main reference on page 176 for details (The Cat Straining to Urinate) on idiopathic lower urinary tract disease.

Clinical signs

Inappropriate urination, pollakiuria, stranguria and hematuria commonly occur.

Idiopathic disease is more common **in cats younger than 10 years of age.**

Clinical signs typically last between 3 and 7 days.

Diagnosis

The diagnosis of idiopathic lower urinary tract disease is based on clinical signs and exclusion of other causes of lower urinary tract disease.
- **Urinalysis reveals hematuria** (> 5 RBC/hbf).
- **Pyuria and bacteruria are not present** (i.e. < 5 WBC/hbf).
- Abdominal radiography and ultrasonography, and contrast urethrocystography are normal or only show mild thickening of the bladder wall.

Complete blood cell counts and serum biochemical analysis are normal, and FeLV and FIV are negative.

UROLITHIASIS**

Classical signs

- Inappropriate urination is usually associated with stranguria and hematuria.

See main reference on page 184 for details on urolithiasis.

Clinical signs

Inappropriate urination due to urolithiasis is usually associated with **stranguria, pollakiuria and hematuria.**

Most uroliths occur in **middle-aged to older cats.**

Urethral obstruction may also occur, therefore, post-renal uremia may also be present (vomiting, anorexia, oral ulceration).

If **urate uroliths** develop in association with a portal vascular anomaly, tremors, seizures, salivation, depression and stunted growth may also be observed. **Signs are usually present before 2 years of age.**

Diagnosis

Diagnosis is based on radiography and/or ultrasonography of the urinary tract.
- Because uroliths composed of **struvite and calcium oxalate** account for more than 85% of urocystoliths, they are often **observed on survey radiography**. Contrast cystography will help identify rediolucent uroliths.
  - Uroliths composed of **cystine, urate and xanthine are not usually radiodense**.
  - Uroliths composed of drug metabolites are not usually radiodense.
- **Ultrasonography** may reveal presence of urocystoliths, but not urethroliths.

Urinalysis may reveal abnormalities.
- **Crystalluria** may or may not be present.
- **Hematuria** is often present, but not always.
- Bacterial urinary tract infection may occur, but is usually secondary to presence of uroliths.

Serum biochemical analysis is usually normal.
- **Approximately 35% of cats with calcium oxalate uroliths are hypercalcemic**.
- Urate uroliths associated with hepatic disease may also be associated with increases in liver enzyme activity, increased blood ammonia concentration, and increased bile acid concentrations (pre- or post-prandial).

TRAUMA TO URETHRA AND/OR URINARY BLADDER**

Classical signs
- **Inappropriate urination, hematuria, pollakiuria and stranguria.**
- **Other signs of trauma, such as fractures and skin abrasions, may be present.**

See main reference on page 189 for details on trauma to the lower urinary tract.

Clinical signs

Inappropriate urination, hematuria, pollakiuria and stranguria may be present because of trauma to the urinary bladder or urethra.

Other signs of trauma, such as fractures and skin abrasions, may be present.

Trauma to the caudal abdomen may result in rupture or **perforation of the urinary bladder.**
- Post-renal uremia may be present.
- **Only a small quantity** or **no urine at all may be passed despite attempts at urination.**
- **Abdominal effusion** may be present due to urine leakage from the damaged bladder.

Diagnosis

Microscopic examination of urine reveals an inflammatory reaction.

Serum biochemical analysis may reveal azotemia.

Contrast cystography is necessary to determine the integrity of the urinary bladder.
- Ultrasonography may reveal abdominal effusion.
- Survey abdominal radiography may have decreased contrast due to abdominal effusion.
- Abdominocentesis may reveal urine.

Other laboratory parameters may be abnormal depending on the extent of the trauma.

POLYURIC STATES**

Classical signs

- Polyuria, polydipsia and inappropriate urination.
- ± Systemic signs such as anorexia or polyphagia, vomiting, weight loss, poor hair coat quality and/or diarrhea.

See main references on page 235 for details (The Cat With Polyuria and Polydipsia) on chronic renal failure, page 236 for details on diabetes mellitus, and page 304 for details (The Cat With Weight Loss and a Good Appetite) on hyperthyroidism.

Clinical signs

Polyuria and polydipsia may result in the cat being unable to adequately retain urine resulting in inappropriate urination.

History of drinking and urinating a greater volume then normal (polyuria and polydipsia).

Inappropriate urination may occur because of the inability to retain larger quantity of urine.

Other clinical signs are variable depending on the underlying disease process.
- The most common causes of polyuria and polydipsia in cats are **renal failure, diabetes mellitus and hyperthyroidism.**
  - Renal failure may be associated with inappetance anorexia, vomiting, poor body condition and oral ulcers.
  - Diabetes mellitus may be associated with weight loss despite a good appetite; vomiting and anorexia may occur if associated with ketoacidosis.
  - Hyperthyroidism may be associated with weight loss despite polyphagia, poor body condition and intermittent vomiting.
- Other causes of polyuria and polydipsia may occur, but are less common.

Diagnosis

Polyuria is confirmed by a **low urine specific gravity** (<1.030).

Polydipsia may be difficult to confirm in cats because measurement of fluid intake may be difficult.

- Cats normally are not observed to drink very much, particularly if consuming canned diets. Cats eating a mix of canned and dry food drink < 20 ml/kg/24 h.
- Owners may notice cats drinking out of water sources, such as sinks and bowls, when the cat has not done so previously. **Water intake of > 100 ml/kg/24 h is abnormal,** even if cats are eating dry food.

Serum biochemical analysis and serum thyroxine concentrations should be performed, in addition to a complete urinalysis, in all cats that may have polyuria and polydipsia to aid in localizing the problem further.

CATHETERIZATION OF THE URINARY BLADDER OR URETHRA*

Classical signs

- Inappropriate urination, stranguria, pollakiuria and hematuria.

See main references on page 187 for details on bacterial urinary tract infection and page 181 for details on urinary catheretization.

Clinical signs

The **urethra or urinary bladder mucosa** may be **traumatized during catheterization** performed to clear an obstruction from the urethra or for diagnostic procedures; therefore, there is a history of urinary catheterization.

Indwelling urinary catheters may predispose to bacterial urinary tract infection.

Inappropriate urination, stranguria, pollakiuria and hematuria may occur following catheterization of the urinary tract if mucosal damage occurs, or if a secondary bacterial infection occurs. Occasionally a urethral or urinary bladder diverticulum is formed by traumatic catheterization, predisposing to recurrent bacterial infection.

Diagnosis

The diagnosis is made based on clinical signs and a history of urethral catheterization.

A **urinalysis and urine culture should be performed** to rule-in or rule-out an iatrogenic bacterial urinary tract infection.

If a polypropylene catheter is placed too far into the urinary bladder, perforation may occur.
- Post-renal azotemia may be found on serum biochemical analysis.
- **Abdominal effusion, if present, will have a composition similar to urine.**
- Contrast cystography is necessary to confirm the perforation although abdominal ultrasonography or survey abdominal radiography will demonstrate abdominal effusion if present.

BACTERIAL URINARY TRACT INFECTION*

Classical signs

- Inappropriate urination occurs together with pollakiuria, stranguria and hematuria.

See main reference on page 187 for details (The Cat Straining to Urinate) on bacterial urinary tract infection.

Clinical signs

Bacterial urinary tract infections often occur as a **consequence of an underlying disease of the urinary bladder, polyuric states or immunosuppressive states**; therefore, other clinical signs may be present.
- Any disease that disrupts the cat's normal defenses may result in a bacterial urinary tract infection.
- Systemic illness may be seen if the underlying disease process is a systemic disease such as diabetes mellitus, chronic renal failure, FeLV or FIV infection.

Urination in inappropriate places usually occurs together with signs of **pollakiuria, stranguria and hematuria.**
- Clinical signs of other lower urinary tract diseases are similar to those observed with bacterial urinary tract infections.

Diagnosis

Diagnosis is made by examination of urine.
- **Pyuria** (> 5 WBC/hpf) and bacteriuria are often observed on microscopic examination of urine, but a bacterial urinary tract infection may be present with an inactive urinary sediment on microscopic examination, especially in older cats with concurrent disease(s).

- **Alkaluria** (pH > 7) may occur with **urease-producing bacteria**, such as *Staphylococcus* spp. and *Mycoplasma* spp.
- Urine culture is necessary to identify the species of bacteria and its antibiotic sensitivity pattern.
  - Urine should be collected by cystocentesis.
  - Nitrite and leukocyte esterase test pads on urine dipsticks are not reliable indicators of bacterial urinary tract infection, and should not be used.

Abdominal radiography or ultrasonography, or contrast studies of the urinary tract may be necessary to detect anatomic defects, and uroliths or neoplasms, that predispose the cat to a bacterial urinary tract infection.

Systemic diseases resulting in dilute urine, such as renal failure or diabetes mellitus, or in immunosuppression, such as FeLV, FIV or diabetes mellitus, may result in a bacterial urinary tract infection.

Drugs resulting in a diuresis, such as furosemide, or in immunosuppression, such as corticosteroids, may **predispose to bacterial urinary tract infection.**

Urethral catheterization may result in iatrogenic bacterial urinary tract infection, particularly if antibiotics are administered concurrently.

NEOPLASM INVOLVING URINARY BLADDER OR URETHRA

Classical signs

- Inappropriate urination may occur with pollakiuria, stranguria and hematuria.
- Typically occurs in cats older than 10 years.

See main reference on page 191 for details on neoplasia.

Clinical signs

Although uncommon, lower urinary tract neoplasia typically occurs in **cats older than 10 years.**

Inappropriate urination associated with neoplasia may occur with other signs of lower urinary tract disease such as **stranguria, pollakiuria and hematuria.**

Urethral obstruction may occur if neoplasm occurs at the trigone region, urethra or prepuce.

If urinary outflow obstruction occurs, signs of **post-renal uremia** may occur (**vomiting, anorexia, depression**).

Diagnosis

Some urinary bladder neoplasms may be palpated on abdominal palpation; urethral neoplasm may be palpated on rectal examination.

Transitional cell carcinoma of the urinary bladder is the most common lower urinary tract neoplasm; other types of neoplasia that may occur include **squamous cell carcinoma, lymphoma, fibrosarcoma, and leiomyoma or leiomyosarcoma.**

Ultrasonography and/or contrast urethrocystography may be necessary to identify the neoplasm.

Diagnosis may require biopsy or fine-needle aspiration of the mass.
- Occasionally, neoplastic cells may be found on microscopic examination of urine sediment.
- Fine-needle aspiration may be accomplished by palpation or by ultrasound guidance.
- Cystoscopy may also be used to identify and aspirate or biopsy a mass.
- It may be necessary to obtain a biopsy using surgery.

VIRAL URINARY TRACT INFECTION

Classical signs

- Lower urinary tract signs including inappropriate urination, pollakiuria, stranguria and hematuria.

See main references on page 187 for details (The Cat Straining to Urinate) on hemorrhagic cystitis and page 225 for details on bacterial urinary tract infection.

Clinical signs

FeLV or FIV infections may result in bacterial urinary tract infections.

A **cell-associated herpesvirus and a urotropic calicivirus have been hypothesized** to be a cause of **idiopathic lower urinary tract disease** in cats resulting in hemorrhagic cystitis (non-obstructive feline lower urinary tract disease, interstitial cystitis).

Inappropriate urination may occur with other clinical signs of lower urinary tract disease including **hematuria, stranguria and pollakiuria**.

FeLV and FIV may be associated with other clinical signs including **gingival disease**, infections of other organs, liver disease or renal disease.

Clinical signs of lower urinary tract disease, if idiopathic in nature (interstitial cystitis), usually resolve in 5–7 days, although a protracted course of clinical signs may occur.

Diagnosis

Hematuria may be observed with or without bacteriuria and pyuria.

FeLV and FIV testing should be performed on cats with lower urinary tract disease or **recurrent bacterial urinary tract infections.**

Viral particles have been observed by electron microscopy in some matrix-crystalline plugs retrieved from male cats with urethral obstruction.

CONGENITAL ANATOMIC DEFECTS OF BLADDER OR URETHRA

Classical signs

- Inappropriate urination usually occurs with other clinical signs such as pollakiuria, stranguria and possibly hematuria.
- Usually evident as a young kitten.

See main references on page 201 for details (The Incontinent Cat) on patent urachus and page 198 for details on ectopic ureters.

Clinical signs

Inappropriate urination is first observed at an early age. It may not be noticed until the kitten is older and litter box training is undertaken.

Pollakiuria, stranguria and/or hematuria may also be present.

Defects of the bladder or urethra may be associated with other congenital anomalies, especially of the vagina.

Diagnosis

Diagnosis is made by historical information concerning age of cat, physical examination of the urinary tract, and radiology including contrast studies and ultrasonography of the lower urinary tract.

Many congenital anomalies are possible, but congenital anomalies are uncommon in cats.
- Patent urachus and ectopic ureters are the most common congenital anomalies.
- Other anomalies include, but are not limited to:
  - Bladder agenesis.
  - Bladder duplication.
  - Vaginal defects such as septal defects.
  - Urethral dysgenesis.
  - Urethral strictures.
  - Bladder and urethral diverticulae.

MENINGIOMA

> ### Classical signs
> - Inappropriate urination.
> - Neurological deficits (altered mentation, abnormal proprioception or spinal reflexes).

See main reference on page 914 for details on meningioma.

Clinical signs

Meningiomas may be associated with urinary incontinence and inappropriate urination.

Inappropriate urination is usually due to incontinence related to a **spinal cord meningioma** but may be associated with cerebral meningioma.

Other neurologic deficits, such as proprioceptive deficits or abnormal spinal reflexes, may or may not be present.

Typically occurs in **old cats > 10 years.**

Diagnosis

Diagnosis is difficult.
- Meningiomas involving spinal cord may require myelography for diagnosis.
- Meningiomas that occur intracranially require computerized tomography or magnetic resonance imaging for diagnosis.

Laboratory evaluation is normal.

INCONTINENCE (INCLUDING HORMONALLY RESPONSIVE INCONTINENCE)

> ### Classical signs
> - Unconscious urination usually occurs when asleep.
> - Cats with congenital disease may continuously pass small drops of urine whether awake or asleep.

See main reference on page 193 for details (The Incontinent Cat) on incontinence.

Clinical signs

Incontinence may be due to an underlying congenital or acquired anatomic problem.

Incontinence is urination that is uncontrolled or unconsciously done.
- **Unconscious urination usually occurs when asleep**.
- Cats with **congenital disease** may **continuously pass small drops of urine** whether awake or asleep.

Pollakiuria, dysuria and stranguria may also occur if a secondary bacterial urinary tract infection occurs.

Urinalysis is usually normal unless a secondary bacterial urinary tract infection is present.

Diagnosis

Diagnosis is usually made on the basis of historical and physical examination findings.

Incontinence must be **differentiated from consciously controlled inappropriate urination** as might be observed with bacterial urinary tract infection, urolithiasis, bladder or urethral neoplasia or other causes of lower urinary tract disease.
- **With lower urinary tract disease, cats appear to have urgency or discomfort when urinating**.
  - Hematuria and/or pyuria with or without crystalluria is usually present.
  - Laboratory and radiological evaluation may be abnormal.

- With incontinence, these signs are not present, instead cats urinate without being aware that they are doing so.
  - Urinalysis is typically normal.

FUNGAL URINARY TRACT INFECTION

Classical signs

- Usually asymptomatic.
- Pollakiuria, stranguria, hematuria and inappropriate urination may occur.
- Systemic clinical signs may be present.

Pathogenesis

Fungal urinary tract infections are **often associated with impaired systemic or local host defenses such as glucosuria, indwelling urinary catheters, urethrostomy and urolithiasis.**

Cats with immunosuppressive diseases such as **FeLV and FIV** infection are also at risk for development of fungal urinary tract infections.

Candida and *Torulopsis* are normal saprophytic inhabitants of the gastrointestinal tract and are the most common fungi observed to occur in urine.

Clinical signs

Fungi are not normally found in urine of healthy animals.
- Cats with funguria **may be asymptomatic.**
- However, clinical signs of systemic disease may be present.

Symptomatic fungal urinary tract infections are associated with **pollakiuria, hematuria, stranguria** and **inappropriate urination** if the infection occurs in the **lower urinary tract**, or **fever, inappetence, vomiting** and **septicemia** if it occurs in the **upper urinary tract.**

Rarely, bezoars (fungal balls) may form.
- **Bezoars are clusters of intertwined fungal hyphae** which may aggregate.
- Bezoars may be present in patients with symptomatic or asymptomatic fungal urinary tract infections.
- They are **sources of persistent funguria**.
- Large bezoars may result in urethral obstruction.

Diagnosis

Diagnosis of funguria is based on results of urinalysis and urine cultures.
- Microscopic examination of urine sediment reveals budding yeasts or elongated hyphae, and inflammation.
- Urine culture is necessary to definitively diagnose fungal urinary tract infections.
  - The **absolute number of fungal organisms does not correlate with infection**; however, fungi are not normal inhabitants of the urinary bladder.
  - A cystocentesis sample should be evaluated.
  - Use of **fungal culture media facilitates isolation and identification of the organism.**

Other diagnostic **tests should be directed at identifying abnormalities in local or systemic host defenses**.
- Serum biochemical analysis may reveal azotemia consistent with **renal failure**, or **hyperglycemia** consistent with diabetes mellitus.
- **FeLV and FIV** testing should be performed.
- Abdominal radiography, including contrast studies, and ultrasonography are necessary to determine if an abnormality of the lower urinary tract is present such as **urolithiasis or neoplasia.**

Differential diagnosis

Any disease of the lower urinary tract may present with similar signs.

Most common diseases with similar signs are non-obstructive idiopathic lower urinary tract disease and urolithiasis. **Differentiation is based on finding yeast or hyphae in the urine**. Urolithiasis may occasionally be concurrent with fungal infection.

Treatment

Some patients have asymptomatic funguria.
- No treatment may be necessary as some spontaneously clear the fungi if predisposing factors can be resolved.
- **Urinary catheters should be removed** or used intermittently.
- If possible, antibacterial and immunosuppressive medication should be discontinued.
- **Alkalinization of urine may aid in clearing of the fungal urinary tract infection.**

- *Candida* species survive poorly at alkaline pH.
- Alkalinization therapy has not been very successful.
- **Potassium citrate** may be administered at 50–75 mg/kg PO q 12 h.
- **Sodium bicarbonate** may also be used at 12 mg/kg PO q 8 h.

More aggressive treatment is warranted in patients that have symptomatic fungal urinary tract infections.
- An attempt should be made to **correct predisposing risk factors**.
- Antifungal drugs should also be used.
  - Flucytosine has a narrow range of antifungal activity, limited primarily to yeast-like fungi such as *Candida*, *Torulopsis* and *Cryptococcus*.
  - **Flucytosine** is deaminated to 5-fluorouracil in fungal cells which **interrupts intracellular protein synthesis** resulting in death of the cell.
  - Flucytosine is excreted largely unchanged in urine which makes it a good first-line treatment.
  - Dosage is 200 mg/kg/day PO divided into three or four sub-doses.
  - Resistance may occur.
  - Flucytosine should be **continued 2–3 weeks beyond clinical resolution** of fungal urinary tract infection.
- **Amphotericin-B** is also effective in the treatment of fungal urinary tract infection and can be used with **flucytosine** or an **imidazole**.
  - Occurrence of **nephrotoxicity** is a major disadvantage to its use.
  - Amphotericin-B disrupts fungal cell membranes making it effective.
  - Resistance is uncommon.
  - Dosage is 0.1–0.25 mg/kg IV (administered in 30 ml of 5% dextrose in water over 15 min) q 48 h for up to 6 weeks. It may be also given **subcutaneously** (see page 26, The Cat With Signs of Chronic Nasal Disease).
  - Amphotericin B may also be administered by **irrigation into the urinary bladder**.
  - A concentration of 200 mg of amphotericin-B per liter of sterile water is recommended.
  - This solution is infused at 5–10 ml/kg into the urinary bladder lumen **daily for 5–15 days**.
- **Imidazole derivatives** may be used as treatment for funguria.

- Ketoconazole and itraconazole are not very effective because they have limited urinary excretion.
- Fluconazole may be a viable alternative.
- This imidazole is smaller, more water soluble, and less protein bound than other commonly used imidazoles.
- Active **fluconazole is excreted primarily in urine**.
- Use a dosage of 50–100 mg/cat PO with food.
- **Intravesicular clotrimazole**
  - Instillation of 1% clotrimazole intravesicularly has been successful in treating fungal cystitis.
  - Instillation can be accomplished by anesthesia or sedation and urinary catheterization or by cystocentesis.
  - Three to four treatments may be necessary.

Prognosis

Prognosis for asymptomatic funguria in cats is unknown.
- Funguria may spontaneously resolve.
- Funguria may also progress to symptomatic infection or to bezoar formation.
- Some animals may have persistent asymptomatic funguria without discernible harm.

Symptomatic funguria carries a variable prognosis.
- **If systemic fungal infection is present, prognosis is guarded**.
- If fungi are limited to the lower urinary tract, the prognosis is fair; however, **complete clearance of the fungal urinary tract infection may be difficult**.

Bezoar formation may require surgical removal if it causes urethral obstruction or persistent or recurrent funguria, and it cannot be disrupted by medical means.

Prevention

Because fungal urinary tract infection usually occurs as a result of a problem with local or systemic host defenses, identification and correction of risk factors may prevent it from occurring.

Urine from cats with indwelling urinary catheters should be examined periodically, particularly if the animal is receiving antibiotics or immunosuppressive therapy.

RECOMMENDED READING

Bartges JW. Diseases of the urinary bladder. In: Birchard S, Sherding R (eds) Saunders Manual of Small Animal Practice. Philadelphia, WB Saunders, 2000; 943–957.

Lulich JP, Osborne CA, Bartges JW, et al. Canine lower urinary tract disorders. In: Ettinger SJ, Feldman EC (eds) Textbook of Small Animal Internal Medicine. Philadelphia, WB Saunders, 2000, pp 1747–1781.

Lulich JP, Osborne CA. Fungal urinary tract infections. In: Kirk RW, Bonagura JD (eds) Current Veterinary Therapy XI. WB Saunders, Philadelphia, 1993, pp 914–919.

Osborne CA, Lulich JP, Kruger JM (eds). Feline lower urinary tract disorders I and II. Vet Clin North Am Small Anim Pract 1996; 26 (2, 3).

Simpson BS. Feline housesoiling part I: Inappropriate elimination. Compend Contin Educ Pract Vet 1998; 20: 1319–1329.

Simpson BS. Feline housesoiling part II: Urine and fecal marking. Compend Contin Educ Pract Vet 1998; 20: 1331–1339.

Toll J, Ashe CA, Trepanier LA. Intravesicular administration of clotrimazole for treatment of Candiduria in a cat with diabetes mellitus J Am Vet Med Assoc 2003; 223:1156–1158.

15. The cat with polyuria and polydipsia

Jacquie Rand

KEY SIGNS

- Drinking more than normal.
- Increased frequency of urination and increased volume and/or nocturia.
- Urinating outside litter box.

MECHANISM?

- Polyuria and polydipsia usually occur in cats because of an inability to concentrate urine.

WHERE?

- Kidney (the kidney controls urine production, but it is influenced by many other organs).

WHAT?

- Most cats with polyuria and polydipsia (PU/PD) have renal failure, diabetes mellitus or hyperthyroidism.

QUICK REFERENCE SUMMARY

Diseases causing polyuria and polydipsia

DEGENERATIVE

- **Chronic renal failure*** (p 235)**
  Inappetence or anorexia, weight loss, PU/PD, vomiting, increased or decreased renal size.

METABOLIC

- **Diabetes mellitus*** (p 236)**
  Usually older than 6 years of age, PU/PD of 1–12 weeks duration, weight loss, polyphagia or inappetence, may have been previously obese.

- **Hyperthyroidism*** (p 242)**
  Older than 7 years of age, weight loss, polyphagia or inappetence, palpable cervical mass, vomiting, tachycardia, restlessness.

- **Diabetes insipidus* (p 243)**
  Central form is rare, nephrogenic form is common, and associated with renal failure, hyperthyroidism, pyometra, etc. Urine specific gravity often <1.007.

continued

continued

- Hyperadrenocorticism (p 251)

Very rare; poorly controlled diabetes mellitus which may be insulin resistant, poor hair coat, weight loss despite higher than normal doses of insulin, thin fragile skin that bruises easily.

- Acromegaly (growth hormone-producing tumor, hypersomatotrophism) (p 254)

Very rare. Often associated with poorly controlled diabetes mellitus, which is usually insulin resistant, often requiring very high doses of insulin. Typically there is a large blocky cat with weight gain, enlarged tongue, widely spaced teeth, cardiomegaly and thickened soft palate.

- Hypoadrenocorticism (p 252)

Very, rare; lethargy, depression, anorexia, and weight loss are most frequent. Less frequent signs include vomiting, polyuria and polydipsia.

- Hyperparathyroidism P (p 256)

A rare cause of hypercalcemia in cats. Usually results from a solitary adenoma, but can be from solitary or bilateral adenocarcinoma or hyperplasia. Older cats (mean age 13 years) and Siamese are overrepresented. Clinical signs are of hypercalcemia and more than half of the cats have a palpable parathyroid mass.

- Primary hyperaldosteronism (p 256)

Rare cause of polyuria and polydipsia. Typically occurs in older cats (10–20 years) and is associated with an adrenal mass. Signs are of intractable hypokalemia and hypertension, and include muscle weakness, cervical ventroflexion, inappetence, weight loss, blindness and polyuria and polydipsia.

- Primary sex hormone-secreting adrenal tumor (p 258)

Very rare cause of polyuria, polydipsia. Progesterone-producing tumors result in signs indistinguishable from hyperadrenocorticism. Typically there is thin fragile skin that bruises easily, patchy symmetrical alopecia, secondary skin infections such as demodicosis and polyuria, polydipsia from poorly controlled diabetes mellitus.

- Pheochromocytoma (p 257)

Very rare cause of polyuria, polydispsia. Typically occurs in older cats (> 8 years of age) and associated with an adrenal mass. Signs are vague and include polyuria and polydispsia. Systemic hypertension is characteristic, and presents as sudden blindness from retinal hemorrhage or retinal detachment, or dyspnea from heart failure. Diabetic cats may be insulin resistant.

- Polycythemia

Dark pink or purple mucosae, bleeding, PU/PD, neurological signs including abnormal behavior and seizures.

- **Hypokalemia* (p 244)**

Lethargy, inappetence, weakness, ventroflexion of neck, stiff/stilted gait, impaired renal function. PU/PD are not prominent signs unless associated with chronic renal failure or hyperthyroidism.

NEOPLASTIC

- Neoplasia (renal neoplasia or. lymphoma) (p 250)

PU/PD results from either renal neoplasia causing chronic renal failure, or lymphoma causing hypercalcemia (very rare in cats).

● Hypercalcemia (p 245)

Associated with renal failure, lymphoma or squamous cell carcinoma, primary hyperparathyroidism, cholecalciferol rodenticide, infectious disease, diabetes mellitus, hyperthyroidism, liver disease or idiopathic. Vomiting, weight loss, inappetence and in some cats, signs associated with calcium oxalate urolithiasis (dysuria and inappropriate urination) may be present. In some cats, signs are those of the primary disease process, e.g. renal failure or lymphoma.

PSYCHOLOGICAL

● Psychological polydipsia

This syndrome is not yet reported in cats.

INFLAMMATION INFECTIOUS (BACTERIAL)

● Pyelonephritis

Chronic form causes chronic renal failure with weight loss, inappetence. The acute phase may be associated with fever, lethargy and pain on palpation of the kidneys. Bacteriuria, pyuria, casts (especially WBC casts) may be present during the active infection, and occasionally leukocytosis occurs.

● Cystic endometrial hyperplasia/pyometra complex (p 259)

Causes nephrogenic diabetes insipidus and PU/PD; vaginal discharge, inappetence, and weight loss.

INFECTIOUS (IMMUNE)

● Chronic renal failure (glomerulonephritis or amyloidosis) (p 235)

Causes chronic renal failure and associated signs of PU/PD, weight loss, inappetence, lethargy, and in the later stages, vomiting.

TREATMENT

● Drug induced* (p 244)

Drugs such as diuretics, phenobarbitol, amphotericin, gentamicin, thyroxine, corticosteroids, and megestrol acetate may be associated with PU/PD through a number of mechanisms.

INTRODUCTION

MECHANISM?

Polyuria and polydipsia in cats usually occurs because of a primary inability to concentrate urine. This is referred to as **primary polyuria and leads to compensatory polydipsia.** Although not reported in cats, the kidney may also be overloaded with water from primary polydipsia, termed psychogenic polydipsia. **Mechanisms for primary polyuria are as follows:**

● **The solute load in the renal tubule is higher than the capacity to reabsorb it, resulting in osmotic diuresis.** This is characterized by isotonic urine with a SG 1.007–1.030. This occurs in the following circumstances:
– Glomerular filtration of an **absorbable solute in excess of the renal tubular ability to reabsorb it**, e.g. glucose in diabetes mellitus. This may also occur when the glomerular filtration rate (GFR) is reduced, as the increased solute load on the remaining functioning nephrons may overwhelm their absorptive capacity.

- – **Glomerular disease** resulting in **leakage of albumin and other poorly absorbable solutes** into the renal tubule.
- – **Impaired tubular reabsorption** of glomerular filtrate solutes such as urea, creatinine, and phosphorus as occurs in renal failure and Fanconi syndrome.
- – **Diuretics which act as a non-absorbable solute**, e.g. Mannitol.
- The **medullary osmotic gradient is compromised**, which decreases the concentrating ability of the kidney, producing urine with a SG of 1.007–1.030. Causes include:
  - – **Interference with the NaCl pump in the loop of Henle.** This leads to a decrease in reabsorption of ions, which is followed by a decrease in medullary hyperosmolality. These effects result in the reduced movement of water out of the lumen of the distal tubules and collecting ducts and hence an increased excretion of water and solutes. Diuretics such as furosemide act via this mechanism.
  - – **Rapid fluid flow through the tubules or rapid blood flow through the vasa recta** washes out the high concentration of solutes within the medulla interstitium, referred to as medullary washout. This impairs the countercurrent system, which normally generates a hyperosmotic environment in the renal medulla interstitium to promote the movement of water out of the lumen of distal tubules and collecting ducts. Medullary washout can occur secondary to marked polyuria, for example from diabetes insipidus, or following diuretic use.
  - – **Disruption to urea recycling through the body** decreases the urea concentration in the medullary interstitium and hence decreases medullary osmolality. Disruption to urea cycling can be the result of decreased tubular response to antidiuretic hormone (ADH) leading to the reduced permeability of collection ducts to urea, or from decreased plasma urea concentration (cirrhosis, protein depletion). Urine specific gravity is 1.007–1.030.
- **Collecting ducts become impermeable to water**. This is characterized by urine with a SG 1.001–1.006, and is due to either:
  - – **Deficiency of ADH** (central diabetes insipidus).

- – **Renal insensitivity to ADH** (nephrogenic diabetes insipidus). Renal cells may not respond to adequate concentrations of ADH because of insufficiency of functioning nephrons, competitive inhibition for ADH receptors, or bacterial endotoxins. Altered cellular concentrations of Ca^{++}, Mg^{+}, prostaglandin E, and corticosteroids interfere with ADH receptor binding and render renal cells unresponsive to ADH (e.g. hyperadrenocorticism, hypercalcaemia). Endotoxins such as *E. coli* render nephrons insensitive to ADH (e.g. in pyometra–endometritis complex).

Polyuria should be differentiated from pollakiuria, which is increased frequency of urination of small quantities of urine, and is typically associated with bladder disease, especially cystitis. Inappropriate urination associated with behavioral disorders should also be differentiated from polyuria.

WHERE?

Primary polyuria is most common, and occurs when the ability to concentrate urine is decreased. Polydipsia is compensatory for polyuria.

Polyuria commonly results from structural and functional renal pathology, such as:
- Loss of functioning nephrons.
- Increased solute loading per nephron.
- Disruption of the medullary countercurrent system.
- Decreased renal responsiveness to ADH.

Polyuria may also be influenced by many **other organs and non-renal etiologies.**

Primary polydipsia (psychogenic polydipsia) has not been reported in the cat.

WHAT?

Renal disease (acute and chronic renal failure), **diabetes mellitus, hyperthyroidism and nephrogenic diabetes insipidus** are the most common causes of polyuria and polydipsia.

Hyperadrenocorticism, hypoadrenocorticism, acromegaly and central diabetes insipidus are uncommon causes.

Psychogenic polydipsia has not been reported.

DISEASES CAUSING POLYURIA AND POLYDIPSIA

CHRONIC RENAL FAILURE***

Classical signs

- Inappetence, anorexia, weight loss.
- Lethargy.
- Vomiting.
- Polyuria, polydipsia.
- Small ± irregular kidneys, occasionally enlarged kidneys.

See main reference on page 333 for details (The Thin, Inappetent Cat).

Clinical signs

Inappetence or anorexia is the most common sign and occurs in 80% of cats.

Weight loss is frequent, together with poor body condition.

Lethargy or depression are common signs.

Polyuria and polydipsia are reported by owners in 40% of cats. Nocturia or urination in inappropriate places may also be observed and must be differentiated from other causes including behavioral.

Weakness occurs in nearly 50% of cats and is often associated with hypokalemia. Cats may appear reluctant to jump or unsteady with jumping, and be less active.

Constipation is common and results from dehydration.

Vomiting is less common, and if present, is usually intermittent and often low grade.

Diarrhea is rare, but very occasionally is hemorrhagic from uremic enterocolitis.

Halitosis, ulcers on the oral mucosa or tongue, brownish discoloration of dorsal surface of tongue, or sloughing of anterior of tongue may occur in advanced disease.

Pale mucous membranes from anemia may be evident.

Dehydration is commonly present because of inadequate water intake to balance the excessive fluid loss in urine.

Ocular signs related to hypertension are common, e.g. scleral or conjunctival injection, hyphema or retinal hemorrhage, retinal edema, retinal vessel tortuosity, retinal detachment.

Terminally, seizures, stupor or coma may occur.

Small and/or irregular kidneys may be palpable but occasionally kidneys are enlarged (associated with amyloid deposition, neoplasia or cystic kidneys).

Diagnosis

Increased blood urea (BUN) and creatinine (azotemia) concentrations together with a urine specific gravity of 1.007–1.030 (usually 1.007–1.015) **is considered presumptive evidence of renal failure**.

Other findings that may or may not be present are the following:

Hyperphosphatemia
- Serum phosphorus concentration increases when glomerular filtration rate (GFR) is below approximately 20% of normal, and **tends to parallel BUN concentration**.

Hypokalemia (< 3.5 mmol/l) occurs in 20% of cats.
- Clinical signs of **inappetence** and **generalized muscle weakness** (such as wobbliness, inability to jump, stiff, stilted gait and **ventroflexion of the neck**) may occur when potassium < 3 mmol (mEq)/L.
- Respiratory muscle failure and death may occur at < 2 mmol (mEq)/L.

Hyper- and hypocalcemia are infrequent abnormalities, and result from derangements of calcium metabolism associated with renal secondary hyperparathyroidism.
- Most cats have normal or low calcium; 10–20% have mild to moderate hypercalcemia (≤ 3.1 mmol/L, 12.5 mg/dl).

Acidosis is common (approximately 80% of cats), and is evident as decreased bicarbonate and increased anion gap.

Normochromic, normocytic, non-regenerative anemia is common when chronic renal failure is advanced.

● It occurs mainly from erythropoietin deficiency, but other factors contribute, such as decreased red cell lifespan.

Proteinuria is typically mild to moderate (1.5–2 times increase in protein excretion occurs).

Radiographs of kidneys may show small irregular kidneys; size may be normal or increased in some cats especially if renal failure is due to amyloid, neoplasia or polycystic kidneys.

Ultrasound examination frequently shows small hyperechoic kidneys.

Differential diagnoses

Pre-renal azotemia. This occurs secondary to dehydration or circulatory collapse; azotemia results from reduced renal blood flow; **typically urine specific gravity is ≥ 1.035,** in contrast to renal failure where SG is < 1.035.

Pre-renal azotemia together with concomitant primary disease that affects renal concentrating ability can mimic renal failure, e.g. a dehydrated cat with central or nephrogenic diabetes insipidus may have azotemia with a urine specific gravity < 1.035.

Treatment

See main reference on page 336 for details.

Correct dehydration, reduce uremia, and improve quality of life.

DIABETES MELLITUS***

Classical signs

● Older than 6 years of age, most > 8 years of age.
● Moderate to marked PU/PD, usually of 2–8 weeks duration.
● Weight loss, but may be normal weight, obese or underweight.
● Polyphagia or inappetence.

Pathogenesis

Most diabetic cats appear to have **type 2 diabetes mellitus**, previously called adult-onset diabetes or non-insulin-dependent diabetes.

● Type 2 diabetes is characterized by decreased insulin secretion, insulin resistance and amyloid deposition in the pancreatic islets.

Risk factors include old age, male gender, obesity, physical inactivity, confinement indoors, Burmese breed (in Australia, New Zealand and UK), and repeated or long-acting steroid or megestrol acetate administration.

At diagnosis, **endogenous insulin secretion is usually very low**.

● This is probably because of the combined effects of:
  – Impaired insulin secretion associated with the beta cell defect causing type 2 diabetes.
  – Amyloid deposition in the islets which replaces beta cells.
  – Suppression of insulin secretion by glucose toxicity.

Glucose toxicity is defined as suppression of insulin secretion by persistently (> 24 h duration) high blood glucose.

● Suppression of insulin secretion by glucose toxicity is **initially functional and reversible**, later it results in structural changes in beta cells. **With time (weeks) changes become irreversible,** and beta cells are lost.

Some cats (5–20%) have other specific types of diabetes. Their diabetes results from another disease process causing decreased insulin secretion or impaired insulin action (insulin resistance).

● **Pancreatic neoplasia** is a significant cause of diabetes in cats referred to specialists, accounting for as many as 18% of cases recorded at referral institutions in USA.
● **Pancreatitis** is commonly associated with feline diabetes (50% of diabetic cats have pancreatitis lesions at necropsy).
  – In most cats, pancreatitis is not severe enough to cause diabetes alone, but probably contributes to loss of beta cells.
● **Hyperadrenocorticism** and **growth hormone-producing tumors (acromegaly)** are rare causes of other specific types of diabetes associated with insulin resistance.

Clinical signs

Earliest signs are **polyuria and polydipsia;** nocturia and urinary incontinence may occur.

Weight loss occurs and is accompanied by increased appetite.
- At the time of diagnosis, some cats are **underweight**, some **normal weight** and others are **obese**.

At diagnosis, some cats have **decreased appetite** and are depressed, others are **polyphagic**.

Lethargy or depression may be present. Other cats are alert at presentation.

Muscle wasting and **weakness** are often present and may be evidenced as reluctance or inability to jump.

Dehydration is common in cats that are lethargic and inappetent.

Vomiting occurs in one third of cats, but is usually infrequent.

Hepatomegaly from hepatic lipidosis, and occasionally jaundice may be present.

Rear limb weakness or plantigrade posture (hocks touching the ground) occur occasionally secondary to diabetic neuropathy.

Acetone odor on breath may be evident on average 5 days before ketonuria is detected.

Poor unkempt scurfy hair coat.

Diagnosis

In most cats, **blood glucose greater than 20 mmol/l (360 mg/dl) is diagnostic** of diabetes.

If **blood glucose is 12–20 mmol/l (216–360 mg/dl), the presence of typical clinical signs** (polyuria, polydipsia, polyphagia with weight loss), significant **glycosuria**, and **increased plasma fructosamine** or **betahydroxybutyrate** or **ketonuria** must be used to differentiate diabetes from stress-induced hyperglycemia.
- Plasma **fructosamine > 406 umol/L** is indicative of diabetes mellitus. However, some diabetic cats have a normal fructosamine concentration, and occasionally, non-diabetic sick cats have mildly increased fructosamine concentrations.
- Persistent hyperglycemia over 24 h is highly suggestive of diabetes, but may also occur with illness.

If persistent hyperglycemia is present in a sick cat, begin treatment with insulin, even if it is not clear if the hyperglycemia is illness-associated. Illness-associated stress hyperglycemia rarely results in blood glucose concentrations higher than 19 mmol/L (342 mg/dl).
- **Plasma betahydroxybutyrate** > 1 mmol/L (10 mg/dl) is indicative of diabetes mellitus. However, some diabetic cats have normal plasma betahydroxybutyrate.
  - A urine dipstick may be used in serum or heparinized plasma to detect ketonemia. A positive test indicates ketonemia. It detects mainly oxaloacetate rather than the predominant ketone in cats, β-hydroxybutyrate.

Differential diagnoses

Stress hyperglycemia from struggling or illness. Beware of misdiagnosis in cats with stress hyperglycemia from illness or struggling, which also have concomitant disease that produces similar signs to diabetes mellitus, e.g. renal failure or hyperthyroidism.
- In stress hyperglycemia associated with struggling, blood glucose concentration is generally < 12 mmol/L (216 mg/dl) within 4 h if the cat is hospitalized and further struggling does not occur.
- Stress hyperglycemia associated with illness may persist for several days and exceed 20 mmol/L (360 mg/dl). If in doubt, treat these cats with insulin and closely monitor blood glucose.

Hyperthyroidism may produce similar signs, i.e. old cat with weight loss, polyphagia and polyuria/polydipsia. Generally the polydipsia in hyperthyroidism is less pronounced. Glucose may be elevated but less than 20 mmol/L (360 mg/dl), from stress and insulin resistance. Elevated thyroxine concentration is diagnostic.

Treatment

General principles

For initial management, most cats have **better glycemic control using insulin** rather than oral hypoglycemic agents.
- **Insulin is more potent in decreasing blood glucose**; this enables beta cells to overcome the effects of glucose toxicity.

Approximately **5–30% of cats have good glycemic control using oral hypoglycemic drugs** which stimulate insulin secretion. The sulfonylurea, glipizide, is the most widely used oral hypoglycemic drug for cats.

Oral hypoglycaemic drugs are most useful as sole treatment when:
- Beta cells are not markedly suppressed by glucose toxicity (e.g. blood glucose is < 16 mmol/L (< 290 mg/dl)) or
- The owner refuses to give insulin injections.

Lente and NPH (Isophane) insulin must be given twice daily in all cats; most cats (up to 90%) require ultralente twice daily.
- In general, **lente and NPH insulin** have too **short a duration of action** to achieve excellent glycemic control in cats, although clinical control is often good, and signs of diabetes resolve in the majority of cats.
- For approximately 4 hours twice a day there is minimal exogenous insulin action when using these insulins. This means that most diabetic cats have episodes of hyperglycemia > 16 mmol/L (> 288 mg/dl) twice daily, which exacerbates glucose toxicity, and makes diabetic remission less likely than when using longer-acting insulins.

Long-acting insulins such as glargine, detemir and PZI in most cats provide better glycemic control and higher remission rates than lente, NPH and ultralente, and best results are obtained when they are administered twice daily.

Because of the small doses used in cats, 40 U/ml insulin is preferable to 100 U/ml insulin. However, expected duration of action is more important than concentration. Using 0.3 ml insulin syringes is advantageous when using 100 U/ml insulin. Syringes with $\frac{1}{4}$ u gradations are available.

Beef or pork insulins have a longer duration of action than human insulin. Most insulins for veterinary use are pork or beef/pork mixes. Human-use insulin is either identical to amino acid sequence in human insulin, or has substitutions to alter duration of action.

Eating does not need to be coordinated with insulin administration, because the postprandial increase in blood glucose is very prolonged (18+ h) in cats. Evidence suggests that a high-protein, low-carbohydrate diet (6–12% of calories from carbohydrate) is best for dia-

betic cats, because it lowers blood glucose and insulin requirement, and may increase the diabetic remission rate.

Underweight and normal bodyweight cats need a high-quality, calorie-dense feline diet that is palatable.

Obese cats should have their weight reduced by 1–2%/week (see page 454 The Cat With Abdominal Distention or Abdominal Fluid for treatment details). Use a high-protein, low-carbohydrate diet.

Transient diabetes.
- **Approximately 20–90% of diabetic cats will undergo remission** of their diabetes in 1–4 months, if good glycemic control is achieved.
- Remission is more **common in diabetic cats recently treated with insulin-antagonistic drugs**, such as megestrol acetate or long-acting steriods.
- Excellent glycemic control facilitates diabetic remission, by enabling beta cells to recover from glucose toxicity. Excellent glycemic control is aided by use of **long-acting insulin, especially glargine** administered twice daily, and a low-carbohydrate diet.
- **Remission rates increase with increasing duration of action of insulin**, and highest rates are obtained using glargine. PZI produces higher remission rates than lente insulin, when both are administered twice daily.

Hypoglycemia kills cats.
- Teach owners to recognize signs (**dazed drunken look, dilated pupils, wobbliness, weakness, head or body tremors, twitching, seizures or coma**). Signs may occur with little warning in cats that have apparently excellent clinical control of their diabetes.
- The owner should immediately start treatment with honey, or a glucose syrup designed for human diabetic patients, given per os. If the cat is seizuring, rub honey or syrup into the gums, or give per rectum using the lubricated insulin syringe, if the needle can be removed.
  - Cats with **severe signs require intravenous glucose or glucagon.**
  - Give 50% dextrose at 0.5–1.0 ml/kg IV.
  - If intravenous access is not possible, 50% dextrose (0.5–1.0 ml/kg) or corn syrup (0.25–0.5 ml/kg) administered per os, or rubbed on the gums may be effective, but glucagon 0.25–1.0 mg IM is superior. Glucagon must be followed

by intravenous dextrose once seizures have stopped to maintain blood glucose.

- **Re-evaluate the cat;** usually the insulin dose needs to be decreased by 50–70%. Some cats will no longer require insulin, because their diabetes is in remission.
- It is important to **check if the cat is being inadvertently overdosed**. This can occur when different syringes have been dispensed with a different volume per gradation than was previously used. For example, for many brands of syringes, the **gradations on a 1 ml 100 U/ml syringe represent 2 U, whereas on a 0.5 ml syringe represent 1 U**. If owners are switched to 1 ml syringes, the dose may be inadvertently doubled, if the same number of graduations is used to dose the insulin. Similarly, a switch from syringes designed for U100 insulin to those for U40 insulin may result in an inadvertent 2.5 times increase in dose.

Treatment of "healthy" diabetic cats.

- If the cat is not very depressed or dehydrated, start **lente, ultralente, PZI or insulin glargine subcutaneously**.
  - Use an initial dose of 0.25 U/kg **ideal body weight q 12 h**, if blood glucose is between 12–19 mmol/L (220–350 mg/dl).
  - Use an initial dose of **0.5 U/kg ideal body weight q 12 h, if blood glucose is 20 mmol/L (360 mg/dl) or more**.

Glycemic control should be monitored using **clinical parameters (water intake, urine glucose concentration, body weight),** and at each **major recheck,** measurement of **glucose concentration** every 2 h (lente, ultralente) or 4 h (PZI, glargine). **Water drunk, urine glucose and blood glucose concentrations are the most useful parameters for adjusting insulin dose.**

- Water drunk of ≤ 20 ml/kg/24 h on canned food or ≤ 60 ml/kg/24 h on dry food indicates exemplary glycemic control.
- Water drunk is a better indicator of mean blood glucose and level of clinical control than is fructosamine concentration.
- **Water drunk** should be measured at home on at least two consecutive days prior to measurement of blood glucose concentration. Ideally, an owner should keep a daily diary of water drunk.

Monitoring urine glucose is very useful. This can be accomplished using poorly absorbent litter material such as silicon beads or shredded paper, which allows collection of urine for testing with a dipstick, or a litter box glucose detector system such as Glucotest (Purina) which is added to the box filler, and reacts to urine with color changes to indicate the level of glucosuria. Some owners are able to train the cat to tolerate a dipstick applied to the urine stream during urination. Alternatively, some of the urine-soaked litter can be mixed with water and tested with a dipstick after straining through a cloth.

- Weekly urine **glucose monitoring** is helpful for **detecting diabetic remission**, especially in cats treated with lente, NPH or ultralente insulin. Cats with negative urine glucose should be evaluated for remission.
- With the long duration of action of glargine, there should be minimal periods when blood glucose is > 14 mmol/L (240 mg/dl), and hence stable cats should almost always be 0 or 1+ for urine glucose. A value 2+ or greater likely indicates that an increase in dose is required.
- Because cats treated with lente, NPH or ultralente insulin usually have hyperglycemia within 6–8 h after insulin administration, which persists until the next dose, it is not recommended to use urine glucose measurements to increase the dose of these insulins.

Monitoring **fructosamine or glycated hemoglobin** concentration can be a useful indicator of glycemic control in cats susceptible to stress hyperglycemia, if the owner is unable to measure water intake. Fructosamine concentrations > 500–550 μmol/L (normal < 400 μmol/L) or glycated hemoglobin > 3–4% (normal < 2.6%) are consistent with poor glycemic control.

Adjusting insulin dose.

- In general, increase the dose by $^1/_2$–1 U/cat q 12 h every **1–4 weeks** to achieve a nadir glucose concentration of **7–9 mmol/L (126–162 mg/dl)**. Once clinical signs have resolved, and the blood glucose is relatively controlled, a nadir of 5–6 mmol/L can be achieved. Rebound hyperglycemia is a common consequence of aiming for a low nadir too early in the stablization process, especially if using lente, ultralente or NPH insulin.

If using **lente, NPH or ultralente insulin, adjust dose based on nadir (lowest) glucose concentration** and **clinical signs.** Do not use pre-insulin blood glucose concentration to increase the dose, only to decrease the dose. There is little appreciable insulin action after 8–12 h, so for most cats on these insulins, the pre-insulin glucose concentration cannot be decreased by increasing insulin dose. In general, aim for a glucose nadir of 7–9 mmol/L (126–162 mg/dl) in the first 1–2 months. Later a nadir of 5–6 mmol/L (90–108 mg/dl) can be achieved in cats that are well controlled.

If using **glargine or PZI, adjust the dose based on nadir** (lowest) glucose and **pre-insulin glucose concentration** (concentration immediately before next insulin injection).

The following criteria can be used for adjusting insulin dose.

- **Indications for increasing dose of insulin** (recommendations assume insulin is being given twice daily):
  - If pre-insulin glucose concentration is > 12 mmol/L (216 mg/dl), then increase dose by 0.5–1 U/cat/injection provided nadir glucose is also high (**glargine and PZI only**) AND / OR
  - If nadir glucose concentration is > 10 mmol/L (180 mg/dl) then increase dose by 0.5–1 U/cat/injection. For well controlled cats after several weeks of therapy, an upper cut–point of > 7 mmol/L (126 mg/dl) can be used.
  - If water intake is > 40 ml/kg on wet food or > 100 ml/kg on dry food and glargine or PZI are being used, then increase dose by 0.5–1 U/cat/injection. Dose may need to be increased or decreased if water intake is excessive when using lente insulin.
- **Indications for maintaining the same dose:**
  - If pre-insulin glucose concentration is ≥ 10–12 mmol/L (≥ 240–360 mg/dl) AND/OR
  - If nadir glucose concentration is 5–9 mmol/L (90–162 mg/dl). For well controlled cats aim for a nadir of 4–7 mmol/L (72–126 mg/dl).
- **Indications for decreasing the dose of insulin**:
  - If pre-insulin glucose concentration is ≤ 10 mmol/L (≤ 180 mg/dl) decrease dose 0.5 U/cat/injection.

  - If cat has been treated with insulin for more than 2 weeks, and total dose is 1 U/cat q 12 h or less, and pre-insulin glucose is ≤ 10 mmol/L (≤ 180 mg/dl), withhold insulin and check subsequent blood glucose concentrations to determine if the cat is in diabetic remission.
  - If nadir glucose concentration < 3 mmol/L (< 54 mg/dl) decrease dose by 1 U/cat/injection.
  - If clinical signs of hypoglycemia develop, then reduce dose by 50%.
- **Insulin dose may be maintained, increased or decreased depending on the water intake, urine glucose, clinical signs and length of time the cat has been treated with insulin.**
  - If pre-insulin glucose concentration 11–14 mmol/L (198– 252 mg/dl) or
- If nadir 3–4 mmol/L (54–72 mg/dl) clinical parameters are essential for adjustment of insulin dose.

Most cats are well controlled on:
- 0.2–0.9 U/kg q 12 h of lente insulin (median dose of porcine lente was 0.5 U/kg q 12 h); only 10–15% require 1 U/kg or more. Most cats are controlled on 2–3 U/cat q 12 h.
- 0.3–1.2 U/kg q 12 h of PZI (average dose of PZI is 0.9 U/kg q 12 h); only about 10% of cats require more than 2 U/kg q 12 h. Most cats are controlled on 4–5 U/cat q 12 h .
- 0.25–0.5 U/kg q 12 h of glargine (average dose is < 0.5 U/kg q 12 h). Most cats are controlled on 1–2 U/cat q 12 h, only a few cats require doses of 4–6 U/cat q 12 h, and the requirement for these high doses may resolve within weeks.
- Using glargine, cats with exemplary control have nadir glucose concentrations of 4–7 mmol/L (72–126 mg/dl) and peak glucose concentrations of ≥ 11 mmol/L (200 mg/dl).

Diabetic remission usually occurs in the first 4 months of therapy, and occurs most often in the first month of treatment in cats on glargine. Impending remission is suggested by a negative urine glucose measurement, and a pre-insulin blood glucose concentration of < 12 mmol/L (216 mg/dl). Decrease insulin dose gradually to 0.5–1 U q 12 h or even q 24 h. If urine glucose is still negative and pre-insulin blood glucose is still low on a minimal dose of insulin, stop insulin and monitor blood glucose for 12–24 h. If it remains low, send the cat home on a low-carbohydrate diet and re-evaluate in 1 week. The owner should closely monitor water intake and urine glucose, and if either increase, the cat should be reassessed immediately and reinstituted if blood glucose ≥ 10 mmol/L (180 mg/dL).

Treatment of "sick" diabetic cats

Fluids are as important as insulin in dehydrated diabetic cats.

- Balanced electrolyte solutions or 0.9% sodium chloride is the best initial fluid depending on the initial potassium concentration, with 0.9% sodium chloride preferred in hyperkalemic cats.
- Once initial fluid and electrolyte deficits are corrected, use 0.45% NaCl with 30–40 mEq (mmol)/L of KCl added.

Serum potassium rapidly falls with treatment and potassium supplementation should be immediately instituted in fluids and orally, if potassium concentration is initially normal. Cats with hyperkalemia at presentation usually require potassium within 12–24 h.

- Supplement potassium in intravenous fluids at 20–80 mmol/L (or mEq/L); do not exceed 0.5 mmol//kg/h.
- Supplement potassium orally using potassium gluconate 2–3 mmol (or mEq), q 8–24 h.

Serum phosphorus falls rapidly with treatment. Hypophosphatemia causes hemolysis, muscle weakness and neurological signs. To supplement phosphate and potassium in intravenous fluids, give potassium as 50% potassium dihydrophosphate and 50% potassium chloride.

Bicarbonate is rarely required, because acidosis improves rapidly with fluids and insulin therapy. If bicarbonate is < 10 mmol/L (10 mEq/L), it can be added to the intravenous fluids using the formula: Body weight × 0.4 × [12 – patient's bicarbonate].

Cats which have **normal hydration** or are only **mildly dehydrated** and not in shock can be started immediately on insulin given **subcutaneously** (0.25 U/kg if glucose is < 20 mmol/L (360 mg/dl); 0.5 U/kg ideal body weight if glucose is ≥ 20 mmol/L).

Subcutaneous insulin is poorly absorbed in significantly dehydrated cats. These cats need intramuscular or intravenous insulin.

For intramuscular dosing of insulin:

- **Dilute regular insulin** with saline or manufacturer's diluent to increase accuracy of dosing. Give 0.2 U/kg intramuscular initially, then continue with **hourly injections** at 0.1 U/kg.
- **Adjust the dose up or down** to achieve a decrease in glucose of 3–6 mmol/L (54–110 mg/dl) per hour.
- Once blood glucose is **16 mmol/L (288 mg/dl),** give 0.1–0.4 U/kg **every 4–6 h** to achieve a blood glucose of 11–14 mmol/L (200–252 mg/dl) in the first 24 h.

For intravenous dosing of insulin:

- Use an infusion pump and add 25 IU of regular insulin to a 500 ml bag of 0.9% saline, to produce an insulin concentration of 0.05 IU/ml.
- Infuse the insulin/saline mix using a pump into the maintenance fluid line via a Y piece, at an initial rate of 1 ml/kg/h (0.05 IU/kg/h). Be sure to flush both sets of tubing before beginning the infusion, as insulin adheres to plastic.
- When blood glucose reaches 180 mg/dl (10 mmol/L), decrease the insulin infusion to 0.5 ml/kg/h. At the same time replace the maintenance fluids with 0.45% NaCl supplemented to contain 2.5% dextrose and 30 mmol/L KCl.

With either intramuscular or intravenous therapy, aim for a glucose drop of 54–72 mg/dl/h (3–4 mmol/L/h) and do not exceed a decrease of 108 mg/dl/h (6 mmol/L/h). In the first 24 h, aim for a glucose concentration of 11–14 mmol/L (200–252 mg/dl). Long-term adaptations to chronic hyperglycemia have occurred, and glucose should not be normalized for 24–48 hours.

If glucose falls below 8 mmol/L (144 mg/dl) in the first 24 h, add 50% dextrose to intravenous fluids to make a 5% **solution.**

Continue regular insulin until dehydration is corrected, and then swap to subcutaneous glargine, PZI, lente, or ultralente insulin administered q 24 h.

Prognosis

Prognosis is relatively good. Reported median survival time is 17 months, considering the average age at diagnosis is 10–13 years.

Prevention

Obesity, physical inactivity and repeated **long-acting steroid or megestrol acetate** administration are preventable risk factors for type 2 diabetes.

Individuals predisposed to type 2 diabetes by low insulin sensitivity (as evidenced by increased fasting glucose concentrations) or reduced beta cell function (evidenced as impaired glucose tolerance) should not become obese, and may benefit from a high-protein, low-carbohydrate diet.

HYPERTHYROIDISM***

> ### Classical signs
> - Weight loss.
> - Hyperactive, restless, aggressive.
> - Polyphagia.
> - Tachycardia.
> - Polyuria/polydipsia.

See main reference on page 304 for details (The Cat With Weight Loss and a Good Appetite).

Clinical signs

Polyuria/polydipsia is present in approximately 50% of hyperthyroid cats, and may be the major presenting complaint.
- Renal blood flow and glomerular filtration rate are increased in hyperthyroidism, leading to an increased water and solute load on the renal tubule. This may exceed the tubular reabsorptive capacity and cause medullary washout. In hyperthyroid humans, impaired concentrating ability is present.
- Because of the advanced age in many hyperthyroid cats, concurrent renal failure is also common.

Typically, a disease of old cats, as the average age is 12–13 years. It is very rare in cats < 8 years of age.

Weight loss is present **in nearly all cats**.

Two major presenting forms occur; either **restless, hyperactive, and polyphagic** (approximately 80% of cats), or **depressed and anorexic** (10–30% of cats).

Signs suggest **cardiac, GIT or renal disease**.

Typical signs of hyperthyroidism:

- Weight loss (95–98% of cats).
- Polyphagia (65–75%), decreased appetite (19–28%).
- Hyperactive, restless, aggressive (68–81%), lethargy (15–25%).
- Tachycardia (57–65%), heart murmur (10–54%).
- Polyuria/polydipsia (45–55%).
- Vomiting (33–50%), diarrhea (30–45%).
- Panting (13–28%).
- Muscle weakness/tremors (15–20%).

An enlarged thyroid gland or glands are palpable in more than 80% of cats.
- These are located anywhere from the larynx to the thoracic inlet.
- Most are 0.5–1 cm in size, although occasionally they are up to 3 cm.

Diagnosis

Increased **plasma total thyroxine (T_4) concentration (> 64 nmol/L (5 µg/dl)) is considered diagnostic of hyperthyroidism**.

2–10% of hyperthyroid cats have a total T_4 concentration between 26–64 nmol/L (2–5 µg/dl), and require additional testing for diagnosis.

In mild (early) hyperthyroidism, total T_4 may be within the normal range.

Severe concurrent illness will also suppress total T_4 concentration.

If clinical signs suggest hyperthyroidism or a mass is palpable in the neck, **but** total T_4 is normal, either:
- Repeat total thyroxine measurement in 1–3 weeks, or
- Measure free T_4 (best option, but must use assay validated for cats), or
- Perform a T_3 (triiodothyronine) suppression test (hyperthyroid cats have little or no suppression), or
- Perform a TRH stimulation test (hyperthyroid cats have **no** increase in total T_4 after TRH).

Urine specific gravity ranges from **1.006–1.060** in hyperthyroid cats.

Approximately one third of hyperthyroid cats have **mild to moderate azotemia**. Many of these cats have underlying renal failure, but others have pre-renal azotemia associated with thyrotoxic cardiac failure.

Increased protein catabolism may also contribute to the azotemia.

See main reference on page 346 for details (The Thin, Inappetant Cat).

Differential diagnosis

Renal failure and diabetes mellitus both cause weight loss with PU/PD in aged cats. The PU/PD is more pronounced in diabetes and occurs with glycosuria. In renal failure, appetite is usually reduced rather than increased as in hyperthyroidism. The apathetic form of hyperthyroidism may be difficult to distinguish clinically from renal failure but measurement of urea, creatinine and thyroxine usually distinguishes these diseases.

Treatment

There are three treatment options: chronic administration of antithyroid drugs, surgical thyroidectomy, radioactive iodine. **See main reference on page 347 for details (The Thin Inappetant Cat).**

DIABETES INSIPIDUS*

Classical signs

- Any age cat.
- Mild to marked polyuria and polydipsia, often present for weeks to months.
- Nocturia or urinary incontinence may occur.
- Urine specific gravity is typically < 1.007, but in some dehydrated cats may be 1.007–1.020.

Pathogenesis

Diabetes insipidus (DI) occurs in two forms, central and nephrogenic.

Central diabetes insipidus is **very rare in cats**, and occurs when vasopressin (antidiuretic hormone, ADH) secretion from the hypothalamic-pituitary system is inadequate.

- Central DI is most commonly idiopathic (i.e. no cause identified on necropsy).

- The most frequent known causes are head trauma, neoplasia, hypothalamic-pituitary malformations (e.g. cystic structures), or following surgery to the hypothalamic-pituitary area.
- Rarely, central diabetes insipidus occurs in kittens, suggesting a congenital form.

Nephrogenic diabetes insipidus occurs when the renal tubules are unresponsive to vasopressin.

Unresponsiveness to vasopressin may result from problems either at the receptor or with postreceptor mechanisms, including inadequate hypertonicity of the renal medulla.

- Primary (familial) nephrogenic DI has not been reported in cats.
- **Secondary (acquired) nephrogenic DI is common.**
  - It occurs with **renal failure, hyperthyroidism, pyelonephritis, pyometra, hypercalcemia, hypokalemia and drugs**.

Clinical signs

Polyuria and polydipsia occur ranging from mild to severe, depending on cause, and is often present for weeks to months.

Nocturia or urinary incontinence may result because of the large volume of urine produced.

Weight loss may occur as a result of the underlying disease, or when the water intake is huge.

Neurologic signs may occur if DI is associated with a hypothalamic-pituitary neoplasia, e.g. stupor, disorientation, ataxia, seizures, circling.

Diagnosis

Urine specific gravity is usually < 1.007, and often 1.001 or 1.002 in classical DI.

- **Urine specific gravity may be 1.007–1.020 if the cat is very dehydrated, or has partial DI.**
- Partial DI frequently occurs with acquired nephrogenic DI such as renal failure, hypercalcemia, hypokalemia, pyometra and pyelonephritis.
- **Urine, hematologic and serum biochemistry analyses must be performed to exclude causes of acquired nephrogenic DI. Renal failure, hyperthyroidism, pyelonephritis, pyometra, hypercalcemia,**

hyperadrenocorticosteroidism, hypokalemia and drugs causing PU/PD (see page 244) must be ruled out.

Trial synthetic vasopressin (DDAVP) therapy to determine if PU/PD resolves. Pretreatment water intake is measured for 2–3 days, and then again following DDAVP therapy. A greater than 50% reduction of water intake suggests central or partial nephrogenic DI, but is rarely indicated.

A modified water deprivation test can be performed if the cat is not dehydrated, azotemic and laboratory tests do not indicate nephrogenic DI.

- Ignoring these contraindications may kill the cat, or make renal failure worse. The cat must be carefully monitored.
- Rarely is a water deprivation test required in feline medicine, because central diabetes insipidus is very rare and psychogenic polydipsia has not been reported.
- The main use of a water deprivation test is to determine if the kidney can concentrate urine when water is unavailable (indicating psychogenic polydipsia), and whether vasopressin therapy can increase urine concentration (central or partial nephrogenic DI) after medullary washout has resolved with water deprivation.
- Only consider performing a water deprivation test if there is massive polyuria and polydipsia, urine SG is < 1.008, and nephrogenic diabetes inspidus has been ruled out.
- Details of the test and interpretation are found in many standard textbooks.

Differential diagnosis

It is important to differentiate central DI from secondary nephrogenic DI, which is much more common. Test for renal failure, hyperthyroidism, hyperadrenocorticosteriodism, pyelonephritis, pyometra, hypercalcemia and hypokalemia.

Treatment

Ensure water is freely available at all times.

If nephrogenic DI, manage the underlying disease, e.g. renal failure, hyperthyroidism. Thiazide diuretics may be useful for reducing water consumption if the underlying disease is not treatable.

If central DI, administer synthetic vasopressin (desmopressin, DDAVP, SC, intranasal or conjunctival). Thiazide diuretics are less expensive, but less effective than desmopressin.

Prognosis

Prognosis depends on cause. The best prognoses occur with reversible nephrogenic DI (e.g. hyperthyroidism) and non-neoplastic central DI.

DRUG INDUCED*

> ### Classical signs
>
> - PU/PD following initiation of drug therapy.

Clinical signs

Common drugs causing polyuria and polydispsia include: diuretics, anticonvulsants (e.g. phenobarbital), thyroxine, salt supplementation, sodium bicarbonate, amphotericin B (from renal toxicity and hypokalemia), corticosteroids and megestrol acetate.

Polyuria and polydipsia occur following initiation of drug therapy.

Other clinical signs relate to the underlying disease process.

Diagnosis

Diagnosis is rarely a problem. If polyuria and polydipsia occur with phenobarbital or thyroxine, check dose is not excessive by measuring trough serum concentration.

Although cats are more resistant to the side effects of corticosteroids, polyuria and polydipsia does occur, but is usually less dramatic than in dogs.

HYPOKALEMIA*

> ### Classical signs
>
> - Acute onset of muscle weakness, neck ventroflexion, a stiff, stilted gait, and muscle pain.

Classical signs—Cont'd

- Decreased activity and inappetence for weeks to months.
- Dyspnea in severe cases.
- Signs relating to the underlying disease, e.g. polyuria and polydipsia in chronic renal failure.
- Occurs in older cats and Burmese kittens.

See main reference on page 893 for details (The Cat With Neck Ventroflexion).

Clinical signs

Acute onset of weakness. However, decreased activity and inappetence are often present for weeks to months prior to presentation.

Ventral neck flexion, **stiff, stilted gait**, and a reluctance to walk or jump are typical.

Larger muscle groups may appear sensitive or palpation.

Dyspnea occurs when the potassium is very low (2.0–2.5 mmol/L), because of weakness of the respiratory muscles. It may occur after **fluid administration** because volume dilution and increased urinary potassium loss induced by diuresis may lead to further worsening of the hypokalemia.

Polyuria, polydipsia may result from hypokalemia or be the result of the underlying disease causing hypokalemia, such as renal failure or hyperthryoidism.

Diagnosis

Decreased serum potassium concentrations (usually < 3.5 mmol/L) in association with clinical signs are required for diagnosis. The severity of signs varies between cats when potassium is 2.5–3.5 mmol/L. Below 2.5 mmol/L and especially below **2.0 mmol/L, signs are life threatening**, with death occurring from **respiratory muscle failure**.

Serum creatine kinase (CK) may be elevated reflecting the mypoathy associated with hypokalemia.

HYPERCALCEMIA (HYPERCALCEMIA ASSOCIATED WITH MALIGNANCY, CHOLECALCIFEROL TOXICITY, CHRONIC RENAL FAILURE, HYPERPARATHYROIDISM AND IDIOPATHIC)

Classical signs

- Anorexia and lethargy.
- Vomiting.
- Weight loss.
- Dysuria, inappropriate urination, pollakiuria, stranguria.
- Respiratory signs.
- Lymphadenopathy.
- Palpable cervical mass.

Pathogenesis

Calcium is important for formation of **bones and teeth**, and is essential for **blood coagulation**. It is important for **muscle function**, including cardiac muscle, as well as **nervous system function** where it stabilizes nerve cell membranes. As a cation, it is important for **cell membrane permeability.**

Calcium is regulated in the body via:
- Gastrointestinal absorption.
- Renal excretion.
- Binding to plasma proteins.
- Tissue deposition, especially into bone.

Parathyroid hormone (PTH) and calcitriol (active form of vitamin D) **maintain calcium homeostasis.** Serum calcium concentration regulates parathyroid hormone secretion and their serum concentrations have an inverse linear relationship.
- **PTH is produced in the parathyroid gland** and acts to increase serum calcium. It stimulates bone resorption by increasing osteoclastic activity, which mobilizes calcium into the bloodstream. PTH promotes renal reabsorption of calcium and excretion of phosphorus.
- **Cholecalciferol (vitamin D)** is a fat-soluble vitamin that is metabolized by the liver and kidney to produce calcitriol (1,25 [OH]$_2$ vitamin D), which acts to increase serum calcium. Calcitriol enhances

intestinal calcium uptake and calcium resorption from bone.

- **Calcitonin** acts to decrease high calcium concentrations, but does not appear to be important in small day-to-day corrections of calcium concentration, which is the role of PTH and calcitriol. Calcitonin decreases osteoclast activity and formation of new osteoclasts.

Hypercalcemia occurs when there is some derangement of the interaction between parathyroid hormone, vitamin D and organs such as the gut, bone, kidneys and parathyroid glands.

Malignancy (lymphoma and squamous cell carcinoma), **renal failure and primary hyperparathyroidism** are the **most common causes** of hypercalcemia in cats. In many cats, the cause of the hypercalcemia is not identified, and is termed idiopathic hypercalcemia.

Hypercalcemia of malignancy is the most common cause of hypercalcemia in cats. It results from secretion of locally acting or humorally acting osteoclast-activating substances.

- In cats, **lymphoma and squamous cell carcinoma are most often associated with hypercalcemia** but multiple myeloma and adenocarcinoma have also been reported.
- In some tumors, for example lymphoma, there is autonomous secretion of a humorally acting PTH-related protein, which activates osteoclasts, increases intestinal absorption and increases renal tubular reabsorption of calcium and excretion of phosphorus. Endogenous PTH secretion is suppressed.
- Some neoplastic cells invade bone or bone marrow and secrete products that act locally to activate osteoclasts, such as prostaglandins, osteoclast-activating factor, calcitriol, interleukin-1, and PTH-related protein or PTH.

Chronic renal failure is the second most common cause of hypercalcemia in cats. A number of mechanisms associated with chronic renal failure lead initially to reduced extracellular calcium. In a few cats, compensatory mechanisms eventually result in hypercalcemia.

- Extracellular calcium concentration is decreased in renal failure because reduced renal mass and hyperphosphatemia reduce formation of calcitriol (active vitamin D), leading to reduced calcium absorption

from the GIT. Phosphate retention also reduces extracellular calcium.
- Chronic stimulation of the parathyroid glands to maintain serum calcium concentrations in renal failure leads to hyperplasia (renal secondary hyperparathyroidism). **In some cats, autonomous function** develops because some hyperplastic cell lines are very deficient in calcitriol receptors. **Calcitriol regulates synthesis of calcium receptors,** so these cells are also poorly sensitive to calcium concentrations, and **produce large amounts of PTH.** Uremia also reduces formation of calcium receptors in parathyroid gland cells, leading to inappropriate PTH secretion.

The diuretic phase of acute renal failure may also be associated with hypercalcemia via other mechanisms.

Primary hyperparathyroidism is a less common cause of hypercalcemia, and is the result of an autonomous adenoma producing excess PTH. It is usually a **solitary functional adenoma**, although bilateral cystadenomas and solitary or bilateral adenocarcinomas have been reported.

Vitamin D toxicosis may be acute and associated with **cholecalciferol (vitamin D) rodenticides,** or chronic due to **excess supplementation or plant ingestion.** In some countries, cholecalciferol rodenticides have been withdrawn from the market because of their potential for irreversible nephrotoxicity in children.

- **Acute toxicity occurs at 5 g of bait/kg body weight** and hypercalcemia occurs within 24 h of ingestion.
- At lower doses of vitamin D, the maximal effect on calcium and phosphorus may not be evident for 1–2 weeks after ingestion.
- Cats requiring supplementation with vitamin D and calcium following thyroidectomy are at risk of vitamin D toxicity and nephrocalcinosis, if calcium and phosphorus is not monitored carefully.
- **Some plants contain active metabolites of vitamin D** such as the houseplant *Cestrum diurnum* (day-blooming jasmine). *Solanum malacoxylon* and *Trisetum flavescen* also contain vitamin D metabolites.

Fungal and bacterial granulomatous disease is a rare cause of hypercalcemia. The inflammatory process may or may not directly involve the bone. The mechanism may involve local osteolysis or secretion of factors from inflammatory cells such as prostaglandins and osteoclast-activating factors, which lead to bone resorption.

Hypoadrenocorticism is a very rare cause of hypercalcemia in cats (<2% of hypercalcemic cats). It is likely multifactorial, and in dogs is related to the severity of hyperkalemia. Mechanisms include hyperproteinemia from dehydration and increased renal resorption of calcium.

Other rare associations with hypercalcemia include **hyperthyroidism, diabetes mellitus, liver disease** (hepatic lipidosis, bilary fibrosis), **and bone marrow diseases** (myelodysplasia, myelofibrosis).

Idiopathic hypercalcemia is common in cats, and has been postulated to be associated with acidifying diets, which increase bone turnover of calcium, but hypercalcemia was not corrected by partial parathyroidectomy or a non-acidifying diet. Many features are similar to familial benign hypercalcemia reported in humans which is associated with a mutation in the calcium-sensing receptor.

Chronic over-supplementation with calcium in the diet increases the intestinal absorption of calcium. It also stimulates bone resorption and results in hypercalcemia and dystrophic calcification. Because the ability to excrete the increased filtered load of calcium is impaired in cats with renal failure, older cats are more sensitive to excess supplementation. Dietary over-supplementation is rarely seen because of the widespread use of balanced commercial diets.

Sequalae to hypercalcemia include:
- **Chronic renal failure.** High levels of **calcium are toxic to the renal tubular cells,** mineralize renal tissue and interfere with ADH action causing renal failure and polyuria/polydipsia. Hypercalcemia can also lead to **calcium oxalate urolithiasis** of the kidney, ureter, bladder or urethra and result in signs of lower urinary tract disease (LUTD).
- **Reduced excitability of smooth muscle** results in altered gastrointestinal function. Chronic vomiting is a common sign of hypercalcemia.
- **Depressed skeletal muscle contractility** and weakness, and altered cardiac contractility and arrhythmias occur with high calcium concentrations.

Clinical signs

Signs associated with hypercalcemia are compounded by signs of the underlying cause of hypercalcemia, such as malignancy, toxicity from cholecalciferol-containing rodenticides and renal failure.

In general there is no breed or gender predisposition, although **Siamese appear predisposed to primary hyperparathyroidism**.
- Cats with hypercalcemia have a **wide range of ages** (1–19 years) reflecting the multitude of causes, but mean age is 9 years old.
- Renal, gastrointestinal or neuromuscular signs occur, and in part may reflect the underlying cause.

Lethargy, anorexia and/or weight loss are typical of hypercalcemia, regardless of the cause.

Polyuria and polydipsia occur in up to **25% of cats** with hypercalcemia, and may be associated with inappropriate urination.

Signs of **lower urinary tract disease,** including dysuria and pollakiuria, occur in approximately 20% of cats. In a high proportion of cats, this is **associated with calcium oxalate urolithiasis** of the urinary bladder. Renal, ureteral, urethral or urolithiasis may also occur.

Vomiting occurs in 20–30% of cats with hypercalcemia, including cats with idiopathic hypercalcemia.

Constipation or diarrhea are infrequently reported.

Neuromuscular weakness evidenced as a **reluctance to jump, or unsteadiness with jumping** is less common.

Shaking, tremors, seizures, stupor and coma have the potential to occur with extremely high calcium concentrations, and are reported in dogs with cholecalciferol toxicity. Cats tend to ingest less toxin and these signs have not been reported.

Cardiac arrhythmias may occur if serum calcium is more than 4.5 mmol/L (18 mg/dL). Prolongation of PR interval and shortening of QT interval may be evident on ECG.

Acute cholecalciferol toxicity is associated with **lethargy, anorexia and polyuria/polydipsia within 24 h of ingestion**. Vomiting may occur, but the hematemesis and bloody stool seen in dogs have not been reported.

Toxicity is less frequently reported and signs are less severe in cats than dogs.

Lower levels of cholecalciferol toxicity result in PU/PD, inappetence and lethargy and low-grade vomiting, and clinically may be indistinguishable from acute or chronic renal failure.

Physical examination findings are dependent on the cause of hypercalcemia. Lymphadenopathy, abdominal organomegaly or dyspnea may be evident in cats with lymphosarcoma. Cats with squamous cell carcinoma-associated hypercalcemia most often have tumors of the head and neck. In contrast to dogs, a palpable cervical mass is present in about 40% of cats with primary hyperparathyroidism.

Diagnosis

Serum calcium concentration greater than 3 mmol/L (12 mg/dl).

- The serum calcium concentration does not fluctuate with age in cats as it does in dogs, where a healthy puppy can have higher calcium and phosphorus levels.

A **non-lipemic fasted blood sample** is required for measurement of serum calcium, phosphorus, urea nitrogen and creatinine concentrations to differentiate between several of the causes of hypercalcemia.

Hypercalcemia of malignancy is a relatively common cause of hypercalcemia in cats and is most often secondary to lymphoma and squamous cell carcinoma, but may be from multiple myeloma or adenocarcinoma. Serum phosphorus concentration is below the midpoint of the reference range, unless renal failure is present. Diagnosis of neoplasia-associated hypercalcemia is based on documenting increased PTH-related protein (PTH-rP) and suppressed PTH concentration in serum, or finding the primary tumor and demonstrating resolution of hypercalcemia with successful tumor therapy.

Primary hyperparathyroidism is rare in cats. It is associated with anorexia and lethargy, an inappropriately high PTH concentration relative to the hypercalcemia. Serum phosphorus is below the midpoint of the reference range unless renal failure is present, and in some cats, a palpable cervical mass is evident.

Cholecalciferol poisoning is associated with acute depression and anorexia, marked hypercalcemia and

hyperphosphatemia, and a history of recent exposure to rodenticide. Polyuria/polydipsia, vomiting and pain on palpation of the kidneys may also be present. PTH and PTH-rP concentrations would be expected to be low if the cat is not dehydrated, but have not been reported. Later there may be evidence of mineralization of abdominal and other soft tissues. Toxicity needs to be distinguished from other causes of hypercalcemia and hyperphosphatemia (renal failure and hypoadrenocorticism) on the basis of history, signs and ionized calcium (often normal or decreased in renal failure).

Chronic renal failure (renal secondary hyperparathyroidism) is associated with normal to elevated PTH concentrations and low to undetectable PTH-rP assay, hyperphosphatemia, but ionized serum calcium is usually normal or decreased. In contrast, ionized serum calcium is increased with other causes of hypercalcemia.

Idiopathic hypercalcemia is increasingly being identified in cats (mean age 5 years). Typically cats are hypercalcemic with normal or slightly low serum phosphorus concentration, and have normal serum concentrations of PTH, calcitriol and 25-hydroxycholecalciferol. Gross and histologic morphology of the parathyroid glands is normal. Subtotal parathyroidectomy does not resolve the hypercalcemia.

Differential diagnosis

Clinical signs of hypercalcemia (anorexia, lethargy, vomiting, weight loss) are **typical of many diseases,** and serum biochemistry analysis is necessary to detect hypercalcemia.

If PU/PD is present in addition to anorexia, vomiting and weight loss, **chronic renal failure would be the most likely differential diagnosis** based on clinical signs. Most cats with chronic renal failure are not hypercalcemic and of those that are, ionized calcium is usually normal or low.

Chronic renal failure with secondary hypercalcemia is usually **differentiated** from **other causes of hypercalcemia causing secondary renal failure** by the presence of anemia, small kidney size on palpation or ultrasound, and normal or low ionized calcium in chronic renal failure. Cats with chronic renal failure and secondary hypercalcemia also tend to have lower calcium concentrations, higher phosphorus concentrations, lower urine specific gravity and higher levels of azotemia than cats with renal failure induced by hypercalcemia.

Treatment

Severe hypercalcemia is a medical emergency as cardiac arrhythmias may occur if serum calcium is more than 4.5 mmol/L (18 mg/dl).

Hypercalcemia with concurrent hyperphosphatemia is associated with **metastatic calcification** and **nephrotoxicity** when the calcium (mg/dl) × phosphorus (mg/dl) product is > 60–80.
- Hypervitaminosis D and hypercalcemia of renal failure are both associated with a high Ca × P product and require early treatment to minimize further nephrotoxicity.

Fluids containing 0.9% NaCl should be used for volume expansion to dilute plasma calcium and to induce sodium diuresis, which causes calcium loss in urine. Avoid calcium-containing fluids.

Diuretics (furosemide) promote renal sodium diuresis and hence renal calcium loss.
- Thiazide diuretics are contraindicated as they can cause calcium retention.

Corticosteroids promote renal calcium loss, and decrease bone resorption and intestinal absorption of calcium, but should only be used once the diagnosis of lymphoma is excluded, as they can conceal the diagnosis.

Vitamin D toxicosis requires intensive therapy to reduce calcium levels and may require therapy to control seizures and arrhythmias.
- **Reduce GIT absorption** using an emetic and activated charcoal with a saline or osmotic cathartic. Do not use emetics in convulsing patients.
  – Xylazine (Rompun) can be used as an emetic in cats (1.1 mg/kg IM or SC).
  – Charcoal 1–4 g/kg combined with saline (5 ml per 1 g of charcoal) as a suspension in water should be administered orally or by gastric tube if ingestion occurred within 3–4 h.
- Reduce hypercalcemia using the **diuretic furosemide** (2–5 mg/kg PO q 8 h).

- **Prednisone** at 2 mg/kg PO q 12 h also increases renal loss of calcium.
- If available, **salmon calcitonin** should be administered until serum calcium levels normalize. Begin with 4–6 IU/kg SC q 2–3 h, and increase the dose up to 10 IU/kg if the lower doses are not effective.
  – Monitor serum calcium, hydration status and renal function via urine output.
  – Complications include soft tissue mineralization, renal failure, seizures and arrhythmias.

Cats with primary hyperparathyroidism are best treated with **surgical removal** of the parathyroid adenoma and **short-term vitamin D** and **calcium therapy** over 2–3 months to prevent post-operative hypocalcemia.

Cats with renal failure causing hypercalcemia, should be started on a low phosphorus diet. If phosphorus is not decreased into the middle of the normal range, add a phosphate binder.
- **Once phosphorus is < 1.9 mmol/L;** (normal range, 0.7–1.8 mmol/L) or < 6 mg/dl (normal range, 2.2–5.6 mg/dl), **begin low-dose calcitiol therapy** (2.5 ng/kg PO q 24 h) to decrease progression of renal failure.
- **Calcitriol decreases PTH concentrations** by inducing formation of the calcium receptor on the parathyroid gland cells membrane. In renal failure, calcium sensing is impaired because of the effect of uremia on formation of calcium receptors. This results in inappropriate PTH secretion. By increasing calcium sensing, PTH secretion is decreased, resulting in decreased serum calcium concentration.
- **PTH is a uremic toxin.** It contributes to **CNS depression** and **EEG abnormalities, appetite suppression and anemia associated with uremia.** It also **promotes progression of chronic renal failure.** Low-dose calcitriol has been shown to slow the progression of renal failure and decrease signs of chronic renal failure.
- At **phosphorus concentrations ≥ 1.9 mmol/L;** (normal range, 0.7–1.8 mmol/L) or 6 mg/dl (normal ≤ 5.6 mg/dl), **calcitriol loses its effectiveness** to suppress PTH secretion. Using higher doses of calcitriol in the face of hyperphosphatemia risks worsening progression of the renal failure, due to mineralization of renal tissue. It is essential to

monitor calcium and phosphate regularly when using calcitriol therapy.

- See Chronic renal failure in The Thin Inappetent Cat (page 336) for details of treatment of chronic renal failure.

In cats with idiopathic hypercalcemia, dietary modification may be partially or fully effective in a minority of cats. Dietary modification is worth trying initially, as the only other reported therapy to be effective is **long-term corticosteroids.**

- Dietary modifications reported to have variable success include use of a **high-fiber diet** (Hills w/d) to reduce availability of calcium for intestinal absorption, or use of a **less-acidifying diet** (Hills k/d) to reduce bone turnover.
- **Prednisone** (2–3 mg/kg PO q 24 h) has been reported to be partially or fully effective in normalizing both total and ionized serum calcium in the small number of cats reported, however therapy was required long term (> 12 months).

Prognosis

If hypercalcemia is unresponsive after aggressive treatment, the prognosis is poor.

In contrast to dogs, cats are reported to have a good prognosis following ingestion of cholecalciferol-containing rodenticide, if appropriate fluid and diuretic therapy are instituted.

Prevention

Do not use calcium-containing intestinal phosphate binders.

Be aware of the **risk of hypercalcemia** and soft tissue calcification when using **calcium supplementation** and **calcitiol therapy** in hypocalcemia.

Avoid inappropriately high doses of calcitriol or other vitamin D preparations, and **monitor calcium and phosphate concentrations** carefully when using these products. Moderately increased ionized calcium does not contraindicate use of calcitriol in chronic renal failure, as low doses of calcitriol (2.5 ng/kg q 24 h) do not significantly increase intestinal calcium absorption. Increased serum phosphate concentration is a contraindication for calcitriol use.

Restrict access to cholecalciferol-based rodenticides.

Avoid diets or dietary supplements that are unusually high in vitamin D, such as liver or cod-liver oil.

NEOPLASIA (RENAL NEOPLASIA OR LYMPHOMA)

Classical signs

- Inappetence, weight loss and lethargy.
- Enlarged kidney/s or abdominal mass on palpation.
- ± Vomiting.
- ± Polyuria, polydipsia.
- ± Dysuria, inappropriate urination, pollakiuria, stranguria.
- ± Respiratory signs.
- ± Lymphadenopathy.
- ± Palpable cervical or abdominal mass.

Clinical signs

Neoplasia is a cause of polyuria in cats.

Lethargy, anorexia and/or weight loss are typical, regardless of the cause.

Renal, gastrointestinal, respiratory or neuromuscular signs may occur, and in part reflect the underlying cause.

Hypercalcemia associated with lymphoma is rare in cats but does occur **(see page 245, Hypercalcemia).** Hypercalcemic cats may have **polyuria and polydipsia** which may be associated with inappropriate urination, and/or have signs of **lower urinary tract disease,** including dysuria and pollakiuria, which is commonly **associated with calcium oxalate urolithiasis.**

Vomiting may occur associated with the underlying neoplasm, hypercalcemia or uremia.

Other signs include unilateral or bilateral renal enlargement on palpation, or an abdominal, cervical or thoracic mass.

Diagnosis

Serum creatinine and urea concentrations may be increased if the neoplasia is associated with renal failure.

Urine specific gravity is usually dilute.

Identification of a mass on palpation or imaging. Biopsy and histology is required for a definitive diagnosis.

HYPERADRENOCORTICISM

Classical signs

- Diabetes mellitus.
- Polyuria and polydipsia.
- Weight loss.
- Fragile skin and poor hair coat.

See main reference on page 324 for details (The Cat With Weight Loss and a Good Appetite).

Pathogenesis

Hyperadrenocorticism is a rare disease in cats.

Usually occurs in **middle-aged to older** cats (average age 10–11 years).

Pituitary-dependent form is most common (approximately 75–80% of cases); a functional adrenocortical tumor is less frequent (20–25%).

Clinical iatrogenic hyperadrenocorticism is less pronounced in cats as they are more resistant to the effects of excess exogenous glucocorticoids than dogs. PU/PD may occur with exogenous steroids, but is less dramatic than in dogs.

Chronic insulin resistance from excess endogenous steroid may result in **diabetes mellitus**.

Clinical signs

Polyuria, polydipsia is typical, which may be marked (>120 ml/kg/24 h) if concurrent diabetes is present.

Weight loss occurs as a result of poorly controlled diabetes.

Lethargy is common.

Many of the common signs are attributable to poorly controlled diabetes mellitus (although not all cats with hyperadrenocorticism have diabetes). The diabetes tends to be insulin resistant. Normal doses of insulin often produce a minimal decrease in glucose concentra-

tion and doses greater than 1.5 U/kg q 12 h are often required. **Poor glycemic control** is often still present despite higher than normal doses of insulin.

Thin, fragile skin that bruises easily is a common sign. Some cats have extremely fragile skin, and normal grooming, or lifting the skin for injection or restraint results in severe skin tears.

Poor unkempt hair coat, patchy alopecia, or skin infections including demodicosis may be evident.

Potbelly, which may be reported by the owner as weight gain or abdominal enlargement.

Muscle wasting.

Hepatomegaly.

Other concomitant infections may occur, e.g. bacterial cystitis, pyothorax.

Diagnosis

Diagnosis is based on consistent clinical signs and an abnormal dexamethasone suppression test, i.e. failure of cortisol to suppress below 41 nmol/L (1.5 µg/dl) at both 4 and 8 h after IV dexamethasone.

- Because up to 20% of normal cats do not suppress using 0.01 mg/kg dexamethasone, a higher dose is recommended in cats, i.e. 0.1 mg/kg.
- It is important not to stress the cat when doing this test.
- Cats with pituitary-dependent hyperadrenocorticism may fail to suppress, or exhibit suppression at 3–4 hours followed by "escape" of suppression at 8 hours. The latter pattern is diagnostic for pituitary-dependent disease, and makes further testing unnecessary.

A normal **urine cortisol:creatinine ratio** is useful for **excluding hyperadrenocorticism**, but lacks specificity for diagnosis.

The **corticotropin (ACTH) stimulation test** is best used to differentiate endogenous from iatrogenic hyperadrenocorticism, rather than as a diagnostic test for hyperadrenocorticism, because 15–30% of cats with hyperadrenocorticism have a normal response.

The **combined dexamethasone suppression/ACTH stimulation test** has been used successfully to diagnose hyperadrenocorticism in cats. The combined test does not appear to be more advantageous than the ACTH stimulation and dexamethasone suppression tests evaluated separately.

Differentiation of pituitary-dependent from adrenal tumors is based on **abdominal ultrasound** (one enlarged adrenal if adrenal tumor) and **ACTH concentration.** Normal to increased ACTH concentrations support a diagnosis of pituitary-dependent disease. Low concentrations support adrenal disease. This test must only be used after hyperadrenocorticism is confirmed, because normal cats often have low ACTH concentrations.

Differential diagnosis

Other causes of poorly controlled diabetes need to be considered, e.g. excessive insulin dose, too short a duration of action of insulin, hyperthyroidism and acromegaly.

Some cats appear to have poorly controlled diabetes based on persistently high blood glucose concentrations measured in hospital, but have good control of clinical signs (e.g. stable weight and water intake < 60 ml/kg). These cats have **stress hyperglycemia** associated with visits to the veterinarian. In contrast, **cats with undiagnosed hyperadrenocorticism and diabetes usually have persisting clinical signs of diabetes,** despite insulin therapy.

Treatment

Medical therapy produces inconsistent results, but is useful in improving the presurgical condition of the cat.
- Drugs which have produced improvement in some cats are **ketaconazole** (15 mg/kg q 12 h) and **metyrapone** (65 mg/kg q 12 h).
- **Trilostane** and L-depronyl have been used in dogs successfully, but there is comparatively little information available on their use in cats. Trilostane ameliorates clinical signs of hyper adrenocorticism in cats based on the studies published.

Surgical **adrenalectomy (unilateral for adrenal tumor and bilateral for pituitary-dependent hyperadrenocorticism)** provides the best response.
- Begin glucocorticoids, fluids and antibiotics just before surgery.
- Fatal post-operative complications are relatively common.

Transsphenoid hypophysectomy may be available in some referral centers.

Prognosis

Prognosis is guarded to grave. Cats that have adrenocortical tumors surgically removed have the longest survival.

HYPOADRENOCORTICISM

> ### Classical signs
>
> - Very rare disease.
> - Lethargy, depression, anorexia and weight loss.
> - Dehydration, hypothermia, ± weakness or collapse.
> - ± Bradycardia.
> - ± Vomiting.
> - ± Polyuria and polydipsia.
> - ± Waxing and waning illness, that responds to fluids or glucocorticoids.

Pathogenesis

Hypoadrenocorticism results from a **deficiency of glucocorticoids and/or mineralocorticoids** produced by the adrenal gland.

It can be **classified as either primary or secondary adrenocortical insufficiency.**
- **Primary adrenocortical** failure occurs rarely in cats as a naturally occurring disease, and is presumed to **result from immune-mediated destruction of the adrenal cortices**.
- **Secondary adrenocortical failure** involves only a **deficiency of glucocorticoid secretion** as a result of reduced secretion of pituitary ACTH.
- Spontaneously occurring secondary hypoadrenocorticism has not been reported in cats.
- Iatrogenic secondary hypoadrenocorticism can be demonstrated with an ACTH stimulation test after withdrawal of potent glucocorticoids or progestins, especially after long-term use. However, clinical signs are rarely seen.

Glucocorticoid (cortisol) deficiency impairs the body's response to stressful situations.

Mineralocorticoid (aldosterone) deficiency directly affects renal function and the body's ionic and water homeostasis.

- Loss of aldosterone secretion results in impaired renal conservation of sodium and chloride and excretion of potassium, leading to **hyponatremia, hypochloremia and hyperkalemia.**
- The loss of sodium and chloride **reduces the extracellular fluid volume**, resulting in hypovolemia, hypotension, reduced cardiac output and decreased renal perfusion.
- Hyperkalemia has deleterious effects on myocardial electrical activity.

For clinical signs to develop there must be a loss of at least 85–90% of the adrenal cortices.

Disease progression varies in severity depending on the degree of stress and the adrenocortical reserve.

An Addisonian crisis is the **most severe presentation** of hypoadrenocorticism. This is the result of severe hyponatremia and hyperkalemia, which are the precursors for hypovolemia, prerenal azotemia and cardiac arrhythmias.

Clinical signs

Very rare disease in cats.

Most common in **young to middle age** 1–9 years (average, 6 years old).

In general, **signs are similar to those in dogs**. It often presents with only vague clinical signs of lethargy, anorexia and weight loss. Vomiting and diarrhea are less common signs in cats, as are changes in the electrocardiogram associated with hyperkalemia.

Signs may be present for only **a few days or up to 4 months** prior to diagnosis.

Lethargy or depression are frequent signs.

Anorexia and weight loss are also common.

On physical examination, most cats (>50%) are **dehydrated, hypothermic or depressed**.

Weakness, weak femoral pulses, and slow capillary refill are common although, unlike dogs, collapse and bradycardia are rare.

Vomiting may be reported.

Polyuria and polydispia are reported in **30% of cats**.

Partial adrenal deficiency is characterized by episodic, non-specific gastrointestinal signs and lethargy or depression, which occur particularly at times of stressful events (travel, boarding, surgery).

A waxing and waning course of illness is typical.

A history of previous response to steroids or fluids is common.

Diagnosis

Diagnosis is based on clinical signs plus a sodium:potassium ratio of < 24:1.

Definitive tests are an ACTH stimulation test combined with measurement of ACTH concentration.

- Synthetic ACTH (Controsyn, Organon) administered at 0.125 mg/cat IM with blood samples collected at 0, 30 and 60 minutes or IV with samples collected at 0, 60 and 90 minutes or ACTH gel (2.2 mg/kg) IM with samples at 0, 60 and 120 minutes.
- Cortisol concentration pre- and post-ACTH < 55 nmol/L (2 µg/dl) is diagnostic.
- Elevated ACTH concentration differentiates spontaneous primary hypoadrenocorticism from iatrogenic steroid administration, because the cause of the spontaneous disease is lack of cortisol response to ACTH.

Hyponatremia occurs in cats, and is usually accompanied by hypochloremia.

Hyperkalemia occurs in 90% of cats, but is less marked (< 7.6 mmol/L or mEq/L) than in dogs.

Azotemia, hyperphosphatemia and dehydration occur in nearly all cats.

Urine specific gravity < 1.030 was present in 70% of cats.

Differential diagnosis

Renal failure is much more common, and also typically presents with azotemia and urine specific gravity of < 1.030, and can have similar signs. The ACTH stimulation test is normal in renal failure and the cats tend to be older.

Chronic glucocorticoid or megestrol acetate administration may result in a similar ACTH stimulation test result. The cortisol increase is suppressed in the ACTH stimulation test. However, ACTH concentration is also suppressed, and electrolytes are normal.

An Addisonian crisis needs to be differentiated from other critical conditions such as **diabetic ketoacidosis, necrotizing pancreatitis and septic shock.**

Mild hypoadrenocorticism displays signs that are relatively non-specific, and are often seen in other gastrointestinal and renal diseases.

Treatment

An acute Addisonian crisis is a medical emergency.

Immediate correction of hypotension, hypovolemia, electrolyte imbalances and metabolic acidosis via fluid administration is essential. Use isotonic fluids (0.9% NaCl) at 40 ml/kg/h IV initially for the first 1–4 hours. Once dehydration is corrected, reduce the fluid rate to 60–90 ml/kg/day, using the higher fluid rate if the cat is not eating.
- Potassium supplementation in fluids is contraindicated, but if the only fluids available immediately have potassium, use them.

Provide an immediate source of **glucocorticoids**.
- Prednisolone sodium succinate (4–20 mg/kg, IV) or dexamethasome (0.1–2.0 mg/kg, IV or IM).
- Mineralocorticoids should be replaced using oral fludrocortisone acetate (0.05–0.1 mg/cat PO q 12 h) or DOCP (deoxycorticosterone pivalate, 2.2 mg/kg, IM q 25 days). In Australia, the long-acting form in oil for intramuscular injection is an acetate product (DOCA).
- If the cat is in shock, higher doses of glucocorticoids may be warranted.

Despite appropriate therapy, lethargy, anorexia and weakness may persist for 3–5 days, unlike the rapid response in dogs.

In the long term, **glucocorticoid and mineralocorticoid replacement** is required lifelong. Use either **fludrocortisone acetate** (0.05–0.1 mg/cat PO q 12 h) or **DOCA** (2.2 mg/kg, IM q 25 days) for mineralocorticoid replacement long term. Some cats require additional glucocorticoid replacement long term or at times of stress, which can be provided using prednisolone/pred-

nisone (0.25–1 mg/cat PO q 12 h) or methylprednisolone (10 mg IM q 1 month).

Stressful events may warrant an increase in medication dose.

Prognosis

Prognosis is good with appropriate treatment, provided the hyperkalemia and electrolyte imbalance is corrected in time. Cats with adrenal insufficiency will have a normal life expectancy provided they are treated appropriately.

Prevention

Secondary adrenocorticism caused by rapid withdrawal of chronic corticosteroid therapy can be prevented via staged withdrawal of steroids and progestins, which allows adrenal gland function to recover from chronic suppression.

ACROMEGALY (HYPERSOMATOTROPISM; GROWTH HORMONE-PRODUCING TUMOR)

Classical signs

- Poorly controlled, insulin-resistant diabetes mellitus requiring high doses of insulin.
- Polyuria, polydipsia, polyphagia.
- Weight gain despite poorly controlled diabetes.
- Large, blocky or coarse body and head.
- Enlarged tongue, widely spaced teeth, thickened soft palate.
- Cardiomegaly.

See main reference on page 322 for details (The Cat With Weight Loss and a Good Appetite).

Pathogenesis

Very rare disease.

Caused by a functional adenoma of the pars distalis which produces excess growth hormone.

Excess growth hormone results in soft tissue and bone overgrowth from the chronic hypertrophic actions of the hormone. These anabolic actions are mediated by insulin-like growth factor-1, a growth factor synthesized in the liver and also locally in the growth plate of bones. The effects of excess growth hormone are chronic and insidious.

Acute catabolic actions of growth hormones result in fat breakdown (lipolysis) and glycolysis. Hyperglycemia results from increased gluconeogenesis in the liver and decreased glucose uptake into tissues as a result of insulin resistance. Long term, the marked insulin resistance results in diabetes mellitus.

Insulin resistance may be extreme with insulin doses between 20–130 U/day required to control blood glucose.

Clinical signs

Cats are typically middle aged to elderly, with a predominance of males.

All cats reported have diabetes mellitus, and in most cats, their diabetes is poorly controlled and insulin-resistant. Normal doses of insulin produce no or minimal decrease in glucose concentration, and in many cats, very large doses of insulin are required to produce an acceptable glucose-lowering effect.

Polyphagia, polyuria and polydipsia are associated with poorly controlled diabetes.

Typically, there is **weight gain despite poorly controlled diabetes**, although sometimes weight loss is present.

A **large, blocky or coarse body** is typical, and cats often have coarse facial features. General coarsening of body type is evident when the cat is compared to pictures taken several years before.

Acromegalic cats often have **thickened enlarged tongues**, sometimes widely spaced teeth and a thickened soft palate. Displacement of lower canine teeth forward (prognathia inferior) may occur.

Cardiomegaly is often evident on radiographs and occasionally congestive heart failure occurs resulting in dyspnea.

Degenerative arthritis may occur resulting in stiffness on rising and walking. Periosteal reaction is evident around the joints on radiographs.

Renal failure occurs in some cats.

Diagnosis

Diagnosis is based on clinical signs and **increased plasma concentrations of insulin-like growth factor-1** (> 1200 U/L).

Growth hormone concentrations can be measured with an assay developed for dogs, available at some research laboratories. Demonstration of persistently elevated GH concentrations, which do not increase with stimulation from GHRH or clonidine, support the diagnosis, but is not readily available to most practitioners.

A pituitary mass on CT or MRI scan supports the diagnosis, and is useful for monitoring response to irradiation therapy.

Differential diagnosis

Other causes of poorly controlled insulin-resistant diabetes need to be distinguished from acromegaly. When insulin resistance is extreme and insulin dose exceeds 20–30 U/cat/injection without causing hypoglycemia, the likely cause is acromegaly. Most other causes of insulin resistance produce less extreme insulin resistance and very high doses of insulin produce severe hypoglycemia.

Hyperadrenocorticism causes poorly controlled insulin-resistant diabetes. Typically, insulin doses required to control hyperglycemia are much lower than for acromegaly. In contrast to acromegaly, cats with hyperadrenocorticism have weight loss. Other signs suggestive of hyperadrenocorticism are a poor hair coat and fragile skin, which may tear with restraint for blood sampling or insulin injection. Many have a potbelly (may also be present in acromegaly) and hepatomegaly.

Other causes of apparent insulin resistance such as **excessive insulin dose resulting in rebound hyperglycaemia or use of an insulin of insufficient duration of action** result in poorly controlled diabetes, but clinical signs of acromegaly are absent.

Treatment

Cobalt radiation has been used successfully, and may result in resolution of the diabetes in some cats.

Pituitary ablation using cryosurgery may be effective (refer to current literature).

The long-acting somatostatin analog, octreotide has the potential to lower GH concentrations, but its use has not been reported in cats.

Prognosis

Without specific treatment for the GH excess, the **long-term prognosis is poor**; most eventually die with congestive heart failure, renal failure or neurologic signs from the expanding pituitary tumor within 1–2 years. Short-term prognosis is reasonable, provided sufficient doses of insulin are administered to control hyperglycemia and resolve the clinical signs of diabetes mellitus.

HYPERPARATHYROIDISM

Classical signs

- Anorexia and lethargy.
- Vomiting.
- Weight loss.
- Dysuria, inappropriate urination, pollakiuria, stranguria.
- Weakness, tremors.
- Palpable cervical mass.

See main reference on page 245 for details of hypercalcemia (The Cat With Polyuria and Polydipsia).

Clinical signs

Primary hyperparathyroidism is an uncommon cause of hypercalcemia, and is usually the result of an autonomous adenoma producing excess PTH. It is usually a **solitary functional adenoma**, although bilateral cystadenomas and solitary or bilateral adenocarcinomas have been reported.

Affected cats are typically old (average age 13 years) and Siamese cats are over-represented.

Clinical signs are of **hypercalcemia** and include **anorexia and lethargy** (50% of cats), **gastrointestinal signs** including vomiting, diarrhea or constipation (27%), polyuria and/or polydipsia (24%), lower uri-nary tract signs including dysuria, inappropriate urination, pollakiuria and stranguria (23%), and weakness and/or muscle tremors (14%).

A **palpable parathyroid mass** is present in more than half the cats.

Diagnosis

A presumptive diagnosis is based on finding **hypercalcemia** and demonstrating a **parathyroid mass** on palpation or cervical ultrasound.

PTH concentrations are **inappropriately high** for the calcium concentration, and are in the normal range or increased.

A definitive diagnosis is by surgical removal of the parathyroid mass and normalization of serum calcium concentrations. Vitamin D and calcium are usually administered following surgical removal to prevent life-threatening hypocalcemia (see page 248, Hypercalcemia).

PRIMARY HYPERALDOSTERONISM

Classical signs

- Weakness, cervical ventroflexion.
- Inappetence and weight loss.
- Polyuria, polydipsia.
- Blindness.

Pathogenesis

Primary hyperaldosteronism is a very rare cause of polyuria and polydipsia, and results from an aldosterone-secreting adrenal tumor.

Aldosterone stimulates reabsorption of sodium in the distal tubule and collecting ducts. To maintain electrical and osmotic neutrality, chloride, bicarbonate and water are reabsorbed, and potassium and hydrogen ions are excreted. Hyperaldosteronism results in hypokalemia, metabolic alkalosis, and systemic hypertension from the sodium and water reabsorption.

Clinical signs

Affected cats are typically old, ranging from **10–20 years.**

Clinical signs are mainly of **hypokalemia** including muscle weakness, ventroflexion of the neck, inappetence and weight loss, or of **hypertension** and include blindness from hypertensive retinopathy. Other signs include ataxia, abdominal enlargement and polyuria and/or polydipsia with two of the five reported feline cases also having **diabetes mellitus.**

Diagnosis

Serum creatinine kinase activity is increased reflecting hypokalemic myopathy.

Urine specific gravity is usually dilute.

A presumptive diagnosis is based on finding **persistent hypokalemia** despite supplementing with high doses of potassium, and **intractable hypertension** in an elderly cat. The finding of an adrenal mass and increased aldosterone concentrations help confirm the diagnosis.

Differential diagnosis

Pheochromocytoma may also cause hypertension in an elderly cat and be associated with an adrenal mass.

Other causes of hypertension in elderly cats including **hyperthyroidism** and **renal disease** need to be ruled out.

Treatment

Clinical signs can be improved or resolved with **potassium supplementation** and **antihypertensive therapy**.
- Use **potassium gluconate** solution, tablets or powder (4–10 mmol (mEq)/cat PO q 24 h in divided doses. See treatment of hypokalemia in The Cat With Generalized Weakness (page 946) and The Cat With Neck Ventroflexion (page 895).
- Use **amlodipine** (0.625 mg or 1/4 of a 2.5 mg tablet, PO q 24 h) for hypertension. Some cats with severe hypertension may require doses as high as 1.25 mg PO q 12 h. Titrate dosage carefully, based upon blood pressure determinations.
- Trilostane has been used in humans with hyperaldosteronism, but its use has not been reported in cats.

Long-term resolution involves **surgical removal** of the adrenal mass.

PHEOCHROMOCYTOMA

Classical signs
- Polyuria, polydipsia.
- Signs of systemic hypertension (blindness, dyspnea from heart failure).

Pathogenesis

Pheochromocytoma is a rare tumor, that develops from the medullary region of the adrenal gland, or occasionally as an extra-adrenal mass.

Functional tumors may produce **adrenaline (epinephrine), noradrenaline (norepinephrine)** and occasionally other hormones such as dopamine.

Signs result from either **elevated catecholamine concentrations** or from a **mass effect** of the tumor, metastasis or local invasion.

Excessive catecholamine concentrations may produce **severe hypertension** and associated signs such as retinal hemorrhage and detachment.

Polyuria and polydipsia may result directly from the excessive catecholamine concentrations, hypertensive renal damage or from insulin resistance. In diabetic cats with unexplained insulin resistance, pheochromocytoma is a rare potential cause.

Clinical signs

Affected cats are typically old, ranging from **10–20 years.**

Clinical signs are vague and diagnosis pre-mortem is rare. Signs include polyuria and/or polydipsia. In diabetic cats, pheochromocytoma may result in poor glycemic control associated with insulin resistance.

Sudden blindness with evidence of retinal hemorrhage and detachment has been reported as well as congestive heart failure.

Differential diagnosis

Primary hyperaldosteronism may also cause hypertension in an elderly cat and be associated with an adrenal mass. Typically there is hypokalemia, which is difficult to control, and increased aldosterone concentrations.

Other causes of hypertension in elderly cats including **hyperthyroidism** and **renal disease** need to be ruled out.

Hyperadrenocorticism may be associated with an adrenal mass and polyuria, polydipsia, but can be ruled out based on clinical signs and a low dose dexamethasone test.

Diagnosis

An index of suspicion is required to make a presumptive diagnosis. **Systemic hypertension** together with an **adrenal mass**, in the absence of signs of hyperadrenocorticism or hypokalemia are suggestive of pheochromocytoma.

The mass can be imaged with ultrasound, MRI or CT. Biopsy may establish a definitive diagnosis.

A definitive diagnosis based on demonstration of increased plasma or 24 h urinary catecholamine excretion is rarely performed.

Treatment

Clinical signs can be improved using **alpha (phenoxybenzamine)** blockers, and if needed beta blockers (e.g. atenolol).

Long-term resolution involves **surgical removal** of the adrenal mass, but perioperative care is critical, and includes use of preoperative alpha blockers for 1–2 weeks prior to surgery. Surgery is best performed where a specialist anesthetic service is available.

PRIMARY SEX HORMONE-SECRETING ADRENAL TUMOR

Classical signs

- Fragile skin and poor hair coat.
- Polyuria and polydipsia.
- Poorly controlled diabetes mellitus.

Pathogenesis

Rarely, adrenal tumors secrete sex hormones. The most common is a **progesterone-secreting** tumor, and

one cat was reported to have an estradiol- and testosterone-secreting tumor.

The few cats reported were **middle-aged to older** cats (aged 7–14 years).

In humans and dogs, progesterone binds to cortisol-binding proteins displacing cortisol and resulting in increased concentrations of free cortisol. Progesterone is also a potent insulin antagonist.

Cats with progesterone-secreting tumors have clinical signs indistinguishable from hyperadrenocorticism, including concurrent diabetes mellitus.

Clinical signs

In cats with a progesterone-secreting tumor, skin and hair coat changes are the most common signs. **Thin, fragile skin that bruised easily**, an **unkempt greasy hair coat**, non-pruritic symmetrical alopecia, and skin infections including demodicosis were the most common signs reported.

Polyuria, polydipsia is typical, and in the majority of cats was attributable to **poorly controlled diabetes mellitus.**

Weight loss occurs as a result of poorly controlled diabetes.

One cat with an **estradiol- and testosterone-secreting tumor,** developed behavioral changes including aggression, had vulval hyperplasia, urine with a strong "tom-cat" smell and an unkempt hair-coat.

Diagnosis

Diagnosis of a progesterone-secreting tumor is based on consistent clinical signs, an abnormal dexamethasone suppression test (0.1 mg/kg), i.e. basal cortisol concentrations are low–normal, but there is failure of cortisol to suppress below 41 nmol/L (1.5 µg/dl) at both 4 and 8 h after IV dexamethasone, increased basal progesterone concentrations and evidence of an adrenal mass on ultrasound. Alternatively, as with dogs, basal cortisol may be low-normal and suppress normally following dexamethasone.

- Cortisol concentrations were below the reference range after ACTH stimulation, but that occurs in 50% of cats with hyperadrenocorticism.

The cat with an **estradiol- and testosterone-secreting** tumor, had **bilaterally enlarged adrenal glands,** and basal estradiol and testosterone concentrations were markedly elevated.

A skin biopsy shows changes consistent with an endocrinopathy.

Differential diagnosis

Hyperadrenocorticism is the most likely differential diagnosis and may appear identical clinically and on hormonal testing to a progesterone-secreting tumor, except for the absence of markedly increased basal progesterone concentrations.

Other causes of poorly controlled diabetes need to be considered, e.g. excessive insulin dose, too short a duration of action of insulin, hyperthyroidism and acromegaly.

Other causes of a poor hair coat need to be considered.

Treatment

Aminoglutethimide (AGT; approximately 6 mg/kg q 12 h PO) was used successfully for 1–2 months in some cats to control signs prior to surgery.
- Aminoglutethimide inhibits the enzyme, which converts cholesterol to prenenolone during synthesis of adrenocortical steroids.
- Mammary gland enlargement following treatment has been reported in a male cat.

Trilostane resulted in a temporary improvement in the cat with the **estradiol- and testosterone-secreting** tumor.

Surgical removal of the **adrenal tumor** is the treatment of choice once signs have been controlled medically. Surgery resulted in long-term survival and resolution of clinical signs including diabetes mellitus.

Prognosis

Prognosis is good for cats that respond to medical therapy and undergo successful surgical removal of the adrenal mass.

CYSTIC ENDOMETRIAL HYPERPLASIA/PYOMETRA COMPLEX

Classical signs
- Low-grade inappetence and lethargy.
- Vaginal discharge or distended uterus palpable.
- ± Fever.
- ± Polyuria, polydipsia.

See main reference on page 269 for details of acute pyometra/metritis (The Cat With Depression, Anorexia or Dehydration).

Clinical signs

Chronic cystic endometrial hyperplasia/pyometra complex presents with **vaginal discharge**, and cats may have **polyuria** and **polydipsia** as a presenting sign. **Pyrexia is rare**.

Stump pyometra is **rarely** a cause of polyuria, polydipsia; it more often presents as vaginal discharge.

Chronic cystic endometrial hyperplasia/pyometra complex occurs in **intact cats** of **any age**, **regardless of whether they have previously had kittens**.

Copious vaginal discharge (watery or thick) is most common.

Low-grade inappetence may be present for weeks or months.

Weight loss, lethargy, unkempt appearance and mild dehydration may be evident.

Depression, listlessness, ± mild dehydration. **Cats are usually not pyrexic**.

Polyuria, polydipsia occurs in some cats.

Diagnosis

Clinical signs that are highly suggestive of cystic endometrial hyperplasia/pyometra complex are vaginal discharge and listlessness in an intact cat, plus a **distended uterus on radiograph**. Radiographically, cystic endometrial hyperplasia/pyometra can only be distinguished from a pregnant uterus after approximately 42 days, when calcification of the fetal skeleton is visible.

Ultrasonography readily distinguishes between pregnancy and pyometra 21 days after last breeding date.

Increased white cell count and/or left shift are found in some cats.

RECOMMENDED READING

Chastin C, Panciera D, Waters C, Savary K, Price G, Vaden S. Hypercalcemia in cats: a retrospective study of 71 cases (1991–1997). Small Anim Endocrinol 2000; 10(3): 9.

Feldman EC, Nelson RW. Hypercalcemia and primary hyperparathyroidism. In: Canine and Feline Endocrinology and Reproduction, 2nd edition. Philadelphia, Saunders, 1996, pp 455–497.

Gunn Moore D. Feline Endocrinopathies. In: Advances in feline medicine. Vet Clin North Am Small Anim Pract 2005; 35(1): 171–210.

Martin GJ, Rand JS. Current understanding of feline diabetes: Part 2, treatment. J Feline Med Surg 2000; 2: 3–17.

Midkiff A, Chew D, Randolph J, Center S, DiBartola S. Idiopathic hypercalcemia in cats. J Vet Intern Med 2000; 14(6): 619–626.

Nelson WN. Diabetes mellitus. In: Ettinger SJ (ed) Textbook of Veterinary Internal Medicine, 5th edition. Philadelphia, Saunders, 2000, pp 1438–1460.

Norman EJ, Mooney CT. Diagnosis and management of diabetes mellitus in five cats with somatotrophic abnormalities. J Feline Med Surg 2000; 2(4): 183–190.

Rand JS, Marshall R. Diabetes mellitus in cats. In: Advances in feline medicine. Vet Clin North Am Small Anim Pract 2005; 35(1): 211–224.

Rand JS, Martin GJ. Management of feline diabetes mellitus. Vet Clin North Am 2001; 31(5): 881–913.

Reusch CE. Hypoadrenocorticism. In: Ettinger SJ (ed) Textbook of Veterinary Internal Medicine, 5th edition. Philadelphia, Saunders, 2000, pp 1488.

Rijnberk A. Acromegaly. In: Ettinger SJ (ed) Textbook of Veterinary Internal Medicine, 5th edition. Philadelphia, Saunders, 2000, pp 1370–1379.

PART 5

Cat with acute illness

16. The cat with acute depression, anorexia or dehydration

Anthony Abrams-Ogg

KEY SIGNS

- Acute lethargy, depression or listlessness.
- Acute inappetence or anorexia.
- Dry mucous membranes, skin tenting.

MECHANISM?

- Depression, anorexia and dehydration are non-specific signs that frequently occur together and accompany most diseases.
- Depression may result from a primary neurologic disorder or be secondary to diseases of other organs.
- Reduced eating behavior may be due to **primary anorexia**, **secondary anorexia** due to an underlying disorder, **pseudoanorexia** and **physiologic anorexia**.
- Dehydration occurs when drinking cannot compensate for water losses.

WHERE?

- Disorders of **any organ system** may cause acute depression, anorexia or dehydration.

WHAT?

- The most common causes of acute depression, anorexia and dehydration without other more specific signs are **pancreatitis, hepatopathies and poisoning.**

QUICK REFERENCE SUMMARY

Diseases causing acute depression, anorexia or dehydration

METABOLIC

- **Acute anemia** (p 270)**

Acute anemia of any cause will result in depression, anorexia and dehydration. Pale mucous membranes are typical, with or without splenomegaly or icterus. Polypnea may be evident, and fever may be present if due to *Mycoplasma haemofelis (Haemobartonella felis)*.

- **Acute renal failure* (p 278)**

This is usually due to renal ischemia or nephrotoxins, and results in progressive depression and anorexia, vomiting, and polyuria, oliguria or anuria. Acute exacerbation of chronic renal failure may also occur.

- **Urethral obstruction*** (p 267)**

Progressive depression and anorexia occur. Dysuria may not be witnessed and non-specific signs predominate due to acute uremia. A turgid bladder is evident on palpation.

- **Hepatic encephalopathy (p 297)**

In young cats this is usually due to a porto-systemic shunt. In mature cats this is usually due to hepatic lipidosis. Intermittent disorientation and ptyalism are the most common signs.

- **Diabetic ketoacidosis* (p 292)**

Insulin deficiency and dehydration lead to hyperglycemia and ketoacidosis. This may occur acutely without a history of weight loss and polyuria/polydipsia. Depression and anorexia are the main signs and a history of infrequent vomiting may be present.

- **Acute hypoglycemia (p 296)**

This is usually due to insulin overdose. Lethargy, disorientation, trembling, ataxia and dilated pupils are often present. Signs may progress to coma or seizures if not treated.

- **Acute hypokalemia** (p 271)**

Hypokalemia has numerous causes including chronic renal failure, post-obstructive diuresis, intravenous fluid therapy with potassium-poor fluids, furosemide therapy, vomiting, hyperaldosteronism (rare) and the treatment of diabetic ketoacidosis. Anorexia may contribute to hypokalemia, which in turn may exacerbate anorexia and depression.

- **Hypophosphatemia* (p 295)**

Severe hypophosphatemia may complicate the treatment of diabetic ketoacidosis and enteral alimentation of an anorexic cat, causing increased depression and anorexia and hemolysis.

- **Hypoparathyroidism* (p 295)**

Hypoparathyroidism is usually caused by parathyroidectomy during thyroidectomy. Idiopathic hypoparathyroidism is uncommon. Hypocalcemia results in anorexia and depression that may progress to muscle fasciculations and seizures.

- **Hypernatremia (p 298)**

Hypernatremia should be considered in a critically ill cat with progressive depression not attributable to other causes.

● **Acute heart failure* (p 292)**

Non-specific signs of lethargy and inappetence may occur prior to dyspnea. An arrhythmia, murmur and/or a weak pulse may be evident. Abnormal lung sounds consistent with edema or pleural fluid may be auscultated.

NEOPLASTIC

● **Neoplasia* (p 293)**

Many tumors may cause acute signs, and non-specific signs of lethargy and inappetence often appear prior to specific signs.

● Central nervous system neoplasia (p 297)

The tumor may acutely affect alertness or appetite. Other neurologic signs may or may not be present.

NUTRITIONAL

● **Unpalatable food* (p 294)**

Primary anorexia may occur due to a change in the diet. History of a diet change, together with normal physical examination findings are suggestive.

● **Alternate food source* (p 294)**

Physiologic anorexia may occur after consumption of an unknown source of food.

PHYSICAL

● **Separation or situation anxiety** (p 270)**

Change in environment and routine may cause primary anorexia and depression. Withdrawal or hiding may occur.

● **Environmental stress* (p 294)**

Temperature extremes may cause primary anorexia and inactivity.

INFLAMMATION

● **Fever*** (p 267)**

Acute fever and its underlying disorder may cause acute depression, anorexia and dehydration. Localizing signs may or may not be present.

● **Pancreatitis* (p 272)**

Non-specific signs of depression and/or anorexia dominate the clinical picture. Unlike the dog, vomiting and abdominal pain are not consistent findings.

● **Gastrointestinal foreign body and inflammation*** (p 268)**

Non-specific signs often predominate and vomiting and diarrhea may or may not be witnessed. Occasionally, a linear foreign body is evident wrapped around the base of the tongue.

● Esophageal foreign body and inflammation (p 299)

Regurgitation and gagging may not be witnessed, and non-specific signs may predominate.

● **Acute intranasal, oral or pharyngeal inflammation ** (p 269)**

Sneezing, nasal discharge and stertor may not be witnessed initially and non-specific signs predominate including depression, anorexia and pyrexia. Careful examination may reveal a mild serous ocular

continued

continued

discharge or tongue ulceration. Acute oral and oropharyngeal inflammation will cause pseudoanorexia. The associated pain and underlying condition may cause non-specific signs. Salivation and halitosis may be evident.

● Central nervous system inflammation (p 297)

Acute meningitis or encephalitis may initially be characterized by non-specific signs. Careful neurological examination may reveal cranial nerve or proprioceptive deficits.

INFECTIOUS

Viral:

● **Panleukopenia** (p 272)**

Non-specific signs of extreme lethargy and anorexia usually appear prior to the onset of vomiting. Diarrhea may occur 1–2 days after vomiting begins. Fever may or may not be present.

● Feline leukemia virus infection (p 299)

Occasionally the only signs of infection are acute depression, anorexia and dehydration.

Bacterial:

● **Bacterial sepsis** (p 269)**

Depression, anorexia and fever are typical of bacterial infection, although fever may not be present, especially in severe sepsis, and hypothermia may herald impending septic shock. Evidence of an internal site of infection may or may not be present on physical examination.

Parasitic:

● **Toxoplasmosis* (p 293)**

Lethargy, anorexia and fever are early signs. Dyspnea is present in the majority of cats, and is associated with increased respiratory sounds over the chest. Neurological signs, icterus, uveitis or evidence of other specific organ involvement may or may not be apparent.

Idiopathic:

● Primary anosmia (p 299)

Reduced sense of smell may cause anorexia. Primary anosmia may be idiopathic or neurologic.

Toxic:

● **Acute poisoning and envenomation* (p 283)**

Poisoning with ingested substances or animal venoms commonly causes acute non-specific signs, although more specific signs are often present as well. Depending on the toxin, these signs include salivation, vomiting, diarrhea, polypnea, arrhythmias, pale mucous membranes, hypothermia, tremors (which may cause hyperthermia), excitability and other behavioral changes, seizures and profound generalized weakness.

● **Ethylene glycol poisoning* (p 287)**

Acute depression in acute ethylene glycol toxicosis is due to direct central nervous system effects. Depression is due later to acute renal failure. Other signs include ataxia, vomiting, tremors, polyuria, painful and swollen kidneys and seizures.

  ● **Lily poisoning* (p 290)**

  Acute depression occurs following ingestion. Later depression is due to acute renal failure. Other signs include vomiting, polyuria, oliguria or anuria and painful and swollen kidneys.

  ● **Snake bite envenomation* (p 291)**

  Acute weakness caused by snake venom neurotoxins may present as acute depression. Other signs depend on the specific snake toxins, which include procoagulants, hemolysins, nephrotoxins, myotoxins and local cytotoxins.

  ● **Drug therapy*** (p 268)**

  Many drugs can cause anorexia.

Traumatic

  ● **Trauma*** (p 266)**

  Trauma may cause primary and secondary depression, anorexia and dehydration. External signs of trauma may be subtle or obvious. Shorn nails are often evident. A fractured jaw and tongue lacerations or puncture wounds cause pseudoanorexia and impede drinking.

  ● **Pain*** (p 268)**

  Pain may contribute to the depression and anorexia seen in many of the disorders listed in all categories above. Other signs of pain include vocalization (spontaneous and evoked by palpation), defensive aggression evoked by palpation, lameness, hunched posture (abdominal pain) and reluctance to move.

INTRODUCTION

MECHANISM?

Depression, anorexia and dehydration are non-specific signs that frequently occur together and accompany most diseases.

- The severity of the signs varies with the primary disease and the temperament of the animal.
- Signs may be stable or progressive.
- Various non-specific (e.g. acute phase response) and specific (e.g. uremia) mechanisms may be involved, depending on the primary disease.

Depression refers to dullness, lethargy and withdrawal from contact (hiding). The animal is less responsive, but not to the extent that it would be considered stuporous or comatose. Depression may result from a primary neurologic disorder or be secondary to diseases of other organs. Weakness, behavioral factors (e.g. anxiety), and depression of the reticular activating system may contribute to depression due to non-neurologic disorders.

- Depressed and critically sick cats may still purr, and the presence of purring should not be interpreted as an indication of mild illness.

Anorexia refers to a reduced appetite. Anorexia may be complete or partial. ("Inappetence" is commonly used to refer to partial anorexia. In this chapter "anorexia" will be used to refer to a reduced appetite regardless of severity.)

- **Primary anorexia** is due to anosmia, behavioral factors or neurologic disorders.
  - The smell of food is important to appetite stimulation, especially in cats.
  - Behavioral (psychologic) factors causing anorexia include fear, change in routine and unpalatable food.
  - Central neurologic disorders may impair the appetite center in the hypothalamus.
- **Secondary anorexia** occurs when a primary disease process affects the cytokine, endocrine and neurologic control of appetite.
  - Most disorders may result in secondary anorexia by various mechanisms.
  - This is the most common cause of anorexia in cats.

- Anorexia may also be due to **pseudoanorexia** and **physiologic anorexia**.
  - In pseudoanorexia the animal has a normal appetite but is reluctant to eat because of oral pain. (If there is a non-painful disorder of prehension, the presenting complaint will be dysphagia not anorexia.)
  - In physiologic anorexia the animal is satiated after eating. This may mimic true anorexia if the animal has an unknown source of food.

Dehydration refers to a reduction in body water other than that present in the transcellular compartment (third space, i.e. the gastrointestinal tract, pleural cavity and peritoneal cavity). It occurs when the animal does not drink and absorb sufficient quantities of water to replace physiologic or pathologic losses. Thirst may be reduced by analogous mechanisms that reduce appetite.

WHERE?

Disorders of **any organ system** may cause acute depression, anorexia or dehydration. The focus of this chapter is diseases where the owner complaint is typically that the cat is suddenly quiet and/or refusing to eat or drink. Specific signs are often not reported and are not obvious on physical examination. Meticulous and repetitive history-taking and physical examinations may be needed to detect subtle signs and development of new signs as the disease progresses. Laboratory assessment and imaging are often required to establish a diagnosis. Acute pyrexia and acute anemia as causes of depression, anorexia and dehydration are discussed in The Pyrexic Cat (page 364) and The Anemic Cat (page 526). The reader should also refer to The Cat With Stupor or Coma (page 821), The Cat With Seizures, Circling and/or Changed Behavior (page 795), and The Cat With Generalized Weakness (page 941). In the absence of a specific diagnosis, treatment should be supportive.

WHAT?

The focus of this chapter is **diseases of acute onset**, as opposed to acute exacerbation of chronic diseases. In most cases the cat will be in **good body condition**.

The most common causes of acute depression, anorexia and dehydration without other more specific signs are **pancreatitis, hepatopathies and poisoning**.

DISEASES CAUSING ACUTE DEPRESSION, ANOREXIA OR DEHYDRATION

TRAUMA***

Classical signs

- Shorn nails, dirty haircoat, dyspnea, pale mucous membranes, weak pulses, lameness or inability to walk.
- Fractured mandible, broken canine teeth, scleral hemorrhages, neurologic signs (head trauma).

Clinical signs

Cats with generalized trauma may be **depressed and anorexic** for a number of reasons including shock, hypovolemia, dyspnea, pain from soft tissue contusions and fractures, herniations and concussion.

Pseudoanorexia may occur from fractures of the jaw and teeth and lacerations to the tongue.

Diagnosis

External signs of trauma are not always obvious. Although shorn nails are usually evident, this sign may be absent. For example, nails may not be shorn on ice following motor vehicle trauma in the winter. Subtle signs of trauma include dried blood around the external nares, blood against the tympanic membranes, bite wounds or lacerations to the ventral surface of the tongue, and pain on palpation of the pelvis of a cat with normal ambulation.

Differential diagnosis

Other causes of acute depression.

Treatment

Intravenous fluids and transfusions to treat hypovolemia.

Surgical and conservative management of injuries.

Injuries to the oral cavity may necessitate placement of an esophagostomy or gastrostomy tube for nutritional support.

FEVER***

Classical signs

- Depression, anorexia.
- Elevated body temperature.

See main reference on page 364 for details (The Pyrexic Cat).

Clinical signs

Febrile cats may be presented for acute depression and anorexia.

Other clinical signs will depend upon cause of fever.

Diagnosis

Fever must be **distinguished from hyperthermia** as a result of environmental stress, activity or anxiety.

To identify the cause of the fever see The Pyrexic Cat (page 364).

Differential diagnosis

Other causes of acute depression and anorexia with superimposed hyperthermia mimicking a febrile condition must be differentiated.

Treatment

Treatment of the underlying cause is of primary importance.

If antipyretic agents are not contraindicated, reducing the fever will usually improve the well-being and appetite of the cat. Dipyrone is the superior agent, but has been discontinued in some countries. Ketoprofen and meloxicam may be used at standard doses.

Hyperthermia is treated by placing the cat in a cool environment.

URETHRAL OBSTRUCTION***

Classical signs

- Straining to urinate (owner reports "constipation").
- Progressive depression and anorexia.

See main reference on page 179 for details (The Cat Straining to Urinate).

Clinical signs

Straining to urinate, vocalizing, growling when handled, difficulty walking, vomiting.

Progressive depression and anorexia.

Pain on abdominal palpation and a turgid bladder are evident.

Whitish, chalky material may be seen blocking the urethral orifice or around the prepucial/perineal area and the cat may be excessively licking the area.

Progressive weakness and bradycardia may occur.

Diagnosis

Palpation of a turgid bladder is diagnostic. Rarely, spontaneous relief of obstruction occurs before examination.

Urinalysis typically reveals blood and struvite crystals.

Blood work reveals elevated urea, creatinine, potassium and phosphorus.

Differential diagnosis

If the owner has only noted non-specific signs, then most other causes of acute depression must be considered. The diagnosis is usually straightforward on the basis of physical examination.

Treatment

Intravenous fluids and correction of hyperkalemia (see Acute renal failure, below).

Urethral catheterization.

Management of urethral spasm, detrusor atony.

Dietary management.

GASTROINTESTINAL FOREIGN BODY AND INFLAMMATION***

> **Classical signs**
>
> - Vomiting and diarrhea.
> - Anorexia and depression.

See main reference on page 636 for details (The Cat With Signs of Acute Vomiting), page 713 (The Cat With Signs of Acute Small Bowel Diarrhea), page 765 (The Cat With Signs of Large Bowel Diarrhea), page 792 (The Constipated or Straining Cat).

Clinical signs

Cats with acute gastritis, acute gastroenteritis or acute gastrointestinal foreign bodies typically have vomiting and diarrhea. However, these signs may be intermittent, so that only non-specific signs such as anorexia and depression are reported by the owners.

Variable more specific findings include **abdominal pain, vomiting following abdominal palpation, dilated loops of intestine** and an **intestinal mass**. A linear foreign body may be evident around the base of the tongue.

Diagnosis

If only non-specific signs are reported, **observation for vomiting and diarrhea** may be of value.

Rule out extra-intestinal causes of vomiting and diarrhea with routine laboratory work.

Diagnostic imaging is required to identify foreign material and intestinal obstruction.

Differential diagnosis

Pancreatitis.

Other causes of acute vomiting and diarrhea. See The Cat With Signs of Acute Vomiting (page 630) and The Cat With Signs of Acute Small Bowel Diarrhea (page 697).

Treatment

Treatment of the underlying cause.

Antiemetic agents will decrease nausea, and thereby reduce depression and anorexia.

DRUG THERAPY***

> **Classical signs**
>
> - Anorexia.

Clinical signs

Anorexia is a side effect of many drugs, including antibiotics, anti-thyroid medications and anti-cancer agents. Anorexia typically develops within the first week of therapy.

Vomiting and diarrhea are the most common concurrent signs.

Some drugs also cause oral irritation.

Diagnosis

Rule out other causes of anorexia.

Improved appetite upon withdrawal of the drug.

PAIN***

> **Classical signs**
>
> - Depression, anorexia and localizing sign of pain.

Clinical signs

Pain may contribute to the depression and anorexia seen in many disorders. Other signs of pain include vocalization (spontaneous and evoked by palpation), defensive aggression evoked by palpation, lameness, hunched posture (abdominal pain) and reluctance to move.

Diagnosis

A cat with acute depression and anorexia should be carefully examined for signs of pain, which may help identify a causative disorder.

ACUTE INTRANASAL, ORAL OR PHARYNGEAL INFLAMMATION

Classical signs

- Partial or complete anorexia and depression.
- Sneezing, nasal discharge.
- Stertor.
- Halitosis, ptyalism.

See main reference on page 5 for details (The Cat With Acute Sneezing or Nasal Discharge), page 32 (The Cat With Stridor).

Clinical signs

Cats with **foreign material** (e.g. **kitty litter, plant material**) in the nose or nasopharynx may be acutely depressed and refuse to eat. Typically there is an acute onset of sneezing or serous nasal discharge. Foreign material in the nasopharynx may result in stertorous respiration.

Cats with **acute viral rhinitis** may also be depressed and anorexic, but these cats usually have a fever. Anosmia may contribute to anorexia; so may concurrent oral inflammation with calicivirus infection. Conjunctivitis may be present.

Cats with oral and oropharyngeal foreign bodies (e.g. needle) will be acutely depressed and refuse to eat. More specific signs include halitosis, ptyalism, unusual jaw motions, gagging, pawing at the mouth and stertorous respiration.

Oral ulcers, acute anorexia and salivation may occur following **exposure to a corrosive substance**.

Uremic ulceration contributes to anorexia in cats with renal failure.

Diagnosis

Acute viral rhinitis is usually diagnosed on the basis of clinical findings.

Foreign material may be evident adhered to the external nares. The nasal cavity may be examined for foreign material by means of an otoscope, rigid endoscope or radiographically. The nasopharynx may be examined under anesthesia with a dental mirror or flexible endoscope.

Ulcers and foreign material in the oral cavity are usually obvious, except for those under the tongue. Anesthesia is often required for thorough evaluation of the tongue and oropharynx.

Differential diagnosis

Other causes of acute depression need to be ruled out.

Treatment

Foreign material should be removed by extraction or lavage.

Antibiotics (e.g. ampicillin or amoxicillin at standard doses) are indicated when secondary bacterial infection is evident with viral, foreign body, corrosive or uremic ulceration.

BACTERIAL SEPSIS**

Classical signs

- Acute anorexia and depression.
- Fever and localizing signs of infection.
- Hypothermia and bradycardia with severe sepsis.

See main reference on page 112 for details (The Fading Kitten and Neonate).

Clinical signs

Cats with a bacterial infection usually have a **fever and localizing signs of infection**, in addition to depression and anorexia.

- Sepsis is defined as presence of a systemic inflammatory response syndrome (SIRS) due to a disseminated bacterial infection. Signs of SIRS include high fever or hypothermia; tachycardia or bradycardia; polypnea; and moderate to marked neutrophilia, neutropenia or left shift.
- Severe sepsis is defined as sepsis accompanied by organ dysfunction, hypoperfusion or hypotension.
- Septic shock is defined as severe sepsis with hypotension that is refractory to adequate fluid resuscitation.

Febrile responses may be blunted in older cats, and the severity of infection may be underestimated based on the magnitude of the fever.

In some cases fever is absent, and this should not be used to rule out bacterial infection. Septic cats without a fever are more likely to have severe sepsis and impending septic shock.

In some cats, the **localizing signs of infection are not readily detectable** on physical examination. This most often occurs when there is **primary neutropenia and secondary infection**.

- Severe sepsis or septic shock should always be considered in the differential diagnoses of cats with acute depression and anorexia without more specific signs.
- Other common signs of severe sepsis are bradycardia, pale mucous membranes, weak pulses, polypnea, diffuse abdominal pain and icterus.

Diagnosis

A complete blood count may reveal **neutrophilia** and a **left shift**. Alternatively, neutropenia may be present from primary bone marrow failure (e.g. FeLV infection) or exhaustion of marrow granulocyte reserve.

Meticulous physical examination, serum chemistries, diagnostic imaging and fine-needle aspiration will help localize the infection (e.g. deep subcutaneous abscess, pyometra, pyelonephritis, peritonitis, pyothorax, pneumonia).

Differential diagnosis

In the absence of a fever and localizing signs, all other causes of acute depression and anorexia should be considered.

Treatment

Treatment is supportive pending a diagnosis.

Systemic antibiotic therapy and **local treatment** of infection if indicated (e.g. drainage of abscess).

Empirical therapy with **broad-spectrum, bactericidal antibiotics** (e.g. cefazolin plus gentamicin, cefoxitin) should be started at standard doses in depressed neutropenic cats.

ACUTE ANEMIA**

Classical signs

- Pale mucous membranes.
- Acute onset of anorexia, depression and physical inactivity.

See main reference on page 526 for details (The Anemic Cat).

Clinical signs

The degree of depression, anorexia and dehydration correlates with the severity and acuteness of the anemia.

Tachypnea and tachycardia may be evident.

Pale mucous membranes with or without splenomegaly or icterus.

If the anemia is due to infectious causes, e.g. *Mycoplasma haemofelis* (*Haemobartonella felis*), the cat may be pyrexic.

Diagnosis

Routine hematology will confirm anemia.

The cause of the anemia can usually be determined by routine work-up (see The Anemic Cat).

Differential diagnosis

Pale mucous membranes due to shock.

Treatment

Treat the cause of anemia; transfusion. See The Anemic Cat.

SEPARATION OR SITUATION ANXIETY**

Classical signs

- Withdrawal or hiding and/or anorexia.

Pathogenesis

Removal of significant persons, or other pets from the cat's environment, or removal of the cat from **familiar surroundings** may **trigger separation or situation anxiety**.

Introduction **to new persons, pets or surroundings** may also trigger anxiety.

The cat's personality is an important risk factor.

Separation/situation anxiety **may exacerbate secondary anorexia** and depression in a hospitalized cat.

Clinical signs

Variable withdrawal, inactivity, anorexia and dehydration.

Other behavioral signs may occur, such as aggression to other pets or persons, and inappropriate elimination.

No signs of another disorder causing depression and anorexia.

Weight loss is dependent on degree and duration of anorexia. Complete anorexia will result in detectable lumbar muscle wasting within one week.

Diagnosis

History of change in environment.

Ruling-out other causes of depression and anorexia.

Differential diagnosis

Other causes of depression and anorexia.

Treatment

No treatment is necessary if signs are mild and it is likely that the cat will adapt.

Return cat to previous environment if possible.

Offer a variety of foods, warm the food, increase palatability of food with clam juice, or canned tuna or salmon juice.

Anxiolytic and/or appetite-stimulant drugs or herbal remedies may be useful if anorexia or anxiety cannot be quickly resolved. **Tricyclic antidepressants** (amitripty-

line, clomipramine) or **selective serotonin re-uptake inhibitors**, together with environmental changes may be effective (see The Cat With Anxiety-Related Behavior Problems, page 1014, for doses). Other treatments that have been used (but some may have undesirable side effects) include hydroxyzine, phenobarbital, megesterol acetate, prednisone, diazepam, oxazepam, cyproheptadine at standard doses and catnip. Dependency can develop with some treatments.

Nasoesophageal, esophagostomy or gastrostomy tube feeding or parenteral nutrition should be instituted for hospitalized cats if anorexia persists for more than 3 days.

Prognosis

The ability of the cat to adapt is dependent upon personality.

Hepatic lipidosis may complicate primary anorexia, especially in an obese cat anorexic for more than two weeks.

ACUTE HYPOKALEMIA**

> ### Classical signs
>
> - Ventroflexion of the neck
> - Stilted forelimb gait.

Pathogenesis

Hypokalemia results from **insufficient potassium intake** and/**or excessive urinary or gastrointestinal potassium loss** and/or **translocation** from extracellular to intracellular fluid.

Hypokalemia may be seen in **numerous disorders** including chronic renal failure, post-obstructive diuresis, intravenous fluid therapy with potassium-poor fluids, furosemide therapy, vomiting, hyperaldosteronism (rare) and the treatment of diabetic ketoacidosis. Anorexia may contribute to hypokalemia, which in turn may exacerbate anorexia and depression.

Clinical signs

Lethargy, muscle weakness, anorexia – increasing risk with decreasing potassium level.

Ventroflexion of the neck and stilted forelimb gait. Severe muscle weakness may lead to respiratory muscle failure (rare).

Polyuria and polydipsia – this is usually due to the underlying disorder, but hypokalemia may impair concentrating ability (hypokalemic nephropathy).

Arrythmias – increasing risk with decreasing potassium level.

Diagnosis

Serum potassium level < 3.5 mmol/L.

Ruling-out other causes of depression, weakness and anorexia.

Differential diagnosis

Other causes of depression, weakness and anorexia related to the primary disorder.

Other causes of cervical ventroflexion include thiamine deficiency and other causes of muscle weakness (including motor neuron disease and myasthenia gravis, which do not cause anorexia).

Treatment

Potassium-rich intravenous fluids. See Diabetic ketoacidosis in The Cat With Polyuria and Polydipsia.

Cats with mild hypokalemia (3.0–3.5 mmol/L) may be treated as outpatients with **potassium gluconate,** 1.0–3.0 mEq/kg/day q 8 h, followed by a maintenance dose of 1.0 mEq/kg/day q 12 h once serum potassium has normalized.

Prognosis

The prognosis for correction of hypokalemia is good and overall prognosis is determined by the underlying disorder.

PANLEUKOPENIA**

Classical signs

- Acute depression, anorexia, dehydration, and fever in kittens or unvaccinated cats.
- Vomiting usually precedes diarrhea.

See main reference on page 650 for details (The Cat With Signs of Acute Vomiting).

Clinical signs

Most common in cats 2–6 months of age.

Typically, there is acute onset of depression and anorexia. Vomiting then appears, followed by the onset of fetid and often bloody diarrhea in 1–2 days. Cats may stand hunched-up, sometimes with the face over a water bowl, but refuse to drink. Dehydration develops with vomiting and diarrhea.

Pain is often evident on abdominal palpation, and loops of intestine may be thickened and contain excess gas and fluid.

Affected kittens are initially **febrile**, but if signs are severe, this progresses rapidly to **hypothermia**. Coma and death usually follow in a few hours.

Diagnosis

Diagnosis is usually suspected when there are consistent clinical signs in a kitten or cat with no history of vaccination.

Complete blood count reveals severe neutropenia and lymphopenia. Fecal tests for parvovirus antigen are sometimes useful.

Differential diagnosis

No other disease mimics classic severe panleukopenia, and this should be the first differential diagnosis in any unvaccinated kitten presented for acute depression.

Many other diseases mimic mild panleukopenia clinically. However, leukopenia is usually present, even in mild cases, which supports the diagnosis.

Treatment

Intravenous fluids and bactericidal antibiotics (e.g. ampicillin plus gentamicin, cefoxitin) at standard doses are required.

PANCREATITIS*

Classical signs

- Acute depression and anorexia.

Pathogenesis

Pancreatitis is typically **classified based on post-mortem pancreatic histopathology**. Classification schemes vary in different reports, but in general the degree of fibrosis and mononuclear cell infiltration correlates with chronicity.

- **Acute pancreatitis is characterized** by variable neutrophil infiltration, edema, hemorrhage, acinar necrosis and peripancreatic fat necrosis, inflammation (steatitis) and saponification. In one series of 40 cats, acute pancreatitis was categorized as necrotizing pancreatitis (some with fibrosis) and suppurative pancreatitis.
- Both acute and chronic pancreatitis can be severe and no clinical, laboratory or diagnostic imaging finding reliably distinguishes the two.

Pancreatitis may occur with or without concurrent disorders. In the absence of a concurrent condition, a specific cause is usually not identified.

- Identified causes of acute pancreatitis include pancreatic neoplasia, hypothermia, virulent systemic feline calicivirus strains, ascending bacterial infection, toxoplasmosis, abdominal trauma and organophosphate intoxication. Ingestion of a high-fat meal is not a cause, unlike in dogs. Pancreatic flukes (*Eurytrema procynonis*) and liver flukes (*Amphimerus pseudofelineus*) have been associated with chronic, but not acute, pancreatitis. The cat has been used extensively as an experimental model of acute pancreatitis, but the methods of inducing pancreatic inflammation have little relevance to the etiology of naturally occurring disease.
- **Associated disorders** include hepatic lipidosis, cholangiohepatitis, inflammatory bowel disease, diabetes mellitus, diabetic ketoacidosis and acute renal failure. Cause and effect between these conditions and pancreatitis is not known, but the disorders are probably related. Other concurrent disorders include chronic renal diseases and neoplasia, which may be related to age rather than pancreatitis. If a concurrent disorder is not identified, pancreatitis is more likely to be acute based on histopathology.
- Obesity is not an independent risk factor, but is a risk factor for conditions associated with pancreatitis, such as hepatic lipidosis and diabetes mellitus. Cats with pancreatitis may be thin, but it is not clear if this is a risk factor or consequence of anorexia.

The **pathogenesis** of acute pancreatitis is believed to be similar to that in other species:

- **Premature zymogen activation occurs** within the pancreas leading to local inflammation, circulating pancreatic enzymes, and systemic inflammatory response syndrome (SIRS). **Potential sequelae include** hypotension, disseminated intravascular coagulation (DIC), pulmonary edema, pleural effusion, pulmonary thromboembolism, encephalopathy, systemic lipodystrophy, acute renal failure and multi-organ failure.
- Neither bacterial infection of the inflamed pancreas nor bacteremia appears to be common in naturally occurring pancreatitis.

Clinical signs

Cat may be of **any age, with no sex or breed predilection**, except perhaps for Siamese cats.

Duration of clinical signs prior to presentation varies from **several days to more than 3 weeks**. Both acute and chronic pancreatitis may present with acute signs, but cats presenting with a longer clinical history are more likely to have pancreatic fibrosis.

Clinical findings are often more subtle than expected for the degree of pancreatic injury. This may explain in part the delay in presentation to a veterinarian.

Depression and/or anorexia are the most common historical signs and may be the only signs present. The **most common physical abnormalities are dehydration and hypothermia** (68% in one study). Fever is uncommon.

Other inconsistent signs include weight loss, vomiting, diarrhea, cranial abdominal pain, cranial abdominal mass, abdominal distention due to ascites, dyspnea, ataxia and disorientation and shock. Polydipsia may be present, but is usually due to concurrent diabetes mellitus. Systemic lypodystrophy is a rare complication of acute pancreatitis, characterized by subcutaneous nodules that may ulcerate.

Diagnosis

Because clinical and laboratory findings are non-specific, diagnosis requires a high index of suspicion.

Pancreatitis should be considered in any cat with unexplained acute depression. Acute pancreatitis should also be considered in any critically ill cat developing pleural effusion, ascites or hypothermia.

Laboratory findings are variable and are most valuable in ruling out other causes of depression and anorexia.

Hematology abnormalities include:
- Mild non-regenerative anemia.
- Neutrophilia, with or without a left shift (inflammatory leukogram).
- Neutropenia.
- Lymphopenia (stress leukogram).
- Thrombocytopenia (consumption).

Serum biochemistry abnormalities include elevations in liver enzymes (with a tendency to be higher in chronic pancreatitis), bilirubin, cholesterol, urea and creatinine, and decreases in potassium, calcium and albumin. Lower concentrations of ionized calcium have been associated with a poor prognosis in acute pancreatitis. Low serum cobalamin levels may be present.

Blood glucose concentration may be increased, normal or low. Mild coagulation abnormalities may be present.
- Serum **amylase and lipase** levels are infrequently elevated in naturally occurring pancreatitis (poor sensitivity).
  - Serum amylase levels may be elevated by **dehydration**, and **amylase and lipase levels may be elevated by renal failure**. An elevated lipase level in the presence of normal renal function is probably highly specific for pancreatitis.
  - There may be a greater likelihood of detecting an elevated lipase level if measured immediately after the onset of clinical signs.
  - In one model of experimental pancreatitis, amylase levels actually decreased from baseline values during the first week of illness.
  - Decreased lipase level usually rules out pancreatitis in the dog; it is not known if this is also true for the cat.
  - The utility of measuring amylase and lipase in peritoneal effusion has not been evaluated in clinical cases.
- A more useful laboratory test is **feline trypsin-like immunoreactivity** (fTLI).
  - **fTLI is a more sensitive test** than amylase or lipase for pancreatitis, but a normal value does not rule out pancreatitis.

  - Elevated fTLI is not specific for pancreatitis. Elevations may also be seen in inflammatory bowel disease, intestinal lymphoma and renal failure.
  - fTLI is not as widely available as other laboratory tests, and delays in reporting reduce its utility.
- The measurement of trypsinogen activation peptide may be useful in the future.
- **Feline pancreatic lipase immunoreactivity** (fPLI) appears to be a very sensitive test for acute pancreatitis, but is currently not widely available.
- Abdominal fluid is usually a modified transudate but may be a non-septic exudate. Pleural fluid is usually a modified transudate.

Diagnostic imaging findings are also variable.

Abdominal **radiography** is most useful in ruling out other causes of vomiting.
- Radiographic findings are often normal and do not rule out pancreatitis.
- If abnormalities are present, they are similar to those of acute pancreatitis in dogs: **decreased cranial abdominal contrast** (due to effusion), a mass effect (displacement of organs) in the right cranial quadrant due to the swollen pancreas), and **localized dilation of loops of intestine** (due to ileus).

Abdominal **ultrasonography** is more useful than radiography. Ideally high-resolution equipment should be used. (Abdominal ultrasonography, fTLI and fPLI are the best non-invasive tests for pancreatitis.)
- Normal findings do not rule out pancreatitis (reported sensitivity is 11–80%).
- **Abnormalities with a high specificity for pancreatitis** include pancreatic regular or irregular enlargement, pancreatic hypoechogenicity, hyperechogenicity of peripancreatic fat (may be difficult to appreciate), dilation of the pancreatic duct in the left lobe and accumulation of peritoneal fluid around the pancreas. Less specific changes include dilated common bile duct and gall bladder, cranial abdominal mass effect, generalized peritoneal effusion and mesenteric lymphadenopathy. If a pancreatic mass is identified, it is most likely a neoplasm, followed by a pseudocyst. Pancreatic abscesses are rare. Hepatic parenchymal and gastrointestinal changes may also be present because of associated conditions.

- CT-scanning has low sensitivity. The diagnostic utility of magnetic resonance imaging is not known. Some cases have had no changes.

Thoracic radiographs should be obtained in dyspneic cats to rule out pleural effusion, which may be caused by pancreatitis. Dyspnea may rarely be due to pulmonary thromboembolism.

Definitive ante-mortem diagnosis requires **biopsy** obtained by exploratory laparotomy or laparoscopy. The pancreas may appear grossly normal (or show only nodular hyperplasia in the older cat).

A cat with pancreatitis may be a poor anesthetic risk. Acute exacerbation of pancreatitis occasionally occurs following biopsy.

Inflammation may be irregularly distributed in dogs and multiple biopsies are recommended; the situation may be the same in cats.

Ultrasound-guided fine-needle aspiration may be used to biopsy pancreatic masses. Amylase and lipase should be measured in cystic fluid – levels above serum levels support a diagnosis of pseudocyst; levels equivalent to serum levels do not rule out a pseudocyst.

Differential diagnosis

Acute anemia.
- Some cats with acute pancreatitis will have **pale mucous membranes** from shock. Routine haematology will confirm severe anemia. Anemia is usually only mild in pancreatitis.

Urethral obstruction.
- A **painful turgid bladder** is palpable. Rarely the obstruction has spontaneously resolved by the time the cat is presented for examination. In the latter case, diagnosis is established by history, prepucial crystal deposits, urinalysis and azotemia.

Acute renal failure.
- Both acute renal failure and pancreatitis may cause depression, anorexia, dehydration, vomiting, azotemia and reduced urine production. In acute renal failure urine will be isosthenuric to minimally concentrated, while in acute pancreatitis urine should be well-concentrated, unless there is pre-existing chronic renal failure. Azotemia is more severe in acute renal failure and will not normalize with rehydration. Acute renal failure may be a complication of acute pancreatitis.

Liver disease.
- Elevations in liver enzymes, bilirubin and cholesterol may characterize both pancreatitis and liver diseases. Furthermore, hepatic lipidosis and cholangiohepatitis are common concurrent disorders with acute pancreatitis. It is often difficult to establish if one disorder preceded the other, and to establish if one is more responsible for clinical signs. Moderate to marked liver enzyme elevations are suggestive of primary hepatic disease, and a disproportionate elevation of ALP compared to ALT and GGT is suggestive of hepatic lipidosis. Elevations in serum bile acids in the absence of cholestasis confirm the presence of hepatocellular dysfunction. Elevated plasma ammonia levels are diagnostic for hepatic encephalopathy. Marked coagulation abnormalities are suggestive of liver disease. Abdominal ultrasound examination of cats with liver disease is recommended in an effort to detect pancreatitis. If laparotomy is performed to obtain a liver biopsy, then a pancreatic biopsy should also be obtained, and vice versa.

Diabetic ketoacidosis (DKA).
- Confirmation of DKA requires demonstration of **hyperglycemia, ketonuria or ketonemia, and acidosis**. DKA may be confused with pancreatitis because urine test strips measure oxaloacetate or acetone, which may be produced in minimal quantities by cats, and cats with pancreatitis may be hyperglycemic. Several drops of hydrogen peroxide may be added to the urine sample in an effort to convert β-hydroxybutyrate to oxaloacetate to increase the concentration of oxaloacetate in urine. Alternatively, β-hydroxybutyrate may be measured in serum using a point-of-care test, or the urine test strip may be used to detect oxaloacetate in heparinized plasma. Using a standard urine test strip, a **negative plasma test rules out ketosis**, and a **positive urine test rules in ketosis**, in cats. It should be remembered that acute pancreatitis and DKA may occur concurrently. Acute pancreatitis, DKA and hypoglycemia should always be considered in an acutely depressed diabetic cat.

Hypoglycemia.
- Cats with acute pancreatitis may be hypoglycemic, but it is not known if this contributes to depression. Clinical hypoglycemia usually results from **insulin overdose**. This is confirmed by measuring blood glucose levels and by prompt resolution of clinical signs following intravenous dextrose or intramuscular glucagon. Portable glucose meters have a tendency to measure falsely low values, so a diagnosis of hypoglycemia should be reconsidered if the cat does not respond to intravenous glucose or glucagon. Lack of response to sugar solutions rubbed on the gums or given by stomach tube does not rule out hypoglycemia, because most absorption of glucose occurs in the small intestine.

Acute gastritis/gastroenteritis.
- This is a differential diagnosis for cats with pancreatitis that are **vomiting**. Indeed, some cases diagnosed with acute gastritis probably have acute pancreatitis. If signs are mild, then distinguishing the two diseases is not important, because both are similarly treated (short-term withholding of food and fluid therapy). The most useful test for distinguishing the two is abdominal ultrasound examination. Abdominal radiography will help rule out foreign material and obstruction as a cause of acute vomiting.

Acute heart failure.
- Potential **overlapping signs** of acute heart failure and pancreatitis include pale mucus membranes, hypothermia, weak pulses, tachycardia, bradycardia, dyspnea and vomiting. Clinical findings of a heart murmur, irregular heart rate, and pulmonary crackles, and radiographic findings of pulmonary edema and cardiomegaly help establish the diagnosis of heart failure. (Note that both heart failure and pancreatitis may be associated with pleural effusion.) Definitive diagnosis of cardiomyopathy requires echocardiography.

Panleukopenia.
- Severe panleukopenia usually affects **immature cats** while pancreatitis usually affects mature cats. A complete blood count will usually reveal severe **neutropenia. Depression and vomiting** are early signs. **Marked diarrhea** typically develops later, but may not be evident at the time of presentation.

Severe sepsis without an externally obvious source of infection.
- Septic cats may not have a **fever**. Meticulous physical examination, serum, chemistries, diagnostic imaging and fine-needle aspiration will help localize the infection (e.g. deep subcutaneous abscess, pyometra, pyelonephritis, peritonitis, pyothorax, pneumonia).

Toxoplasmosis.
- Acute systemic toxoplasmosis typically **affects kittens or immunosuppressed cats**, causes a fever, and uveitis is a common finding. Confirmation is by measuring serum IgM antibodies or demonstrating rising serum IgG antibodies.

Ethylene glycol poisoning.
- The diagnosis of acute poisoning relies on history of ingestion or a high index of suspicion. Both cats with pancreatitis and cats with acute ethylene glycol poisoning may have acute depression without other signs, but cats with acute ethylene glycol poisoning should be **isosthenuric**, while cats with pancreatitis should have well-concentrated urine, unless there is a concurrent disorder causing dilute urine, such as chronic renal failure. Metabolic acidosis, increased anion gap and increased osmolal gap will be more severe than in pancreatitis. Definitive diagnosis relies on measuring ethylene glycol in serum or urine or seeing **oxalate crystals in urine or in a kidney biopsy**.
- In the later stage of poisoning (renal failure), kidneys may be firm and painful on palpation, and the bladder is usually small because of anuria. The elevations in urea and creatinine will be marked.

Lily poisoning.
- The diagnosis of acute poisoning relies on history of ingestion or a high index of suspicion. Cats in the acute stage of lily poisoning should have **poorly concentrated urine**, while cats with pancreatitis should have well-concentrated urine, unless there is a concurrent disorder causing dilute urine, such as chronic renal failure.
- In the later stage of poisoning (renal failure), kidneys may be firm and painful on palpation, and the bladder is usually small because of anuria. The elevations in urea and creatinine will be marked.

Acetaminophen (paracetamol) poisoning.

- Probing for a history of ingestion, and careful observation for appearance of **brown mucous membranes**, and **facial and paw edema**, will establish the diagnosis.

Anticoagulant rodenticide poisoning.

- A careful search for **subcutaneous or internal bleeding** will help establish that a bleeding disorder is present. Clotting times are likely to be normal to minimally elevated in acute pancreatitis, and markedly prolonged in rodenticide poisoning. Note that markedly prolonged clotting times and vitamin K deficiency have been recognized in chronic pancreatitis.

Snake bite envenomation.

- A high index of suspicion should be maintained for cats at risk because of geographical location and season. For North American snakes with cytotoxins, a thorough physical examination should reveal a **bite wound**; there may be associated tissue necrosis. For Australian snakes, acute onset of weakness and depression are early findings. Dilated pupils with slow or absent papillary light reflexes, ataxia and elevated creatine kinase concentration or evidence of a bleeding tendency are frequent findings. Paresis may progress to flaccid paralysis.

Trauma.

- Subtle **external signs of trauma** include car grease on the fur, shorn nails, dried blood around the external nares, blood seen on otoscopic examination, small scleral hemorrhages and lacerations on the ventral surface of the tongue.

The above differential diagnoses are applicable to cats with acute onset of signs. Other than liver diseases, most of the above differential diagnoses will not be applicable to cats with pancreatitis with a longer duration of clinical signs and weight loss. For cats with **pancreatitis and subacute or chronic signs**, the **primary differential diagnoses are neoplasia, chronic renal failure, and inflammatory bowel disease**. Concurrent diabetes mellitus may confuse the clinical picture. See The Thin, Inappetent Cat (page 355).

Treatment

Address the inciting cause if one is identified.

The remainder of therapy is largely **supportive.**

Fluid therapy to correct dehydration and hypotension.

- If crystalloid solutions are insufficient, or pulmonary or peripheral edema is present, colloid solutions should be considered (e.g. plasma, dextrans, hetastarch, pentastarch).

Nutritional support.

- The optimal approach is not known. The tendency to withhold food based on treatment of acute pancreatitis in dogs is tempered by the overlap between acute and chronic pancreatitis in cats, the presence and risk of hepatic lipidosis in cats, the observation that most cats are not vomiting, and the observation that feeding does not appear to aggravate pancreatitis in cats.
- **Cats that are willing to eat should be fed**. Food should be withheld for 2–3 days for cats that are vomiting. For anorexic cats that are not vomiting, an appetite stimulant may also be considered – these include cyproheptidine (may cause unusual behavior), intravenous diazepam and oral oxazepam at standard doses.
- **Parenteral nutrition** may be used if available, especially for cats that are vomiting.
- If exploratory laparotomy is used to make a diagnosis, **a jejunal feeding tube should be placed**. This is best placed as a jejunostomy tube. Transpyloric tubes may also be used, either threaded through a gastrostomy tube, or as a nasojejunostomy tube, but preliminary experience is that such tubes tend to back out into the stomach.
- If laparotomy is not performed, **a gastrostomy or esophagostomy tube** may be placed once the cat has stopped vomiting. Endoscopic placement of a transpyloric tube is difficult.
- If it is desired to avoid anesthesia, a nasoesophageal tube should be used.
- The optimal diet is not known. Low-protein, low-fat and high-carbohydrate diets are recommended for dogs, but may not be appropriate for cats, especially if there is concurrent diabetes mellitus, and may not be sufficiently calorie-dense. Another problem is that the fat content on an energy basis is not provided for many foods. A food with a moderate fat content is a reasonable initial choice, which includes most commercial cat foods.

- **Supplemental B vitamins** should be considered. Specifically, cobalamin treatment should be given (0.5–1 mg SC q 2–3 weeks) if serum level is low.
- **Antiemetics.** Metoclopramide, ondansetron, prochlorperazine and chlorpromazine given at standard doses may be used to control vomiting. The latter two should not be given if the cat is hypotensive.
- **Analgesics.** Although many cats do not show evidence of abdominal pain, it is likely present, and may contribute to depression. Opioid analgesics should be considered at standard doses.
- **Antibiotics** are not indicated in most cases. Antibiotics are recommended if there is a marked inflammatory leukogram or fever (blood culture is recommended), or evidence of pancreatic infection on biopsy (pancreatic and liver biopsies should be cultured). Empirical choices include ampicillin, cefazolin and cefoxitin at standard doses.
- **Corticosteroids** should only be used if needed to treat a concurrent disorder (e.g. inflammatory bowel disease). They may be considered if the cat is presented in shock, but the value of such therapy has been overstated.
- **Fresh-frozen plasma** (10–20 ml/kg) has been advocated in acute pancreatitis to replenish coagulation factors and anti-thrombin III consumed in DIC, and to replenish α-macroglobulins, which are involved in clearing pancreatic enzymes from the circulation. There is no evidence of a beneficial effect in humans, and there are too few reports in dogs or cats to make an assessment. Transfusions are expensive, and any benefit is probably as a colloid solution. (It should be noted that **α-macroglobulins and anti-thrombin III are stable in regular plasma**. The main difference in regular plasma and fresh-frozen plasma are the concentrations of factor VIII and von Willebrand's factor. Fresh-frozen plasma is potentially more beneficial in DIC only if the aPTT is prolonged.)
- **Dopamine** 5 μg/kg/min as a constant rate infusion is beneficial in experimental acute pancreatitis when given within the first 12 hours of injury, but not after that time. Most cats with naturally occurring disease are presented after 12 hours, and it is unknown if there is any benefit.
- Vitamin K – see The Bleeding Cat (page 499).

Surgical debridement of grossly necrotic tissue and abdominal lavage may be performed if a diagnostic laparotomy reveals abnormal pancreatic tissue. For cats with a non-surgical presumptive diagnosis of pancreatitis, similar to dogs, **surgery should be considered if the cat is not improving with conservative management**, if there are worsening pancreatic changes on ultrasound examination, or if peritoneal effusion is an exudate, but there are no firm guidelines. Closed therapeutic abdominal lavage may also be considered if peritoneal effusion is an exudate. Therapeutic abdominocentesis should be considered if there is large-volume ascites, and it should definitely be performed if there is a problem secondary to a volume effect (e.g. dyspnea from diaphragmatic compression), but the benefit of the procedure on the course of the disease is not known.

Prognosis

The true prognosis is not known because of underdiagnosis, mortality due to concurrent disorders, and euthanasia because of the prevailing attitude that feline pancreatitis carries a poor prognosis. **Prognosis is related to the severity of the pancreatitis.**

Cats with mild acute pancreatitis probably have a good prognosis, while cats with severe pancreatitis and an associated disorder have a poor prognosis. Chronic pancreatitis may be subclinical.

In one series of 13 cats with acute pancreatitis and hepatic lipidosis, recovery rate was 20%, versus 50% for cats with hepatic lipidosis alone. In another series of 40 cats with severe acute pancreatitis, all cats died or were euthanized. Successful management of acute pancreatitis has been anecdotally reported and reported in individual case reports and small case series.

ACUTE RENAL FAILURE*

Classical signs

- **Progressive depression and anorexia.**
- **Vomiting.**
- **Polyuria, oliguria or anuria.**

Pathogenesis

Acute renal failure is a syndrome characterized by an abrupt reduction in glomerular filtration rate and resultant dysregulation of water, acid–base and electrolyte balance, and accumulation of uremic toxins. Acute renal failure may be non-oliguric (polyuric), oliguric or anuric.

- **Oliguria** is defined as **< 0.27 ml/kg/h,** and **anuria < 0.08 ml/kg/h** and these definitions may be used as guidelines for cats.

The **central pathophysiologic event** in acute renal failure is **acute tubular necrosis**. This is initiated by **altered hemodynamics** (ischemia), **nephrotoxins** or **miscellaneous primary renal diseases**. In some cases more than one mechanism is involved.

- **Ischemia may be caused by hypotension** (e.g. prolonged anesthesia, shock), **thromboembolism** (e.g. cardiomyopathy), or **acute hydronephrosis** (e.g. prolonged urethral obstruction).
  - **Hemodynamically mediated** acute renal failure may be caused by the same factors that cause pre-renal azotemia, but the reduced perfusion of the kidney is so profound that it leads to acute tubular necrosis.
- **Nephrotoxins** include ethylene glycol and lilies; mercury, lead and other heavy metals; aminoglycoside antibiotics and amphotericin B; NSAIDs, and cholecalciferol (vitamin D_3) rodenticides. The mechanism of NSAID nephrotoxicity is ischemia from vasoconstriction. The chemotherapeutic agents doxorubicin, epirubicin and carboplatin are also nephrotoxic, although the clinical importance of this appears to be low.
- **Primary renal diseases** do not commonly cause acute renal failure in the cat. Glomerulonephritis, amyloidosis, feline infectious peritonitis, bacterial pyelonephritis and bilateral renal lymphoma may cause renal failure with a more acute clinical course than typical chronic renal failure due to age-related chronic tubulointerstitial disease, but true acute renal failure is rare. It is most likely to occur with acute bacterial pyelonephritis. Acute exacerbation of chronic renal failure ("acute on chronic renal failure") may also occur; the mechanism in most cases is probably ischemia.

Acute oliguric renal failure is classically **divided into initiation, oliguric, polyuric and recovery stages.**

The **oliguric stage** is maintained by various factors, including:

- Arteriolar vasoconstriction.

- Intratubular obstruction from desquamated tubular epithelial cells.
- Tubular backleak, where filtrate leaks across the injured tubular epithelium and is thus shunted directly to the peritubular capillaries.
- Reduced glomerular permeability.

Clinical signs

The salient historical findings are **acute depression and anorexia**, which are progressive in nature. Most cats will **vomit**; diarrhea may also occur.

Physical examination findings are variable. **Hypothermia** typically develops within 24–48 hours of the development of oliguria or anuria. **Bradycardia** may be present.

- Body condition is normal in a cat without pre-existing chronic renal failure or other disorder-promoting weight loss.
- **Renal size is normal to large** in a cat without pre-existing renal disease, and kidneys may be painful on palpation. Kidneys are likely to be small in cats with chronic renal failure. Kidneys may also be enlarged in FIP, lymphoma, polycystic kidney disease, chronic hydronephrosis and amyloidosis, but are not painful. It should be noted that hydration status and the quantity of peri-renal fat affects renal size on palpation. Kidneys may feel larger upon rehydration.
- **The bladder is small with oliguria and anuria,** may be large with polyuria, and is large and turgid with urethral obstruction. Owners should be queried as to when the cat was last seen to urinate.
- Halitosis and oral ulceration and dehydration are common findings.

Diagnosis

The diagnosis of acute renal failure is based on:

- **Acute onset** of clinical signs.
- **Elevated serum urea, creatinine and phosphorus levels**.
- Increased **(polyuria),** or reduced **(oliguria/anuria)** production of **inappropriately concentrated urine.**
  - In cats with pre-renal azotemia, urine specific gravity should be > 1.035 unless there is another mechanism present for reducing specific gravity

(e.g. therapy with a diuretic). In **acute renal failure, urine is usually isosthenuric or minimally concentrated.** Some cats with chronic renal failure maintain adequate urine concentrating ability, but this does not appear to happen in acute renal failure.

- If urine specific gravity was not measured prior to initiating fluid therapy, monitoring serum biochemistry abnormalities will help in distinguishing pre-renal from renal azotemia. If azotemia is **pre-renal** in origin, it **will normalize within 24–48 hours upon rehydration** and/or correction of hypotension, whereas renal azotemia will remain elevated during this period (although it may improve).

- In animals with pre-renal azotemia, urine production will increase as the animal becomes rehydrated and/or hypotension is corrected. The volume of urine produced and time to do so will depend on the rate of fluids. Because these animals are usually acutely dehydrated, rehydration is typically performed quickly, so within a few hours urine production is expected. A method **to rapidly detect oliguria or anuria** is to **give a 10 ml/kg bolus of intravenous fluids over 10 minutes**. This should cause sufficient volume expansion and increase in blood pressure to initiate urine production within 10–30 minutes. If there is no urine produced after 30 minutes, another fluid bolus may be considered. **If there is no urine production after two fluid boluses**, then it is likely that **intrinsic oliguric renal failure** is present. Ideally blood pressure should be measured to confirm that reduced urine production is not due to persistent hypotension that is still causing pre-renal azotemia. A normotensive cat receiving maintenance fluid therapy should produce urine at **0.5–2 ml/kg/h.**

- The diagnosis of acute oliguric/anuric renal failure is usually straightforward. Acute non-oliguric renal failure is more difficult to distinguish from subacute chronic renal failure and acute-on-chronic renal failure.

A hemogram typically reveals **hemoconcentration** and a **stress leukogram**. Cats with **acute-on-chronic renal failure may have anemia**, and this finding is highly suggestive of pre-existing chronic renal failure. The anemia may not be evident until the cat is rehydrated.

Other variable serum biochemistry abnormalities include hyperglycemia, hyperkalemia, hyponatremia, hypocalcemia and decreased bicarbonate (total CO_2).

Other variable urinalysis findings include glucosuria, proteinuria, tubular casts, crystalluria, pyuria and bacteruria.

Diagnostic imaging of the kidneys, urinalysis, urine culture and kidney biopsy may be needed to rule in and rule out causes of renal failure. See Ethylene glycol poisoning and Lily poisoning, below.

- **Renal biopsy** may also help determine the **severity and reversibility of the injury**, but there is poor correlation between histopathologic findings and renal function.

Differential diagnosis

Pre-renal azotemia and reduced urine production. Causes of acute depression, anorexia, dehydration and vomiting may cause pre-renal azotemia and reduced urine production. These causes include acute gastritis, gastroenteritis and **pancreatitis**. In acute renal failure, urine will be isosthenuric to minimally concentrated, while in the other disorders urine should be well-concentrated, unless there is pre-existing chronic renal failure. Azotemia is more severe in acute renal failure and will not normalize with rehydration. Acute renal failure may be a complication of a primary disorder, due to the progression from pre-renal to renal azotemia.

Pre-renal azotemia and increased urine production.

- Both acute renal failure and **diabetic ketoacidosis** may cause acute depression, polyuria, vomiting, dehydration, hyperglycemia and glucosuria, and both may be preceded by a history of chronic polyuria and polydipsia (due to chronic renal failure and diabetes mellitus, respectively). Diabetic ketoacidosis is confirmed by detecting ketones in the blood or urine. Acute renal failure is also an uncommon complication of diabetic ketoacidosis. Cats with diabetic ketoacidosis may have concurrent chronic renal failure.

- Other disorders that cause polyuria and polydipsia in the cat include hyperthyroidism (common), and hepatic encephalopathy and central diabetes insipidus (rare) (see The Cat With Polyuria and

Polydipsia, page 231). Dehydrated animals with such a condition will appear to be in renal failure because of concurrent azotemia and poorly concentrated urine (SG < 1.035).

- Cats with hypovolemia from hypoadrenocorticism may also present with pre-renal azotemia, hyperphosphatemia and poorly concentrated urine.

Post-renal azotemia. The conditions will result in azotemia, hyperkalemia and reduced urination.

- **Urethral obstruction.** A painful turgid bladder is palpable. Rarely the obstruction has spontaneously resolved by the time the cat is presented for examination. In the latter case, diagnosis is established by history, preputial crystal deposits, urinalysis and azotemia. Note that prolonged urethral obstruction may rarely lead to acute renal failure.
- **Ruptured bladder.** The bladder is not palpable or, rarely, is palpable but small, and abdominal fluid is present. Creatinine or potassium concentrations higher in the abdominal fluid than that of serum are strongly suggestive of uroperitoneum. A ruptured bladder may be confirmed by a positive contrast cystogram. See page 464, The Cat With Abdominal Distention or Abdominal Fluid.

Treatment

Remove or correct the primary cause. Avoid any nephrotoxic drugs.

Administer intravenous fluid therapy.
- **Weigh the cat prior to fluid therapy** and monitor weight throughout treatment. Weight is one of the most important markers of hydration status. **Daily weight loss of 0.5–1% is expected in anorexic animals**, and this should be taken into account when judging hydration based on weight.
- Establish a **jugular catheter** if possible. This will facilitate fluid therapy, repetitive blood sampling and measurement of central venous pressure.
  - If direct measurement of central venous pressure is not possible, **observe the jugular veins.** Progressive distention of these veins and/or increase in the jugular pulse indicates rising central venous pressure. The medial saphenous veins may also be observed while the hind legs are raised and lowered. **Decreased emptying and increased refilling of the medial saphenous veins indicates volume expansion**.

Monitor for changes in respiratory pattern and auscultate lungs frequently for evidence of pulmonary edema. Observe extremities and intermandibular space for subcutaneous edema.

- Normal saline, lactated Ringer's or other balanced electrolyte solutions.
  - Rehydration. The goal of initial fluid therapy is to **correct dehydration and achieve 3–5% volume** expansion. Replace fluid deficits over 4–6 hours. An initial fluid bolus may be given in an effort to overcome renal arteriolar vasoconstriction. Use **10 ml/kg over 10 minutes in cats with anuria** or rapidly progressive oliguria, and **7–10 ml/kg/h for 4–6 hours** if there is increased concern for pulmonary edema or oliguria is less severe.

The goal of fluid therapy after rehydration is to **maintain 3–5% volume expansion above normal hydration**. More aggressive fluid therapy will not "flush out" or "open up" the kidneys, and overzealous treatment will result in pulmonary edema. Fluid rate must be adjusted based on body weight, central venous pressure, PCV and total protein levels and urine output.

- In cats with anuria or oliguria, place a urinary catheter and attach to a closed collection bag. **Always palpate the bladder** whenever checking urine production because the **catheter may kink**. The **urine should be cultured periodically** to monitor for urinary tract infection.
- In cats with polyuria, while a urinary catheter may be used, frequent palpation of the bladder and measurement of voided urine by weighing the litter pan is usually adequate to estimate urine production.

Monitor electrolytes and acid–base status (initially three times daily) and adjust fluids accordingly.

- **Hyperkalemia** is a potentially life-threatening complication of acute renal failure. Signs of significant hyperkalemia include bradycardia and weakness, which may progress to shock and a moribund state. ECG findings include loss of P waves, spiked T waves, and shortened Q–T interval.
- **Mild hyperkalemia** (above reference range to 6.5 mEq/L) may not require immediate treatment. If no clinical signs are present, one or more of the following treatments will usually suffice: reducing potassium concentration in the fluids, changing fluids to a more alkalinizing fluid, adding 5% dextrose to the fluids, and furosemide (see below).

- **Moderate hyperkalemia** (6.5–8.0 mEq/L) should always be treated promptly.
- **Severe hyperkalemia** (> 8.0 mEq/L) **may be life-threatening** and usually requires aggressive treatment. The higher the potassium level and the worse the clinical signs, the more rapid and aggressive should be the treatment. Treatments include:
  - **Dilution of potassium concentration** by rapid infusion of intravenous fluids (60 ml/kg/h). Potassium-free solutions have the most dilutional effect. Saline is beneficial for this reason although it is acidifying. Note that life-threatening hyperkalemia in acute renal failure is most likely to occur in anuric animals, which may not tolerate a large fluid bolus.
  - **Protect the heart** against the membrane effects of hyperkalemia with 10% calcium gluconate, 0.5–1.0 ml/kg IV, over 5–15 minutes. This should be given if there is a life-threatening arrhythmia. Monitor the ECG during therapy.
  - **Translocate** potassium from the blood into the intracellular fluid. Usually only one of the following treatments is necessary.
  - **NaHCO$_3$**, 0.5 mEq/kg IV over 5 minutes, followed by another 0.5 mEq/kg over the next 30–60 minutes. This treatment is best reserved for cats with HCO$_3^-$ or total CO$_2$ < 12 mmol/L, if measurements are available.
  - **Dextrose:** Severe hyperkalemia or moderate hyperkalemia with clinical signs – give 50% dextrose, 1.0–2.0 ml/kg IV (ideally diluted 1:1 with sterile water or saline), over 30–60 minutes. Moderate hyperkalemia without clinical signs – add 5–10% dextrose to the fluids (100–200 ml 50% dextrose/L). Monitor blood glucose. Note that dextrose may also serve as a diuretic.
  - **Insulin-dextrose:** regular insulin 0.1–0.5 units/kg IV followed by 2–4 ml of 50% dextrose/unit of insulin given (ideally diluted 1:1 with sterile water or saline) and then followed by adding 2.5% dextrose to the fluids (50 ml of 50% dextrose/L of fluids). Monitor blood glucose. Note that NaHCO$_3$ and dextrose should be avoided if effective serum osmolality is > 330 mOsm/kg. (Effective osmolality is calculated as [1.86(Na$^+$ + K$^+$)] + glucose + 9, with all units in mmol/L.) If the cat is hyperosmolar and dehydrated, increase the fluid rate. If dextrose therapy is needed, then it is best used in conjunction with insulin to minimize exacerbation of hyperosmolality.
  - Enhance potassium secretion. Give furosemide as discussed below. This may be used in the management of mild hyperkalemia, or subsequent to emergency management of moderate to severe hyperkalemia, but it will not act rapidly enough to correct hyperkalemia that is causing clinical signs, especially in the presence of oliguria or anuria where the drug may not promote urine production.

Diuretics.
  - **If anuria or oliguria persists after fluid replacement**, administer **furosemide** 2 mg/kg. If diuresis does not occur within 30 minutes, repeat once. Furosemide will not improve glomerular filtration rate, but diuresis **may reduce tubular blockage and tubular back-leak,** and a polyuric animal is easier to manage than an oliguric one. If diuresis does occur, treatment may be given two to three times a day if needed to maintain diuresis. Fluid requirements will be increased. Constant-rate infusions of furosemide have been used in the management of acute renal failure in dogs but there is limited experience with cats. Constant rate infusions of furosemide at 0.25 mg/kg/h have been used in the management of congestive heart failure in cats and may be considered in the management of acute renal failure.
- Osmotic diuretics.
  - **If furosemide fails to induce a diuresis**, consider using **10–20% dextrose** as an osmotic diuretic, **25–50 ml/kg over 1–2 hours**. Monitor urine for glucosuria indicating adequate dosage. Diuresis should occur within 60 minutes of completing infusion. If diuresis results, the treatment may be repeated every 8–12 hours.
  - Mannitol may also be used as an osmotic diuretic at a dose of **0.25–0.5 g/kg over 10 minutes.** Diuresis should occur within 60 minutes of completing infusion. If diuresis results, the treatment may be repeated every 4–6 hours. Mannitol is a more potent osmotic agent than dextrose, but can **only be eliminated by renal excretion**, and carries a **higher risk of causing pulmonary edema**.

- **Osmotic diuretics should not be used in the presence of hyperosmolality** (e.g. ethylene glycol poisoning, diabetic ketoacidosis), dehydration or overhydration.

Monitor urea, creatinine and phosphorus levels (initially once daily).

- **A rapid fall in serum urea and creatinine levels** in the first 24–48 hours of fluid therapy indicates that there was a substantial **pre-renal component** to azotemia. Mild decreases in urea and creatinine levels during the following week are usually due to mild ongoing volume expansion and the cat should be watched closely for over-hydration. **Decreases in urea and creatinine levels due to improved renal function usually take 10–14 days** to appear. After renal function improves and then stabilizes, fluids may be tapered. Urea and creatinine levels will rise when fluids are tapered.

Obtain minimum blood sample sizes. Frequent blood sampling may lead to anemia and hypoproteinemia that will affect use of PCV and total protein values to monitor hydration. Anemia may require correction by transfusion.

Dopamine is not recommended as its effects are uncertain in cats and its benefit in acute renal failure in humans is being questioned.

Antiemetics. Prochlorperazine, chlorpromazine, yohimbine, metoclopramide and ondansetron may be used to control vomiting. Metoclopramide is a less effective antiemetic in the cat than in the dog. It is eliminated via the kidney so an initial dose of 0.2 mg/kg, SC, twice daily is recommended (dose range 0.2–0.5 mg/kg three times a day). It may also be given by constant rate infusion at a dose of 0.005–0.02 mg/kg/h (lower end of the range recommended initially). Prochlorperazine and chlorpromazine may cause hypotension.

Gastrointestinal protectants. Ranitidine and famotidine (H2 blockers) are eliminated via the kidney (about 2/3–3/4 of the dose) so an initial dose of 0.5 mg/kg IV once daily is recommended. Sulcralfate 0.25–0.5 g PO three times a day may be used if it does not increase vomiting.

Nutritional support. This may include **nasoesophageal or esophageal feeding** in cats that are not vomiting, and parenteral nutrition.

Opioid **analgesics** should be considered at standard doses for cats with swollen and painful kidneys or oral ulceration.

Peritoneal dialysis, pleural dialysis, hemodialysis or transplantation should be considered for cats with anuria or severe oliguria.

Prognosis

There are few reports of acute renal failure in cats due to causes other than ethylene glycol or lily poisoning (see below). Most cats with hemodynamically mediated non-oliguric acute renal failure and cats with pyelonephritis will probably recover with appropriate critical care, but may have **residual or worsened chronic renal failure.** In general, the prognosis for non-oliguric renal failure is better than for oliguric or anuric renal failure. Without dialysis, the **prognosis is typically considered poor if there is persistent oliguria or anuria**.

Prevention

Minimize prolonged renal hypoperfusion. Correct fluid deficits and hypotension promptly in cats with chronic renal failure.

Begin intravenous fluids preoperatively in elderly cats undergoing surgery, to prevent acute exacerbation of chronic renal failure.

Minimize exposure to ethylene glycol and lilies. Use aminoglycosides and other nephrotoxic drugs judiciously and avoid in elderly cats and in cats with chronic renal failure.

ACUTE POISONING AND EVENOMATION*

Classical signs

- Acute depression.
- Other specific signs: weakness, tremor, GIT signs.

See main reference on page 594 for details (The Cat With Salivation) and page 481 (The Bleeding Cat) and page 381 (The Pyrexic Cat), page 812 (The Cat With Seizures, Circling and/or Changed Behavior for bromethalin, lead, methaldehyde, strychnine, organo-phosphates, carbamates, organochlorines, pyrethrins, pyrethroids), page 833 (The Cat With Stupor or Coma for lead), page 850 (The Cat With a Head Tilt, Vestibular Ataxia or Nystagmus for blue-tailed lizard), page 861 (The Cat With Tremor or Twitching for hexachlorophene, organophosphate) and pages 947, 950 (The Cat With Generalized Weakness for OP, snakes, spiders, ticks).

Clinical signs

Acute depression and anorexia are signs of most poisonings and envenomations and are not listed with every poison below. Other common signs include hypersalivation, vomiting, diarrhea, polypnea, arrhythmias, pale mucous membranes, hypothermia, tremors (which may cause hyperthermia), excitability, agitation and other behavior changes, seizures, and generalized weakness.

Rodenticides.
- **Anticoagulants:** signs include pale mucous membranes and signs referable to localized bleeding. Acute depression may be the only initial sign of internal bleeding, occurring prior to pale mucous membranes. See page 522, The Bleeding Cat.
- **Cholecalciferol:** signs include vomiting, diarrhea and polydipsia.
- **Bromethalin:** signs include mydriasis, paresis, tremors, hyperthermia, excitability and seizures.
- **Strychnine:** signs include muscle stiffness, extensor rigidity and opisthotonus, and tetanic seizures that may be initiated by physical, visual or auditory stimulation.

Anthelmintics.
- **Ivermectin:** signs include tremors, abnormal behavior, ataxia, blindness, bradycardia, hypothermia, seizures and coma.
- **Piperazine:** signs include weakness, tremors, ataxia, behavior changes, seizures and vomiting and diarrhea.

Insecticides.
- **Organophosphates and carbamates:** signs variably include systemic **parasympathetic** (muscarinic) signs (salivation, lacrimation, urination, defecation, miosis, dyspnea, bradycardia); **sympathetic** (ganglionic) signs (tachycardia, mydriasis); **neuromuscular** (nicotinic) signs (muscle stiffness, tremors, weakness, paralysis); and **CNS cholinergic signs** (hyperactivity, seizures, marked depres-

sion). Chlorpyrifos may cause a delayed toxicosis characterized by cervical ventroflexion and marked hind limb ataxia.
- **Pyrethrins, pyrethroids (phenothrin, etofenprox, and especially permethrin) and rotenone:** signs include hypersalivation, vomiting and agitation from oral irritation and tremors, ataxia, and seizures from systemic toxicoses.
- **Organochlorines (e.g. lindane):** signs include ataxia, tremors and seizures.

Slug and snail bait.
- **Metaldehyde:** signs include hypersalivation, vomiting, diarrhea, tachycardia, polypnea, mydriasis, ataxia, excitability, hyperesthesia and marked muscle tremors progressing to convulsions, with resultant hyperthermia.

Analgesics.
- **Acetaminophen:** signs include depression, anorexia, salivation, vomiting, abdominal pain, polypnea, dark mucous membranes, edema of the face and paws, and dark discolored urine. See page 595, The Cat With Salivation.
- **Aspirin:** signs include hematemesis, melena, polypnea and fever.
- **Ibuprofen** and other non-selective NSAIDs: signs include depression, hematemesis, melena, diarrhea, abdominal pain, polydipsia (renal failure), and seizures and coma with very high doses.

Plants (partial list).
- **Lilies:** signs are described in a separate heading below.
- **Marijuana:** signs include acute depression, ataxia, hypothermia and polyphagia.
- **Azaleas and oleander:** signs include arrhythmias, shock and acute heart failure.
- **Daffodils:** signs include vomiting, hypothermia, hypotension and bradycardia.
- Many other plants result in oropharyngeal and gastrointestinal irritation. **English ivy (*Hedera helix*)** and *Cyclamen* species may cause severe, potentially life-threatening, vomiting (including hematemesis) and diarrhea.
- **Pine** (water in Christmas tree reservoir): signs include vomiting, abdominal pain and icterus.

Heavy metals.
- **Lead:** Anorexia may be the only sign. Other signs include vomiting, diarrhea, abdominal pain, excitability, seizures and blindness.

Miscellaneous.

- **Ethylene glycol:** signs are described in separate headings below.
  - **Venlafaxine** is a human antidepressant medication (serotonin and noradrenaline reuptake inhibitor). It is an emerging toxicosis in that it is one of the few human medications that cats voluntarily ingest. Clinical signs include vomiting, polypnea, tachycardia, ataxia, mydriasis and agitation.
  - **Glow-in-the-dark items** contain dibutyl (n-butyl) phthalate as a luminescent. It is extremely unpalatable and when a cat bites into a glow-in-the-dark item it causes marked hypersalivation, frothing, head-shaking, agitation, hyperactivity, aggression and other behavioral changes. The luminescent is of low toxicity and a sufficient quantity to cause systemic toxicosis would not be ingested.
  - **Liquid potpourri** causes poisoning when there is accidental skin contact and the product is licked off. The product may contain essential oils (irritants and central nervous system depressants), and/or cationic detergents (corrosives) that cause more severe signs. Cutaneous and oral cavity signs vary from erythema to ulceration. Marked hyperthermia may accompany oral inflammation and precede ulceration. Gastrointestinal signs include dysphagia (esophagitis) and vomiting, hematemesis, melena, and abdominal pain (gastritis). Esophageal and gastrointestinal ulceration and perforation may occur.

Envenomation.

- **Tick bite paralysis:** Cats do not appear to be affected by North American ticks. *Ixodes holocyclus* in Australia causes rapidly progressive motor weakness, megaesophagus, mydriasis, tachyarrhythmias and dyspnea (various causes).
- **Spider bites:** *Latrodectus* spp. (black widow spider in North America, red back spider in Australia) live in warm and temperature regions in all continents. Cats are very sensitive to the venom. Signs of envenomation include loud vocalization from pain; restlessness and polypnea; salivation, vomiting and diarrhea; and muscle tremors and spasms that progress to flaccid paralysis.
- **Wasp and bee stings:** Local angioedema and pain are common signs. Anaphylaxis is rare.

- **Toad poisoning:** *Bufo marinus* (cane toad) is found mostly in South America, southeast United States and Hawaii, and Australia. *Bufo alvarius* is found is the southwest United States and northern Mexico. Signs of poisoning include profuse salivation, vomiting, arrhythmias, hindlimb weakness, a fixed trance-like stare and collapse.
- **Poisonous lizards:** Gila monster (*Heloderma suspectum*) and Mexican beaded lizard (*Heloderma horridum*) are found in the southwest United States and Mexico. Envenomation occurs during a tenacious bite with chewing action. Signs of envenomation include painful bite wound, salivation, lacrimation, urination, defecation, and loss of voice. Ingestion of a blue-tailed lizard skink (*Eumece egregius*) found in the southeast United States may cause vestibular signs.

Diagnosis

History is often critical to the diagnosis of intoxication.

Definitive diagnosis can be made by measuring poisonous principles in vomitus, serum or urine.

Anticoagulant rodenticide: prolonged prothrombin, activated partial thromboplastin times, and activated clotting time.

Cholecalciferol rodenticide: hypercalcemia and hyperphosphatemia.

Black widow spider (*Latrodectus*) envenomation: marked elevation in creatinine kinase and aspartate aminotransferase, and myoglobinuria.

Differential diagnosis

Other causes of acute depression are differential diagnoses. Other differential diagnoses should be considered for the more specific signs (e.g. hypocalcemia as a cause of tremors).

Treatment

The most effective treatments vary with the toxin, and **consultation with a toxicology service** is recommended.

Minimize further absorption (cutaneous and gastrointestinal decontamination).

- Bath the cat if there is poison on the skin (e.g. permethrin)
- Remove the source of the poison.
- **Irrigate oral cavity** if there is poison in the mouth (e.g. after mouthing a *Bufo* toad). If clinical signs are due to unpleasant taste or oral irritation (hypersalivation, agitation +/– vomiting) after milk or liquid from a can of tuna.
- **Induction of emesis. Xylazine** 0.44 mg/kg IM reliably causes vomiting in 5–20 minutes. The effect can be reversed with yohimbine 0.1–0.5 mg/kg IV. If xylazine is not available, or for induction of vomiting at home, use fresh 3% **hydrogen peroxide**, 2 ml/kg PO, or syrup of **ipecac**, 3–6 ml/kg diluted 1:1 with water, PO or by gavage (i.e. via stomach tube). Vomiting should occur within 10–30 minutes. Hydrogen peroxide and syrup of ipecac treatments may be repeated once if the initial treatment is ineffective.
- **Induction of emesis is absolutely contraindicated** in the presence of a caustic or volatile poison, impaired gag reflex, laryngeal paralysis, extreme weakness or unconsciousness, and is relatively contraindicated in the presence of seizures or dyspnea.
- **If induction of emesis is ineffective or contraindicated**, perform **gastric lavage**. Establish light general anesthesia if the cat is not unconscious and place a cuffed endotracheal tube extending 2–3 cm beyond the teeth. Position the cat with the head and thorax slightly lowered. Pass a tube the same size or slightly larger than the endotracheal tube into the stomach, deliver 5–10 ml/kg tepid water, and aspirate with a 60 ml syringe or aspiration bulb. Repeat the procedure 10–15 times. Kink the stomach tube as it is removed from the stomach. Addition of activated charcoal at the dose below to the lavage solution will increase its effectiveness.
- Solid poisons (e.g. lead) may be removed by **endoscopy** or **gastrotomy/enterotomy**.
- **Absorption of remaining poison.** Give a slurry of **activated charcoal** by gavage, 1–5 g/kg dissolved in 3–5 ml of tepid water/g charcoal, after induction of emesis or when gastric lavage is complete. Treatment may need to be repeated every 4–6 hours for 2–3 days because the poison may return to the intestinal tract by enterohepatic circulation.

Activated charcoal is an effective absorbent for many poisons including vitamin K antagonist rodenticides, ethylene glycol, alkaloids, organophosphate and other insecticides, acetylsalicylic acid, NSAIDS and barbiturates. It is not effective with most caustic or corrosive agents.

- **Catharsis** is used to promote elimination of the toxin in the stool. It should always be used following the use of activated charcoal and should not be used in the presence of diarrhea. Catharsis may have to be repeated every 4–6 hours as with activated charcoal. Catharsis using non-absorbed salts or sugars will cause dehydration that must be addressed with fluid therapy.
  - Salts: s**odium sulfate** (Glauber's salts, preferred) or **magnesium sulfate** (Epsom salts), 1/2 level teaspoon per kg in 5–10 volumes of tepid water, by gavage. Magnesium sulfate may cause central nervous system depression, should not be repeated, and must be used cautiously in renal failure. These salts are the preferred cathartics in lead poisoning as lead will precipitate as unabsorbable lead sulfate.
  - **Sugars: sorbitol 70% solution** (preferred) or **lactulose**, 3 ml/kg. The **most practical product** to use in the non-specific treatment of poisoning is a commercial product that combines activated charcoal and sorbitol in a suspension.
  - **Colonic lavage** ("high enema"), 20 ml/kg tepid water.

Enhance elimination.

- **Diuresis**. Diuresis will hasten renal elimination of a toxin only if it is reabsorbed by the renal tubules, e.g. ethylene glycol. Diuresis may be achieved with fluid therapy, furosemide, mannitol or dextrose (see Acute renal failure, page 282).
- **Ion trapping**. A toxin must be unionized to be reabsorbed by the renal tubules. Elimination of **acidic toxins** (e.g. aspirin) may be hastened by alkalinizing the urine using sodium bicarbonate. Elimination of **alkaline toxins** (e.g. strychnine) may be hastened by acidifying the urine using saline or ammonium chloride.
- Peritoneal dialysis or hemodialysis.

Specific therapy.

- **Anticoagulant rodenticide** – vitamin K (see page 509, The Bleeding Cat).

- Cholecalciferol rodenticide – treatment of hypercalcemia (saline, furosemide, calcitonin, prednisone, ± biphosphonates).
- Organophosphates and carbamates – atropine (both), pralidoxime chloride (organophosphates only).
- Acetaminophen – acetylcysteine, ascorbic acid, transfusion (see page 596, The Cat With Salivation).
- Aspirin and NSAIDs – Treatment of gastric ulceration (H2 blockers, sulcralfate), treatment of acute renal injury with fluids.
- Lilies – see separate heading below.
- Lead – CaNa$_2$EDTA, D-penicillamine (contraindicated if lead present in intestinal tract), succimer (preferred treatment).
- Ethylene glycol – see separate heading below.
- Venlafaxine – cyproheptadine 2–4 mg/cat PO or per rectum may counteract serotonin effects.
- Ixodid tick paralysis and *Lactrodectus* spider bites – specific antivenin (see pages 954, 975, The Cat With Generalized Weakness).

Treat arrhythmias, e.g. atropine for daffodil-induced bradycardia (**see page 160, The Cat With Tachycardia, Bradycardia or an Irregular Rhythm**).

Treat tremors and seizures – diazepam, methocarbamol, phenobarbital, pentobarbital (**see page 801, The Cat With Seizures, Circling, and/or Changed Behavior**). Beware of hypothermia following correction of hyperthermia, which may cause renewed tremors.

Treat agitation – consider acepromazine (ensure cat is not hypotensive).

Supportive care.

ETHYLENE GLYCOL POISONING*

Classical signs

- Acute depression and anorexia.

Pathogenesis

Ethylene glycol is a solvent used in paints, polishes, inks and antifreeze, which is the most common source of poisoning. It is a colorless liquid – the yellow-green appearance of antifreeze is due to the addition of fluorescein.

It tastes sweet to humans, and is palatable to cats. The **minimum lethal dose of undiluted ethylene glycol in cats is only 1.4 ml/kg.**

Ethylene glycol is **rapidly absorbed from the intestinal tract**.

- **Peak plasma concentration is achieved 1 hour post ingestion** in a fasted cat. Food probably delays peak plasma concentrations, but by at most 1–2 hours.

Following absorption, ethylene glycol is excreted about **50% unchanged in the urine** (peak urine concentration is achieved at 6 hours). Some passive reabsorption occurs in the distal convoluted tubules and collecting ducts. The other **50% is metabolized in the liver** by alcohol dehydrogenase to glycoaldehyde, which in turn is metabolized by aldehyde dehydrogenase to glycolic acid. Glycolic acid is further metabolized to glyoxylic acid, which is then metabolized to final metabolites including **oxalic acid.** Oxalic acid combines with calcium to form **calcium oxalate crystals**. The serum half-life of ethylene glycol in untreated cats is 2–5 hours.

- Acute tubular necrosis is caused by **cytotoxic effects of glycolic, glyoxalic and oxalic acids**. Deposition of crystals in the kidneys has a minor role.

Clinical signs

Signs of **acute ethylene glycol poisoning** (<12 hours) are due to direct effects of the poison and metabolites on the central nervous system and gastrointestinal tract, and include **depression, ataxia, tremors, vomiting, and a sweet odor to the breath. Polyuria** occurs due to osmotic diuresis. Polydipsia is uncommon in cats.

Later signs (> 12 hours) are due to acute renal failure and include progressive depression, anorexia, oral ulceration, hypothermia, painful and swollen kidneys, seizures, oliguria and anuria.

Diagnosis

The **diagnosis** of acute poisoning **relies on history of ingestion or a high index of suspicion**.

- Acute ethylene glycol poisoning should be considered in **any cat at risk with acute depression.**

A **hemogram** typically reveals hemoconcentration and a stress leukogram.

A **serum biochemistry** profile will reveal **decreased bicarbonate (total CO_2)** and an **increased anion gap**. Blood gases, if available, will reveal **severe metabolic acidosis** with or without partial respiratory compensation. Measured osmolality, if available, will be increased in parallel with ethylene glycol concentration, resulting in an increased **osmolal gap**. Other variable findings are **hyperglycemia** (stress and reduced metabolism by aldehydes), **hypocalcemia** (chelation by oxalic acid), and **hypophosphatemia** (binding by rust-inhibitors in antifreeze). In the later stage of poisoning serum chemistry findings are typical of acute renal failure.

Urinalysis will reveal persistent **isosthenuria to minimally concentrated urine** and aciduria within 3 hours of ingestion. **Oxalate crystals** are usually present at some point during the acute phase of intoxication, and may appear as early as 3 hours. Glucosuria and proteinuria may be present. A **Wood's lamp** may be used in an effort to detect **fluorescence** from fluorescein in stomach contents and on the muzzle and paws. However numerous products contain fluorescents and absence of fluorescence does not rule-out exposure, so the diagnostic utility of fluorescence may be limited. Similarly examination of urine for fluorescence is likely of limited values as cat's urine normally fluoresces and a potential increase in fluorescence from a small amount of excreted fluorescein may be difficult to detect.

Definitive diagnosis can be made by **measuring ethylene glycol in serum or urine**, but cats are very sensitive to ethylene glycol poisoning and may develop signs at concentrations below that detected by the assays. Serum is preferred because concentration of the poison is higher than in urine. Ethylene glycol is usually not detectable in serum or urine after 72 hours. Propylene glycol (present in diazepam injection) causes a false positive reaction in some assays.

Ultrasound may reveal hyperechoic renal cortices. The kidney may feel very firm when advancing a percutaneous biopsy needle.
- **Kidney biopsy** will reveal acute tubular necrosis, with the presence of oxalate crystals.

Differential diagnosis

Both ethylene glycol and **lily intoxication** cause acute depression and acute renal failure. The laboratory features of lily poisoning have not been as well characterized as those of ethylene glycol poisoning therefore it is difficult to use these to differentiate the two poisonings. **Ethylene glycol poisoning** is more **likely in outdoor cats and lily poisoning in indoor cats.** Vomiting is more consistent in lily poisoning and there is evidence of plants being chewed. Detectable serum or urine **concentrations of ethylene glycol, oxalate crystalluria, and oxalates on kidney biopsy are diagnostic for ethylene glycol poisoning**. If these findings are absent, other causes of acute renal failure must be ruled out.
- Both cats with **pancreatitis** and cats with acute ethylene glycol poisoning may have acute depression with or without vomiting, but cats with acute ethylene glycol poisoning will be **isosthenuric**, while cats with **acute pancreatitis should have well-concentrated urine**. Azotemia, metabolic acidosis, increased anion gap and increased osmolal gap will be more severe than in pancreatitis. Definitive diagnosis relies on measuring ethylene glycol in serum or urine or seeing **oxalate crystals** in urine or a kidney biopsy.
- Both ethylene glycol poisoning and **diabetic ketoacidosis** may cause acute depression, polyuria, vomiting, dehydration, hyperglycemia, azotemia, increased anion gap metabolic acidosis, and increased osmolality. The former is confirmed by detecting ethylene glycol in serum or oxalate crystals and the latter by **detecting ketones in the blood or urine**. Ethylene glycol poisoning invariably causes acute renal failure (unless treated within 3 hours), while acute renal failure is an uncommon complication of diabetic ketoacidosis, although cats with diabetic ketoacidosis may have concurrent chronic renal failure.

Ethanol ingestion may cause depression, polyuria, ataxia and increased osmolality. Diagnosis relies on history of ingestion and **measurement of ethanol in the serum.**

Certain abnormalities in the acute phase of ethylene glycol poisoning (depression, tremors, hypocalcemia) may resemble acute hypoparathyroidism. Other historical and physical abnormalities, and the presence of hyperphosphatemia in the latter, will distinguish the two.

Treatment

Immediate **induction of emesis and activated charcoal or gastric lavage** if ingestion is witnessed. Ethylene glycol is rapidly absorbed and intestinal decontamination is unlikely to be of any benefit after two hours or once clinical signs have appeared.

Prevent ethylene glycol metabolism. This may be achieved using either ethanol or fomepizole as competitive inhibitors of alcohol dehydrogenase. Treatment must be initiated within 3 hours of ingestion to prevent acute renal failure. The unmetabolized ethylene glycol is eliminated via the kidneys.

- Cats are usually treated with **ethanol;** several protocols exist. Prepare 20% (20 g/100 ml, 200 mg/ml) ethanol my mixing 1 part of 95–100% ethanol with 4 parts saline. (An alternative is to mix 1 part vodka [40% ethanol] with 1 part saline.) Give 3 ml/kg 20% ethanol (600 mg/kg) over 1 hour further diluted to a minimum of 1 part 20% solution and 2 parts saline for a final ≈7% maximum concentration solution. (Additional dilution is needed in these protocols as the ethanol solutions are hyperosmolar). This is followed by a constant rate infusion of 20% ethanol, 0.5 ml/kg/hr (100 mg/kg/hr), in a minimum of 2 ml/kg/hr saline (again for a final ≈7% maximum concentration). (The dose may be increased with close monitoring up to 1.0 ml [200 mg]/kg/hr in 4 ml/kg/hr fluids.) Treatment is continued for 10 hours after a negative serum ethylene glycol test, or 18 hours after correction of metabolic acidosis without ongoing need for $NaHCO_3$ treatment. An alternative protocol is to give 5 mL/kg 20% ethanol, diluted into IV fluids, by constant rate infusion over 6 hours for 5 treatments, then over 8 hours for 4 treatments. (The serum half-life of ethylene glycol for cats receiving ethanol is 29 hours.)
- **Begin IV fluids** (do not use Ringer's or lactated Ringer's) **at 1.5–3 times maintenance** based on patient requirements and adjusted to account for volume delivered with ethanol solutions. Monitor hydration status, body weight, and urine output; observe respiration and auscultate lungs frequently to monitor for pulmonary edema.
- Ideally **measure serum ethanol concentrations** and maintain at 100 mg/dL. **Treatment will increase central nervous system depression and serum osmolality.** The cat may become comatose during therapy. Observe very closely for life-threatening respiratory depression, which should prompt reduction of ethanol treatmet. Monitor body temperature and rewarm if hypothermia develops.
- Ideally monitor **acid-base status.** If pH < 7.25 and/or $HCO_3^- $ < 8 mmol/L, give $NaHCO_3$ (mmol = 0.2 × kg × base deficit) over 4 hours IV. Repeat as necessary.
- **If intravenous therapy is not possible**, give the ethanol doses above intraperitoneally, and additional fluids subcutaneously.
  - If the cat cannot be hospitalized immediately for ethanol therapy, the owner can attempt to give a **40% alcoholic beverage by mouth** (e.g. rum, vodka), 2.5 ml/kg, although a cat is less likely to tolerate this than a dog.
- **Fomepizole (4-methylpyrazole)** is the treatment of choice in dogs. The drug causes minimal central nervous system depression and does not increase serum osmolality or metabolic acidosis. Although initially considered ineffective in cats, recent studies suggest that higher doses are effective.
  - Give 125 mg/kg 5% solution IV initial dose, followed by 31.25 mg/kg IV at 12, 24 and 36 hours post-ingestion. The dose should be given over 15–30 minutes.

Multiple B-vitamins containing pyridoxine and thiamine may enhance the metabolism of glyoxylic acid to non-toxic metabolites and protect the nervous system during ethanol therapy. Compatability of B-vitamins with ethanol solutions is not known, so administration via a separate IV line is recommended.

See Acute renal failure, above.
- Most ingestion is not witnessed, and, without dialysis, the prognosis for cats with oliguric or anuric renal failure is grave. Hemodialysis has been used successfully to support cats through oliguric and anuric renal failure until tubular regeneration occurred. **Peritoneal dialysis** may be considered, especially if oliguria has not progressed to anuria, as the chances for recovery of renal function are perhaps somewhat better with oliguria than with anuria.
- **Renal transplantation** may be considered in cats with oliguric or anuric renal failure.

LILY POISONING*

Classical signs

- Acute depression and anorexia.
- Vomiting.

Pathogenesis

Lily poisoning is caused by ingestion of plants in the genera *Lilium* and *Hemerocallis,* and all plants within these genera should be considered potentially toxic. Plants with proven toxicity include the Easter lily (*L. longiflorum*), tiger lily (*L. tigrinum*), rubrum lily (*L. speciosum*), Japanese show lily (*L. lancifolium*), *Lilium* hybrids and daylilies (all *Hemerocallis* spp.). Calla lilies (*Zantedeschia aethiopia*) and peace lilies (*Spathyphyllum wallis*) are not toxic.

Leaves, flowers and stems are toxic; only small quantities have to be ingested to result in intoxication. The flowers are most toxic.

The toxic principles have not been fully characterized and it is not known if *Lilium* and *Hemerocallis* toxins are the same.

Poisoning results in acute renal failure, which initially is non-oliguric.

Dehydration appears to be a critical factor in the progression of non-oliguric to oliguric renal failure.

Clinical signs

Signs of **acute lily poisoning** (< 24 hours) are probably due to direct effects of the uncharacterized poison and include **depression, anorexia, polyuria with or without polydipsia, hypersalivation and acute vomiting.** Hypersalivation and vomiting typically **begin within 3 hours of ingestion and lasts for 4–6 hours**. Cases have been presented without a history of vomiting. Polyuria typically begins within 12–30 hours and lasts for 12–24 hours. Ataxia, tremors and seizures have also been reported .

Later signs (> 24 hours) are due to acute renal failure and include persistent depression and anorexia, hypothermia, recurrent vomiting, painful and swollen kidneys, and polyuria, oliguria or anuria.

Diagnosis

The diagnosis of acute poisoning relies on history of ingestion or a high index of suspicion.

- Acute lily poisoning should be considered in any cat at risk with acute depression and vomiting. Indoor cats with access to newly introduced plants are at highest risk.
- Vomitus should be examined for plant material. Plants should be examined for evidence of having been chewed.

A **hemogram** typically reveals hemoconcentration and a stress leukogram.

Acid-base and osmolality values in the acute phase of poisoning have not been well characterized. In the later phase of poisoning serum chemistry findings are typical of acute renal failure, but there may be a **disproportionate elevation in creatinine compared to urea. Liver enzyme and creatinine kinase values may also increase.**

Urinalysis will reveal **isosthenuria to minimally concentrated urine.** Glucosuria and proteinuria may be present.

Ultrasound may reveal **hyperechoic renal cortices.** The kidney may feel very firm when advancing a percutaneous biopsy needle.

Kidney biopsy will reveal acute tubular necrosis and intact basement membranes. Low numbers of birefringent crystals may be present.

Differential diagnosis

Other causes of acute renal failure.

Other causes of **acute vomiting.**

- Both cats with **acute pancreatitis** and cats with acute lily poisoning may have acute depression and vomiting, but cats with **lily poisoning** will have **minimally concentrated urine**, while cats with acute pancreatitis should have **well-concentrated urine** unless there is a concurrent disorder causing dilute urine, such as chronic renal failure.

Treatment

Induction of emesis, activated charcoal and **catharsis** if recent ingestion.

Prompt intravenous fluid therapy. This is critical for a good prognosis.

Dehydration is an important mechanism in the development of renal failure. Prompt initiation of intravenous fluids will halt progression of non-oliguric to oliguric/anuric renal failure and hasten recovery. Deliver **fluids at 2–3 times maintenance** for a minimum of 24 hours (48 hours preferred).

Gastrointestinal decontamination and intravenous fluid therapy within 6 hours of ingestion is likely to prevent renal failure. If such treatment is delayed for more than 18–24 hours, acute renal failure will likely occur.

If renal failure occurs, see Acute renal failure, above.
- Hemodialysis and peritoneal dialysis have been used to support cats through oliguric/anuric renal failure until tubular regeneration occurs. Without dialysis, the prognosis for oliguric/anuric renal failure is grave. Cats with non-oliguric acute renal failure may develop chronic renal failure.

SNAKE BITE ENVENOMATION*

Classical signs

- Flaccid paresis/paralysis with mydriasis (most Elapidae, some Crotalidae and Viperidae snakes).
- Bleeding tendency (some Elapidae and Viperidae snakes).
- Bite wound on cranial half of body ± local swelling or bleeding (Viperidae snakes).

See main reference on page 950 for details (The Cat With Generalized Weakness).

Clinical signs

Cats are less likely to be bitten than dogs.

Venoms from **Elapidae** snakes (all Australian snakes) are predominantly **neurotoxic**. Initial signs may be acute depression and weakness. More specific signs include areflexic dilated pupils, dysphagia (salivation), dyspnea (respiratory paralysis), hindlimb ataxia and flaccid quadraplegia. Local reaction to the bite is minimal, and the bite wound is rarely located. Some

Elapidae also have hematoxins that activate and deplete clotting factors resulting in bleeding, myotoxins that cause rhabdomyolysis, or hemolysins that cause intravascular hemolysis.

Venoms from **Viperidae** are predominantly **hematoxic**, although some have **neurotoxic properties. Edema ± bleeding/bruising around the bite is typical.**

Venoms from **Crotalidae** are predominantly **hematoxic**, although some are **potent neurotoxins**. Acute depression may occur from hypotension or neurotoxicity.

Venoms from most **Colubridae** are mild and clinical reports of bites to cats lacking.

Diagnosis

Diagnosis is based on **history of** possible **exposure** to a snake and physical examination findings.

CBC may reveal hemoconcentration, echinocytosis and thrombocytopenia. Serum chemistry profile may reveal hypokalemia and elevated CK, ALT, urea and creatinine levels. Urinalysis may reveal myoglobiunuria or hemoglobinuria and glucosuria.

Differential diagnosis

See The Cat With Generlized Weakness (page 952) and for differential diagnosis of neurologic signs and The Bleeding Cat (page 503) for differential diagnosis of hematologic signs.

Differential diagnoses for the local reaction include angioedema from insect envenomation, animal bite wounds, sharp and blunt trauma.

Treatment

Keep the animal calm.

Supportive care. See page 953, The Cat With Generalized Weakness.

Specific antivenin therapy.

Transfusions for clinically significant hemostatic or hematologic abnormalities.

ACUTE HEART FAILURE*

Classical signs

- Acute dyspnea.
- Lethargy and inappetence.

See main reference on page 124 for details (The Cat With Abnormal Heart Sounds and/or an Enlarged Heart).

Clinical signs

Acute onset of depression, anorexia and dyspnea. In severe cases, collapse may occur, especially if stressed.

Pulmonary crackles, a heart murmur, arrhythmia and/or weak pulses may be found on physical examination.

Some cats have a history of vomiting.

Diagnosis

Pulmonary edema and cardiomegaly are evident on radiographs. The radiographic appearance of pulmonary edema is variable in cats.

Furosemide may be given and radiographs repeated in one hour to see if the pulmonary changes have improved. Definitive diagnosis of cardiomyopathy requires echocardiography.

Differential diagnosis

Other causes of depression and dyspnea. See The Dyspneic or Tachypneic Cat (page 47).

Treatment

Furosemide and nitroglycerin ointment at standard dosages. See details of additional treatment page 130 (The Cat With Abnormal Heart Sounds and/or an Enlarged Heart).

DIABETIC KETOACIDOSIS*

Classical signs

- Polyuria, polydipsia, and weight loss.
- Recent onset of acute depression and anorexia.

See main reference on page 236 for details (The Cat With Polyuria and Polydipsia).

Clinical signs

Typically there is a history of **weight loss, polyuria and polydipsia**, together with a normal appetite or polyphagia in the preceding weeks or months prior to an acute onset of anorexia, vomiting, dehydration, and depression. Other signs that may be evident with the onset of depression include icterus and dyspnea.

Diagnosis

Diagnosis requires **demonstration of ketonemia or ketonuria, and hyperglycemia**. Ketones may be falsely negative in urine because urine test strips measure primarily oxaloacetate (and to a lesser extent acetone), which may be present in concentrations in urine below the limit of detection by the test strip in cats. Several drops of hydrogen peroxide may be added to the urine sample in an effort to convert β-hydroxybutyrate to oxaloacetate to increase the concentration of oxaloacetate in urine. Alternatively, β-hydroxybutyrate may be measured in serum using a point-of-care test, or the urine test strip may be used to detect oxaloacetate in heparinized plasma. Using a standard urine test strip, a **negative plasma test rules-out ketosis**, and a **positive urine test rules-in ketosis**, in cats. Finally, bicarbonate (total CO_2) concentrations in plasma may be used to demonstrate acidosis.

Differential diagnosis

Acute pancreatitis or sepsis (depression), hepatic lipidosis or cholangiohepatitis (depression and icterus), ethylene glycol or lily intoxication (depression and polyuria), acute heart failure (depression and dyspnea) may all cause vomiting and dehydration and appear similar to diabetic ketoacidosis.

Treatment

Intravenous fluids are required to correct dehydration and electrolyte imbalances.

Regular insulin should be administered using intravenous, intramuscular or subcutaneous administration protocols depending on the status of the cat's peripheral perfusion.

Appropriate antibiotics should be administered if urine has evidence of bacteria or inflammation. Many diabetic cats have urinary tract infection at the time of admission (culture urine).

NEOPLASIA*

Classical signs

- Usually chronic depression, anorexia and weight loss.
- Occasionally acute signs.

Clinical signs

Neoplasia **typically causes chronic signs**, but depending on location and growth rate, a **tumor may cause acute signs**, which may include acute depression, anorexia, and dehydration.

Diagnosis

Routine **history-taking, physical examination**, and **diagnostic work-up** is required to identify specific signs and localize organ involvement. Definitive diagnosis requires biopsy.

Differential diagnosis

Other causes of acute depression and anorexia.

Treatment

Surgery, radiation therapy, chemotherapy and other treatment modalities may be indicated, depending upon the neoplasm.

NUTRITIONAL SUPPORT

TOXOPLASMOSIS*

Classical signs

- Fever, anorexia and depression.
- Uveitis, dyspnea, icterus, or neurologic signs.

See main reference on page 432 for details (The Yellow Cat or Cat With Elevated Liver Enzymes), page 375 (The Pyrexic Cat).

Clinical signs

Cats of any age may be affected, but **70% of cats are less than 2 years of age**.

Toxoplasmosis may affect any organ system resulting in a wide variety of clinical signs. Uveitis, **pneumonia, hepatitis and encephalitis** are the most common syndromes. Most cats with systemic toxoplasmosis have a fever.

Lethargy, anorexia and fever are early signs.

Uveitis or other forms of intraocular inflammation are present in about 80% of cases.

Dyspnea is present in the majority of cats, and associated with increased respiratory sounds over the chest.

Abdominal signs may occur associated with hepatitis or pancreatitis and include abdominal pain on palpation, infrequent vomiting, and enlarged mesenteric lymph nodes.

Neurologic signs are more common in older cats.

Diagnosis

Acute systemic toxoplasmosis typically affects kittens, or immunosuppressed cats, which usually have a history of chronic disease.

Confirmation is **by measuring serum IgM antibodies or** demonstrating **rising serum IgG antibodies.**

The organism occasionally may be seen in airway wash cytology of cats with pneumonia.

Differential diagnosis

Rule out **other diseases** causing **acute lethargy, anorexia and fever**, which in the cat are usually **infectious causes**. Physical examination will often identify localizing signs, which can be pursued diagnostically.

Treatment

Clindamycin at standard doses (10–12 mg/kg orally q 12 h for 4 weeks).

Other drugs with potential efficacy include trimethoprim-sulfas, doxycycline, minocycline, azithromycin and clarithromycin.

UPALATABLE FOOD*

Classical signs

- Partial anorexia.

Pathogenesis

Change in diet to unpalatable food may precipitate total or partial anorexia.

Stale food or spoiled food may cause anorexia.

Clinical signs

Complete or partial anorexia.

Diagnosis

History of change in diet.

History of feeding from a large, slowly consumed bag of dry food, or providing several days of rations in one meal.

Ruling out other causes of anorexia.

Differential diagnosis

Other causes of depression and anorexia.

Treatment

Resume previous diet or offer other more palatable food.

Prognosis

Excellent provided anorexia is not protracted in obese cats resulting in hepatic lipidosis.

ALTERNATE FOOD SOURCE*

Classical signs

- Partial anorexia.

Pathogenesis

The cat has another food source in addition to its usual source, causing physiologic anorexia.

Clinical signs

Partial or complete anorexia is observed with respect to the cat's normal food source.

No weight loss or other signs of illness are apparent.

Diagnosis

Diagnosis is based on confirming that another food source is being used, e.g. neighbors, successful hunting.

Ruling out other causes of anorexia.

Differential diagnosis

Other causes of anorexia.

Treatment

Eliminate the alternate food source if indicated.

ENVIRONMENTAL STRESS*

Classical signs

- Inactivity and/or anorexia.

Pathogenesis

Hot weather may cause inactivity and withdrawal to cool locations.

Cold weather may cause withdrawal to warm locations.

The cat may not be eating because of discomfort or because of inactivity and withdrawal.

Clinical signs

Variable withdrawal, inactivity, anorexia and dehydration.

During hot weather periods the cat may be more active than usual at night when it is cooler.

No signs of another disorder causing depression and anorexia.

Diagnosis

History of temperature extremes.

Ruling-out other causes of depression and anorexia.

Differential diagnosis

Other causes of depression and anorexia.

Treatment

Provide a thermoneutral environment.

Place food in withdrawal location.

Prognosis

This is usually a short-term problem with no adverse consequences.

HYPOPHOSPHATEMIA*

> ### Classical signs
>
> - Weakness.
> - Pallor and hemoglobinuria (hemolysis).

Pathogenesis

Hypophosphatemia results from **insufficient phosphorus intake** and/or **excessive urinary phosphorus loss** and/or **translocation** from extracellular to intracellular fluid.

Mild to moderate hypophosphatemia (serum phosphorus level 0.5–0.8 mmol/L) may be seen in **numerous disorders** where anorexia is a feature. It is seen most often with hepatic lipidosis and chronic renal failure. Anorexia may contribute to hypophosphatemia, which in turn may exacerbate anorexia and depression.

Severe hypophosphatemia (serum phosphorus level < 0.5 mmol/L) is most likely to be seen in the **treatment of diabetic ketoacidosis** and within 3 days of initiating tube feeding in an anorexic cat.

Clinical signs

Lethargy, muscle weakness, anorexia – increasing risk with decreasing phosphorus level.

Severe muscle weakness may lead to respiratory muscle failure (rare).

Pale mucous membranes, hemoglobinemia and hemoglobinuria from **hemolysis** – most likely to occur with serum phosphorus level < 0.3–0.5 mmol/L, but has occurred at higher levels.

Diagnosis

Serum phosphorus level < 0.8 mmol/L.

Ruling out other causes of depression, weakness, anorexia and hemolysis.

Differential diagnosis

Other causes of depression, weakness and anorexia related to the primary disorder.

Treatment

Intravenous **potassium phosphate** or sodium phosphate. See Diabetic ketoacidosis in The Cat With Polyuria and Polydipsia (page 236).

Transfusion with fresh red blood cells if hemolysis occurs.

Prognosis

The prognosis for correction of hypophosphatemia is good and overall prognosis is determined by the underlying disorder.

HYPOPARATHYROIDISM*

> ### Classical signs
>
> - Anorexia and depression.
> - Muscle tremors and seizures.
> - History of thyroidectomy.

Clinical signs

Anorexia and depression are consistent findings.

Muscle tremors have been reported in 83%, and **seizures** in 50%, of cases of idiopathic hypoparathyroidism.

Diagnosis

Hypocalcemia (**serum calcium level usually < 1.6 mmol/L** in the presence of normal serum albumin level) and hyperphosphatemia.

History of **thyroidectomy** within the previous 2 weeks.

Differential diagnosis

Acute poisoning is main differential diagnosis for acute anorexia and depression progressing to muscle tremors and seizures.

Hypoglycemia may cause similar signs.

Treatment

Tremors or seizures:
- 10% calcium gluconate 0.5–1.0 ml/kg, or 10% calcium chloride 0.15–0.5 ml/kg, given IV over 10–15 min. Temporarily stop administration if bradycardia, QT-interval shortening or vomiting occur. Both solutions are caustic (calcium chloride >> calcium gluconate) if extravasated.
- If severe initial signs or recurrent signs, follow with 10% calcium gluconate 0.25–0.375 ml/kg/h CRI.

Long-term management:
- Vitamin D and oral calcium preparations – see The Cat With Tremor or Twitching (page 864).
- Cats with post-thyroidectomy hypoparathyroidism typically regain parathyroid function within 2 weeks to 6 months.

ACUTE HYPOGLYCEMIA

> ### Classical signs
>
> - Acute depression in an insulin-treated cat.
> - Weak wobbly gait.
> - Muscle fasciculations.
> - Dilated pupils.

See main reference on page 236 for details (The Cat With Polyuria and Polydipsia).

Clinical signs

Clinical signs of hypoglycemia most often occur in insulin-treated diabetic cats.

Signs may be mild and include lethargy or increased somnolence, a weak wobbly gait and mydriasis, or be more severe and include **seizures**, stupor or coma.

Other signs that are sometimes observed include muscle tremors, vomiting, vocalizing, circling, panting, diarrhea or urination.

Hypoglycemia is unlikely to stimulate eating behavior in a cat; it is more likely to cause anorexia.

Diagnosis

Clinical hypoglycemia usually results from insulin overdose in a diabetic cat. This is confirmed by measuring blood glucose levels and by prompt resolution of clinical signs following intravenous dextrose or intramuscular glucagon.

Portable glucose meters have a tendency to measure falsely low values. A diagnosis of hypoglycemia should be reconsidered if the signs do not improve once blood glucose increases in response to intravenous glucose or glucagon. **Lack of response to sugar solutions rubbed on the gums or given by stomach tube does not rule out hypoglycemia**, because most absorption of glucose occurs in the small intestine. Cats with severe signs such as coma may not respond if there is irreversible brain damage.

Differential diagnosis

Other causes of neurologic disease. See The Cat With Stupor or Coma (page 821) and The Cat With Seizures, Circling and/or Changed Behavior (page 809).

Some poisonings may cause similar signs, e.g. vocalizing, mydriasis, vomiting, diarrhea, polypnea, tremors, seizures and stupor (see Acute poisoning and envenomation, above).

Hypocalcemia may also cause lethargy and anorexia progressing to muscle tremors and seizures.

Hypoglycemia may also be a finding in acute pancreatitis, porto-systemic shunts, hepatic lipidosis, cholangiohepatitis, and overwhelming sepsis, but it is usually a marker of disease rather than a cause of clinical signs.

Treatment

A Somogyi reaction should not be relied upon to rescue a cat from hypoglycemia.

Give **50% dextrose** at 0.5–1.0 ml/kg IV.

If intravenous access is not possible, 50% dextrose (0.5–1.0 ml/kg) or corn syrup (0.25–0.5 ml/kg) PO and rubbed on the gums may be effective, but **glucagon 0.25–1.0 mg IM is superior**. Glucagon must be followed by intravenous dextrose once seizures have stopped and intravenous access is possible.

CENTRAL NERVOUS SYSTEM NEOPLASIA OR INFLAMMATION

Classical signs

- Acute depression and anorexia.
- Stupor, coma, and specific neurological signs.

See main reference on page 795 for details (The Cat With Seizures, Circling and/or Changed Behavior), page 821 (The Cat With Stupor or Coma), page 835 (The Cat With a Head Tilt, Vestibular Ataxia or Nystagmus), page 852 (The Cat With Tremor or Twitching) and page 941 (The Cat With Generalized Weakness).

Clinical signs

Acute meningitis, encephalitis or **central nervous system neoplasia** may initially be characterized by non-specific signs such as acute onset of anorexia and depression.

Depression may then progress to stupor, coma, behavior change or other specific neurological signs. See The Cat With Stupor or Coma, The Cat With Seizures, Circling and/or Changed Behavior, and The Cat With a Head Tilt.

- Acute depression may be the only finding in a cat in the prodromal phase of clinical rabies, but fever spikes are typical. The prodromal phase typically only lasts one to two days in cats before proceeding to the furious phase (most often) or the paralytic phase. Rabies is highly unlikely if there is persistent depression and anorexia without the development of other behavior changes or specific neurologic signs.
- Acute depression is a consistent initial sign in pseudorabies (Aujesky's disease, mad itch), but typically progresses to severe pruritus, voice change and anisocoria with 1–2 days.

Diagnosis

The cat with unexplained acute depression should be carefully examined repetitively for neurological signs.

Differential diagnosis

In the absence of specific neurologic signs, all other causes of acute depression and anorexia should be considered.

If neurologic signs develop, poisoning should be considered.

Treatment

Treat the underlying disease.

In the absence of a specific diagnosis, treatment should be supportive.

HEPATIC ENCEPHALOPATHY

Classical signs

- Disorientation and ptyalism.
- Intermittent central nervous system (CNS) signs often associated with eating.
- Usually in young cats (< 1 year).
- Affected cats are often stunted in size.

See main reference on page 588 for details (The Cat With Salivation) and page 425 (The Yellow Cat or Cat With Elevated Liver Enzymes).

Clinical signs

Porto-systemic shunts usually cause signs in young cats that are small in size. Copper-colored irises may be evident. Intermittent central nervous system signs including disorientation and behavioral changes, and occasionally seizures occur, often associated with eating. Ptyalism may occur alone or associated with neurological signs. Occasionally urethral obstruction results from ammonium biurate uroliths. Prolonged post-anesthetic recovery may be reported.

Mature cats with hepatic lipidosis and cholangio-hepatitis typically have anorexia, weight loss, vomiting and icterus. In severe cases, collapse, disorientation and ptyalism may occur.

Diagnosis

Elevated plasma ammonia level confirms hepatic encephalopathy; but a normal fasting concentration does not rule it out.

Porto-systemic shunts have variable hematologic and biochemical findings, which may include low normal to low MCV, low urea, albumin, glucose and cholesterol concentrations, and elevated globulin and bile acid concentrations. Imaging may reveal a small liver and the shunt. Definitive diagnosis may require an exploratory laparotomy.

Hepatic lipidosis and cholangiohepatitis are typically associated with increased ALT and/or ALP. A disproportionate elevation of ALP compared to ALT and GGT is suggestive of hepatic lipidosis. Elevations in serum bile acids in the absence of cholestasis confirm the presence of liver dysfunction. Coagulation abnormalities may be present. Imaging may reveal an enlarged, hyperechoic liver. Definitive diagnosis relies on liver biopsy.

Differential diagnosis

The main differential diagnosis for ptyalism is oral cavity ulceration.

The main differential diagnoses for icteric depressed cats are acute pancreatitis and diabetic ketoacidosis.

The main differential diagnosis for transient depression and disorientation is poisoning.

Treatment

Hepatic encephalopathy treatment includes lactulose, enema, lactulose retention enema, correction of hypokalemia, and antibiotics (neomycin, metronidazole, ampicillin/amoxicillin).

Porto-systemic shunts can often be reduced or closed by partial or complete surgical ligation or placement of an ameroid constrictor.

Hepatic lipidosis requires nutritional support.

Cholangiohepatitis treatment includes nutritional support, antibiotics if an organism is cultured, and corcorticosteroids if lymphocytic-plasmacytic inflammation is evident on biopsy.

HYPERNATREMIA

> ### Classical signs
> - Coma, twitching, seizures.

Pathogenesis

Hypernatremia results from excessive sodium intake and/or inadequate water intake and/or excessive water loss.

Hypernatremia in cats is most likely to occur in critically ill cats receiving sodium-rich fluids that have concurrent sodium-poor water loss (e.g. diabetes mellitus, head-trauma induced central diabetes insipidus).

Clinical signs

Acute progressive lethargy in a critically ill cat.

May progress to coma, twitching, and seizures.

Dehydration.

Weak pulse, prolonged capillary refill time and hypothermia may be present.

Diagnosis

Serum sodium level > 160 mmol/L.

Ruling out other causes of depression and anorexia.

Urine specific gravity < 1.035 may indicate diabetes insipidus.

Differential diagnosis

Other causes of depression and anorexia related to the primary disorder causing critical illness.

Treatment

Sodium-poor intravenous fluids. Hypernatremia should be corrected at the same rate at which it developed, i.e. serum sodium concentration should be lowered rapidly in acute hypernatremia, and slowly in chronic hypernatremia. Overly rapid correction of hypernatremia will result in signs similar to hypernatremia. Idiogenic osmols form in hypernatremia to protect the brain against dehydration; these osmols result in cerebral edema if serum sodium concentration is lowered too quickly. Because the rate at which hypernatremia developed is often not known, a general recommendation is to **lower serum sodium level by 1–2 mmol/L/h.**

Assess percent dehydration and replace using 0.9% saline over 4–8 hours if acute dehydration and over 8–12 hours if chronic dehydration.

Once the cat is rehydrated, **calculate free water deficit**:

Deficit (L) = 0.6 × body weight (kg) × ([Na ÷ 140] – 1).

Give this volume over 12–24 h if the cat's mentation is normal, and over 24–48 h if mentation is abnormal.

Give furosemide 0.5 mg/kg IV if hypernatremia persists and the cat is normally hydrated.

Consider antidiuretic hormone therapy (e.g. DDAVP) if there is diabetes insipidus (see The Cat With Polyuria and Polydipsia, page 231).

Prognosis

The prognosis for hypernatremic cats with head trauma is poor; the prognosis for uncomplicated correction of hypernatremia with other disorders is good and overall prognosis is determined by the underlying disorder.

ESOPHAGEAL FOREIGN BODY AND INFLAMMATION

Classical signs

- Regurgitation.
- Anorexia and depression.

See main reference on page 616 for details (The Cat With Signs of Regurgitation (Acute or Chronic)).

Clinical signs

Cats with esophageal foreign bodies or esophagitis (e.g. secondary to treatment with tetracyclines) are typically presented for **regurgitation** (or vomiting as perceived by the owner), **dysphagia** or **gagging**. However, this may be intermittent, so that only non-specific signs such as anorexia and depression are reported by the owners. Anorexia and depression may be due to esophageal pain.

Diagnosis

Diagnostic imaging or **endoscopy** is required to identify foreign material. The latter is required to identify esophagitis.

PRIMARY ANOSMIA

Classical signs

- Anorexia.

Clinical signs

Anorexia and cat may sniff less.

Diagnosis

History of olfactory tractotomy for inappropriate elimination behavior.

No reaction to placement of noxious stimuli in front of nose.

FELINE LEUKEMIA VIRUS INFECTION

Classical signs

- Fever.
- Signs of secondary infections, hematologic disorders, or neoplasia.

Clinical signs

Feline leukemia virus infection usually causes fever; anemia and other hematologic disorders; immunosuppression leading to secondary infections; lymphoma, myeloproliferative disorders, and fibrosarcomas and neurologic disorders.

Occasionally the only sign of infection is acute depression, anorexia and dehydration.

Diagnosis

A feline leukemia virus test should be considered in the work-up of a cat with acute depression and anorexia.

RECOMMENDED READING

Akol KG, Wachabau RJ, Saunders HM, Hendrick MJ. Acute pancreatitis in cats with hepatic lipidosis. J Vet Intern Med 1993; 7: 205–209.

Brady CA, Otto CM, Van Winkle TJ, King LG. Severe sepsis in cats: 29 cases (1986–1998). J Am Vet Med Assoc 2000; 217: 531–535.

Connally HE, Thrall MA, Hamar DW. Safety and efficacy of high dose fomepizole as therapy for ethylene glycol intoxication in cats. Proceedings of the 8th International Veterinary and Emergency and Critical Care Symposium, 2002, p 777.

Ferreri JA, Hardam E, Kimmel S, Saunders HM, Van Winkle TJ, Robatz KJ, Washabau RJ. Clinical differentiation of acute necrotizing from chronic nonsuppurative pancreatitis in cats: 63 cases (1996–2001). J Am Vet Med Assoc 2003; 223: 469–474.

Forman MA, Mark SL, De Cock HE, Hergesell EJ, Wisner ER, Baker TW, Kass PH, Steiner JM, Williams DA. Evaluation of serum feline pancreatic lipase immunoreactivity and helical computed tomography versus conventional testing for the diagnosis of feline pancreatitis. J. Vet. Intern. Med., 2004; 18: 807–815.

Frenier SL, Dhein CR. Diagnosis and management of acute renal failure. In: August FR (ed) Consultations in Feline Internal Medicine. Philadelphia, WB Saunders, 1991, pp 281–288.

Hill RC, Van Winkle TJ. Acute necrotizing pancreatitis and acute suppurative pancreatitis in the cat. J Vet Intern Med 1993; 7: 25–33.

Holzworth J. Diseases of the Cat. W.B. Saunders, Philadelphia, 1987.

Mathews KA (ed) Veterinary Emergency and Critical Care Manual. 2 Edition, Guelph, Ontario, Lifelearn Inc., 2006.

Mathews KA. Acute renal failure: what's new in treatment and prevention. Proceedings of the 8th International Veterinary and Emergency and Critical Care Symposium, 2002, pp 399–403.

Rumbeiha WK, Francis JA, Fitzgerald SD, Nair MG, Holan K, Bugyei KA, Simmons H. A comprehensive study of Easter lily poisoning in cats. J. Vet. Diagn. Invest., 2004; 16: 527–541.

Simpson KW, Michel KE. Medical and nutritional management of feline pancreatitis. Proceedings of the 18th Annual Veterinary Medical Forum. American College of Veterinary Internal Medicine, 2000, pp 428–430.

Steiner JM. Diagnosis of pancreatitis. Vet Clin North Am Small Anim Pract 2003; 33: 1181–1195.

Tefft KM. Lily nephrotoxicity in cats. Comp Cont Edu Pract Vet 2004: 26: 149–156.

Temo K, Rudloff E, Lichtneberger M, Kirby R. Hypernatremia in critically ill cats: evaluation and treatment. Comp Cont Ed Pract Vet 2004; 26: 434–444.

Wisner T. Top feline toxicities. Veterinary Information Network, 2005.

PART 6

Cat with weight loss or chronic illness

17. The cat with weight loss and a good appetite

Danièlle Gunn-Moore and James B Miller

KEY SIGNS

- Thin cat eating well.
- Weight loss and a good appetite.

MECHANISM?

- Weight loss with a good appetite occurs when the cat is unable to gain sufficient nutrition from its diet.

WHERE?

- Diseases involving many body systems can lead to weight loss with a good appetite.

WHAT?

- In older cats the most common causes of weight loss with a good appetite are hyperthyroidism, diabetes mellitus and inflammatory bowel disease. In younger cats, inflammatory bowel disease and intestinal parasites are the most common causes.

QUICK REFERENCE SUMMARY

Diseases causing weight loss and a good appetite

METABOLIC

● Hyperthyroidism*** (p 304)

Usually seen in cats greater than eight years of age. Weight loss, good appetite, tachycardia, restlessness and/or intermittent vomiting and diarrhea.

● Diabetes mellitus** (p 310)

Usually seen in older cats. Increased risk in fat cats and some Burmese. History of polyuria, polydipsia and polyphagia, plus variable weight changes.

● Acromegaly (p 322)

Rare condition of older, typically males, cats. Slow increase in body size, especially affecting the head and feet. Usually diabetic; so polyuric, polydipsic and polyphagic.

● Hyperadrenocorticism (p 324)

Rare condition of middle-aged and older cats. Poor coat condition and pot-bellied appearance. Often diabetic; so polyuric, polydipsic and polyphagic.

● Glomerulonephritis (protein-losing nephropathy) (p 326)

Weight loss with a good appetite may be seen early in disease, accompanied by ascites, subcutaneous edema, polydipsia and polyuria, ± vomiting and diarrhea.

NEOPLASTIC

● Alimentary lymphosarcoma* (p 317)

Usually older cats. Weight loss with variable appetite. History of acute, or more commonly, chronic vomiting and/or diarrhea.

NUTRITIONAL

● Inadequate nutrition** (p 316)

Weight loss with a good appetite, few other signs. History of inadequate or inappropriate diet. Seen in kittens from poor conditions or cats that have recently changed environment.

INFLAMMATORY

● Inflammatory bowel disease*** (p 307)

Can affect any age but most typically seen in middle-aged cats. Any combination of chronic weight loss, vomiting and/or diarrhea.

● Chronic pancreatitis/exocrine pancreatic insufficiency* (p 318)

Typically seen in middle-aged to older cats with a history of episodic anorexia, lethargy, vomiting and/or diarrhea. If also diabetic; polyuria and polydipsia.

● Lymphocytic cholangiohepatitis* (p 320)

Typically seen in younger to middle-aged cats. Often polyphagic, may have mild generalized lymphadenopathy. May be associated with inflammatory bowel disease.

INFECTIOUS

● Intestinal parasites** (p 314)

Usually seen in young cats from poorly cleaned multi-cat environments. Weight loss or failure to gain weight, usually with a good appetite, may have diarrhea and/or vomiting.

INTRODUCTION

MECHANISM?

While weight loss is a common presenting problem in feline medicine, weight loss in association with a good appetite is seen less frequently. This occurs when the cat is unable to gain sufficient nutrition from its diet.

This can result from **inadequate nutrition** (feeding insufficient food or a diet of inadequate nutritional content), or **an inability to derive nutrient from the diet**. The latter can result from:

- **Inability to digest or absorb nutrients** (malassimilation syndromes), e.g. parasitism, inflammatory bowel disease, pancreatitis/exocrine pancreatic insufficiency, lymphocytic cholangiohepatitis, alimentary lymphosarcoma or lymphangectasia.
- **Inability to utilize absorbed nutrients** – as seen with diabetes mellitus, or endocrinopathies which result in diabetes, e.g. acromegaly or hyperadrenocorticism.
- **Increased utilization of absorbed nutrients** (hypermetabolic states), e.g. hyperthyroidism, pregnancy, lactation, congestive heart failure, excessive physical activity or neoplasia.
- **Excessive nutrient loss,** e.g. diabetes mellitus, protein-losing nephropathy or lymphangectasia.

WHERE?

Weight loss with a good appetite may be seen when the **intestinal tract** is **unable to digest and/or absorb food** (malassimilation syndromes, hyperthyroidism), **the body tissues are unable to utilize nutrition** that has been absorbed (diabetes mellitus), the **body loses essential nutrients** through the **intestines or kidneys** (diabetes, protein-losing nephropathy, lymphangectasia), or the **demands of the body have been raised** beyond the level that the diet can supply (hyperthyroidism, pregnancy, lactation).

Weight loss with a good appetite **indicates a gastrointestinal problem, renal problem or a problem-involving tissue metabolism** (either metabolic demands have increased, or the tissues are unable to utilize nutrients).

WHAT?

The **most common cause** of weight loss with a good appetite is **hyperthyroidism.** Other common causes include various **malassimilation syndromes** including combinations of inflammatory bowel disease, pancreatitis and/or lymphocytic cholangiohepatitis (in combination termed **"triaditis"**). **Intestinal parasitism, diabetes** and **alimentary lymphosarcoma** are seen reasonably commonly, while hyperadrenocorticism, acromegaly, protein-losing nephropathy and lymphangiectasia are seen very rarely.

Disorders which may occasionally present with weight loss with a good appetite, but more typically present with a poor appetite are discussed elsewhere, e.g. congestive heart failure, congenital portosystemic shunts.

DIAGNOSIS

Initial diagnostic evaluation should include history, physical examination, hematology, serum biochemistry, serum thyroxin if > 8 years of age, urinalysis, and fecal examination for parasites.

Age of cat is an important consideration. Younger cats are more likely to develop parasitism, inappropriate nutrition, or protein-losing nephropathy. **Middle-aged cats** have a greater risk of hyperadrenocorticism, while **older cats** develop hyperthyroidism, diabetes mellitus, alimentary lymphosarcoma or acromegaly. Inflammatory bowel disease can affect cats of any age, but most typically affects middle-aged or older individuals.

The history is essential. Determine the cat's environment (inside or outside, competition over food supplies), what and how much is fed, whether nutritional requirements have changed (pregnancy, going outside in cold weather), or whether diabetogenic drugs have been given.

Other clinical signs are important to consider. These signs may result from underlying or concurrent disease processes. **Polyuria and/or polydipsia** are suggestive of an endocrinopathy or protein-losing nephropathy. **Vomiting and/or diarrhea** are suggestive of enteric disease, hyperthyroidism, lymphocytic cholangiohepatitis or protein-losing nephropathy. **Feces becoming bulky or fatty** suggest malassimilation syndromes or hyperthyroidism, and increased **aggression or restlessness** are suggestive of hyperthyroidism.

Careful physical examination is essential for diagnosis. Careful palpation of the ventral cervical region is required to detect thyroid mass(es). **Thorough abdominal palpation** is essential to detect anterior **abdominal pain** (pancreatitis, hepatopathy), **liver enlargement** (diabetes-associated hepatopathy, hyperadrenocorticism, lymphocytic cholangiohepatitis), **thickened bowel loops** (inflammatory bowel disease, alimentary lymphosarcoma), **mesenteric lymphadenopathy** (alimentary lymphosarcoma, occasionally eosinophilic or suppurative inflammatory bowel disease), **ascites** (lymphocytic cholangiohepatitis, protein-losing nephropathy) or an **enlarged uterus** (late pregnancy). **General physical examination** is important to detect mild **generalized lymphadenopathy** (lymphosarcoma, lymphocytic cholangiohepatitis), an **ill-kept coat** (hyperthyroidism), a **greasy coat** (exocrine pancreatic insufficiency), **alopecia and thin skin** (hyperadrenocorticism), **subcutaneous edema** (protein-losing nephropathy), or **extremities that appear disproportionately enlarged** (acromegaly).

DISEASES CAUSING SIGNS OF A THIN CAT WITH A GOOD APPETITE

HYPERTHYROIDISM***

> ### Classical signs
>
> - Older cats (usually > 8 years).
> - Progressive weight loss, often with a ravenous appetite.
> - May also show restlessness, a lack of grooming, vomiting ± diarrhea, ± polyuria/polydipsia.

Pathogenesis

99% of cases of hyperthyroidism result from benign nodular hyperplasia/adenoma.

- Disease results from autonomous secretion of thyroxine (T4) and triiodothyroxinine (T3). Negative feedback on the pituitary suppresses release of thyroid-stimulating hormone (TSH) and normal thyroid tissue atrophies.
- **Cause is unknown** but may involve diet (iodine content, frequent changes, food additives), environmental causes (in cat litter, toxins, pollution,

exposure to allergens), genetic mutation, abnormal immune and/or hormonal responses.

- **70% of the cats have both thyroid glands affected.**

1% of cases result from mild to moderately malignant thyroid carcinoma.

GIT signs may result from polyphagia, malabsorption or intestinal hypermotility.

Polyuria/polydipsia may result from diuretic effects of T4, increased renal blood flow, associated renal insufficiency or compulsive polydipsia.

Cardiac effects result from a high output state, induced, in part, by a demand for increased tissue perfusion to meet the needs of increased tissue metabolism. Cardiovascular changes include left ventricular hypertrophy, left atrial and ventricular dilation, increased myocardial contractility, and decreased peripheral vascular resistance. Other contributors are the direct effect of thyroid hormones on cardiac muscle and the nervous system.

Associated cardiac hypertrophy may cause congestive heart failure with tachycardia, a gallop rhythm, systolic murmurs, dyspnea, apathy, hindlimb weakness due to aortic thromboemboli or collapse.

Associated hypertension may be seen as ocular hemorrhage, or may cause clinical signs associated with cerebrovascular accidents, dementia and/or renal failure.

- Up to 85% of cats with hyperthyroidism may develop systemic hypertension, either initially or even some time after apparently successful treatment.

Clinical signs

Hyperthyroidism is the most common endocrinopathy in cats; affecting ~1 in 300 pet cats.

It is seen mainly in older cats (>8 years of age); it is occasionally seen in cats as young as 4 years, and has even been documented in an 8-month-old kitten.

There is no sex or breed predisposition, but Siamese cats appear to be under-represented.

Most cats have a history of weight loss and polyphagia.

Weight loss usually occurs over several months.

10–20% of cats will present with signs of inappetence with weight loss.

Cats may have a **history of restlessness, aggression and a lack of grooming.**

Cats may also show **tachycardia ± a gallop rhythm, vomiting and/or diarrhea** (feces may become bulky) and/or **polyuria/polydipsia**.

GIT signs may result from polyphagia, malabsorption or intestinal hypermotility.

Polyuria/polydipsia may result from diuretic effects of T4, increased renal blood flow, associated renal insufficiency or compulsive polydipsia.

Associated cardiac hypertrophy may cause congestive heart failure with tachycardia, a gallop rhythm, systolic murmurs, dyspnea, apathy, hindlimb weakness due to aortic thromboemboli or collapse.

Associated hypertension may be seen as ocular hemorrhage, or may cause clinical signs associated with cerebrovascular accidents, dementia and/or renal failure.
- Up to 85% of cats with hyperthyroidism may have signs of systemic hypertension.

Many hyperthyroid cats are presented for their routine vaccination with no owner complaints.

Diagnosis

Hyperthyroidism should be suspected when any older cat presents with weight loss, and especially when the weight loss is associated with a good appetite. However, inappetence should not rule out hyperthyroidism.

Physical examination usually reveals a thyroid nodule on either or both sides of the trachea in the ventral cervical region (80–90%).

Tachycardia and/or a gallop rhythm are usually present.

Liver enzymes (ALT and/or SAP) are often raised. Hepatopathy may be secondary to a direct toxic effect of thyroid hormones, hepatic lipidosis, malnutrition or hepatic hypoxia resulting from cardiac failure.

Definitive diagnosis is based on detecting elevated serum concentrations of total T4 (and/or T3).

Some cats with hyperthyroidism have a T4 concentration that is within the normal range. This may be due to:
- Early or mild hyperthyroidism.

- T4 concentrations varying during the day.
- Severe systemic illness causing a reduction in T4 (euthyroid sick syndrome).

If hyperthyroidism is suspected despite a high normal T4 concentration:
- **Retest the cat** – either immediately, or in a few weeks time.
- **Check free T4** – by equilibrium dialysis.
- **T3 suppression test** – Collect blood sample, give 7×25 mg doses of T3 PO every 8 h, then collect blood 2–4 h after the 7th dose (i.e. on day 3). An increase in T3 concentration confirms successful medication. Suppression of T4 concentration (below 50% of baseline, <20 nmol/l [1.5 ug/dl] does not usually occur in hyperthyroid cats.
- **Thyrotropin-releasing hormone** (TRH) **stimulation test** – Collect blood, give 0.1 mg/kg TRH IV, then collect second blood sample 4 hours later. Assess both samples for serum T4 concentration. Stimulation to > 50% does not occur in hyperthyroid cats. Side effects of TRH include transient salivation, vomiting, tachypnea and defecation.
- **Thyroid-stimulating hormone** (TSH) **response test** – The usefulness of this test has been questioned and TSH may be difficult to obtain.
- **Nuclear isotope scanning** detects hyperactive thyroid tissue. Procedure is relatively safe and simple to perform, but requires access to a licensed facility, which is not always available.
- **Trial course of anti-thyroid therapy** (see below) of approximately 30 days is not without risk of toxic side effects.

Differential diagnosis

These include most other causes of weight loss with a good appetite. However, hyperthyroidism typically occurs in older cats and presents with polyuria, polydipsia, vomiting and/or diarrhea, so diabetes, renal disease, malassimilation syndromes (including IBD, pancreatitis/exocrine pancreatic insufficiency, and early intestinal lymphosarcoma), acromegaly and hyperadrenocorticism are perhaps the most important differentials.

Treatment

Hyperthyroidism can be treated medically, surgically, or with radioiodine (I^{131}).

Prior to deciding which treatment to use the cat should be assessed for concurrent disease, especially renal disease, systemic hypertension and heart disease, all of which occur commonly in association with hyperthyroidism.

- The interplay between systemic blood pressure and renal function is complex. While **systemic hypertension is detrimental to kidney function**, a sudden fall in blood pressure or a reduction in glomerular filtration rate (e.g. associated with a sudden fall in T4) can exacerbate renal dysfunction by causing a sudden fall in renal blood flow. **Changes in T4 need to be made gradually** so there are no sudden changes in renal blood pressure.
- By maintaining renal blood pressure, hyperthyroidism can mask low-grade renal insufficiency. It is essential to check serum urea and creatinine concentrations and urine specific gravity prior to inducing irreversible reduction of T4 (i.e. by thyroidectomy or I^{131} treatment). A short course of medical therapy may reveal the presence of masked renal insufficiency.

Medical therapy tends to be given to stabilize the cat prior to surgical treatment, to check for masked renal disease prior to thyroidectomy or I^{131} treatment, or when neither I^{131} nor surgery are possible.

Methimazole and carbimazole block T3 and T4 synthesis. It takes 1–3 weeks before a significant decrease in T4 concentrations occur after beginning treatment.

- Carbimazole is broken down to methimazole in vivo. Bioavailability and volume of distribution of methimazole is highly variable between cats.
- Dose for both is 1.25–5.0 mg PO every 8–24 hours initially, reducing to every 12–24 hours. If the cat has concurrent renal insufficiency, start with a low dose and monitor renal values as dose is gradually increased. Preliminary studies with topical transdermal applications show promise.
- When cat and owner compliance is good, the successful response rate is approximately 85% with medical treatment.
- **Poor compliance results** from:
  - The need for **frequent medication**.
  - The need for **frequent blood samples** to look for possible side effects. Blood dyscrasias occur in 2–10% of cats and include eosinophilia, lymphocytosis, leukopenia, thrombocytopenia

and/or agranulocytosis, hepatopathy and, rarely, immune-mediated hemolytic anemia (IMHA).
  - **Frequent side effects**. Up to approximately 20% of cats develop anorexia, vomiting, lethargy, hepatopathy ± jaundice, cutaneous reactions (typically pruritus of the head and neck), bleeding tendencies or, very occasionally, myasthenia gravis, or IMHA.
  - Mild side effects may resolve despite continued treatment.

Other medical therapies include:
- **Atenolol (selective β_1 adrenoceptor blocking agent)** may be added to reduce tachycardia, arrhythmias and hypertension (6.25 mg/cat PO every 24 hours).
- **Stable iodine** helps to decrease T3 and T4 synthesis and reduce thyroid gland vascularity, but the effect can be transient and inconsistent. Give potassium iodide 30–100 mg/cat/day PO for 10–14 days prior to surgery using 100 g potassium iodide/100 ml solution, or potassium iodate ~20 mg/cat every 12 hours PO.
- **Calcium or sodium ipodate** is a radiopaque iodine agent that reduces T3 concentrations. Its effect can be transient, and it may be difficult to obtain (15 mg/kg PO every 12 hours).

Surgical thyroidectomy. The success depends on the stability of the patient, the expertise of the surgeon (a bilateral thyroidectomy is usually performed), and the expertise of the anesthetist (e.g. do not give atropine).
- Successful response rate is > 95%. Ectopic overactive thyroid tissue is a cause of failure, as it is usually missed at surgery.
- Reduce the risks of surgery by making the cat euthyroid prior to surgery (see Medical therapy, above).
- Surgical risks include anesthetic risks in older patients (often with concurrent renal ± cardiac disease), iatrogenic damage to parathyroid tissue leading to transient or permanent hypocalcemia, or to the local nerves leading to laryngeal paralysis or Horner's syndrome.

Radioiodine (I^{131}) is taken up by and destroys the overactive thyroid tissue, but spares the normal tissue.
- Successful response rate is > 95%, but it may take a few weeks, or occasionally months, for the normal tissue to recover function.

- Availability of facilities and length of stay in hospital varies from 2 days to 4 weeks depending on country and state, as it often depends on the interpretation of radiation safety laws.
- Side effects are few and include transient dysphagia or dysphonia, or permanent hypothyroidism (~2%).

Prognosis

Without treatment, cats with hyperthyroidism will usually die of concurrent renal disease, heart disease, liver disease or systemic hypertension.

With **treatment, prognosis varies from very good to guarded**, dependent on the presence of heart disease, renal disease and systemic hypertension, whether or not any damage has become permanent prior to treatment of the hyperthyroidism, and which treatment options are available.

Prevention

Since it is not known what triggers the development of hyperthyroidism, it is currently not possible to prevent its onset.

INFLAMMATORY BOWEL DISEASE***

Classical signs

- Any age, sex or breed of cat.
- Any combination of progressive weight loss, vomiting and/or diarrhea.

Pathogenesis

Inflammatory bowel disease (IBD) is a group of chronic idiopathic gastrointestinal tract disorders that are characterized by **infiltration with inflammatory cells**. The infiltration may consist of lymphocytes, plasma cells, neutrophils, eosinophils and/or macrophages, and the inflammation may involve the stomach, small intestine and/or colon.

The etiology is probably multifactorial and appears to involve host hypersensitivity responses to antigens within the bowel lumen or mucosa. Suspected antigens include food, bacteria, parasites or self-antigens.

- The hypersensitivity may result from a primary, possible genetic, disorder, or arise secondary to mucosal injury incurred by a number of different disorders including bacterial, viral, protozoal or fungal infections, bacterial overgrowth, food hypersensitivity, drug administration, metabolic disease, neoplasia, pancreatitis or cholangiohepatitis.
- Regardless of the initial cause of the hypersensitivity, it results in **increased mucosal permeability** which allows **luminal antigens to cross the mucosa**, leading to inflammation and further mucosal damage.

Clinical signs

IBD can occur in any age, sex or breed of cat. While it is most commonly seen in middle-aged to older cats, a third of cases occur in cats of less than 2 years of age. Some purebred cats may be predisposed.

Clinical signs include any combination of progressive weight loss, and/or vomiting and/or diarrhea.

Weight loss may result from malabsorption and/or inappetence (which usually occurs late in the disease). Not all cases show significant enteric signs, so some cats present with only weight loss and a variable appetite.

Vomiting is often intermittent and may occur every few days to weeks, often accompanied by anorexia and lethargy. Vomiting is rarely associated with feeding. It may contain froth, bile-stained fluid and food or, occasionally, blood.

Diarrhea can vary in consistency from almost well formed to liquid. Some cats may show evidence of large bowel involvement with mucus and/or blood and increased frequency.

Clinical signs may wax and wane, and tend to vary with the type and severity of inflammation.

Physical examination is often unremarkable, but may reveal a thin cat, palpably thickened intestines, enlarged mesenteric lymph nodes and/or abdominal discomfort.

Concurrent pancreatitis and/or cholangiohepatitis may result in jaundice, a palpably enlarged liver and/or anterior abdominal discomfort.

When lymphangectasia is present, severe hypoproteinemia may lead to subcutaneous edema and/or ascites.

Diagnosis

Before a diagnosis of IBD can be made, all other causes of enteropathy must be ruled out. These include bacterial enteritis (*Helicobacter* spp., *Salmonella* spp., *Campylobacter* spp., *Clostridium perfringens*, *E. coli*), intestinal parasites (helminths, cestodes, protozoans), fungal enteritis, GI neoplasia (lymphosarcoma, adenocarcinoma) and viral enteritis (feline leukemia virus, feline immunodeficiency virus, feline coronavirus, feline panleukopenia). **IBD is diagnosed by documenting histopathological evidence of GI inflammation and excluding all of other causes of it.**

Baseline laboratory tests include hematology, serum biochemistry (including total T4 concentration in older cats), FeLV and FIV tests, urinalysis, fecal culture for pathogenic bacteria and a full examination for fecal parasites.

- Performing all of these investigations can be expensive so the investigation should, where possible, be tailored to the patient, and many clinicians start with a dietary trial (see below).
- Since the investigations are being performed to rule out other causes of enteropathy they are frequently unremarkable. However, IBD may be associated with a number of non-specific findings:
  - **Hematology** may reveal an inflammatory response; neutrophilia, eosinophilia, lymphopenia or monocytosis. Microcytic anemia may result from chronic blood loss associated with severe IBD.
  - **Hyperglobulinemia** may result from chronic inflammation. **Panhypoproteinemia** may be seen with severe protein-losing enteropathies.
  - **Increases in liver enzymes** may result from associated hepatic inflammation (see below).

Non-invasive screening tests may provide additional information. These include abdominal radiography, ultrasound examination, assessment of serum folate and cobalamine (B12) levels, examination of fecal smears for the presence of undigested fats or starch, fat absorption tests, breath hydrogen analysis and sugar permeability studies (where available).

- **Survey radiographs** tend to be unrewarding, but may reveal gas- or fluid-filled loops of intestines. **Barium studies** may reveal flocculation or persistent adherence of the barium to the mucosa, irregular mucosal surfaces or delayed transit times.
- **Ultrasound examination** may reveal intestinal wall irregularity or echogenicity. It may also be used to examine the mesenteric lymph nodes and other intra-abdominal structures.
- **Serum folate and cobalamin** levels may be reduced because of malabsorption.
- **Serum feline trypsin-like immunoreactivity (fTLI)** and **feline pancreatic lipase immunoreactivity (fPLI)** may be helpful in the diagnosis of exocrine pancreatic insufficiency (EPI) and pancreatic inflammation, respectively.
- **Breath hydrogen analysis and sugar permeability studies** may be used to try to demonstrate malabsorption and/or small intestinal bacterial overgrowth (SIBO)/antibiotic-responsive diarrhea.

A dietary trial should be performed in all except very ill patients prior to more invasive investigation.

- Feed a single highly digestible source of protein for at least 3–4 weeks and see if the clinical signs resolve.

It is inadvisable to carry out treatment trials with antibiotics or corticosteroids prior to making a definitive diagnosis.

- This delays making the correct diagnosis, and may cause complicating intestinal bacterial overgrowth (antibiotics) or potentiate secondary infections (corticosteroids).

Definitive diagnosis requires the collection of intestinal biopsies.

- **Mucosal biopsies** may be collected by endoscopy. Unfortunately, it is not always possible to make a definitive diagnosis from these biopsies, so in some cases, full-thickness biopsies must be collected via laparotomy or laparoscopy.
- IBD often causes no gross mucosal changes, but changes that may be seen include increased granularity and friability, the presence of erythema, ulcerations, and/or mass lesions and poor distensibility.
- **Multiple biopsies should be taken** since the inflammatory infiltrates may not be spread diffusely throughout the gastrointestinal tract.

- When performing laparotomy or laparoscopy it is advisable to **collect biopsies of the mesenteric lymph nodes, liver** and, if possible, **pancreas**, as well as from **multiple intestinal sites**. Part of the liver and/or mesenteric lymph node biopsy, and bile aspirated from the gall bladder can be sent for culture.
- Collection of **duodenal aspirates for quantitative culture** may help to determine the bacterial load of the small intestine.
- **Gastric biopsies** should always be assessed for the presence of *Helicobacter* spp.
- **Histopathology reveals inflammatory cells infiltrating the lamina propria**, plus variable degrees of epithelial abnormality and glandular distortion.
  - **Lymphocytic-plasmacytic IBD** is the most common form of IBD in the cat. It may occasionally progress to intestinal lymphosarcoma.
  - **Granulomatous enterocolitis** is less common, and often presents as GI obstruction.
  - **Eosinophilic IBD** is rare. It may be associated with eosinophilia and/or hypereosinophilic syndrome where tissues other than the GI tract are also affected.
  - **Suppurative IBD** is usually associated with an infectious etiology.
  - Other forms also exist and many cats have mixed populations of inflammatory cells.
- Unfortunately, when lymphangectasia is present, severe hypoproteinemia may render these patients a poor anesthetic and surgical risk. It may therefore be necessary to make a presumptive diagnosis based on the presence of diarrhea, panhypoproteinemia and lymphopenia in the absence of finding other diseases on hematology, serum biochemistry, fecal evaluation, abdominal ultrasound examination ± mucosal biopsies.

Differential diagnosis

These include most of the other causes of weight loss with a good appetite. However, since cats with IBD usually develop vomiting and/or diarrhea, **other causes of enteropathy, cholangiohepatitis, pancreatitis, hyperthyroidism and the other malassimilation syndromes** (including alimentary lymphosarcoma) should be considered as important differentials.

Treatment

The basic aims of treatment are to remove the source of antigenic stimulation and to suppress the inflammatory response within the GI tract.
- **Treatment typically involves dietary management, ± metronidazole, ± prednisolone**.
- Treatment should be tailored to each patient.
- Relapses warrant critical reassessment of the case, and often require repeated intensification of treatment and/or the addition of more potent immunosuppressive drugs.

The diet should contain a single highly digestible source of protein, ideally that the cat has not eaten before.
- The diet should preferably contain few food additives, be gluten-free, lactose-free, low residue, not too high in fat, and adequately supplemented with vitamins and minerals, especially B vitamins and potassium.
- High-fiber diets may help when the large bowel is affected.
- No other foods should be fed concurrently.
- During the **initial phase of treatment**, when the bowel is recovering, it may be preferable to **feed either a home-cooked diet**, a "sacrificial protein" which the cat will then not be fed again, or **protein hydrolysate** which has reduced molecular weight protein and is supposed to be less antigenic. This should be fed for 1–2 months, after which time the cat can then be fed a commercial "hypoallergenic" diet, or further protein sources can be gradually reintroduced. If feeding homemade diets long-term, great care should be taken to ensure they are balanced.

Metronidazole often forms the mainstay of treatment. Its effect against **anaerobic bacteria** helps to reduce secondary bacterial overgrowth. It is also effective against **protozoa** (e.g. *Giardia* spp.), has positive effects on **brush border enzymes levels**, and is believed to **alter the immune function** of the GI tract, perhaps by altering neutrophil chemotaxis and inhibiting cell-mediated immunity. Administer 7.5–15 mg/kg PO q 8–12 hours for 2–4 weeks, then taper gradually over 1–2 months. Some authors suggest that it is inadvisable to give very prolonged courses.

Immunosuppressive agents:
- **Immunosuppressive doses of corticosteroids** are usually required. Administer prednisolone 2–4 mg/kg q 12–24 hours PO, then taper over 1–3

months and maintain on every other day doses, if needed. Use of budesonide (1 mg/cat PO q 24 hours) instead of prednisolone may help to reduce systemic signs of corticosteroid administration.

- Other immunosuppressive agents may be considered. While they all have potential side effects and warrant regular monitoring **chlorambucil** (2–5 mg/m^2 PO up to once every 48 h) is often very well tolerated. Other less favorable options include **cyclophosphamide** (50 mg/m^2 PO up to four times a week), **cyclosporine** (0.5–8.5 mg/kg every 12–24 hours, indefinitely) or, in the cases of **colonic disease**, **sulfasalazine** (10–20 mg/kg/day PO for 7–10 days).

Supportive therapies are often recommended. However, few have been assessed using controlled studies in cats.

- **Tylosin** may be effective for its antibiotic actions as well as other, as yet undefined, effects (5–20 mg/kg every 6–12 hours PO).
- **Motility modifiers** may give short-term palliative relief in cases of very watery diarrhea (**loperamide** 0.04–0.2 mg/kg every 8–12 hours PO).
- **Metoclopramide** may be useful for its anti-emetic and prokinetic effects (0.2–0.5 mg/kg PO up to four times a day, being given just prior to feeding, or as a constant IV infusion 1–2 mg/kg over 24 hours).
- **Cisapride** is a good prokinetic, but it is now more difficult to obtain (0.3–1.0 mg/kg every 8–12 hours PO).
- **Cobalamin and folate** may be needed as they are often reduced by malabsorption (cobalamin 125–250 μg/week SC or IM for 6–8 weeks then q 2–4 weeks [50–100 μg/cat/day PO]; folate 0.5–1.0 mg/cat/day PO for 1 month).
- **Vitamin K1** is often required because fat malabsorption results in poor absorption of fat-soluble vitamins like vitamin K, and this can result in abnormal hemostasis (0.5 mg/kg/day SC for 3–4 days, then once weekly).
- **Glutamine** may be given as an energy source for the GI mucosal cells (250–5000 mg/cat/day PO, indefinitely).
- *Lactobacillus acidophilus* may be given as a probiotic to help restore intestinal flora (50–500 M organisms/cat/day PO until feces return to normal).
- Various nutritional supplements may be given for their potential anti-inflammatory properties. These include **vitamin E** (50–200 IU/cat/day PO), **vitamin A** (1000–5000 IU/cat/day PO), **vitamin C** (50–80 mg/kg/day PO), **zinc** (7.5 mg/cat/day PO), and **N-acetyl glucosamine** (125–1500 mg/cat/day PO).

Prognosis

The prognosis depends on the nature and severity of the GI infiltration, and the presence of concurrent and/or associated disease, such as pancreatitis or cholangiohepatitis. In general, the prognosis for control is reasonably good, but the condition cannot be cured, and many cats will need treatment for the rest of their life.

Prevention

Since it is not known what triggers IBD to develop, it is not currently possible to prevent its onset.

DIABETES MELLITUS**

Classical signs

- Usually seen in older, obese, neutered male cats, and Burmese cats may be over-represented.
- History of polyuria, polydipsia and polyphagia.
- Possible initial weight gain, followed by weight loss.

Pathogenesis

Diabetes results from a variety of mechanisms that cause an absolute or relative lack of insulin.

Classification of diabetes in cats is best made by cause, rather than whether or not they require exogenous insulin.

Type 1 diabetes, previously called juvenile-onset diabetes, is due to **immune-mediated destruction** of pancreatic islet beta cells. It appears to be very rare in cats.

Type 2 diabetes results from impaired insulin secretion, and peripheral resistance to the action of insulin. Hyperglycemia results from decreased glucose uptake in tissues and increased hepatic glucose production. Many cats with diabetes appear to have type 2 diabetes.

- This is often associated with **accumulation of islet-specific amyloid polypeptide** (IAPP), which occurs in aggregates around pancreatic islets. While

IAPP is co-secreted and accumulates as amyloid in normal cats as they age, it accumulates more extensively in cats with diabetes. The accumulation of islet amyloid eventually leads to loss of beta cells.

- **Obesity** is a significant risk factor for diabetes because it results in peripheral insulin resistance.

Other specific types of diabetes, previously called **type 3** or secondary diabetes, results from diseases which destroy beta cells or cause marked insulin resistance, such as:

- Beta cell destruction due to **pancreatitis** or neoplasia. Pancreatitis may be more common than previously thought, as >50% of diabetic cats have evidence of past or current pancreatitis at necropsy (see below under pancreatitis/exocrine pancreatic insufficiency).
- Insulin resistance resulting from unrelated endocrinopathies, e.g. **acromegaly** or **hyperadrenocortisim** (see below under Acromegaly and Hyperadrenocorticism).
- Insulin resistance from **drug administration**, e.g. corticosteroids, megestrol acetate.

60–70% of cats with diabetes require exogenous insulin, at least temporarily.

10–80% of cats with diabetes may lose the need for exogenous insulin. This may result from:

- Correction of **'glucose toxicity'**. Prolonged hyperglycemia causes impaired insulin and increased peripheral insulin resistance, termed glucose toxicity. Exogenous insulin administration and reduction of hyperglycemia can result in resolution of this toxicity and return of sufficient insulin secretion to maintain normoglycemia. Long-acting insulin administered twice daily and a low-carbohydrate, high-protein diet appear to facilitate this.
- Reduction of obesity which deceases insulin resistance.
- Resolution of pancreatitis.
- Treatment of underlying disease, e.g. acromegaly or hyperadrenocortisim.
- Removal of diabetogenic drugs, e.g. progestogens (megestrol acetate) or exogenous corticosteroids.

Clinical signs

Diabetes is the second most common endocrinopathy in cats following hyperthyroidism. However, while it used to affect ~1 in 400 pet cats, in Great Britain this has risen to ~1 in 200.

It can occur in any age, sex or breed of cat, but is seen most frequently in older obese neutered male cats.

In Australia, New Zealand and Great Britain, Burmese cats appear to be predisposed, with ~1 in 50 affected.

The most consistent signs are polyuria, polydipsia and polyphagia. In the early stages these signs may go unnoticed by the owners, possibly because of free choice feeding and outdoor toileting habits.

Possible initial weight gain is followed by weight loss.

Urinary tract infections are common, and cats may present with signs of cystitis and/or renal failure.

The coat may be ill kept and a pot-bellied appearance may result from hepatomegaly.

Hindlimb weakness and a plantigrade stance due to diabetic neuropathy are seen quite frequently, but cataracts occur rarely.

Cats are frequently presented only when they become systemically ill with signs of anorexia, vomiting and/or diarrhea, jaundiced and depression (see page 261, The Cat With Depression, Anorexia or Dehydration).

Cases of diabetes that result from chronic pancreatitis may have a history that includes episodes of depression, anorexia, vomiting, diarrhea and/or abdominal pain. Since diabetes is most likely to occur when most of the pancreatic mass has been destroyed, it may be accompanied by signs of exocrine pancreatic insufficiency, evidenced by large quantities of voluminous fatty feces and a voracious appetite (see below under pancreatitis/exocrine pancreatic insufficiency).

Diagnosis

Diagnosis of diabetes mellitus is based on documenting persistent fasting hyperglycemia (> 11 mmol/l [200 mg/dl]) and glucosuria in a cat with appropriate clinical signs (polyuria, polydipsia and polyphagia).

Stress-induced hyperglycemia can result in glucose levels above the renal threshold and hence glucosuria, so a single documentation of these findings is not diagnostic of diabetes.

Allowing the cat to settle down then re-testing it after a few hours may help to determine whether or not the hyperglycemia is stress-induced. Alternately, the owner can be asked to test the cat's urine for the presence of glucose when it is at home.

Assessing serum fructosamine or glycosylated hemoglobin concentrations will give an indication of how high the blood glucose concentration has been during the preceding 2–3 weeks, and 1–2 months, respectively.

Many cats with diabetes have mild to moderate increases in serum concentrations of cholesterol and liver enzymes. However, more severe changes such as bilirubinemia, acidemia, uremia and electrolyte disorders are unlikely to be present in a cat that is maintaining a good appetite, that is, a cat with uncomplicated diabetes.

Ketones may or may not be present in the urine. Their presence further confirms the diagnosis of diabetes. By the time a cat has developed diabetic ketoacidosis it is unlikely to be maintaining a good appetite (see page 355, The Thin, Inappetent Cat).

Differential diagnosis

These include most of the other causes of weight loss with a good appetite. However, since cats with diabetes develop polyuria and polydipsia, hyperthyroidism and renal disease (particularly protein-losing nephropathies) should be considered as important differentials, as should underlying causes of diabetes, such as acromegaly and hyperadrenocorticism.

Treatment

Treatment consists of various combinations of weight loss, dietary modification, oral hypoglycemic agents and insulin administration.
- While the signs of diabetes in obese cats may resolve with dietary modification alone, most cats need at least temporary medical intervention.
- Oral hypoglycemic agents may be successfully used in some cases of uncomplicated diabetes, or once glucose toxicity has resolved following insulin therapy.
- Insulin is required for most diabetics, at least initially.

Obese cats usually benefit from weight loss. However, this should be done very gradually, restricting calorie intake to no more than 75% of maintenance requirements and monitoring for changes in insulin requirement. Aim for no more than 2% weight loss per week.

Dietary modification – all cats with diabetes benefit from being fed a well-balanced diet on a regular, consistent, feeding schedule.
- Obese cats may benefit from being fed a low-calorie, high-fiber diet to help them lose weight. However, a low-carbohydrate, high-protein diet may be more beneficial to minimize demand for insulin secretion and minimize post-prandial hyperglycemia.
- Non-obese cats benefit from being fed a low-carbohydrate, high-protein diet. The choice of diet may be affected by concurrent illness, especially renal disease.
- Regular feeding is essential. Cats on once-daily insulin are usually fed just before their morning insulin, then again in the early evening. Cats on twice daily insulin are usually fed just before both insulin injections. Free-choice feeding can be beneficial, but it is important to monitor the amount of food eaten on a daily basis.

Oral hypoglycemic agents act to increase insulin secretion, decrease peripheral insulin resistance, and/or decrease absorption of glucose from the intestinal tract. They may successfully control some non-ketotic, uncomplicated diabetic cats, either temporarily or longer term, particularly when given in conjunction with dietary modification. There are several different types of drugs that have been shown to be at least somewhat effective in cats.
- **Sulfonylureas, e.g. glipizide** (0.25 mg/kg PO q 8–12 h, adjust dose as needed). Side effects include vomiting, anorexia and hepatopathy. Periodic checks for serum biochemistry and hematology are recommended. It may take a few weeks of medicating to see the full effect of the drug.
- **Alpha-glucosidase inhibitors, e.g. ararbose** (12.5–25 mg/cat with meals). Side effects include flatulence, soft feces and diarrhea.
- **Transition metals, e.g. vanadium** (0.2 mg/kg/day in food). Side effects include anorexia, vomiting, diarrhea and renal disease; **chromium** (200 µg/cat/day PO). Side effects are unknown.

Insulin: There are a number of different types of insulin, and the choice is often based on personal preference.

- **Most cats with uncomplicated diabetes respond well to once- or twice-daily subcutaneous administration of lente, protamine zinc insulin (PZI) or glargine**.
- The source of the insulin does not appear to be important in cats, as anti-insulin antibodies do not cause many problems.
- The duration of action of the different preparations varies between cats (lente – peak 2–10 h, duration of action 6–16 h; PZI – peak effect at 3–12 h, duration of action 6–24 h; glargine peak effect at 16 h, duration of action > 24 h). In general, PZI and glargine are preferred because of their longer duration of action, improved glycemic control and increased remission rates.
- Start at ~0.25–0.5 IU insulin/kg/per injection, then adjust as necessary, usually by 0.5–1.0 IU per dose. See page 239, Diabetes mellitus in The Cat With Polyuria or Polydipsia, for detailed criteria for adjusting the insulin dose.
- The aim of therapy is to prevent the clinical signs of diabetes and, if possible, maintain blood glucose concentration between 5.5–14 mmol/l (100–250 md/dl).
- It takes 2–3 days for glucose homeostasis to adjust after starting or altering insulin doses. Any changes in dose should therefore be based on recurring effects, not a single urine (or blood) glucose determination. Owners can monitor water intake, urine glucose and ketone levels at home. Ideally glucose will be negative or trace, and ketones will be negative. Glucose curves can also be performed at home by obtaining a drop of blood for glucose testing via ear vein pricking.
  - It is generally recommended that glucose curves be performed every 1–2 weeks until the diabetes is stable. After this time they need be performed less frequently, and the dosage can be adjusted in response to changed clinical signs, ± serum fructosamine concentrations.
  - The usefulness of glucose curves can be very limited in easily stressed cats that become hyperglycemic whenever they are hospitalized. Anorexic cats may have a lower blood glucose concentration in the hospital than at home when eating.
  - A glucose curve is performed by giving the cat its usual breakfast and dose of insulin, then determining blood glucose level every 1–2 h

during a 12–24 h period. The level of the blood glucose at its nadir (lowest point) determines whether or not the dose of insulin needs to be changed, while the duration of insulin action determines how frequently it needs to be given.

Water drunk measured at home on at least two consecutive days is better correlated with mean blood glucose than is fructosamine concentration. If water intake is < 20 ml/kg on wet food or < 70 ml/kg on dry food, it indicates good glycemic control.

At all times, but especially after altering the insulin dosage, the owners should be warned to look for signs of hypoglycemia (weakness, lethargy, shaking, ataxia, collapse and coma). If these signs occur, the cat's gums should be rubbed with sugar water, jam or honey, and immediate veterinary attention sort.

- **Reasons for apparent insulin resistance** include ineffective insulin (out of date, poor storage, incomplete mixing), poor injection technique, out-of-date urine test strips and insulin overdose leading to insulin-induced hyperglycemia. The Somogyi over-swing occurs when hypoglycemia induces counter-regulatory hormones such as epinephrine and glucagon to induce hyperglycemia. True insulin resistance can result from recent weight gain, infection, acromegaly, hyperadrenocorticism, hyperthyroidism, the administration of diabetogenic drugs, renal or hepatic insufficiency, anti-insulin antibodies or presence of certain types of tumor.

Prognosis

The prognosis is very variable. It depends on the owner's commitment, the presence of concurrent and interacting disease and the ease of glycemic control. If diabetes arises secondary to chronic pancreatitis it can be particularly difficult to control.

Prevention

The risk of developing diabetes can be reduced by not allowing cats to become obese or physically inactive and not giving long courses of diabetogenic drugs. A low-carbohydrate, high-protein diet may also help to reduce the demand on beta cells to produce insulin.

INTESTINAL PARASITES**

Classical signs

- Usually in kittens or young adult cats.
- Weight loss or failure to gain weight, usually with a good appetite.
- Diarrhea and/or vomiting may be present.

Pathogenesis

Intestinal parasites that can infect cats and, at least occasionally, cause weight loss associated with a good appetite include **nematodes** (large ascarid roundworms *Toxocara cati* and *Toxascaris leonina*), and **hookworms** (*Ancylostoma braziliense, A. tubaeforme* and *Uncinaria stenocephala*), cestodes (tapeworms *Dipylidium caninum* and *Taenia taeninaeformis*), and **protozoans** (coccidians, *Isospora felis, I. rivolta*, and *Cryptosporidium parvum* and flagellates *Giardia lamblia* and *Tritrichomonas foetus*).

T. cati and *Isospora* spp. are the most common parasites of kittens. *D. caninum, T. taeninaeformis* and *G. lamblia* are the most common parasites of adult cats.

Adult *T. cati* live in the **small intestine** of cats. Eggs are passed into the environment with the feces to be ingested by other cats, in which they **migrate via the liver and lungs** to the small intestine.

- Larvae can be **transmitted lactationally** to kittens, but prenatal infection does not occur.
- Rodents can act as transport hosts.
- Infection can cause *visceral larva migrans* in humans.

Adult *T. leonina* live in the **small intestine of cats**. Eggs are passed into the environment with the feces to be ingested by other cats where they **mature in the wall of the small intestine**.

- Lactational and prenatal infections do not occur.
- Rodents can act as transport hosts.
- Does not cause *visceral larva migrans* in humans.

The prevalence of **hookworms** varies. *Ancylostoma* **spp. prefer warm, humid climates**, while *U. stenocephala* can live in **colder climates**. Severe hookworm infections are usually seen in warm, moist climates.

- Adults hookworms live in the **small intestine** of cats. Eggs are passed into the environment with the feces and then hatch. They can be ingested by other cats or infect them by **skin penetration**.

- Lactational and prenatal infections do not occur.
- Rodents can act as transport hosts.
- Infection can cause *cutaneous larva migrans* in **humans**.

Adult **tapeworms** live in the **small intestine** and both *D. caninum* and *T. taeninaeformis* require an **intermediate host** to complete their life cycle. Gravid proglottids containing many eggs are released from the adult worms. They may rupture within the intestines, or remain intact and pass out in the feces and be seen around the cat's anus.

- **Dog and cat fleas are the intermediate hosts for *D. caninum*.**
- **Rodents are the intermediate hosts for *T. taeninaeformis*.**

Isospora **spp.** live in **intestine** of cats and shed oocysts into the environment via the feces. Sporulated oocysts can be directly ingested by other cats.

- Rodents harboring cyst stages can act as transport hosts.
- Infection and clinical disease is seen most commonly in cats kept in large unhygienic groups.

C. parvum lives in the **small intestine** and sheds oocysts that can either break open to release sporozoites into the intestine resulting in chronic infection or be passed out into the environment where they can remain viable for many months.

- Infection can cause severe disease in immuno-deficient humans.

In cats, *G. lamblia* lives in the **jejunum and ileum**. Environmentally resistant cysts are shed in feces, contaminate drinking water or food, and are then ingested by other cats.

- Infection and clinical disease are seen most commonly in **cats kept in large unhygienic groups**.
- *Giardia* spp. do not appear to be host-specific and have a world-wide distribution in tropical and temperate areas.

In cats, *T. foetus* lives in the **colon** and sheds flagellated protozoa into the feces. Infection and clinical disease are seen most commonly in young cats kept in large unhygienic groups.

Clinical signs

The prevalence of intestinal parasites **varies** with **geographic location, the level of sanitation, whether or**

not the cat is an indoor or outdoor animal, and whether or not it **hunts and eats its prey**.

While infection is common, disease is seen most commonly in **young cats living in poorly cleaned multi-animal environments.**

In these situations, episodes of **disease** may be seen in kittens or cats of similar ages, and may **be preceded by a stressful event** such as an environment change, addition of new cats, or weaning, etc.

Clinical signs vary but typically include **diarrhea and vomiting** (especially with *T. cati* infections), but anorexia is not often present.

- **Ascarids:** In adult cats, infections are usually subclinical, but kittens and young cats may develop vomiting, small bowel diarrhea, a pot-bellied appearance, poor coat condition and a failure to thrive.
- **Hookworms:** Infections cause less disease in cats than dogs, and most disease is seen in young adult cats that live in poorly cleaned, crowded conditions. A heavy infection can cause weight loss, poor coat condition and melena.
- **Tapeworms:** Infections are usually subclinical, but heavy infections can cause anal pruritus, vomiting, diarrhea, weight loss and, occasionally, intestinal obstruction.
- **Isospora spp.:** Infections rarely cause clinical disease in adult cats unless they are stressed or immunocompromised. In kittens, infections can range from subclinical through to severe hemorrhagic diarrhea.
- **C. parvum:** Infections are usually subclinical, but can also cause acute or chronic small bowel diarrhea, or result in lymphocytic-plasmacytic duodenitis.
- **G. lambia:** Infections can be subclinical, or cause acute, chronic or episodic small bowel diarrhea where intestinal malabsorption may result in mucoid, soft, foul-smelling feces.
- **T. foetus:** Infections can be subclinical or cause chronic large bowel diarrhea.

Diagnosis

Intestinal parasites should be suspected in any cat, but especially those coming from a poorly cleaned multi-animal environment in a geographic region with a high prevalence of intestinal parasites.

Since some parasites can be transmitted lactationally (*T. cati*), and infections are frequently more severe in young cats, all young cats should be evaluated for intestinal parasites or treated against the common parasites of the region.

Infection rarely causes systemic changes. However, hematology may reveal an eosinophilia and, in severe cases, low serum proteins may be found on serum biochemistry.

With the exception of tapeworm segments, most intestinal parasites are not noticed in the feces.

Fecal floatation techniques are used to diagnose most intestinal parasites (round worms, hook worms and *Isospora* spp.). However, special techniques may be necessary for some parasites, such as *C. parvum* (special stains or, possibly, fecal antigen tests), *Giardia* spp. (direct saline fecal smears or fecal antigen tests), or *T. foetus* (PCR, 'In Pouch' culture or direct saline fecal smears).

Rather than confirming the presence of an infection with fecal tests, a therapeutic trial with a suitable drug may be considered.

Differential diagnoses

Differential diagnoses include most of the other causes of weight loss with a good appetite. **Inadequate nutrition** becomes the most likely differential when there are no signs other than weight loss. However, the variable presence of **gastrointestinal signs is more suggestive of some of the malassimilation syndromes such as IBD, exocrine pancreatic insufficiency, or early alimentary lymphosarcoma.**

Treatment

Roundworms and hookworms may be treated with **pyrantel pamoate** (20 mg/kg/day – two doses need to be given 2–3 weeks apart) or **fenbendazole** (20–50 mg/kg/day usually given for 3–5 days, then repeated 2–3 weeks later) which are both safe and effective in cats.

Tapeworms may be treated with **praziquantel** (3.5–7.5 mg/kg SC, PO) or **epsiprantel** (2.75 mg/kg PO). One dose is effective against *D. caninum* and *T. taeninaeformis.*

Isospora spp. may be treated with **trimethoprim/sulfonamide** (15 mg/kg q 12 hours PO for 10–14 days), plus improved sanitation.

C. parvum can be difficult to treat, but **tylosin** (10–15 mg/kg q 12 hours PO for 28 days, but may need higher doses), **paromycin** (125–165 mg/kg q 12 hours PO for 5 days), or **azithromycin** (7–15 mg/kg q 12 hours PO for 5–7 days) may be effective.

Giardia **spp.** may be treated with **fenbendazole** (10–30 mg/kg/day PO for 5 days) or **metronidazole** (10–25 mg/kg q 12–24 hours PO for 5–7 days). Repeated treatment may be needed. The possibility of vaccination is currently being studied.

T. foetus may be treated with **ronidazole** (10–30 mg/kg q 12 hours PO for 14 days).

Prognosis

If given the correct treatment, the prognosis for full recovery is usually very good.

Severe infections can occasionally result in permanent intestinal damage and chronic clinical signs.

Resistant *C. parvum*, *Giardia* spp. and/or *T. foetus* infections can occasionally result in chronic disease.

Prevention

Severe infections can usually be prevented by having a good preventative worming policy, giving prompt and effective treatment to any animals found to be infected or carrying these organisms, improving sanitation, and reducing stocking densities.

INADEQUATE NUTRITION**

> **Classical signs**
>
> - Seen in any age, sex or breed of cat, but mostly typically in kittens from poor environments.
> - Weight loss, often in association with a voracious appetite.
> - Few other signs until terminal stages of malnutrition.

Pathogenesis

Disease due to inadequate nutrition is caused by feeding an inadequate or inappropriate diet.

Clinical signs

Disease can be seen in any age, sex or breed of cat, but is seen **most commonly in kittens from poor environments**.

It may also be seen in **pregnant or lactating queens**, or in **cats that have recently changed environments**: e.g. changed from having a sedentary life in a warm environment, to having an active life in adverse weather conditions.

Affected cats show a **generalized loss of body condition** despite a good appetite.

They are usually bright and active until terminal stages of malnutrition.

There are few specific findings, but severe cases may show lethargy, muscle weakness, depression, diarrhea, neurological signs, blindness and/or ascites.

Diagnosis

Diagnosis is based on resolution of clinical signs following correction of diet. If necessary, rule out other likely differentials.

Differential diagnosis

These include most other causes of weight loss with a good appetite. However, given the lack of other clinical signs, the most likely differentials include **intestinal parasites** and **some of the malassimilation syndromes including IBD, exocrine pancreatic insufficiency, early alimentary lymphosarcoma.**

Treatment

Changing the diet to a suitable well-balanced diet is usually all the treatment that is necessary. Very severe cases may need supportive care and nursing.

Prognosis

Provided that the malnutrition was not too severe or prolonged, the prognosis for recovery is very good.

Prevention

Cats should always be fed appropriate amounts of a suitable well-balanced diet that has been designed to be fed to cats.

ALIMENTARY LYMPHOSARCOMA*

Classical signs

- Usually older cats.
- Anorexia and weight loss, ± vomiting, ± diarrhea.
- Early in disease may have a good appetite.

Pathogenesis

Lymphosarcoma is the most common GI neoplasia of cats.

Alimentary lymphosarcoma can occur isolated to the intestine, or as part of multicentric disease.

It can occur as a **focal lesion or diffuse intestinal thickening**. It can arise in the stomach, small intestines and/or colon, and involvement of the ileocolic junction is common.
- Concurrent involvement of mesenteric lymph nodes, liver and/or spleen is not uncommon.

The cells may be lymphocytic, lymphoblastic, of B or T cell origin or, occasionally, large granular lymphocytes or globular leukocytes.

Lymphoblastic lymphosarcoma are more likely than lymphocytic lymphosarcoma to present as an abdominal mass.

Alimentary lymphosarcoma may arise secondary to chronic lymphocytic-plasmacytic IBD.

Clinical signs

Typically seen in older cats of any sex or breed.

History usually includes anorexia and weight loss, but early in the disease the appetite may be good. Vomiting and/or diarrhea may or may not be present.

Some cats develop fever, ascites or jaundice, and at this stage they rarely maintain a good appetite.

Physical examination typically reveals a thin cat with a palpable abdominal mass(es) and/or thickened intestines.

Diagnosis

Hematology may reveal non-specific changes including neutrophilia and lymphopenia. Lymphoblasts may occasionally be seen in the circulation.

Serum biochemistry may reveal panhypoproteinemia and/or hyperbilirubinemia.

Most cats test negative for FeLV infection.

Survey radiographs may reveal gas- or fluid-filled loops of intestines. Barium studies may reveal flocculation or persistent adherence of the barium to the mucosa, irregular mucosal surfaces, luminal narrowing or intramural thickening.

Ultrasound examination may reveal intestinal wall irregularity, thickening, or altered echogenicity, and/or enlarged mesenteric lymph nodes, liver or spleen.

Diagnosis is made by examination of a **GI tract fine-needle aspirate or biopsy**, with or without biopsies from mesenteric lymph nodes and/or other abdominal organs.

Differentiating lymphocytic (small cell) alimentary lymphosarcoma from lymphocytic-plasmacytic IBD can be very difficult.

Determining which types of cells are involved can aid in treatment and prognosis (see below).

Differential diagnosis

These include most of the other causes of weight loss with a good appetite. However, since cats with alimentary lymphosarcoma usually develop vomiting and/or diarrhea, **other causes of enteropathy, IBD, cholangiohepatitis, pancreatitis, hyperthyroidism** and the **other malassimilation syndromes** should be considered as important differentials.

Treatment

Localized alimentary lymphosarcoma may respond to **surgical resection** and adjunct chemotherapy.
- Large masses involving the entire thickness of the bowel wall should not be treated with chemotherapy alone as this may result in **gut perforation**.

Diffuse lymphosarcoma are best treated with combination chemotherapy.

- Lymphoblastic lymphosarcoma and lymphosarcoma affecting more than just the GI tract are best treated with combinations of cyclophosphamide, vincristine and prednisolone, ± doxorubicin, ± l-asparaginase (see page 676, for protocols and doses).
- Lymphocytic lymphosarcoma may respond more favorably to a combination of only prednisolone (10 mg/cat/day PO) and chlorambucil (2–5 mg/m^2 PO up to once every 48 h or 15 mg/m^2/day for 4 days PO, every 3 weeks).

Prognosis

The prognosis is guarded. The best prognostic indicators are response to therapy and the duration of the first remission.

Response rates to chemotherapy range from 30–70%, with median remissions of 4–23 months.

Being **FeLV positive or having lymphoblastic lymphosarcoma are negative indicators**, while having lymphocytic lymphosarcoma is a positive indicator.

- **Lymphoblastic lymphosarcoma** has a complete remission rate of 18%, and median survival time of 2.7 months.
- **Lymphocytic lymphosarcoma** has a complete remission rate 69%, median survival time 22.8 months.

Prevention

Since it is not known what triggers lymphosarcoma to develop, it is not currently possible to prevent its onset. However, since lymphocytic IBD has been seen to progress to lymphosarcoma, it would appear sensible to try to control lymphocytic IBD as well as possible, to try to prevent its progression.

CHRONIC PANCREATITIS/EXOCRINE PANCREATIC INSUFFICIENCY*

Classical signs

- Typically seen in middle-aged to older cats.
- History of episodic anorexia, lethargy, vomiting and/or diarrhea.
- If also diabetic; polyuria and polydipsia.

Pathogenesis

Pancreatitis develops when there is **activation of digestive enzymes** within the pancreas, which results in some degree of auto-digestion. While there are many possible causes of pancreatitis in cats, over 90% are idiopathic.

In cats, the **most common forms** of pancreatic disease are **chronic non-suppurative** (lymphocytic/plasmacytic or, occasionally, eosinophilic) pancreatitis and **suppurative** (neutrophilic) pancreatitis, while acute septicemic pancreatitis and exocrine pancreatic insufficiency (EPI) are seen less frequently.

It is the presence of exocrine pancreatic insufficiency that results in weight loss with a good, often ravenous, appetite.

- Primary exocrine pancreatic insufficiency is uncommon in cats. However, exocrine pancreatic insufficiency secondary to chronic, often episodic, pancreatitis is being recognized more frequently.
- In exocrine pancreatic insufficiency the lack of pancreatic digestive enzymes leads to maldigestion and malabsorption.

In cats, pancreatitis is often seen in association with idiopathic inflammatory bowel disease (IBD), cholangitis/cholangiohepatitis complex, or both (termed "triaditis").

- This association may occur because the **pancreatic duct in some cats enters the common bile duct** before it opens into the duodenum. In other cats, the pancreatic and bile ducts enter the duodenum separately.
- When disease occurs in the small bowel it may ascend the common bile duct and from there affect the pancreas and the rest of the biliary tree, or it may ascend both ducts from their opening in the duodenum. For the same reason, disease of the biliary tree or pancreas may affect the other two regions.
- Regardless of which organ is affected first, the other two organs tend to become involved as inflammatory mediators, infectious agents, bile and/or pancreatic secretions pass from one area to another.

Clinical signs

Chronic pancreatitis can occur in **any sex or breed of cat,** and is typically seen in middle-aged or older cats.

Burmese cats in Great Britain may be predisposed to pancreatitis.

History and clinical signs of chronic pancreatitis tend to be **very variable and non-specific.**

They usually include **episodes of anorexia or variable appetite, with or without vomiting and/or diarrhea, weight loss and/or possible abdominal pain.**

Once exocrine pancreatic insufficiency develops the cat is usually **thin, has a greasy coat** and produces large quantities of voluminous, fatty, foul-smelling feces or has severe diarrhea.

Cats with chronic pancreatitis **may also develop episodic or persistent diabetes mellitus**, which is seen as polyuria and polydipsia.

When both exocrine pancreatic insufficiency and diabetes occur concurrently the **polyphagia** can be profound.

Physical examination is often unremarkable, but may reveal anterior abdominal discomfort, a palpably irregular and enlarged pancreas, or hepatomegaly associated with cholangitis/cholangiohepatitis complex.

Diagnosis

Chronic pancreatitis is very difficult to diagnose.

Hematology and serum biochemistry may reveal non-specific changes.

- **Hematology** may show neutrophilia, neutropenia (associated with sequestration during acute exacerbation), monocytosis and/or a mild non-regenerative anemia.
- **Serum biochemistry** may show hyperglobulinemia, bilirubinemia and raised liver enzymes (depending on the degree of associated cholangitis/cholangiohepatitis complex), and/or hypercholesterolemia, hypertriglyceridemia and hyperglycemia (often associated with concurrent diabetes). Hypocalcemia may be associated with severe disease.
- **Serum amylase and lipase tests** are **rarely useful** in the diagnosis of pancreatitis in cats, although a raised lipase level may be seen occasionally.

Serum cobalamin and folate levels are usually decreased.

A number of older tests are very unreliable and are now rarely used. These include staining fecal smears to demonstrate undigested fat (Sudan III or IV stain) and starch (iodine stain), and fat absorption tests.

Abdominal radiographs are usually unremarkable.

Ultrasound examination may reveal pancreatic enlargement, irregularity or heterogeneity, evidence of peripancreatic fat necrosis, enlargement of mesenteric lymph nodes, and/or evidence of post-hepatic biliary obstruction (enlarged gall bladder, thickened bile or tortuous common bile duct).

Evaluation of serum **trypsin-like immunoreactivity** (TLI) may be helpful.

- The species-specific assay must be performed on a fasted serum sample.
- Serum TLI may be increase with pancreatitis and decrease with exocrine pancreatic insufficiency.
- While it consistently diagnoses exocrine pancreatic insufficiency, it often fails to confirm pancreatitis, possibly because chronic inflammation has reduced the overall ability of the pancreas to produce TLI.

Evaluation of serum **pancreatic lipase immunoreactivity** (PLI) may be helpful.

- The species-specific assay must be performed on a fasted serum sample.
- Serum PLI may increase with pancreatitis and appears to be more sensitive than TLI.

A therapeutic trial with replacement pancreatic enzymes may be considered (see under treatment).

- Providing that any associated IBD and/or cholangitis/cholangiohepatitis complex has been addressed, the response to treatment may be dramatic. However, a positive response is not diagnostic of chronic pancreatitis and/or exocrine pancreatic insufficiency.

Pancreatic biopsy is required to confirm a diagnosis of pancreatitis.

- Because triaditis is common, it is advisable to collect liver and intestinal biopsies at the same time, and send part of the liver biopsy and a sample of bile for culture.

Differential diagnosis

These include most of the other causes of weight loss with a good appetite. However, since cats with chronic pancreatitis and exocrine pancreatic insufficiency usually develop diarrhea and/or vomiting, other **causes of enteropathy, IBD, cholangiohepatitis, alimentary** lymphosarcoma, hyperthyroidism and the other malassimilation syndromes should be considered as important differentials.

Treatment

(For treatment of acute pancreatitis see page 277, The Cat With Depression, Anorexia or Dehydration)

Replace pancreatic enzymes by adding pancreatic enzyme replacement to food (~ half a teaspoonful of powder per meal, or to effect), or add fresh-frozen then defrosted pig pancreas (~20–40 g per meal, or to effect).

Immunosuppression: In the non-suppurative form of pancreatitis, immunosuppressive doses of **corticosteroids** may be needed to reduce ongoing inflammation (prednisolone 1–4 mg/kg q 12–24 hours PO, then taper over 1–3 months and maintain on every other day doses if needed). Alternately, **chlorambucil** could be considered (2–5 mg/m^2 PO up to once every 48 h).

Supportive therapies:
- **Feed a highly digestible, "bland enteric diet"**, which is low in fat. Feed small meals frequently.
- **Cobalamin** is often reduced by lack of pancreatic intrinsic factor and malabsorption and should be supplemented (125–250 µg/week SC or IM for 6–8 weeks or 50–100 µg/cat/day PO).
- **Vitamin K1** is often required because fat malabsorption results in poor absorption of fat-soluble vitamins like vitamin K, and this can result in abnormal hemostasis (0.5 mg/kg/day SC for 3–4 days, then once weekly).
- **Vitamin E** may be given for its anti-oxidative properties (50–200 IU/cat/day PO).

Surgical intervention may be required if complete biliary obstruction occurs (cholecystotomy or cholecystoduodenostomy), or if a focal pancreatic mass is detected (partial pancrectomy to remove a pancreatic pseudocyst, abscess, fibrotic mass or tumor).

Diabetes that develops secondary to chronic pancreatitis can be very difficult to stabilize. Insulin requirements may vary widely because of the ongoing pancreatic pathology, and treatment is complicated further when corticosteroids also need to be given.

It is essential to diagnose and treat any concurrent disease (e.g. IBD and/or cholangitis/cholangiohepatitis complex).

Prognosis

Prognosis depends on the severity of damage. Many cats live with low-grade smoldering pancreatitis for many years, however, once exocrine pancreatic insufficiency and/or diabetes has developed the prognosis is worse.

In rare cases of congenital exocrine pancreatic insufficiency, the prognosis is good, as long as the cat receives pancreatic supplementation.

Prevention

Since it is not known what triggers pancreatitis to develop, it is not currently possible to prevent its onset. However, since chronic pancreatitis can progress to exocrine pancreatic insufficiency, it would appear sensible to try to control it as well as possible to try to prevent its progression.

LYMPHOCYTIC CHOLANGIOHEPATITIS*

Classical signs

- Typically seen in middle-aged cats, and Persian cats may be over-represented.
- Weight loss, inappetence, some cats may be polyphagic,
- ± mild generalized lymphadenopathy,
- ± vomiting and/or diarrhea.
- In some cats, is associated with IBD and/or pancreatitis.

Pathogenesis

The **cholangitis/cholangiohepatitis complex** comprises chronic non-suppurative (lymphocytic) cholangitis/cholangiohepatitis, suppurative cholangitis/cholangiohepatitis and biliary cirrhosis.
- The pathogenesis and interaction of the three conditions is poorly understood and it is highly probably that each of these conditions incorporates a number of different diseases.
- Cholangitis describes inflammation of the biliary tract, while cholangiohepatitis describes inflammation of the peribiliary hepatocytes as well as the biliary tract.

- **The only condition that may be associated with polyphagia is lymphocytic cholangitis/cholangiohepatitis.**

Pathogenesis of lymphocytic cholangitis/cholangiohepatitis complex is unknown. It is probably immune-mediated, but is possibly associated with progression of the suppurative form. **It is often associated with IBD and/or pancreatitis, and when all three occur together it is termed "triaditis".**

Clinical signs

Cats of any age may be affected, but disease is seen most typically in **middle-aged cats. Persian cats** may have an increased risk.

Clinical signs are usually chronic and insidious in nature.

Affected cats are **typically jaundiced, but bright, and are often polyphagic.**

Vomiting and/or diarrhea may be present.

Cats may have a **palpably enlarged liver and mild generalized lymphadenopathy.**

Cats may show **intermittent signs of systemic illness**, with **fever**, **anorexia**, weight loss, and vomiting. Systemic signs are sometimes associated with secondary infections, typically of the liver and/or pancreas.

The disease may progress to causing chronic biliary cirrhosis with ascites, hepatic encephalopathy, and bleeding tendencies.

Diagnosis

Serum biochemistry often reveals mild to moderately (occasionally severely) increased liver enzymes, increased bile acids, hyperbilirubinemia, hyperglobulinemia and hypoalbuminemia.

Hematology may reveal mild anemia, lymphopenia or lymphocytosis, monocytosis and/or thrombocytopenia. **Blood clotting times are frequently prolonged.**

Ascitic fluid, if present, is typically high in protein.

Radiographs typically reveal **hepatomegaly** and occasionally choleliths (gallstones), while **ultrasound** examination may also show blotchy hepatic hyperechogenicity, "sludging" of bile, and evidence of common bile duct obstruction. Associated findings may include enlarged mesenteric lymph nodes, pancreatic irregularity, and/or thickening of the duodenal walls.

A **definitive diagnosis** is made by **histopathological examination of a liver biopsy**.

- A fine-needle aspirate is rarely diagnostic, so a **percutaneous needle biopsy or surgical wedge biopsy** is required. Blood clotting times and/or a PIVKA test (protein induced by vitamin K absence or antagonism) should be assessed first, and a platelet count should be performed.
- Typical gross findings include a **very firm often rather irregular liver**, and a thickened and distended gallbladder and common bile duct, which often contains inspissated bile. Enlarged mesenteric lymph nodes, pancreatic irregularity and/or thickening of the duodenal walls may also be present.
- If performing an exploratory laparotomy, it is sensible to check the patency of the biliary outflow, then collect biopsies from the mesenteric lymph nodes, small intestines and pancreas as well as liver. Send bile and part of the liver biopsy for culture.
- Histopathology of the liver reveals **lymphocytic and/or plasmacytic periportal inflammation, bile ductule hyperplasia**, and **periportal fibrosis**. Very chronic cases may have biliary cirrhosis.

Differential diagnosis

These include most of the other causes of weight loss with a good appetite. However, since cats with lymphocytic cholangitis/cholangiohepatitis complex often develop vomiting and/or diarrhea enteropathies (including IBD), **pancreatitis**, **and the other malassimilation syndromes** should be considered as important differentials. In cases that develop ascites, the **wet form of feline infectious peritonitis (FIP)** should also be considered. This is because both conditions produce a protein-rich ascitic fluid and have similar biochemical and hematological changes. However, the presence of polyphagia usually differentiates the two conditions as cats with FIP are usually anorexic.

Treatment

Treatment is largely empirical.

Antibiotics, if needed:

- Ampicillin (10–40 mg/kg q 8 hours PO), amoxicillin (11–22 mg/kg q 8–12 hours PO), or cephalexin (10–35 mg/kg q 8–12 hours PO)
- Add **metronidazole** for its effect against anaerobes and its immune-modulating effects (7.5–10 mg/kg every 12 hours PO). Do not use higher doses, as these can be hepatotoxic.

Immunosuppressive agents:
- Immunosuppressive doses of **corticosteroids** (prednisolone 2–4 mg/kg q 12–24 hours PO), then taper over 1–3 months, and maintain on every other day doses if needed.
- Other immunosuppressive agents may be considered, e.g. **methotrexate** (0.13 mg/cat every 12 hours × 3 doses PO, repeated once weekly) or **chlorambucil** (2–5 mg/m² PO up to once every 48 h).

Supportive therapies:
- **Ursodeoxycholic acid** aids bile flow and is believed to have hepatoprotective effects (10–15 mg/kg q 24 hours PO).
- **Vitamin K1** is often required because fat malabsorption results in poor absorption of fat-soluble vitamins like vitamin K and this can result in abnormal hemostasis (0.5 mg/kg q 24 hours SC for 3–4 days, then once every 7–14 days).
- **Vitamin E** may be given for its anti-oxidative properties (50–200 IU/cat/day PO).
- **S-adenosylmethionine** (SAMe) may be given for its hepato-protective and anti-oxidative properties (18 mg/kg/day PO).
- Some authors suggest feeding either hypoallergenic or high-fiber diets.
- **Milk thistle**, 7–50 mg/kg q24h PO.

Surgery will be required where **complete biliary obstruction** occurs (cholecystotomy or cholecystoduodenostomy).

It is important to address any associated or underlying conditions, such as IBD, pancreatitis, extrahepatic bile duct obstruction or cholecystitis.

Prognosis

Prognosis is **very variable and often unpredictable**. Some cases respond well and only need temporary treatment, others require continued therapy to maintain remission, while others progress relatively rapidly and require euthanasia. Once severe fibrosis, cirrhosis or ascites has developed the prognosis is usually guarded.

Prevention

Since it is not known what triggers the development of lymphocytic cholangitis/cholangiohepatitis complex, it is currently not possible to prevent its onset.

ACROMEGALY

Classical signs

- Rare condition of older, typically, male cats.
- Slow increase in body size, especially affecting head and feet.
- Variable weight change with a good appetite.
- Usually diabetic; so polyuric and polydipsic.

Pathogenesis

In cats, most cases of acromegaly are caused by the development of a **growth hormone-secreting tumor within the pituitary gland.**

Unlike the situation in the dog, increased levels of circulating progestogens or progesterone do not stimulate growth hormone secretion in the cat.

Clinical signs

Acromegaly is seen most typically in older, male, mixed-breed cats.

Affected cats slowly increase in size, with somewhat disproportionate enlargement and thickening of the head and feet.
- Growth of the jaw bones may result in obvious interdental spaces and/or prognathism.
- A mild increase in respiratory noise may result from increased soft tissue thickness around the airways.
- Distortion of the joints can lead to destructive arthritis.

Acromegalic cats develop insulin-resistant diabetes because excess growth hormone causes peripheral insulin resistance. However, early cases may have unstable diabetes rather than being truly resistant.

- They therefore develop polyuria, polydipsia and polyphagia.
- They may either gain or lose weight.

While all organs undergo growth and hypertrophy, hepatomegaly and renomegaly are the easiest to detect on palpation. Enlargement of the abdominal organs often results in a pot-bellied appearance.

Organ enlargement may lead to organ failure. The clinical signs will therefore reflect the particular organ systems that have been affected; e.g. cardiac hypertrophy and eventual congestive heart failure, liver failure and/or kidney failure.

Concurrent hypertension may result in clinical signs, typically ocular hemorrhages, sudden blindness and/or neurological signs.

Only rarely do neurological signs result from the pituitary tumor compressing and invading the hypothalmus.

Diagnosis

Acromegaly should be considered in any large-sized cat which develops insulin-resistant or unstable diabetes.
- Hyperglycemia and glycosuria will be present, but ketosis is rare.
- Affected cats may also show azotemia, hypercholesterolemia, hyperphosphatemia, hyperproteinemia, erythrocytosis and mildly raised liver enzymes.

Comparing the cat to a previous photograph of itself can be helpful in confirming the disproportionate enlargement and thickening of its head.

A definitive diagnosis can be made by measuring growth hormone levels (where available) **or insulin-like growth factor-1** (IGF-1) assay, which gives similar results. Unfortunately, the degree of elevation does not always correlate with the clinical signs, and IGF-1 will also be increased in most cats treated long-term with insulin.

The presence of acromegaly can be confirmed by evaluating the **growth hormone response** to a **glucose suppression test**.

Other tests can be used to gain supportive evidence.
- Radiography may show organomegaly, increased interdental spaces, hyperostosis of the skull and/or degenerative arthritis.

- Ultrasonography and, where available, computed tomography (CT) or magnetic resonance imaging (MRI) can also be used to detect organomegaly. CT and MRI may be used to determine the location and extent of the tumor within the brain.

Differential diagnosis

Differential diagnoses include most of the other causes of weight loss with a good appetite. However, since all cats with acromegaly develop diabetes with polyuria and polydipsia, other causes of **diabetes, hyperadrenocorticism, hyperthyroidism and renal insufficiency** are the most important differentials.

Treatment

Acromegaly can be **treated three ways; surgery, external-beam radiotherapy or medically**.
- **Surgical excision of the growth hormone-secreting tumor** is usually a rapid and effective treatment for affected humans. However, the procedure has rarely been performed in cats, and mapping of the tumor is essential prior to considering surgery.
- **In humans, external-beam radiotherapy is often effective**, although clinical improvement may be slow to develop. The few cats that have been treated in this way have shown variable results. Treatment requires repeated anesthetics and suitable facilities are limited.
- Although they require frequent administration and usually cause side-effects, **somatostatin analogs** (e.g. octreotide) and **dopamine agonists** (e.g. bromocriptine) are sometimes used in the treatment of humans with acromegaly. Unfortunately, limited trials with octreotide in acromegalic cats have not been promising, and dopamine agonists have not yet been evaluated in this species.

Temporary management consists of **trying to treat the diabetes** and any other concurrent or related diseases (e.g. hypertension, heart failure, renal disease).
- Control of the diabetes can usually be achieved by giving extremely **high doses of exogenous** insulin (20–130 IU/day), sometimes in various combinations of short-, intermediate- or long-acting insulin. However, because the severity of the insulin resistance can fluctuate, the dose should not exceed 12–15 IU/injection so the risk of iatrogenic hypoglycemia is reduced.

- Very rarely, spontaneous necrosis of the tumor can result in temporary or permanent remission of clinical signs.

Prognosis

The long-term prognosis is poor. However, because the tumors grow very slowly, the short-term prognosis may be good to guarded with **survival times of 4–48 or more months reported**.

Prevention

Since acromegaly is usually caused by a slow growing pituitary tumor, its development cannot be prevented.

HYPERADRENOCORTICISM

Classical signs

- A rare condition of middle-aged and older cats.
- Poor coat condition and pot-bellied appearance.
- Polyuric, polydipsic, polyphagic and often diabetic.

Pathogenesis

In cats, hyperadrenocorticism, more correctly termed **hypercortisolism, can be caused by:**
- **Adrenocorticotropin (ACTH)-secreting pituitary tumors**;
  - Approximately 80% of cats with hyperadrenocorticism have a pituitary tumor and most are microadenomas.
- **Adrenal tumors that autonomously secretes cortisol**;
  - Represent about 20% of cases, and approximately 50% of adrenal tumors are benign adenoma, and 50% are malignant.
- **Iatrogenic hyperadrenocorticism** can be caused by giving long courses of exogenous corticosteroids (parenteral, oral or topical) or megestrol actetate.

Clinical signs

Hyperadrenocorticism is typically seen in middle-aged to older cats. Females may be over represented.

History is often vague, but usually includes **polyuria, polydipsia, polyphagia, weight loss and lethargy**, and affected cats may have a history of recurrent infections and/or abscesses.

Since cortisol antagonizes insulin, **approximately 80% of cases develop diabetes**, which may or may not be insulin resistant, based on the insulin dose administered.

Cats with hyperadrenocorticism typically have **poor coat condition, spontaneous alopecia, very fragile thin skin that bruises easily** and a **pot-bellied appearance**. Hepatomegaly is often palpable.

Diagnosis

Hyperadrenocorticism should be suspected in any cat with the clinical signs described above, particularly if it has **unstable diabetes**, and/or **a long history of exogenous corticosteroids administration**.

Since hyperadrenocorticism is frequently associated with diabetes, serum biochemistry and urinalysis often reveal persistent **hyperglycemia, glucosuria ± ketonuria**.

Unlike in dogs, a stress leukogram is rarely present, although lymphopenia may be seen.

Increased liver enzymes and **hypercholesterolemia** may be seen regardless of whether or not the cat has diabetes.

Making a diagnosis of hyperadrenocorticism can be very difficult:
- Few of the tests have well-established specificity and sensitivity in cats.
- It is usually necessary to use a combination of tests.

In cats, the **most useful screening tests** are:
- **Adrenocorticotropic hormone (ACTH) stimulation test** – Collect baseline blood sample, give 0.125 mg of synthetic ACTH IV, collect blood after 1 ± 2 hours. Normal basal serum cortisol concentration is 10–110 nmol/L (0.36–3.6 µg/dl); at 1 h and/or 2 h after ACTH is 210–330 nmol/L (7.6–11.9 µg/dl); > 330 nmol/L (> 11.9 µg/dl) is

consistent with hyperadrenocorticism. False negatives and positives occur.

- **Low-dose dexamethasone suppression test** – Collect baseline blood sample, give dexamethasone 0.01 mg/kg IV, collect blood after 4 and 8 hours. In normal cats serum cortisol should be < 30 nmol/L (< 1.0 µg/dl) at 4 h and 8 h after dexamethasone. Lack of suppression is seen in most cats (95%) with hyperadrenocorticism, and some cats with non-adrenal illness.
- **Urine cortisol to creatinine ratio (UC/CR)** – Collect urine sample, centrifuge and submit supernatant. A normal ratio almost always rules out hyperadrenocorticism. Unfortunately, an increased ratio is commonly caused by non-adrenal illness. The test is more reliable if the sample is collected at home.

Additional tests may be used to try to differentiate pituitary-dependent hyperadrenocorticism (PDH) from adrenal neoplasia. These include:

- **High-dose dexamethasone suppression test** – Performed as low-dose dexamethasone suppression test but give 0.1 mg/kg. Lack of suppression at 8 h is seen in most cats (80%) with hyperadrenocorticism. Suppression at 4 h but not at 8 h is consistent with PDH. False negatives may occur in mild cases of hyperadrenocorticism.
- **Ultra-high-dose dexamethasone suppression test** – Performed as low-dose dexamethasone suppression test but give 1.0 mg/kg. Suppression at 4 h or 8 h to < 30 nmol/l (< 1.0 µg/dl) or <50% of baseline is consistent with PDH, but lack of suppression may be seen with PDH and adrenal tumors.
- **Combination test** – Collect blood sample, give 1.0 mg/kg dexamethasone IV, collect blood after 4 h, then immediately perform ACTH stimulation test as above. Interpretation is as for ACTH stimulation test and ultra-high-dose dexamethasone suppression test (taking ultra-high-dose dexamethasone suppression test result as result at 4 h).
- **'At home' protocol** – Collect urine on the morning of Days 1 and 2; give two oral doses of dexamethasone at 8 hour intervals at 4 pm and 12 pm; then collect a third urine sample on the morning of Day 3. All three samples are assessed for UC/CR. The mean of the first two UC/CR = basal value and acts as a screening test. Suppression < 50% basal on Day 3 is not seen in cats with adrenal-

dependent hyperadrenocorticism, but may be seen in cats with PDH.

- **Measurement of endogenous ACTH** – Collect blood sample in EDTA, spin immediately, transfer plasma to a plastic tube, ship overnight on ice or freeze for storage. Plasma ACTH is high normal or above (>15 pg/ml) with PDH, and low (<10 pg/ml) with adrenal tumors.
- **Radiography, ultrasonography and, where available, CT or MRI**. Use to determine adrenal size and shape. The presence of adrenal mineralization should not be over-interpreted as it occurs in ~30% of normal cats. Unilateral adrenal enlargement is typical of an adrenal tumor. While bilateral enlargement usually indicates PDH, it can occasionally result from bilateral adrenal tumors. Hepatomegaly is found in ~75% of all cats with hyperadrenocorticism. CT and MRI can be used to image the pituitary gland as well as the adrenal glands.

Differential diagnoses

Differential diagnoses include most of the other causes of weight loss with a good appetite. However, since most cats with hyperadrenocorticism develop polyuria, polydipsia and diabetes, **other causes of diabetes, acromegaly, hyperthyroidism and renal insufficiency** are the most important differentials.

Treatment

While there are a number of different treatment options, there have been few good studies into their use in cats.

Medical therapies have generally given poor results, and safe dosages have not been established. They may be given pre-surgically to reduce the operative risks.

- **Trilostane** has produced promising results in a very small number of cases and warrants further investigation, particularly given that side effects have not been significant.
- **Mitotane** gave poor results in early trials, and it has been suggested that higher doses and/or longer courses may be needed.
- **Ketoconazole** has given mixed results and considerable toxicity.

- **Metyrapone** has given mixed results and is difficult to obtain.
- **L-depronyl** has little information available on use in cats, and no proven efficacy.

Radiation therapy with ablation of the pituitary tumor has given mixed results.

Adrenalectomy. Because of the difficulties of medical therapy, **surgery has been considered the treatment of choice**. However, this is changing with the success of trilostane treatment. Where a single adrenal tumor is present, the removal of the affected adrenal gland is recommended. With PDH or bilateral adrenal tumors, bilateral adrenalectomy is recommended. While surgery can provide successful treatment, the **risk of a fatal peri-operative hypoadrenal crisis, renal failure or surgical complications are great**. The procedure should only be performed by an **experienced surgeon**. Consideration of the diabetic state must be given, and peri-operative and post-operative treatment with glucocorticoids is essential. **Glucocorticoids are needed in all cases**. Short-term treatment will be needed after unilateral adrenalectomy, because the contralateral gland will be temporarily atrophied. Long-term treatment will be needed after bilateral adrenalectomy, and should also include mineralocorticoids.

Prognosis

Without successful treatment, the prognosis is poor. Where PDH is present, successful bilateral adrenalectomy will reduce the signs of hyperadrenocorticism, but the risk of a hypoadrenal crisis is high and tumor expansion will eventually lead to neurological signs. If adrenal tumors are successfully removed the hyperadrenocorticism should resolve, and the diabetic state may become less insulin resistant or even resolve. Early studies with trilostane appear to show that while it may ameliorate signs of hyperadrenocorticism, it may not alter the need for exogenous insulin in cats that are also diabetic.

Prevention

Since hyperadrenocorticism is usually caused by pituitary or adrenal tumors, its development cannot be prevented. Iatrogenic hyperadrenocorticism can be prevented by not giving long courses of exogenous corticosteroids.

GLOMERULONEPHRITIS (PROTEIN-LOSING NEPHROPATHY)

Classical signs

- Rare disease seen most frequently in young male cats.
- Weight loss with a good appetite early in disease.
- Often marked subcutaneous edema and ascites.
- ± polydipsia and polyuria.
- ± vomiting and/or diarrhea.

Pathogenesis

Glomerulonephropathy can arise from **one of two mechanisms**:

- **Primary glomerulonephritis** has **antibodies** targeted directly against the **glomerular basement membrane**.
- **Secondary glomerulonephritis** has **deposition of immune complexes** within the glomeruli that have arisen elsewhere in the body.
  - This is the most common form in cats.
  - It tends to be **membranous or membrano-proliferative** in nature.
  - It may be associated with many different conditions (see below), but in most cases the underlying cause cannot be found.
- **Diseases** that may be **associated with secondary glomerulonephritis** in cats include infection with FeLV, FIV, FIP, *Mycoplasma* spp., or *Ehrlichia* spp., chronic pyoderma, chronic gingivitis, dirofilariasis, endocarditis, pancreatitis, pyometra, neoplasia or other immune-mediated diseases.

Deposition of immune complexes within the glomerulus leads to the initiation of inflammation and this results in proteinuria (protein-losing nephropathy).

Clinical signs

Rare condition seen most typically in **young male cats**.

Clinical signs may be non-specific. Typically in the later stages there is anorexia, depression, weight loss, lethargy and poor coat condition. More specific signs include **subcutaneous edema, ascites, and polyuria and polydipsia**.

It tends to takes one of two clinical forms:
- **Nephrotic syndrome** with ascites and subcutaneous edema, usually affecting the hind legs, ventral body wall and neck. This form may or may not be associated with signs of renal failure (polyuria, polydipsia).
- **Renal failure with no signs of nephrotic syndrome.**

Cats with early nephrotic syndrome may present with weight loss with a good appetite.

Edema affecting the intestines can exacerbate the protein loss and result in **malabsorption, diarrhea, vomiting and weight loss**.

Systemic hypertension may arise secondary to the renal dysfunction and result in **acute blindness, ocular hemorrhages** or signs of CNS dysfunction.

Other clinical signs may result from any primary disease conditions.

On abdominal palpation, the **kidneys may appear small and/or irregular or, occasionally, enlarged.**

Diagnosis

Cats with nephrotic syndrome have marked proteinuria, hypoalbuminemia and hypercholesterolemia.

Other findings may include hypertriglyceridemia, hypocalcemia, non-regenerative anemia and neutrophilia.

Increased concentrations of blood urea and creatinine (azotemia) and a low urine specific gravity (<1.035) will indicate whether or not renal insufficiency is present.

Persistent proteinuria is the hallmark of glomerulonephritis.
- This should be quantified by determining the **urine protein to creatinine ratio (UPC ratio)**.
- UPC ratio: < 0.4 = normal, > 0.4–2 suggestive of glomerulonephropathy or tubular disease, > 2 consistent with glomerulonephropathy.

Urinalysis may reveal an inactive sediment, with or without hyaline and/or granular casts.

It is important to try to determine an underlying cause. This may involve screening radiography and ultrasonography, tests for immune-mediated disease, and numerous tests for infectious disease (see above for the list of possible diseases).

Systemic blood pressure should be **assessed**.

Abdominal radiographs and ultrasound examination rarely reveal obvious renal changes.

Renal biopsy is necessary to confirm the diagnosis and find which type of glomerular disease is present.
- Blood clotting times, platelet number, and systemic blood pressure should be assessed prior to biopsy.
- **Ultrasound-guided percutaneous biopsy** is relatively safe but **laparotomy or laparoscopy** reduces the risk of post-operative bleeding. Renal hemorrhage is a risk, especially if hypertensive.
- Sample must **contain >5 glomeruli** to make a diagnosis; this usually means **multiple needle biopsies or a wedge biopsy** are required.
- Routine **histopathology** (fix sample in buffered normal formalin), **electromicroscopy** (fix sample in paraformaldehyde-glutaraldehyde), ± **immunohistochemistry** (keep fresh and paraffin embed) are needed to confirm a diagnosis.
- **On gross inspection** kidneys may appear normal, be slightly small, firm and pale, or show irregular pitting and fibrosis.
- Light microscopy typically shows **diffuse thickening of the glomerular basement membrane**, with variable degrees of **cellular proliferation** in the affected glomeruli. Special stains can help to define the changes, but electromicroscopy and immunohistochemistry are needed to define the exact nature and extent of the disease.

Differential diagnosis

Chronic renal failure, diabetes, acromegaly, hyperadrenocorticism and hyperthyroidism are important differentials in those cats that develop polyuria and polydipsia. However, the presence of ascites in combination with polyphagia is suggestive of **lymphocytic cholangitis/cholangiohepatitis complex**. Once hypoalbuminemia is detected, then a **protein-**

losing enteropathy or severe liver failure should be considered.

Treatment

Treatment for nephrotic syndrome is controversial and usually empirical.

Monitor response to treatment by assessing changes in body weight, serum and urinary protein levels.

Where an underlying cause can be found it should be treated.

Alter the level of dietary protein:
- High protein diets may help to correct hypoalbuminemia and reduce protein malnutrition.
- However, they may exacerbate proteinuria, glomerular hypertension and glomerular damage.
- High-protein diets should not be fed if serum urea is elevated.
- Some cats benefit from mild protein addition while others benefit from mild protein restriction. Feed the chosen diet for ~ 2 weeks then reassess.

Angiotensin-converting enzyme (ACE) inhibitors help to reduce proteinuria and any associated systemic hypertension (e.g. benazepril 0.25–0.5 mg/kg/day PO).

If systemic hypertension is significant, the calcium channel antagonist amlodipine (0.625 mg/cat/day PO) should be given.

Use of corticosteroids and immunosuppressive drugs is controversial. They may or may not help to reduce immune complex formation, will worsen any azotemia, and are contraindicated once renal failure is evident.

Very careful use of diuretics can help to reduce fluid retention and improve the patient's well-being (e.g. frusemide 1–2 mg/kg q 8–12 hours PO, reducing to as low dose as possible and monitoring closely for side-effects).

Thromboembolic disorder is rare in cats, but if present consider giving low doses of aspirin (10–25 mg/kg every 3 days PO).

Prognosis

Very variable and often unpredictable. Some undergo spontaneous complete or partial remissions (~30%), others need temporary or continuous therapy, while others progress relatively rapidly to require euthanasia.

Approximately 50% survive for 2.5–6 years.

Cats with nephrotic syndrome that do not originally have renal insufficiency, may or may not progress to develop renal insufficiency.

Prognosis is poor with worsening clinical signs or progression to renal failure.

Prevention

Prompt recognition and treatment of underlying disease may prevent the development of secondary glomerulonephritis. However, since it is not usually possible to detect the underlying cause, it is not usually possible to prevent the onset of glomerulonephritis.

RECOMMENDED READING

Arthur JE, Lucke VM, Newby TJ, Bourne FJ. The long-term prognosis of feline idiopathic membranous glomerulonephropathy. J Am Anim Hosp Assoc 1986; 22: 731–737.

Fondacaro JV, Richter KP, Carpenter JL, et al. Feline gastrointestinal lymphoma: 67 cases (1988–1996). Eur J Comp Gastroenterol 1999; 4: 5–11.

Foster DM, Gookin JL, Poore MF, Stebbins ME, Levy MG. Outcome of cats with diarrhea and *Tritrichomonas foetus* infection. J Am Vet Med Assoc 2004; 225: 888–892.

Gookin JL, Breitschwerdt EB, Levy MG, Gager RB, Benrud JG. Diarrhea associated with tritrichomonas in cats. J Am Vet Med Assoc 1999; 215: 1450–1454.

Gookin J, Copple C, Papich M, Poore M, Levy M. Efficacy of ronidazole *in vitro* and *in vivo* for treatment of feline *Tritrichomonas foetus* infection. Proceedings of the ACVIM, 2005, Abstract 131.

Gookin J, Stebbins ME, Hunt E, et al. Prevalence of and risk factors for feline *Tritrichomonas foetus* and *Giardia* infection. J Clin Micro 2004; 42: 2707–2710.

Goossens M, Nelson RW, Feldman EC, Griffey SM. Response to insulin treatment and survival in 104 cats with diabetes mellitus (1985–1995). J Vet Intern Med 1998; 12: 1–6.

Lees GE, Brown SA, Elliot J, et al. Assessment and management of proteinuria in dogs and cats. 2004 ACVIM Forum Consensus Statement (small animal). J Vet Intern Med 2005; 19: 377–385.

Lucke VM. Glomerulonephritis in the cat. Vet Ann 1982; 22: 270–278.

Lutz TA, Rand JS. Pathogenesis of feline diabetes mellitus. Vet Clin North Am Small Anim Pract 1995; 25(3):527–552.

Neiger R, Witt AL, Noble A, German AJ. Trilostane therapy for treatment of pituitary-dependent hyperadrenocorticism in 5 cats. J Vet Intern Med 2004; 18: 160–164.

Peterson ME, Taylor RS, Greco DS, et al. Acromegaly in 14 cats. J Vet Intern Med 1990; 4: 192–201.

Rand JS, Bobbermien LM, Hendrikz JK, Copland M. Over representation of Burmese cats with diabetes mellitus. Aust Vet J 1997; 75: 402–405.

Vail DM, Moore AS, Ogilvie GK, Volk LM. Feline lymphoma (145 cases): Proliferation indices, cluster of differentiation 3 immunoreactivity, and their association with prognosis in 90 cats. J Vet Intern Med 1998; 12: 349–354.

Zwahlen CH, Lucroy MD, Kraegel SA, Madewell BR. Results of chemotherapy for cats with alimentary malignant lymphoma: 21 case (1993–1997). J Am Vet Med Assoc 1998; 213: 1144–1149.

18. The thin, inappetent cat

Penny Barber[†], James B Miller and Jacquie Rand

KEY SIGNS

- Thin cat or cat with weight loss and a poor appetite.

MECHANISM?

- Weight loss occurs when nutrient loss or metabolic utilization exceeds intake. Weight loss results from one or more of the following mechanisms: inadequate intake; impaired ability to digest or absorb; inability to utilize; increased utilization or the increased loss of nutrients.
  A lack of appetite is associated with suppression of the appetite center in the hypothalamus.

WHERE?

- Diseases involving most body systems can cause weight loss and affect appetite.

WHAT?

- The most common causes of a thin, inappetent cat are chronic renal failure, neoplasia and several of the viral diseases (FIV, FeLV, FIP). Many other diseases will cause weight loss, but inappetence will frequently occur late in the disease process.

QUICK REFERENCE SUMMARY
Diseases causing signs of a thin, inappetent cat

ANOMALY

- Portosystemic shunts (p 361)
May be congenital or acquired. In congenital portosystemic shunts, growth may be stunted. Neurological signs of hepatic encephalopathy (behavioral, seizures, blindness) may occur and hypersalivation is a frequent sign.

METABOLIC

- **Chronic renal failure*** (p 333)**
Chronic history of gradual weight loss, polyuria and polydipsia. Systemic signs such as inappetence and vomiting are common.

- ### Septic focus/persistent fever ** (p 344)
Anorexia is associated with the pyrexia. Anorexia and a hypermetabolic state lead to weight loss. Fluctuating pyrexia, poor appetite and weight loss are present, along with other clinical signs dependent on the etiology of the pyrexia. Common sites of bacterial infection include pyothorax, upper urinary tract infections and bite wounds, with peritonitis, osteomyelitis, endocarditis and pneumonia occurring less commonly.

- ### Apathetic hyperthyroidism* (p 346)
Weight loss, poor appetite, tachycardia and intermittent vomiting and diarrhea are common. Usually affects cats greater than 6 years of age.

- ### Cholangiohepatitis complex* (p 348)
Anorexia or poor appetite, weight loss and depression. Icterus and hepatomegaly are common. Ascites occasionally occurs.

- ### Cardiac cachexia (p 356)
Clinical signs relating to the cardiac disease including murmurs, gallop rhythm and arrhythmias. Dyspnea caused by pleural effusion or pulmonary edema may also be present.

- ### Diabetes mellitus (p 355)
Polyuria and polydypsia. Frequently history of good appetite with weight loss prior to inappetence.

NEOPLASTIC

- ### Cancer cachexia** (p 342)
Paraneoplastic syndrome characterized by anorexia, wasting and weight loss. Occurs with a variety of malignancies, and more specific signs will relate to the site of the neoplasm.

INFECTIOUS

- ### Feline immunodeficiency virus (FIV)*** (p 339)
Chronic weight loss, stomatitis, lymph node enlargement and neurologic signs. Signs may be vague and variable. Immunosuppression resulting in secondary, opportunistic infections is common.

- ### Feline leukemia virus (FeLV)* (p 350)
A variety of clinical signs depending on the system(s) of the body affected. Neoplasia, particularly lymphoma, and chronic anemia or pancytopenia occur. Immunosuppression resulting in secondary, opportunistic infections is common.

- ### Feline infectious peritonitis (FIP)* (p 352)
Chronic, fluctuating pyrexia with anorexia and weight loss. The non-effusive ("dry") form frequently leads to clinical signs associated with the organs involved (liver, kidney, ocular or central nervous system). The effusive ("wet") form of the disease causes ascites, pleural or occasionally pericardial effusions.

- ### Chronic bacterial rhinitis and sinusitis (p 356)
Chronic sneezing, and mucopurulent nasal discharge may be associated with a poor appetite and weight loss.

- ### Toxoplasmosis (p 359)
Muscle hyperesthesia, respiratory distress, fever, uveitis and neurological signs including seizures occur variably.

continued

continued

● Cryptococcosis (p 360)

Chronic mucopurulent or hemorrhagic nasal discharge, sneezing and distortion of the dorsum of the nose are typical. Central nervous system signs including seizures are less common.

● Systemic mycoses (p 361)

Blastomycosis and histoplasmosis may cause depression, anorexia and weight loss in endemic areas. The most common clinical sign is dyspnea, but signs vary with the organ systems affected.

INFLAMMATION

● **Oral inflammatory disease* (p 353)**

Usually lymphocytic-plasmacytic in nature. Causes reluctance to eat, dysphagia and drooling of saliva with associated weight loss.

● **Inflammatory bowel disease* (p 349)**

Chronic weight loss, intermittent vomiting and/or diarrhea. Cats may have minimal clinical signs other than weight loss.

● Protein-losing nephropathy (p 358)

Results from glomerulonephritis (rare) and amyloidosis (familial disease in Abyssinian). Marked weight loss occurs initially, followed by decreased appetite, polyuria and polydipsia associated with the development of renal failure. Ascites and peripheral edema occur if protein loss is severe.

IDIOPATHIC

● Chylothorax (p 357)

Respiratory distress. Decreased appetite may occur late in the disease.

INTRODUCTION

MECHANISM?

Weight loss of greater than 10% of body weight is significant and should be investigated.

Any cause of weight loss may present as failure to grow or stunting if affecting an immature cat.

Weight loss occurs when there are one or more of the following:

● Inappetence (inadequate caloric intake).
● Inability to digest or absorb nutrients (e.g. pancreatic exocrine insufficiency, inflammatory bowel disease).
● Inability to utilize absorbed nutrients (e.g. diabetes mellitus).
● Increased utilization of absorbed nutrients (e.g. hyperthyroidism, fever).

● Increased loss of nutrients (e.g. protein-losing enteropathy or nephropathy).

Maintenance energy requirements in the adult cat are approximately 50–70 kcal/kg body weight/day. Intakes below maintenance will result in weight loss.

Anorexia has a diverse etiology including stress, pain, fear, trauma, disease or neoplasia.

Causes of anorexia may broadly be categorized as:
● Pseudoanorexia (e.g. oral cavity disease, dental pain).
● Primary anorexia (e.g. central nervous system disorders affecting appetite center).
● Secondary anorexia (e.g. metabolic diseases such as renal failure).

It is important to note that many diseases leading to a thin inappetent cat involve more that just loss of appetite. When weight loss appears to exceed that which can be accounted for by decreased intake, other mechanisms need to be considered.

WHERE?

Signs of a thin inappetent cat may be the result of any disease process that can cause decreased body weight and/or suppression of appetite.

The appetite center is in the hypothalamus.

Diseases affecting the oral cavity and pharynx may cause pain or dysphagia and so decrease nutrient intake. Such animals will often show interest in food but cannot eat. Inability to smell food (anosmia) will frequently cause anorexia (e.g. chronic nasal disease).

Diseases of the gastrointestinal tract, liver and pancreas may cause anorexia, maldigestion or malabsorption of nutrients, and therefore weight loss.

Careful history taking regarding the animal's environment (inside, outside; single-, multiple-cat household) may aid in deciding a diagnostic approach.

Good history taking and complete physical examination are essential, due to the lack of specificity of these clinical signs.

WHAT?

The most common causes of the thin innappetent cat with few other clinical signs are chronic renal failure, neoplasia and, depending on geographical location, several viral diseases (FIV, FeLV and FIP).

Weight loss followed by inappetence tends to be a terminal event in many disease processes.

Many other causes will usually have other significant clinical problems that will aid the clinician in formulating a diagnostic plan.

DISEASES CAUSING SIGNS OF A THIN INAPPETENT CAT

CHRONIC RENAL FAILURE***

Classical signs

- Polyuria, polydipsia.
- Weight loss, inappetence.
- Vomiting.

PATHOGENESIS

Chronic renal failure is defined as primary renal failure that has persisted for an extended period (usually greater than 2 weeks).

Chronic renal failure is associated with irreversible structural lesions in the kidney.

Chronic renal failure is the end result of many disease processes affecting the kidney:
- Anomaly: Familial renal disease, polycystic kidney disease.
- Metabolic: Hypercalcemia (from cholecalciferol rodenticide, granulomatous disease or neoplasia), ischemic injury.
- Mechanical: Chronic urinary tract obstruction (e.g. urolith) resulting in hydronephrosis.
- Neoplastic: Lymphoma, primary neoplasia.
- Infectious: Feline infectious peritonitis, upper urinary tract infection (pyelonephritis).
- Immune: Secondary to glomerulonephritits, amyloidosis.
- Toxic: Therapeutic agents (e.g. gentamicin, amphotericin B, NSAIDs), intravenous contrast agents, heavy metals (e.g. lead), hemaglobin, ethylene glycol and plants (lilies).

The initiating cause of chronic renal failure is often not identified.

At the time of diagnosis there is usually diffuse pathology of the renal parenchyma termed chronic generalized nephropathy.

Polycystic kidney disease is a common cause of renal failure in some breeds of cats and has the following characteristics:
- Renal cysts may be congenital or acquired and may affect one or both kidneys.
- Polycystic kidney disease is characterized by multiple cysts occurring in both kidneys.
- **Polycystic kidney disease occurs as an autosomal dominant inherited renal disease of Persian and Persian-related cats,** with a prevalence of at least 45% in some Persian populations.
- Renal cysts are fluid-filled sacs lined with epithelium, that generally originate in existing nephrons and may therefore occur in the renal cortex or medulla. Cystic structures have also been noted in other organs, such as the liver, in cats with polycystic kidney disease.

- Cysts vary in size and tend to increase in number and size with time. Eventually progressive cyst enlargement compresses the adjacent renal parenchyma and if sufficient renal mass is affected renal failure will develop. **Renal failure may occur at any age**, however affected Persian cats typically present at approximately 7 years.
- Renomegaly may be obvious with the kidneys being irregular in outline. Laboratory evaluation is necessary to determine the extent of the renal dysfunction. Ultrasonographic examination is non-invasive and a very sensitive diagnostic technique for this condition. Cysts are seen as multiple, round anechoic regions.

In chronic renal failure resulting from many of the disease processes, **renal function often slowly deteriorates over months or years**, but the rate of deterioration is very variable between cats. Deterioration is not necessarily linear and many cats are stable for long periods of time with intermittent acute decrements. The postulated causes of progression include:

- Primary disease process; the inciting cause may lead to ongoing renal damage.
- Systemic and metabolic derangements of chronic renal failure.
- Renal compensatory mechanisms (increase in single nephron glomerular filtration rate).

In chronic renal failure, **surviving functional nephrons undergo compensatory changes** including glomerular hypertension, hypertrophy and hyperfiltration (leading to an increase in single nephron glomerular filtration rate).

- These adaptive mechanisms compensate for the loss of nephrons and so minimize the overall decrease in glomerular filtration rate.
- However, it is postulated, based on extrapolation from other species, that these compensatory changes are maladaptive and represent a final common pathway for the progression to eventual glomerular sclerosis and end stage renal failure.

Clinical signs

Chronic renal failure is mainly a disease of older cats, with Persian, Abyssinian, Maine coon, Siamese and Burmese breeds of cat being identified to be at increased risk.

Early cases may be asymptomatic.

Signs associated with chronic renal failure result from failure of excretory, regulatory and synthetic functions of the kidney.

Polydipsia is the most commonly reported clinical sign. The polydipsia is compensatory to an obligatory polyuria. If fluid intake is insufficient, dehydration will result. Polyuria results from:

- Increased solute load in surviving functional nephrons (solute diuresis).
- Disruption of medullary anatomy.
- Impaired response to antidiuretic hormone.

Inappetence or anorexia, weight loss and poor body condition are common clinical signs as the disease progresses.

Lethargy, weakness and depression.

Vomiting (with possible hematemesis) is usually **intermittent and often low grade**. Vomiting and nausea may be associated with:

- The action of uremic toxins on the medullary emetic chemoreceptor trigger zone.
- Uremic gastritis and gastrointestinal ulceration.

Constipation is common and results from dehydration.

Severe uremia associated with an acute exacerbation of chronic renal failure (acute on chronic) or end-stage chronic renal failure may be associated with extreme clinical signs including:

- **Halitosis, ulceration of oral mucosa or tongue** and brownish discoloration of dorsal surface and sloughing of anterior tip of tongue (due to fibinoid necrosis, arteritis and bacterial degradation of urea to ammonia).
- Occasionally diarrhea, which may be hemorrhagic from uremic enterocolitis.
- Terminally, seizures, stupor or coma may occur.

Clinical signs relating to systemic arterial hypertension are common. **Hypertension is reported in 29–61% of cats with chronic renal failure.** Clinical signs which may be associated with hypertension include:

- **Ocular signs** include sudden blindness with dilated pupils, **hyphema or retinal hemorrhage**, retinal edema, retinal vessel tortuosity, retinal detachment.
- Systolic **heart murmurs** and a gallop rhythm.
- **Neurological** signs including seizures and stupor.

Small and/or irregular kidneys may be palpable, occasionally kidneys are enlarged (for example in neoplastic or cystic kidney disease).

Diagnosis

Diagnosis is based on demonstration of persistently decreased renal excretory function.
- **Persistently elevated blood urea and creatinine concentrations (azotemia) are indicative.**
- **Chronicity and stability is based on two assessments, ideally at a 2–4 week interval.**

Diagnosis is further supported by demonstration of tubular dysfunction:
- **Urine specific gravity of less than 1.030 (typically less than 1.020).**

Any factors contributing to the progression of the renal failure, including the initiating disease, and any systemic complications of renal failure should be identified by diagnostic tests.

Attempt to identify the renal disease initiating the failure using all or any of the following tests:
- Routine hematology and biochemistry.
- Routine urinalysis (including microscopic sediment examination).
- Assessment of proteinuria by urine protein:creatinine ratio. Proteinuria is typically very low (1.5–2 times increase in protein excretion), unless there is significant glomerular disease.
- Quantitative urine bacterial culture.
- Imaging, either radiography to assess renal size and shape, and/or ultrasound examination to assess renal architecture.
- Renal cytology (fine needle aspiration biopsy) and biopsy.
  - However, due to the high risk and low diagnostic yield of histopathology in CRF, biopsy is rarely indicated unless atypical features such as renomegaly, proteinuria or hematuria are present. **Biopsy is only indicated in cases where the result of histopathology will influence the treatment options and therefore, outcome of the case.**

Secondary hyperparathyroidism, hypokalemia, anemia and systemic hypertension are all possible complications of chronic renal failure.

Renal secondary hyperparathyroidism is characterized by excess circulating concentrations of parathyroid hormone (PTH) resulting from altered mineral homeostasis in renal failure, and is present in approximately 80% of cats with chronic renal failure.
- Chronically increased PTH concentrations are toxic to the kidney and contribute to ongoing loss of renal function.
- Factors involved in the pathogenesis of renal hyperparathyroidism leading to increased PTH concentrations include phosphate retention with declining glomerular filtration rate, hypocalcemia and decreased synthesis of 1,25-dihydroxycholecalciferol (calcitriol) by proximal tubular cells.
- Diagnosis is based on elevated PTH concentrations in a cat with chronic renal failure, and normal or slightly low serum calcium concentrations. Measurement of ionized calcium is a better indicator of calcium levels than total calcium. Cats with chronic renal failure and hyperphosphatemia will be hyperparathyroid.
  - Samples for PTH assay require special handling, therefore contact the diagnostic laboratory.
- **Hypokalemia occurs in many cats (20–30%) with polyuric renal failure.**
- Hypokalemia may be a consequence or cause of chronic renal failure in the cat.
- The mechanism is unknown but increased renal losses of potassium, decreased dietary intake and decreased gastrointestinal absorption are implicated.
- Clinical signs of inappetence and generalized muscle weakness (such as ataxia, inability to jump, stiff, stilted gait and ventroflexion of the neck) may occur.

Normochromic, normocytic, nonregenerative anemia is common when chronic renal failure is advanced.
- Occurs mainly from relative erythropoietin deficiency, but other factors contribute, such as decreased red cell life span, uremic suppression of erythropoiesis and gastrointestinal blood loss.
- Routine hematology should be used to monitor anemia and rule out other causes.

Systemic hypertension is present in many cats with chronic renal failure.
- Diagnosis is based on serial blood pressure measurements.

- Systemic hypertension is usually measured using a Doppler technique (Doppler ultrasonic sphygmomanometry) to assess systolic blood pressure.
- Normal range is technique dependent, however systolic pressures > 200 mmHg indicate severe hypertension.
- Retinal examination to detect end organ damage should also be carried out.

Proteinuria is a risk factor for progression of chronic renal insufficiency in cats, and may be a marker of glomerular hypertension. Median survival times are significantly reduced if the urine protein/creatinine ratio is > 0.43.

All chronic renal failure cases should receive regular monitoring, involving full clinical examination (including assessment of body weight), measurement of systemic arterial blood pressure and analysis of blood and urine samples. This allows early detection of problems, and assessment of efficacy of therapy and tailoring of treatment to the individual.

Differential diagnosis

Pre-renal azotemia occurs secondary to dehydration or circulatory collapse, and the azotemia results from reduced renal perfusion.

- Typically urine specific gravity is greater than 1.035.
- Pre-renal azotemia concurrent with primary disease affecting renal concentrating ability can mimic renal failure, for example a dehydrated cat with diabetes insipidus.

Acute renal failure.

- Therapeutically and prognostically it is important to distinguish between chronic and acute renal failure.
- Evidence of chronicity is usually obvious from the history (polydipsia, weight loss), physical examination (small kidneys), and diagnostic tests (non-regenerative anemia).
- Due to the gradual decline in glomerular filtration rate in chronic compared to acute renal failure, clinical signs in chronic renal failure tend to be less dramatic relative to the metabolic derangements.

Treatment

Treatment of chronic renal failure is aimed at:

- Ameliorating the clinical signs and systemic complications associated with renal dysfunction.
- Prevention of further deterioration of renal function (progression).
  - Management of end-stage renal failure by renal replacement therapy (dialysis or transplant) is generally prohibitive because of cost, technical and ethical considerations.

Although chronic renal failure is irreversible, many cats presented in a uremic crisis have superimposed prerenal azotemia or acute renal failure (so called acute on chronic).

- It is very important that appropriate therapy be used to correct reversible azotemia.
- Once reversible azotemia is corrected, more accurate assessment of the severity of the underlying irreversible chronic renal failure can be made.

Treatment of progression of chronic renal failure involves:

- Identifying and eliminating the inciting cause of the renal damage.
- Correcting the systemic and metabolic derangements of chronic renal failure.
- Preventing the intrinsic progression of renal failure (if such progression occurs in the cat).
  - A number of therapeutic maneuvers may be effective slowing intrinsic progression. These include dietary protein restriction, angiotensin-converting enzyme (ACE) inhibitors, modification of dietary lipid intake and phosphate restriction. Evidence for a beneficial effect on survival for each of these treatments is limited and therefore currently each case should be assessed on an individual basis.

Maintenance of hydration.

- Unrestricted access to water is essential in any cat with chronic renal failure to allow thirst to compensate for the obligatory polyuria. Additional fluids (oral, subcutaneous or intravenous) may be required when intake fails to keep pace with diuresis. Home administration of subcutaneous fluids are indicated when the cat is unable to maintain hydration. Typically, cats require 75–150 ml SQ q 12–72 h. Begin a 4–5 kg cat on 150 ml twice weekly, and use normal saline with 35 mmol (mEq)/L of KCl added. Education of the owner on proper administration and sterile technique is vital.

Dietary management of chronic renal failure.

- Treatment of cats with chronic renal failure by dietary modification has been proven to significantly increase survival. Generally, commercially available "renal diets" are recommended. These diets have restricted protein, calcium, sodium, phosphorus and acid-load, and added potassium.

Dietary protein restriction is frequently advocated.

- In moderate to severe chronic renal failure, controlled restriction of non-essential protein will reduce the accumulation of nitrogenous waste products that are believed to contribute to the uremic syndrome.
- More controversially, the use of a restricted protein diet in early CRF may slow the rate of progression to end-stage renal failure by preventing maladaptive changes in surviving nephrons. However, evidence for a beneficial effect of protein restriction on renal function in cats with early renal failure is not available.
- Poor appetite and the decreased palatability of restricted protein diets make mal-nutrition a serious problem in renal-failure patients. Monitor carefully for weight loss and decreasing muscle mass.
- Dietary protein intake should be tailored to the metabolic needs of the individual cat. Usually a diet containing at least 21% of gross energy as protein is required (usual maintenance diets contain 35–55% gross energy as protein). The goal is to maintain a BUN of ≤ 29 mmol/L (80 mg/dl). In general, the more severe the renal dysfunction, the greater the protein restriction required, but protein should not be decreased below 19–20% of gross energy (metabolizable energy).

A number of other dietary components have been studied for their effect to modify the rate of progression including calorie intake and fatty acid composition. Dietary phosphate restriction is discussed under the section on renal secondary hyperparathyroidism.

Angiotensin-converting enzyme (ACE) inhibitors may have a renoprotective effect, which is independent of any effect on systemic blood pressure. **ACE inhibitor therapy may also be useful in reducing the degree of proteinuria in cats with chronic renal failure.** benazepril 0.25–0.5 mg/kg PO q 24 h.

- The mechanisms of these effects are unclear, but may be hemodynamically mediated by causing renal vasodilation especially of the efferent arteriole, and reducing glomerular capillary pressure.
- Preliminary studies of ACE inhibitor use in naturally occurring chronic renal failure in cats have shown significantly increased survival times for the subgroup of renal-failure cats with urine protein/creatinine ratios > 1.
- By reducing glomerular pressure, ACE inhibition would be expected to cause a decrease in glomerular filtration rate and so may increase azotemia. A rise in creatinine of > 50% warrants withdrawal of the drug.

Treatment of renal secondary hyperparathyroidism should be instituted in a staged manner.

The cornerstone of therapy is dietary phosphate restriction.

- After initiation of phosphate restriction, plasma phosphate levels usually stabilize at a lower level by 2–8 weeks, however PTH concentrations may continue to decline without additional intervention.
- Proteinaceous foods are the main source of phosphate in the diet, so phosphate restriction is generally combined with protein restriction.
- The aim of dietary phosphate restriction is to reduce plasma phosphorus to the lower limit of the reference range, the point at which the most effective control of PTH secretion is usually attained.

If after 4 weeks dietary management alone is not achieving this, or if PTH concentrations are not decreasing, then **intestinal phosphate-binding agents should be introduced to further restrict phosphate intake.**

- Intestinal phosphate-binding agents form non-absorbable salts of phosphate, binding phosphate in both the diet and intestinal secretions. To achieve efficient phosphate binding, the medication should be given, ideally mixed through the food or immediately before feeding.
- **Aluminum hydroxide** should be dosed at 30–100 mg/kg/day PO in divided doses with each meal, titrated to effect based on plasma phosphate concentrations. Dose can be increased to 200–300 mg/kg if necessary to control phosphate. If the cat refuses to eat it with food, a compounding pharmacy can formulate

it in capsules to administer immediately after a meal. Calcium-containing phosphate binders such as calcium acetate (60–90 mg/kg/day divided with meals) or calcium carbonate (90–150 mg/kg/day divided with meals) can be used, but serum calcium must be monitored carefully. Do not use if there is hypercalcemia.

- High dietary phosphate limits the effectiveness of phosphate-binding agents, so preferably these should be used in combination with a low-phosphate diet.

Treatment with an active form of vitamin D directly inhibits PTH secretion. This group of drugs has **a very narrow therapeutic index**.

- **Calcitriol or alphacalcidol** 1.5–3.5 ng/kg/day PO on an empty stomach (maximum 10 ng/kg/day). Because of the very low dose, the human preparations must be re-formulated by a compounding pharmacy for use in cats.
- All active vitamin D preparations enhance intestinal absorption of calcium and phosphorus, and so are contraindicated unless plasma concentrations of calcium and phosphate are normal. In addition, they are ineffective in decreasing PTH concentrations if phosphorus is elevated. Phosphorus concentration must be below 2 mmol/L (6 mg/dl) before calcitriol use is optimal. Between serum phosphorus of 2–2.25 mmol/L (6–7 mg/dl), the effectiveness of calcitriol is decreased, and above a phosphorus of 2.5 mmol/L (8 mg/dl) it is ineffective in reducing PTH concentration.
- Plasma calcium must be closely monitored, initially weekly. If possible measure ionized calcium rather than total calcium. The dosage should be titrated to maintain normocalcemia, not merely to decrease PTH concentrations, and therapy should be discontinued if hypercalcemia occurs. If hypercalcemia does not resolve within 7–10 days of stopping calcitriol, begin intermittent dosing of calcitriol. For cats with mild hypercalcemia based on the ionized calcium concentration, give calcitriol every other day at twice the daily dose, so the total amount per week is the same. If calcium levels do not decrease, try twice weekly dosing at 3.5 times the daily dose (8 pm one day and 8 am 4 days later). Do not use less than twice weekly. PTH concentrations should be measured to document successful control of renal secondary hyper-para-thyroidism.

- The long-term advantages of this form of therapy are as yet unproven. The aim is to decrease progression of renal failure through a reduction in PTH concentrations. If there is marked hypercalcemia based on measurement of ionized calcium, care should be taken to rule out other causes of hypercalcemia, because the hypercalcemia of renal failure is usually only mild to moderate in severity (total calcium <3.4 mmol/L or 13.5 mg/dl).

Treatment of hypokalemia.

Hypokalemia may be treated with oral potassium gluconate (2–6 mmol/cat/day PO). The exact dose is dependent on the response to therapy, determined by monitoring plasma potassium concentrations.

Treatment of the anemia.

Management of the anemia of CRF should include an initial assessment of the cat to rule out and treat other potential causes of anemia, such as flea infestation and gastrointestinal ulceration.

Nutritional and iron deficiencies will impair the erythropoietic potential, and should be corrected prior to initiating other treatment.

Blood transfusions (limited availability), androgen (poor efficacy) and recombinant erythropoietin therapy have all been used to treat the anemia of CRF.

Recombinant human erythropoietin (rHuEPO) is the most effective therapy.

- Therapy should be started only if clinical signs relating to the anemia are present, such as weakness, inactivity or lethargy, which is usually when the packed cell volume (PCV) is less than 18%. Because of potential side effects of treatment, it is usually only commenced once PCV is <15%.
- Initial dosage is 50–100 U/kg injected subcutaneously three times weekly, with PCV monitored at least twice weekly. Once the PCV has increased to the lower end of the reference range, the dosage is usually reduced to once or twice weekly.
- Adverse effects of rHuEPO include polycythemia, seizures, hypersensitivity reactions and systemic hypertension. Absolute failure to respond to rHuEPO is usually due to iron deficiency.
- After an initial response, many treated cats develop antibodies to rHuEPO, which leads to a severe refractory anemia greater than that present prior to

treatment. This anemia is usually reversible when therapy is discontinued. For this reason rHuEPO should not be initiated too early in the course of progressive CRF.

Treatment of systemic hypertension.
- Treatment is usually carried out on a trial basis, monitoring for a decrease in blood pressure without adverse effects or the development of hypotension. Generally a period of about 2 weeks is sufficient to document a response. If severe clinical signs are present, therapy may need to be more aggressive.
- Classically, a staged therapeutic response is recommended, starting with dietary sodium restriction, followed by the use of various pharmacological agents.

The current treatment of choice for the cat is amlodipine besylate. An initial dose of 0.625 mg/cat PO q 24 h is recommended and may be increased cautiously if the response is poor, to 1.25 mg daily.

Combination therapy is required in some cases, with the addition of an ACE inhibitor or beta blocker.

Treatment of proteinuria involves protein restriction to maintain a BUN of ≤ 29 mmol/L (80 mg/dl) and use of an ACE inhibitor to reduce glomerular pressure.

Treatment of anorexia associated with chronic renal failure.
- Anorexia is usually associated with moderate to severe uremia, and contributes to further uremia by resulting in catabolism of tissue protein for energy.
- Change food gradually over 1–2 weeks in a renal diet, and increase palatability by warming to just below body temperature.

Reduce gastric hyperacidity from hypergastrinemia.
- H2-receptor antagonists such as famotidine (0.5–1 mg/kg PO q 24 hours).
- Gastric mucosal protectant, sucralfate (250 mg/cat q 8–12 hours, on an empty stomach).

Modify doses of drugs if excreted by kidneys.

Prognosis

Chronic renal failure tends to be progressive and the long-term prognosis is poor, although with careful management some cats will live for years.

Prevention

Since the majority of cases of chronic renal failure are of unknown primary cause, there are currently no preventative recommendations.

Avoid any potential renal insults, particularly in cats with pre-existing comprise of renal function or renal perfusion. For example, avoid using NSAIDs in dehydrated cats, and use intravenous fluids prior to induction of anesthesia and during surgery, to maintain renal perfusion in elderly cats and cats with compromised renal function. Remember that minor renal insults may summate to cause clinically significant renal damage.
- Promptly and appropriately treat conditions causing decreased renal perfusion including dehydration, shock and hypotension associated with anesthesia and surgery.

Pre-renal and post-renal azotaemia, if not corrected, may lead to renal damage and renal failure.

FELINE IMMUNODEFICIENCY VIRUS (FIV)***

> ### Classical signs
> - Middle-aged to older cats, particularly entire males and feral cats.
> - Clinical signs variable, often vague.
> - Weight loss, inappetence.
> - Pyrexia, lymphadenopathy.
> - Immunosuppression (cat flu, diarrhea, neoplasia).
> - Gingivitis/stomatitis.

Pathogenesis

Feline immunodeficiency virus (FIV) is a lymphotrophic lentivirus, which causes an acquired immunodeficiency syndrome (AIDS) in cats.
- FIV is morphologically and biochemically similar to human immunodeficiency virus (HIV), however it is antigenically distinct and the viruses are species specific.

Infectious virus is found in the saliva of FIV-positive cats and transmission occurs primarily though inoculation of the virus through saliva or blood.

- **Bite wounds are considered a primary source of infection.**
- Vertical transmission either transplacentally or via infected milk occurs experimentally but is of questionable significance in natural settings.
- Horizontal transmission in multiple cat households via food bowls, mutual grooming appears rare.
- Sexual transmission is not thought to be a significant route of infection.

The prevalence of FIV infection varies with the population studied:

- FIV infection in healthy cats in the United States and United Kingdom ranges from 2–3%, compared to rates approaching 30% in sick cats or cats with a high risk of exposure.
- **Male cats are three times more likely to be infected than female, especially male entire cats.**
- **Risk of infection is greater in free-roaming and feral cats than indoor cats.**

FIV has a worldwide distribution in domestic cats.

The course of the disease following FIV infection is dependent on a number of host- and virus-related factors, such as the age and health status of the cat and the strain and dose of the virus.

Acute infection involves rapid replication of virus in lymphoid organs and salivary glands.

Although CD4+ (helper) and CD8+ (cytotoxic) T lymphocytes may be infected by FIV, FIV selectively destroys CD4+ cells.

- The ratio of CD4+ to CD8+ becomes "inverted" in cats with FIV because of the relative lack of CD4+ cells.
- The lack of CD4+ leads to the immunosuppression associated with many of the clinical signs of FIV infection.

Many cats remain completely asymptomatic for years, despite severe lack of CD4+ lymphocytes.

Clinical signs

Clinical signs are very variable from cat to cat, and may be a direct effect of the virus or secondary to immunosuppression.

The infection can be divided into stages: acute, asymptomatic carrier, persistent generalized lymph-

adenopathy, AIDS-related complex (ARC), and AIDS. However it may be difficult to distinguish these stages clinically.

- The **acute** phase begins about 4 weeks following infection and may persist for up to 4 months.
  - Mild lymphadenopathy, neutropenia, fever, malaise and diarrhea may occur.
  - These signs may be mild and go completely unnoticed by the owner.
  - These cats will usually test seronegative for the virus.
- The **asymptomatic carrier** phase may last for months to years.
  - Despite being asymptomatic, significant immune aberrations may be present
- **Persistent generalized lymphadenopathy** lasts for less than 2–4 months.
  - Poor hair coat, fever and leukopenia may be noted.
- **The terminal clinical phase can sometimes be divided in to ARC and AIDS.**
- ARC is the presence of clinical disease that does not fulfill the criteria for AIDS.
- **AIDS is the final stage of the infection.**
  - **Profound weight loss (> 20% of body weight) and a variety of opportunistic infections.**
  - **Frequently there is persistent leukopenia and anemia.**
  - **Additionally, cats may have neurological disease or malignancy.**
  - **Average life expectancy is less than 1 year.**

Many diseases found in the asymptomatic phase may or may not be related to the virus.

Immunosuppression leads to opportunistic infections with bacterial, fungal or protozoal agents.

- Little good statistical evidence is available to show that there is a higher incidence of many of these diseases in FIV-infected cats.
- Some studies indicate that these diseases may be more severe in the FIV-infected cat.

Certain disease processes have been directly associated with the terminal clinical phase of the disease.

- **Chronic ulceroproliferative stomatitis is common,** and may be associated with concurrent calicivirus infection.
- **Ocular disease** including uveitis, glaucoma, infiltration of inflammatory cells in the posterior chamber

(pars planitis), focal retinal chorioretinitis and retinal hemorrhages have been reported.

- **Neoplasia** including lymphoma (often extra-nodal), leukemia, and several others have been associated with the terminal stage of the disease. However, the exact role of FIV in the neoplastic process is unclear.
- **Central and peripheral nervous system disease** has been associated with FIV infections. These signs may be transient. Clinical signs include behavior changes, seizures, paresis and anisocoria. Concomitant infections (cryptococcosis, toxoplasmosis or FIP) may contribute to neurologic signs.
- **Renal disease** and failure may have an association with the FIV virus. Since many older cats suffer from chronic renal failure, the exact association between the virus and renal failure has yet to be determined.

Diagnosis

Diagnosis of FIV infection is based on serological evidence of the presence of FIV specific antibodies.
- **In practice, diagnostic kits are available to detect antibody to either p24 core protein or gp41 envelope protein using enzyme-linked immunosorbent assay (ELISA) or rapid immunomigration (RIM).**

Interpretation of a positive antibody result:
- Vaccinated cats will test positive with all current testing methods.
- In unvaccinated cats, FIV antibodies are associated with lifelong viral infection. A positive test implies a persistently infected cat.
- Passive transfer of antibody via milk will result in a positive test in kittens nursed by an infected queen. Such kittens should not be tested until at least 6 months of age.
- False-positive results occur with ELISA or RIM tests, but at a low frequency. A positive test should be confirmed using a western blot if it will influence management of the cat.

Interpretation of a negative antibody result:
- The cat is not infected with FIV.
- The cat is infected but no antibodies are present.
  - This occurs in early stages of infection, usually 2–4 weeks after infection.

- Small numbers of cats (up to 10–20%) have delayed seroconversion or may never seroconvert.
- The cat is in the terminal stages of the disease, when antibody production declines.

Detection of FIV infection does not prove that the clinical signs are necessarily related to the infection.
- Since cats can live for years in the "asymptomatic" stage of the disease, the clinician should try to decide if the virus is a cause, contributing factor, or just incidental to the cat's problem.

Immunoflourescent antibody or western blot techniques may be used to confirm the presence of FIV antibody, particularly in ELISA-positive cats from low-risk populations, or if initial test results were equivocal.

Non-specific findings on routine hematology and biochemistry include:
- Various cytopenias including neutropenia, thrombocytopenia, lymphopenia, and anemia.
- Mild non-regenerative anemia.
- A polyclonal hyperglobulinemia.

Differential diagnosis

Feline leukemia virus infection (FeLV) may be clinically very similar to FIV infection, as many signs are associated with the immunosuppression which is common to both conditions.
- Most cats that are tested for FeLV probably should be tested for FIV.

The dry form of feline infectious peritonitis (FIP) may lead to signs of wasting, neurologic signs, renal failure and ocular disease. The "dry" form of FIP is extremely difficult to diagnose without histologic examination of tissue.

Toxoplasmosis causes neurologic and ocular signs as well as wasting. FIV and toxoplasmosis may also occur concurrently.

Treatment

The FIV status of the cat should not necessarily preclude treatment for other diseases.

No specific therapy has proven effective against the virus in the long term, but reverse transcriptase inhibitors and immunomodulating drugs may provide some benefit in rescuing severely ill cats in the short-term. Although some drugs can reduce viral load (AZT and PMEA), there are no studies showing a proven clinical benefit long term, or resolution of infection, and long-term use is hindered by side effects.

Reverse transcriptase inhibitors may suppress viral replication.
- **Zidovudine (3′-azido-3′-deoxythymidine, AZT)** (5–15 mg/kg PO or 5 mg/kg subcutaneously q 12 hours) has been shown to improve clinical signs, but does not eliminate the virus.
  - Increased numbers of CD4+ cells and improvement in CD4+:CD8+ ratios have occurred in naturally infected FIV cats.
  - Remission in stomatitis has been reported.
  - The virus may become resistant to AZT
  - Anemia and hepatotoxicity are potential side effects.

Immunomodulating drugs to potentiate the immune response against the virus include:
- **Evening primrose oil (550 mg PO q 24 hours).**
- **Low-dose oral human recombinant alpha interferon** (30 IU/cat PO q 24 hours, 7 days on, 7 days off).
- **Acemannan, *Propionibacterium acnes* and staphylococcal protein A** have been suggested as immunomodulating agents in FIV infection.

Aggressive supportive care and management of secondary infections are essential in FIV-positive cats. All infections should be fully assessed in terms of extent and appropriate treatment administered, ideally based on culture and sensitivity results. Response to treatment may be slower in FIV-infected cats, and so sufficient duration of antibiotic must be administered.

Appropriate preventative medicine is important in immunosuppressed cats.
- Inactivated vaccines should be used against respiratory or enteric pathogens.
- However the ability of an FIV-infected cat to produce an adequate immune response to a vaccine is unknown.

Prognosis

In the acute or asymptomatic phases of the disease, it is not possible to predict the short- or long-term prognosis.

Many cats appear to live for years with no or minimal problems.

In the terminal clinical phase, the prognosis is poor to grave with average life expectancy of less than 1 year.

Prevention

One vaccine has been approved for the prevention of FIV. There are still questions on its efficacy and the American Association of Feline Practitioners (AAFP) has yet to recommend its use.

Until a proven effective vaccine is developed and the ability to differentiate a false positive vaccine titer from infection, prevention is achieved by avoiding exposure to infected cats.
- FIV-positive cats should be neutered to reduce the tendency to fight.
- Confinement of FIV-positive cats to indoors will reduce the spread of the virus, and will also reduce the exposure of the affected cat to secondary infectious diseases.
- In single-cat households or multiple-cat households where all cats are seronegative for the virus, the animals are at negligible risk if they are kept as indoor cats.
- FIV is readily killed by disinfectants and survives only a few hours in the environment, so risk of fomite transmission is low.

The FIV status of new cats should be determined prior to introduction to a group. Ideally these cats should be rechecked in 4–6 weeks because of the latency period between exposure and production of antibody.

CANCER CACHEXIA**

> ### Classical signs
> - Anorexia, muscle wasting and weight loss.
> - Weakness, lethargy.
> - Clinical signs associated with the neoplastic lesion.

Pathogenesis

Cancer cachexia is probably the most common paraneoplastic syndrome.

It is associated with a variety of malignancies.

Although many cats with neoplasia are cachexic, little information is available on the metabolic derangements present. Care must be taken extrapolating data from the dog and man, given the differing nutritional requirements of these species.

Weight loss occurs in patients with neoplasia because:
- **Nutrient intake is reduced.**
  - This is related to tumor size and location. For example, intraoral masses cause dysphagia, and infiltrative intestinal neoplasia may reduce nutrient assimilation.
  - Decreased appetite may be a consequence of therapy.
- **Metabolic and hormonal changes secondary to neoplasia lead to inefficient energy utilization.**

Clinical signs

Inappetence and weight loss are common clinical findings in many cats with varying malignancies.

Weight loss is frequently associated with muscle wasting, and consequent lethargy and weakness.

Poor hair coat, delayed wound healing and impaired immune function are associated with cachexia.

Other clinical signs will vary with the nature and location of the neoplasia.

Diagnosis

Neoplasia should be suspected in any cat showing inappetence and weight loss, with no obvious other cause.

A thorough clinical examination, including palpation of all lymph nodes, may provide an indication of the site of the lesion and direct further investigation.

Principal diagnostic efforts are aimed at establishing the nature and extent of the neoplastic lesion. The exact diagnostic investigation will depend on the location and type of lesion being investigated but may include:

- **Diagnostic imaging** (radiography, ultrasound examinations and computed tomography) of the thorax and abdomen.
  - Evaluation of pulmonary neoplasia should include two lateral and ventrodorsal radiographic views.
- Cytological or histopathological evaluation of tissue is required to confirm the diagnosis.

Cats with neoplastic lesions should be monitored closely for evidence of malnutrition. A detailed dietary history and physical examination are important for monitoring. Regularly assess body weight and use a body condition scoring system.

Hematological and biochemical parameters are relatively insensitive markers of nutritional status, but may provide additional information. However these markers may be affected by the neoplasia itself.
- Creatine kinase concentrations may increase rapidly in response to anorexia.
- Protein malnutrition may lead to hypoalbuminemia.
- Malnutrition may also cause anemia and lymphopenia.

Differential diagnosis

Differential diagnoses include **most causes of inappetence and weight loss.**

Other differentials to be considered depend on the site, location and nature of the tumor.

Treatment

Treatment specific to the neoplastic lesion will depend on the nature, extent and location of the tumor, but may include excisional surgery, radiotherapy or chemotherapy.

Dietary recommendations postulated to prevent or ameliorate cancer cachexia include:
- **Palatable, highly digestible, complete and balanced diets.**
- Tumor cells have an obligate requirement for glucose and are unable to utilize significant amounts of lipid for energy. Therefore, **energy-dense diets, which are relatively high in fat** and restricted in carbohydrate, may theoretically have beneficial effects.

Appropriate treatment of associated symptoms such as nausea, diarrhea or vomiting.

Pharmacological appetite stimulation may be considered but objective evidence of their efficacy is not available.

In cats which are unable or unwilling to eat, enteral or parenteral feeding may be considered.
- **Enteral nutrition should be used wherever possible**, as this prevents intestinal mucosal atrophy
  - Nasoesophageal, esophageal, gastrostomy and jejunostomy tubes may be used
  - Esophagostomy and gastrostomy tubes are preferable in cats requiring more long-term nutrition.
- Parenteral feeding is more technically complex and expensive, and should only be used when feeding via the gastrointestinal tract is impossible.

Prognosis

The prognosis for each individual case will be dependent on the nature of the neoplasm and the response to therapy.

Cachexia and hypoalbuminemia tend to be poor prognostic indicators.

Prevention

Cats with neoplastic lesions should **be monitored closely for evidence of malnutrition**.

SEPTIC FOCUS/PERSISTENT FEVER**

Classical signs

- Fluctuating pyrexia and associated inappetence.
- Weight loss.
- Clinical signs associated with the etiology of the fever.

See main references on page 364 for details (The Pyrexic Cat).

Pathogenesis

The thermoregulatory center is located in the preoptic region of the anterior hypothalamus.

Hyperthermia describes a core body temperature above that considered normal in the cat. **In fever, the set point of the thermoregulatory center is increased.**

Fever may be caused by exogenous pyrogens such as infectious agents, immune complexes and tissue inflammation or necrosis.
- **Exogenous pyrogens** principally act by causing the host to release endogenous pyrogens.
- **Endogenous pyrogens** act on the thermoregulatory center, alter the set point and induce a febrile response.

Weight loss frequently occurs in cats with prolonged fever because:
- **Febrile cats are frequently inappetent.**
- **A febrile cat is in a hypermetabolic state.**
- **Weight loss may be associated with the fever per se, or more often with the disease causing the fever.**

The differential diagnosis list for causes of fever is extensive but may be broadly categorized:
- **Localized infection.**
  - Including urinary tract infection, pyometra, pyothorax, peritonitis, abscess, bronchopneumonia, endocarditis, suppurative cholangitis/cholangiohepatitis, dental disease, retrobulbar or pulmonary abscess and osteomyelitis.
- **Systemic infection.**
  - Including FeLV, FIV, feline infectious peritonitis (FIP), feline panleukopenia, respiratory tract virus infection, bacteremias, toxoplasmosis, mycobacterial infection and systemic mycoses.
- **Immune-mediated disorders.**
  - Including primary immunodeficiencies, systemic lupus erythematosus, polyarteritis nodosa, chronic progressive polyarthritis, immune-mediated hemolytic anemia and immune-mediated thrombocytpenia.
- **Neoplasia**.
  - Including lympho- and myeloproliferative diseases and large neoplastic lesions with central necrosis.
- **Miscellaneous conditions.**
  - Including drug reactions.

Clinical signs

Principal clinical signs will be **fever, weight loss and inappetence**.

Fever may be **sustained or fluctuating**.

Other clinical signs will vary with the nature of the disease causing the fever.

Diagnosis

A thorough history and clinical examination is vital to identify any localizing signs that would narrow the differential diagnosis list.

Monitoring the cat's temperature **three or four times daily** over a period of 48–72 hours confirms the presence and nature of the fever.

Routine hematology often reveals a **neutrophilia with or without a regenerative left shift**.
- Occasionally a degenerative left shift occurs when the bone marrow is unable to make an adequate response, and neutropenia develops in the face of a left shift. This has a poor prognosis.

In the absence of localizing signs a series of initial screening tests are carried out to identify the septic focus:
- Routine hematology and biochemistry.
- Routine urinalysis including bacterial culture and sensitivity.
- Thoracic and abdominal radiographs.
- Fecal analysis and culture for enteric pathogens.

Further diagnostic investigation may be required depending on the cause of the fever, this may include:
- Blood culture.
- Synovial fluid aspirates.
- Echocardiography.
- Bone marrow aspirates.
- Immunological tests such as Coomb's, antiplatelet antibody and antinuclear antibody tests.
- Serum protein electrophoresis.
- Serology.

If a bacterial cause is suspected, strenuous attempts should be made **to obtain a sample of infected material for bacterial culture and sensitivity testing prior to administering antibiotics**.

Differential diagnosis

Differential diagnoses include **most causes of inappetence and weight loss.**

Other differentials to be considered depend on the site, location and nature of the disease causing fever.

Treatment

Effective treatment is based on accurate assessment of the cause of the fever, followed by appropriate management.

Use of antibiotics, corticosteroids and NSAIDs prior to diagnosis should be avoided where possible, as it will mask the clinical signs and interfere with diagnostic testing.

If a septic focus is identified, treatment involves **drainage where appropriate (e.g. placement of thoracic drains in pyothorax) and use of antibiotic therapy based on the results of culture and sensitivity testing.**

Mild fever is unlikely to be fatal and may be beneficial in inhibiting viral and bacterial replication and increasing leukocyte function.

Fever in excess of 41.0°C often results in significant organ damage and may initiate disseminated intravascular coagulation.

Symptomatic therapy for fever includes:
- Oxygen.
- Crystalloid fluid therapy.
- **Antipyretic drugs** (NSAIDs) – these act directly on the thermoregulatory center and should be tried before surface cooling, unless the fever is life-threatening, when they may be instituted together.
- **Surface cooling.** Core temperature will continue to decrease after surface cooling has ceased, so to avoid large oscillations in temperature, aggressive cooling should stop just prior to reaching the desired temperature.
  - With cool, not cold, water (avoid inducing shivering).
  - Fans.
  - Ice packs over large blood vessels.

Prognosis

The prognosis for each individual case will be dependent on the etiology of the fever and the response to therapy.

APATHETIC HYPERTHYROIDISM*

Classical signs

- Older cats (usually > 8 years).
- Weight loss and inappetence.
- Weakness and depression.
- Palpable goiter.
- Tachycardia ± gallop rhythm.

See main references on page 304 for details (The Cat With Weight Loss and a Good Appetite).

Clinical signs

Hyperthyroidism is a disease of older cats, with only 5% being under 10 years of age at first diagnosis.

The majority of cats with hyperthyroidism present with weight loss and polyphagia.

In approximately 5% of cases, apathetic or masked hyperthyroidism occurs.
- **Weight loss is accompanied by a decreased appetite.**
- Cats tend to be depressed.
- Muscle weakness may be evident as ventroflexion of the neck.
- Cats with apathetic hyperthyroidism may show **signs of concurrent disease including congestive cardiac failure, renal failure or neoplasia.**

Other clinical signs are those typical for hyperthyroidism.
- **Unilateral or bilateral palpably enlarged thyroid (goiter).**
- Polyuria and polydipsia.
- Vomiting and diarrhea (bulky feces).
- Tachycardia, gallop rhythm, murmur and arrhythmia may be noted.
- Poor coat condition with decreased grooming.

Diagnosis

Although clinical signs of inappetence and depression are atypical for hyperthyroidism, **the presence of a thyroid goiter or tachycardia** should alert the clinician to the possibility of hyperthyroidism.

As apathetic hyperthyroidism typically **occurs in hyperthyroid cats with significant concurrent disease,** a thorough investigation is required to establish the presence of such disease.

Routine hematology may reveal a mild erythrocytosis.

Serum biochemistry frequently shows elevations of hepatic enzymes (alanine amino transferase and alkaline phosphatase).

A definitive diagnosis of hyperthyroidism is made on the basis of **high serum basal total thyroxine (T_4) concentrations.**

Normal serum thyroid hormone concentrations are occasionally found in hyperthyroid cats due to:
- Day-to-day fluctuation in hormone levels.
- Early or mild hyperthyroidism.
- The presence of concurrent non-thyroidal disease that suppresses serum thyroid levels.

Given that concurrent disease is common in cats with apathetic hyperthyroidism, suspect hyperthyroidism despite normal Total T_4 concentrations if the cat is older than 8 years and has signs consistent with hyperthyroidism. e.g. tachycardia or thyroid goitre.

If hyperthyroidism is suspected despite normal total T_4 concentrations, diagnostic possibilities include:
- **Repeat basal total T_4 measurement in 1–2 weeks.**
- **Identify and treat concurrent disease, then repeat basal total T_4 measurement.**
- Measure basal free T_4 concentrations, although euthyriod cats with non-thyroidal illness may have an elevated concentration.
- Dynamic thyroid testing may also be used:
  - Triiodothyronine (T_3) suppression test.
  - Thyrotropin (TRH) stimulation test, although the usefulness of this test in cats with non-thyroidal illness to distinguish those with and without hyperthyroidism has recently been questioned.
- Radionucleotide uptake and imaging.

Concurrent disease may be present and should be investigated, in particular:
- Evidence of concurrent renal failure with increased creatinine and urea concentration may also be present. Urine specific gravity will also provide further information regarding renal function.
- Hypertrophic cardiomyopathy secondary to hyperthyroidism (thyrotoxic cardiac disease) is frequently seen on echocardiography. This may be reversible with resolution of the hyperthyroid state but may progress to congestive cardiac failure.

Differential diagnosis

These include most other causes of inappetence and weight loss.

As tachycardia (with or without cardiac failure) is often present, cardiac disease should be placed high on the differential diagnosis list.

For cats with polydipsia and polyuria in addition to inappetence and weight loss, the main differential diagnoses would include chronic renal failure and diabetes mellitus.

Treatment

Hyperthyroid cats may be treated by surgical thyroidectomy or radioactive iodine (^{131}I), which are curative, or alternatively the condition may be controlled using antithyroid therapy.

The ideal form of treatment for each case will depend on a number of factors:
- Age of the cat.
- Presence of concurrent disease, particularly chronic renal failure or cardiovascular disease.
- Availability of appropriate nuclear medicine facilities.
- Owner's wishes, including ability to medicate cat and cost.

Cats with apathetic hyperthyroidism frequently have concurrent disease, and it is essential that this is thoroughly investigated and considered prior to embarking on therapy.
- Cardiac disease may preclude safe anesthesia and surgical thyroidectomy.
- **Glomerular filtration rate declines with resolution of the hyperthyroid state.** Therefore, any cat suspected of having underlying renal disease (azotemia, creatinine and urea concentrations in the upper part of the reference range, or lack of urine-concentrating ability) should be treated with antithyroid medication until it can be determined if induction of euthyroidism would have detrimental effects.

Medical therapy for hyperthyroidism is used in the short term to stabilize a hyperthyroid cat prior to surgical thyroidectomy, as trial therapy assesses the effect on renal function prior to curative treatment, or for long-term management if surgery or radioiodine therapy are not suitable.
- Medical management merely blocks thyroid hormone synthesis and so requires continuous life-long treatment.
- **Carbimazole** (5 mg PO q 8 hours for 2–3 weeks, then 5 mg PO q 12 hours to maintain euthy-

roidism) and **methimazole** (10–15 mg/day PO divided q 8–12 hours for 2–3 weeks, then 7.5–10 mg/day PO divided q 12 hours to maintain euthyroidism) are the drugs of choice for both short- and long-term medical management of hyperthyroidism. Transdermally absorbed methimazole may be obtained from a compounding pharmacist, and may be useful if the owners are unable to give oral medication.
  - Exact dosage should be adjusted on the basis of basal total T_4 concentrations.
  - Failure of efficacy is usually due to poor compliance.
  - Adverse effects appear to be less common with carbimazole than methimazole and usually occur in the first 3 months of therapy.
  - Transient vomiting, anorexia and lethargy have been reported, and usually resolve without withdrawal of the drug.
  - Serious hematological adverse effects may occur, and so routine monitoring is required.
  - Hepatopathy and self-induced facial excoriation may rarely occur.
- Other medical therapies may be considered including atenolol (to reduce the cardiac effects of hyperthyroidism), **stable iodine** (preoperatively to reduce gland vascularity) and **ipodate**.

Surgical thyroidectomy is curative when it is possible to remove all abnormal thyroid tissue.
- **Medical stabilization, ideally for 3 weeks preoperatively significantly reduces the anesthetic and surgical complications.**
- The most common complication is post-operative hypoparathyroidism, although Horner's syndrome and laryngeal paralysis may also occur.

Radioactive iodine therapy is the treatment of choice for most hyperthyroid cats when suitable facilities for treatment are available.
- This is the treatment of choice for cats with hyperthyroidism induced by thyroid carcinoma.
- Complications include the induction of permanent hypothyroidism and incomplete ablation requiring an additional treatment.
- The principal disadvantage is a period of isolation is required to comply with local radiation safety regulations. This makes treatment of intercurrent disease difficult or impossible during this time.

CHOLANGIOHEPATITIS COMPLEX*

Classical signs

- Inappetence and weight loss.
- Lethargy.
- Jaundice.
- Hepatomegaly and/or ascites.

See main references on page 427 for details (The Yellow Cat or Cat With Elevated Liver Enzymes).

Clinical signs

The most consistent clinical signs in these cases are **weight loss, variable anorexia, lethargy and depression**.

Fever may occur, particularly in the acute or suppurative form of the disease.

Vomiting, diarrhea and abdominal pain may also occur.

Clinical signs more specific to hepatic disease such as **hepatomegaly and jaundice** are common, particularly in the early stages of the condition.

Occasionally polyphagia or a normal appetite may be seen, particularly associated with lymphocytic cholangiohepatits.

Ascites, hepatic encephalopathy and a generalized lymphadenopathy are uncommon clinical signs.

In some cats, cholangiohepatitis is associated with inflammatory bowel disease and pancreatitis.

Diagnosis

Routine serum biochemistry findings include **mild to severe elevations in hepatic enzymes** (especially **alanine amino transferase (ALT)**). Hyperbilirubinemia and elevated bile acids are often also present.

Elevated **serum globulin concentrations** are common in the chronic stage of the disease.

A **neutrophilia**, often with **left shift** may be present in acute cases on routine hematology. More chronic cases often have a lymphocytosis.

If there is significant biliary stasis, intestinal absorption of vitamin K may be impaired leading to impaired secondary hemostasis and a **coagulopathy**.

Abdominal radiography may be normal or reveal:
- Hepatomegaly.
- Loss of abdominal contrast due to the presence of ascites, or if more localized, due to pancreatitis.
- Occasionally, choleliths may be noted.

Hepatic parenchymal changes on **abdominal ultrasound** are not specific to cholangiohepatitis, varying from normal parenchymal architecture, to diffuse increases (particularly if cirrhosis is present), or decreases (especially in acute or suppurative inflammatory disease) in echogenicity. Ultrasonography is helpful to demonstrate:
- Abnormalities of the biliary tract including biliary stasis or sludging, cholecystitis, biliary tract distention and obstruction.
- Concurrent pancreatic or intestinal disease.

A definitive diagnosis requires histopathological examination of hepatic tissue. Although as a diffuse disease, cholangiohepatitis should be amenable to diagnosis by percutaneous fine-needle aspiration techniques, blood contamination and the inability to assess hepatic architecture make definitive diagnosis of inflammatory disease difficult. Tissue core biopsy or surgical wedge biopsy yield improved diagnostic accuracy.
- Surgical exploration and wedge biopsy are required if there is evidence of extra-hepatic biliary stasis, severe biliary sludging or clinically significant choleliths.
- In addition, surgical exploration permits a complete evaluation of the biliary tree and pancreas, aspiration of bile for culture (although this may be carried out percutaneously by ultrasound guidance), biopsy of pancreas, and intestine and placement of feeding tubes.

Differential diagnosis

Differential diagnoses for inappetence and weight loss associated with suspicion of hepatic pathology includes hepatic lipidosis, hepatic neoplasia, feline infectious peritonitis affecting the liver and hyperthyroidism.

Feline infectious peritonitis is an important differential diagnosis for cholangiohepatitis, as both may present with hyperglobulinemia or ascites.

Treatment

Acute or suppurative cholangiohepatitis is treated primarily with antibiotics, ideally based on the results of culture and sensitivity testing.

- Ampicillin (10–40 mg/kg PO q 8 hours), amoxycillin (11–22 mg/kg PO q 8–12 hours), amoxycillin clavulanate (12.5–25 mg/kg PO q 12 hours), or cephalexin (10–30 mg/kg PO q 8–12 hours) are good empirical choices.
- Metronidazole in combination with the above antibiotics, provides broader anaerobic cover. Use at a lower dose (7.5–10 mg/kg PO q 12 hours) because of hepatotoxicity and the increased potential for neurological signs in animals with pre-existing hepatic disease. In addition it may have immunomodulating properties.

Immunosuppressive therapy is used if there is a lymphocytic component to the pathology, and in more chronic cases, although definitive evidence of efficacy is lacking.

- Prednisolone (2–4 mg/kg q 12–24 hours), gradually tapering the dose.
- Other immunosuppressive agents may be considered in non-responsive cases.

Fluid therapy and nutritional support will be required if anorexia is present.

Supportive and adjunctive therapy is often recommended on an empirical basis.

- **Ursodeoxycholic acid** (10–15 mg/kg PO q 24 hours) is a hydrophilic bile acid which has cytoprotective properties.
- **Parenteral vitamin K1** (0.5 mg/kg SC q 12 hours for 3 days) may be provided for those cases showing evidence of a coagulopathy.
- **S-adenosylmethionine** (18 mg/kg PO q 24 hours) and **vitamin E** have antioxidant properties and may be useful supplements.

INFLAMMATORY BOWEL DISEASE*

Classical signs

- Weight loss.
- Chronic vomiting and/or diarrhea.
- Variable appetite.

See main references on page 307 for details (The Cat With Weight Loss and a Good appetite).

Clinical signs

Clinical signs vary with the type and severity of the inflammation, and with the anatomical extent of the disease, although the correlation is poor.

Characteristically, any combination of **weight loss, vomiting or diarrhea** may be seen.

Vomiting is particularly evident **if the pathology involves the stomach or proximal small intestine** and may occur every few days to weeks. Vomiting is usually **unrelated to feeding**, and is more frequently composed of **fluid** rather than food.

Diarrhea may be soft and semi-formed to watery in consistency, with or without steatorrhea. Occasionally large bowel diarrhea with tenesmus, mucus and hematochezia may be present.

Clinical signs are usually chronic and may initially be intermittent.

Weight loss initially results from malabsorption and later from inappetence. In some cases, progressive weight loss is the only clinical sign.

Flatus and borborygmi may be reported.

Initially, **polyphagia or a normal appetite** may be seen, but this frequently **progresses to inappetence** as the disease increases in severity.

Intestinal thickening, mesenteric lymphadenopathy or abdominal pain may be revealed by abdominal palpation.

Occasionally, severe small intestinal disease leading to protein leakage into the gut lumen (**protein-losing enteropathy**) leads to extreme weight loss and hypoproteinemia. Although usually polyphagic, if the condition is associated with severe inflammatory or malignant disease, anorexia may occur. Vomiting and diarrhea may rarely be accompanied by ascites and peripheral edema.

Diagnosis

The diagnosis of inflammatory bowel disease is made based on exclusion of all other causes of the clinical signs in association with appropriate histopathology.

- Intestinal infiltration with inflammatory cells is non-specific.

- Inflammatory bowel disease is an idiopathic condition.

Initial diagnostic investigation should aim to exclude other causes of gastrointestinal signs and may include:
- Routine hematology and biochemistry and serum basal total T_4 concentrations.
  - Stress leukogram and occasionally eosinophilia.
  - Serum globulins may be increased as part of the chronic immune stimulation. In severe cases hypoproteinemia may result from protein-losing enteropathy.
- Fecal analysis and culture to exclude fecal parasites and enteric pathogens.
- Radiography and ultrasonography should be performed.
  - Radiography is frequently unremarkable, although increased gas may be present in intestinal loops.
  - Ultrasonography may show evidence of thickened or abnormal intestinal walls. Abdominal lymph node enlargement may be present.
- A dietary trial is a valuable tool to determine if signs resolve when the cat is fed a novel single protein and carbohydrate diet.

Assessment of serum cobalamin and folate concentrations, breath hydrogen analysis and sugar permeability studies may be supportive of inflammatory bowel disease.

Definitive diagnosis requires multiple intestinal biopsies either by endoscopy, laparoscopy or laparotomy:
- Gastrointestinal endoscopy permits visual evaluation of the mucosa, but the superficial nature of the mucosal biopsies obtained by this technique limits their diagnostic value.
- Laparotomy allows the collection of full-thickness biopsies, and gross evaluation and biopsy of other abdominal organs if required.

Differential diagnosis

The principal differential diagnoses are those conditions causing inappetence and weight loss in conjunction with gastrointestinal signs, namely other causes of enteropathy, chronic pancreatitis, cholangiohepatitis, gastrointestinal neoplasia and apathetic hyperthyroidism.

Treatment

As the etiology of the immune response in inflammatory bowel disease is unknown, the **principal form of treatment involves immunosuppressive therapy in combination with dietary management**.

A therapeutic dietary trial may be undertaken as part of the diagnostic evaluation (to eliminate dietary sensitivity), as the initial stage of treatment, or in combination with immunosuppressive therapy, depending on the severity of the clinical signs.
- A nutritionally balanced, highly digestible diet should be used.
- Usually a single protein, single carbohydrate source diet is used (hypoallergenic), preferably one to which the cat has not previously been exposed.
- Use of diets with hydrolized protein (e.g. Hill's z/d or Royal Canin HA) may be efficacious in some cats. Hydrolization reduces the molecular weight of dietary proteins to < 10 000 so they are not detected by the immune system.
- A high-fiber diet has proven beneficial in cases with large intestinal involvement.
- Minimum duration of the trial should be 3 weeks, but may be longer. If an improvement is seen, the cat should then be challenged with the original diet to confirm sensitivity.

Immunosuppressive therapy is required in the majority of cases:
- Prednisolone (2–4 mg/kg PO q 12–24 hours) is used at higher initial doses, which are gradually reduced to the lowest maintenance dose.
- Metronidazole (7.5–15 mg/kg PO q 12 hours) is used either as sole therapy in mild cases, or in addition to prednisolone for those cats in which the response to prednisolone is inadequate. Metronidazole has activity against anaerobic bacteria, protozoa and may be anti-inflammatory and influence cell-mediated immunity.
- Other more potent immunosuppressive therapy may be required in some cases.

FELINE LEUKEMIA VIRUS (FELV)*

Classical signs

- Younger cats, often less than 6 years of age, clinical signs variable.
- Inappetence, weight loss and lethargy.
- ± Neoplasia (lymphoma) – lymph node enlargement, organomegaly, solid masses.
- ± Anemia – pica, lethargy, pale mucous membranes, tachycardia.

Classical signs—Cont'd

- Immunosuppression – abscesses, cat flu, vomiting, diarrhea, neoplasia.
- Ocular signs – uveitis.
- Neurological signs – ataxia, behavioral changes.

See main references on page 540 for details (The Anemic Cat).

Clinical signs

There are no "classical signs" in a FeLV infection. A variety of clinical signs may be noted dependent on the body system affected. No one clinical sign is found in all cats with persistent viral infection.

The most consistent clinical signs are **weight loss, variable anorexia, lethargy and depression**.

Early infection with the virus is usually characterized by **submandibular lymph-adenopathy and fever**. This usually resolves in several days to weeks.

Pale mucous membranes, weakness and anorexia are seen if the virus causes anemia or bone marrow suppression. Hematological disease may be a primary viral effect on the bone marrow or secondary (e.g. neoplastic infiltration, hemobartonellosis)

Respiratory distress occurs if the virus leads to development of an **anterior mediastinal lymphoma** with or without pleural effusion.

Signs of **vomiting, diarrhea, and weight loss** may be evident if there is **gastro-intestinal infiltration** with malignant lymphocytes.

Signs of **liver or renal failure** occur if these organs are involved in lymphoma.

Gingivitis/stomatitis.

Ocular signs are relatively common, primarily uveitis, although neuro-ophthalmic signs, such as anisocoria may occur.

Various neurological signs may also be noted including ataxia and behavioral changes.

Immunosuppression may cause recurrent bacterial infections, especially subcutaneous abscesses, which recur or fail to respond to appropriate therapy.

Many of the clinical signs relate to the presence of concurrent disease such as toxoplasmosis or hemobartonellosis.

Diagnosis

When clinical disease warrants evaluation for FeLV, testing should be performed.
- **However a positive test does not prove that the disease process is caused by the virus.**

Diagnosis is usually based on the detection of viral antigen (usually the p27 core protein) by immunoassay. The ELISA test is recommended by the American Association of Feline Practitioners.
- **Serum or plasma** is preferred over whole blood when ELISA testing because there are reported to be fewer false positives.

A **positive result may indicate**:
- **Transient viremia** in the early viremic state; the cat may become negative later if a successful immune response is mounted.
- **Persistent viremia**; such cats are likely to develop FeLV-related disease.
- **Discordant results** (positive antigen test and negative on virus isolation) may occur early in the course of the infection or may indicate focal infection with no virus present in the circulation.
- **False-positive result**.

Confirmatory tests should be considered in cats with a positive ELISA result, especially if the cat is asymptomatic.
- **Immunoflorescent antibody test** (IFA) detects **p27 antigen** within **neutrophils and platelets**.
  - A positive result indicates that the **bone marrow is infected** and such cats are likely to be persistently infected. The **IFA** test is considered **more specific**, although slightly **less sensitive**, than the ELISA.
- **Virus isolation is considered the gold standard test for confirmation of FeLV infection.**
- Polymerase chain reaction (PCR) assays have been recently developed, however testing protocols require further validation.

Certain forms of diseases (abdominal visceral lymphoma) may be negative for the virus, although FeLV may have played a role in their development.

Other diagnostic tests should be carried out as required to investigate the presenting signs.

Differential diagnosis

The differential diagnoses will vary depending on the clinical manifestation(s) of the FeLV-related disease.

Because the clinical signs in a cat having disease caused by this virus are so extremely diverse, FeLV-associated disease must be considered in any chronically ill cat.

FIV infection is a principal differential diagnosis, as this may also be a cause of immunosuppression and neoplasia.

Treatment

The FeLV status of the cat should not necessarily preclude treatment for other diseases.

Chemotherapy has been used to treat a variety of lymphomas caused by the FeLV virus. Certain forms (mediastinal) seem to be more chemoresponsive than others (abdominal visceral).

Blood transfusions can give temporary help for the anemic patient.

Aggressive supportive care and management of secondary infections are essential in FeLV-positive cats. All infections should be fully assessed in terms of extent, and appropriate treatment administered, ideally based on culture and sensitivity results. Response to treatment may be slower in FeLV-infected cats, and so sufficient duration of antibiotic must be administered.

A variety of immunomodulator and antiviral therapies have been tried. As with FIV, the efficacy of these agents to clear the virus completely is questionable, although there is evidence that they may decrease total viral load.

FELINE INFECTIOUS PERITONITIS (FIP)*

Classical signs

- Younger cats, pedigree cats with variable clinical signs.
- Inappetence, weight loss and depression.

Classical signs—Cont'd

- Fever.
- Pleural and/or peritoneal effusions (abdominal enlargement and respiratory difficulties).
- Uveitis and neurological signs.

See main references on page 372 for details (The Pyrexic Cat).

Clinical signs

Most common in pure-bred cats from multi-cat households.

FIP is primarily seen in cats from 3 months to 3 years of age, although a second peak in incidence may occur in geriatric cats.

FIP occurs in two main forms, wet (or effusive) and dry (non-effusive). Weight loss, variable appetite, fever, lethargy and depression occur in both forms and may be the only clinical signs in early disease.

The **wet form** tends to progress more rapidly, and is characterized by combinations of **abdominal, pleural** or **pericardial effusions**.
- Non-painful abdominal enlargement is the main clinical sign if ascites is present. Vomiting and diarrhea may occur as the disease advances.
- **Dyspnea** is characteristic of pleural effusions.

The **dry form** leads to clinical signs associated with **pyogranulomatous perivascular disease** in **multiple organs** and clinical signs vary with the affected body system.
- This form of the disease tends to be more chronic (months) and progressive.
- **Neurological** (seizures, nystagmus, behavioral changes, peripheral neuropathies) and **ocular** (posterior and anterior uveitis) involvement is common.
- The liver, kidney and abdominal lymph nodes may also be involved.

Diagnosis

Definitive diagnosis is difficult, if not impossible, without histopathological examination of affected tissues.

- Histologic evaluation revealing typical pyogranulo-matous is diagnostic.

By combining clinical signs with other testing, a high suspicion of FIP may be obtained.

In the wet form, **evaluation of the fluid is helpful.**
- Fluid is typically yellow, viscous, and may have fibrin clots.
- Fluid is high in protein (> 35g/L or 3.5 g/dl and usu-ally 50–120g/L or 5–12 g/dl) with moderate numbers of non-degenerate neutrophils and macrophages, although lower than usual for an exudate.
- If the albumin:globulin ratio of the fluid is > 0.81, FIP is an extremely unlikely diagnosis.

Aspiration of affected organs (liver, lymph nodes, kidney) will often reveal a pyogranulomatous response.

Increased serum globulin concentration (polyclonal gammopathy) is present in the majority of cats with FIP.
- Other biochemical findings will vary, dependent on the organ system involved.

Complete blood count usually often reveals a normo-cytic, normochromic, nonregenerative anemia, a neu-trophilic leukocytosis and lymphopenia.

"FIP titers" reported by laboratories are either **corona-virus titers** or **titers to the 7B protein in coronavirus. Neither are specific for the mutated FIP-coronavirus virus.** Although claimed that 7B protein was specific for FIP strains, subsequent studies have shown that it is not present in some FIP strains, and that non-FIP coro-navirus may have an active 7B component. Currently there is no serological test that is specific for FIP-coro-navirus.

Differential diagnosis

FIV, FeLV and toxoplasmosis are the three most com-mon differentials for the non-effusive form of FIP. All three can lead to fever, inappetence and weight loss. Toxoplasmosis and FeLV can both present with ocular and neurological signs.

Abdominal neoplasia, liver disease (especially cholan-giohepatitis), **pancreatitis, peritonitis** and **diseases causing hypoproteinemia** can lead to abdominal effu-sion. Fluid analysis and cytology of the fluid can fre-quently distinguish between these diseases.

Heart failure, diaphragmatic hernias, neoplasia and chylothorax may all present signs similar to effusive FIP in the thorax. Fluid analysis and thoracic radi-ographs will help in differentiating the cause of fluid accumulation.

Treatment

Clinical FIP is invariably fatal, and no effective treat-ment has been found in cats.

Anti-inflammatory and immunosuppressive ther-apy may increase life span by controlling the comple-ment mediated vasculitis, but will not cure the condition.
- **Prednisolone** (2–4 mg/kg PO daily).
- **Cyclophosphamide** and **chlorambucil** may be used for more potent immunosuppression, but cytotoxic agents should be avoided in debilitated cats.
  - Broad-spectrum antibiotic cover should be given if immunosuppressive drugs are used to prevent secondary infections.
  - Therapy should be re-evaluated regularly, including monitoring for myelosuppression.

Other immunomodulating drugs (recombinant **human interferon-α**) and **anti-viral agents** have been promis-ing in vitro but have limited efficacy in *in vivo* studies.

Supportive care should be provided if the cat is not euthanized.

ORAL INFLAMMATORY DISEASE*

Classical signs

- Inappetence associated with dysphagia.
- Weight loss.
- Ptyalism, halitosis and oral pain.
- Oral inflammatory, ulcerative and proliferative lesions.

See main references on page 585 for details (The Cat With Salivation).

Clinical signs

Pure-bred cats may be predisposed.

Continuum of disease from mild gingivitis to chronic, severe, intractable oral inflammation.

- **Most cases are due to lymphoplasmacytic gingivitis/stomatitis.**

The condition may be waxing and waning in nature but in some cases is progressive.

Oral examination reveals erythema, swelling, ulceration and proliferative lesions (giving a cobblestone appearance) of varying severity. The tissue is friable and therefore tends to bleed easily.

- These lesions may involve the **gingiva, glossopalatine arches** (fauces), **pharynx, buccal mucosa** and less commonly the tongue, hard palate and lips.
- Many cats have significant dental disease but it is not clear whether the inflammation precedes, contributes to, or results from this.

Submandibular lymphadenopathy is also common.

A poor hair coat may be noted due to decreased grooming. It is usually accompanied by varying degrees of dental disease.

A particular form of oral inflammatory disease is **feline juvenile hyperplastic gingivitis**.

- This condition affects young cats at the **time of eruption of adult teeth.** Abyssinian and Persian cats may be predisposed.
- There is a tendency for spontaneous remission with maturity.
- Lesions consist of a very proliferative, hyperemic gingivitis.

Diagnosis

The identification of this condition is usually obvious on **oral examination.**

- A complete history and clinical examination is essential to ensure evidence of concurrent disease or additional lesions are not overlooked.

The investigation should aim to identify any possible predisposing causes of oral inflammation.

- Perform routine hematology, biochemistry and urinalysis to assess for systemic predisposing disease.
  - Approximately half the cats have a polyclonal gammopathy.
- Test for FeLV, FIV and respiratory tract viruses.

- Perform a full oral examination under general anesthesia to assess for periodontal disease and feline odontoclastic resorptive lesions, including a full mouth radiographic dental survey.

Biopsy and histopathological examination of affected areas is required for **definitive diagnosis** of the lymphoplasmacytic nature of the lesions.

Differential diagnosis

Other diseases that may appear clinically similar on examination include neoplasia (squamous cell carcinoma and fibrosarcoma), eosinophilic granuloma complex and autoimmune disease (pemphigus vulgaris and systemic lupus erythematosus).

FIV, FeLV and the respiratory tract viruses, particularly feline calicivirus, may be associated with oral ulceration or stomatitis.

Stomatitis may be found in association with severe uremia.

Dental disease may be associated with oral inflammatory lesions. If the oral inflammation does not resolve with treatment of the dental disease, lymphoplasmacytic gingivitis/stomatitis should be considered.

Treatment

Initial management involves removing or treating any underlying etiology identified.

Attention should be given to the nutritional status of the cat, including other forms of feeding, if the severity of the lesions is preventing the oral intake of food.

- A dietary trial of a novel protein source should also be considered to exclude hypersensitivity as a cause.

Pivotal to management is thorough dental management. The aim is to improve the overall oral hygiene by scaling and polishing, followed by extraction of any anatomically compromised teeth which may be acting as foci of inflammation.

- Repeated dental prophylaxis may be required to maintain oral hygiene.
- In a number of cases the condition resolves or can be more effectively managed after extraction of all

the teeth caudal to the canines. Occasionally removal of the canines and incisors is also required.

Systemic antibiotics frequently produce only a transient improvement.
- Effective antibiotics include clindamycin, clavulanate potentiated amoxycillin, metro-nidazole and spiramycin (which is concentrated in saliva).

Immunosuppressive therapy appears to produce the most reliable responses in chronic cases.
- Prednisolone (2–4 mg/kg PO once daily) on a tapering regime to the lowest maintenance dose.
- In cases failing to respond to corticosteroid therapy, alternative immunosuppressive or immunomodulating therapies should be considered.
  - Including chlorambucil, cyclosporin A, gold salts, human recombinant interferon alpha and topical application of bovine lactoferrin. There have been few studies evaluating these drugs and most have more potential side effects, requiring closer monitoring.

DIABETES MELLITUS

Classical signs

- More common in older cats, especially neutered males.
- Polyuria and polydipsia.
- Usually polyphagia and weight loss.
- May progress to decreased appetite.

See main references on page 236 for details (The Cat With Polydipsia and Polyuria).

Clinical signs

Although diabetes mellitus may occur in any cat, it is more frequent in older cats, especially neutered males.
- In some regions Burmese cats may be predisposed.

The classic clinical signs are those of polydipsia, polyuria, polyphagia and weight loss.
- These signs are frequently unnoticed by cat owners.
- Therefore many cats do not present until the cat develops more severe clinical signs such as inappetence, vomiting and depression.
  - These clinical signs may be associated with the development of ketoacidosis.

Body condition varies from obese to thin.

Coat condition is often poor, with seborrhea and scales.

Hepatomegaly is common. If diabetes mellitus is associated with pancreatitis, abdominal discomfort may be present.

A plantigrade stance may be noted due to diabetic neuropathy.

If the diabetic cat is ketoacidotic, dehydration, depression and weakness may also be present.

Diagnosis

Documenting a persistent fasting hyperglycemia (blood glucose > 12 mmol/L, 217 mg/dl) and glucosuria in a cat with appropriate clinical signs is required to establish a diagnosis of diabetes mellitus.
- It is important to distinguish diabetes mellitus from stress hyperglycemia.
  - Glucosuria rarely results from stress hyperglycemia because the hyperglycemia is usually below the renal threshold or only transient, however glucosuria does not exclude this possibility.
  - Monitoring for glucosuria at home may aid differentiation.

Blood glycosylated hemoglobin and serum fructosamine concentrations represent the average blood glucose concentrations over the preceding 4–6 weeks and 2–3 weeks respectively.
- They may be helpful to distinguish diabetes mellitus from stress hyperglycemia.
- They also provide further information regarding glycemic control when monitoring patients under treatment.

Further investigation is required to assess for concurrent disease or systemic complications of diabetes mellitus.
- Routine hematology and biochemistry, including assessment of electrolytes.
  - Diabetic cats frequently have mild to moderate increases in hepatic enzymes and cholesterol.
  - Concurrent renal failure or pre-renal azotemia may be present.
- Complete urinalysis should be carried out.
  - The presence of ketones in the urine confirms the diagnosis of diabetes mellitus. Sick ketoacidotic cats require aggressive monitoring and management.

– Symptomatic or asymptomatic **urinary tract infections** are frequently present in diabetes mellitus.

CARDIAC CACHEXIA

Classical signs

- Decreased appetite and weight loss.
- Lethargy.
- Signs relating to cardiac disease – tachycardia, cardiac murmurs and arrhythmias.
- Dyspnea if pleural effusion or pulmonary edema present.

See main references on page 124 for details (The Cat With Abnormal Heart Sounds and/or an Enlarged Heart).

Clinical signs

Inappetence and weight loss may occur, associated with cardiac disease.

- The remaining clinical signs will vary with the nature of the cardiac disease, although cardiac cachexia usually only occurs in cats with cardiac disease sufficient to cause failure.
- **Generally it is seen in cats with chronic, severe right-sided congestive cardiac failure.**

Lethargy and exercise intolerance are present.

Dyspnea due to the presence of pleural effusion or pulmonary edema may be present.

Rarely **ascites** may be present.

Physical examination may reveal poor peripheral pulses or evidence of venous congestion (jugular distention and pulses, hepatojugular reflux).

Cardiac auscultation may reveal tachycardia, arrhythmias or cardiac murmurs.

Diagnosis

Diagnosis is based on documenting the presence of severe cardiac disease in a cat with weight loss.

Evidence of cardiac disease may be provided by thoracic radiography, electrocardiography, measurement of systemic blood pressure and echocardiography.

- Thoracic radiography may show cardiomegaly, vascular congestion and possibly pleural effusion or pulmonary edema.
- **Echocardiographic examination is usually required to make a definitive diagnosis of the type of cardiac disease.**

CHRONIC BACTERIAL RHINITIS AND SINUSITIS

Classical signs

- Chronic sneezing and snuffling.
- Chronic, persistent or intermittent, mucopurulent nasal discharge.
- Stertorous respiration.

See main references on page 21 for details (The Cat With Signs of Chronic Nasal Disease).

Clinical signs

Usually there is a history of chronic upper respiratory tract disease following an acute episode of signs.

- Typically there is serous to mucopurulent, unilateral or bilateral oculonasal discharge, often associated with sneezing.
  - Signs may be persistent or intermittent, but are usually gradually progressive.
  - Rarely epistaxis may be noted, but this is more frequently associated with neoplasia.
- Stertorous respiration may be audible.

If chronic and severe, in rare cases, bone destruction may lead to nasal distortion.

Inappetence, which is often associated with inability to smell food, and weight loss may occur.

Systemic signs such as depression and anorexia are often associated with intermittent exacerbation of disease.

Diagnosis

Appropriate clinical signs and a history of previous acute upper respiratory tract disease are supportive of the diagnosis, however a full investigation is required to exclude other causes of nasal discharge including neoplasia and fungal disease.

- Neoplasia and fungal causes are unlikely if the clinical signs have been constant for a protracted period (1–2 years).

A **thorough examination of the oral cavity** and pharynx should be made whilst the cat is anesthetized to exclude congenital and traumatic palate defects, dental disease, nasopharyngeal polyps and neoplasia as a cause.

Radiographic evidence of bilateral fluid density in nasal passages often extending into the frontal sinuses is typical.
- Occasionally bone destruction is seen on radiographs.

Cytology of the nasal discharge reveals neutrophils, bacteria, and the absence of neoplastic or fungal elements.

Rhinoscopy (anterior and posterior) will permit visual examination and flushing of the nasal cavity, and facilitate nasal biopsy.
- Blind biopsy or traumatic flushing may be used to obtain biopsy material from the nasal cavity.
- **It is extremely difficult to definitively exclude neoplasia in these cases.**
  - A diagnosis should not be made on cytology alone, because both neoplasia and fungal disease frequently reveal only neutrophils and bacteria on cytologic examination.
  - Rhinotomy and biopsy may be necessary to definitively exclude neoplasia, particularly in cases with suggestive clinical signs.

Respiratory virus status may be evaluated by virus isolation from oropharyngeal and nasal swabs.

FeLV and FIV status should be assessed and other causes of immunosuppression should be excluded.

CHYLOTHORAX

Classical signs

- Respiratory distress – tachypnea, dyspnea and open mouth breathing.
- Weight loss.
- Inappetence.

See main references on page 77 for details (The Cat With Hydrothorax).

Clinical signs

Although signs of respiratory distress may appear acute, the disease process is often more chronic.

Clinical signs will vary with the quantity of fluid present.
- Cats adjust to the decreased lung volume, and distress is not usually apparent until late in the disease.
- **Tachypnea and dyspnea** are often present.
- If ventilation is severely impaired, cyanosis may be noted.

Auscultation usually reveals **decreased breath sounds** (muffled and dull) ventrally.
- Occasionally fluid may accumulate in focal areas, and unilaterally rather than bilaterally.
- Heart sounds may be muffled.

The thorax may be dull on percussion.

Weight loss in usually present, accompanied by inappetence as the respiratory difficulty increases.

Clinical signs to a certain degree will depend on the underlying cause of the pleural effusion.
- **Possible causes of chylothorax include** neoplasia, heart failure, trauma and hyperthyroidism, although in many cases the underlying etiology is not determined despite extensive investigation (termed idiopathic chylothorax).

Diagnosis

The presence of a pleural effusion may be confirmed radiographically or ultrasonographically.
- **Care should be taken in handling and positioning cats with respiratory distress, and thoracocentesis may be required to stabilize the cat prior to these procedures.**
- Radiographic evidence of a pleural effusion includes:
  - Presence of pleural fissure lines.
  - Separation of lung borders from the thoracic wall and rounding of edges of the lung lobes.
  - Loss of cardiac silhouette.

Thoracocentesis with biochemical and cytological analysis of thoracic fluid is required for definitive diagnosis:
- Chylous fluid is usually a white "milky" fluid.
  - It may be slightly pink on repeated aspirations.

- If the cat has not eaten recently, the fluid may appear only slightly opaque.
- Lymphocytes are usually the predominant cell type, with some non-degenerate neutrophils.
- **The concentration of triglycerides in the fluid exceeds that of the serum in a true chylous effusion.**

It is important that, where possible, the underlying cause is investigated, as this will influence the treatment and prognosis.

PROTEIN-LOSING NEPHROPATHY

Classical signs

- Marked weight loss.
- Initially polyphagia may be present but progresses to inappetence.
- Polydipsia and polyuria.
- Subcutaneous edema and/or ascites.

Pathogenesis

The most common causes of protein-losing nephropathy are glomerulo-nephritis and renal amyloidosis.

Renal amyloidosis is characterized by the extracellular deposition of fibrillar proteins arranged in a beta-pleated sheet configuration.

- **Reactive (secondary) systemic amyloidosis is the form of amyloidosis occurring in cats.**
  - It is considered to be **secondary to inflammatory, neoplastic and chronic infectious** disease, although in many cases the predisposing disease is not found.
- Severe proteinuria occurs when amyloid deposits in the glomerulus cause glomerular damage.
  - Most domestic cats with amyloidosis and at least 25% of Abyssinian cats with familial amyloidosis have medullary amyloid deposits, without significant glomerular deposits.
  - In cases of medullary amyloidosis, proteinuria may be mild or absent, although the deposits will interfere with renal concentrating ability.

Glomerulonephritis is caused by antibody–antigen complexes present in the glomerulus that lead to immune-mediated glomerular damage.

- Initially the glomerular injury is characterized by proteinuria, but as the condition progresses, the entire nephron may become non-functional, with decreased glomerular filtration rate and azotemia.
- **Glomerulonephritis** may be found in association with any **chronic antigenic stimulus**, including **infectious, inflammatory** and **neoplastic diseases**.
  - In the cat, glomerulonephritis has been particularly associated with infectious diseases including FeLV, FIV and FIP, and hemolymphatic neoplasia.
  - In the majority of cases an underlying antigen source is not identified and the disease is classed as idiopathic.

Glomerular proteinuria is characteristically massive, and in many cases may lead to clinical signs related to protein loss and eventually the nephrotic syndrome.

The nephrotic syndrome is characterized by massive proteinuria, hypoalbuminemia, hyperlipidemia and subcutaneous edema and/or ascites.

- The proteinuria leads to hypoalbuminemia and subsequent development of edema.

Clinical signs

Protein-losing nephropathies are uncommon conditions in the cat.

- **Glomerulonephritis** usually affects **young adult cats** (average age 3–4 years), with males being predisposed. The condition is rare.
- Most cats with **amyloidosis** are **over 5 years** of age at diagnosis. Systemic reactive amyloidosis occurs as a familial disease in Abyssinian cats.

Clinical signs in early disease are principally weight loss with a good appetite and even polyphagia.

- Signs frequently progress to inappetence and depression.
- Continued protein loss eventually leads to the **nephrotic syndrome** with subcutaneous edema and/or ascites.

Polyuria and polydipsia are common if the condition progresses to renal failure and uremia.

- Polyuria and polydipsia are also common if there are medullary amyloid deposits.
- Clinical signs of uremia may also be noted (see page 334, chronic renal failure).

The **kidneys** are usually **small, firm and irregular on palpation**.

Both conditions are associated with an underlying chronic antigenic stimulus, including infectious, inflammatory and neoplastic diseases. Clinical signs may also relate to the underlying disease.

Systemic hypertension may occur and result in hypertensive retinopathy, acute-onset blindness or neurological signs.

The prognosis is variable depending on the cause of the protein-losing nephropathy, although is generally considered poor if actual renal failure is present.
- Clinical signs in glomerulonephritis may wax and wane, and occasionally undergo complete or prolonged periods of remission.
- Amyloidosis tends to be slowly progressive, and is generally fatal.

Diagnosis

Diagnosis of protein-losing nephropathy is made on the documentation of proteinuria, in the absence of pre- and post-renal causes. A complete urinalysis should therefore be carried out.
- **Urinalysis typically reveals proteinuria with a benign sediment.** A benign sediment excludes lower urinary tract disease as a cause of the proteinuria.
- Hyaline casts may be noted on sediment examination.
- In the early stages of disease, urine-concentrating ability may be retained.
- Proteinuria is usually detected on qualitative screening tests, such as urine dipstick reagent strips.

The protein:creatinine ratio should be evaluated to further quantify the urinary protein loss.
- Although the magnitude of the proteinuria can be used to predict the site of protein loss, there is great variability in ratios with different diseases.
- The quantity of protein loss in glomerular disease is massive compared with that in pre-renal and post-renal proteinuria. Protein:creatinine ratios of greater than 13 commonly occur in glomerular proteinuria, although ratios generally range from mild to severe (ratio of 5–13).

Routine biochemistry should be evaluated.
- **Plasma protein concentrations** may be variable, with hypoalbuminemia occurring if the protein loss is severe. Conversely, hyperglobulinemia may occur associated with the chronic inflammatory focus initiating the lesion.
- **Hypercholesterolemia** is reported as a characteristic feature of the nephrotic syndrome, however it is a common non-specific finding in cats with any form of renal disease.
- **Azotemia** and a **low urine specific gravity** will indicate the presence of **renal failure.**

Abdominal radiography and ultrasound may provide information on renal architecture and size.

Renal biopsy is the only definitive method of distinguishing between glomerulonephritis and amyloidosis.
- Complete morphological classification of glomerular lesions may require light, electron and immunofluorescence microscopy.
- Amyloid deposits demonstrate characteristic green birefringence after Congo red staining when viewed under polarized light.
  - The diagnosis is frequently difficult to achieve if glomerular involvement is minimal or absent, requiring medullary biopsies.

A thorough investigation for an underlying inflammatory focus should be made, including assessment of FeLV and FIV status.

TOXOPLASMOSIS

Classical signs

- Especially in immuno-compromised individuals, particularly free-roaming cats.
- Weight loss, lethargy and inappetence.
- Fever.
- Respiratory distress.
- Icterus.
- Uveitis.
- Neurological signs including ataxia and seizures.
- Muscle hyperesthesia.

See main references on page 376 for details (The Pyrexic Cat).

Clinical signs

Self-limiting small bowel diarrhea is common after primary exposure, although it is often unrecognized.

Acute fatal toxoplasmosis is recognized in kittens and immuno-compromised cats.

Chronic toxoplasmosis is characterized by diverse clinical signs depending on the tissue affected.

Respiratory distress due to pneumonia is common in kittens and cats with acute infection.

Central nervous system disease, including ataxia and seizures, may occur either with acute or chronic infection.

Icterus is common due to infection involving the liver.

Anterior or posterior uveitis may be the only obvious sign present in some cats.

Muscle stiffness or hyperesthesia.

The disease may be chronic with weight loss and lack of appetite. Occasionally, toxoplasma granulomas (tissue cysts) form in the gastrointestinal tract or pancreas causing chronic vomiting.

Diagnosis

Routine laboratory testing is not specific for toxoplasmosis.

Diagnosis of toxoplasmosis may be made on:
- **Rarely tachyzoites or bradyzoites may be identified in tissues, broncho-alveolar lavage fluid, cerebrospinal fluid and effusions.**
- Oocysts in the feces do not provide definitive diagnosis due to difficulties of identification.
  - **Shedding** only occurs for **1 or 2 weeks** following initial infection, **usually prior to illness**.
- Serologic testing for antibodies is helpful, but not definitive because clinically normal cats frequently have significant titers. The magnitude of the titers is not proportional to severity of the disease.
  - **IgG titers may last for years and are common in normal cats indicating previous infection.** A four-fold rise in IgG titer over 2–4 weeks suggests active infection.
  - **A positive IgM titer persists for approximately 3 months, so tends to indicate recent infection** but may persist for much longer.

- A positive response to appropriate treatment provides a presumptive diagnosis.

Routine hematology and biochemistry findings are variable dependent on the tissues affected.

Thoracic radiography may reveal a pleural effusion and diffuse interstitial or alveolar patterns.

CRYPTOCOCCOSIS

> **Classical signs**
> - Progressive chronic nasal discharge and sneezing.
> - Soft tissue swelling over the nose, polypoid masses in the nasal cavity.
> - Neurological and ocular signs.

See main references on page 25 for details (The Cat With Signs of Chronic Nasal Disease).

Clinical signs

Cryptococcosis is the most common systemic fungal disease of the cat, and has a worldwide distribution.

It is most commonly **acquired by inhalation,** and so clinical signs are often localized to the respiratory tract.
- Immune response leads to **granuloma formation**, leading to **facial swellings** and **polypoid mass** lesions within the nasal cavity.
- Stertor and inspiratory dyspnea may occur.
- Typically there is **sneezing and mucopurulent nasal discharge** (unilateral and bilateral), which is commonly blood tinged.

The **central nervous system and eyes** may be affected by direct extension from the nose.
- Signs include depression, behavior changes, ataxia and seizures.
- Ocular signs include granulomatous chorioretinitis and uveitis.

Depression, inappetence (which occurs as a result of the inability to smell the food) and weight loss are common.

Skin involvement (papules and draining nodules) with peripheral lymphadenopathy may occur.

Diagnosis

Diagnosis based on cytological identification of cryptococcal organisms in nasal discharge, exudates, fine-needle aspiration of masses and lymph nodes and cerebrospinal fluid.

Histopathology may be required if cytology is not diagnostic.

Using a latex agglutination test to identify cryptococcal capsular antigen (on serum, urine or cerebrospinal fluid) provides a non-invasive, sensitive and specific diagnostic test.

Nasal radiography may reveal increased soft tissue density and bone destruction.

PCR (polymerase chain reaction) assays are now available to detect cryptoccal antigens in biopsy material.

SYSTEMIC MYCOSES

Classical signs

- Vague, non-specific signs of weight loss, inappetence and depression.
- Dyspnea.

See main references on pages 371, 388 for details (The Pyrexic Cat).

Clinical signs

The most common systemic mycoses (excluding cryptococcosis) are **histoplasmosis** and **blastomycosis.**
- Both are geographically restricted infections.
  - *Histoplasma capsulatum*, the agent causing histoplasmosis, is endemic throughout large areas of the temperate and subtropical regions of the world.
  - Blastomycosis (caused by *Blastomyces dermatitidis*) is principally a disease of North America, but has occurred in Africa and Central America.

History tends to be vague and chronic, including weight loss, inappetence and weakness.

Mild to moderate **fever.**

Infection is commonly acquired by inhalation, and so clinical signs are often localized to respiratory tract.

- **Dyspnea** and occasionally coughing may occur, with increased respiratory noise on auscultation.
- Absence of respiratory signs does not exclude significant lung involvement.

Involvement of the gastrointestinal tract causes **diarrhea and weight loss.**

Peripheral lymphadenopathy and granulomatous, ulcerating skin lesions may be noted.

Ocular involvement is common, and may cause a granulomatous retinitis, uveitis and panophthalmitis.

Hepatomegaly, splenomegaly and neurological signs may also be seen.

Cats with disseminated disease are generally extremely ill.

Diagnosis

Diagnosis is based on cytological identification of the organisms in exudates, fine-needle aspiration of lesions and lymph nodes, cerebrospinal fluid and bronchoalveolar lavage fluid.
- Fungal culture may assist, but is not required for identification of the organism.

Histopathology may be required if cytology is not diagnostic, and shows pyogranulomatous lesions.

Serology may be useful in the diagnosis of blastomycosis, but false-negative results may occur both early and late in the infection. It should be used in cases where there is a high level of suspicion of the disease, but organisms can not be demonstrated.

Thoracic radiography may show varying changes, however a **diffuse interstitial or nodular interstitial pattern** is most commonly seen.

Hematological changes tend to be non-specific, and include the presence of a mild non-regenerative anemia in some cases.

PORTOSYSTEMIC SHUNTS

Classical signs

- Congenital shunts usually show clinical signs by 6 months of age.
- Weight loss or stunting (congenital shunts).

continued

Classical signs—Cont'd

- Neurological signs – hypersalivation, seizures, ataxia, blindness and behavioral changes.
- Inappetence, vomiting or diarrhea.

See main references on page 588 for details (The Cat With Salivation).

Clinical signs

Portosystemic shunts are vascular **communications between the portal and systemic** venous circulation, and may be a congenital anomaly or acquired.

- **Congenital portosystemic shunts** in cats are usually **single extrahepatic shunts** resulting from developmental anomalies of the vitelline system.
  - Persian and Himalayan cats are predisposed.
  - A predilection for male cats has been suggested, and such cats are often crypt-orchid.
  - Cats with congenital shunts will usually show clinical **signs by 6 months of age,** however a congenital portosytemic shunt should not be excluded on the basis of age alone.
- Multiple **extrahepatic acquired portosystemic shunts** are formed secondary to portal hypertension, and are extremely uncommon in the cat.
  - Acquired shunts usually occur in cats with chronic, severe, diffuse hepatic disease.

Signs are often vague or non-specific and episodic.

Cats with congenital shunts may show **stunting** (smaller than littermates) or **weight loss**.

Clinical signs of **hepatic encephalopathy predominate** in cats with portosystemic shunts.

- Vague anorexia, depression and weakness.
- Ataxia, behavioral changes (bizarre and aggressive behavior), aimless pacing, blindness and seizures may occur.
- **Hypersalivation,** often profuse, is also common.

There are often intermittent episodes of vomiting, diarrhea and inappetence with normal periods between.

Lower urinary tract signs are present in cats with concurrent urate urolithiasis.

Copper- or golden-colored irises have been noted in some cats with portosystemic shunts.

Heart murmurs have also been noted in some affected cats.

Ascites and signs of primary hepatic disease may be seen in cats with acquired portosystemic shunts.

Diagnosis

Routine hematology and biochemistry may be unremarkable in cats with congenital portosystemic shunts however:

- Routine hematology may reveal a **mild non-regenerative, microcytic anemia** often with **poikilocytosis**.
- **Hypoglycemia, hypoalbuminemia, hypocholesterolemia and decreased blood urea concentrations** may indicate hepatic dysfunction.

Pre- and post-prandial serum bile acids should be assessed.

- Pre-prandial bile acid concentrations may be normal or elevated.
- **Post-prandial bile acids are typically elevated, frequently exceeding 100 µmol/L (39.2 mg/L).**

Hyperammonemia, particularly post prandial is commonly present.

Abdominal radiographs may demonstrate microhepatica, but in many cats hepatic size is normal.

Ammonium biurate crystals may be present on urine sediment examination.

- Ammonium urate calculi are often radiolucent.

Portosystemic shunts may be identified and localized on abdominal ultrasound.

Other techniques may be required to definitively demonstrate the presence of shunting vessels.

- Transcolonic portal scintigraphy is a non-invasive technique but requires specialist equipment.
  - It may produce false-negative results when the shunt connects the gastric vein to the caudal vena cava, a common type of shunt in the cat.
- **Venous portography, although requiring surgery, is the definitive method for identifying shunts.**

RECOMMENDED READING

Elliott J, Rawlings JM, Markwell PJ, Barber PJ. Survival of cats with naturally occurring chronic renal failure: Effect of dietary management. J Small Anim Pract 2000: 41: 235–242.

Levy JK CVT Update: Feline immunodeficiency virus. In: Bonagura (ed) Kirk's Current Veterinary Therapy XIII. W.B. Saunders, Philadelphia, 2000, pp 284–288.

Nagode LA, Dennis JC. Frequently Asked Questions RE: Use of Calcitriol Versus Renal Secondary Hyperparathyroidism. Veterinary Information Network, June 8, 2001. Retrieved June 20, 2003 from www.vin.com/Members/SearchDB/misc/m05000/m01284.htm

Polzin DJ, Osborne CA, Jacob F, Ross S. Chronic renal failure. In: Ettinger, Feldman (eds) Textbook of Veterinary Internal Medicine, 5th Edition. W.B. Saunders, Philadelphia, 2000, pp 1634–1662.

PART 7

Sick cat with specific signs

19. The pyrexic cat

Kristy L Dowers and Michael R Lappin

KEY SIGNS

- Temperature > 39.2°C (102.5°F).

MECHANISM?

- True fever results from a cascade of events, which starts with activation of leukocytes. Pyrogenic factors released from the leukocytes increase the thermoregulatory set point in the hypothalamus.
  Signs that may be associated with fever include:
- Elevated body temperature.
- Reluctance to move.
- Anorexia.
- Depression.
- Hyperpnea.
- Muscle or joint stiffness/discomfort.
- Shivering.

WHERE?

- Inflammation anywhere in the body can result in elevation of core body temperature above 39.2°C (102.5°F).

WHAT?

- The most common etiology for fever in the cat is percutaneous cellulitis or abscess. Viral diseases such as FIV, FeLV and FIP are important diseases to consider.

QUICK REFERENCE SUMMARY

Diseases causing a pyrexic cat

METABOLIC

- Hyperthyroidism (p 389)

Occasionally mild fever occurs from the increased metabolic rate. Typical signs are history of weight loss despite good appetite, unkempt hair coat, change in temperament and vomiting/diarrhea.

NEOPLASTIC

- Neoplasia (p 385)

Fever associated with antibody stimulation from tumor antigens, tissue necrosis or destruction of bone marrow. Lymphoma is the most common neoplasia in cats.

INFLAMMATION

INFECTIOUS

Viral:

- **Feline leukemia virus (FeLV)***** (p 374)**

Fever may occur in any age cat but is primarily seen initially in the viremic stage or later in response to neoplastic, inflammatory or immunosuppressive effects. Signs include chronic infections, anemia, thrombocytopenia, elevated MCV and lymphoma.

- **Feline immunodeficiency virus (FIV)** (p 378)**

Fever in adult cats is associated with the acute stage and in older cats with the chronic terminal stage. Signs include chronic infections, especially upper respiratory and skin infections, gingivitis, weight loss and diarrhea.

- **Feline infectious peritonitis (FIP)***** (p 372)**

Tends to occur in very young or very old cats. Signs include fever, anorexia, lethargy, weight loss, pleural effusion and dyspnea, peritoneal effusion, vomiting/diarrhea, ocular changes (uveitis, in particular), neurologic signs, hyperglobulinemia, leukopenia.

- **Panleukopenia* (p 382)**

Acute onset of fever in young cats with vomiting, anorexia, depression, dehydration and profound leukopenia. Diarrhea usually follows 1–2 days later.

- **Feline viral rhinotracheitis (herpesvirus-1)*** (p 370)**

Paroxysms of sneezing followed by severe conjunctivitis with serous to mucopurulent nasal discharge, fever, anorexia and lethargy. Ocular signs (corneal ulcerations) may follow 1–2 weeks later.

- **Calicivirus*** (p 370)**

Inconsistent fever, anorexia, lethargy, mild upper respiratory signs with a serous to mucopurulent oculonasal discharge, oral ulcers predominately on the anterior or lateral margins of the tongue and salivation.

Bacterial/rickettsial:

- **Percutaneous cellulitis/abscess*** (p 368)**

Fever, anorexia, depression, localized swelling/pain in area of abscess.

continued

continued

● *Chlamydophila felis** (p 381)

Conjunctivitis is the predominant sign and is often initially unilateral and becomes bilateral. Ocular discharge is serous initially then mucopurulent, but is usually mild. Fever, anorexia and lethargy may occur.

● *Yersinia pestis* (feline plague)* (p 383)

Acute onset of a high fever, anorexia and depression. Lymphadenopathy, with marked swelling over submandibular or cervical lymph nodes, which may abscess. Pneumonic form is less common and may have upper and lower respiratory signs with sneezing, nasal discharge, dyspnea or cough.

● *Salmonella* spp. (songbird fever)

Signs occur in outdoor cats which hunt. Acute onset of fever, anorexia and depression, and 50% of cats have GI signs with vomiting and diarrhea.

● *Francisella tularensis* (tularemia)* (p 382)

Occurs in outdoor cats which hunt and have recent exposure to rabbits. Signs include fever, depression, anorexia, peripheral lymphadenopathy, oral ulcerations and hepatomegaly.

● *Ehrlichia* spp. and *Anaplasma phagocytophilum** (p 385)

Chronic intermittent fever, weight loss and anorexia occur. Hyperesthesia, joint pain or irritable disposition is common. Exposure to ticks may or may not be documented.

● *Mycoplasma haemofelis* and Candidatus *'M. haemominutum'* (*Haemobartonella felis*)** (p 374)

Pale mucous membranes, anorexia and depression. Fever occurs in approximately 50% of cats and icterus may be evident.

● *Bartonella henselae* (cat-scratch fever)

Mild, self-limiting fever occurs in experimentally infected cats. Naturally infected cats are usually subclinical and fever is not well documented.

Parasitic/protozoal:

● *Toxoplasma gondii** (p 375)

Fever, anorexia and depression are often present. Dyspnea is common. Kittens and cats may also have icterus, abdominal distension or pain/discomfort, ocular signs (uveitis, retinochoroiditis) or neurologic signs.

● *Cytauxzoon felis*

Rapid onset of fever with lethargy, anorexia, pale mucous membranes, dehydration, icterus and splenomegaly.

Fungal:

● *Blastomyces dermatiditis* (blastomycosis)

Fever, anorexia, depression and lymph-adenopathy occur together with respiratory signs (dyspnea, coughing). Ocular signs are frequent. Signs are more common in dogs than cats.

● *Coccidioides immitis*

Clinical disease is uncommon in cats. Fever, anorexia and depression are common. Skin lesions occur in 50% of cats with nodules progressing to abscesses. Respiratory, musculoskeletal and ocular signs are less common.

- *Cryptococcus neoformans* **(cryptococcosis)** (p 379)**

Low-grade fever, malaise, anorexia and weight loss are typical. Most common form presents with chronic mucopurulent or hemorrhagic nasal discharge, sneezing, stertorous respiration, distortion over bridge of nose (Roman nose) or polyp-like mass in nasal opening.

- *Histoplasma capsulatum* **(histoplasmosis)** (p 371)**

Signs are often non-specific with fever, depression, and weight loss. Dyspnea, lymphadenopathy, pale mucous membranes, gastrointestinal signs or ocular signs may be present.

Non-infectious:

- **Pancreatitis** (p 377)**

Signs are often vague and non-specific with anorexia and depression predominating. Fever is inconsistent and may be accompanied by abdominal pain, vomiting and dehydration.

- **Cholangiohepatitis** (p 378)**

Typically anorexia and depression are present together with icterus or increased liver enzymes. Vomiting may be evident and fever is present in about 1/3 of cats.

- **Non-suppurative meningoencephalitis** (p 379)**

Signs are chronic, of 1–4 weeks duration and include fever in some cats and variable CNS signs, especially seizures and focal or multifocal neurologic signs.

- **Myocarditis/diaphragmitis** (p 380)**

Uniphasic or biphasic fever together with depression and lethargy are typical. Mild generalized lymphadenopathy may be present and in a few cats overt cardiac failure occurred.

- **Immune-mediated disease**

Primary immune-mediated disease, such as systemic lupus erythematosus, is extremely rare in cats. Secondary immune-mediated disease can occur due to primary infection, vaccination or neoplasia. Anorexia, weight loss, fever and signs specific for the disease occur, such as bleeding, pale mucous membranes, skin lesion or lameness.

Toxins/drugs:

- **Drug-induced fever* (p 381)**

Tetracyclines, amphotericin B and other drugs may cause a fever. The severity of fever is out of proportion with the mild clinical signs. There is a history of antibiotic or antifungal therapy.

Trauma:

- **Trauma** (p 380)**

Mild fever associated with pain and inflammation often occurs 10–14 h after injury. There is evidence of external or internal trauma. Sterile surgical trauma causes fever in some cats for 24 hours post-surgery.

INTRODUCTION

MECHANISM?

True fever must be differentiated from hyperthermia, which can be caused by increased muscle activity, increased environmental temperature and stress.

True fever results from **activation of leukocytes** that release factors (pyrogens) such as interleukin-1 and tumor necrosis factor.

- These factors cross the blood–brain barrier and increase the **thermoregulatory set point** in the hypothalamus.

- Leukocytes are activated by a multitude of **infectious agents**, **neoplasia**, **tissue necrosis** and **immune-mediated diseases**.

WHERE?

Fever is defined as systemic elevation of **core body temperature above 39.2˚C (102.5˚F)**.

The most accurate measurement of core body temperature is obtained **rectally**.

Aural temperature is approximately −17.2˚C (0.5˚F) lower than the rectal temperature.

WHAT?

Fever is a general clinical sign that can be associated with many different diseases.

The **most common** disease causing fever in the cat is **percutaneous cellulites or abscess**.

Many **viral and bacterial diseases** cause fever because leukocytes are recruited and activated as part of the general immune response.

Organ inflammation, such as pancreatitis, cholangiohepatitis and myocarditis, can be associated with an elevated temperature even when an infectious agent is not present.

DISEASES CAUSING AN ELEVATED TEMPERATURE

PERCUTANEOUS CELLULITIS/ABSCESS***

Classical signs

- Fever.
- Anorexia (partial or complete).
- Reluctance to move, lethargy and depression.
- Pain, heat or swelling at site of abscess or cellulitis.

Pathogenesis

Percutaneous abscesses and cellulitis are caused by puncture wounds, most typically from cat bites or scratches, but can be from other animal bite wounds, or foreign bodies such as grass awns.

Tissue trauma results in decreased blood flow to the area, and therefore selects for those bacteria which are facultative or obligate anaerobes.

Common bacteria isolated from cat abscesses are **obligate anaerobes** (*Fusobacterium*, anaerobic cocci, *Bacteroides*, *Eubacterium*, *Peptococcus* and *Peptostreptococcus*) **and/or microaerophilic or facultative organisms** (*Pasteurella*, *Corynebacterium*, *Actinomyces* and *Micrococcus*); abscesses commonly contain more than one isolate.

Abscesses resulting from cat bites are often infected with *Pasteurella* spp.; L-forms and *Mycoplasma* spp. are occasionally involved.

Proliferation of injected organism results in infiltration of tissue by neutrophils and other phagocytes and eventual pus production.

The body generally walls off infection, and purulent products build up to form a soft, fluccuant swelling, usually associated with hair loss over the area.

The abscess may **rupture spontaneously**.

Persistent cellulitis can be a consequence of long-standing abscess.

Bone involvement may also occur with long-standing abscesses. Osteomyelitis should be suspected if the abscess heals but repeatedly breaks as a draining tract.

Clinical signs

Owners will report that cats are **indoor/outdoor** or recently escaped up to a week prior to appearance of the clinical signs.

Pyrexia may occur within 12 hours of a fight. Cats may be quite depressed following a fight, even prior to the onset of fever.

Some cats present without systemic signs and only a mild swelling in the fore- or hindlimbs, neck, face or head.

If limbs are involved, the only complaint may be progressive lameness.

Reluctance to move and anorexia may be a consequence of pain, fever or systemic response to infection.

Cellulitis usually precedes an abscess, and if treated appropriately, the abscess may not even form. **Cellulitis** may be the only evidence of a previous abscess.

An abscess may rupture spontaneously, and the owner may notice **foul-smelling, purulent discharge** on the fur.

● Some abscesses resolve on their own with or without rupture, if they have been present long enough.

Regional lymphadenopathy may occur near the affected site.

L forms produce cellulitis 4–5 days after injury. Cellulitis spreads rapidly with the development of multiple fistulae and a febrile response.

● Lameness from septic arthritis is a common sequelae to infection with L forms. Joints are affected by the hematogenous route and may be distant to the initial site. Lower limbs (tarsus and carpus) are most commonly affected. The joints often ulcerate with a grayish mucinous exudate. Infection remains confined to subcutaneous tissues and joints without systemic spread to internal organs.

Diagnosis

History supports access to outdoors or conflict with other cats indoors.

Palpation reveals a tender area or fluctuant swelling, with or without evidence of puncture wounds.

Microscopic examination of a fine-needle aspirate of the abscess **reveals a heterogeneous population of bacteria**, numerous degenerate neutrophils and intracellular bacteria.

A complete blood count will generally show neutrophilia.

L forms are not visible in tissue samples even with special stains, nor do they grow on culture. On electromicroscopy, organisms are visible intracellularly within phagocytes. Diagnosis is often made by response to tetracyclines in a therapeutic trial (doxycycline 10 mg/kg PO, q 24 h). Response is rapid and evident within 48 h.

Non-healing abscesses should have **histopathology and culture of tissue.** Causes include nocardia, fungi, mycobacteria, and tumors. See page 1081, The Cat With Non-Healing Wounds.

Differential diagnoses

In plague-endemic regions, *Yersinia pestis* **(plague) must be considered**, if the swelling is predominately in the neck region and the cat's fever is in the region of 40.5°C (105°F). Cautionary measures such as gloves, masks and isolation of the suspect cat should be taken until diagnosis established. (See below for discussion of *Y. pestis* infections).

Fracture.

Ligament/tendon injury.

Cellulitis.

Neoplasia.

Treatment

Clip area looking for evidence of puncture wounds.

Drainage of the purulent material is the key to treatment. Surgical drainage can be done under sedation or general anesthesia with a #15 blade. Make a 1/4–1/2" incision over the dependent area, or the area most likely to allow for continued drainage.

Flush the wound thoroughly with sterile saline or a saline/betadine mixture.

Explore the wound with a sterile cotton swab or hemostats to assess the extent of dead-space and to look for a possible foreign body.

Leave the wound open to allow drainage of further purulent material. Do not suture incision closed, as this will only allow the abscess to reform. A Penrose drain may be placed for 2–3 days to allow maximum drainage for abscesses that close too early.

Antibiotic therapy for 7–10 days directed against anaerobes: penicillins, cephalosporins, clindamycin and metronidazole are reasonable choices. Most abscesses respond extremely well to drainage and amoxicillin at 10–20 mg/kg PO q 12 hours for 7 days or amoxicillin/clavulonic acid (12.5 mg/kg PO q 12 hours).

L-forms and *Mycoplasma* spp. respond to doxycycline or tetracycline within 48 hours, but not other antibiotics.

If the wound is not healing well, or the cat has had recurrent abscesses, FeLV/FIV testing is recommended to rule out an underlying immunodeficiency. Further considerations are inappropriate antibiotics (consider culture and sensitivity testing) or the presence of an undetected foreign body (consider surgical exploration of the area) or involvement of underlying bone (osteomyelitis).

Prognosis

Prognosis is good unless there is an underlying immuno-deficiency.

Prevention

Restrict the cat to an **indoor environment** only; although less effective, confine cat indoors at least from dusk to dawn.

Neuter male intact animals to decrease territorial behavior.

FeLV and FIV serology should be repeated 2–4 months following bite wounds.

FELINE VIRAL RHINOTRACHEITIS (FVR)*** (FELINE HERPESVIRUS INFECTION (FVH-1))

Classical signs

- Sneezing.
- Conjunctivitis.
- Punctate corneal ulceration.
- Ocular discharge.
- Anterior uveitis.
- Nasal discharge.
- Fever, anorexia and depression.

See main reference on page 7 for details (The Cat With Acute Sneezing or Nasal Discharge).

Clinical signs

Acute onset of sneezing followed by oculonasal discharge.

Discharge progresses from **serous to mucoid to mucopurulent.**

Severe **conjunctivitis** with tearing, photophobia and chemosis.

Hypersalivation may occur as an initial sign before the classic signs of upper respiratory tract appear.

Punctate corneal ulcers that may coalesce to larger ulcers or perforation.

Fever of 1–2 days duration, anorexia and depression.

Retching or coughing may occur.

Cats with anterior uveitis have occasionally have herpes-virus 1 in the aqueous humor.

Diagnosis

Presumptive diagnosis can be made on the basis of history and clinical signs because treatment for feline herpes virus-1 and calicivirus are similar.

Ocular ulcerations and chemosis are more suggestive of **FHV-1.**

Definitive diagnosis is by **direct IFA** of cells obtained from conjunctival or nasal scrapings, or by **viral isolation or polymerase chain reaction assays** from **oropharyngeal or nasal swabs.**

CALICIVIRUS***

Classical signs

- Mild conjunctivitis and ocular discharge.
- Serous to mucoid nasal discharge.
- Stomatitis, oral ulcerations.
- Fever.
- Signs associated with pneumonia.
- Rarely, facial and paw edema, hemorrhage, icterus and rapid death.

See main reference on page 11 for details (The Cat With Acute Sneezing or Nasal Discharge).

Clinical signs

Sudden onset of **serous ocular discharge and mild conjunctivitis**; these signs may begin unilaterally, but often progress bilaterally.

Initial signs are rapidly followed by **sneezing,** which are not paroxysmal and are less prominent than in herpesvirus.

Nasal discharge is primarily serous to mucoid and rarely progresses to purulent.

Oral ulcerations are common, especially on the tongue, and may be associated with drooling or hypersalivation. Ulcers may also occur at the mucocutaneous junction, hard palate and nose.

Fever generally spikes initially after infection prior to onset of signs, and returns with onset of clinical signs.

Viral pneumonia occurs occasionally with certain strains, and may produce significant mortality. Death is often sudden and preceded by **laboured respiration**.

A rare variant strain (FCV-Ari) reported from the United States, produces a high fever, facial and paw edema (50% of cats), ocular and nasal discharge, conjunctivitis and ulcerative stomatitis (50% of cats), hemorrhage from the nose, GIT, etc. (30–40% of cats), icterus (20% of cats) and rapid death. Mortality is high (30–50%).

Diagnosis

Presumptive diagnosis can be made on basis of **history and clinical signs** because treatment for feline herpesvirus-1 and calicivirus are similar.

Oral ulcerations or clinical signs of **pneumonia** are more suggestive of calicivirus.

Definitive diagnosis is by **viral isolation or reverse transcriptase polymerase chain reaction** assays from swabs taken from the **oropharynx,** ideally in the first week of illness.

Demonstration of **increasing serum antibody titers** to feline calicivirus in paired samples is also useful, whereas measurement of a single titer is not useful because many cats have titers from vaccination.

Identification of FCV-Ari is based on the clinical syndrome, pathology and culture of virus from blood, nasal or ocular discharge, spleen or lungs.

HISTOPLASMA CAPSULATUM (HISTOPLASMOSIS)*–***

Classical signs

- Fever.
- Weight loss.
- Anorexia.
- Pale mucous membranes.
- Dyspnea.
- Lymphadenopathy.

See main reference on page 755 for details (The Cat With Signs of Chronic Small Bowel Diarrhea).

Clinical signs

Clinical signs are often non-specific and include fever, anorexia and weight loss.

Dyspnea and harsh lung sounds without coughing is common.

Peripheral and visceral **lymphadenopathies** are frequently present.

Pale mucous membranes, icterus, hepatomegaly or splenomegaly may be evident.

Ocular signs are uncommon, but can occur.

Gastrointestinal signs are uncommon in cats compared to dogs, and include chronic diarrhea, mesenteric lymphadenopathy and anorexia.

Osseous lesions produce soft tissue swelling and lameness.

Diagnosis

Diagnosis is by **demonstration of the organism** in lymph nodes, draining tracts, bone lesions or vitreous humor.

The organism has a **thin capsule** and is **intracellular within macrophages**.

No reliable serologic test available.

FELINE INFECTIOUS PERITONITIS (FIP)*–***

Classical signs

- Fever.
- Weight loss, anorexia.
- Lethargy.
- Abdominal effusion.
- Dyspnea from pleural effusion.
- Ocular and/or neurologic signs.
- Hepatic, intestinal and/or renal signs.

Pathogenesis

Feline coronaviruses (FCoV) are divided into:
- **FIP-inducing strains**, which are **mutated strains** that infect macrophages and can be distributed to many organ systems.
- **Feline enteric coronavirus (FECV)** which are mildly pathogenic strains producing signs limited to the intestinal lumen.

Mutations of FECV that lead to FIP can **occur in the host within about 18 months** of contracting the virus.

The chance of developing FIP decreases the longer the cat has high coronavirus titers.

Immune responses play a large role in the development of this disease:
- If a **cell-mediated response is not mounted** to mutated FCoV, **effusive FIP** generally results, producing abdominal, thoracic, pericardial and/or scrotal effusions.
- A **partial cell-mediated response** to mutated FCoV generally results in non-effusive FIP, and clinical signs are due to formation of **granulomas,** with signs depending on the organ affected.
- A strong cell-mediated response results in clearance of the virus.

Stress may contribute to development of disease, as stress can interfere with the immune response. Multiple-cat households, surgery, illness and pregnancy may be part of the history in a cat with clinical signs of FIP.

Typically, cats have been in **multi-cat environments** (cat breeders or rescue facilities) within the previous year.

Genetic predisposition appears to play a role.

FIP is most common in catteries and multi-cat households.

Clinical signs

There are **two clinical forms of FIP, effusive or wet form and non-effusive or dry form**. Both are characterized by a **fluctuating fever unresponsive to antibiotics, anorexia, lethargy** and weight loss.

Typical age of onset is **6 months to 2 years**, but any age can be affected.

The effusive form may have any of the following signs:
- **Abdominal effusion** that is non-painful but progressive. The amount of effusion varies from volumes causing abdominal enlargement, to amounts only detectable by abdominocentesis. **Fluid is straw-colored and highly viscous**, like egg white.
- **Pleural effusion** resulting in **dyspnea** occurs in 30% of cats with the effusive form. **Pericardial fluid** may be evident on ultrasound. Usually it not associated with clinical signs, but occasionally can produce cardiac tamponade.
- Male cats may present with **scrotal swelling**.

The non-effusive form may have any of the following signs:
- **Ocular signs** result from pyogranulomatous inflammation of the iris and ciliary body. They include bilateral uveitis, perivascular exudates (cuffing), retinal hemorrhage, retinal detachment.
- **Neurologic signs** include **cerebral and cerebellar-vestibular signs** such as seizures, personality changes, nystagmus, head tilt, circling, head tremor and hyperesthesia.
- **Dysfunction of any organ system** may result from **granuloma formation** within the tissue of that organ, e.g., **liver, kidney, spleen, intestines, lungs**, etc., however, organ failure producing clinical signs only rarely occurs, and most dysfunction is only detected on biochemical tests.
- **Granulomatous masses may be palpable** in abdominal viscera especially mesentery, mesenteric lymph nodes and omentum as tender, irregular masses. **Occasionally vomiting or diarrhea** results from extensive lesions on the bowel wall.

Jaundice may occur with either form of the disease.

Diagnosis

Histopathology of affected tissues provides the only definitive antemortem diagnosis. The classic FIP lesion is **pyogranulomatous infiltration around venules**.

The following are **typical abnormalities associated with FIP**. All asterisked items must be present for a high likelihood of FIP; if any one parameter is not present, FIP is unlikely. A negative coronavirus ("FIP") titer suggests FIP is not the cause of the fever, although a few cats with the effusive form of the disease are titer negative.

Lymphopenia ($< 1.5 \times 10^3$ cells/µl).* Occurs in many cats with FIP, and many cats without FIP.

Hyperglobulinemia > 51 g/L [> 5.1 g/dl].* Present in 50% of cats with effusive FIP and 70% with non-effusive FIP.

High coronavirus/FIP titers (>= 1:160).* Present in most cats with FIP and many healthy cats without FIP.

The effusive or wet form of FIP has pleural and/or abdominal effusion with:
- Protein 35 g/L [> 3.5 g/dl].
- Albumin:globulin ratio < 0.8.
- Protein electrophoresis should demonstrate a polyclonal gammopathy with gamma globulins representing > 32%.
- Cell count varies from low to moderate (1500 to more than 25 000 cells/µl) and mainly non-lytic neutrophils, lymphocytes and macrophages.

"FIP titers" reported by laboratories are either **coronavirus titers** or **titers to the 7B protein in coronavirus**. **Neither are specific for the mutated FIP-coronavirus.** Although it had been claimed that 7B protein was specific for FIP strains, subsequent studies have shown that it is not present in some FIP strains, and that non-FIP coronavirus may have an active 7B component. Currently there is no serological test that is specific for FIP-coronavirus.
- **30% of household pet cats and 80–90% of cattery cats carry coronavirus and have positive coronavirus titers.**
- Although a few cats with effusive FIP have a negative coronavirus titer, cats with a negative coronavirus titer are unlikely to have FIP.

Reverse transcriptase, polymerase chain reaction (PCR) is available for detection of viral RNA. Positive results correlate with a diagnosis of FIP when fluid from an effusion is used for analysis. Note that when whole blood is used for analysis, positive results do not correlate to FIP.
- To date, **no nucleoprotein sequences specific for FIP-coronavirus have been identified.** Some non-pathogenic coronaviruses have systemic spread, therefore finding coronavirus nucleoprotein by PCR in the systemic circulation or tissue is not indicative of FIP-coronavirus infection.

Except where the classical effusive fluid is present, **definitive diagnosis of FIP requires organ biopsy** and demonstration of classical histopathological lesions.

Various non-specific abnormalities may be evident on laboratory tests, including increased total white cell count, mild to moderate anemia, and increased concentrations of bilirubin, liver enzymes, BUN, creatinine, fibrinogen, globulin and mild proteinuria.

Disseminated intravascular coagulopathy (DIC) is evident in some cats.

CSF typically has **increased protein (> 2 g/L) and cell counts (>100 cells/µl)** which are predominantly non-lytic neutrophils.

Differential diagnosis

Ocular signs: toxoplasmosis, fungal agents.

Neurologic signs: toxoplasmosis, neoplasia (e.g., lymphoma), trauma, congenital abnormalities in young cats.

Other clinical signs: rule out other diseases associated with the apparent organ dysfunction.

Lymphocytic, plasmocytic cholangiohepatitis occasionally produces a high protein abdominal fluid similar to that of effusive FIP.

Treatment

FIP is a **fatal disease with no known treatments**. The therapies listed below have been used in an attempt to slow progression and/or to improve quality of life.

Glucocorticoids at immunosuppressive doses (prednisolone 4 mg/kg/day).

Cyclophosphamide (200–300 mg/m² q 2–3 weeks or 2.2 mg/kg daily for 4 days each week) or chlorambucil (20 mg/m² q 2–3 weeks).

+/– Broad-spectrum antibiotics to control secondary bacterial infections while the cat is immunosuppressed.

+/– Interferon-alpha (see FeLV/FIV section for recommended dosages).

Prognosis

Prognosis is poor. The mortality is > 95%.

Transmission

Fecal–oral transmission is most likely; transplacental transmission is rare.

Fomites, e.g., **food bowls and litter trays**, may be an important mode of transmission, as some strains of FCoV survive in dried secretions for **several weeks**.

About 1/3 of cats seropositive for coronavirus shed virus for up to 10 months; 40–75% of cats with FIP shed virus.

A seronegative cat introduced into a household where coronavirus is endemic has a **1 in 6 chance of developing FIP**; a seropositive cat under the same conditions has a 1 in 12 chance.

Both young and old animals seem to be most susceptible due to vulnerable immune systems.

Maternal antibodies that protect kittens wane at approximately 5–6 weeks of age.

Prevention

Reduce fecal–oral contamination by providing one litterbox for every 1–2 cats, cleaning litterboxes daily, and placing litterboxes away from feeding areas.

Minimize stress, especially crowding in catteries.

Do not introduce FcoV-positive cats into a multi-cat household.

Wean kittens at 5 weeks and remove from the queen's environment if she is seropositive.

An **intranasal vaccine** is available for use in seronegative cats. However, efficacy has not yet been demonstrated against wild strains.

FELINE LEUKEMIA VIRUS (FELV)*–***

> **Classical signs**
> - Opportunistic infections.
> - Weight loss/cachexia.
> - Chronic fever.
> - Neoplasia.

See main reference on page 540 for details (The Anemic Cat).

Clinical signs

Onset of illnesses occurs over an extended period of time (months to years), although young kittens can become acutely ill.

Chronic, opportunistic infections occur that **do not respond to appropriate antibiotic therapy** and are primarily due to immunosuppression.

Fever may occur in any age cat but is primarily seen **initially in the viremic stage** or later in response to neoplastic, inflammatory or immunosuppressive effects. **Chronic fever** occurs in later stages of disease.

Weight-loss/cachexia.

Non-regenerative anemia.

Thrombocytopenia.

Lymphoma is associated with FeLV-positive cats, especially thymic and multicentric forms.

Diagnosis

History and clinical signs may be suggestive.

Complete blood count showing anemia, thrombocytopenia, leukemias, increased MCV and leukopenia are supportive.

Bone marrow aspirate may show myeloproliferation and arrested erythroid differentiation.

A positive FeLV antigen test (viral core antigen p27) on whole blood using an IFA (can also be done on bone marrow sample) or an ELISA test (also on serum, plasma, saliva, tears). See page 543 for interpretation.

Polymerase chain reaction is available from some laboratories.

MYCOPLASMA HAEMOFELIS AND CANDIDATUS 'M. HAEMOMINUTUM' (HAEMOBARTONELLA FELIS)**

Classical signs

- Pale mucous membranes.
- Depression.
- Anorexia.
- Icterus.
- Splenomegaly.
- Fever.

See main reference on page 530 for details (The Anemic Cat).

Clinical signs

Classical signs are **pale mucous membranes and/or icterus** primarily from **extravascular hemolysis** due to complement binding of infected erythrocytes.

Severe, regenerative hemolytic anemia may ensue.

Anorexia and depression are typical.

Fever occurs in **50% of cats** in the acute phase, and may occur intermittently in chronic infections.

Diagnosis

History and clinical signs are suggestive, especially if an immunosuppressive disorder is present concurrently.

Diagnosis is via **demonstration** of the **organism on the surface of erythrocytes.** Use a marginated blood sample for diagnosis, e.g., ear vein. Multiple blood smears over a number of days may be required as most of the organisms are removed from circulation by the time clinical signs are apparent.

Infected cats may be Coomb's positive.

A **polymerase chain reaction** test is available in some laboratories for diagnosis.

TOXOPLASMA GONDII**

Classical signs

- Fever.
- Anorexia/weight loss.

Classical signs—Cont'd

- Anterior uveitis, retinochoroiditis.
- Seizures, ataxia.
- Dyspnea/polypnea.
- Icterus.
- Abdominal discomfort.
- Small bowel diarrhea.

Pathogenesis

Gastrointestinal signs, primarily abdominal discomfort and small bowel diarrhea, are due most likely to replication of the organism (tachyzoites) in enteroepithelial cells resulting in necrosis.

Clinical signs in the acute, fatal form of **extraintestinal disease** are caused primarily by tissue damage from the rapidly dividing tachyzoites.

Tachyzoites begin to disappear from tissues approximately 3 weeks after infection. The organism may persist in tissues as **tissue cysts containing bradyzoites.**

Chronic disease may be a result of delayed hypersensitivity reactions and tissue reaction to antibody–antigen complex deposition.

Concomitant illness, such as FeLV, FIV and immunosuppression with glucocorticoids, has been reported in some cases.

Clinical signs

Gastrointestinal disease.
- Mild, **self-limiting small bowel diarrhea** may occur in the definitive host (cats), but only after ingestion of tissue cysts, oocysts or sporulated oocysts.
- **Young kittens** are more likely to have gastrointestinal signs, although mild clinical disease has been reported in adult cats as well. All newborn kittens experimentally infected developed severe diarrhea 5–6 days later.

Fatal extraintestinal disease (acute course).
- Fatal extraintestinal disease is most likely to occur in **transplacentally infected kittens**.
- Kittens may be **stillborn** or **exhibit signs that are severe and rapidly progressive** and reflect involvement of the **lungs**, **liver** and **CNS tissues**.

These signs may also be observed in **postnatally infected kittens** and include:
- A **distended abdomen** from an enlarged liver and/or ascites.
- **Icterus** from hepatitis or cholangiohepatitis.
- **Dyspnea** is present in most kittens and cats with signs of acute infection.
- **Neurologic deficits; continuous vocalization; excessive sleeping.**
- **Fever, anorexia, depression** often accompanies the tissue-specific signs.

Non-fatal extraintestinal disease (chronic, intermittent course).
- Cats may have a **moderate fever, lethargy and depression** that waxes and wanes.
- **Hyperesthesia and stiff painful joints or shifting lameness** may be evident, presumably due to an immune-mediated process.
- Unilateral or bilateral **anterior or posterior uveitis** may occur with possible sequelae of lens luxation, glaucoma or retinal detachment.
- **Seizures and ataxia** may be present if CNS tissues are involved.
- Rarely, a **toxoplasma granuloma (tissue cyst)** forms in the **gastrointestinal tract or pancreas** causing chronic vomiting.

Diagnosis

Clinical signs consistent with toxoplasmosis are **suggestive**, especially when other causes of the signs have been ruled out.

IgM titers > 1:64 and **a four-fold increase in IgG:IgM titers** within 2 weeks correlate best with clinical toxoplasmosis. However, some cats do not develop detectable IgM titers, and in other cats, positive IgM titers can persist for months to years after infection.

Elevated ocular and CSF titers relative to serum titers in cats with ocular or neurologic signs, respectively, are very suggestive. Coefficient values > 1.0 are highly suspect and > 8.0 strongly suggest local production of *T. gondii* antibodies.

Response to therapy for toxoplasmosis is a useful indicator of infection.

Definitive diagnosis requires demonstration of the organism in inflamed tissues by histology, immunohistochemistry or polymerase chain reaction assay.

Differential diagnosis

Rule out diseases associated with affected organs, e.g., FIP for neurologic and ocular signs.

Treatment

Clindamycin at 10–12 mg/kg orally q 12 hours for 4 weeks is usually effective.
- Cats should respond within several days of treatment.
- If no response is evident after 3 weeks of antibiotic therapy, reconsider the diagnosis.
- The chronic form may recur even after successful treatment, as drugs tend to suppress replication rather than kill the parasite.

Other systemic drugs with potential efficacy include the trimethoprim sulfas combination, doxycycline, minocycline, azithromycin and clarythromycin.

Cats with **ocular lesions** should also be treated with **corticosteroids**, either topically (e.g. topical 0.5% Prednisolone acetate drops applied q 6–12 h) or systemically to control inflammation and its sequelae (glaucoma, lens luxation).

Prognosis

Gastrointestinal disease has a good prognosis, although it may lead to inflammatory bowel disease in rare cases.

Acute extraintestinal disease has a guarded to poor prognosis.

Chronic extraintestinal disease has a fair to good.

Transmission

Infection in cats can occur via:
- The placenta or milk with tachyzoites.
- Ingestion of meat infected with tissue bradyzoites, e.g., rodents.
- Ingestion of sporulated oocysts in food or water.

***T. gondii* has a zoonotic potential.** Infection of humans can occur via:
- Ingestion of **undercooked meat** containing tissue bradyzoites (most common mode of transmission).
- Ingestion of sporulated oocysts from the environment.

- Transplacentally, if first-time exposure to the organism occurs during pregnancy.

Only cats host the sexual replication that results in oocysts in the feces.
- Oocysts are shed for 1–2 weeks.
- Most seropositive cats do not shed oocysts on repeat exposure.

Oocysts must sporulate to be infectious:
- Sporulation occurs 1–5 days after environmental exposure, thus handling individual cats rarely results in infection of humans.

Transplacental transmission occurs in cats and people after primary exposure.

Prevention

Discourage cats from going outdoors and hunting behavior.

Do not feed cats undercooked meat.

To prevent human infection:
- **Cook meat** at 80°C (176°F) for 15 minutes.
- Use **gloves when gardening** or changing the litterbox, and wash hands well.
- **Change litterboxes daily**. Use litterbox liners or clean with scalding water.

PANCREATITIS**

Classical signs

- Lethargy and anorexia.
- Fever.
- Vomiting.
- Dehydration.
- Tachycardia.
- Hypothermia.
- Abdominal pain.

See main reference on page 272 for details (The Cat With Depression, Anorexia or Dehydration).

Clinical signs

The **classical signs** are **not as well-defined for cats** as for dogs for the following reasons:

- Cats tend to have intermittent bouts of **chronic pancreatitis**.
- Diagnostic tests for pancreatitis are not as reliable in cats.
- There is poor correlation of biochemical parameters with pancreatitis in the cat.

Lethargy and anorexia is variable depending on chronicity.

Vomiting only occurred in **35%** of cases in one study.

Dehydration occurred in **50%** of cases in the same study.

Abdominal pain is quite **variable**.

Fever is variably present, and generally mild. In severe acute pancreatitis it may progress to hypothermia, which is a poor prognostic sign.

Diagnosis

Diagnosis is unreliable based on a biochemistry panel. Lipase may be increased or normal in pancreatitis.
- **Hyperbilirubinemia** and **elevated liver enzymes** may be present.
- **Hypocalcemia** occurs in 40% (total serum calcium) or 60% (plasma ionized calcium concentration) of cats due to soponification of fat. Cats with a plasma ionized calcium concentration < 1.00 mmol/L (< 4.00 mg/dl) have a grave prognosis (77% mortality) and aggressive medical treatment is indicated.

Pancreatic lipase immunoreactivity is probably a **more sensitive diagnostic tool** for confirming pancreatitis in cats than measurement of plasma lipase concentration or trypsin like immunoreactivity. A feline-specific assay must be used.

Abdominal ultrasound to visualize an enlarged pancreas or heterogeneous echogenicity in the area of the pancreas is considered by many to be most sensitive.

Demonstration of higher lipase levels in abdominal fluid compared to those of the serum is suggestive. Diagnostic peritoneal lavage may be necessary to obtain a fluid sample.

CHOLANGIOHEPATITIS**

Classical signs

- Anorexia.
- Vomiting.
- Icterus.
- Dehydration.
- Fever.
- Weight loss.

See main reference on page 427 for details (The Yellow Cat or Cat With Elevated Liver Enzymes).

Clinical signs

Clinical signs may be acute, chronic or intermittent.

Typically, there is **anorexia and depression** together with **icterus** or increased bilirubin and **liver enzymes on a biochemistry panel.**

Vomiting and dehydration may be present.

Fever, especially in the suppurative form occurs in approximately 38% of the cases.

Chronic cholangiohepatitis may lead to **end-stage liver disease** and the cat may present with **ascites and hepatic encephalopathy.**

Multiple causes include bacterial, protozoal (*T. gondii*) and immune-mediated disease.

Diagnosis

Complete blood count may show neutrophilia with a left shift, and mild non-regenerative anemia.

Biochemistry panel shows **hyperbilirubinemia, elevated liver enzyme activities** (ALP, ALT, GGT), +/- **elevated serum bile acids.**

- Signs of late-stage liver disease are occasionally present, such as decreased BUN, glucose and albumin concentrations.

Abdominal ultrasound should be performed to evaluate the gall bladder and bile duct for cholelithiasis, bile sludging and cholecystitis.

Liver aspirates/biopsy allows for differentiation of suppurative from non-suppurative forms of cholangiohepatitis.

Culture and sensitivity of the **liver biopsy** should be performed if suppurative cholangiohepatitis suspected.

Lymphocytic, plasmocytic cholangiohepatitis occasionally produces **a high protein abdominal fluid** similar to that of **effusive FIP**.

FELINE IMMUNODEFICIENCY VIRUS (FIV)**

Classical signs

- Opportunistic infections.
- Gingivitis.
- Weight-loss/cachexia.
- Diarrhea.
- Chronic fever.

See main reference on page 339 for details (The Thin, Inappetent Cat).

Clinical signs

Clinical signs are primarily due to **immunosuppression**, i.e., chronic recurring infections that do not respond to appropriate therapy.

Gingivitis, stomatitis and peridontitis are more common findings in FIV infections than in FeLV, although one study suggests that these signs may be to an effect of age, rather than a consequence of FIV infection.

Fever is chronic and is related to production of tumor necrosis factor and/or IL-1 in infected cats.

Weight loss/cachexia are common in the late stages of FIV, as in human HIV infections.

Diarrhea resembles a panleukopenia-type syndrome that may be due to actual enterocyte infection by the virus or secondary to inflammation.

Cats are often thin and scruffy with an **unkempt haircoat**, and may have miliary dermatitis.

Diagnosis

Diagnosis may be suspected based on history and clinical signs, but requires antibody or antigen tests for confirmation.

Diagnosis of FIV infection is by demonstration of **FIV-specific antibody titers via ELISA, IFA or Western blot**.

Virus isolation and polymerase chain reaction for virus detection is available at some research facilities.

Cats infected with FIV can be co-infected with FeLV.

*CRYPTOCOCCUS NEOFORMANS (CRYPTOCOCCOSIS)***

> ### Classical signs
>
> - Sneezing.
> - Stertorous breathing.
> - Chronic nasal discharge.
> - Facial deformity.
> - Low-grade fever.
> - Regional lymphadenopathy.
> - Neurologic signs: ataxia, seizures, blindness.
> - Skin form: ulcerated lesions.

See main reference on page 25 for details (The Cat With Signs of Chronic Nasal Disease).

Clinical signs

Chronic nasal discharge can be unilateral or bilateral and is generally serosanguineous. Sneezing and stertorous breathing is often present.

Facial deformity may occur due to invasion of the surrounding bone.

Chronic low-grade fever may be present.

Depression, anorexia and weight-loss are signs of disseminated disease.

Neurologic signs occur via hematogenous spread or invasion into the CNS through the cribiform plate but are uncommon. Signs include seizures, blindness, depression and ataxia.

The skin form typically produces nodules which often ulcerate.

Diagnosis

Diagnosis is by **demonstration of narrow-based budding yeast** with a **very thick capsule** from affected tissue or by culture of affected tissue or CSF.

Demonstration of *Cryptococcus* **antigen** in serum, urine or CSF is also diagnostic.

NON-SUPPURATIVE MENINGOENCEPHALITIS**

> ### Classical signs
>
> - Seizures.
> - Focal or multifocal neurologic signs.
> - Fever.
> - Lethargy.
> - Inappetence.

See main reference on page 803 for details (The Cat With Seizures, Circling and/or Changed Behavior).

Clinical signs

Occurs in cats of all ages, with and without outdoor access.

Progressive clinical signs occur over a period of 1–4 weeks.

Recurrent seizures may be the only clinical sign, while other cats exhibit multifocal neurologic abnormalities including:
- Progressive spinal cord signs.
- Vestibular signs.
- Cerebellar signs.
- Cranial nerve signs.

According to one study, non-supportive meningo-encephalitis may be the most common cause of seizures in cats.

Systemic signs, which are not present in all cats, include **fever, anorexia, lethargy, vomiting, diarrhea and lymphadenopathy.**

Viral or immune-mediated etiology is suspected. The condition, however, does not appear to be contagious to other cats.

Diagnosis

CSF tap can be very useful to **rule out other causes of CNS signs**, specifically toxoplasmosis and FIP; CSF analysis reveals a normal or mild protein elevation (typically < 1 g/L) and/or an increased white cell count (< 50 cells/μl).

Complete blood count findings are non-specific and may include leukopenia or leuko-cytosis, eosinophilia and anemia.

MYOCARDITIS/DIAPHRAGMITIS**

> **Classical signs**
>
> - Uniphasic or biphasic fever.
> - Depression.
> - Lethargy.
> - Mild generalized lymphadenopathy.
> - +/– Signs of cardiac failure.

Pathogenesis

Several different **infectious agents have been implicated** in cats:

- Viral, e.g., FIP has been shown to cause cardiac infection.
- *Trypanosoma cruzi*, which causes Chagas' disease in humans.
- *Streptococcus* and *Borrelia* (Lyme's disease) in certain geographic areas.

No single agent has been identified, and the disease **may be multifactorial**.

Clinical signs

Fever is biphasic in 50% of the cats; if biphasic:

- **First fever** occurs approximately 10 days after exposure, lasts 1–3 days and peaks at 39.3–40.7°C (102.7–105.2°F).
- **Second fever** occurs 1–2 weeks after the first fever (at 3–4 weeks post-exposure), lasts 5 days and peaks at 39.9–40.9°C (103.8–105.6°F).

Depression and lethargy lasts 5–10 days.

Appetite is mildly decreased in some cats, but most continue to eat and drink.

Some animals exhibit **mild generalized lymphadenopathy**.

Irritable disposition and **hyperesthesia** may occur, and are most likely due to fever and malaise.

In a few case reports, cats have died from **peracute cardiac failure**, but this outcome is not common.

Diagnosis

Myocarditis/diaphragmitis is a **diagnosis of exclusion**.

Biochemistry and complete blood counts are unremarkable, except for a mild to moderate increase in CK in less than 50% of experimentally infected cats.

Definitive diagnosis can only be made at **necropsy**.

Histopathology shows a neutrophilic infiltrate with a foci of myonecrosis in myocardium and diaphragm.

Differential diagnosis

Any **other causes of fever should be ruled out** including infectious, inflammatory, immune-mediated, drugs, neoplasia and metabolic.

Other causes of cardiac failure that should be ruled out include congenital deformities, hypertrophic cardiomyopathy, restrictive cardiomyopathy and dilatative cardiomyopathy.

Treatment

Supportive therapy is indicated if dehydration or cardiac disease are present.

Broad-spectrum antibiotics are indicated if complete blood count supports an infectious cause.

Prognosis

Fever and depression **resolve spontaneously in the majority of cats**.

Prognosis is poor if peracute cardiac failure is present with systemic signs of fever and depression.

Prevention

Although an infectious agent is suspected, no single etiologic agent has been identified, making recommendations for prevention difficult.

TRAUMA**

> **Classical signs**
>
> - Cardiovascular or respiratory compromise.
> - External signs of injury.

- Pain on palpation.
- Moderate fever approx. 39.2°C–40.0°C (102.5–104.0°F).

See main reference on page 52 for details (The Dyspneic or Tachypneic Cat).

Clinical signs

Cardiovascular compromise may result in **tachycardia, hypovolemia or hypotension.**

Respiratory compromise may produce **dyspnea/tachypnea** due to pneumothorax, hemothorax or pyothorax.

External injuries including abrasions/bruising, degloving injuries, bite wounds and open fractures may be evident.

Internal injuries may result in abdominal pain from organ rupture, bone/joint pain or focal swelling.

Fever from inflammation may occur but often lags behind acute injury by 10–14 hours.

Diagnosis

Diagnosis is based on **clinical signs and history**.

Radiographs of the chest, abdomen and/or limbs may be required to characterize the injury.

Complete blood count and biochemistry panel is indicated to rule out specific organ injury and primary infection.

DRUG-INDUCED FEVER*

Classical signs

- Alert, febrile cat being treated with antibiotics or antifungal agents.

Clinical signs

History of treatment with **antibiotics** or **antifungal agents**.

Fever does not correspond to clinical appearance of animal. Cats are bright, alert and responsive, despite a temperature in the range of 39.4–40°C (103–104°F).

Onset of **fever is idiosyncratic** and variable, but the fever is generally present for the duration of the drug treatment.

Tetracycline is the most common antibiotic cause of drug-induced fever in cats.

Amphotericin B can cause fever by disrupting cell membranes and releasing pyrogens into circulation.

Be aware that other drugs (griseofulvin, chloramphenicol and chemotherapeutic drugs) can cause bone marrow suppression leading to a cat with fever, neutropenia and secondary bacterial infection. These cats are obviously sick, whereas the drug-induced fever animals are bright and alert in comparison.

Diagnosis

Diagnosis is based on history and clinical signs.
- History is of treatment with fever-inducing drugs, especially tetracycline and amphotericin B.
- Clinical signs are inappropriate, that is, the cat appears bright and alert although febrile.

Temperature normalizes after drug is discontinued.

CHLAMYDOPHILA FELIS*

Classical signs

- Sneezing.
- Conjunctivitis and ocular discharge.
- Nasal discharge.
- Fever.

See main reference on page 13 for details (The Cat With Acute Sneezing or Nasal Discharge).

Clinical signs

Marked conjunctivitis is the predominant sign, which often starts unilaterally, but usually progresses to both eyes.

Classic triad of upper respiratory infection signs including oculonasal discharge and sneezing.

Serous ocular discharge accompanied by blepharospasm, chemosis and conjunctival hyperemia are initial signs. Discharge becomes mucopurulent over the course of the disease.

Mild to moderate **fever can be seen in the acute phase**.

Pneumonia is rarely associated with this infection.

Diagnosis

History and clinical signs are highly suggestive.

Cytology of conjunctival scrapings reveal dark blue inclusion bodies (Giemsa stain).

Immunofluorescent antibody staining or polymerase chain reaction assay to demonstrate the organism in conjunctival scrapings is available from some laboratories.

PANLEUKOPENIA*

Classical signs

- Acute onset of depression.
- Acute onset of vomiting.
- Diarrhea usually 1–2 days later.
- Dehydration.
- Fever or hypothermia.
- In utero infection can result in cerebellar signs.

See main reference on page 722 for details (The Cat With Signs of Acute Small Bowel Diarrhea).

Clinical signs

Rapid onset of depression, anorexia, and vomiting especially in peracute and acute disease. Fetid diarrhea (may be hemorrhagic) typically follows 1–2 days after initial onset of signs.

Severe dehydration and electrolyte abnormalities.

Initial fever followed by hypothermia as the disease progresses.

High mortality rate when signs are severe.

Diagnosis

The disease should be suspected in cats less than one year of age with no history of vaccination and a rapid clinical course.

Panleukopenia evident on hematology.

Parvoviral antigen can be detected in feces using the canine parvoviral antigen tests or electron microscopy.

Histopathologic changes include denuded intestinal crypts and blunted villi (often a post-mortem diagnosis).

FRANCISELLA TULARENSIS (TULAREMIA)*

Classical signs

- Fever.
- Anorexia.
- Lethargy.
- Lymphadenopathy.
- Oral ulcers.
- Icterus.

Pathogenesis

Francisella tularensis is a Gram-negative coccobacillus. Clinical signs are associated with **Gram-negative endotoxins** and **bacteremia**.

There are two main strains of the organism, both of which have been isolated from cats.

Type A strain is:
- Associated with **tick–rabbit cycle**.
- Found only in North America.
- Highly virulent for laboratory rabbits.
- Associated with more severe disease in humans.

Type B strain is:
- Associated with a more complex cycle involving rodents, ticks, mosquitoes, mud and water.
- Found throughout the northern hemisphere.
- Avirulent for laboratory rabbits.

Clinical signs

History of **contact with rabbits**, especially if the cat is a hunter.

Any age of cat can be infected, but younger cats are more susceptible to developing septicemia.

The spectrum of **illness varies** from severely affected to asymptomatic.

Fever is generally > 40°C (104°F).

Marked depression, anorexia and lethargy, with or without vomiting are typical.

On physical examination, **peripheral lymphadenopathy, icterus and palpable splenomegaly and hepatomegaly** are reported.

Oral, lingual or pharyngeal ulcers may be present.

Diagnosis

Clinical signs together with a history of exposure to wild rabbits is highly suggestive.

Hematologic and serum biochemical abnormalities may include **panleukopenia**, with **severe toxic changes in neutrophils**, high band neutrophil count, thrombocyto-penia and hyperbilirubinemia.

Definitive diagnosis is via identification of the bacterial agent by **IFA or bacterial culture**, but should only be performed in a qualified laboratory.
- Samples can be obtained from affected **lymph nodes, bone marrow, urine or blood**.

Serum antibody titers > 1:120 or a four-fold increase in serum antibodies in samples collected during acute and convalescent phases (10–14 days) are considered diagnostic.

Differential diagnosis

FIP, FIV, panleukopenia.

Plague (*Yersinia pestis*).

Toxoplasmosis.

Cytauxzoon felis.

Multicentric lymphoma.

Treatment

Antimicrobial efficacy studies have not been done in the cat, therefore therapy is derived from case reports and/or human therapy regimens.

Enrofloxacin (5 mg/kg q 12 hours IV or PO).

Tetracycline and chloramphenicol may be effective, but because they are bacteriostatic for *F. tularensis*, relapses can occur.

In humans, the drugs of choice are streptomycin and gentamycin.

Prognosis

Prognosis is poor to fair as mortality rate varies across case reports.

Transmission

F. tularensis has a **serious zoonotic potential** if there is **contact with infected animal tissue**.

Bites from infected ticks, deer flies or mosquitoes are the most common method of transmission.

Infection can also occur via ingestion of infected meat.

Transmission may occur via a **bite or scratch from an infected mammal**.
- This is the most common method of transmission to humans in cat-associated cases.
- The infected cat may have no obvious signs of illness, but have a history of hunting wild animals, especially rabbits.

Inhalation of aerosolized organisms may also transmit the disease. **Care should be taken by veterinary and laboratory personnel handling suspected animals** or samples being prepared for IFA or culture.

Prevention

Discourage hunting behavior in cats.

Ectoparasite control, especially tick control.

YERSINIA PESTIS (FELINE PLAGUE)*

Classical signs

- Acute onset of signs.
- Moderate to high fever (39.4–41.2°C; 103–106°F).
- Submandibular lymphadenopathy.
- Depression.
- Anorexia.

Pathogenesis

Onset of **illness occurs 24–72 hours after exposure** to the organism.

Transmission to cats is either **via ingestion** of **infected rodents** or a **fleabite** from infected fleas.

Rapid multiplication of organism causes tissue damage and necrosis. The host immune response contributes to pathology.

Three forms of the plague exist: **bubonic (local infection), bacteremic/septicemic and pneumonic**.

Bacteremia occurs in many cases, resulting in the **septicemic** or **pneumonic form** of plague.

Endemic regions of the world include the western USA, South America, Africa, Asia, eastern Europe.

Clinical signs

History of hunting rodents, especially in known endemic areas.

Current **flea infestation** is evident.

Acute onset of fever, anorexia, depression over a period of 2–6 days. The clinical course may last 6–20 days.

Submandibular or cervical swelling associated with lymph nodes (can be unilateral or bilateral). The inflamed, swollen lymph node is referred to as a **bubo**.

Subcutaneous abscessation may occur and appear similar to a cat bite abscess.

In the **pneumonic form** (~10% of cases), upper and lower respiratory signs may be present, including **sneezing, nasal discharge, coughing**, dyspnea/tachypnea.

Diagnosis

Initially, **microscopic examination of a lymph node aspirate**, especially a markedly swollen lymph node (bubo) should reveal a homogeneous population **of bipolar-staining coccobacilli**.
- Blood should be examined in cats with the bacteremic/septicemic form.

Fluorescent antibody testing of sample provides a definitive diagnosis.

Culture of organism should be performed by a qualified laboratory only.

A **four-fold rise in antibody titers** (taken 10–14 days apart) is suggestive of plague. These results must be

interpreted carefully, as high titers can persist for up to one year after infection.

Chest radiographs may reveal patchy, nodular lesions if the pneumonic form is present.

Be aware that the **risk of exposing other staff members to the disease** should be weighed against the benefit of the diagnostic test.

Differential diagnosis

Reactive lymph nodes from a percutaneous abscess or tooth-root abscess.
- Aspirates of cat bite abscesses contain a mixed bacterial population compared to *Y. pestis*, which is homogeneous.

Neoplasia, although it is less common in the US for cats with lymphoma to have peripheral lymphadenopathy.

Respiratory signs may be due to other upper respiratory infections (**calicivirus, herpesvirus,** *Chlamydophila*) or lower respiratory disease (parenchymal lung disease, pleural disease).

Other diseases which cause high fever (**tularemia, toxoplasmosis, FIP**, etc.).

Treatment

Absolute caution must be practiced in all suspect plague cases. Cautionary measures include gloves, mask, isolation of animal and limited exposure to other staff members.

Doxycycline/tetracycline: (1) Doxycycline at 5 mg/kg q 12 hours PO for 14–21 days or (2) tetracycline 25 mg/kg q 8 hours PO.
- Begin treatment immediately after samples for diagnosis have been collected.
- Doxycycline is preferred as tetracycline has been associated with relapse.

Consider aminoglycosides or enrofloxacin (5 mg/kg IM q 8 hours) **for the first 3 days** to avoid placing hands into the cat's mouth (see Transmission section below).

Prognosis

Prognosis for **bubonic plague** is fair to good.

Prognosis for the **pneumonic form** is guarded to fair.

Prognosis for **septicemic form** is guarded.

Persistent fever > 40°C (104°F) despite treatment is associated with a poor prognosis.

Transmission

Y. pestis **has a serious zoonotic potential**, and great care should be taken in suspect cats to prevent transmission to humans and other cats.

- Infected cats are no longer a zoonotic risk after 3 days of antibiotic therapy.

Transmission occurs via **rodent flea bites or ingestion of infected animals**.

Infection can also occur via **inhalation of aerosolized organism**, either from **aspirates** of infected tissue or **nasal discharge/sneezing** of cats with pneumonic form.

Prevention

Confine cats indoors in endemic areas.

Discourage hunting behavior especially during the peak flea season (April to October).

Provide effective flea control to prevent flea bites.

EHRLICHIA SPP. AND ANAPLASMA PHAGOCYTOPHILUM*

Classical signs

- Anorexia and weight loss.
- Fever.
- Lymphadenopathy.
- Lameness.
- Non-specific hyperesthesia.

See main reference on page 547 for details (The Anemic Cat).

Clinical signs

This disease is **uncommonly reported in cats** and is difficult to diagnose because of its vague and variable clinical signs.

Age range of cats with documented disease was **2–10 years of age,** with no breed or sex predilection reported.

Infection has a variable effect on appetite, from **mild inappetence to anorexia** and mild to moderate weight loss.

Chronic intermittent fever in the moderate range is common.

Lymphadenopathy was reported in three of 23 cats.

Hyperesthesia, **joint pain** or irritable disposition is common.

Complete blood counts may show a **non-regenerative anemia** with a leukopenia or a leukocytosis; **thrombocytopenia** is present in about **25%** of the cats.

Biochemistry abnormalities are uncommon, except for **hyperglobulinemia** in about **33%** of documented cases.

Diagnosis

A complete blood count and biochemistry panel consistent with chronic *Ehrlichia* spp. infection is suggestive.

Diagnosis is by demonstrating *E. canis* and/or *Anaplasma phagocytophilum* serum **antibody titers** or a positive IFA test.

Demonstration of **morulae in mononuclear cells, neutrophils** or eosinophils (rare) is diagnostic.

PCR assays can be positive.

NEOPLASIA

Classical signs

- Anorexia, lethargy, weight loss.
- ± Fever.
- Signs depend on tumor type and organ system involved.

Clinical signs

Anorexia, lethargy and weight loss.

Poorly groomed coat.

Some cats have a fever associated with neoplasia, which is generally a secondary neoplastic syndrome. **Tumors which destroy the bone marrow** and result in neutro-penia are classically associated with fever. Fever may occur with other tumors via other mechanisms, including antibody stimulation from tumor antigens, and tissue necrosis which activates leukocytes to release pyrogenic factors.

Signs are specific to the organ system involved.

Lymphoma (mediastinal, GI, renal), **mammary adenocarcinoma, squamous cell carcinoma** (nasal, oral) and **mast cell tumor** are the most common tumors in cats.

Diagnosis

Hematology, biochemistry panel, radiology, ultrasound and/or bone marrow aspirates may be necessary to **provide evidence that a tumor is present**, especially if it involves the hematopoietic system (leukemia) or is located internally (splenic mast cell tumor).

Identification of the tumor type is via fine-needle aspirates and/or biopsies.

Differential diagnosis

Organ dysfunction due to infectious or degenerative disease process.

FeLV/FIV or other immunosuppressive illness.

Benign masses (granulomas, abscesses, reactive lymph nodes, benign tumors).

Treatment

Treatment involves **surgical excision of identifiable masses** +/– regional lymph nodes, especially for mammary adenocarcinoma, nasal squamous cell carcinoma, splenic mast cell tumor, etc.

Chemotherapy may be effective and needs to be based on tumor type, e.g., COP (cyclophosphamide, vincristine, prednisolone) protocol in lymphoma cases.

Radiation therapy is used for local disease only, and response to radiation therapy is tumor dependent (e.g., squamous cell carcinoma).

- Radiation therapy is most effective after surgical debulking of the primary mass. The effectiveness of radiation therapy may be enhanced with concurrent chemotherapy.

SALMONELLA SPP. (SONGBIRD FEVER)

Classical signs

- Vomiting/diarrhea.
- Fever (40.0–40.6°C [104.0–105.0°F]).
- Depression.
- Anorexia.

See main reference on page 719 for details (The Cat With Signs of Acute Small Bowel Diarrhea).

Clinical signs

Acute onset of fever and malaise are initial clinical signs.

Vomiting, diarrhea and abdominal pain may occur, however, approximately 50% do not have gastrointestinal signs.

Dehydration.

Shock may occur if **septicemia/bacteremia** develops.

Mortality rate approaches 10% and may be higher if the cat is concurrently immunosuppressed.

Diagnosis

Typically, the cat is an **outdoor cat with a history of hunting behavior**, especially of birds.

Complete blood count and biochemistry panel supports infectious diarrhea or septicemia, e.g., neutropenia with a left shift, bacterial rods in blood leukocytes if overwhelming sepsis present, hypoglycemia, hypoproteinemia, pre-renal azotemia.

Blood cultures provide the **best definitive diagnosis if positive**. Three separate samples over a 4–6 hour period should be taken during febrile episodes using aseptic techniques.

Fecal cultures may isolate *Salmonella* organisms, but because **many animals are subclinical carriers**, positive culture does not prove that the organism is the cause of the clinical signs.

COCCIDIODES IMMITIS

Classical signs

- Skin lesions.
- Respiratory signs.
- Ocular lesions.
- Fever, anorexia, depression.

Pathogenesis

The geographical distribution includes **south-west USA**, **Central America** and **South America** in areas that have **sandy soil with low rainfall** and high temperatures.

Soil is the **reservoir for infection,** and the highest frequency of cases occur when the soil is dry and dusty, and organisms are disseminated in the wind.

Most humans and animals in endemic areas become infected, but the **majority of infections are subclinical** or cause only mild, transient clinical signs.

Cats are more resistant to infection and signs are less common than in dogs.

Infection is contracted via inhalation, and only a few organisms are required to produce signs, which occur after 1–3 weeks.

Initial infection is confined to the respiratory tract, but **dissemination may occur** resulting in chronic disease over months or years with signs referable to bones, eyes, central nervous system and abdominal organs.

Localized infection following a penetrating skin wound appears to be rare.

Clinical signs

Cats appear to be resistant to clinical disease.

Skin lesions are the most frequent types of infection in cats and were reported in 56% of cats in one study.
- Lesions begin as small bumps and progress to abscesses, ulcers or draining tracts.
- In cats, underlying bone involvement is uncommon.

Systemic signs such as **fever, anorexia and depression** are commonly reported (44% of cats) and can be seen with skin lesions.

Respiratory signs such as coughing and wheezing are less common in cats and occur in approximately 25% of cases.

Musculoskeletal signs such as lameness, with or without painful bone swelling, were reported in 19% of cats.

Ocular lesions are seen infrequently and include chorioretinitis and anterior uveitis. **Ocular or CNS signs** were reported in 19% of cats.

Most cats have clinical **signs for less than 4 weeks prior to diagnosis.**

Diagnosis

Hyperproteinemia is present in approximately 50% of cats.

Definitive diagnosis is by identification of the organism via biopsy of lesions.

Antibody detection is available using latex agglutination (IgM), AGID (IgM) or ELISA (IgM or IgG).

Tube precipitin (TP) for IgM and complement fixation (CP) for IgG were previously thought to be less reliable in cats, but have been subsequently demonstrated to detect feline infections.

Treatment

Itraconazole (10 mg/kg PO if possible, q 24 h or 5 mg/kg q 12 h) is the treatment of choice. Treatment is required for **4–6 months** and must be continued for at least 2 months after all signs have resolved.
- Some cats develop anorexia, and less commonly vomiting or diarrhea. Stop the drug for a few days until the cat is eating, and then restart at 1/2 the dose for 7–10 days, before increasing back to the full dose, which is usually then tolerated.

Amphoteracin B is also effective (0.25 mg/kg in 30 ml dextrose 5% IV over 15 minutes q 48 h or given subcutaneously) – see page 26, for Cyptococcosis in The Cat With Signs of Chronic Nasal Disease. Continue amphotericin B therapy until a cumulative dose of 4 mg/kg is given or until BUN > 17.9 mmol/L (50 mg/dl). Amphotericin has the disadvantage of requiring frequent parenteral or subcutaneous administration and causes significant nephrotoxicity.

- Because of its quick onset of action, **amphoteracin B in combination with itraconazole is useful in cats with severe pulmonary signs** that are rapidly deteriorating. If the cat survives, after a few weeks treatment can be continued with itraconazole alone.
- **Lipid-complexed amphoteracin** formulations allow **higher dosages with less toxicity**, and should be used in cats with severe pulmonary signs, although the cost is higher. Dose at 2–3 mg/kg IV 3 days per week for a total of 9–12 treatments (cumulative dose of 24–27 mg). Dilute to a concentration of 1 mg/ml in dextrose 5% and infuse over 1–2 hours.

If the **titer has decreased four-fold** and there is a similar **improvement in physical and radiographic signs**, treatment can be stopped after 4–6 months. Antibodies may persist for long periods and obtaining a zero titer is not a useful treatment goal.

BLASTOMYCES DERMATIDITIS (BLASTOMYCOSIS)

Classical signs

- Fever.
- Respiratory signs.
- Ocular signs.
- Lymphadenopathy.

Pathogenesis

The geographical distribution includes **North America**, **Central America** and **Africa**.

Soil is believed to be the **reservoir for infection**, and living near a lake or river increases the risk of infection in dogs.

Signs are more common in dogs than in the cats.

Disseminated disease is primarily contracted via **inhalation**.

Clinical signs

Respiratory signs include coughing, dyspnea and harsh lung sounds.

Ocular disease, such as uveitis, glaucoma and retinal detachment, is a frequent finding.

Fever, anorexia, depression, weight loss and lymphadenopathy are systemic signs associated with disseminated disease.

Draining skin lesions may occur and are usually a manifestation of systemic disease rather than local disease.

Neurological signs are associated with CNS involvement of the brain or spine and include circling, disorientation, anisocoria, paresis, decreased conscious proprioception, or upper motor neuron signs, hyperesthesia and extensor rigidity.

Diagnosis

Definitive diagnosis is by demonstration of an **extracellular, broad-based budding yeast** in aspirates or biopsies from lymph nodes, draining tracts, bone lesions or vitreous humor.

An **antibody detection** test is available, but may be negative.

Treatment

Itraconazole (10 mg/kg PO if possible, q 24 h or 5 mg/kg q 12 h) is the treatment of choice. Treatment is required for **4–6 months** and must be continued for at least 2 months after all signs have resolved.

- Some cats develop anorexia, and less commonly vomiting or diarrhea. Stop the drug for a few days until the cat is eating, and then restart at 1/2 the dose for 7–10 days, before increasing back to the full dose, which is usually then tolerated.

Amphoteracin B is also effective (0.25 mg/kg in 30 ml dextrose 5% IV over 15 minutes q 48 h or given subcutaneously) – see page 26, for Cyptococcosis in The Cat With Signs of Chronic Nasal Disease. Continue amphotericin B therapy until a cumulative dose of 4 mg/kg is given or until BUN > 17.9 mmol/L (50 mg/dl). Amphotericin has the disadvantages of requiring frequent parenteral or subcutaneous administration and causing significant nephrotoxicity.

- Because of its quick onset of action, **Amphoteracin B in combination with itraconazole is useful in cats with severe pulmonary signs** that are rapidly deteriorating. If the cat survives, after a few weeks treatment can be continued with itraconazole alone.
- **Lipid-complexed amphoteracin** formulations allow **higher dosages with less toxicity**, and should be

used in cats with severe pulmonary signs, although the cost is higher. Dose at 2–3 mg/kg IV 3 days per week for a total of 9–12 treatments (cumulative dose of 24–27 mg). Dilute to a concentration of 1 mg/ml in dextrose 5% and infuse over 1–2 hours.

CYTAUXZOON FELIS

Classical signs

- Fever.
- Anorexia.
- Dyspnea.
- Pale mucous membranes.
- Icterus.
- Collapse.

See main reference on page 534 for details (The Anemic Cat).

Clinical signs

Primarily found in the south-central and southeast United States. The North American **bobcat** is the natural host.

There is usually a history of **exposure to ticks** in the previous 5–20 days (incubation period is 5–20 days).

The clinical course of disease is approximately 1 week and **often ends in death**.

Clinical signs are the result of an overwhelming **hemolytic crisis**.

Rapid onset of fever, dyspnea, anorexia, pale mucous membranes, icterus and dark-colored urine are typical.

Collapse and **death occur 2–3 days after the fever peak**. Hypothermia occurs in the terminal stages.

There appear to be non-pathogenic strains as well.

Diagnosis

A **complete blood count** reveals **regenerative anemia**, hemoglobinemia and neutrophilia or neutropenia.

The biochemistry panel commonly has **hyperbilirubinemia**.

Urinalysis may show evidence of **hemoglobin and bilirubin**.

Demonstration of the **organism in erythrocytes (merozoite stage)** is possible only **relatively late in the disease**, approximately 1–3 days before death. Parasitemic cats usually have only 1–2% of RBCs affected, and up to 50% of cats have parasitemias that are very low or undetectable.

Demonstration of the organism in macrophages from **bone marrow, spleen, liver or lymph node aspirates** may be possible even when organisms are not evident in blood.

Serum antibody levels and **direct FA test** for detection of tissue phase are available through some labs.

HYPERTHYROIDISM

Classical signs

- Weight loss.
- Polyphagia.
- Polyuria/polydipsia.
- Behavioral changes.
- Unkempt appearance.
- Mild elevations in temperature.

See main reference on page 304 for details (The Cat With Weight Loss and a Good Appetite).

Clinical signs

Weight loss in spite of normal to increased appetite.

Polyuria/polydipsia.

Behavioral changes which often include hyperactivity and aggression.

Unkempt, rough hair coat and sometimes overgrown nails.

Tachycardia accompanied by a "gallop" rhythm and/or a systolic murmur.

Mild fever which may be intermittent in nature and reflect the increased metabolic rate in this disease. These cats are easily stressed and may present dyspneic and tachycardic with a mildly elevated temperature, usually not greater than 39.4°C (103.0°F).

Enlarged thyroid glands are often evident on palpation of the neck.

Diagnosis

Diagnosis is based on clinical signs and history and confirmed by demonstrating increased thyroid hormone concentrations (**total T4, free T4**).

Thyroid glands can be palpated in approximately 80% of cats with hyperthyroidism, and are unilaterally or bilaterally enlarged.
- Enlarged thyroid glands may not be palpable if the abnormal thyroid tissue is within the thoracic inlet.

Complete blood count and a biochemistry panel are required to rule out diseases such as diabetes mellitus, renal disease, etc.

A TRH stimulation test may be necessary when clinical signs are highly suggestive and total and free T4 are in the upper region of the reference range for normal cats.

Thyroid radionuclide uptake and imaging with pertechnetate (^{99m}Tc) is also available at some institutions.

Response to therapy with anti-rickettsial drugs (tetracycline or doxycycline) is highly suggestive.

BARTONELLA HENSELLA (CAT-SCRATCH FEVER)

Classical signs

- Subclinical or mild fever and occasional ocular signs.

Pathogenesis

Bartonella henselae is an intracellular bacterium within erythrocytes.

Bacteremia is present in many healthy cats in the population, and cats are reservoirs for infection.

B. henselae is an important pathogen because of its **zoonotic potential in immunocompromised humans**.
- **Humans** may develop **fever, malaise, lymphadenopathy and skin eruptions following cat scratches or bites**.
- *B. henselae* causes bacillary angiomatosis, bacillary peliosis and encephalitis in human AIDS patients.

Clinical signs

Naturally infected cats usually only develop **subclinical infection**.

Mild, **self-limiting fever** lasting 48–72 hours has been documented in some experimentally infected cats.

Anterior uveitis and fever were documented in naturally exposed cats.

Lymphadenopathy.

Stomatitis and gingivitis have been proposed as clinical manifestations.

Atypical seizures occur in some cats.

Diagnosis

Antibody titers are prevalent in healthy cats, but there is a **poor correlation with blood culture and PCR assay results**.

Intermittent bacteremia may occur for longer than one year following infection, with 25–41% of healthy cats bacteremic for up to 22 months.

The organism is present within erythrocytes, therefore, **hemolyzing red blood cells** increases the sensitivity of the culture.

Differential diagnosis

Other causes of mild transient fever need to be considered, such as mild cellulitis following a cat fight.

Other infectious causes of anterior uveitis need to be ruled out, such as toxoplasmosis, fungal diseases, FeLV, FIV, Cuterebra or dirofilaria.

Treatment

Antimicrobial efficacy has not been clearly demonstrated.

Clinical signs of disease have resolved when the cats are administered **doxycycline** at 25–50 mg PO q 12 h for 28 days.

Azithromycin is used in humans and is a safe alternative in cats when administered at 10 mg/kg PO q 24 h for 28 days

Fluoroquinolones also may be effective.

While clinical signs resolve, bacteremia is usually only temporarily suppressed.

Prognosis

B. henselae has very low pathogenicity in cats.

Once cleared of infection, cats are resistant to re-infection by innoculation, but are still susceptible if transmitted via blood transfusion.

Transmission

Transmission is via **arthropod vectors**. In endemic areas, cats infested with **fleas and/or ear mites** are more likely to be seropositive.

The organism survives in flea feces for at least 9 days.

Because of the frequency of bacteremia in healthy cats, blood transfusions are a likely route of infection.

IMMUNE-MEDIATED DISEASE

Classical signs

- Fever.
- Anemia or thrombocytopenia.
- Cutaneous lesions.
- Polyarthritis.

Clinical signs

Primary immune-mediated disease is **extremely rare in cats.**

Stimulation from primary infectious disease antigens is the most common cause of immune-mediated disease in cats, and is most often associated with **hemobartonella** (mycoplasma) and **calicivirus.**

Systemic lupus erythematosus is rare in cats. A multitude of signs may occur including fever, weight loss and cutaneous lesions.

Immune-mediated hemolytic anemia is most commonly associated with hemobartonellosis. Signs include anemia, icterus, fever and anorexia. Cats with immunosuppressive disorders such as FeLV may be more susceptible.

Immune-mediated thrombocytopenia is rarely reported in cats. FeLV-positive cats, however, may have thrombocytopenia that is thought to be the result of an immune-mediated response.

Immune-mediated polyarthritis is uncommon in cats, but has been documented in kittens and adult cats with post-calicivirus vaccination.

RECOMMENDED READING

Dobbinson SS, Tannock GW. A bacteriologic investigation of subcutaneous abscesses in cats. NZ Vet J 1985; 33: 27–29.

Eidson M, Thilsted JP, Rollag OJ. Clinical, clinicopathologic, and pathologic features of plague in cats: 119 cases (1977–1988). JAVMA 1991; 199: 1191–1197.

Greene CE. Bacterial diseases; fungal diseases; and protozoal diseases. In: Greene CE (ed) Infectious Diseases of the Dog and Cat. 2nd edn. Philadelphia, WB Saunders Co., 1998, pp 179–509.

Lappin MR. Feline toxoplasmosis: interpretation of diagnostic test results. Sem Vet Med Surg Sm An 1996; 11: 154–160.

Lappin MR, Jensen W, Kordick DL, Karem K, Breitschwerdt EB. *Bartonella* spp. antibodies and DNA in aqueous humor of cats. Fel Med Surg 2000; 2: 61–68.

Lindsay DS, Blagburn BL, Dubey JP. Feline toxoplasmosis and the importance of the *Toxoplasma gondii* oocyst. Compendium 1997; 19: 448–461.

McReynolds C, Macy D. Feline infectious peritonitis. Part I. Etiology and diagnosis. Compendium 1997; 19: 1007–1016.

McReynolds C, Macy D. Feline infectious peritonitis. Part II. Treatment and prevention. Compendium 1997; 19: 1111–1116.

Neer TM, Breitschwerdt EB, Greene RT, Lappin MR. Consensus statement of ehrlichial disease of small animals from the infectious disease study group of the ACVIM. J Vet Int Med 2002; 16: 309–315.

Pedersen NC. Feline infectious myocarditis/diaphragmitis. In: August JR (ed) Consultations in Feline Internal Medicine. Philadelphia, WB Saunders Co., 1997, pp 31–33.

Quesnel AD, Parent JM. Diagnostic approach and medical treatment of seizure disorders. In: August JR (ed) Consultations in Feline Internal Medicine. Philadelphia, WB Saunders Co., 1997, p 393.

Sparks AH. An appraisal of the value of laboratory tests in the diagnosis of feline infectious peritonitis. J AAHA 1994; 30: 345–349.

Woods JP, et al. Tularemia in two cats. JAVMA 1998; 212: 81–83.

20. The cat with enlarged lymph nodes

Anthony Abrams-Ogg

> **KEY SIGNS**
>
> - Hyperplasia, neoplasia, lymphadenitis most common.
> - Edema, vascularization, infarction less common.
> - Biopsy and culture lymph node.

MECHANISM?

- Reactive lymphoid **hyperplasia, neoplasia or lymphadenitis** are the most common causes of lymphadenopathy.

WHERE?

- Peripheral (superficial) lymph nodes – enlargement may be confined to a solitary/local node, or be regional or generalized.
  There may be accompanying internal (deep) lymphadenopathy.

WHAT?

- The most common causes of **generalized lymphadenopathy** are generalized skin diseases, retroviral infections and lymphoma. The most common causes of **local and regional lymphadenopathy** are bacterial and fungal infections in the area drained by the node(s). All causes may result in mild to marked lymphadenopathy.

QUICK REFERENCE SUMMARY

Diseases causing enlarged lymph nodes

MECHANICAL

- **Obstructive edema* (p 411)**

Local or regional lymphadenopathy occurs due to nodal edema and/or hyperplasia, secondary to obstructive edema from a tumor or other mass involving the head, neck or a limb.

NEOPLASTIC

- **Nodal lymphoma* (p 403)**

Regional (head and neck) or generalized (multicentric) lymphadenopathy occurs with predominance of lymphoblasts on biopsy. Average age of cats with multicentric lymphoma is 4 years. Age

continued

393

continued

of most cats with Hodgkin's-like lymphoma is > 6 years. Cats may be presented for nodal enlargement without concurrent signs, with non-specific signs of illness (lethargy, inappetence and weight loss), and with specific signs due to internal organ involvement (e.g. icterus with hepatic involvement).

● **Metastatic neoplastic lymphadenopathy: mast cell tumor, other tumors (carcinomas, sarcomas, plasma cell tumors, myeloid leukemias, malignant histiocytosis, melanoma)* (p 409)**
Local to generalized lymphadenopathy occurs with malignant cells and hyperplasia found on biopsy. Most metastatic neoplasia occurs in older cats. Cats usually have localizing signs of the primary tumor or non-specific signs of illness.

NUTRITIONAL

● Steatitis (p 412)
Regional to generalized lymphadenopathy results from hyperplasia. Other clinical signs include fever, anorexia, depression, reluctance to move, pain on handling, ascites and firm subcutaneous and abdominal fat.

IDIOPATHIC

● Plexiform vascularization of lymph nodes (p 414)
Solitary or regional lymphadenopathy in neck or inguinal area occur due to capillary vasoproliferation. Tracheal compression may occur causing dyspnea. No other signs are present.

INFLAMMATION

● **Parasitic, immunologic and miscellaneous skin disorders** (p 400)**
Regional or generalized lymphadenopathy results from hyperplasia. Signs of skin disease are present, such as erythema, pruritus, alopecia, excoriations, scales, crusts, papules, nodules, plaques, vesicles, pustules, erosions and ulcers.

● Idiopathic atypical hyperplasia (p 412)
Generalized lymphadenopathy occurs due to atypical hyperplasia. Cats are ~ 4 years of age. Cats are usually presented for nodal enlargement without other signs, but variable non-specific and specific signs may be present.

● Non-cutaneous immunologic/inflammatory disorders (p 416)
Regional or generalized lymphadenopathy results from hyperplasia associated with polyarthritis (lameness), systemic lupus erythematosus (cutaneous signs) or certain forms of lymphocytic cholangitis (icterus and ascites).

● Hypereosinophilic syndrome (p 416)
Generalized lymphadenopathy results from eosinophilic lymphadenitis. Other clinical signs are usually present, including lethargy, inappetence, weight loss, vomiting and diarrhea.

● Post-vaccinal lymphadenopathy (p 416)
Local or generalized lymphadenopathy results from hyperplasia, associated with a history of vaccination in the preceding few weeks.

● **Cutaneous/subcutaneous foreign body reaction* (p 406)**

Local lymphadenopathy occurs due to hyperplasia or lymphadenitis, secondary to aseptic or septic inflammation around the foreign body. Other localizing clinical signs include erythema, warmth and pain on palpation, swelling or thickening of tissue, and wounds.

● **Oral cavity diseases* (p 406)**

Mandibular lymphadenopathy results from hyperplasia or lymphadenitis. Signs of oral cavity disease are present, including halitosis, gingivitis, ulceration and masses.

INFECTIOUS

Viral:

● **Feline leukemia virus (FeLV) infection** (p 398)**

Generalized lymphadenopathy occurs due to hyperplasia during acute and persistent viremia. Lymphadenopathy may also result from lymphoma or secondary infection. Cats may otherwise be normal, or have lethargy, inappetence and fever. Localizing signs of infection or neoplasia may also be present.

● **Feline immunodeficiency virus (FIV) infection** (p 398)**

Generalized lymphadenopathy occurs due to hyperplasia during acute and chronic clinical stages of infection. Lymphadenopathy may also result from lymphoma or secondary infection. Cats may otherwise be normal, or have lethargy, inappetence and fever. Localizing signs of infection or neoplasia may also be present.

Bacterial:

● **Acute cat-bite wound cellulitis/abscess** (p 401)**

Local to regional lymphadenopathy occurs due to hyperplasia. Other localizing clinical signs include erythema, warmth and pain on palpation, swelling or thickening of tissue, and wounds. Systemic signs may be present including lethargy, inappetence and fever.

● Juvenile streptococcal lymphadenitis (p 415)

Cervical lymphadenopathy occurs due to lymph node abscessation in kittens. Kittens are depressed, inappetent and febrile.

● **Mycobacterial infections* (p 407)**

Generalized lymphadenopathy results from granulomatous lymphadenitis in tuberculosis, and accompanies chronic vomiting, diarrhea and weight loss. Regional lymphadenopathy due to hyperplasia may accompany cutaneous nodules in leprosy, and occur with chronic ulcerated subcutaneous lesions in atypical mycobacteriosis.

● **(Pyo)granulomatous bacterial infections*, mycoplasma and L-form infections, miscellaneous bacterial infections* (p 408)**

Local to generalized lymphadenopathy results from hyperplasia or lymphadenitis and often accompanies an acute or chronic wound. Systemic signs may be present including lethargy, inappetence and fever.

● **Plague* (p 404)**

Fulminant disease with head and neck lymphadenopathy resulting from abscessation and/or necrosis. Cats are highly susceptible to plague. Cats typically have acute onset of high fever, depression and anorexia.

continued

continued

● Tularemia* (p 410)

Fulminant disease with peripheral and internal lymphadenopathy. Cats are moderately susceptible to tularemia, Cats typically have acute onset of high fever, depression and anorexia.

● Anthrax (p 418)

Fulminant disease sometimes presenting as acute death with no promontory signs. Rare in cats because they are resistant to anthrax. Cervical lymphadenopathy and edema of the tongue and pharynx.

● Ehrlichiosis and bartonellosis (p 417)

Regional to generalized lymphadenopathy occur due to hyperplasia. Cats with ehrlichiosis usually have non-specific signs of illness, while cats with bartonellosis are asymptomatic.

● Bacteremia (p 416)

Variable lymphadenopathy due to hyperplasia may occur in chronic bacteremia, accompanied by chronic signs of fever, lethargy and inappetence.

Fungal and algal:

● Dimorphic fungal infections**, prototheocosis (p 418)

Local to generalized lymphadenopathy occurs due to hyperplasia or lymphadenitis. Concurrent localizing signs include nasal discharge, dyspnea, lameness, cutaneous nodules and ulcers, seizures and uveitis. Concurrent systemic signs include fever, weight loss and inappetence.

● Miscellaneous fungal infections* (p 411)

Local to generalized lymphadenopathy results from hyperplasia or lymphadenitis. Cats typically have chronic ulcerating cutaneous or subcutaneous lesions.

Protozoal:

● Cytauxzoonosis, American and African trypanosomiasis (p 418, 419)

Fulminant diseases where generalized lymphadenopathy may be present. Cats with cytauxzoonosis and African trypanosomiasis are febrile. Cats with American trypanosomiasis have signs of acute heart failure.

● Toxoplasmosis (p 419)

Acute toxoplasmosis may cause reactive peripheral lymphadenopathy and mesenteric lymph node necrosis.

INTRODUCTION

MECHANISM?

Lymphadenopathy refers to **enlarged lymph nodes**. Lymphadenopathy may accompany a number of common and uncommon diseases, but it is uncommonly the chief complaint.

Reactive lymphoid hyperplasia, neoplasia and lymphadenitis are the usual causes of lymphadenopathy. Lymphadenopathy is infrequently due to vascularization, edema or infarction.

- Lymph node biopsy (fine needle, incisional or excisional) for cytology, histology and culture is required to identify these mechanisms.

Hyperplasia is the most common cause of lymphadenopathy. It represents the immune response of normal lymphoid cells to antigenic stimulation.

- It is characterized **cytologically** by a predominance of **small mature lymphocytes** with or without increased numbers of immature lymphocytes, plasma cells and macrophages.
- Some distinguish between **lymph node hyperplasia** and **reactive lymphadenopathy**. The former is

characterized by a clinically enlarged node but normal cellular composition on biopsy; the latter is characterized by a mild to marked increase of plasma cells, with or without a mild increase of immature lymphocytes and/or macrophages. These two patterns have the same etiologies, will not be distinguished here, and will be referred to as "hyperplasia".

- Based on lymph node **histology**, patterns of lymph node hyperplasia may vary, e.g. as follicular center expansion (B-cells), paracortical expansion (T-cells), combined B- and T-cell hyperplasia, and sinusoidal cell hyperplasia (macrophages). In most disorders lymph node architecture is preserved.
- **Hyperplasia is generally a non-specific finding**.
- Some tendencies for specific cytologic and histologic patterns occur with certain diseases, e.g. increased numbers of **eosinophils in parasitic skin diseases**. Communicating with the pathologist may assist the clinician in determining etiology.
- Hyperplasia may be the initial finding before the development of detectable neoplasia or lymphadenitis.
- Hyperplastic nodes without a diagnosis should be **cultured for bacteria and fungi**.

Neoplastic lymphadenopathy is characterized by **proliferation or invasion of malignant cells**.

- Lymphoma and lymphoid leukemia are due to proliferation and invasion of malignant lymphocytes.
- On histology, lymphoid neoplasia typically **disrupts lymph node architecture** and **demonstrates a uniform cell-type and chromatin pattern**.
- Other **hematopoietic tumors and solid tumors may metastasize** to local, regional or distant nodes.

Lymphadenitis is characterized by a **cellular infiltrate of neutrophils** (suppurative) macrophages (pyogranulomatous), or **eosinophils** (eosinophilic), focal necrosis or abscessation. It usually results from an **extension of an inflammatory process into the node**.

- Severe, peracute infectious lymphadenitis may cause hemorrhage and necrosis with destruction of architecture, minimal inflammatory infiltrate, and nodal and perinodal edema.

Lymphadenopathy may be mild to marked with any cause.

- Lymphadenopathy tends to be more prominent in younger animals compared to older animals.

Lymph nodes may be **painful, warm and soft with bacterial and fungal lymphadenitis**. Lymph nodes are painless, firm and at body temperature with most other diseases.

Lymph nodes may be fixed (instead of mobile) with lymphadenitis, metastatic neoplasia and lymphoma with extracapsular invasion.

Lethargy, inappetence, weight loss and fever may be present, especially with generalized lymphadenopathy.

Local or regional enlargement is usually due to a disorder in the area drained by the node(s).

WHERE?

The focus of this chapter is **peripheral lymphadenopathy** (e.g. mandibular, prescapular, axillary, inguinal and popliteal nodes). There may be accompanying internal lymphadenopathy (e.g. hilar and mesenteric nodes).

- **Inguinal fat should not be mistaken** for enlarged inguinal nodes and contracted muscles of the caudal aspects of the hindlimb should not be mistaken for popliteal nodes.

Diseases causing primarily internal lymphadenopathy are discussed in The Dyspneic or Tachypneic Cat, The Cat With Chronic Diarrhea and The Thin Inappetent Cat.

WHAT?

The most common causes of **generalized lymphadenopathy** are chronic generalized skin diseases (dermatopathic lymphadenopathy), FeLV/FIV infections and lymphoma.

- The most common causes of **marked generalized lymphadenopathy** are chronic flea allergy dermatitis, lymphoma, idiopathic atypical hyperplasia and acute FIV infection.

The most common causes of **local and regional lymphadenopathy** are bacterial and fungal infections in the area drained by the node(s).

- The most common cause of **marked solitary lymphadenopathy** is abscessation.

DISEASES CAUSING PERIPHERAL LYMPHADENOPATHY

FELINE LEUKEMIA VIRUS (FELV) INFECTION**

> **Classical signs**
>
> - Lethargy, inappetence, weight loss, unkempt haircoat.
> - Fever, gingivitis, recurrent upper respiratory infections, opportunistic infections.
> - Anemia.
> - Generalized lymphadenopathy may occur in viremic cats.

See main reference, page 540 (The Anemic Cat).

Pathogenesis

FeLV infection may cause **solitary, regional and generalized lymphadenopathy** by several mechanisms. These include:

- Lymphoid hyperplasia during primary viremia (initial infection).
- Lymphoid hyperplasia during persistent viremia.
- Atypical hyperplasia.
- Lymphoma.
- Metastatic neoplasia.
- Immunosuppression causing bacterial infections (e.g. gingivitis/stomatitis, pyoderma) and fungal infections (e.g. cryptococcosis), and reactive hyperplasia or lymphadenitis.
- Immune-complex diseases (e.g. polyarthritis) and reactive hyperplasia.

Clinical signs

Mild to moderate generalized lymphadenopathy may occur during **primary viremia**.

- Cats may otherwise be normal or have **variable lethargy, inappetence and fever**.

Mild to moderate generalized lymphadenopathy may occur during **persistent viremia**.

- Mandibular nodes may be more affected.
- Cats may otherwise be normal or have variable lethargy, inappetence and fever.

Mild to marked lymphadenopathy and various associated signs may occur with other **FeLV-associated disorders** (e.g. neoplasia and fungal infection).

Diagnosis

FeLV tests.

- **ELISA, FA and rapid immunomigration (RIM) tests detect p27 protein** produced by the virus.
  - ELISA test may be weakly positive during primary viremia; FA test is negative. Because primary viremia may be terminated by an effective immune response, the ELISA test should be repeated in 4–6 weeks.
  - ELISA and FA tests are usually both positive during persistent viremia.
  - RIM test results correlate closely to ELISA test results.
- Some PCR tests are available to detect viral DNA. PCR may be positive during primary viremia. PCR is positive during persistent viremia, and is more sensitive than either ELISA or FA. **It should be noted that PCR testing has not been standardized and is more likely to give false-positive results than ELISA and FA if the laboratory does not maintain the highest standards of quality control.**
- If FeLV tests on peripheral blood are negative and another cause of lymphadenopathy has not been determined, obtain a **FA or PCR test on a bone marrow or lymph node aspirate, or immunohistochemistry test on a bone marrow core or lymph node biopsy.**

Lymph node biopsy reveals follicular or paracortical lymphoid hyperplasia.

Differential diagnosis

Lymphoma, metastatic lymphadenopathy, atypical hyperplasia, and possibly hyperplasia from other causes may be distinguished from FeLV-induced hyperplasia by **lymph node histology.**

Lymphoma may be present at other sites – e.g. bone marrow, liver, spleen.

A primary tumor should be identifiable with metastatic lymphadenopathy.

Signs of infections, skin diseases or immune-mediated disorders should be present if lymphadenopathy is due to hyperplasia from a cause other than retroviral infection.

An FIV antibody test or PCR test for FIV DNA may be used to rule out FIV infection.

Treatment

Treat neoplasia, infection, skin disease or immune-mediated disease as discussed elsewhere.

There is no specific treatment for lymphadenopathy that is not due to these conditions.

Supportive care as needed.

Immunomodulation with agents such as *Staphylococcus protein A or interferon-α* may improve subjective impression of the cat's well-being, but will not accelerate resolution of lymphadenopathy.

Prognosis

Lymphadenopathy of primary viremia will resolve with resolution of viremia.
- Lymphadenopathy usually resolves within 4 months.
- Cats with more pronounced signs during primary viremia are more likely to become persistently viremic.

In most cases, **lymphadenopathy of persistent viremia** not due to neoplasia, infection, skin disease, or immune-mediated disease **will resolve spontaneously.**
- Some cases will progress to lymphoma.

Long-term prognosis is determined by other FeLV-associated disorders.

FELINE IMMUNODEFICIENCY VIRUS (FIV) INFECTION**

Classical signs

- Lethargy, inappetence, weight loss, unkempt haircoat.
- Fever, gingivitis, diarrhea, dermatitis, recurrent upper respiratory infections.
- Opportunistic infections.
- Neurologic signs, uveitis.
- Generalized lymphadenopathy usually occurs during symptomatic phases.

See main reference, page 378 (The Pyrexic Cat).

Pathogenesis

FIV infection can cause solitary, regional and generalized lymphadenopathy by several mechanisms. These include:
- Hyperplasia during the acute phase (initial infection).
- Hyperplasia during the chronic symptomatic phase of infection (encompassing the phases of progressive generalized lymphadenopathy, AIDS [acquired immunodeficiency syndrome]-related complex and terminal AIDS). Some of the hyperplastic changes may be reactions to secondary infections.
- Increased risk for lymphoma, which may cause lymphadenopathy.
- Increased risk for non-lymphomatous neoplasia, which may cause metastatic lymphadenopathy.
- Immunosuppression causing bacterial infections (e.g. gingivitis/stomatitis, pyoderma) and fungal infections (e.g. dermatophytosis), and subsequent reactive lymph node hyperplasia or lymphadenitis.
- **Immune-mediated disorders** (which may have associated lymphadenopathy) have been described in FIV-positive cats, but the role of FIV in pathogenesis is not known.

Clinical signs

Mild to moderate generalized lymphadenopathy is common during the **acute phase.**
- Concurrent signs include variable lethargy, inappetence, fever and signs of gingivitis/stomatitis, enteritis, conjunctivitis, respiratory tract infections, dermatitis and neurologic disorders.
- Although other clinical signs are usually only present for several days to weeks, **lymphadenopathy may persist for over a year.**
- **Internal lymphadenopathy occurs concurrently.**

Mild to moderate generalized lymphadenopathy is common during the **chronic symptomatic phase.**
- Concurrent signs include variable lethargy, inappetence, fever, and signs of gingivitis/stomatitis, enteritis, conjunctivitis, uveitis, respiratory tract infections, dermatitis, neurologic disorders and other signs due to secondary infections.
- Internal lymphadenopathy occurs concurrently.
- **In the terminal phase** of infection, lymphadenopathy may disappear and **lymph nodes may become small** due to marked follicular involution.

Mild to marked lymphadenopathy and various associated signs may occur with **other FIV-associated disorders** (e.g. neoplasia and fungal infection).

- In the **terminal phase of FIV infection**, appropriate lymphadenopathy due to hyperplasia may not occur in response to secondary infection because of **marked follicular involution.**

Diagnosis

FIV antibody test (ELISA, RIM, FA, western blot).

- Antibody is usually detectable within 2 months of infection, but may take up to 6 months, therefore a negative test should be repeated.

PCR test for FIV DNA. The sensitivity of PCR for viral DNA compared to antibody tests is not known. **It should be noted that PCR testing has not been standardized and is more likely to give false-positive results than antibody tests if the laboratory does not maintain the highest standards of quality control.**

During the **acute phase**, lymph node biopsy reveals **marked follicular hyperplasia** with or without dysplasia, and less intense parafollicular hyperplasia.

During the **chronic symptomatic phase**, lymph node biopsy reveals **follicular hyperplasia** with or without follicular involution, **follicular plasmacytosis**, and variable erythrophagocytosis by macrophages. These changes are not specific for FIV infection. **Lymph node histology progresses** from **follicular hyperplasia**, through mixed **hyperplasia/involution**, to follicular involution, corresponding to generalized lymphadenopathy, AIDS-related complex and terminal AIDS.

Neutropenia and lymphopenia are common hematologic abnormalities in symptomatic cats.

Differential diagnosis

Lymphoma, metastatic lymphadenopathy, atypical hyperplasia and possibly hyperplasia from other causes may be distinguished from FIV-induced hyperplasia by **lymph node histology**.

Lymphoma may be present at other sites – e.g. bone marrow, liver or spleen.

A **primary tumor** should be identifiable with metastatic lymphadenopathy.

Signs of infections, skin diseases or immune-mediated disorders should be present if lymphadenopathy is due

to hyperplasia from a cause other than retroviral infection.

A FeLV antigen test may be used to rule-out FeLV infection.

Generalized lymphadenopathy is a more prominent feature of FIV, compared to FeLV, infection.

Treatment

Treat neoplasia, infection, skin disease or immune-mediated disease as discussed elsewhere.

There is no specific treatment for lymphadenopathy that is not due to these conditions.

Supportive care as needed.

Prognosis

Lymphadenopathy is not a distinct disorder in FIV-positive cats, but rather a **marker of the symptomatic phases of infection.** There is no specific prognosis attached to lymphadenopathy, except that **disappearance** during the chronic symptomatic phase **correlates with progression to terminal illness.**

Prognosis is determined by other FIV-associated disorders.

PARASITIC, IMMUNOLOGIC AND MISCELLANEOUS SKIN DISORDERS**

Classical signs

- Skin lesions typical of the primary disease (e.g. miliary dermatitis).
- ± Mild to marked lymphadenopathy.

See The Cat With Miliary Dermatitis (page 1022), The Cat With Skin Lumps and Bumps (page 1067) and The Cat With Non-healing Wounds (page 1081).

Clinical signs

Mild to marked lymphadenopathy may be present with disorders of the skin and subcutis, especially chronic ones, but it is not the salient feature.

Mandibular lymphadenopathy may be present with acne, mosquito bite hypersensitivity, notoedric mange, poxvirus infection, discoid lupus erythematosus and auricular chondritis.

Regional and generalized lymphadenopathy may be present with flea allergy dermatitis, eosinophilic granuloma complex, food hypersensitivity, neoplasia (including cutaneous lymphoma), dermatophytosis, demodicosis, pemphigus complex, panniculitis, vasculitis, systemic lupus erythematosus, drug eruption, erythema multiforme/toxic epidermal necrolysis, mechanobullous skin disease and steatitis.

Diagnosis

Work-up of the primary disease will usually identify the reason for the lymphadenopathy. Skin biopsy is often required for a definitive diagnosis.

Lymph node biopsy will reveal **hyperplasia** with or without metastasis with neoplastic disorders.

Differential diagnosis

Chronic bacterial and other fungal infections. Differentiation is on the basis of biopsy and culture.

Treatment

Treat the primary disease.

ACUTE CAT BITE WOUND CELLULITIS/ABSCESS**

> **Classical signs**
>
> - Acute onset fever, lethargy, inappetence.
> - Puncture wounds or abscess(es) from bite.
> - ± Mild local lymphadenopathy.

See main reference on page 368 (The Pyrexic Cat).

Clinical signs

Acute-onset fever, lethargy and inappetence.

The wound area is usually swollen and/or painful; bites to limbs cause acute lameness.

Gentle passage of a finger back and forth through the fur over a painful area will reveal puncture wounds.

Abscesses may spontaneously rupture, at which time systemic signs usually improve.

Mild local non-painful lymphadenopathy may occur.

Diagnosis

Diagnosis is based on **physical examination findings**.

Culture is not routinely performed, but numerous common organisms have been isolated.

Lymph node biopsy is rarely warranted but reveals hyperplasia.

Wound and lymph node should be examined cytologically and cultured if there is painful local lymphadenopathy.

Differential diagnosis

Foreign body cellulitis and abscessation.

Lymph node abscessation due to juvenile streptococcosis or bubonic plague.

Infection with atypical organism that may progress to a chronic condition.

Differentiation is on the basis of clinical progression, cytology and culture.

Treatment

Treat the primary disease. See The Pyrexic Cat (page 369).

DIMORPHIC FUNGAL INFECTIONS**

> **Classical signs**
>
> - Fever, weight loss, inappetence and localizing signs of infection.

See main references on page 25 for details of cryptococcosis (The Cat With Signs of Chronic Nasal Disease), page 1095 for sporothricosis (The Cat With Non-Healing Wounds), and page 62 for histoplasmosis and blastomycosis (The Cat With Dyspnea or Tachypnea).

Clinical signs

Non-specific signs are common.

Common localizing signs of infection include:

- **Respiratory signs,** including nasal discharge (cryptococcosis), and dyspnea due to fungal pneumonia; hilar lymphadenitis. More than 50% of cats with histoplasmosis are dyspneic.
- **Lameness** from bone or joint infection, especially with coccidioidomycosis.
- **Skin lesions:** nodules, ulcers and abscesses that have not resolved with typical wound treatment, i.e. drainage, irrigation and antibiotic therapy. Skin lesions are the salient feature of sporotrichosis.
- **Neurologic signs,** including seizures.
- **Ocular signs,** including uveitis and chorioretinitis.

Solitary, regional, generalized peripheral and internal lymphadenopathy may be present. Peripheral lymphadenopathy is common with sporotrichosis.

Diagnosis

Exposure history is important for diagnosis. Endemic areas include: eastern North America (blastomycosis); southwest North America, northern and south central South America (coccidioidomycosis). Others are world-wide.

Blastomycosis is uncommon in cats compared to dogs.

Lymph node biopsy reveals hyperplasia or less commonly lymphadenitis.

Definitive diagnosis is by identification of the organisms in biopsy specimens of affected tissues by cytology or histology. **Cytologically**:

- *Cryptococcus neoformans* appears as large, encapsulated, narrow-based budding yeasts. With the capsule most organisms are the same size or larger than surrounding inflammatory and epithelial cells. India ink stain helps identify the capsule.
- *Sporothrix schenkii* appears as a cigar-shaped yeast inside macrophages.
- *Blastomyces dermatitidis* appears as broad-based budding yeasts, slightly larger than surrounding neutrophils. With new methylene blue stain the organism has an obvious double wall and green tinge.
- *Coccidioides immitis* appears as solitary large non-budding yeasts three times the size of surrounding neutrophils, but it is present in low numbers and hard to find.

- *Histoplasma capsulatum* appears as numerous small round yeasts with a dark center and surrounding halo inside macrophages.

Serology is useful for identifying cryptococcosis, coccidioidomycosis, blastomycosis and sporotrichosis.

Organisms can be cultured, but this requires special media and biohazard containment.

Differential diagnosis

Neoplasia – signs of neoplasia and systemic mycoses are similar because both are due to invasion and proliferation of eukaryotic cells.

Tuberculosis, nocardiosis and other chronic bacterial infections.

Differentiation is based on cytology, histology and culture.

Treatment

Itraconazole 5 mg/kg q 12 h for weeks to months is effective against most dimorphic fungi. Treat a minimum of 30 days beyond clinical resolution. Amphotericin B and liposomal-encapsulated amphotericin B are alternate treatments. Ketoconazole may be substituted for itraconazole in some cases to reduce cost of therapy, but is often less effective.

Fluconazole is the drug of choice for **central nervous system infections**.

Iodides are the older standard treatments for sporotrichosis. Supersaturated solution of **potassium iodide** or **20% sodium iodide** may be used at a dose of 20 mg/kg PO once or twice daily, with food.

Zoonotic potential:

- *Sporothrix schenkii* is highly contagious from lesions.
- *Coccidioides immitis* may revert from tissue yeast phase to mycelial phase on bandage surfaces and release highly contagious arthrospores. Avoid bandaging wounds or change dressings frequently.

Other dimorphic fungi are not contagious.

NODAL LYMPHOMA*

Classical signs

- Painless lymphadenopathy.

Pathogenesis

Based on the histological classification in humans, lymphoma in cats may be classified as **non-Hodgkin's lymphoma** and **Hodgkin's-like lymphoma**. The latter has been recently recognized.

- **Non-Hodgkin's lymphoma** includes the most commonly recognized forms of lymphoma in cats, including **mediastinal, alimentary, multicentric, other extra-nodal lymphomas and lymphocytic leukemia.**
- Primary **multicentric nodal lymphoma** (initial site of disease is a lymph node) causes generalized peripheral lymphadenopathy from malignant lymphoid cell proliferation.
- The disease may metastasize to the bone marrow (leukemic lymphoma) and liver and spleen.
- Primary **lymphocytic leukemia** (initial site of disease is the bone marrow) may metastasize to peripheral nodes and cause lymphadenopathy.
- Non-Hodgkin's nodal lymphoma **less commonly involves solitary or regional nodes,** and occasionally solitary to generalized nodal involvement accompanies other forms (e.g. mediastinal lymphoma).
- Historically, **multicentric nodal lymphoma and lymphocytic leukemia** in most cats has been **associated with FeLV infection**. However, as the prevalence of FeLV declines in some regions, the incidence of FeLV-negative nodal lymphoma is increasing.
- FIV infection increases the risk of non-Hodgkin's lymphoma.

Hogkin's-like lymphoma histologically resembles "lymphocyte-predominance Hodgkin's disease" in humans.

- Most cases involve a **solitary mandibular or cervical node**. Solitary inguinal, regional cervical and generalized lymphadenopathy have also been recognized.
- Most cats tested are **FeLV and FIV negative**.

Clinical signs

Solitary, regional (especially mandibular or cervical) **or generalized**, moderate to marked painless peripheral lymphadenopathy.

- Non-Hodgkin's lymphoma may occur at any age. The **average age** for cats with multicentric lymphoma is **4 years**.
- Most cats with **Hodgkin's-like lymphoma are > 6 years of age** (range 1–14 years).

Cats may not have other historical signs, or may have lethargy, inappetence and weight loss.

Hepatosplenomegaly may be present.

Mediastinal lymphoma and alimentary lymphoma are not typically associated with peripheral lymphadenopathy, although nodal involvement occasionally occurs.

Diagnosis

Diagnosis requires finding lymph node cytology consistent with lymphoma, and biopsy-confirmed lymphoma (cytology or histology) at another site, e.g. bone marrow, liver, spleen.

If lymphoma cannot be confirmed at another site, **excisional lymph node biopsy and histology are mandatory** to distinguish from atypical hyperplasia and to characterize the lymphoma.

FeLV and FIV tests should be obtained.

Differential diagnosis

Differential diagnoses for generalized lymphadenopathy include atypical hyperplasia, hyperplasia in response to generalized skin diseases, immunologic disorders and systemic infections, widely metastatic neoplasia, and generalized bacterial or fungal lymphadenitis.

Differential diagnoses for solitary or regional lymphadenopathy include plexiform vascularization of lymph nodes, atypical hyperplasia, hyperplasia in response to local tumors, oral cavity and skin diseases, and infections, metastatic lymphadenopathy, and bacterial or fungal lymphadenitis.

These are distinguished on the basis of lymph node cytology, histology and culture and work-up for an underlying disease.

Treatment

Multicentric lymphoma should be treated with **chemotherapy** as described in Chapter 31.

Some cats with **solitary nodal lymphomas** have been cured by **surgical excision** alone.
- Because of the tendency for lymphoma to be a systemic disease, chemotherapy is usually recommended following excision.
- If work-up fails to identify lymphoma at another site, then surgery (or radiation therapy) without subsequent chemotherapy may be considered, especially for Hodgkin's-like lymphoma.

Prognosis

Reported response rates to therapy provide general information, but it is difficult to give a prognosis for an individual cat.

Providing a prognosis is even more difficult for a cat with multicentric nodal lymphoma.
- In some studies "multicentric" included extra-nodal lymphomas involving multiple sites.
- Some cats with only peripheral lymph node disease and long-term remissions may have had atypical hyperplasia or Hodgkin's-like lymphoma.

Providing a prognosis for leukemic cats may be complicated by difficulty in distinguishing nodal leukemic lymphoma and primary leukemia, which carries a worse prognosis.

The best predictor of response is response itself, i.e. the longer a cat is in remission, the more likely it is to remain in remission.

FeLV and FIV status does not affect initial response to therapy. It does negatively affect long-term survival, mostly because of the occurrence of other FeLV- and FIV-related disorders.

Cats with a small tumor burden have a better prognosis.

With these caveats, using combination chemotherapy protocols for the treatment of non-Hodgkin's nodal lymphoma:
- **For multicentric nodal lymphoma**: rate of **complete remission is 60–80%**, 1-year survival is 10%, and 2 and 3 year survival 5%. These figures are based on older studies where the majority of cats were FeLV positive. In a more recent study

where the majority of cats were **FeLV-negative, rate of remission was 86% and 1-year survival was 57%.**
- **For solitary or regional nodal lymphoma**: **rate of complete remission is > 80%,** 1-year survival is 35%, and 2 and 3 year survival is 20–30%.
- **For primary lymphocytic leukemia**: rate of complete remission is 25%, 1-year survival is 10%, and 2 and 3 year survival 5%. Cats with acute pancytopenia have a worse prognosis.

It appears that many cats with solitary Hodgkin's-like lymphoma may be cured with surgical excision alone.

PLAGUE*

Classical signs
- Acute high fever.
- Cranial body regional lymphadenopathy.

See main reference page 383 (The Pyrexic Cat).

Pathogenesis

Infection with *Yersinia pestis*. Cats are uniquely sensitive among carnivores.

Most cats appear to be infected by ingestion of an infected rodent. The organism spreads rapidly to the regional nodes (mandibular and cervical nodes). Cats may also be infected by a **bite from an infected flea**, where the organism spreads rapidly to the local lymph node.
- The **organism replicates in the local/regional nodes** and from there may progress to other nodes, **bacteremia and pneumonia**.

Clinical signs

Signs appear within **1–7 days of infection**.

High fever (> 40°C), lethargy, inappetence, dehydration.

Minimal reaction at site of innoculation.

Bubonic plague is characterized by **marked solitary or regional painful mandibular**, **retropharyngeal and cervical lymphadenopathy** due to **severe lymphadenitis**.

The lymphadenitis is characterized by hemorrhage, necrosis and perinodal edema, and later by lymph node abscessation. **Abscesses may rupture** and drain thick, creamy pus. The severely swollen, inflamed nodes are referred to as "bubos".

- This distribution of lymphadenopathy results from oral exposure during hunting.
- Flea bites may occur elsewhere resulting in a different distribution, e.g. solitary inguinal bubo formation.

Other possible signs include **oral ulcers, tonsillar enlargement, ocular and nasal discharges** and **abdominal distention**. Cats may initially present with less severe signs.

Septicemic plague, characterized by fever and septic shock may occur with or without bubo formation.

Pneumonic plague in cats, characterized by **fever, dyspnea**, oral or nasal discharges, and coughing or sneezing occurs occasionally and is usually a sequel to bubonic or septicemic plague.

Diagnosis

History of exposure to **infected rodents**.

Cytology of lymph node biopsy/exudate reveals neutrophils and a **monomorphic population of Gram-negative, bipolar staining, coccobacilli**.

FA test of air-dried smears of tissues or exudate.

Culture of organism from lymph nodes or other affected tissues (e.g. tonsils).

Acute (as early as possible once illness is detected) and convalescent (14 days later) **antibody titers demonstrating a four-fold rise in titer** are diagnostic for plague. Titers are useful to confirm a zoonotic disease when treatment is based on a tentative diagnosis.

All plague suspects should have **thoracic radiographs** taken to **rule-out pneumonia**.

Differential diagnosis

Cat bite abscess.

- Most **cat bite wounds** result in **cellulitis and subcutaneous abscessation rather than lymph node abscessation**. However, subcutaneous/muscle

abscesses have been reported in plague, with lymphadenopathy due to hyperplasia.

- *Pasteurella multocida*, a frequent organism found in bite wounds, resembles *Y. pestis* cytologically. However, **bite wounds usually contain a mixed bacterial population** while bubos usually contain a monomorphic population of bacteria.

Anthrax.

- Rare.
- Lymph node abscessation probably does not occur as with plague.
- Lingual, pharyngeal and cervical edema may be more pronounced than with plague.

Tularemia.

- A papule may be present at the site of innoculation.
- Lymphadenopathy is not as prominent, and abscessation does not occur.

Other causes of bacterial lymphadenitis.

- Unlike most other causes of bacterial lymphadenitis, there is usually minimal reaction at the site of innoculation with plague organisms.
- Culture of organism is required to definitively differentiate.

Acute infection with FeLV or FIV and regional lymphadenopathy.

- Retroviral infections have clinically a more subacute to chronic course.
- Lymph node biopsy with retroviral infections will reveal hyperplasia.

Treatment

Treat early on the basis of tentative diagnosis.

Antibiotics (optimal treatment is not known).

- Recommended antibiotics include **tetracycline, doxycycline, chloramphenicol, trimethoprim-sulfonamide, streptomycin, gentamicin, and kanamycin** at standard recommended doses. Fluoroquiniolones have been effective experimentally.
- Recommended duration of therapy is 10–21 days.
- Use **parenteral treatment initially** to minimize contact of nursing personnel with oral cavity. Use follow-up treatment with oral antibiotics to minimize hospitalization and aminoglycoside toxicoses.

Treat animal and environment for fleas.

Strict isolation and barrier nursing procedures must be followed.
- Treat in an isolation area using isolation gowns, high-density filter masks and gloves.
- Clean and decontaminate all surfaces with usual hospital disinfectants.
- Lance and irrigate abscessed lymph nodes.
- Place all contaminated material in double-layer bio-hazard bags and incinerate.

Notify public health officials; veterinary personnel should contact a physician.

Prognosis

Mortality of plague is **50% in untreated cats.**

There are a number of reports of successful treatment of cats with bubonic plague.

Cats with septicemic and pneumonic plague have the worst prognosis.

Transmission

Cats become infected by ingesting, or being bitten by fleas from infected rodents or other wild animals.

The disease is highly zoonotic.
- **Humans may be infected by flea-bites** and **contact with infected animals or their tissues**.
- There is a high risk for developing **primary pneumonic plague** following inhalation of *Y. pestis*-infected droplets expelled from cats with secondary pneumonic plague.

Prevention

Minimize cat contact with rodents and fleas in endemic areas.
- Eliminate rodents indoors; control rodent habitats near domestic dwellings (e.g. garbage piles).
- Keep cats indoors; neuter outdoor cats to reduce roaming and hunting.
- Flea control.

Use post-exposure prophylaxis for other cats: tetracycline or doxycycline at standard doses for 7 days.

ORAL CAVITY DISEASES*

> **Classical signs**
> - **Oral lesions typical of the primary disease.**
> - **± Mild to moderate mandibular lymphadenopathy.**

See The Cat With Bad Breath or Oral Lesions. (page 602)

Clinical signs

Mild to moderate mandibular lymphadenopathy may be present with lymphocytic-plasmacytic stomatitis/gingivitis, periodontal disease, and oral neoplasia, but it is not the salient feature of the disorders.

Diagnosis

Work-up of the primary disease will usually identify the reason for the lymphadenopathy. Biopsy of lesions may be necessary.

Lymph node biopsy is recommended if lymphadenopathy is present, and bilateral lymph node biopsy should always be performed in the staging of oral cancer.

Biopsy reveals hyperplasia with or without metastasis with neoplastic disorders.

Differential diagnosis

Differential diagnoses for mandibular lymphadenopathy include hyperplasia due to regional skin disorders, FeLV/FIV infection, lymphoma, metastatic lymphadenopathy and atypical hyperplasia.

Treatment

Treat the primary disease.

CUTANEOUS/SUBCUTANEOUS FOREIGN BODY REACTION*

> **Classical signs**
> - **Lymphadenopathy in local node draining from foreign body region.**

See main reference on page 1073 (The Cat With Skin Lumps and Bumps.

Clinical signs

Signs of aseptic or septic inflammation are present at the foreign body site (cutaneous, subcutaneous or deeper) and local lymphadenopathy may or may not be present.

Diagnosis

Exploration of area reveals foreign body.

Lymph node biopsy reveals **hyperplasia** or uncommonly lymphadenitis.

Differential diagnoses

Bite wound cellulitis, chronic bacterial and fungal infections, neoplasia and eosinophilic granuloma complex.

Differentiation is based on cytology, histology and culture.

Treatment

See The Cat With Skin Lumps and Bumps (page 1074).

MYCOBACTERIAL INFECTIONS*

Classical signs

- Chronic vomiting, diarrhea, mesenteric lymphadenopathy (tuberculosis).
- Multiple chronic ulcerated fleshy cutaneous nodules on head and limbs (leprosy) and regional lymphadenopathy.
- Chronic ulcerated subcutaneous lesions on caudal abdomen, inguinal and groin regions (atypical mycobacteriosis) ± local or regional lymphadenopathy.

See main reference, page 1085 (The Cat With Non-Healing Wounds).

Clinical signs

There are three categories of *Mycobacterium* sp. infection in cats: tuberculosis, leprosy and atypical.

Tuberculosis is caused by *M. tuberculosis, M. bovis, M. tuberculosis-bovis* variant, and *M. microti*. It may be subclinical or cause chronic weight loss, vomiting, diarrhea and mesenteric lymphadenopathy.

- The infection **occasionally disseminates** to virtually all organs with corresponding systemic and local signs.
- **Peripheral lymphadenopathy** occurs with disseminated disease.

Leprosy is caused by *M. lepraemurium* and is characterized by chronic single to multiple, freely moveable, non-painful intact or ulcerated and abscessed **fleshy cutaneous nodules**, with or without subcutaneous lesions. Systemic signs are rare.

- **Painless regional lymphadenopathy** is typical.

Atypical mycobacteriosis is caused by several non-tubercular, non-lepromatous *Mycobacterium* sp., and is usually characterized by **chronic, local or regional subcutaneous lesions** with multiple draining tracts. Lesions are most often found on the caudal abdomen, inguinal region or lumbar region, but also on the thorax. Systemic signs are uncommon but may occur.

- **Disseminated infection** (systemic non-tuberculous mycobacteriosis), which is clinically similar to tuberculosis, **is most likely with organisms from the** *M. avium* complex,
- Local, regional or generalized lymphadenopathy may occur.

Diagnosis

Cytology and histology of affected tissues reveal **granulomatous to pyogranulomatous inflammation.**

Lymph node biopsy reveals hyperplasia (all clinical forms) or granulomatous lymphadenitis (tuberculosis, systemic non-tuberculous mycobacteriosis).

Acid-fast bacteria are **usually detectable** in affected tissues with tuberculosis and leprosy, but may be difficult to find with atypical mycobacteriosis.

Culture is possible at selected laboratories, and particularly **useful for identifying fast-growing mycobacteria**, the most common causes of atypical mycobacteriosis.

Tuberculin testing is not reliable in cats.

Immunoassays may be available for some organisms.

Differential diagnosis

Differential diagnoses for disseminated mycobacterial infections include multicentric lymphoma, widely metastatic tumors, other pyogranulomatous bacterial infections and systemic fungal infections.

Differential diagnoses for leprosy include neoplasia, eosinophilic granuloma complex, other chronic bacterial infections and fungal infections.

Differential diagnoses for local or regional atypical mycobacteriosis include neoplasia, foreign body reaction, eosinophilic granuloma complex, panniculitis, pansteatitis, other chronic bacterial infections and fungal infections.

Differentiation is based on cytology, histology and culture.

Treatment

Tuberculosis.

- **Notify public health officials.** Euthanasia is often advised because of the zoonotic risk. If treatment is attempted, drug doses are provided in the reference at the end of the chapter.

Treatment of leprosy and atypical mycobacteriosis are discussed in The Cat With Non-Healing Wounds (page 1086).

(PYO)GRANULOMATOUS BACTERIAL INFECTIONS*

> **Classical signs**
>
> - Chronic ulcerating cutaneous/subcutaneous lesions.
> - ± Local, regional or generalized lymphadenopathy.

See main reference, page 1086 (The Cat With Non-Healing Wounds).

Clinical signs

Chronic ulcerating lesions occur with a number of bacteria, including *Rhodococcus equi*, *Actinomyces* sp., *Nocardia* sp., and *Dermatophilus congolensis*.

These organisms typically produce chronic ulcerating lesions or masses (abscesses and mycetomas) that are cutaneous or subcutaneous. The lesions have usually developed at sites of penetrating wounds and have **not resolved with typical wound treatment**. Localized infections in other organs and disseminated infections may also occur. Accompanying signs vary with organ involvement.

Local, regional, generalized peripheral and internal lymphadenopathy may occur.

Systemic signs may be absent or mild with local cutaneous and subcutaneous infections. Mild to severe signs occur with internal or disseminated infections.

Diagnosis

Pyogranulomatous-granulomatous inflammation is evident on cytology and histology of exudates and biopsy specimens.

Cytology may reveal Gram-positive bacteria in macrophages (*Rhodococcus equi*), mats of Gram-positive filamentous organisms (*Actinomyces* sp.), Gram-positive, weakly acid-fast beaded filamentous organisms (*Nocardia* sp.), or Gram-positive branching filamentous organisms with transverse longitudinal divisions resulting in paired rows of coccoid spores (*Dermatophilus congolensis*).

Lymph node biopsy reveals hyperplasia or lymphadenitis.

Definitive diagnosis is by culture of the organism from lesions.

There may be a history of exposure to horses with rhodococcosis.

Differential diagnosis

Eosinophilic granuloma complex, mycobacterial infections, fungal infections, neoplasia, panniculitis and steatitis.

Differentiation is based on cytology, histology and culture.

Treatment

Treat the primary disease. See page 1087 (The Cat With Non-Healing Wounds).

METASTATIC NEOPLASTIC LYMPHADENOPATHY: MAST CELL TUMOR*

Classical signs

- Firm cutaneous nodule (cutaneous form).
- Marked splenomegaly (lymphoreticular form).

See main reference, page 1074 (The Cat With Skin Lumps and Bumps).

Clinical signs

Most primary cutaneous mast cell tumors present as single, or less commonly, multiple dermal **nodules** without other clinical signs.

- Histologically they may be classified as compact mastocytic, diffuse mastocytic and histiocytic. The **average age of cats** with mastocytic tumors **is 10 years**, while the average age with histiocytic tumors is 2.4 years.

Cutaneous mast cell tumors may **infrequently metastasize** to local, regional and distant peripheral lymph nodes causing lymphadenopathy. **This is most likely with diffuse mastocytic tumors and tumors with > four mitoses/ten high-power fields.**

Cutaneous and lymphoreticular (splenic) mast cell tumors may occur together with variable involvement of internal and peripheral lymph nodes. The average age of cats with lymphoreticular tumors is 10 years.

Diagnosis

Biopsy of the cutaneous mass and/or spleen reveals numerous normal or atypical mast cells.

Lymph node biopsy reveals hyperplasia and increased numbers of mast cells.

Differential diagnosis

Other neoplasia, eosinophilic granuloma complex, chronic bacterial infections, fungal infections, and prototothecosis.

Differentiation is based on cytology, histology and culture.

Treatment

See page 1075 (The Cat With Skin Lumps and Bumps).

METASTATIC NEOPLASTIC LYMPHADENOPATHY: OTHER TUMORS*

Classical signs

- Signs of primary tumor.
- ± Local, regional or generalized lymphadenopathy.

See main reference, page 1067 (The Cat With Skin Lumps and Bumps).

Clinical signs

The cat is usually presented for signs of the primary tumor.

Occasionally the cat is presented because of local, regional or rarely generalized lymphadenopathy.

Most metastatic neoplasia occurs in older cats.

Diagnosis

Lymph node biopsy reveals hyperplasia and infiltration by carcinoma, uncommonly sarcoma, and rarely non-lymphoid, non-mast cell round cell tumors.

- **Carcinomas include** squamous cell carcinoma, bronchogenic carcinoma, mammary carcinoma and others.
- **Sarcomas include** fibrosarcoma, osteosarcoma and others.
- **Round cell tumors include** plasma cell tumors, myeloid leukemia, malignant histiocytosis and melanoma.

If the cat is presented for lymphadenopathy, reviewing the history and physical examination, and performing routine laboratory evaluation, and **thoracic and abdominal radiographs** and **ultrasound** examinations, will help **identify and stage the primary tumor**.

Normal and enlarged regional lymph nodes should be biopsied as part of clinical staging of the cat with cancer.

Differential diagnosis

For a cat presented for lymphadenopathy, differential diagnoses include lymphoma and most chronic causes of hyperplasia.

Differentiation is based on cytology, histology and culture.

Treatment

See page 1067 (The Cat With Skin Lumps and Bumps).

TULAREMIA*

> **Classical signs**
>
> - Acute high fever.
> - Peripheral and internal lymphadenopathy

See main reference, page 382 (The Pyrexic Cat).

Clinical signs

Signs appear within 2–7 days of infection with *Francisella tularensis* subsp. *tularensis* or *palaearctica*.

High fever (> 40°C), lethargy, inappetence, dehydration.

Moderate to marked painful lymphadenopathy due to lymphadenitis is common; site of infection affects distribution:
- Cats exposed by **mouthing or ingesting a rabbit or rabbit tick** will have initial mandibular, cervical or mesenteric lymphadenopathy.
- Cats exposed by **a mosquito, tick bite or innoculation** will have initial lymphadenopathy in the **node draining the region**.

Other variable signs include multifocal white oral ulcers, abdominal pain, hepatosplenomegaly, vomiting and diarrhea.
- Localized tularemia causing a chronically draining subcutaneous mass has also been reported.

Diagnosis

History of exposure to wild rabbits (North America, *F. tularensis tularensis*).

History of exposure to infected rodents, ticks and mosquitoes, or contaminated soil and water (Northern hemisphere, *F. tularensis palaearctica*).

Lymph node cytology reveals hyperplasia; histology reveals multifocal necrosis.

The organism, a **small Gram-negative coccobacilli**, is difficult to see on routine cytology and Gram-stain.
- **FA test** of air-dried smears of tissues or exudate helps identify the organism.

The organism may be **cultured from an aspirate of lymph node**, bone marrow (not blood), or other tissue.
- Not all laboratories will attempt culture and special media is required – check before submitting.

A **single titer ~ 1:80 gives a presumptive diagnosis**, while acute (as early as possible once illness is detected) and convalescent (14 days later) antibody titers demonstrating a four-fold rise give a confirmatory diagnosis. Titers are useful to confirm a zoonotic disease when treatment is based on a tentative diagnosis.

Differential diagnosis

Other acute viral, bacterial, fungal and parasitic (e.g. toxoplasmosis) infectious processes.
- These are distinguished on the basis of exposure risk, serologic testing and organism identification.
- Acute Gram-negative bacteremia, e.g. secondary to myelosuppression, is not usually associated with lymphadenopathy.

Treatment

Treat early on the basis of tentative diagnosis.

Antibiotics (optimal treatment is not known).
- **Recommended antibiotics include** tetracycline, doxycycline, chloramphenicol, streptomycin and gentamicin at standard recommended doses. Fluoroquinolones have been effective experimentally.
- Recommended duration of therapy is 7–14 days.
- **Use parenteral treatment** initially to minimize contact of nursing personnel with oral cavity. **Use follow-up treatment with oral antibiotics** to minimize hospitalization and aminoglycoside toxicoses.

Treat animal for ticks.

Highly zoonotic from tissues and ticks – strict isolation and barrier nursing procedures must be followed.

- Treat in an isolation area using isolation gowns, high-density filter masks and gloves.
- Clean and decontaminate all surfaces with usual hospital disinfectants.
- Place all contaminated material in double-layer bio-hazard bags and incinerate.

Notify public health officials; veterinary personnel should contact a physician.

OBSTRUCTIVE EDEMA*

Classical signs

- Localized edema.
- ± Local or regional lymphadenopathy.

Clinical signs

Lymphatic obstruction due to a tumor or other mass causes edema (e.g. head and neck, limb).

Local or regional nodes may be enlarged.

Diagnosis

Biopsy of the primary lesion.

Lymph node biopsy reveals edema with or without hyperplasia, metastasis or infection.

MISCELLANEOUS BACTERIAL INFECTIONS*

Classical signs

- Localizing signs of inflammation.
- Local, regional or generalized lymphadenopathy.

Clinical signs

Solitary to generalized lymphadenopathy.

Oral or skin wounds may be present indicating the site of entry. Infection may also be via the intestinal tract and cause mesenteric lymphadenopathy.

Systemic signs are usually present, and more severe with more generalized infections.

Diagnosis

Lymph node biopsy reveals **hyperplasia** or **lymphadenitis**.

Culture of bacteria from lymph node or other lesions. Bacteria include *Pseudomonas mallei* (glanders), *Burkholderia pseudomallei* (meliodosis), *Yersinia enterocolitica*, *Yersinia pseudotuberculosis*, *Serratia marscecens*, *Listeria monocytogenes,* and *Chriseomonas luteola*.

With glanders there is a history of exposure to diseased horses or other solipeds, or contaminated meat, and there may be respiratory tract nodules similar to tuberculosis.

MISCELLANEOUS FUNGAL INFECTIONS*

Classical signs

- Chronic ulcerating cutaneous/subcutaneous lesions.
- ± Local, regional or generalized lymphadenopathy.

Clinical signs

Chronic ulcerating lesions or masses that are cutaneous or subcutaneous. Usually they have developed at sites of penetrating wounds and have **not resolved with typical wound treatment**.

Infections of mucosal surfaces, localized infections in other organs and disseminated infections may also occur with accompanying signs varying with organ involvement. Internal infections are more common with certain organisms.

Local, regional or generalized lymphadenopathy may occur.

Systemic signs may be absent or mild with local cutaneous and subcutaneous infections, and mild to severe with internal or disseminated infections.

Diagnosis

Culture of the organism and histologic demonstration of tissue invasion in biopsy specimens. **Organisms include** *Pythium insidiosum* (oomycete), *Trichosporon* sp. (yeastlike fungus), *Candida* sp. (dimorphic fungus), dermatophytes (pseudomycetoma) and numerous hyphae-producing organisms. The latter infections are termed zygomycosis, hyalohyphomycosis and phaehypho-mycosis based on characteristics of fungal hyphae, and eumycotic mycetoma if pyogranulomatous nodules containing tissue grains are formed.

Lymph node biopsy reveals hyperplasia or lymph-adenitis.

Rule out immunosuppression (diabetes mellitus, hyperadrenocorticism, lymphoma, FeLV/FIV infection, immunosuppressive therapy) and neutropenia, especially if internal or disseminated mycosis is present.

STEATITIS

> ### Classical signs
>
> - Depression, anorexia, reluctance to move and pain on landing.
> - ± Lymphadenopathy.

Clinical signs

Depression, anorexia, reluctance to move because of pain, and pain upon handling.

Firm and lumpy subcutaneous fat with or without accompanying lymphadenopathy.

Other clinical signs include **fever** and **abdominal distention** from fluid and firm abdominal fat.

Diagnosis

History of a diet high in oxidized unsaturated fats (e.g. rancid tuna) and/or deficient in vitamin E. Rare in cats fed commercial foods.

Biopsy of fat confirms steatitis – the fat may be grossly yellow to brown.

Lymph node biopsy reveals hyperplasia.

IDIOPATHIC ATYPICAL HYPERPLASIA

> ### Classical signs
>
> - Moderate to marked generalized lymphadenopathy in young cats.

Pathogenesis

Two forms have been described.
- In cats ~ 2 years of age, lymphadenopathy was due to a **distinctive hyperplasia resembling that seen in experimental FeLV infection**.
  - Some cats were FeLV positive.
  - It was postulated that lymphadenopathy was due to FeLV infection.
- In cats ~ 4 years of age, marked lymphadenopathy was due to **hyperplasia resembling lymphoma**.
  - Tested cats were FeLV negative.
  - Cats were recovering from urinary tract, upper respiratory, and FeLV infections.
  - It was postulated that lymphadenopathy was due to an immune response to infection.
- A follow-up report used **silver staining** to identify tiny bacteria in the nodes of some cats from both studies. These bacteria may have been *Bartonella henselae*, the causative agent of cat-scratch disease in humans. Cats harboring *B. henselae* are usually young and recent studies show that *Bartonella henselae* may induce lymph node hyperplasia in cats.
  - Could the acute phase of FIV infection have been responsible for some of the cases?
  - FIV status was not known – reports antidated routine testing for FIV infection.
  - A recent study shows that co-infection with *Bartonella henselae* and FIV increases the risk for lymphadenopathy.
  - Unusual infections in some of the cases suggest immunodeficiency.
  - However, no cases of atypical hyperplasia have been reported in FIV-infected cats.

Clinical signs

Moderate to marked, regional to generalized **non-painful peripheral lymphadenopathy** in a cat ~ 4 years of age.
- **Lymphadenopathy is usually the chief complaint**; most cats are otherwise normal.

Other signs variably present include lethargy, inappetence, weight loss, fever, pale mucous membranes, hepatosplenomegaly (first case series) and signs due to concurrent infections (e.g. sneezing, hematuria).

Diagnosis

Lymph node cytology consistent with **hyperplasia, lymphoma, or suspicious for lymphoma**.

Lymph node histology reveals marked hyperplasia with disruption of lymph node architecture.
- Characteristic findings in the first case series were paracortical hyperplasia with histiocytes, lymphocytes, plasma cells, and immunoblasts, and post-capillary venular proliferation.
- Characteristic findings in the second case series were paracortical, follicular or diffuse lymphoid expansion, but other findings typical of lymphoid malignancy were variably absent.

Idiopathic lymphadenopathy is not a diagnosis in itself. Lymph node hyperplasia is an immune reaction to a cause. Atypical hyperplasia represents either an unusual cause or an atypical response to a usual cause. Aggressive diagnostic evaluation should be performed to reveal infection or neoplasia, especially since multi-system immune-mediated diseases such as systemic lupus erythematosus are rare in cats. **Work-up includes**:
- **FeLV test**.
- If an ELISA (enzyme-linked immunosorbent assay) test on blood is negative, and another cause of lymph-adenopathy has not been found, obtain a FA (fluo-rescent antibody) or PCR (polymerase chain reaction) test on blood. If negative, obtain a FA or PCR test on a bone marrow or lymph node aspirate, or immunohistochemistry test on a bone marrow core or lymph node biopsy. It should be noted that PCR testing has not been standardized and is more likely to give false-positive results than ELISA and FA if the laboratory does not maintain the highest standards of quality control.
- **FIV test**.
- Search for other infections and neoplasia.
  - Detailed review of history of physical examination for subtle signs, including ophthalmologic examination.
  - Further work-up will depend on clinical signs, exposure risks for infectious agents and financial considerations.
  - Diagnostic evaluation may include complete blood count, serum chemistry profile, urinalysis, blood culture, urine culture, abdominal and thoracic radiographs, cardiac and abdominal ultra-

sound examinations, bone marrow biopsy, lymph node bacterial/fungal culture, biopsies of other abnormal organs (submit for cytology/histology and culture), tests for *Bartonella henselae* and *Ehrlichia* sp. infection (see page 417), serologic tests for fungal agents, and antinuclear antibody and lupus erythematosus cell tests.
  - Although FIP may cause mesenteric lymph-adenopathy, peripheral lymphadenopathy has not been reported.

Differential diagnosis

Lymphadenopathy is a problem and not a diagnosis, and as such this discussion of idiopathic generalized lymphadenopathy is an extension of the Introduction.

The most common causes of generalized lymph-adenopathy are generalized skin diseases, FeLV/FIV infections and lymphoma.
- Skin lesions are usually obvious if lymphadenopathy is due to a skin disease.
- If a cat is FeLV- and/or FIV-positive, the possibility of concurrent neoplasia or infection contributing to lymphadenopathy should be considered.
- **Nodal lymphoma** is one of the **less common forms of lymphoma.**
  - It may be solitary, regional or generalized, similar to cats with atypical hyperplasia.
  - Cats may have no historical signs other than lymphadenopathy, similar to cats with atypical hyperplasia.
  - **Excisional biopsy is mandatory** and communication with the pathologist essential to rule in or rule out lymphoma.
  - There may be evidence of lymphoma at another site, e.g. bone marrow, liver, spleen or the disease will progress to involve these sites. Hepatosplenomegaly was not reported in the case series where lymph node histology resembled lymphoma.

Treatment

Treatment should be supportive if needed pending a diagnosis.

If the owner refuses a work-up, and the cat is otherwise normal, encourage observation rather than euthanasia.

Pending a diagnosis, or if owner refuses a work-up, if the cat is febrile or has localizing signs of infection, consider **empirical antibiotic treatment.** Acceptable choices include amoxicillin 10–20 mg/kg PO bid, amoxicillin-clavulanate 62.5 mg (combined dose) PO bid, doxycycline 5 mg/kg PO bid, enrofloxacin 5 mg/kg PO once daily, orbifloxacin 2.5–7.5 mg/kg once daily, and marbofloxacin 2.5–5.0 mg/kg once daily, for 2 weeks. Cats receiving fluoroquinolones should be monitored for visual disturbances.

Do not treat for lymphoma unless lymph node histology is unequivocal or there is evidence of lymphoma at another site.
- Waiting to treat is probably not harmful.
- An indolent lymphoma is unlikely to respond to aggressive chemotherapy.

Do not treat with corticosteroids.
- Corticosteroids may allow an infectious process to worsen that may otherwise resolve spontaneously.
- Corticosteroids may induce lymphoma cell resistance to other anticancer drugs.

Prognosis

Dependent on cause of lymphadenopathy.

In the two case series, **lymphadenopathy resolved within 4 months in 60% of cats** with follow-up in the first study, and all cats with follow-up in the second study.

PLEXIFORM VASCULARIZATION OF LYMPH NODES

Classical signs

- Unilateral cervical mass.
- Unilateral or bilateral inguinal mass(es).

Pathogenesis

A single case series and individual cases have been reported.

Pathogenesis is not known.
- An **ischemic pathogenesis has been postulated**, but cats have not been evaluated with respect to thromboembolic disease nor have other thromboembolic events been identified.

FeLV/FIV status has not been reported in most cases, but cats have not had signs of such infections.

Clinical signs

Unilateral cervical, or unilateral and bilateral inguinal masses.

Mass has been painless on palpation in 2/3 of cases.

No sex predilection; the majority of cases have been reported in **cats 3–8 years of age**.

Cervical mass may cause **dyspnea from tracheal compression**.

No other clinical signs.

Diagnosis

Histology of excised lymph node reveals **capillary vasoproliferation, lymphoid atrophy** and preservation of architecture.

Differential diagnosis

Differential diagnoses for superficial masses include benign and malignant solid tumors of skin, subcutaneous tissue, and muscle; epidermal cyst, granuloma, abscess, hematoma, and scar tissue; typical and atypical lymph node hyperplasia, lymphoma, metastatic lymphadenopathy, and lymphadenitis.

Additional diagnoses for cervical masses include enlarged thyroid or parathyroid gland, and salivary mucocele.

Additional diagnoses for inguinal masses include prominent inguinal fat pads.

Differentiation is based on biopsy for cytology, histology and culture.

Presence of other clinical signs, laboratory findings, radiographs and ultrasound examination of the mass may help narrow the list of differential diagnoses prior to biopsy, and in some cases exclude biopsy (e.g. hyperthyroidism).

Treatment

Surgical excision of the affected node(s).

Prognosis

Complete resolution reported for all cats.

Local edema for several weeks may occur post-operatively.

JUVENILE STREPTOCOCCAL LYMPHADENITIS

Classical signs

- Kittens.
- Fever.
- Cervical lymphadenopathy.

Pathogenesis

Streptococcus canis (**Group G β-hemolytic strepto-cocci**) may cause a variety of infections in cats including bacteremia, wound sepsis, pyoderma/cellulitis, pyothorax, pneumonia, urogenital infections, arthritis, discospondylitis, acute neonatal death, and fading kittens.

In **3–7-month-old kittens, streptococcal lymphadenitis** may occur.
- The organism colonizes the tonsils (pharyngeal trauma is not necessary) and then disseminates along lymphatics to the lymph nodes of the head and neck.

In mature cats **necrotizing fasciitis** has been reported. The pathogenesis of increased streptococcal virulence is not known.

In dogs, the use of fluoquinolones has been incriminated as a risk factor for streptococcal infections.

Clinical signs

Juvenile lymphadenitis is characterized by **acute fever, lethargy and inappetence**.
- **Marked unilateral or bilateral cervical lymphadenopathy** with or without generalized lymphadenopathy occurs.
- **Single to multiple kittens** in a litter may be affected; they are usually litters from a young queen.

Necrotizing fasciitis in mature cats is characterized by **multifocal ulcerative purulent skin lesions and lymph-adenopathy.** Unlike in other species, **minimal systemic signs** have been noted.

Diagnosis

Lymph node biopsy reveals lymphadenitis with or without abscessation; chains of cocci are seen.

Biopsy of distant nodes reveals hyperplasia.

Culture of organism from lymph nodes, or skin (fasciitis) and tonsil (cervical lymphadenitis).

Differential diagnosis

In the initial febrile phase, **other infections** could mimic juvenile streptococcosis, and lymphadenitis from other organisms could rarely occur. **Acute FeLV/FIV infection** can also cause fever and lymphadenopathy, although cats are not usually as ill and nor is lymphadenopathy as prominent. Differentiation is on the basis of lymph node culture and FeLV/FIV tests.

Differential diagnoses for necrotizing fasciitis include eosinophilic granuloma complex, other chronic bacterial (e.g. nocardiosis) and fungal infections, panniculitis and steatitis. Differentiation is based on cytology, histology and culture.

Treatment

Reported treatments include procaine penicillin 50 000 IU SC once daily, or **procaine and benzathine penicillin** 75 000–100 000 IU (combined dose) q 48–72 hours, or penicillin V 20 mg/kg PO q 8 h, for 5 days. Penicillin G, ampicillin, amoxicillin and amocillin-clavulanate should also be effective.

Lance and irrigate abscesses.

Prognosis

Prognosis is excellent with early treatment.

Untreated cases of juvenile lymphadenitis may progress to **pyothorax, pneumonia and acute death**, likely due to streptococcal toxic shock syndrome.

Transmission

Streptococci do not live in the environment; the **source of infection is other cats** harboring streptococci in a carrier state.

Juvenile streptococcal lymphadenitis is **usually a cattery problem**, with concurrent neonatal infections.

- **Vaginal colonization in young nulliparous queens** is the **main source of neonatal infection;** older queens eliminate the infection and pass colostral antibodies to their young.
- Epidemics may occur following introduction of an **infected queen or tom** (preputial colonization) into a naïve cattery.

Transmission with juvenile lymphadenitis is presumably from **oral to oral contact** (e.g. grooming) with carrier cats with pharyngeal/tonsillar colonization.

Prevention

The **carrier state cannot be eliminated by antibiotic therapy**. While short-term penicillin treatment of queens at parturition will reduce neonatal mortality, chronic treatment in a cattery as prophylaxis against juvenile infections is not recommended as this will promote resistant organisms. As herd immunity increases, epidemics will resolve.

POST-VACCINAL LYMPHADENOPATHY

> **Classical signs**
>
> - Mild incidental lymphadenopathy.
> - History of recent vaccination.

Clinical signs

Mild generalized lymphadenopathy or local lymphadenopathy draining the vaccination site may be noted for **several weeks post-vaccination**.

Diagnosis

History of vaccination and no other clinical signs.

Lymph node biopsy reveals hyperplasia.

NON-CUTANEOUS IMMUNOLOGIC/ INFLAMMATORY DISORDERS

> **Classical signs**
>
> - Signs of polyarthritis.
> - Signs of systemic lupus erthematosus.
> - Signs of lymphocytic cholangitis.

Clinical signs

Lymphadenopathy may be present but is not the salient feature of **chronic progressive polyarthritis**.

Lymphadenopathy is one of the "minor signs" of **systemic lupus erythematosis**.

Lymphadenopathy was present in a series of cats with progressive **lymphocytic cholangitis**.

Diagnosis

- Work-up of the primary disease.
- Lymph node biopsy reveals hyperplasia.

HYPEREOSINOPHILIC SYNDROME

> **Classical signs**
>
> - Lethargy, inappetence, weight loss, vomiting, diarrhea.

See main reference page 758.

Clinical signs

Most cats are presented for chronic lethargy, inappetence, weight loss, vomiting and diarrhea.

Other clinical signs include fever, pruritus and seizures.

Abdominal palpation may reveal thickened intestines, mesenteric lymphadenopathy and hepatosplenomegaly.

Peripheral lymphadenopathy is present infrequently.

Diagnosis

Marked mature eosinophilia, increased synchronous eosinopoiesis on bone marrow biopsy, and exclusion of other causes of eosinophilia.

Lymph node biopsy reveals hyperplasia with or without eosinophilic infiltration.

BACTEREMIA

> **Classical signs**
>
> - Fever, lethargy, inappetence.

Clinical signs

Lymphadenopathy is not usually present in acute bacteremia or endotoxemia due to conventional Gram-negative (e.g. *Escherichia coli*), Gram-positive (e.g. *Staphylococcus* sp.) and anaerobic (e.g. *Clostridium perfringens*) organisms unless lymphadenitis occurs.

Mild–moderate generalized lymphadenopathy may be present with **chronic bacteremia** regardless of origin.

Diagnosis

Documenting infection and identifying the site may require routine laboratory tests, imaging, and blood, urine and lymph node cultures.

Lymph node biopsy reveals hyperplasia or lymphadenitis.

MYCOPLASMA AND L-FORM INFECTIONS

Classical signs

- Chronic limb wound and lameness.
- ± Local or regional lymphadenopathy.

Clinical signs

Non-healing bite wound (cellulitis) and **lameness** due to (poly)**arthritis/synovitis**.

Local or regional lymphadenopathy may be present.

Diagnosis

Cytology of skin lesions or joint fluid lesions reveals **suppurative inflammation but no organisms**.

Lymph node biopsy reveals hyperplasia or lymphadenitis.

Culture of organism is necessary for a definitive diagnosis. Culture requires special transport and culture media – contact the laboratory prior to submitting specimen.

Response to a tetracycline or a fluoroquinolone gives a presumptive diagnosis. Failure to respond does not rule-out the diagnosis.

EHRLICHIOSIS

Classical signs

- Lethargy, inappetence, weight loss.
- ± Lymphadenopathy.

Clinical signs

Most cats have lethargy, inappetence and weight loss.

Other signs variably present include fever, anemia, hyperesthesia, arthralgia, irritable disposition, lymphadenopathy and splenomegaly.

Diagnosis

Variable laboratory findings include **non-regenerative anemia**, neutropenia, neutrophilia, lymphopenia, lymphocytosis, monocytosis, thrombocytopenia and hyperproteinemia due to polyclonal gammopathy.

Lymph node biopsy reveals hyperplasia.

A positive FA test for antibodies against *Ehrlichia canis* and *Ehrlichia risticii* or positive PCR test for ehrlichial DNA is diagnostic of infection. Preliminary evidence suggests that cats may be PCR positive but FA negative.

Resolution of clinical signs with treatment with tetracyclines.

BARTONELLOSIS

Classical signs

- Asymptomatic cats.
- ± Lymphadenopathy.

See main reference page 530 (The Anemic Cat).

Clinical signs

Cats usually harbor ***Bartonella henselae***, the main causative agent of human cat-scratch disease, without clinical signs.

Mild popliteal lymphadenopathy occurs during acute experimental infection.

Lymph nodes are normal during chronic experimental infection.

Bacteria resembling *B. henselae* have been seen in some clinical cases with moderate to marked lymphadenopathy due to **atypical hyperplasia**.

Diagnosis

Lymph node biopsy reveals **follicular hyperplasia** in grossly normal lymph nodes during chronic experimental infection.

Silver staining of lymph nodes of cats with lymphadenopathy may reveal bacteria. In such cases blood culture and/or serologic testing and/or PCR testing for *B. henselae* should be performed.

PROTOTHECOSIS

> ### Classical signs
> - Firm cutaneous nodule on foot.

Clinical signs

Large firm **cutaneous nodule(s)**, which may be ulcerated, on foot, limb, head or base of tail. Nodules are not painful on palpation, but may cause discomfort and other signs from local mass effect.

Local lymph node is usually normal.

No systemic signs.

Diagnosis

Cytology and histology of biopsy specimens reveal granulomatous inflammation.

Lymph node biopsy may reveal hyperplasia or lymphadenitis.

Identification of *Prototheca* sp. (algae), in specimens by cytology, histology or culture.
- Mature organisms are round, have a hyaline cell wall, small central nucleus, may show internal cleavage into endospores, and vary from smaller to larger than neutrophils.

CYTAUXZOONOSIS

> ### Classical signs
> - Fulminant disease with fever and hemolytic anemia.

See main reference page 389 (The Pyrexic Cat).

Clinical signs

Acute onset of fever, lethargy, inappetence, dyspnea, **anemia** and **jaundice**.

Lymphadenopathy is usually identified at necropsy.

Diagnosis

Exposure history (tick exposure in south-central or south-eastern North America).

Identification of the protozoan, *Cytauxzoon felis*, **on red cells**, as tiny dot, tetrad, safety-pin or signet ring forms.

Lymph node histology reveals hemorrhage and edema.

ANTHRAX

> ### Classical signs
> - Edema of the head and neck.
> - Acute death with no promontory signs.

Clinical signs

Rare – cats are resistant to anthrax.

Lingual and pharyngeal edema cause oral serosanguineous discharge and dyspnea.

Cervical regional lymphadenopathy due to edema, hemorrhage and necrosis may occur.

In one case acute death occurred with no promontory signs and there were no significant necropsy findings other than congested lungs and unclotted blood.

Diagnosis

History of **ingesting potentially contaminated raw meat or animal by-products**.

Do not perform necropsy if anthrax suspected.

Identification of a large bacillus on stained blood smear from marginal ear vein or other peripheral vein, or on stained smear from aspiration biopsy of tissue.

Culture of *Bacillus anthracis* from aspirated material.

AMERICAN TRYPANOSOMIASIS

> **Classical signs**
> - Acute and chronic right-sided heart failure.

Clinical signs

The cat is susceptible to infection in South America and may act as a reservoir host.

Clinical disease has not been formally described but is stated to be similar to dogs.

Generalized lymphadenopathy is present during acute infection in dogs, in addition to signs due to **myocarditis** (acute death, collapse, hypothermia, pale mucous membranes, weak pulses, arrhythmias, dyspnea).

Diagnosis

Diagnosis is based on exposure history (*Triatomae* [kissing bugs] vectors), clinical signs, serologic testing for antibodies to *Trypanosoma cruzi*, and identification of trypomastigotes in buffy coat smears.

AFRICAN TRYPANOSOMIASIS

> **Classical signs**
> - Fulminant disease resembling overwhelming sepsis.

Clinical signs

Fever, generalized edema, purulent nasal and ocular discharges, signs of disseminated intravascular coagulation, lymphadenopathy, splenomegaly and neurologic signs.

Diagnosis

Exposure history (*Glossina* spp. **[tsetse flies]** vectors), clinical signs, serologic testing for antibodies to *Trypanasoma* sp.

The cat is highly susceptible to experimental infection with certain African *Trypanasoma* sp., but natural infection is rarely encountered clinically.

TOXOPLASMOSIS

> **Classical signs**
> - Anorexia, fever, dyspnea and signs of ocular inflammation in mature cats.
> - Fading neonate.

See main reference on page 432 for details (The Yellow Cat or Cat With Elevated Liver Enzymes), page 375 (The Pyrexic Cat).

Clinical signs

Common signs include **fever, uveitis, dyspnea** (pneumonia), **vomiting, diarrhea, icterus** (hepatitis and hepatic necrosis), **mesenteric lymphadenopathy, muscle pain** and **neurologic signs**.

Generalized peripheral lymphadenopathy may be present, which is due to reactive lymphoid hyperplasia and not *Toxoplasma*-induced lymphadenitis.

Diagnosis

Acute systemic toxoplasmosis typically affects kittens, or immunosuppressed cats, which usually have a history of chronic disease.

Confirmation is **by measuring serum IgM antibodies or** demonstrating **rising serum IgG antibodies.**

The organism occasionally may be seen in airway wash cytology of cats with pneumonia.

Peripheral lymph node biopsy may reveal hyperplasia. Mesenteric lymph node biopsy may reveal necrosis.

RECOMMENDED READING

Greene CE (ed) Infectious Diseases of the Dog and Cat, 2nd edn. London, W.B. Saunders Company, 1998.

Lucke VM, Davies JD, Wood CM, Whitbread TJ. Plexiform vascularization of lymph nodes: An unusual but distinctive lymphadenopathy in cats. J Comp Path 1987; 97: 109–119.

Mooney SC, Patnaik AK, Hayes AA, MacEwen EG. Generalized lymphadenopathy resembling lymphoma in cats: Six cases (1972–1976). J Am Vet Med Assoc 1987; 190: 897–900.

Moore FM, Emerson WE, Cotter SM, DeLellis RA. Distinctive peripheral lymph node hyperplasia of young cats. Vet Pathol 1986; 23: 386–391.

Teske E, Van Straten G, Van Noort R, Rutteman GR. Chemotherapy with cyclophosphamide, vincristine, and prednisolone (COP) in cats with malignant lymphoma: new results with an old protocol. J Vet Intern Med 2002; 16: 179–186.

Walton RM, Hendrick MJ. Feline Hodgkin's-like lymphoma: 20 cases (1992–1999). Vet Pathol 2001; 38: 504–511.

21. The yellow cat or cat with elevated liver enzymes

Albert E Jergens

> ## KEY SIGNS
> - Jaundiced cat.

MECHANISM?

- Jaundice occurs when serum bilirubin values exceed 2.0 mg/dl.
  Jaundice results from either increased erythrocyte hemolysis or hepatobiliary disease.

WHERE?

- **Pre-hepatic** (hemolytic processes), **hepatic** (parenchymal disease), or **post-hepatic** (extra-hepatic biliary obstruction).

WHAT?

- Most cats with jaundice have hepatic lipidosis, cholangiohepatitis syndrome (CHS), or extrahepatic biliary obstruction (EHBO).
  Non-jaundiced cats with elevated liver enzymes may or may not have liver disease. The degree of dysfunction is assessed by bile acid analysis and the cause determined by liver cytology and/or biopsy if indicated.

QUICK REFERENCE SUMMARY

Diseases causing a yellow cat or cat with elevated liver enzymes

PRE-HEPATIC

- Hemolytic processes causing clinical signs are usually associated with PCV < 18%.

INFLAMMATION

INFECTION

- ***Mycoplasma haemofelis *(Hemobartonella felis)* (p 424)***
  Bacterial (Mycoplasma) parasite which infects red blood cells and causes RBC destruction.
  Jaundice, lethargy, inappetance and occasional vomiting.

continued

continued

IMMUNE

- Immune-mediated anemia (p 424)

Jaundice, lethargy, inappetance, occasional vomiting, and respiratory distress with severe anemia.

HEPATIC

- Jaundice caused by primary hepatic parenchymal diseases.

DEGENERATIVE

- Cirrhosis (p 435)

Rare and usually follows severe chronic hepatopathy. Jaundice, anorexia, weight loss and/or hepatomegaly.

METABOLIC

- Diabetes mellitus (p 436)

Polyuria, polydipsia, increased appetite, weight loss, plantigrade stance with neuropathy.

- Hyperthyroidism (p 437)

Generally seen in cats greater than 8 years old. Often have an increased appetite, weight loss, poor hair coat, vomiting.

- **Hepatic lipidosis*** (p 425)**

Often previous history of obesity and/or anorexia. Jaundice, weight loss, and anorexia are common.

NEOPLASTIC

- **Lymphosarcoma* (p 431)**

Usually a manifestation of multicentric lymphosarcoma. Jaundice, anorexia, weight loss, vomiting and/or diarrhea.

- Non-hematopoietic liver tumors (biliary cyst adenoma, hepatocellular carcinoma) (p 436)

Vast majority are benign tumors seen in old cats. Anorexia, lethargy, and weight loss predominate.

INFLAMMATION

- **Feline cholangitis (cholangitis/cholangiohepatitis syndrome)*** (p 427)**

The neutrophilic form is seen most commonly in male cats. It may be associated with other inflammatory disorders (IBD, pancreatitis) concurrently affecting the gastrointestinal tract. It occurs as an acute phase associated with signs of systemic illness such as fever, anorexia, lethargy, vomiting and jaundice. Signs in the chronic phase are milder and weight loss dominates. The lymphocytic form is associated with jaundice, hepatomegaly, vomiting, diarrhea and/or ascites.

INFECTIOUS

Mycotic:

● Histoplasmosis (p 438)
Of regional significance in the central US. Seen primarily in young cats with depression, weight loss, fever and anorexia. Dyspnea, tachypnea and abnormal lung sounds seen in 50% of cats.

Viral:

● **Feline infectious peritonitis (FIP)* (p 430)**
Progressive anorexia, weight loss, jaundice, fever and/or ascites with effusive forms of disease.

● **Feline leukemia virus* (p 437)**
May cause pre-hepatic jaundice, immunosuppression and/or lymphosarcoma. Salient signs include mucus membrane pallor, anorexia, weight loss, lymphadenopathy and/or jaundice.

Protozoan:

● **Toxoplasmosis* (p 432)**
Jaundice, cyclical fever, and anterior uveitis are commonly observed. Dyspnea and central nervous system signs may or may not occur concurrently.

Toxic:

● Acetaminophen (paracetamol) toxicity (p 433)
Acetaminophen toxicity causes cyanosis, dyspnea and facial edema.

● Diazepam toxicity (p 434)
Diazepam toxicity causes anorexia, depression and jaundice.

POST-HEPATIC

Jaundice caused by decreased or impaired biliary excretion.

Mechanical:

● **Extrahepatic biliary obstruction (EHBO)** (p 439)**
May be caused by pancreatic diseases, neoplasia or extrinsic compression. Jaundice, anorexia, weight loss, vomiting and abdominal pain seen with pancreatitis.

Inflammation:

● **Pancreatitis** (p 439)**
Anorexia, lethargy and abdominal pain predominate. Jaundice may occur several days after mild signs.

● Cholecystitis (p 440)
Uncommonly recognized, but may cause abdominal pain, fever, vomiting and jaundice.

Trauma:

● Ruptured bile duct (p 441)
Low-grade abdominal pain, malaise, weight loss and/or effusion.

INTRODUCTION

MECHANISM?

Jaundice results when serum bilirubin is increased above 2 mg/ml.

Most bilirubin originates from senescent erythrocytes and is processed in the liver for excretion in the bile.

Jaundice results from either increased erythrocyte hemolysis, which exceeds the processing capacity of the liver, or hepatobiliary disease.

WHERE?

Pre-hepatic jaundice is due to hemolytic processes. Erythrocyte hemolysis causes release of increased heme pigments, which overwhelm hepatic processing/excretion of bilirubin.

Hepatic jaundice is seen with severe diffuse hepatic cholestasis (via inflammation) or major bile duct obstruction. Inflammation in portal or periportal areas causes jaundice early in the disease course; whereas, parenchymal injury away from periportal areas results in jaundice development late in the disease course.

Post-hepatic jaundice is caused by intraluminal or extraluminal disorders that mechanically occlude the biliary tree (e.g., gall bladder and common bile duct).

Post-hepatic (extrahepatic biliary obstruction).

WHAT?

Pre-hepatic causes for jaundice are primarily attributable to erythrocyte parasitemia (hemobartellosis), infectious disease (FeLV), and immune-mediated hemolysis (rare).

Hepatic causes for jaundice may be caused by hepatic lipidosis, cholangiohepatitis syndrome and hepatic lymphosarcoma.

Post-hepatic causes for jaundice are caused by pancreatitis and neoplasms involving the gallbladder and biliary tree (less common).

Non-jaundiced cats with elevated liver enzymes may or may not have significant hepatic disease. An underlying defect in bilirubin metabolism affecting conjugation reactions or cytosolic pigment transport

or storage is suspected. This phenomena is observed with a variety of non-hepatic primary disorders (e.g., renal and gastrointestinal diseases) which may cause these cats to later develop primary liver disease. Bile acid analysis determines hepatic function and the need to obtain cytologic/biopsy specimens for definitive diagnosis.

INCREASED BILIRUBIN PRODUCTION (PRE-HEPATIC CAUSES OF JAUNDICE OR INCREASE\D LIVER ENZYMES)

MYCOPLASMA HAEMOFELIS (HEMOBARTONELLA FELIS)* IMMUNE-MEDIATED ANEMIA

> **Classical signs**
>
> - Pale mucus membranes, PCV usually < 18%; hemoglobin < 10 g/dl.
> - Lethargy, in appetence, and anorexia may be observed.
> - +/− fever.
> - Occasional vomiting.

See main reference on page 530 for details (The Anemic Cat).

Pathogenesis

Rapid destruction of red cells exceeds the liver's capacity to metabolize increased hemoglobin breakdown products (bilirubin).

Most commonly associated with *Mycoplasma haemofelis* infection and less commonly with immune-mediated anemia. Hemolysis may also be caused by feline leukemia viral (FeLV) infection.

Pre-hepatic causes for jaundice in the cat are uncommon.

Clinical signs

Pale mucus membranes, PCV< 18% and often 12–15%; hemoglobin < 10 g/dl.

Lethargy, inappetance, anorexia.

+/– fever and vomiting.

Lymphadenopathy, or skin, respiratory, and gastro-intestinal infections secondary to immunosuppression are seen with FeLV infection.

Diagnosis

Typically anemia is moderate to severe (PCV 12–17%) with a reduced hemoglobin < 10 g/dl.

Examine blood smears closely with a reduced PCV for presence of red cell parasites (hemobartonellosis).

Saline agglutination and direct Coomb's tests confirm immune-mediated anemia but the Coomb's test requires feline specific antibody to be meaningful.

Liver enzymes (ALT, ALP) are often normal or insignificantly elevated.

Serologic testing (ELISA or fluorescent antibody) for FeLV infection.

Polymerase chain reaction assays may be of great benefit in documenting infection if available.

Differential diagnosis

Hepatic and post-hepatic disorders are often chronic diseases and are associated with some anemia. In these instances, the anemia is mild (PCV of 18–27%), non-regenerative and is attributable to anemia of chronic disease.

Hemolytic anemia is usually regenerative unless it is detected early (< 4 days) or if stem cells are involved; as may occur with *Mycoplasma haemofelis* infection or immune-mediated red cell destruction.

Hemolytic anemia associated with FeLV infection may or may not be regenerative.

Treatment

Supportive care and antibiotics (doxycycline 5 mg/kg PO q 12 h for 21 days or enrofloxacin 5 mg/kg PO q 12 h for 7–14 days) for cats with hemobartonellosis.

Whole blood/packed red cell transfusions, cortico-steroids (prednisone 1–2 mg/kg PO q 12 h as needed), and supportive care for immune-mediated anemia. Clinical parameters which suggest the need for transfu-

sion include increased heart and respiratory rates which usually occur when the PCV < 15–18% for acute loss and < 12% for more chronic loss. See page 531 (The Anemic Cat).

Antivirals and immunotherapy for FeLV infection.

HEPATOCELLULAR DISEASES (JAUNDICE OR INCREASED LIVER ENZYMES CAUSED BY HEPATIC PARENCHYMAL DISEASES)

HEPATIC LIPIDOSIS***

Classical signs

- Obese anorectic female cats are predisposed.
- Progressive anorexia, vomiting, and diarrhea are common.
- Severe jaundice and hepatomegaly are present.

Pathogenesis

The etiopathogenesis is poorly understood and ill-defined.

Triglycerides accumulate in the liver as a consequence of imbalanced fat metabolism which is likely multifactorial in origin. These imbalances may include uptake of fatty acids, use of fatty acids for energy (e.g., ketone production and fatty acid oxidation), production and dispersal of lipoproteins throughout the body, and de novo synthesis of triglycerides. Many metabolic conditions, nutritional factors, drugs and toxins can cause excessive hepatic fat accumulation (see below). Approximately 50% of cats have idiopathic (primary) hepatic lipidosis in which no underlying medical condition is detected.

- History of previous obesity is observed in nearly all cats.
- Anorexia or rapid weight reduction contributes to hepatic fat accumulation. Anorexia may be preceded by a stressful event such as a move to a new house.
- Imbalanced nutrition using caloric- or protein-restricted diets, especially if unpalatable, can trigger marked weight loss. Experimentally, dietary

energy must be restricted 50–75% for at least 2 weeks to induce hepatic lipidosis.

- Hepatic lipidosis occurs either as a primary idiopathic event or secondary to another disease process. Frequently it occurs secondary to underlying diseases, most commonly cholangiohepatitis, inflammatory bowel disease, and acute or chronic pancreatitis. A recent study for 30% of cats had acute pancreatitis.
- Acquired carnitine deficiency may be related to the development of hepatic lipidosis. Carnitine is primarily synthesized in the liver and is essential for enzyme-mediated uptake of fatty acids into mitochondria. In health, it also facilitates fatty acid product transport and the oxidation of long-chain fatty acids. Starved cats have diminished capacity for fatty acid beta-oxidation or export of VLDL, leading to hepatic triglyceride sequestration.
- Less commonly observed in association with diabetes mellitus and toxicity (e.g., aflatoxins, bacterial toxins).

Fat accumulation in hepatocytes results in cholestasis and hepatic jaundice.

Progressive liver dysfunction causes anorexia, vomiting and dehydration.

Signs of overt hepatic encephalopathy (ptyalism, seizures) are uncommon.

Clinical signs

Most commonly seen in middle-aged to older cats of either sex. There is no breed predisposition.

The most common early signs are progressive anorexia and depression with intermittent vomiting over several weeks.

Common presenting complaints include, weight loss, prolonged (> 2 weeks) anorexia, vomiting and lethargy.

Jaundice, hepatomegaly and dehydration are detected on physical examination.

Ascites, fever and ptyalism are uncommon.

Diagnosis

Cytologic examination of hepatic parenchyma obtained via fine-needle aspirate, or histologic examination of a liver biopsy specimen is usually diagnostic for hepatic lipidosis. Histologic confirmation is the preferred modality, as recent reports have noted poor correlation between cytologic interpretation and histologic findings in cats with liver disease.

Histopathologic confirmation requires specialized processing to assess.

- Both hematoxylin/eosin and specific staining for fat should be performed.
- Greater than 50% of hepatocytes contain lipid vacuolation.

Abdominal ultrasonography may suggest hepatic lipidosis versus extrahepatic biliary obstruction, cholangiohepatitis and neoplasia.

- Cats with hepatic lipidosis have diffuse hyperechogenicity, hepatomegaly, and an absence of biliary tract abnormalities.

Non-regenerative anemia is seen in 30% of cats.

Biochemical liver parameters are often suggestive of hepatic lipidosis.

- Marked but discrepant increases of serum ALP in comparison to ALT and AST.
- Total bilirubin values exceed 2 mg/dl as most cats are severely jaundiced.

Approximately 30% of cats are hypokalemic.

Abnormal coagulation tests are observed in > 50% of cats. Approximately 20% have clinical evidence of excessive bleeding. Vitamin K deficiency is the most common coagulation abnormality.

- Carefully appraise coagulation status prior to liver aspirate or biopsy.

Differential diagnosis

Cats with inflammatory liver disease (cholangiohepatitis) are often febrile and may have ascites. Increased ALT +/− AST and hyperglobulinemia are prominent features in these cats and are not observed in cats with hepatic lipidosis.

Sonographic abnormalities to the biliary excretory pathway or hepatic parenchyma are evident in most cats with extrahepatic biliary obstruction and neoplasia, respectively.

Treatment

Cats must be fed 65–90 kcal/kg/day until eating.

- Gastrostomy or jejunostomy tube alimentation with high-energy commercial enteral diets is necessary if vomiting is frequent.
- Esophagostomy tubes can be used when vomiting is not frequent, and may be simpler and safer to place than gastrostomy tubes.
- Nasoesophageal tubes are indicated in cats too ill for a gastrostomy tube.
- They are often used for short-term support until placement of gastrostomy tube.
- Nasoesophageal and some esophageal tubes require liquified commercial diets (Iams Nutritional Recovery Formula, Clinicare, or Hill's A/d mixed with water).
- It takes several days before the caloric requirements can be fed in 3–4 meals per day without inducing vomiting. Initially small volumes, e.g., 5 ml, should be fed every 2 hours, and the volume is increased while reducing the frequency over several days. Alternatively, feeding can begin with a constant rate infusion over 24 hours using a syringe infusion pump with the volume increased gradually until the daily caloric requirements are met. Cats can then be transitioned to bolus feeding four times daily. Tubes should be left in place until the cat is voluntarily eating its full caloric requirements for 2 weeks and has a stable and increasing weight.

Avoid benzodiazipines as they are inadequate to stimulate appetite and may aggravate CNS signs.

Vomiting is controlled with metoclopramide (0.2–0.5 mg/kg q 8 h or using a constant rate infusion 1–2 mg/cat/24 h). Two periods of exercise totaling 45–60 min/day help reduce vomiting and high gastric residual volumes. This can be accomplished by letting the cat free in a consulting room, preferably with a window.

Correct dehydration and electrolyte imbalances with fluid therapy.

- Monitor serum potassium and phosphorous and supplement with KCl and potassium dihydrophosphate as needed to combat hypokalemia and hypophosphatemia.

Ursodeoxycholic acid (10–15 mg PO q 24 h) for intrahepatic cholestasis.

Vitamin K_1 is often given (3–5 mg per cat q 12 h initially) due to the frequency of coagulation disturbances.

Thiamine supplementation (100 mg of thiamine hydrochloride, q 12 h by oral, subcutaneous or IM routes) is generally advised.

The potential value of carnitine (1250 mg L-carnitine/cat q 24 h) and taurine (250–500 mg q 24 h) supplementation has not been critically assessed but is unlikely to be harmful.

Prognosis

Survival rates are up to 60% with aggressive therapy.

Evaluate closely for concomitant diseases (pancreatitis) as they warrant a more guarded prognosis.

Prevention

It is important to use sensible restriction diets for obese cats. Feed 60–75% of maintenance requirements (60 kcal/kg) to promote slow but steady weight loss. Food intake should be adjusted monthly for the individual cat to produce a weight loss of 1–2% per week.

- A variety of commercial, nutritionally balanced but reduced caloric rations are available.

FELINE CHOLANGITIS (CHOLANGITIS/ CHOLANGIOHEPATITIS SYNDROME)***

Classical signs

- Anorexia, weight loss, and vomiting.
- Jaundice, +/− fever, +/− ascites.
- Often palpable hepatomegaly.

Pathogenesis

Cholangitis is the cause of jaundice in 30% of cats.

Etiology is unknown but may involve causative factors such as bacterial infection. The different forms of cholangitis **may** represent different stages of the same disease process. One hypothesis suggests that the unique anatomic relationship in which the bile duct and major pancreatic duct form a short common duct entering the duodenum may predispose cats to inflammatory hepatic disease. This connection might favor the ascension of luminal bacteria or the entrance of pancreatic enzymes into the biliary tract. Supporting this theory is the observation that inflammatory disease of other alimentary organs, such as pancreatitis and inflammatory bowel disease, are associated with cholangitis.

A new classification scheme by the World Small Animal Veterinary Association Liver Diseases and Pathology Standardisation Research Group recognizes three distinct forms of cholangitis in cats.

In the traditional classification scheme, cholangitis denoted inflammation of the biliary tree and cholangiohepatitis referred to inflammation around bile ducts and peribiliary hepatocytes.

However, with the new classification scheme, the term cholangitis is used in preference to cholangiohepatitis, because inflammatory disruption of the limiting plate to involve hepatic parenchyma is not always a feature and, when present, is an extension of a primary cholangitis, and inflammation is centered on intrahepatic bile ducts.

Three separate syndromes occur as defined by clinical and histologic criteria: **neutrophilic cholangitis, lymphocytic cholangitis and chronic cholangitis**.

Cirrhosis may occur as an end-stage of cholangitis but is rare.
- The lymphocytic form is more common than the neutrophilic form of cholangitis in the UK and Australia, but the neutrophilic form appears to be the most common form in some other locations.

Neutrophilic cholangitis.
- This is usually referable to ascending bacterial infection but is also rarely reported in protozoal infections. *E. coli* is sometimes cultured from the bile, and occasionally Gram-positive anaerobes are cultured.
- **Two phases of neutrophilic cholangitis** are recognized; an acute phase and a chronic phase.

Neutrophilic cholangitis – Acute phase.
- Neutrophils are within walls and lumina of intrahepatic bile ducts and within portal areas. Bile duct epithelial degeneration and necrosis is present. There is variable extension of inflammation through the limiting plate to involve periportal parenchyma. Bacteria may be visible. There is usually minimal biliary hyperplasia or periductal fibrosis.
- Generally, there is an acute onset of signs with marked systemic illness (fever, anorexia, lethargy, vomiting).

Neutrophilic cholangitis – Chronic phase.
- Mild to severe infiltration of portal areas by plasma cells, lymphocytes and neutrophils, without or without macrophages is present. Leukocytes are within walls and/or lumina of bile ducts, and are associated with biliary epithelial degeneration or necrosis. Lymphoid aggregates may be present in portal areas. Biliary hyperplasia, periductal fibrosis or bridging portal fibrosis may be present.
- It is usually associated with partial or complete biliary obstructive lesions resulting in cholestasis.
- Signs and liver enzyme elevations tend to be milder than with the acute neutrophilic phase, and reflect a smoldering inflammatory hepatic disease. Weight loss is a dominant sign. Signs may wax and wane. Jaundice may or may not be present. Ascites is not a feature of the acute or chronic phase. In general, the chronic phase appears less common than the acute phase.

Lymphocytic cholangitis.
- Lymphocytic cholangitis is postulated to be immune-mediated in origin.
- Histologically there is moderate to marked infiltration of portal areas by small lymphocytes. With chronicity, the intensity of portal infiltration tends to abate. Lymphocytic infiltrates may also be present that are centered on and infiltrating walls of bile ducts, but this is an inconsistent feature, especially in the chronic phase. Inflammation may or may not extend into the periportal parenchyma. Histologic evidence of intrahepatic cholestasis may be present.
- It occurs primarily in middle-aged cats with chronic (> 3 weeks) signs. Recurrent episodes of clinical signs are often interspersed with weeks or months of normalcy, with a normal or even increased appetite.
- Cats are often less ill than with the acute neutrophilic form, and may have ascites.

Chronic cholangitis associated with liver fluke infestation.
- Lesions result from infection by liver flukes such as *Amphimerus pseudofelineus*, (*Opisthorchis pseudofelineus*), *Opisthorchis tenuicollis*, *Metorchis albidus*, *M. conjunctus* (*M. complexus*), *Platynosomum concinnum* (*page fastosum*).

Clinical signs

Often observed in middle-aged cats.

Intermittent episodes of inappetance or anorexia and lethargy.

Weight loss.

Fever occurs with neutrophilic cholangitis.

Ascites is sometimes observed with lymphocytic cholangitis. Ascitic fluid had a high total protein content attributable primarily to globulins.

Jaundice +/– hepatomegaly occur with both types.

Diagnosis

Definitive diagnosis requires histologic evaluation of liver biopsy specimens.
- Tissues may be obtained via ultrasound-guided percutaneous biopsy, laparoscopically or by laparotomy. However, 18-gauge needle biopsies are less reliable than wedge biopsies. In one study, less than 60% of cats with cholangitis had needle biopsy results that were in accordance with the diagnoses based on the wedge biopsy.
- Perform coagulation tests (ACT or APTT/OSPT or PIVKA) prior to hepatic biopsy. Initiate vitamin K_1 therapy if abnormal (see dosage below).

Bile and liver culture are recommended in cats with suspected neutrophilic cholangitis.

Survey abdominal radiographs are usually normal but are useful to confirm hepatomegaly and the presence of peritoneal effusion. Abdominal sonography shows biliary tract thickening and distention (neutrophilic cholangitis) or increased parenchymal echogenicity (lymphocytic cholangitis).

Biochemical liver parameters show high ALT, ALP and total bilirubin concentrations. Total bilirubin concentrations may increase 2–10 times normal values, with ALT concentration increased to a greater extent relative to ALP.

Increased plasma globulin and decreased albumin are often present in the lymphocytic form.

Leukocytosis may be present in suppurative form.

Biliary obstruction should be suspected in cats with lethargy, intermittent fever and progressive jaundice. These cats will require surgical correction for obstructive jaundice.

Differential diagnosis

Cholangitis produces greater increases of serum ALT as compared to HL.
- Cats with lymphocytic cholangitis may have concurrent inflammation involving pancreatic, intestinal and renal tissues.

Fever and ascites are common with cholangitis but are not observed with HL.

Cats with HL have higher ALP activity as compared to cholangitis-affected cats.

Feline infectious peritonitis (FIP) may appear similar to the lymphocytic form, particularly if there is ascitic fluid with a high protein content. The syndromes clinically look similar, although fever is more common with FIP. Liver biopsy, especially a wedge section, is usually diagnostic.

Treatment

Specific treatment is dictated by results of hepatic biopsy.

Neutrophilic cholangitis.
- Empiric antibiotic choices are amoxicillin (22 mg/kg PO q 12 h) and metronidazole (10 mg/kg PO q 12 h) or enrofloxacin (2.2 mg/kg bid PO) until bile culture results are known.
- Continue antibiotic therapy for 6–8 weeks.
- Ursodeoxycholic acid (10–15 mg/kg PO q 24 h) may be useful for choleresis following correction of biliary obstruction.
- S-adenosylmethionine (20 mg/kg PO q 24 h) is recommended to replenish glutathione stores and scavenge free radicals.
- Surgical correction (biliary diversion) is indicated in cats with clinical signs or imaging features (e.g., distended and tortuous common bile duct, large gall bladder and/or prominent intrahepatic bile ducts) indicative of obstructive biliary tract lesions.

Lymphocytic cholangitis.
- Use immunosuppressive doses of steroids (prednisone 2 mg/kg PO q 24 h) for 4–6 weeks to reduce hepatic inflammation. If a favorable response is observed, then steroids may be tapered at 25% of the dose q 2 weeks as determined by clinical signs, liver enzymes and/or bile acid tests.

- Administer ursodeoxycholic acid for choleresis and modulation of "noxious" bile acids.
- Long-term immunosuppressive therapy (steroids +/– metronidazole) is often required in cats with persistent clinical signs or abnormal laboratory values. Some cats that fail to respond to prednisone may respond to chlorambucil (0.2 mg/kg PO q 48 h).

Supportive care as dictated by the animal's needs.
- Vitamin K_1 for coagulopathy (3–5 mg per cat PO q 24 hours as needed).
- Fluid therapy to combat dehydration and electrolyte disturbances.
- Nutritional therapy is important to reduce the hepatic workload and augment recovery.
  - Jejunostomy or gastrostomy tubes and feeding a pureed commercial or esophagostomy tubes and feeding a commercial liquified diet are best tolerated.
  - Feed a protein-modified diet as dictated by the status of renal function and signs of hepatic encephalopathy (rare).
  - Control vomiting with famotidine (0.2 mg/kg SID PO) or metoclopramide (0.2–0.5 mg/kg q 8 h) or constant rate infusion at 1–2 mg/cat/24 h.

Prognosis

Long-term follow-up on a large number of cats with cholangitis has not been performed.

The prognosis with neutrophilic cholangitis is less favorable than for cats with lymphocytic cholangitis.

Cats with the neutrophilic form that survive the initial treatment period of several months have a reasonable chance for long-term survival.

Cats with lymphocytic cholangitis may survive comfortably for months to years with appropriate therapy.

Prevention

Medical/surgical correction of biliary obstructive lesions when recognized.

Treatment of inflammatory (lymphocytic-plasmacytic) lesions involving the intestinal mucosa (i.e., inflammatory bowel disease).

FELINE INFECTIOUS PERITONITIS (FIP)*

> **Classical signs**
>
> - **50% of cats are < 2 years of age.**
> - **Weight loss, anorexia, vomiting and lethargy.**
> - **Jaundice +/– cyclical fever.**
> - **Protein-rich ascites in "effusive" form.**

See main reference, page 372 (The Pyrexic Cat).

Clinical signs

Young cats (< 2 years old) and from a multicat environment are most susceptible.

Signs are referable to chronic inflammation of the kidneys, liver, visceral lymph nodes, intestines, lungs, eyes and brain.

Chronic, progressive inappetance, weight loss, fever and depression.

Signs may be cyclical at first.

Jaundice and ascites may occur in cats with chronic liver involvement.

Dyspnea from pleural effusion occurs in about one in five cats.

CNS signs include seizures, personality changes, nystagmus, head tremor and hyperesthesia.

Vomiting may occur with granuloma formation in the intestines, or inflammation in other organs such as the liver.

Ocular signs include bilateral uveitis, perivascular exudates, retinal hemorrhage or detachment.

Diagnosis

Diagnosis is based on history, clinical signs and characteristic histologic lesions on tissue biopsy.
- Parenchymal lesions are characterized by multifocal hepatic necrosis with pyogranulomatous inflammation.
- Pyogranulomas may be grossly evident on the capsule of the liver.

Increased activities of ALT and ALP are common. Total bilirubin values may be increased above 2–3 mg/dl (jaundice).

Diagnostic sampling of effusions is useful as they are generally high protein but low to moderate cellularity (modified transudate) with non-lytic neutrophils.

Serologic testing for FIP antibodies may give confounding results. Coronaviral antibodies are widespread in the general cat population and the new 7B FIP antibody test appears to have problems with false negatives and false positives in the field.

- Reverse transcriptase-PCR detection of coronaviral antigens in effusion fluid or tissues presently lacks high diagnostic accuracy. False positives occur because enteric coronavirus may be present systemically, and false-negative results also occur.
- Immunocytochemistry demonstrating coronavirus antigen within circulating monocytes or tissue macrophages appears to be specific, but low numbers of infected cells in tissue samples limit the sensitivity for use in biopsy samples. The technique is only available at some laboratories.

Differential diagnosis

Abdominocentesis in FIP-infected cats may yield a protein-rich exudate which is dissimilar from other inflammatory/degenerative hepatopathies except lymphocytic cholangiohepatitis. Histopathology of the liver is diagnostic. Also, differentiate FIP from cardiomyopathy and neoplasia which may cause chronic illness similar to FIP or cavity effusion.

Cats with FIP will often have involvement of multiple organ systems (eyes, lungs, CNS).

Treatment

There is no definitive therapy for FIP and the disease is almost uniformly fatal in cats with signs.
- Supportive care is palliative at best.
  - Immunosuppressive doses of steroids (2–4 mg/kg PO q 24 h) +/– other cytotoxic drugs (e.g., cyclophosphamide 2.2 mg/kg/day on four consecutive days each week or chlorambucil 20 mg/m² every 2–3 weeks) are recommended for vasculitis.
  - Administer broad-spectrum antimicrobials for secondary bacterial infections.

  - Give human interferon-β 30 IU/day for 7 days at alternate weeks to boost immunity.
  - Nutritional support via force feedings, esophagostomy or gastrostomy tube, or naso-esophageal catheter.
- Because of the extremely poor prognosis, euthanasia is recommended if there is no response to palliative therapy.

LYMPHOSARCOMA*

Classical signs

- **Most cats > 10 years of age.**
- **Lethargy, anorexia, weight loss.**
- **Jaundice may be present.**
- **Hepatomegaly +/– effusion (ascites or hemoperitoneum).**

Pathogenesis

Generally presents as a manifestation of multicentric lymphosarcoma. Lesions may occur in conjunction with neoplastic infiltrates involving other lymphoid organs, such as peripheral lymph nodes, or the alimentary mucosa.

Neoplastic lymphocytes gradually replace normal hepatocytes causing organ enlargement and hepatic failure.
- Cholestasis and jaundice result from involvement of intrahepatic biliary structures.

Clinical signs

Mostly seen in middle-aged and older cats.

Lethargy, anorexia, and weight loss predominate.

Hepatomegaly +/– jaundice are common.

Diagnosis

Suspicion of hepatic neoplasia is raised by older age, history of chronic illness and suggestive clinical signs.

Increased serum ALT and ALP activities are common. In general, relatively greater increases in ALT versus ALP are observed.

Radiographic imaging may aid diagnosis.
- Symmetrical hepatomegaly is often observed on survey radiographs.
- Hepatic sonography shows generalized hyper-echogenicity or multifocal hypoechogenicity to the liver parenchyma.

Definitive diagnosis requires cytologic or histologic evaluation of liver specimens.

Differential diagnosis

Rule out benign conditions, such as hepatic cysts, hepatocellular/bile duct adenomas, and regenerative nodules which may mimic hepatic lymphosarcoma. These other diseases may be definitively ruled out by performance of liver biopsy with histologic interpretation.

Treatment

Combination chemotherapy using cyclophosphamide (300 mg/m^2 PO q 3 weeks), vincristine (0.75 mg/m^2 IV weekly for 4 weeks), and prednisone (2 mg/kg/day) is recommended. See page 676 for treatment details.

Provide supportive therapy (including provision of enteral feeding if needed) as needed.

Prognosis

The prognosis is guarded. Approximately 50% of cats with hepatic lymphosarcoma will respond to multi-drug chemotherapy.

Concurrent FeLV infection shortens survival times but does not influence response to chemotherapy.

TOXOPLASMOSIS*

Classical signs

- Anorexia, lethargy, neurologic signs and dyspnea.
- Cyclical fever.
- +/− icterus, vomiting and diarrhea.
- Anterior or posterior uveitis.

See main reference, page 375 (The Pyrexic Cat).

Clinical signs

Infection with the obligate intracellular coccidia causes inflammation and cell necrosis in affected tissues. Lung, brain, gut, liver and eye are most affected.

Diverse but are generally referable to respiratory, neuromuscular or gastrointestinal systems.

Anorexia, cyclical fever, dyspnea and lethargy are common.

Uveitis may involve one or both eyes.

Cystic involvement of the CNS may cause pronounced neurologic deficits (with the type of observed CNS deficit dependent upon involvement of the brain, brain stem and/or spinal cord), or may be rapidly fatal with advanced disease.

Cysts located within skeletal muscles are painful, and often cause hyperesthesia on muscle palpation, stiffness of gait and shifting leg lameness.

Hepatic involvement may follow dissemination causing jaundice due to hepatitis or cholangiohepatitis. Cystic involvement of the intestinal mucosa may cause lymphocytic-plasmacytic enteritis.

Diagnosis

Non-regenerative anemia and leukopenia.

Marked increases in serum ALT and AST activities occur with hepatic infection.

Hyperproteinemia occurs in some cats with chronic toxoplasmosis.

Thoracic radiographs may demonstrate diffuse interstitial to alveolar opacities.

Serologic testing provides useful diagnostic information.
- IgM and IgG titers are assessed by ELISA techniques.
  - A high (> 256) IgM titer is suggestive of active infection.
  - A 4 × rise in IgG titer over 2–3 weeks is suggestive of active infection.

Demonstration of the organism (cysts) in affected biopsy/necropsy tissues is helpful in making a diagnosis.

Differential diagnosis

Toxoplasmosis should be differentiated from other feline systemic infections including feline leukemia and immunodeficiency viral infections and feline infectious peritonitis.

Treatment

Available drugs suppress replication of *T. gondii* but do not completely kill the parasite.

- Use clindamycin (12.5 mg/kg PO q 12 h) for 3 weeks.
- Cats with ocular inflammation should be judiciously treated with topical glucocorticoids (topical 0.5 % prednisolone acetate drops q 6–12 h).

ACETAMINOPHEN (PARACETAMOL) INTOXICATION

Classical signs

- **Often history of recent drug exposure.**
- **Acute onset of cyanosis, dyspnea and facial edema.**
- **+/− jaundice occurs several days post-ingestion.**

Pathogenesis

Cats have impaired ability to readily metabolize acetaminophen. Ingestion of 50–60 mg/kg may be fatal for cats. This is equivalent to one child tablet or half an adult tablet.

Large doses of acetaminophen produce toxic intermediates which cause oxidative damage in cells, especially erythrocytes and hepatocytes.

- Oxidative damage to hemoglobin leads to methemoglobinemia and reduced oxygen-carrying capacity.
- Tissue hypoxia and vascular injury occur.

Hepatic injury is characterized by hepatocellular necrosis.

Clinical signs

Pale mucous membranes or acute cyanosis with blue-tinged mucous membranes, dyspnea, facial edema, salivation and depression are typical signs of poisoning.

Increasing depression, weakness and panting occur. Increasing harsh lung sounds are secondary to worsening pulmonary edema.

Vomiting and generalized weakness are less common.

Jaundice may occur 3–6 days post-ingestion.

Hemoglobinuria occurs in some cats or a dark brown urine containing increased amounts of hemoglobin, bilirubin and protein may be seen.

Death occurs within 18–36 hours of ingestion of a toxic dose.

Diagnosis

Diagnosis is based on a history of recent drug exposure and the presence of "unique" clinical signs.

Anemia is typically non-regenerative within 4–6 days of intoxication.

- Heinz-bodies may be visualized with new methylene blue stain.
- Increased numbers of nucleated red cells reflecting hypoxemia may be evident.

Neutrophilic leukocytosis reflects stress.

Unexplained and rapid increase in liver biochemical parameters are observed.

- ALT, AST, ALP and total bilirubin concentrations may be elevated.

Histologic examination of hepatic biopsy specimens reveals hepatocellular necrosis, lipid accumulation and/or biliary duct proliferation.

Differential diagnosis

The features of acetaminophen toxicosis (drug exposure classic signs, clinico-pathologic findings and acute hepatic injury) make most other diseases unlikely.

Treatment

Attempt to minimize drug absorption in acute (< 4 hours) intoxications.

- Perform orogastric lavages (several cycles each at 5–10 ml/kg of tepid water) to mechanically remove gastric contents.
- Give activated charcoal (2 g/kg body weight) to bind residual luminal toxicants via orogastric tube.

Fluid therapy may be required to correct dehydration, acid–base imbalances and electrolyte abnormalities occurring from vomiting.

Specific antidotal therapy.
- N-acetylcysteine (Mucomyst, Mead Johnson & Co.) helps to neutralize toxic intermediates.
  - Administer a loading dose of 140 mg/kg orally, followed by doses of 70 mg/kg every 4–6 hours for upto 3 days.
- Ascorbic acid is used in combination with N-acetylcysteine.
  - Its use is controversial. It works slowly and is used as adjunctive therapy.
  - Give 30 mg/kg q 6 h PO for seven or more treatments.
- Cimetidine inhibits hepatic production of toxic intermediates.
  - Give 5 mg/kg q 8 h PO or parenterally for 3 days minimum.

Blood transfusions and oxygen therapy should be given as needed.

Prognosis

The prognosis is guarded and is highly dependent on severity of intoxication and time lapse prior to treatment.

Prevention

Avoid drug overdosage.

Store medication safely away from pets.

DIAZEPAM INTOXICATION

Classical signs

- Lethargy, ataxia and anorexia < 3–4 days post-ingestion.
- Jaundice commonly observed.

Pathogenesis

Idiosyncratic hepatotoxicity is suspected. The dosage causing toxicity may range from 1 mg once daily to 2.5 mg twice daily.

Prior sensitization to diazepam is **not** required.

Clinical signs

Most cats become lethargic, ataxic and anorectic within 96 hours following ingestion.

Jaundice is common and occurs during the first 11 days of illness.

Diagnosis

History of recent drug exposure.

Unexplained and rapid increase in liver biochemical parameters.
- Profound increases in ALT, AST and total bilirubin are present.
- Hypoglycemia/hypocholesterolemia indicates severe hepatic insufficiency.
- Abnormal coagulation tests (OSPT, APTT) suggest disseminated intravascular coagulation.

Death occurs from acute hepatic failure.
- Histologic review of tissue specimens reveals profound hepatocellular necrosis.

Differential diagnosis

A history of diazepam administration associated with fulminate hepatic failure make most other diseases unlikely.

Treatment

Supportive care as dictated by the patient.

Fluid therapy for hydration maintenance.
- Add dextrose to combat hypoglycemia.

Meet nutritional needs to facilitated hepatic regeneration.
- Total parenteral nutrition or nasoesophageal catheter feeding.

Plasma transfusions to replace consumed coagulation factors.

Prognosis

Poor: cats presented in an obtunded condition warrant a grave prognosis.

Prevention

Evaluate baseline ALT and AST activities in cats prior to initiating daily oral treatment with diazepam.

- Retest again 1 week after initiating therapy.
- Discontinue diazepam therapy in cats with unexplained increases in liver enzyme activities.

Peractin is a more effective appetite stimulant, and has not been reported to have serious idiosyncratic reactions.

CIRRHOSIS

Classical signs

- Anorexia, weight loss, lethargy and jaundice.
- Hepatomegaly or a normal-sized liver may be palpated.

Pathogenesis

Cirrhosis is a relatively uncommon disease in the cat but may occur as a progression of specific feline hepatopathies (e.g cholangiohepatitis, chronic biliary obstruction), systemic disorders (e.g., pancreatitis, inflammatory bowel disease, chronic renal disease), and possibly vascular and immune-mediated diseases.

Cirrhosis would appear to occur most frequently with diseases affecting the portal areas, specifically the bile ducts.

Cirrhosis is characterized by both fibrosis and the conversion of normal hepatic architecture into structurally abnormal (regenerative) nodules.

Clinical signs

Anorexia, weight loss and lethargy predominate.

Hepatomegaly and intermittent diarrhea may also be observed.

Ascites is uncommon.

Jaundice is often present.

Diagnosis

Cats usually have a previous diagnosis of chronic hepatopathy, such as cholangitis (cholangitis/cholangiohepatitis).

Liver enzyme activities are variably increased depending upon the relative magnitude of cholestasis or hepatocellular inflammation.

Ultrasound may reveal diffuse parenchymal nodules and an irregular liver margin.

Histologic evaluation of liver biopsy specimens is required for definitive diagnosis.

- Microscopic lesions show both fibrosis and abnormal regenerative nodules.
- Tissues may be obtained by ultrasound-guided biopsy, laparoscopy or via laparotomy.
- Cirrhosis may be difficult to confirm by needle biopsy unless multiple sites are sampled. In practice, a small laparotomy incision and wedge biopsy of the liver gives a better diagnostic sample and is quick and simple. In cats with chronic hepatitis/cirrhosis, less than 40% of paired needle biopsy results may be in accordance with the wedge biopsy diagnosis.
- Patients with cirrhosis may have occult bleeding tendencies. Screen for the presence of coagulopathy prior to liver biopsy by performing evaluation of a PIVKA assay or APTT/OSPT.

Differential diagnosis

Cirrhosis is the end result of many **different chronic** liver disorders. Therefore, differentiation of the primary parenchymal disease leading to cirrhosis is generally not clinically relevant.

Treatment

Strategies for therapeutic support in cats with cirrhosis are first prioritized as to severity, and approached in a logical step-wise fashion. The presence of jaundice or ascites does not indicate a hopeless situation for medical treatment.

Feed adequate calories (1.25–1.50 MER) to prevent further malnourishment. Use of enteral nutrition is strongly recommended in anorectic cats. Reduce dietary protein intake in cats with overt signs of hepatic encephalopathy (HE).

Supplement water-soluble vitamins as needed at twice the normal dose. Use vitamin K in cats with biliary occlusion and elevated PIVKA or APTT/OSPT assays.

Control signs of HE with antimicrobials, reduced protein diets and mucosal protectants (e.g., sucralfate). Vitamin K therapy may reduce GI bleeding which also contributes to HE.

Correct hydration deficits with intravenous fluids. Fluid choices are based on the presence of ascites and electrolyte status.

Use low-salt diets, cage rest and diuretics for control of ascites.

Antibiotics are indicated in patients with suppurative inflammation, fever and/or leukocytosis.

Use anti-inflammatory (e.g., prednisone, azathioprine) drugs to reduce mononuclear cellular infiltrates.

Anti-fibrotic agents, such as colchicine, D-penicillamine, may reduce hepatic fibrosis.

Actigal may cause choleresis and promote a more beneficial bile acid milieu.

Reduce free radical damage to hepatocytes by administration of S-adenosyl.

Prognosis

The prognosis in most animals with cirrhosis is poor.

DIABETES MELLITUS

Classical signs

- Polyuria and polydipsia.
- Increased appetite.
- Weight loss with palpable hepatomegaly.

Clinical signs

Polyuria/polydipsia (PU/PD) are common.

Increased to ravenous appetite, although terminally it may be decreased.

Weight loss with or without hepatomegaly.

Jaundice is an uncommon complication of diabetes. It is more commonly associated with sulfonylurea (e.g., glipizide) therapy. Approximately 20% of cats on sulfonylurea therapy develop increased liver enzymes and a small percentage become jaundiced.

Diagnosis

Suggested by salient clinical signs (PU/PD, alterations in appetite, weight loss).

Persistent hyperglycemia observed on 2–3 occasions at least 3 hours apart over 24 hours.

Urinalysis shows glucosuria, +/– ketonuria, +/– proteinuria and +/– bacteriuria.

Liver biochemical parameters (ALT, ALP) are mildly to moderately increased.

NON-HEMATOPOIETIC LIVER TUMORS (BILIARY CYST ADENOMA, HEPATOCELLULAR CARCINOMA)

Classical signs

- Most cats are > 10 years old.
- More common in DSH.
- Hepatomegaly +/– mass lesion is often palpable.

Pathogenesis

Most (60%) of cats have benign tumors.

Bile duct tumors may progress from benign to malignant lesions.

- Benign lesions are usually focal and cystic; malignant tumors often involve multiple lobes.

Hepatomegaly is associated with extensive infiltrative disease.

Metastasis is common with bile duct carcinomas.

Clinical signs

Generally seen in geriatric cats (> 10 years old).

More common in DSH than in Siamese.

Anorexia, lethargy and weakness are seen.

Hepatomegaly +/– mass lesion is often palpable.

Diagnosis

Variable elevation in hepatic biochemical parameters. In general, relative increases in ALP versus ALT activity are observed. However, dramatic increases in either liver enzyme may not be present even with moderately sized tumors.

Abdominal imaging (survey radiographs, sonography) confirms hepatomegaly or mass.

- Ultrasonography is useful in detecting involvement of multiple hepatic lobes and in obtaining a guided core biopsy of lesions.

Definitive diagnosis requires histologic evaluation of liver biopsy specimens.

Differential diagnosis

It is important to distinguish benign from malignant hepatic tumors, as treatment and prognosis are widely divergent. Differentiation may only be made by histologic interpretation of hepatic biopsy specimens.

Treatment

Surgical resection (lobectomy) of benign hepatocellular or biliary tumors is recommended.

Chemotherapy is not useful for treatment of malignant neoplasia.

Prognosis

The prognosis for cats with benign tumors after resection is good. Most cats are disease free at least 1 year later.

The prognosis for malignant neoplasia is poor.

HYPERTHYROIDISM

Classical signs

- Rarely seen in cats < 8 years of age.
- Weight loss, polyphagia and unthrifty appearance predominate.
- Polyuria/polydipsia +/– vomiting/diarrhea may be seen.

See main reference, page 304 (The Cat With Weight Loss and a Good Appetite).

Clinical signs

Clinical signs result from overproduction/secretion of thyroid hormones. Malignant thyroid tumors are rare.

More than 70% of hyperthyroid cats have bilateral thyroid adenomas or adenomatous hyperplasia.

Weight loss, polyphagia and unkempt haircoat are common.

Vomiting and small bowel diarrhea may be observed.

A reduced appetite is seen in about one in ten cats with hyperthyroidism.

Panting and respiratory distress are observed with concomitant cardiac disease.

Seen primarily in middle-aged and older cats.

Physical examination is suggestive.
- Palpable thyroid gland enlargement is evident in 90% of cats if the examiner is experienced.
- Patchy alopecia/unkempt haircoat, overgrown toe nails are often present.
- Reduced muscle mass; most cats are thin.

Cardiac auscultation may reveal cardiac disturbances.
- Tachycardia (>240 bpm), murmurs and/or a gallop rhythm suggest cardiac manifestations of thyrotoxicosis.

Diagnosis

Increased liver enzyme (ALT, ALP) activities are seen in > 75% of hyperthyroid cats.

Closely assess renal parameters (BUN, creatinine, urinalysis) as concomitant renal disease may be present.

Demonstration of elevated basal serum thyroxine (T_4) concentration provides definitive diagnosis.
- Suspicious cats with a "borderline" T_4 value should be retested.
- Increased free T_4 may be observed in some cats with high normal total T_4 concentrations.
- Alternatively, performance of a T_3 suppression test may discriminate between normal and mildly hyperthyroid cats.

Perform thoracic radiography, electrocardiography (ECG), +/– echocardiography to rule out cardiac disease.

FELINE LEUKEMIA VIRUS

See page 424 under pre-hepatic causes for jaundice and page 432 for hepatic causes for jaundice (e.g. lymphosarcoma).

HISTOPLASMOSIS

Classical signs

- Young, outdoor cats (< 4 years old).
- Lethargy, anorexia and weight loss.
- Pale mucous membranes.
- Mild to moderate respiratory signs (fever, dyspnea, tachypnea).
- Occurs in central United States.

Pathogenesis

The etiologic agent is a soil-borne dimorphic fungus, *Histoplasma capsulatum*. The organism is likely inhaled and disseminates from the respiratory tract to multiple other sites in the body (e.g. liver).

Granulomatous inflammation occurs in response to fungal infection.

The disease is of regional significance in the central United States, especially the Mississippi and Ohio River Valleys and Texas.

Clinical signs

Primarily disease of young (< 4 years of age) outdoor cats.

Cats present with a vague history of an insidious chronic illness.

Lethargy, anorexia, weight loss and pale mucous membrane color are common.

Respiratory distress (dyspnea/tachypnea) is seen in 50% of infected cats and occasionally coughing.

Lymphadenopathy, splenomegaly and hepatomegaly are common.

Mild to moderate fever is usually present, but the temperature may be normal.

Intestinal involvement may result in diarrhea and weight loss. On palpation thickened intestinal loops, mesenteric lymphadenopathy and/or hepato/splenomegaly may be evident.

Ocular involvement may cause granulomatous chorioretinitis, retinal detachment with blindness and optic neuritis.

Diagnosis

Non-regenerative anemia is typically present and neutrophilic leukocytosis. Severe pancytopenia is occasionally observed when there is bone marrow involvement.

Hyperproteinemia, hyperglobulinemia, +/− mild elevations of ALT may be observed.

Radiographic imaging may aid diagnosis.
- Survey thoracic radiographs show a diffuse pulmonary interstitial pattern suggesting fungal pneumonia.
- Symmetrical hepatomegaly is observed on survey abdominal radiographs/ultrasonography.

Definitive diagnosis requires demonstration of organisms in infected tissues.
- Potential diagnostic modalities include bronchoalveolar lavage, fine-needle aspiration and exfoliative cytology, and tissue biopsy.

Serologic tests for antibodies directed against *Histoplasma* antigens are not recommended, as false-negative results are common in cats with naturally occurring disease.

Differential diagnosis

Neoplasia and other systemic mycoses may produce similar signs to histoplasmosis.
- Cats with histoplasmosis (and other mycoses) tend to be younger than cats with neoplasia.
- Serologic testing may be useful in detecting cats with cryptococcosis.

Treatment

Combination chemotherapy with amphotericin B and itraconazole (5 mg/kg PO q 12 h), or high loading doses (10 mg/kg PO q 12–24 h) of itraconazole.

Generally treat for 4–6 months but dependent on remission of signs.

See page 26 for details of amphotericin treatment in cats (Cryptococcus in The Cat With Signs of Chronic Nasal Disease).

Prognosis

Fair to good with disseminated disease depending on the severity of fungal involvement and the chronicity.

Emaciated cats with advanced disseminated disease have a poor prognosis and they may not live long enough for the treatment to take effect.

POST-HEPATIC CAUSES OF JAUNDICE OR INCREASED LIVER ENZYMES

EXTRAHEPATIC BILIARY OBSTRUCTION (EHBO)** PANCREATITIS**

> **Classical signs**
> - Progressive anorexia, lethargy and marked jaundice.
> - Vomiting and fever may be episodic.
> - Hepatomegaly.
> - +/– acholic feces.

Pathogenesis

Obstruction of the extrahepatic biliary system has diverse causes, including pancreatic disease, neoplasia, cholelithiasis and extrinsic compression (masses). Consequences of biliary obstruction include cell membrane and organelle injury due to stagnation of bile acids and other injurious substances. Pancreatitis and neoplasia are the most common causes.

- Pancreatitis may cause obstructive jaundice through direct cholangiohepatic injury via refluxed pancreatic secretions, pancreatic fibrosis and/or obstruction of the common bile duct within a few weeks following pancreatic injury.
- Neoplasia (e.g., pancreatic adenocarcinoma) may cause slowly progressive external compression of the major bile ducts, resulting in obstructed biliary flow and jaundice.

Complete occlusion leads to cholestasis, hepatomegaly and dilatation of intrahepatic biliary structures.

Obstruction of bile flow incites biliary tract/hepatocellular inflammation and injury.

- Permanent biliary tract dilatation and hepatic fibrosis may be seen with chronic extrahepatic biliary obstruction.

Clinical signs

Anorexia, lethargy and marked jaundice which are progressive.

Cyclical vomiting and fever.

Hepatomegaly may be palpable.

Acholic feces are occasionally seen with complete obstruction.

Acute pancreatitis may cause anorexia, lethargy, abdominal pain and jaundice as a consequence of extrahepatic biliary obstruction.

Pancreatic abscesses, cysts and neoplasia may cause signs of extrahepatic biliary obstruction.

Diagnosis

Non-regenerative anemia and possibly a neutrophilic leukocytosis are seen.

Increased liver biochemical parameters are commonly observed.

- Dramatic elevations in serum total bilirubin concentration. Elevations may occur as rapidly as 4 hours following complete biliary obstruction.
- Increased ALP and GGT activities occur secondary to cholestasis. A 3–5-fold increase in GGT and 2–10-fold rise in ALP are often present.
- Increased ALT (up to 10-fold) and 3–10-fold increased AST activities reflect hepatocellular injury.

An antemortem diagnosis of pancreatitis causing obstructive jaundice is elusive.

- Variable leukocytosis with elevation of liver biochemical parameters (total bilirubin, ALP, ALT) are present.
- Recent studies show that elevation in feline pancreatic-like immunoreactivity assay (fPLI) may provide presumptive serologic evidence of pancreatitis. Serum fPLI appears to be more sensitive and more specific than serum feline trypsin-like immunoreactivity assay (fTLI) or abdominal ultrasonography.
- Ultrasonography demonstrates a generalized loss of pancreatic echogenicity with pancreatitis in most cases.

Ultrasonography may confirm the presence of a pancreatic mass and/or extrahepatic biliary obstruction causing extrahepatic biliary obstruction.

- Diagnosis of extrahepatic biliary obstruction is confirmed on ultrasonographic evaluation or exploratory surgery.

- Sonography shows a distended/tortuous common bile duct, large gall bladder and distended intrahepatic biliary ducts. These findings may be observed as early as 5–7 days post-obstruction when viewed by an experienced sonographer.

Differential diagnosis

The historical, clinical and laboratory features of extrahepatic biliary obstruction may be indistinguishable from other severe cholestatic hepatopathies.

Abdominal ultrasonography is the quickest and least invasive means to confirm extrahepatic biliary obstruction.

Treatment

First stabilize the patient with fluid and electrolyte therapy.

Perform a laparotomy for inspection/correction of the biliary tract obstructive lesion.
- Prompt correction of complete obstruction via performance of cholecystoduodenostomy or cholecystojejunostomy is recommended.
- Broad-spectrum antibiotics are indicated if biliary-enteric anastomosis is performed.

Extrahepatic biliary obstruction caused by pancreatitis may be amenable to medical therapy (dietary modification, IV fluids, antiemetics, etc.).
- Biliary decompression is recommended in pancreatitis patients with rising hype bilirubinemia or sonographic evidence of worsening gall bladder distention.

Specific therapy for hepatocellular inflammation (confirmed by biopsy) and intrahepatic cholestasis may be required.
- Use ursodeoxycholic acid (10 mg/kg PO q 12 h) for 5–7 days post-operatively to reduce cholestatic injury.

Prognosis

Guarded to good depending upon the underlying cause.

Biochemical abnormalities associated with extraheptic biliary obstruction subside quickly following successful surgery.

CHOLECYSTITIS

Classical signs

- Abdominal pain, fever, vomiting.
- +/- jaundice.
- Palpable right cranial abdominal mass.

Clinical signs

Abdominal pain, fever, vomiting and jaundice.

A mass lesion may be palpable in the cranial abdomen.

Animals may present in endotoxic shock with gall bladder rupture.

Pathogenesis

Inflammation of the gall bladder is uncommon.

Inflammation may occur from occlusion of the cystic duct, with resultant gall bladder inflammation resulting from bile stasis. Occlusion may occur due to extraluminal compression (e.g., mass, adhesion) or intraluminal obstruction as seen with cholelithiasis.

Emphysematous cholecystitis is most commonly observed in association with diabetes mellitus, acute cholecystitis with/without cholelithiasis, and traumatic ischemia of the gall bladder.

E. coli bacteria are most commonly cultured from the biliary tree of affected cats.

Diagnosis

Most animals have a variable leukocytosis.

Hepatic biochemical parameters (total bilirubin, ALT and ALP) are modestly increased.

Ultrasonography or laparotomy is usually necessary for a diagnosis.
- Gas accumulation within the biliary tree/gall bladder indicates cholecystitis.
- Choleliths may be an uncommonly recognized incidental finding.
- Cranial abdominal fluid accumulation indicates biliary rupture and peritoneal inflammation. Analysis of peritoneal effusion reveals the presence of inflammatory cells (e.g., neutrophils, macrophages) and bilirubin crystals in a turbid golden-brown or green fluid.

Laparotomy allows for cholecystectomy and treatment of peritonitis.

Treatment

Surgically remove calculi causing clinical signs of hepatobiliary disease.

Assess patency of biliary tree during surgery. If the gallbladder appears inflamed, consider cholecystectomy.
- Administer vitamin K 12–24 hours prior to surgical intervention.
- Perform concurrent liver biopsy to assess the extent of hepatic inflammation.

Culture bile fluid for the presence of aerobic/anaerobic bacterial pathogens.
- Use broad-spectrum antibiotic therapy effective against enteric pathogens. Good first-choice drugs which reach therapeutic biliary concentrations include cephalosporins, penicillins, doxycycline, metronidazole, clindamycin and the quinolones. Base antimicrobial therapy on the results obtained from biliary culture and susceptibility testing.

Fluid therapy is administered to hypovolemic cats or those requiring correction of electrolyte derangements.

Prognosis

The prognosis in most cases is guarded. Those cats which are not extremely debilitated or that have necrotizing cholecystitis have a more favorable prognosis.

RUPTURED BILE DUCT

Classical signs
- Malaise, weight loss.
- Low-grade abdominal pain.
- Abdominal effusion +/- jaundice.

Clinical signs

There is often a history of trauma.

General malaise, weight loss and abdominal pain predominate.

Abdominal effusion +/– jaundice may be present. Intervals ranging from 3 days to 3 weeks before the presentation may be observed.

Pathogenesis

Rupture of the extrahepatic biliary tree may occur with blunt or penetrating abdominal trauma, necrotizing cholecystitis and cholelithiasis (rare). Leakage of significant volumes of bile into the peritoneal cavity induces tissue inflammation. Unconjugated bile acids are most irritating, as they alter the permeability of vascular structures within the peritoneal membranes.

Altered membrane permeability promotes transmural bacterial migration into the peritoneal cavity, septic inflammation and septicemia.

Non-septic inflammation causes intra-abdominal fluid sequestration, contraction of circulating blood volume and dehydration which may induce hypovolemic shock.

Diagnosis

Suggestive history with other evidence of trauma.

Liver enzymes (ALP, ALT) are mildly to moderately increased. Moderate-to-severe hyperbilirubinemia is often present.

Cytologic examination of abdominal effusion confirms the diagnosis.
- The effusion is turbid and golden brown-to-green in appearance. Inflammatory cells (macrophages and neutrophils) and bilirubin crystals are generally seen.

Treatment

Immediate surgical correction of bile leakage.
- Perform cholecystectomy if concurrent necrotizing cholecystitis is present.
- Provide adequate post-operative drainage.

Correct fluid and electrolyte derangements intravenously using a balanced electrolyte solution with electrolyte supplements as needed. Colloids may be needed for correction of hypoalbuminemia if present.

Broad-spectrum antibiotic therapy, as per cholecystitis, if septicemia is present.

Prognosis

A guarded prognosis is warranted in most cats. Cats having pronounced effusion, chronic debilitation, or clinical evidence of sepsis at the time of diagnosis have a poor prognosis.

RECOMMENDED READING

Addie DD, Jarrett O. Feline coronavirus infection. In: Greene CE (ed) Infectious Diseases of the Dog and Cat, 2nd edn. Philadelphia, PA, W.B. Saunders, 1998, pp. 58–69.

Bunch SE. Hepatobiliary diseases in the cat. In: Nelson RW, Cuoto CG (eds) Small Animal Internal Medicine, 3rd edn. St. Louis, MO, Mosby, 2003, pp. 506–524.

Center SA, Warner K, Corbett J, et al. Proteins invoked by vitamin K absence and clotting times in clinically ill cats. J Vet Intern Med 2000; 14: 292–297.

Charles JA, Histologic Classification of Cholangitis in Cats Proceedings of 12th ECVIM - CA/ESVIM Congress.

Ogilvie GK, Moore AS. Lymphoma in cats. In: Ogilvie GK, Moore AS (eds) Managing the Veterinary Cancer Patient. Trenton, NJ, Veterinary Learning Systems Co, 1995, pp. 249–259.

WSAVA Standards for Histological and Clinical Diagnosis of Canine and Feline Liver Diseases. Elsevier, 2005

22. The cat with abdominal distention or abdominal fluid

Anthony Abrams-Ogg

KEY SIGNS

- Abdominal distention or pendulous abdomen.
- Fluid wave on ballotment.
- Abdominal mass.

MECHANISM?

- In the "8F" classification scheme the causes of abdominal distention are **fluid, fat, food, feces, flatus, fetus, formidable** organomegaly and **feeble** abdominal musculature.

WHERE?

- Abdomen. The primary disease process may be intra-abdominal, extra-abdominal or systemic.

WHAT?

- The most common causes of moderate to marked abdominal distention in cats are physiologic – pregnancy and obesity. The most common pathologic cause is abdominal fluid.

QUICK REFERENCE SUMMARY

Diseases causing abdominal distention or abdominal fluid

ANOMALY

- Intrahepatic arteriovenous fistula (p 474)

The pressure differential between the artery and portal vein leads to ascites (transudate) secondary to portal hypertension.

- Portal vein atresia or hypoplasia (p 475)

Congenital underdevelopment of the portal vein leads to ascites (transudate) secondary to portal hypertension.

- Inherited coagulation defects (p 473)

Inherited coagulation factor deficiencies or deficiencies in vitamin K metabolism may cause spontaneous abdominal bleeding and re-bleeding after trauma.

continued

continued

● Umbilical or inguinal hernia* (p 478)

Owners may misinterpret a change in abdominal contour due to herniation of abdominal fat or organs as abdominal distention.

METABOLIC

● Obesity*** (p 452)

A round abdominal contour results from excessive intra-abdominal and abdominal subcutaneous fat.

● Pregnancy*** (p 455)

Abdominal distention is usually apparent by the last 2 weeks of gestation.

● Hepatic lipidosis* (p 472)

Ascites (usually transudate or modified transudate) occasionally occurs with hepatic lipidosis. Abdominal bleeding may occur secondary to coagulopathy.

● Juvenile abdominal fluid** (p 465)

A mild increase in normal peritoneal fluid compared to a mature animal may be encountered during laparotomy of an immature animal. Fluid is a transudate.

● Hyperadrenocorticism* (p 470)

A pendulous abdomen results from feeble abdominal musculature and increased abdominal fat.

NEOPLASTIC

● Abdominal lymphoma*** (p 458)

Alimentary lymphoma may cause abdominal distention due to marked intestinal thickening, mesenteric lymphadenopathy or obstructive effusion. Splenic or hepatic lymphoma may spontaneously bleed.

● Visceral mast cell tumor** (p 461)

Marked splenic enlargement with a mast cell tumor may cause abdominal distention. Abdominal mast cell tumors may spontaneously bleed or cause obstructive ascites. Abdominal fluid often contains mast cells.

● Solid tumors*** (p 460)

Hepatic or splenic hemangiosarcoma and other solid tumors may spontaneously bleed. A tumor may cause portal hypertension. Carcinomatosis may cause obstructive effusion.

● Neoplasia obstructing or compressing lower urinary tract (p 474)

Tumors obstructing or compressing the trigone region of the bladder or the urethra and causing paradoxical incontinence may cause abdominal distention secondary to marked enlargement of the bladder.

NUTRITIONAL

● Overeating* (p 471)

An unusually large meal may cause transient abdominal distention.

PHYSICAL

● Aerophagia* (p 471)

Dyspneic or tachypneic cats may swallow sufficient air to cause mild abdominal distention.

IDIOPATHIC

- **Megacolon** (p 465)**

Obstipation results in marked colonic enlargement that may cause abdominal distention.

- Peliosis hepatis (p 476)

Hepatomegaly and/or spontaneous abdominal hemorrhage may cause abdominal distention.

- Hepatic amyloidosis (p 475)

Hepatomegaly, splenomegaly, intestinal dilation and/or spontaneous intra-abdominal hemorrhage may cause abdominal distention.

- Hepatic necrosis (p 475)

Ascites or spontaneous abdominal hemorrhage may occur secondary to hepatic necrosis due to various causes.

- Hepatic cirrhosis (p 472)

Ascites may occur with hepatic cirrhosis. The fluid may be transudate, modified transudate or exudate.

- Gastric-dilation volvulus (p 478)

Gastric dilation with air results in tympanic abdominal distention.

- Perirenal pseudocysts (p 476)

Fluid-filled sacs surrounding the kidneys cause abdominal distention. Chronic renal failure is commonly present.

- **Right heart failure** (p 462)**

Ascites may occur in cats with right heart failure. The fluid is a modified transudate.

- Extra-uterine fetuses (p 477)

Ascites occasionally occurs with "ectopic pregnancy".

- Budd–Chiari-like syndrome (p 477)

Obstruction of the cranial vena cava or venous vasculature of the liver causes ascites. Ascitic fluid is a modified transudate.

- Idiopathic chylous ascites (p 479)

Chylous ascites is usually due to neoplasia. Idiopathic chylous ascites is rare.

INFLAMMATION

- **Gastroenteritis* (p 468)**

Flatus formation and intestinal thickening in cats with diarrhea may cause mild abdominal distention.

- **Non-suppurative cholangiohepatitis* (p 472)**

Ascites occasionally occurs with cholangiohepatitis. The fluid may be a transudate, modified transudate or exudate.

- **Pancreatitis** (p 466)**

Cats with pancreatitis may have abdominal effusion, which is occasionally detectable on physical examination. Fluid may be a modified transudate or exudate.

- Pneumoperitoneum (p 477)

Acute pneumoperitoneum is usually due to gastric perforation or gastrointestinal rupture.

continued

continued

    ● Steatitis (p 472)

Inflammation of abdominal fat may cause peritoneal effusion with high protein content and mature neutrophils (exudate).

    ● Granulomatous urethritis and urethral stricture (p 474)

Chronic narrowing of the urethra leads to massive enlargement of the bladder and urine dribbling from paradoxical incontinence.

    ● Glomerulonephritis (p 473)

Glomerulonephritis may cause nephrotic syndrome and ascites, which is a transudate.

    ● Sclerosing encapsulating peritonitis (p 479)

The abdominal mesothelial lining becomes replaced by fibrous tissue. Ascites may occur.

INFECTIOUS:

Viral:

    ● **Feline infectious peritonitis (FIP)*** (p 456)**

Immune-complex vasculitis results in a marked peritoneal exudate. Fluid is typically straw-colored, viscous like egg white and highly proteinaceous (exudate) with mature neutrophils. Hepatic infection may also cause ascites due to portal hypertension.

Bacterial:

    ● **Septic peritonitis* (p 467)**

Bacterial infection results in a septic suppurative exudate.

    ● **Intestinal tuberculosis* (p 469)**

Effusion may occur secondary to mesenteric lymphadenopathy. The fluid may be a transudate, modified transudate, exudate or chylous effusion and may contain macrophages containing acid-fast bacteria.

    ● Leptospirosis (p 478)

Leptospirosis has been associated with liver disease and ascites in cats.

    ● Hepatic abscess (p 476)

Hepatic abscesses may be associated with septic and non-septic effusions.

Protozoal:

    ● **Toxoplasmosis* (p 469)**

Toxoplasmosis may cause peritoneal effusion secondary to liver and mesenteric lymph node infection. Fluid is a transudate or modified transudate and may contain tachyzooites.

Parasitic:

    ● Abdominal fluke infection (p 479)

Metorchis spp. are bile duct parasites that may cause hepatic cysts and ascites.

Iatrogenic:

    ● **Fluid overload* (p 471)**

Excessive fluid therapy tends to cause pulmonary edema leading to dyspnea or subcutaneous edema.

● Ligation of portosystemic shunt (p 475)

Ligation of a portosystemic shunt may lead to ascites secondary to portal hypertension.

Toxic:

● **Anticoagulant rodenticide poisoning (and other acquired coagulopathies)* (p 473)**

Acquired coagulopathy may cause abdominal hemorrhage.

Trauma:

● **Traumatic hemorrhage*(p 471)**

Abdominal hemorrhage may occur with blunt trauma (e.g. motor vehicle accident, falling from heights), penetrating trauma (e.g. abdominal bite wound), or post-operatively.

● **Traumatic rupture of the urinary bladder or urethra* (p 463)**

The urinary bladder may rupture from motor vehicle trauma, falling from heights, bladder expression, cystocentesis, penetrating trauma and as a complication of urethral obstruction. Abdominal fluid is urine ± blood.

● Umbilical, inguinal and traumatic abdominal wall hernia (p 478)

Owners may misinterpret change in abdominal contour due to herniation of abdominal fat or organs as abdominal distention.

● Ruptured gall bladder or bile duct (p 478)

Motor vehicle trauma, falling from heights, gunshot wounds and cholelithiasis may cause rupture of the gall bladder or a major bile duct. Fluid is dark bile-stained and a modified transudate to exudate.

● **Traumatic abdominal wall hernia* (p 478)**

Owners may misinterpret a change in abdominal contour due to herniation of abdominal fat or organs as abdominal distention.

INTRODUCTION

MECHANISM?

Abdominal distention has several causes. These causes may be present alone or in combination. A mnemonic classifies the causes using an "8F scheme": **fluid, fat, food, feces, flatus, fetus, formidable** organomegaly and **feeble** abdominal musculature.

Fluid accumulation in the peritoneal cavity is the most common cause of pathologic abdominal distention and of marked abdominal distention, but it is not as common in cats as in dogs.

● In broad definitions (used here), fluid in the peritoneal cavity is referred to as **peritoneal effusion** or **ascites**. In terms of clinical pathology, the type of fluid may be a **transudate, modified transudate, septic exudate, non-septic exudate, chyle, blood,** **bile** or **urine**. In narrow definitions, peritoneal effusion and ascites refer to transudates and modified transudates. Characteristics of the various types of fluids vary somewhat with laboratories, but the following definitions are typical.

– **Transudate** – clear and colorless, specific gravity (SG) ≤ 1.013–1.018, total protein <25 g/L (2.5 g/dl), low cellularity (total nucleated cell count < $1.0–1.5 \times 10^9$/L [1000–1500/μl]).

– **Modified transudate** – clear to slightly cloudy, straw-colored to pink-white, SG > 1.013–1.018, total protein between 25 and 50 g/L (2.5–5.0 g/dl), and total nucleated cell count < $5.0–7.0 \times 10^9$/L (< 5000–7000/μl). Nucleated cells consist of mesothelial cells, non-degenerate neutrophils, macrophages and lymphocytes.

– **Exudate** – turbid to opaque white to yellow or red, SG > 1.018, high protein (> 25 g/L [2.5 g/dl]), highly cellular (total nucleated cell count > 5.0×10^9/L [5000/μl]).

- Cell types in a non-septic exudate are similar to a modified transudate, except for feline infectious peritonitis, where the predominant cells are non-degenerate neutrophils, and in some neoplastic effusions, where malignant cells predominate.
- Cells in a septic exudate are predominantly neutrophils. The fluid is further characterized by the presence of intracellular bacteria, degenerate changes in the neutrophils and a foul odor.
- **Degenerate and non-degenerate neutrophils are distinguished on the appearance of their nuclei.** Non-degenerate neutrophils appear similar to peripheral blood neutrophils and have tightly clumped, basophilic nuclear chromatin. As the neutrophils age, the nuclei become hypersegmented, and then pyknotic (tightly clumped sphere), and then eventually break up into several smaller tightly clumped spheres (karyorrhexis). This aging change should not be confused with degenerative change. Degenerate neutrophils have swollen pale eosinophilic nuclei resulting from increased membrane permeability to water. Toxic changes in the cytoplasm (basophilia, vacuolation and Dohle bodies) may also be present.
- In a recent report, a nucleated cell count $> 13 \times 10^9$/L (13 000/μl) was highly sensitive and specific for septic peritonitis, although cats with FIP were not included.
- Protein content characteristic of an exudate may be confirmed by Rivalta's test (see Feline infectious peritonitis).
- **Chyle** – opaque and white to pink (slightly cloudy and straw-colored in fasting animals), SG variable, protein 2.0–7.0 g/L (20–70 g/dl), and total nucleated cell count $< 10 \times 10^9$/L (10 000/μl) containing a large number of small lymphocytes (chyle is comprised of lymph and chylomicrons). The fluid in the tube separates into a cream-like layer when refrigerated. Chylous effusions are also characterized by fluid triglyceride level greater than serum triglyceride level, fluid cholesterol level lower than serum cholesterol level, and a fluid cholesterol:triglyceride ratio < 1 (with the values measured in mg/dl).
- **Blood** – cloudy and red (centrifugation results in a clear supernatant above red sediment), SG, protein and total nucleated cell count consistent with peripheral blood. Effusion may contain clots but does not clot further after withdrawal. Platelets disappear within several hours, and erythrophagocytosis by macrophages begins within 1 day, and this can be used to help age the effusion.
- **Bile** – clear to cloudy and dark yellow with a green or orange tinge, SG > 1.018, protein > 25 g/L (2.5 g/dl), total nucleated cells $> 5 \times 10^9$/L (5000/μl) with cell composition similar to modified transudate, but may become a highly cellular septic exudate. Bilirubin may be confirmed using a urine dipstick or by seeing bilirubin crystals free in the fluid or in macrophages.
- **Urine** – clear to slightly cloudy and pale yellow, variable SG and protein content. It may be a transudate, but total nucleated cells are often $> 3 \times 10^9$/L (3000/μl) with cell composition similar to modified transudate, and it may become a highly cellular septic exudate.

- While in theory a specific disease process causes a specific type of fluid, in reality the type of fluid may vary somewhat. In particular, the disorders that generally cause pure transudates are occasionally associated with modified transudates, and vice versa. This may be due to modification of fluid production by concurrent disorders as well as variable criteria for characterizing the fluids. The implication of this fact is that **a specific differential diagnosis should not be ruled out strictly on the grounds that the type of fluid is not the classic type for that disorder**.
  - Although protein content is one of the classic clinicopathologic values by which to categorize fluids, protein levels were recently reported to be similar in septic and non-septic peritoneal fluids.
- The peritoneal cavity is lined by a serous membrane (serosa) and normally contains a small amount of fluid that serves as a lubricant for the abdominal organs. **Normal peritoneal fluid** is a transudate (ultrafiltrate) that comes from interstitial fluid produced by local capillary beds, which diffuses across the serosa into the peritoneal cavity. The serosa is equally permeable to diffusion of the fluid back into the interstitium, but most is reabsorbed from the abdomen by uptake by lymphatics, especially of the diaphragm. The ultrafiltrate contains protein that is in equilibrium with plasma protein. The mechanisms that promote formation of subcutaneous edema will thus promote formation of peritoneal fluid. These mechanisms are:

- **Reduced plasma colloidal osmotic (oncotic) pressure** due to **hypoalbuminemia**. Hypoalbuminemia occurs by the same mechanisms as in dogs, i.e. reduced hepatic production, or renal, gastrointestinal or cutaneous loss. **Hypoalbuminemia** severe enough to cause spontaneous effusions or edema (typically ≤ 10–15 g/L [1–1.5 g/dl) is **rare in cats**. As albumin levels drop there is a progressive risk for exacerbation of ascites formed by other mechanisms, for example, increased hydrostatic pressure. When spontaneous fluid accumulation occurs, subcutaneous edema may develop preferentially to pleural and peritoneal effusions. Peritoneal fluid is a transudate.
- **Increased capillary hydrostatic pressure.** This may occur from **fluid overload**, decreased arteriolar resistance, and **increased venous pressure**. Cats with fluid overload usually develop pulmonary or subcutaneous edema preferentially to pleural and peritoneal effusions. Fluid overload causes a transudate.
- **Portal venous hypertension** is an increase in venous pressure unique to the abdomen. It is classified anatomically as pre-hepatic (which is also pre-sinusoidal), hepatic (pre-sinusoidal, sinusoidal, or post-sinusoidal), or post-hepatic (which is also post-sinusoidal) in origin. Anatomic location affects protein content of the ascitic fluid and is relevant to differential diagnoses. Pre-sinusoidal disorders usually cause a pure transudate. Sinusoidal and post-sinusoidal disorders increase hepatic sinusoidal pressure, which, in addition to portal hypertension, causes effusion of hepatic lymph from the hepatic lymphatics through the surface of the liver. Hepatic lymph is high in protein. The resulting fluid is a modified transudate, i.e. a transudate modified by increased levels of protein. The fluid may also have a mild increase in red blood cells, resulting in a serosanguineous fluid.
- **Pre-hepatic** portal hypertension results from **obstruction of the portal vein**, usually by a tumor. The fluid is a transudate, but may contain neoplastic cells. Other potential causes include **surgical ligation of a portosystemic shunt** or of the portal vein, portal vein atresia or hypoplasia (anecdotal reports in the cat), and portal vein

thrombosis (not reported in the cat). The fluid is usually a transudate.
- **Pre-sinusoidal hepatic** portal hypertension may be caused by an **arterioportal fistula** and **surgical ligation of a portosystemic shunt**. The fluid is usually a transudate.
- **Sinusoidal hepatic** portal hypertension results from **liver disease**. The most common cause is cirrhosis, which is uncommon in cats. Severe hepatocyte swelling in hepatic lipidosis, and chronic cholangiohepatitis and hepatic neoplasia may also cause sinusoidal hypertension. Other mechanisms contribute to ascites in liver disease, including hypoalbuminemia, water and salt retention (see below) and non-septic peritonitis. The fluid may thus be a transudate, modified transudate or exudate. Although liver diseases are common in cats, ascites sufficient to cause abdominal distention is not.
- **Post-sinusoidal hepatic** portal hypertension is caused by veno-occlusive disease. The fluid is a modified transudate.
- **Post-hepatic (post-sinusoidal)** portal hypertension results from **obstruction of the hepatic veins or caudal vena cava** and **right heart failure**. Increase in vena caval pressure increases hepatic vein pressure, which increases sinusoidal and portal pressures. The fluid is a modified transudate.
- **Obstruction** of the venous outflow of the liver, from the hepatic venules to the right atrium, is referred to as **Budd–Chiari-like syndrome**. It is rare in cats.
- **Reduced lymphatic uptake.** This usually occurs with **tumors** obstructing a substantial portion of the serosal surface or mesenteric lymph nodes (± venous obstruction). The fluid is a transudate to modified transudate, but may contain neoplastic cells. Lymphatic obstruction occurs occasionally with inflammation, in which case the fluid is a modified transudate to exudate.
- **Increased permeability of the capillary endothelium and blood vessels.** This occurs secondary to inflammation.
  - In **feline infectious peritonitis** a type III hypersensitivity reaction leads to leukocytoclastic (neutrophil-mediated) vasculitis. The fluid is a non-septic exudate, containing increased levels

of inflammatory proteins and neutrophils from the vasculitis.

- In **septic peritonitis** the fluid is a septic exudate containing bacteria and increased levels of protein, neutrophils and bacteria.
- In **pancreatitis** the fluid is a modified transudate to non-septic exudate, depending on the increase in protein and cells.
- Ascites may be associated with a **decreased effective plasma volume**, which **promotes salt and water retention** by the renin-angiotensin-aldosterone system, antidiuretic hormone, and the sympathetic nervous system, thereby helping to maintain the ascitic state. (Water retention may result in hyponatremia. Hyperkalemia may also result from a decreased effective plasma volume and other mechanisms in cats with ascites. The combination of hyponatremia and hyperkalemia mimics hypoadrenocorticism.)

Chyle in the peritoneal cavity is an uncommon **non-specific finding** indicating that lymphatic rupture has occurred. Chylous effusion may occur with any of the basic mechanisms that promote peritoneal fluid production except for hypoalbuminemia. Most cases are caused by **neoplasia**, and fewer are caused by **inflammation, right heart failure and liver disease**. Other causes are rare in cats, including **primary abdominal lymphangiectasia and traumatic rupture of a major lymphatic** vessel.

Blood in the peritoneal cavity results from injury to blood vessels, spontaneous or traumatic rupture of abnormal blood-filled spaces, or a coagulopathy. Hemoperitoneum is not as common in cats as dogs, because abdominal trauma does not commonly cause severe abdominal hemorrhage in cats, and hemangiosarcoma is rare. Other causes of hemoperitoneum in the dog such as anticoagulant rodenticide poisoning, perforated gastrointestinal ulcers, and splenic torsions, are also uncommon in cats. Clinical signs due to acute anemia and local effects of hemorrhage vary with the severity of bleeding. Signs of acute hypovolemia, e.g. weakness, lethargy, hypothermia, pale mucus membranes, tachycardia and weak pulses, occur with a smaller volume of blood loss than do abdominal distention. In most cases of hemoperitoneum in cats, abdominal distention is not noted. In converse, cats with abdominal distention due to acute blood loss will have signs of hypovolemia.

Bile in the peritoneal cavity results from traumatic injury to the gall bladder or bile ducts. It is rare in cats. The presence of bile may be associated with septic or non-septic peritonitis, with increases in bacteria and/or protein and neutrophils accordingly.

Urine in the peritoneal cavity usually results from traumatic injury to the urinary bladder. It is uncommon in cats. Rarely direct effusion of urine may occur with severe cystitis. The presence of urine may be associated with septic or non-septic peritonitis, with increases in bacteria and/or protein and neutrophils accordingly. Rupture of the bladder may also cause abdominal hemorrhage.

Fat accumulates because of overeating and underactivity. Fat accumulates within the abdomen as well as within the abdominal subcutaneous tissue, especially of the caudal ventral abdomen.

Food may cause increased distention of the stomach and small intestine after a large meal. This is a physiologic cause of organomegaly.

Feces may cause increased distention of the large intestine after a large meal. This is a physiologic cause of organomegaly. More often, increased accumulation of feces in the large intestine is a sign of constipation. Severe constipation (obstipation, megacolon) may result in marked abdominal distention.

Flatus (gastrointestinal air) is not physiologically common in cats. Flatus may develop secondary to aerophagia in dyspneic cats and as a sign of primary intestinal disorders. Gastric dilation-volvulus is rare. Abdominal distention may also develop from pneumoperitoneum. Sources of air include gastric perforation, gastrointestinal rupture, extension of air from the thoracic cavity, penetrating abdominal wounds and intra-abdominal gas-forming bacteria.

Fetuses are a cause of physiologic organomegaly.

Formidable organomegaly usually results from markedly distended hollow organs (bladder, intestinal tract, uterus) or neoplasia. Granulomatous inflammation, cyst and pseudocyst formation is less common. Rare causes include heterotopic ossification. Acute inflammation of an organ usually causes minimal to moderate organomegaly and does not cause abdominal distention.

Feeble abdominal musculature is caused by hyperadrenocorticism.

WHERE?

Abdominal distention and/or fluid may be signs of:

- A **primary abdominal disorder** or physiologic change. Any abdominal organ may be involved.
- An **extra-abdominal disorder**.
- A **systemic disorder**.

Peritoneal fluid may be accompanied by pleural fluid, pericardial fluid or subcutaneous edema.

A large volume of abdominal fluid, in addition to causing abdominal distention, may cause dyspnea (diaphragmatic compression), anorexia (compression of the stomach), increased frequency of urination (compression of the bladder), abdominal discomfort, and difficulty walking. A large volume of fluid can also compress the caudal vena cava and decrease venous return to the heart.

WHAT?

The chief complaint may be abdominal distention, perceived weight gain, signs due to abdominal distention, or signs of an underlying or associated disease.

Most causes of abdominal distention may result in minimal to marked distention, but most commonly result in minimal to mild distention. The most common causes of abdominal distention in cats are physiologic – pregnancy and obesity. The most common pathologic cause of moderate to marked abdominal distention is abdominal effusion. The most common causes of marked abdominal effusion are right heart failure, feline infectious peritonitis and neoplasia.

DIAGNOSIS

Fat is easily confused with fluid, both peripherally and in the abdomen, and the two cannot always be distinguished by palpation alone. However, cats with severe abdominal distention due to fluid will have a more taught abdomen than severely obese cats, and body contour will change more with position when distention is due to fluid. Fluid is confirmed on physical examination only if a fluid thrill or abdominal organ is noted with ballottement, which requires a large volume of fluid. Smaller amounts of fluid may cause the abdominal organs, especially the loops of intestine, to feel more slippery than usual, or to be less distinct than usual, on palpation.

Organomegaly is easily detected on abdominal palpation, with the exception of hepatomegaly where falciform fat may preclude palpation of the liver.

- Mild distention of the intestines with air may make them less distinct than usual on palpation.
- Free-living toms may have firm abdominal musculature and be more difficult to palpate.

Abdominal pain may be signaled by contraction of abdominal musculature, vocalization on abdominal palpation, attempting to escape, and defensive aggression. Some clinicians believe that cats with abdominal pain may not react, and that inactivity and remaining hunched-up also signify abdominal pain. Abdominal pain may be caused by trauma, inflammation of a specific organ, peritonitis, acute over-distention of the bladder or gastrointestinal tract, and over-exuberant palpation. Abdominal pain may be mimicked by back pain (uncommon in cats), or the cat objecting to veterinary examination. Fluid distention due to transudates and modified transudates is not painful.

Abdominal **radiography**, abdominal **ultrasound** examination, and **abdominocentesis** will reveal the cause of abdominal distention if clinical findings are inconclusive.

- If imaging is planned it should be performed prior to abdominocentesis (1) to identify organomegaly, and (2) because a small amount of air may enter the abdomen during abdominocentesis, which may create imaging artifacts.
  - **Radiography** will not detect small volumes of fluid. There is progressive loss of abdominal detail with increasing amounts of fluid, and large-volume ascites creates a homogeneous soft-tissue density. Radiography is not very useful to distinguish the type of fluid, except that exudates tend to produce a "ground-glass appearance" because the presence of flocculent material produces variation in radiographic density.
  - **Ultrasonography** will detect small volumes of fluid, and may identify flocculent densities in exudates and debris on the serosa.
- **Abdominocentesis** will usually be positive if there is > 4–5 ml/kg of fluid.
  - If fluid is detected during an ultrasound examination, ultrasound-guided aspiration of the fluid is recommended.
  - For blind abdominocentesis, the cat is best supported in the standing position or held in the restrainer's arms with the ventrum parallel to the ground. Ideally the bladder should be empty.

- If a large volume of fluid is known to be present, a regular needle, butterfly needle, intravenous catheter or peritoneal lavage catheter attached to a syringe ± three-way stopcock may be used to remove the desired volume. Following surgical preparation of the skin, the needle or catheter is inserted along the ventral midline caudal to the umbilicus.
- If the procedure is being used to diagnose the presence of a small volume of fluid, a 1-inch, 22-G needle should be inserted along the ventral midline caudal to the umbilicus, and the fluid allowed to drip out by gravity. Samples should be collected into an EDTA (purple top) tube and into a clot tube (red top). If no fluid appears, the needle should be gently twisted, and, if this is unsuccessful, a syringe may be attached and gentle suction applied. If midline abdominocentesis is negative, the abdomen may be "divided" into four quadrants with the umbilicus as the center point, and the procedure repeated in each quadrant, stopping when a sample is obtained.
- Minimal analysis of the fluid consists of visual inspection, specific gravity, packed cell volume and total protein (measured by refractometer or urine dipstick), and cytologic examination using a routine hematology stain. Fluids with high cellularity may be examined using a smear similar to a blood smear or using a squash smear. Fluids with low cellularity should be centrifuged prior to examination and/or examined using a line-smear technique, a technique similar to a blood smear, but where the spreader slide is rapidly drawn back several millimeters before the end of the sample slide, thus concentrating the cells in a line. More extensive evaluation may include cell counts, bilirubin, urea, creatinine, potassium, glucose, bibarbonate, lactate, pH, albumin, globulin, cholesterol, triglyceride, amylase and lipase levels, RT-PCR for feline coronavirus, Gram-stain and microbial culture.
- If abdominocentesis is unsuccessful, **diagnostic peritoneal lavage** may be performed.
  - The bladder is emptied and the cat is restrained in dorsal or left lateral recumbency.
  - The skin is surgically prepared. An intravenous catheter (which may be fenestrated with a scalpel blade, although this may make

the catheter more difficult to advance and more prone to kinking or breakage) or peritoneal dialysis/lavage catheter (preferred) is inserted caudally, or right laterally, to the umbilicus (dissection may be used), and directed caudally and towards the right.
  - 20 ml/kg warm saline is infused by gravity or injected over 2–5 minutes. The cat is gently rolled from side-to-side (catheter in place), and then after 2–5 minutes a diagnostic sample is retrieved by gravity or by aspiration (it is neither necessary nor possible to retrieve all the infused fluid). The catheter is removed and the skin incision sutured.
- Complications from presence of a large volume of ascites may necessitate large-volume abdominocentesis. This is normally a safe procedure, however:
  - The fluid may rapidly re-accumulate, especially if intra-abdominal pressure from the fluid (tamponade) was in equilibrium with the forces promoting fluid accumulation. Very rapid re-accumulation could lead to acute hypovolemia. This is most likely to occur with hypoproteinemia and right-sided heart failure.
  - Repetitive large-volume abdominocentesis will promote hypoproteinemia because of repetitive loss of protein in the ascitic fluid.
  - For these reasons it is recommended to remove enough fluid to resolve secondary problems, but not to try to empty the abdomen.

The prognosis for cats with peritoneal effusion is generally poor, especially if accompanied by pleural effusion.

DISEASES CAUSING ABDOMINAL DISTENTION OR ABDOMINAL FLUID

OBESITY***

Classical signs

- Disproportionately large abdomen compared to head, thorax and distal limbs.

Pathogenesis

Obesity results from **caloric intake in excess of that required for basal metabolism and physical activity**.

Overfeeding prior to maturity may cause adipocyte proliferation predisposing to obesity in maturity.

Adipocyte numbers gradually increase with aging and basal metabolic rate decreases.

Some cats are probably more likely to become obese by genetic predisposition.

Neutering promotes obesity in part because sex hormones affect appetite and protein and fat metabolism. Neutered cats have lower basal energy requirements and are also less likely to roam.

- Neutered male cats are more prone to obesity than neutered female cats.
- Obesity in neutered male cats is primarily due to increased food intake.

Physical activity is reduced in many housecats and with aging. Reduced physical activity reduces caloric needs, and also results in reduced muscle mass, which in turn lowers basal metabolic rate.

Offering **highly palatable foods** and boredom may increase calorie intake.

Appetite stimulation is a **side effect of certain drugs**. This effect is most pronounced with megesterol acetate and benzodiazepines, but may occur occasionally with glucocorticoids and phenobarbital. Various drugs may also reduce physical activity.

Endocrine disorders causing obesity are rare in cats.

- Hypothyroidism is usually caused by treatment of hyperthyroidism. Naturally occurring hypothyroidism in mature cats is rare, but may be idiopathic or immune-mediated as in the dog.
- Acromegaly may cause initial obesity by appetite stimulation and weight gain by stimulation of bone and muscle growth. Cats with acromegaly ultimately develop diabetes mellitus, which causes weight loss.
- Hyperadrenocorticism may cause initial obesity by appetite stimulation. Many cats with hyperadrenocorticism develop diabetes mellitus, which causes weight loss.
- Insulinoma could theoretically promote obesity because of the anabolic effects of insulin, but this has not been reported.

Obesity causes or increases the risk for insulin resistance, impaired glucose tolerance, diabetes mellitus, hepatic lipidosis, feline lower urinary tract disease, musculoskeletal problems, bacterial skin infections, increased risk of surgical and anesthetic complications and impaired immune function. Obesity as a risk factor for cardiovascular disease and neoplasia in cats has not been reported.

Clinical signs

Obesity is typically **most pronounced in the abdominal region**, although the thorax, neck and upper limbs will also have increased subcutaneous fat.

- If abdominal distention is due to intra-abdominal fat, it will be **accompanied by deposition of subcutaneous fat**. Large subcutaneous fat depots may accumulate in the inguinal area.

Signs of adult-onset **hypothyroidism** include lethargy, inappetence, mild hypothermia and heat-seeking behavior, skin changes (dry lusterless hair, scale formation, alopecia, myxedema), bradycardia and reproductive problems. Obesity may be severe.

Signs of **acromegaly** include signs of diabetes mellitus, facial and carpopedal dysmorphism, and cardiomegaly. Signs of **hyperadrenocorticism** include signs of diabetes mellitus, abdominal distention, alopecia and fragile skin. The signs of **insulinoma** are those of hypoglycemia.

Diagnosis

Diagnosis of obesity is usually made on the basis of physical examination. Abdominal radiography or ultrasound examination can be used to confirm obesity as a cause of abdominal distention if necessary.

There is usually a **history of a highly palatable, high-calorie** diet being consumed and **physical inactivity**.

There is absence of other clinical signs of other causes of abdominal distention.

If there are signs of endocrinopathy, it should be confirmed by appropriate testing. Endocrinopathies are rare causes of obesity.

- Hypothyroidism may be suspected on the basis of clinical signs, a low T4 and/or free T4 (measured by equilibrium dialysis validated for cats), and absence of evidence for a concurrent disorder causing euthyroid sick syndrome.

- If there is a history of treatment for hyperthyroidism, the above findings plus response to therapy are sufficient for a diagnosis.
- If naturally occurring hypothyroidism is suspected, additional testing is recommended. Similar to testing for hypothyroidism in dogs, interpretation of tests is controversial.
- TSH response tests using animal-origin TSH have been used in the past, but such TSH is no longer widely available. Recombinant human TSH is now available, and protocols using this preparation should be defined in the future.
- TRH response test may be used: Obtain baseline serum sample, give 0.1 mg/kg IV, obtain post serum sample at 4 hours. A normal response is a > 50% increase from baseline.
- The assay for canine TSH has been used anecdotally but has not been validated for the cat.
- Thyroid biopsy may be obtained, demonstrating atrophy or thyroiditis.
- If there is a response to therapy, thyroid supplement can then be withdrawn to observe for recurrence of signs.

Differential diagnosis

The principal cause of abdominal distention that may be confused with fat is **fluid**. However, **many cats with ascites are chronically ill and have muscle wasting.**

Pregnancy – in pregnant cats the degree of abdominal distention may be disproportionate to the amount of subcutaneous fat.

Obesity is a common disorder and may make diagnosis of other concurrent causes of abdominal distention difficult by interfering with palpation.

Treatment

For successful management of obesity, it is **essential that the owner is committed to the goal** that their cat achieves a healthy body weight. The owner needs to understand and believe that appropriate management of obesity leads to a more active and healthier pet, and a longer life of their pet. The evidence that only **53% of obese cats were alive after 4 years** compared to 83% of cats with optimum body weight may help to convince some owners of the importance of weight loss.

Primary obesity is best treated by offering a **hypocaloric diet** designed for weight loss in cats. These diets generally have reduced fat and higher carbohydrate than maintenance diets, and a higher concentration of essential nutrients. Some are also high in fiber. Newer weight-loss diets for cats have restricted carbohydrate (<25% ME) and are high in protein.

A satiety effect of insoluble fiber (e.g. cellulose) used as a bulking agent has not been proven in cats, and foods rich in such fiber increase the risk of constipation. Fermentable fiber may promote satiety.

Because some obese cats have very low metabolic rates, it is best to calculate the amount of energy being consumed by the cat, and then **reduce energy fed to 80% of current consumption.** Using current energy consumption as a basis for restricting calories, makes it more likely that successful weight loss will be achieved in the first month of the program, which makes it more likely the owner will continue the program.

- If current energy consumption cannot be determined, a guideline is to offer 60–75% of energy theoretically required for maintenance of ideal body weight (i.e. **60–75% of 60 kcal/kg ideal body weight/day**) and **adjust every 2–4 weeks** to achieve a loss of about 1% of body weight per week.

At 1% weight loss per week, about 90% of weight will be lost from fat and <10% from lean body tissue. More severe calorie restriction decreases the proportion lost from fat and increases the proportion of weight lost from lean body tissue. Losses of body weight greater than 2% per week are dangerous as hepatic lipidosis may develop. During a weight loss program it is important to verify that the cat is eating regularly. Fasting will increase the risk for developing **hepatic lipidosis.**

It is important not to restrict calories by restricting protein.

Dietary additives may help promote weight loss and/or ameliorate secondary glucose intolerance, and are being added to commercial diets for cats.

- **l-carnitine** increases fatty acid oxidation and promotes fat loss, while preserving muscle mass. It also appears beneficial in treating cats with hepatic lipidosis. Supplemental l-carnitine can be dosed orally (250 mg/cat q 24 h of pharmacological grade product added to food or formulated as aqueous suspension).
- **Vitamin A** promotes weight loss by stimulating uncoupling protein formation, which increases

energy loss as heat. Vitamin A also decreases leptin (a hormone involved in fat metabolism) concentrations, which may improve insulin sensitivity.

- **Chromium, fermentable fiber and low glycemic index starch sources** (corn, sorghum) may improve glucose tolerance status by improving insulin sensitivity, increasing insulin secretion and decreasing post-prandial glucose concentrations, respectively.
- **Increasing physical activity is also beneficial,** but is not as easy to achieve in cats as in dogs. The most practical approach is to encourage the owner to engage in regular active play with the cat, such as having the cat chase an object on a string or a light spot, although it is not known what constitutes a proper "feline exercise program". Other alternatives for indoor cats are to provide an outdoor enclosure or leash-controlled outdoor activity sessions.
  - Cats given **environmental enrichments** such as additional food dishes, water bowls and litter boxes, plus climbing towers, window perches, scratching posts, cat spas, grooming supplies and toys, had **increased activity levels and greater weight loss** compared to cats that did not have an enriched environment

Surgical debulking of fat or liposuction has not been reported in cats and is not recommended.

The **use of drugs is currently not recommended**. Dehydroepiandrosterone may cause severe adverse reactions in cats. Thyroid hormone should only be used in cases of proven hypothyroidism. The initial dose is 0.05–1.0 mg once a day, with a goal of maintaining serum T4 between 20–40 nmol/L 4–6 hours after dosing.

Prognosis

The prognosis for weight reduction is dependent upon compliance.

The prognosis for complications of obesity depends upon the severity of obesity and other factors affecting the complicating disorder.

The prognosis for hypothyroidism is excellent.

Prevention

The ration should be restricted or a hypocaloric diet offered as soon as the propensity for obesity is noticed. Physical activity should be encouraged.

PREGNANCY***

Classical signs

- Mild to marked abdominal distention in breeding cats.

Pathogenesis

Intentional or unintentional breeding.

Clinical signs

Previous signs of estrus.

Abdominal distention usually does not become apparent until the **last 1–2 weeks of gestation**. It is easiest to detect in queens that are thin, have a short haircoat, have had previous pregnancies, and have large litters.

Mammary gland development ("milk bar") usually **does not become apparent until the last week of gestation**, although pinking of the nipples may be noted sooner. Abdominal distention is usually noted before development of a milk bar.

Nesting behavior does not begin until **1–2 days before delivery**.

Diagnosis

History of estrus, indoor/outdoor lifestyle, escape from indoors, or intentional breeding.

Fetal membranes can usually be **palpated from day 17–25 of gestation**, and occasionally up to day 35. The fetuses palpate as distinct water-filled spheres ("tiny bladders"). An enlarged uterus is palpable as a tubular organ between the colon and bladder from day 25 of gestation and on.

Fetuses can be seen by **ultrasound examination** beginning day **11–14 of gestation**; **fetal heartbeats** can be **seen by day 22–24**.

Fetal mineralization is first detectable by radiography beginning day 38 of gestation, but is most reliable for identifying **fetal skeletons after day 45 of gestation**. This corresponds to the period that abdominal distention becomes apparent.

- The above times are based on breeding dates and are not as reliable as times based on days prior to parturition. In a recent report, fetal mineralization was first detectable 25–29 days prior to parturition, and the vertebral column detectable by day 22–27 prior to parturition. The pattern of progressive mineralization was used to accurately predict day of parturition.

Differential diagnosis

Cats with uncomplicated pregnancies are healthy, and as such the **main differential diagnosis is obesity**. However, obese cats are more often neutered, and obese cats also have evidence of increased subcutaneous inguinal fat. Palpation of an enlarged uterus is usually possible in pregnant cats, and palpation findings can be confirmed by imaging.

If a **sick cat with abdominal distention with an unknown pregnancy** is presented for examination, all other causes for abdominal distention should be considered. If the only cause of abdominal distention found during work-up appears to be an enlarged uterus, then **acute metritis or spontaneous abortion should be considered**, as well as an unrelated disorder complicating pregnancy.

Treatment

Ovariohysterectomy if the pregnancy is unwanted.

Prognosis

Good – dystocia is uncommon in cats.

Prevention

Ovariohysterectomy; isolate from toms during heat.

FELINE INFECTIOUS PERITONITIS (FIP)***

Classical signs

- Depression, anorexia, weight loss, fever, pleural or peritoneal effusion.

Pathogenesis

FIP is caused by strains of **feline coronavirus (FCoV)**. These virulent stains have the **ability to replicate in macrophages as well as in epithelial cells**. The viru-

lent FIP strains arise from mutations in the avirulent (enteric) strains during replication of the latter. Both type I (genuine) FCoV and type II FCoV (which result from recombination between FCoV and canine coronavirus) can give rise to FIP strains.

The virus initially replicates in epithelial cells of the pharynx, respiratory system and intestinal tract.

Antibodies are produced, which fail to eliminate the virus and facilitate its uptake by macrophages, where the virus further replicates.

Macrophages migrate in the blood to venules of various tissues, e.g. the serosa of the abdomen. The macrophages exit the venules, and virus replication continues. **Antigen–antibody complexes form around the venules, attracting neutrophils**. The result is a **pyogranulomatous vasculitis, resulting in effusion.**

FIP is **more common in cats infected with feline leukemia virus** (FeLV) in areas where FeLV is frequent.

Clinical signs

Most common in cats **3 months to 3 years old**. There may also be an **increased prevalence in geriatric cats**.

FIP occurs in **two main forms: wet (effusive) and dry. Non-specific signs (depression, anorexia, weight loss, fever)** are common in both forms.

In **wet FIP, pericardial, pleural and/or peritoneal effusions** occur.
- Initially abdominal organs, especially the **intestines, may not feel as distinct as usual**.
- Later, as fluid accumulates, **marked painless distention of the abdomen** occurs.

In **dry FIP**, signs are referable to the organ involved.
- FIP may cause **chronic hepatitis**, which could result in abdominal distention from hepatomegaly and ascites from portal hypertension.
- Massive mesenteric lymphadenopathy has also been reported.

Diagnosis

No routinely performed test has 100% sensitivity or specificity, and diagnosis always relies on a combination of clinical signs and laboratory test results.

A complete blood count may reveal a mature **neutrophilia** (chronic inflammation), lymphopenia (stress), and **high plasma total protein** (increased globulins and fibrinogen).

A serum chemistry profile may reveal hyperglobulinemia and a decreased albumin to globulin ratio. (Total serum protein is less than plasma protein because of the absence of fibrinogen.) Liver enzymes ± bilirubin will be elevated if there is hepatic involvement.

"FIP tests", which include various **serum antibody tests and RT-PCR assays for FCoV viral antigens, are often non-contributory**. Positive tests indicate exposure or presence of FCoV and not necessarily the FIP strains. Tests are likely to be positive with classic effusive FIP, but a negative test result does not rule out the disease if the clinical, laboratory and pathologic findings are typical of the disease. Cats with very high titers are likely to have FIP. Furthermore, because the negative predictive value of the antibody test is high overall, cats with abdominal effusion and a negative antibody test result are unlikely to have FIP (although serum antibody titers may be low because of binding by the large viral load in the effusion).

Abdominal radiography or ultrasonography will demonstrate peritoneal fluid, typically containing echogenic debris.

Abdominocentesis. Cytologic, biochemical and immunologic **tests on the abdominal fluid are more useful than blood tests**. These tests include:

● **Cytology.** Peritoneal fluid from a cat with wet FIP will typically reveal a non-septic exudate. The **fluid is pale to straw-colored**, may contain white flecks (fibrin) and may clot upon standing. Cytology reveals a **high-protein** background (stippling, crescent formation) and **mature neutrophils**. Chylous effusion may also occur.

● **Total protein, albumin and globulin levels**. As in serum, but of more diagnostic value: the higher the total protein and globulin level, and lower the albumin to globulin ratio, the more likely the cat has FIP. Total protein ≥ 120 g/L (12 g/dl) had a specificity of 99% and positive predictive value of 89% in one study, while gamma-globulins ≥ 30 g/L (3.0 g/dl) and gamma-globulin content >32% in the fluid as demonstrated by protein electrophoresis have been reported to have 100% specificity and positive predictive values for FIP. An albumin to globulin ratio

of 1 was reported to have a negative predictive value of 91% (and a higher ratio would presumably have a higher negative predictive value.)
 – Rivalta's test is useful to confirm that the fluid is an exudate, by testing for coagulation of protein in an acetic acid solution. Five ml of distilled water and one drop of 98% (glacial) acetic acid are mixed in a test tube. Vinegar should be a practical alternative to use as a point-of-care test. One drop of the effusion is carefully layered on the surface of the solution. If the drop disappears and the solution remains clear, the test is negative and the fluid is a transudate. If the drop retains its shape, remains on the surface, or slowly floats down, the test is positive and the fluid is an exudate. Rivalta's test may also be positive in septic peritonitis and lymphoma (i.e. other causes of exudates), but these disorders can usually be ruled in or out with other tests.
 – Glucose may be detected with a urine dipstick but the diagnostic value of glucose level is not known.
 – **Direct immunofluorescence of FCoV antigen** in the peritoneal fluid macrophages. This has been reported to have a specificity and positive predictive value of 100%, and negative predictive value of 57–89%.
 – **Utility of measuring FCoV antibody in the effusion varies**, but it is at least as good as, and probably better, than a serum test.
 – Preliminary results indicate that RT-PCR for FCoV in the effusion is of high sensitivity and specificity.
 – Adenosine deaminase activity. The level in the fluid is usually higher than with other causes, but the test is not routinely available.

An FeLV test should be performed.

Exploratory surgery or laparoscopy with reveal multifocal small (e.g. 1–5 mm) white serosal plaques. Biopsies of abdominal lesions seen at surgery or laparascopy reveal **pyogranulomatous to granulomatous inflammation**. Immunohistochemistry may be used to demonstrate FCoV antigen within tissues. Viral culture may be available through research facilities.

Differential diagnosis

Differential diagnoses for cats with non-specific signs and peritoneal fluid include **neoplasia, pancreatitis** and **right heart failure**.

The main differential diagnoses for abdominal distention due to a **non-septic exudate are steatitis** and cholangiohepatitis. With steatitis, the abdomen is usually painful on palpation and abdominal fat is yellow to brown.

Differential diagnoses for liver disease include cholangiohepatitis, lipidosis and neoplasia.

Treatment

Supportive care.

Large-volume abdominocentesis.

Corticosteroids and immunosuppressive agents at standard doses have been used with limited success.

Antiviral drugs have been used with limited success.

Recombinant human and recombinant feline interferons appear to prolong survival in some cats. Recombinant feline interferon has been used at a dose of 1 million U/kg SC every other day until remission of clinical signs, followed by 1 million U/kg SC once a week. Prednisolone has been given concurrently at an initial dose of 2 mg/kg once a day and then tapered to 0.5 mg/kg every other day. A common recommendation is to use low-dose human recombinant interferon-alpha at 30 U/cat/day PO for 7 days on alternate weeks, although there are little firm data documenting benefit.

The **thromboxane synthetase inhibitor ozagrel hydrochloride**, 5–10 mg/kg, **combined with prednisolone**, 2 mg/kg, dramatically improved clinical signs in two cases, but ozagrel is not readily available.

Dapsone is effective in the treatment of vasculitis but has not been evaluated for FIP.

Prognosis

Effusive FIP is **almost always fatal within a few days to months** of onset of signs.

Transmission

FIP is most **common in multiple cat households** where cats are exposed to FCoV.

FCoV transmission occurs by **inhalation** of virus shed from oronasal secretions or **ingestion** of virus shed in feces.

An important time of transmission is from asymptomatic queens to kittens at 5–7 weeks of age.

In utero infection may occur, but this usually leads to abortion or neonatal loss.

Prevention

Routine disinfection is important because the virus is readily inactivated.

Do not introduce FCoV test-positive cats into a household. Identifying FCoV carriers prior to introduction in a multi-cat facility is the main value of FIP tests.

For catteries with a history of FCoV infections, isolate queens 2–3 weeks before parturition, quarantine queen and kittens after parturition, and then wean kittens at 4–5 weeks of age and isolate.

Modified-live intranasal vaccine is recommended for open multiple-cat households.

FeLV vaccination is recommended for open, multiple-cat households.

ABDOMINAL LYMPHOMA***

> ### Classical signs
>
> - Painless lymphadenopathy (multicentric lymphoma).
> - Anorexia, weight loss, vomiting, diarrhea (alimentary lymphoma).

Pathogenesis

Multicentric nodal lymphoma, characterized by **peripheral lymphadenopathy, frequently involves the liver and/or spleen**. This form is often associated with **FeLV infection** and is occasionally associated with **FIV infection**.

Alimentary lymphoma may affect various sites in the **gastrointestinal tract and mesenteric lymph nodes**, and may extend into the **liver, spleen or kidneys**. Extra-abdominal sites (e.g. lung, bone marrow) may also be involved. Alimentary lymphoma is infrequently associated with FeLV infection, and is occasionally associated with FIV infection.

- It has long been believed that chronic inflammatory bowel disease may progress to lymphoma.

Alternatively, severe inflammatory bowel disease may actually represent an indolent lymphoma. A progressive course of disease is more consistent with lymphoma while a waxing and waning course is more consistent with inflammatory bowel disease.
- Alimentary lymphoma has historically been considered to be primarily of B-cell origin. There is increasing evidence of T-cell alimentary lymphoma, especially with low-grade lymphomas.

Solitary hepatic, splenic or renal lymphoma may also occur.

Abdominal lymphoma may cause abdominal distention by **hepatomegaly, splenomegaly, gastrointestinal thickening or dilation, or fluid.**
- Abdominal lymphoma may cause ascites by portal vein compression, lymphatic obstruction, septic peritonitis secondary to intestinal perforation and spontaneous hemorrhage.

Clinical signs

Multicentric nodal lymphoma:
- Variable lethargy, inappetence and weight loss. Some cats have no systemic signs.
- Generalized moderate to marked painless **peripheral lymphadenopathy**.
- Variable hepatomegaly and icterus, splenomegaly, abdominal distention (uncommon).

Alimentary lymphoma:
- Anorexia, inappetence and weight loss.
- **Variable vomiting and diarrhea**, but absence of these signs does not rule out alimentary lymphoma.
- Variable intestinal mass or thickening, organomegaly, icterus and abdominal distention.
- Peripheral lymphadenopathy is uncommon.

Other abdominal extra-nodal lymphoma:
- Signs of specific organ failure, e.g. icterus with hepatic lymphoma.
- Variable organomegaly and abdominal distention.

Diagnosis

Abdominal radiography or ultrasonography may demonstrate an intestinal mass or intestinal thickening, splenomegaly, hepatomegaly, lymphadenopathy or peritoneal fluid.

Biopsy of gastrointestinal tract or other abdominal organ.
- In addition to making a diagnosis, the biopsy should be used to grade the lymphoma with respect to its aggressiveness. High-grade lymphomas are poorly differentiated and may be further characterized as immunoblastic or lymphoblastic. Low-grade lymphomas are well differentiated and may also be referred to as lymphocytic. Intermediate forms also occur. The percentage of cell types varies between studies, but overall low-grade lymphomas are less common than intermediate and high-grade lymphomas.
- Lymphocytic gastrointestinal lymphoma may have a tendency to be epitheliotropic (to involve the mucosa) and to be of T-cell origin.

FeLV and FIV tests should be obtained.

Iron-deficiency anemia from chronic gastrointestinal hemorrhage may occur with alimentary lymphoma.

Peritoneal fluid may be a **transudate, modified transudate, septic exudate, chylous** or **hemorrhagic effusion**, and may contain neoplastic cells.

Differential diagnosis

Differential diagnoses for generalized lymphadenopathy include atypical hyperplasia, hyperplasia in response to generalized skin diseases, immunologic disorders and systemic infections, widely metastatic neoplasia, and generalized bacterial or fungal lymphadenitis.

Differential diagnoses for lethargy, anorexia, weight loss, vomiting and diarrhea include inflammatory bowel disease, other gastrointestinal neoplasia, pancreatitis, systemic mycoses and cholangiohepatitis. Other than inflammatory bowel disease, these disorders may also cause lethargy, anorexia and weight loss without vomiting and diarrhea.

Differential diagnoses for marked splenomegaly include mast cell tumor and other tumors.

Treatment

Chemotherapy as described in Chapter 31 Aggressive lymphomas should be treated aggressively and indolent lymphomas should be treated more conservatively.

Cats with **high-grade lymphoma** should be treated with a **multi-agent protocol**.

Cats with **low-grade lymphoma** (usually alimentary) may be treated with less aggressive protocols such as **prednisone and chlorambucil**.

Splenectomy may be considered for splenic lymphoma if there is no evidence of lymphoma at another site. Because there is always the possibility of undetected microscopic lymphoma at another site, surgery should be reserved **for cats where there is poor response** to, or **unacceptable side effects with**, **chemotherapy**.

Surgical removal of a gastrointestinal lymphomatous mass should be reserved for cats where the tumor is causing gastrointestinal obstruction or perforation. **Surgical removal in addition to chemotherapy in other cases does not appear to be of added benefit.**

Prognosis

Response to chemotherapy in several case series provides general information, but it is difficult to give a prognosis for an individual cat. Ultimately the only way to determine prognosis is to treat the cat and observe response.

The prognosis for multicentric lymphoma is discussed in The Cat With Enlarged Lymph Nodes.

In recent reports, about **one-third to two-thirds of cats with alimentary lymphoma achieved a complete remission** with chemotherapy, many of the other cats achieved a partial remission (with overall response rates up to 90%), and **1-year survival about 20–40%**. Some of these cats will become long-term survivors and are considered to be cured.

Regardless of anatomic location, usually only cats that achieve a complete remission with induction chemotherapy have the possibility of being cured.

FeLV status, FIV status, sex, tumor burden and location, histologic grade and immunophenotype do not independently consistently predict achievement of remission, duration of remission or survival. Some of the weakness of prognostic factors may reflect different criteria for anatomic location and histologic grade as well as the poor statistical power of relatively small case series. Certain combination of factors may affect prognosis. For example, cats with well-differentiated

intestinal epitheliotropic lymphoma have a better prognosis than with other forms of abdominal lymphoma. In one report, 69% achieved complete remission with a median survival of 22.8 months.

Most cats tolerate chemotherapy for lymphoma and fatal complications of chemotherapy are rare.

Solid tumors***

> ### Classical signs
>
> ● Chronic anorexia, lethargy, weight loss.

Clinical signs

Anorexia, lethargy and weight loss.

Variable fever, vomiting, diarrhea, icterus, palpable mass, depending upon the location of the tumor.
● Absence of vomiting or diarrhea does not rule out a gastrointestinal tumor.

Abdominal fluid ± abdominal distention may be present because of **pre-hepatic or hepatic portal hypertension, lymphatic obstruction or hemorrhage**. A **large abdominal mass** may contribute to abdominal distention.
● **Splenic or hepatic hemangiosarcoma** is the most common neoplastic cause of **hemoperitoneum**, but it is much less common than in the dog. Other tumors may also spontaneously bleed.
● **Abdominal fluid** has been recognized with **many solid tumors**, including those of the **liver, pancreas, kidney, intestinal tract and peritoneum** (mesothelioma).

Iron-deficiency anemia from chronic gastrointestinal hemorrhage may occur with gastrointestinal adenocarcinomas.

Diagnosis

Abdominal radiography or ultrasonography may demonstrate an abdominal mass, organomegaly or peritoneal fluid.

Biopsy of suspected neoplastic tissue.

Abdominal fluid may be a transudate, modified transudate, chylous or hemorrhagic effusion, and may contain neoplastic cells.

Differential diagnosis

Differential diagnoses for a cat with subacute to chronic non-specific signs and peritoneal fluid include cholangiohepatitis, pancreatitis, tuberculosis, pyogranulomatous bacterial infections, systemic mycoses and toxoplasmosis.

Differential diagnoses for an abdominal mass include cyst, focal necrosis, abscess, granulomatous inflammation, intussusception and heterotopic ossification of the liver. Most of these will not commonly cause abdominal distention or fluid.

Differential diagnosis for a thickened peritoneum or peritoneum covered with multiple plaques or nodules other than mesothelioma or metastatic neoplasia include FIP, tuberculosis and sclerosing encapsulating peritonitis.

Treatment

Most solid tumors are best treated by surgical excision, but they are often unresectable by the time ascites develops.

Benefit of chemotherapy for most abdominal solid tumors is not known, but effect is likely to be poor in most cases, and anorexia is common with aggressive combination protocols. Use of **carboplatin or lomustine** as single agents may be considered in that side effects in most cats are minimal.

Radiation therapy may be considered, but in many cases will not be feasible.

Abdominocentesis may be used to reduce signs attributable to marked abdominal distention.

Rutin, 50 mg/kg PO tid, may be considered to reduce effusion if it is chylous. (It may also be used to help alleviate chylous effusions due to other causes.)

Intracavitary chemotherapy with carboplatin or thiotepa may be considered in an effort to alleviate effusion due to widespread metastasis or mesothelioma.

Diuretics may reduce malignant ascites in some cases. Furosemide, 1 mg/kg PO/SC/IV once to twice daily, or spironolactone, 1–2 mg/kg PO, bid may be tried.

VISCERAL MAST CELL TUMOR**

Classical signs

- Depression, anorexia, weight loss, marked splenomegaly (splenic mast cell tumor).
- Depression, anorexia, weight loss, vomiting, diarrhea (intestinal mast cell tumor).

Pathogenesis

Mast cell tumor is a spontaneously arising neoplasm and is not related to FeLV or FIV infection.

Splenic mast cell tumor **frequently metastasizes**; organs involved, in decreasing order of frequency, are **liver, abdominal or thoracic lymph nodes, bone marrow** and peripheral blood, lung and intestine.

Intestinal mast cell tumor most commonly involves the **small intestine**, and may involve multiple sites. Metastasis to liver and mesenteric lymph nodes is common; metastasis to spleen, lung and bone marrow may also occur.

Visceral mast cell tumor may cause abdominal distention by **splenomegaly**, effusion or spontaneous hemorrhage.

Clinical signs

Splenic mast cell tumor:
- Variable depression, anorexia, weight loss, intermittent vomiting, dyspnea.
- Marked splenomegaly.
- Abdominal fluid may be detectable on physical examination.

Intestinal mast cell tumor:
- Variable depression, anorexia, weight loss, fever, dyspnea, intermittent vomiting, diarrhea. Melena or hematochezia may be present.
- Intestinal mass(es) or thickened intestines may be palpable.
- Peritoneal fluid may be detectable on physical examination.

Diagnosis

Abdominal radiography or ultrasonography may demonstrate splenomegaly, hepatomegaly, intestinal mass, lymphadenopathy or peritoneal fluid.

- Sonographic abnormalities of the spleen include splenomegaly, irregular contour, mottled appearance, and hyperechoic and hypoechoic nodules. Lymph nodes may be hypoechoic. Intestinal masses are hypoechoic and there is loss of normal wall layering. Effusion is anechoic.

Fine-needle biopsy of spleen, gastrointestinal mass or other organ based on clinical signs will often reveal neoplastic mast cells. Surgical biopsy of intestinal masses may be required for diagnosis. Intraoperative cytology is recommended, so that wide surgical excision of the tumor(s) may follow.

- **Abdominal fluid usually contains mast cells with or without eosinophils.** Occasionally no mast cells are present.

Fifty percent of cats with splenic mast cell tumor will have **mast cells in the peripheral blood** on cytologic examination of direct smear or buffy coat smears. Other laboratory findings include **hyperglobulinemia** and coagulation abnormalities.

Iron-deficiency anemia from chronic intestinal hemorrhage may occur with intestinal mast cell tumor.

Eosinophilia may occur with visceral mast cell tumors.

Differential diagnosis

The main **differential diagnosis for marked splenomegaly** is **lymphoma**, but it does not typically cause the massive splenomegaly seen in cats with mast cell tumor.

The main differential diagnoses for an **intestinal mass and abdominal distention** are **adenocarcinoma** and **lymphoma**. Chronic intussusceptions are rare, and would not typically be associated with abdominal distention or fluid.

The **presence of eosinophils in peritoneal fluid** is not specific for mast cell tumor, and has also been seen with **lymphoma, septic peritonitis** and **pneumothorax**. However, the presence of mast cells is highly specific for visceral mast cell tumor.

Treatment

Splenectomy or excision with 5–10 cm margins of intestinal masses.

The benefit or detriment of chemotherapy in addition to surgery is not known. Prednisone alone or protocols used to treat lymphoma may be considered.

Prognosis

The prognosis for **splenic mast cell tumor** is good, even with evidence of widespread dissemination. **Median survival post-splenectomy is 12–19 months**, and peripheral mastocytosis declines.

The **prognosis for intestinal mast cell tumor is poor**, with most cats being euthanized soon after diagnosis or treatment.

RIGHT HEART FAILURE**

> **Classical signs**
>
> - Dyspnea due to pleural effusion.

Pathogenesis

Cats with right heart failure usually develop pleural effusion. Peritoneal effusion is a less common occurrence.

- Peritoneal effusion has been observed with **congenital tricuspid valve dysplasia, patent ductus arteriosus and intrapericardial heterotopic liver**.
- Peritoneal effusion has been observed with **acquired pericardial effusion** (which in-itself may be a sign of right heart failure), **persistent atrial standstill**, traumatic tricuspid valvular insufficiency, tricuspid valvular endocarditis, myocarditis, **heartworm disease**, severe chronic anemia, and **dilated, hypertrophic and restrictive cardiomyopathy**. Of these various disorders, dilated cardiomyopathy is most likely to cause peritoneal effusion.

Pulmonary edema may also be present due to left heart failure.

Clinical signs

Peritoneal effusion is usually accompanied by pleural effusion. Pleural effusion ± pulmonary edema will cause dyspnea.

- Most peritoneal effusion due to right heart failure causes undetected to minimal abdominal distention.

- Marked abdominal distention is occasionally the predominant clinical sign.

Other signs of heart disease variably present include jugular distention, murmur, gallop rhythm, tachycardia, bradycardia and irregular rhythm.

Diagnosis

Radiography is useful to demonstrate pleural effusion and large-volume peritoneal effusion.

Echocardiography will assess myocardial function, and valvular competency, and may demonstrate trans-diaphragmatic peritoneal effusion. If echocardiography is not available, non-selective angiocardiography is useful to diagnose dilated and hypertrophic cardiomyopathy.

Electrocardiography will characterize arrhythmias.

Abdominal ultrasonography will demonstrate peritoneal fluid.

Abdominocentesis usually reveals a **modified transudate**.

Differential diagnosis

The **main differential diagnosis** for a cat presented in **acute heart failure** characterized by cardiogenic shock, dyspnea and abdominal fluid is **acute abdominal hemorrhage**. Pulmonary crackles will usually be present in heart failure.

The main differential diagnosis for a cat with **chronic heart failure** characterized by **pleural and peritoneal effusions is neoplasia**. Other differential diagnoses include iatrogenic volume overload, hypoalbuminemia, feline infectious peritonitis and systemic bacterial and mycotic infections.

Treatment

The treatment of heart failure is discussed in The Cat With an Enlarged Heart or Abnormal Heart Sounds.

Specific treatment of peritoneal effusion is usually not required.

Diuretic therapy (e.g. furosemide, initial dose 1–2 mg/kg bid) will help reduce abdominal fluid.

Large-volume abdominocentesis should be considered for ascites not responsive to diuretic treatment that is causing diaphragmatic compression, stomach compression or abdominal discomfort.

Prognosis

The prognosis for cats with ascites due to right heart failure is poor, because of the poor prognosis of most of the underling heart diseases.

For a specific heart disease, it is not known if the presence of peritoneal effusion in addition to pleural effusion changes prognosis.

TRAUMATIC RUPTURE OF THE URINARY BLADDER OR URETHRA**

> ### Classical signs
> - Acute depression, anorexia, dehydration, vomiting, anuria.

Pathogenesis

Causes are listed in approximate decreasing order of frequency. These causes include:

- **Blunt abdominal trauma.**
  - **Motor vehicle trauma** is the most common cause, followed by **falling from heights**, although a ruptured urinary bladder is not a common injury, especially compared to other traumatic injuries (e.g. pelvic fractures, facial injuries). **Trauma usually causes rupture at the apex of the bladder.**
- **Urethral catheterization**.
  - This is most likely to occur when treating urethral obstruction. Rupture usually occurs in the **urethra or neck of the bladder**. Urethral obstruction may also spontaneously lead to urethral rupture without catheterization.
- **Expression of the urinary bladder.**
  - This is most likely to occur when trying to express the bladder in an unsedated cat with urethral spasm following relief of urethral obstruction, or following cystocentesis.
- **Cystocentesis.**
  - This rarely causes rupture of the bladder, but has occurred when performing cystocentesis on cats

with a severely distended bladder following urethral obstruction.

● **Penetrating abdominal trauma.**
  – Bite wounds, staking injuries and bullet wounds are uncommon causes of urinary tract trauma.

Acute bladder rupture occasionally causes marked hemorrhage into the abdomen or into the bladder (with massive clot formation).

Clinical signs

Clinical signs are due to **post-renal uremia** and associated disorders.

Non-specific signs of uroperitoneum include variable **depression, lethargy, anorexia and dehydration**. Body temperature and heart rate may be elevated, normal or low. Vomiting is common. Abdominal pain may be present.

Many cats are not urinating, but **presence of urination does not rule out urinary tract rupture**. (If urination is present, there may be hematuria.)

Similarly, a **palpable bladder does not rule out rupture of either the bladder or urethra**.

Abdominal distention and a fluid wave are occasionally evident. Urethral rupture may also cause inguinal subcutaneous edema (there may also be signs of inflammation due to cellulitis).

Diagnosis

A serum chemistry profile will reveal mild to **marked elevations in urea and creatinine levels** unless the animal is tested shortly after injury. Hyperkalemia may also be present.

Abdominal ultrasonography will demonstrate peritoneal fluid.

Peritoneal fluid is initially a pale yellow to serosanguineous transudate, and cytology will be unremarkable, unless the cat is a tom, where sperm may be present. Cell counts may increase with time (> 3×10^9/L, 3000/µl) resulting in a modified transudate. Secondary septic peritonitis will result in an exudate with degenerate neutrophils and bacteria.

● **Creatinine or potassium levels** in the abdominal fluid **greater than that of the serum** are strongly suggestive of uroperitoneum. (It is not sufficient to simply measure those parameters in the peritoneal fluid because azotemic animals with ascites will also have creatinine and potassium in the ascitic fluid.) The higher the abdominal fluid:serum creatinine and potassium ratios, the more likely the cat has uroperitoneum. In one study of cats with uroperitoneum, the abdominal fluid:serum creatinine ratio ranged from 1.1:1 to 4:1, with a mean of 2:1, and the abdominal fluid:serum potassium ratio ranged from 1.2:1 to 2.4:1, with a mean of 1.9:1. Abdominal fluid:serum urea ratios are not as reliable because of more rapid equilibration of urea.

Contrast radiography will demonstrate a rupture of the bladder or urethra. To demonstrate a rupture of the bladder, the **radiograph should be obtained just as the final amount of contrast material is injected**. If only a small amount of contrast material leaks out of the bladder, it may be rapidly diluted in the peritoneal fluid resulting in a false-negative study.

Differential diagnosis

Differential diagnoses for a cat presented for **no urination** include **ethylene glycol** or **lily poisoning**, or **urethral obstruction**.

Differential diagnoses for a cat presented with **acute depression and peritoneal fluid** include **right heart failure, acute pancreatitis, liver disease** with ascites and hepatic encephalopathy, and **acute abdominal hemorrhage** (mucous membranes will be pale).

Other rare causes of **uroperitoneum** include spontaneous leakage at the site of a bladder tumor, traumatic avulsion of a ureter, transudation of urine through a severely inflamed bladder wall and leakage post-nephrotomy. Radiographic contrast studies will facilitate diagnosis. An excretory urogram may be required to demonstrate an avulsed ureter.

Treatment

Fluid therapy to correct dehydration and reduce uremia.

Antibiotics if there is secondary septic peritonitis, e.g. ampicillin, cefoxitin at standard doses.

Large-volume abdominocentesis to reduce uremia. Peritoneal dialysis will further reduce uremia but is not usually required.

Ruptured urinary bladders are usually surgically repaired.

Non-surgical management (catheterization to keep the bladder empty) has been described in other species. It may be considered if the cat is too unstable for surgery, but will not usually reduce costs because of the longer hospitalization period.

Ruptured urethras may be treated by **surgical repair** or by **placement of an ante-pubic urinary catheter**, or less optimally by chronic urethral catheterization.

Prognosis

Uroperitoneum in-itself carries a good prognosis. Uremia will rapidly resolve once the urinary tract is repaired. Chemical peritonitis from urine also usually rapidly resolves. Prognosis is largely determined by associated injuries.

MEGACOLON**

> **Classical signs**
>
> - Chronic straining to defecate.

See main reference on page 783 for details (The Constipated or Straining Cat).

Clinical signs

Variable anorexia, lethargy, weight loss, unkempt haircoat and vomiting.

Straining to defecate, with the resultant minimal passage of feces that may be dry or mucoid.

Large volume of firm feces in the colon on abdominal palpation. Digital rectal examination may reveal **narrowing of pelvic canal** secondary to fractures or tumor. Neurologic examination may reveal **sacral nerve injury.**

Marked colonic dilation may occur causing abdominal distention.

Diagnosis

Abdominal radiography will demonstrate marked accumulation of feces in the colon.

Differential diagnosis

The main differential diagnosis for a cat with chronic dyschezia, tenesmus and abdominal distention is colonic neoplasia with metastases resulting in obstructive ascites.

Treatment

For the cat with megacolon sufficiently severe to cause abdominal distention, subtotal colectomy is recommended.

If medical therapy is desired, correct dehydration, administer parenteral antibiotics (e.g. ampicillin) to protect against bacterial translocation, and administer multiple small volume enemas with lactulose prior to anesthetizing the cat for manual disimpaction. Use of enema soap will facilitate the latter (do not use chlorhexidine soaps). If disimpaction is successful, chronic therapy consists of a low-residue diet, lactulose and prokinetic agents (e.g. cisapride).

JUVENILE ABDOMINAL FLUID**

> **Classical signs**
>
> - Mild excess in abdominal fluid encountered during pediatric ovariohysterectomy.

Clinical signs

More peritoneal fluid may be encountered when spaying a cat at an early age (e.g. 3 months) than at a traditional age (e.g. 6 months).

Diagnosis

The fluid is a **transudate**.

Differential diagnosis

FIP, where the fluid is a non-septic exudate.

Treatment

None required.

PANCREATITIS**

> **Classical signs**
>
> - Acute depression and anorexia.
> - Ascites may develop.

See main reference on page 272 (The Cat With Depression, Anorexia or Dehydration).

Clinical signs

Cat may be of **any age, with no sex or breed predilection**, except perhaps for Siamese cats.

Duration of clinical signs prior to presentation varies from **several days to more than 3 weeks**.

Depression and/or anorexia are the most common historical signs and may be the only signs present. The **most common physical abnormalities are dehydration and hypothermia**. Fever is uncommon.

Other inconsistent signs include weight loss, vomiting, diarrhea, cranial abdominal pain, cranial abdominal mass, dyspnea, ataxia and disorientation, and shock. Polydipsia may be present, but is usually due to concurrent diabetes mellitus.

- **Peritoneal effusion** may occur, and in some cases may be of sufficient quantity to cause abdominal distention. Peritoneal effusion may be more likely to occur when there is concurrent liver disease. Pleural effusion may also occur.

Diagnosis

Because clinical and laboratory findings are non-specific, diagnosis requires a high index of suspicion.

Pancreatitis should be considered in any cat with unexplained acute depression. Pancreatitis should also be considered in any critically ill cat developing ascites, pleural effusion or hypothermia.

Laboratory findings are variable and are most valuable in ruling out other causes of depression and anorexia. The most sensitive and specific tests are elevations in feline trypsin-like immunoreactivity and feline pancreatic lipase immunoreactivity. No laboratory abnormality appears to be correlated with the development or severity of effusion.

- Peritoneal effusion is usually a modified transudate, but may be a non-septic exudate.

Diagnostic imaging findings are also variable.

- On abdominal radiographs, **decreased contrast** may be present due to effusion. This may be restricted to the cranial abdomen or be more generalized.
- Other radiographic findings supportive of pancreatitis include a mass effect in the right cranial quadrant (displacement of organs), and localized dilation of loops of intestine (ileus). Normal findings do not rule out pancreatitis.
- On abdominal ultrasonography, accumulation of **peritoneal fluid around the pancreas** is a highly specific finding for pancreatitis. Generalized peritoneal effusion is a less specific finding.
- Other ultrasonographic findings with a high specificity for pancreatitis include pancreatic regular or irregular enlargement, pancreatic hypoechogenicity, hyperechogenicity of peripancreatic fat (may be difficult to appreciate), and dilation of the pancreatic duct in the left lobe. Normal findings do not rule out pancreatitis.
- Definitive ante-mortem diagnosis requires **biopsy** obtained by exploratory laparotomy or laparoscopy.

Differential diagnosis

Differential diagnoses for cats with **pancreatitis causing acute depression and abdominal fluid** include septic peritonitis, acute abdominal hemorrhage, right heart failure, ruptured urinary bladder, ruptured gall bladder, steatitis, toxoplasmosis, ligation of a portosystemic shunt and, uncommonly, hepatic encephalopathy where liver disease is also causing ascites.

For cats with **pancreatitis causing subacute depression and abdominal fluid**, the primary differential diagnoses are neoplasia, feline infectious peritonitis and right heart failure.

Treatment

Address the inciting cause if one is identified.

The remainder of therapy is largely **supportive**.

Antiemetics and analgesics.

Surgical debridement of grossly necrotic tissue and therapeutic abdominal lavage, or closed therapeutic abdominal lavage using a technique similar to diagnostic peritoneal lavage, should be considered if peritoneal fluid is an exudate.

If there is a large volume of ascites that is a modified transudate, therapeutic abdominocentesis should be considered, and it should definitely be performed if there is a problem secondary to a volume effect (e.g. dyspnea from diaphragmatic compression), but the benefit of the procedure on the course of the disease is not known.

SEPTIC PERITONITIS*

Classical signs

- Acute depression, anorexia, fever, abdominal pain.

Clinical signs

Acute onset of depression and anorexia; the cat may be moribund.

Variable vomiting and diarrhea. These are most likely if the cause is a perforating intestinal foreign body.

Initial fever, tachycardia ± dark pink mucous membranes, but these signs may **progress rapidly to normothermia** or **hypothermia**, **bradycardia** and **pale mucous membranes with severe sepsis or septic shock** (see The Cat With Acute Depression, Anorexia and Dehydration).

Pain is present on abdominal palpation in about 2/3 of cases. The cat is probably less likely to react if it is moribund. Mild abdominal distention may be present.

Polypnea and icterus may be present.

Diagnosis

History or signs of **abdominal surgery**, sharp or blunt **trauma to abdomen**, linear or sharp gastrointestinal **foreign body**, pre-existing **infection of abdominal organ** (e.g. hepatic abscess, pyometra), pre-existing abdominal neoplasia, pre-existing disorder with ascites, pre-existing infection outside of abdomen causing peritonitis by extension or hematogenous spread, ingestion of raw meat (source of *Salmonella* spp.), or inappropriate use of NSAIDs. In some cases no cause can be found. Septic peritonitis is less common in cats than dogs.

A complete blood count usually reveals **hemoconcentration and a left shift and toxic neutrophils**. The total neutrophil count may be elevated, normal or low, depending upon the severity and acuteness of inflammation. Mild anemia may be present.

A serum chemistry profile may reveal **hyperalbuminemia (dehydration), hypoalbuminemia (abdominal exudation), hyperglycemia (stress)** or **hypoglycemia (severe sepsis).**

Abdominal radiography may demonstrate loss of detail and **"ground-glass" appearance and/or free gas** in the abdomen. Abdominal ultrasonography may demonstrate peritoneal fluid and ileus. Imaging may also reveal evidence of pleural fluid.

Abdominocentesis may yield fluid. The **fluid is a septic exudate**, although intra-cellular bacteria may not be seen. Sensitivity of cytology is reported as approximately 60–90%, although in a recent case series peritoneal fluid cytology and a nucleated cell count $> 13 \times 10^9/L$ (13 000/µl) had a diagnostic accuracy of 100% in cats. Abdominal fluid should be Gram-stained and cultured for aerobic and anaerobic bacteria. The most frequently isolated organisms are *Escherichia coli, Enterococcus* spp and *Clostridium* spp.

- In a recent report, glucose levels in septic peritoneal fluid were usually lower than blood glucose levels, and a difference of > 1.1 mmol/L (20 mg/dl) was highly specific for septic peritonitis. In contrast, glucose levels in non-septic effusions were equal or higher than blood levels. (This study did not include cats with FIP.) In addition, septic effusions tended to have a lower pH and higher lactate levels than non-septic effusions.
- Food particles may be seen with gastrointestinal perforation.
- If abdominocentesis is unsuccessful, and pre-surgical confirmation of septic peritonitis is desired, diagnostic peritoneal lavage should be performed.

Differential diagnosis

Differential diagnoses for an **acutely depressed cat** with abdominal distention and/or pain include **trauma,** urethral obstruction, panleukopenia and other causes of acute enteritis, acute pancreatitis and acute pyelonephritis.

Differential diagnoses for a moribund cat with abdominal distention include urethral obstruction, hepatic encephalopathy, feline infectious peritonitis, advanced neoplasia, heart failure and hemoperitoneum.

Treatment

Supportive care and treatment for hypotension or shock, including intravenous fluids, is required.

Broad-spectrum intravenous antibiotics, e.g. ampicillin and gentamicin; cefoxitin (second-generation cephalosporin); cefazolin (first-generation cephalosporin) combined with enrofloxacin and metronidazole or clindamycin; or imipenem-cilastatin as a single agent. It should be remembered that enrofloxacin is not licensed for parenteral use in the cat, and there are anecdotal reports of blindness following a single injection. If "sulfur granules" are seen suggestive of *Actinomyces* spp. or *Nocardia* spp., then initial empirical therapy should consist of penicillin G or ampicillin and trimethoprim-sulfa, or imipenem-cilastatin.

Exploratory laparatomy to address underlying cause of peritonitis and to lavage abdomen. Post-operative open-abdomen management or closed-suction drainage systems are often required to treat severe generalized peritonitis. With such management, the prognosis for cats appears to be similar to dogs, with average survival rates of 60–80%.

GASTROENTERITIS*

Classical signs

- Vomiting and/or diarrhea.

Clinical signs

Cats with acute or chronic gastroenteritis will have vomiting and/or diarrhea of variable frequency and severity.

Other variable clinical signs include depression, anorexia, dehydration, weight loss, reduced growth rate in kittens, abdominal pain, melena and hematochezia.

Abdominal distention may occur because of ileus, with intestinal fluid retention, flatus (especially in acute gastroenteritis), thickening of the intestinal wall (especially in chronic gastroenteritis, e.g. inflammatory bowel disease), or rarely because of ascites due to protein-losing enteropathy. Enlarged intestines contribute to the prominent abdominal contour characteristic of malnourished kittens with a heavy roundworm burden.

- Abdominal distention is usually mild except in neonatal kittens where it may be severe.
- Distended loops of intestine may feel more or less distinct than usual. Palpation may yield a "squishy" or spongy sensation and create borborygmus.
- Thickened loops of intestine will feel more prominent on abdominal palpation.

Diagnosis

Abdominal radiographs will always demonstrate dilation of the intestines with air, and may demonstrate dilation of the intestines with fluid. Neither plain nor contrast radiographs are very useful to evaluate thickness of the intestinal walls.

Abdominal ultrasonography is very useful to rule out peritoneal fluid, to demonstrate intestinal wall thickening and to evaluate intestinal motility.

Differential diagnosis

Differential diagnoses for cats with vomiting, diarrhea and abdominal distention include acute pancreatitis, cholangiohepatitis, hepatic lipidosis, gastrointestinal neoplasia and acute renal failure with volume overload.

Treatment

Treatment of the primary disease.

Severe gastrointestinal distention by flatus in neonates should be relieved by intubation (stomach air) or trans-abdominal enterocentesis (intestinal air).

Simethicone is not of proven value to reduce flatus formation in humans, and is likely of no benefit in cats.

TOXOPLASMOSIS*

Classical signs

- Anorexia, fever, dyspnea and signs of ocular inflammation in mature cats.
- Fading neonate.

See main references on page 375 for details (The Pyrexic Cat).

Clinical signs

Non-specific signs of **depression, anorexia, weight loss and fever** are common.

Specific clinical signs vary with the various organs involved.
- Common signs include **uveitis, dyspnea** (pneumonia) and **muscle pain**.
- All abdominal organs may be infected by *Toxoplasma gondii*. Specific clinical signs of abdominal infection are usually due to **hepatitis** and **hepatic necrosis** (icterus), and **mesenteric lymphadenopathy** (palpable nodes). Vomiting, diarrhea and pain on abdominal palpation may be present. Peritoneal fluid may also be present, but is unlikely to cause abdominal distention.

Specific signs may also be due to concurrent disorders causing immunosuppression.

Diagnosis

Routine laboratory results are variable. **Neutrophilia** is common with systemic infection. Hepatitis is common, causing **elevations in liver enzymes and bilirubin**.

Abdominal imaging may reveal hepatomegaly, changes consistent with pancreatitis (see The Cat With Acute Anorexia, Depression or Dehydration), mesenteric lymphadenopathy and peritoneal fluid.

Peritoneal fluid is presumably a **transudate or modified transudate, which may contain tachyzooites**.

Abnormalities at exploratory laparatomy include hepatomegaly, reticular pattern to the surface of the liver with **multiple 1–3 mm spots**, **thickened pancreas** with **saponification of peripancreatic fat**, **lymphadenopathy** and focal thickening of the intestines.

Biopsies of abdominal organs may reveal **mixed inflammation, tachyzooites**, and **occasionally cysts**. Histology will also reveal multifocal necrosis.

Elevated IgM titer; **four-fold rise in IgG titers 3 weeks apart**. Serology gives the most interpretable information if both acute and convalescent IgM and IgG titers are obtained.

Differential diagnosis

Differential diagnoses for cats with hepatopathy, mesenteric lymphadenopathy and peritoneal fluid include concurrent inflammatory bowel disease and pancreatitis, alimentary lymphoma, FIP, tuberculosis and systemic fungal infections. Of these, only the infectious diseases are likely to also cause pleural fluid, pneumonia (except for FIP), or uveitis.

Treatment

Clindamycin 10–25 mg/kg PO, IM, IV bid continuing at least 2 weeks beyond resolution of clinical signs.

Sulfadiazine (30 mg/kg PO bid) and **pyrimethamine** (0.5 mg/kg PO bid) may be used if clindamycin is not available or not tolerated. **Folinic acid** (5 mg/day) or **brewer's yeast** (100 mg/kg/day) may be required to correct myelosuppression resulting from folinic acid deficiency caused by therapy.

Trimethoprim-sulfonamide 30 mg/kg bid may be considered if these are the only drugs available.

Supportive care.

INTESTINAL TUBERCULOSIS*

Classical signs

- Chronic weight loss, vomiting, diarrhea, mesenteric lymphadenopathy.

Clinical signs

Cats with the intestinal form of tuberculosis (caused by *Mycobacteria tuberculosis, M. bovis, M. tuberculosis-bovis* variant, and *M. microti*) and intestinal involvement with non-tubercular mycobacteria (*M. avium* complex) may show signs varying from **subclinical infection to chronic enteritis** characterized by **weight loss, fever, vomiting, diarrhea and mesenteric lymphadenopathy**.

Cats with advanced disease may develop obstructive ascites.

Diagnosis

Laboratory results are variable, but **non-regenerative anemia** is common.

Abdominal radiographs may reveal **mesenteric lymphadenopathy** and **peritoneal fluid**. Abdominal ultrasonography may reveal **intestinal thickening**, **mesenteric lymphadenopathy**, and peritoneal fluid. Lymph nodes may be calcified.

Peritoneal fluid may presumably be a **transudate, modified transudate, chylous or exudate. Macrophages containing acid-fast bacteria may be seen**.

Cytology and histology of a biopsy of the intestinal tract and mesenteric lymph nodes reveal **granulomatous to pyogranulomatous inflammation**. Acid-fast bacteria are usually detectable in biopsies.

Culture is possible at selected laboratories, but may take weeks for a positive result.

Differential diagnosis

Differential diagnoses for **intestinal tuberculosis include alimentary lymphoma**, widely metastatic tumors, other pyogranulomatous bacterial infections and systemic fungal infections.

Treatment

Notify public health officials. Euthanasia is often advised with true tuberculosis because of the zoonotic risk. If treatment of a mycobacterial infection is attempted, drug doses are provided in references in The Cat With Non-Healing Wounds and The Cat With Enlarged Lymph Nodes.

HYPERADRENOCORTICISM*

> **Classical signs**
>
> - Polyuria, polydipsia, polyphagia.
> - Abdominal distention, alopecia, fragile skin.

See main reference on page 251 for details (The Cat With Polyuria and Polydipsia).

Clinical signs

Many cats with hyperadrenocorticism have diabetes mellitus, which causes the polyuria and polydipsia. **Polyphagia** may be due to both diabetes and hyperadrenocorticism, and may be severe.

Muscle wasting is due to both disorders. This contributes to **abdominal distention**, which is manifested as a **"pot-bellied" appearance**, similar to the dog.

Dermatologic signs include **unkempt haircoat, patchy alopecia, and skin that tears and bruises easily**.

Diagnosis

Confirmatory testing and distinguishing a pituitary tumor from an adrenal tumor is similar to the dog, involving urine cortisol:creatinine ratio, ACTH stimulation test, dexamethasone suppression tests, plasma ACTH level, abdominal ultrasonography and CT-scanning or magnetic resonance imaging.

Differential diagnosis

Other causes of insulin-resistant diabetes mellitus.

Muscle wasting from another chronic disease plus marked obesity or **peritoneal fluid** can mimic the pot-bellied appearance of hyperadrenocorticism.

Treatment

Hypophysectomy and adrenectomy have historically provided the most consistent results.

Trilostane has alleviated clinical signs of pituitary-dependent hyperadrenocorticism in all reported cases.

Mitotane and ketoconazole have inconsistent results.

Pituitary irradiation has inconsistent results.

FLUID OVERLOAD*

Classical signs

- Dyspnea due to pulmonary edema, and/or subcutaneous edema.

Clinical signs

Excessive fluid therapy **tends to cause pulmonary or subcutaneous edema** more than pleural or peritoneal effusions.

Fluid therapy may exacerbate pre-existing ascites by causing increased hydrostatic pressure or exacerbating hypoalbuminemia. The presence of a mechanism for ascites formation may divert fluid away from the lungs or subcutaneous tissue into the peritoneal space.

Diagnosis

History of fluid therapy and improvement of ascites with decreasing fluid rates or diuretic therapy.

OVEREATING*

Classical signs

- Abdominal distention following a large meal.

Clinical signs

Mild abdominal distention is commonly noted in **kittens following nursing or drinking**.

Occasionally a mature cat may eat an unusually large quantity of food sufficient to cause noticeable abdominal distention. This is most likely to happen when offering a new, highly palatable food, in cats that have fasted, and in cats with polyphagia.

Diagnosis

History of consuming a large meal.

Palpable distention of gastrointestinal tract.

Radiography will demonstrate a large quantity of ingesta.

AEROPHAGIA*

Classical signs

- Mild abdominal distention in a dyspneic cat.

Clinical signs

Dyspnea.

Mildly distended stomach or loops of intestine on abdominal palpation. Loops of intestine may feel more or less distinct than usual. **Palpation may yield a "squishy" or spongy sensation** and **create borborygmus**.

Diagnosis

History of dyspnea.

Palpable distention of gastrointestinal tract by air.

Radiography will confirm air in the gastrointestinal tract and rule out dyspnea due to diaphragmatic compression by a large volume of fluid causing abdominal distention.

TRAUMATIC HEMORRHAGE*

Classical signs

- Pale mucous membranes, weak pulses, tachycardia.
- External signs of trauma.

Clinical signs

With blunt trauma in cats (e.g. motor vehicle accidents, falling from heights), thoracic injuries and resulting dyspnea are more common or clinically important than abdominal injuries. Abdominal hemorrhage may occur but is rarely life threatening.

- Signs of blunt trauma may be present, including shorn nails, excoriations of the skin, fractured teeth and mandible, epistaxis and pelvic fractures.

Penetrating trauma is less common than blunt trauma, and includes bite wounds, staking injuries and bullet wounds. Bacterial peritonitis is more common or clinically important than acute abdominal hemorrhage.

- The wound may be difficult to visualize or palpate, but palpation of the abdominal wall at the wound site will usually incite a painful response. The severity of bleeding varies with the organs and blood vessels that are injured.

Abdominal hemorrhage may occur following surgery or external biopsy procedures (e.g. percutaneous liver biopsy).

Regardless of the type of trauma, the signs of abdominal hemorrhage are those of acute hypovolemia. Abdominal distention is unlikely.

Diagnosis

Abdominal ultrasonography will usually demonstrate peritoneal fluid. Abdominocentesis may yield blood.
- Following percutaneous biopsy of an abdominal organ, tachycardia is the first sign of hemorrhage and this finding is more sensitive than ultrasound or abdominocentesis to detect active bleeding.

HEPATIC LIPIDOSIS, NON-SUPPURATIVE CHOLANGIOHEPATITIS AND HEPATIC CIRRHOSIS*

Classical signs

- Anorexia, lethargy, weight loss, icterus.

See main reference on page 425 for details (The Yellow Cat or Cat With Elevated Liver Enzymes).

Clinical signs

Anorexia, lethargy and weight loss.

Variable icterus, vomiting, diarrhea.

Ascites is uncommon, especially ascites sufficient to cause abdominal distention.
- Ascites is reported more frequently in some case series, which may represent distinct sub-types of chronic liver diseases.

Hepatomegaly is common with lipidosis, but is usually not sufficient to cause abdominal distention.

Diagnosis

These liver diseases may be **suspected on the basic of clinical signs and variably elevated liver enzymes**.

Abdominal ultrasonography may reveal a normal or enlarged liver, altered hepatic echogenicity and peritoneal fluid.

Peritoneal fluid is **usually a transudate or modified transudate**. Occasionally, high protein fluid typical of an exudate occurs with non-suppurative cholangiohepatitis.

Definitive diagnosis requires liver biopsy.

Differential diagnosis

Differential diagnoses for a cat with signs of liver abnormalities and peritoneal fluid include hepatic neoplasia and other chronic liver diseases, acute pancreatitis, right heart failure, feline infectious peritonitis and toxoplasmosis.

Treatment

Nutritional support.

Corticosteroids for cholangiohepatitis.

Therapeutic abdominocentesis is not required.

STEATITIS

Classical signs

- Depression, anorexia and reluctance to move.

Clinical signs

Depression, anorexia, fever and reluctance to move because of pain.

Abdominal distention may occur from fluid and firm abdominal fat, and the abdomen may be tense because of pain.

Other clinical signs include fever and firm and lumpy subcutaneous fat with or without accompanying lymphadenopathy.

Diagnosis

History of a **diet high in oxidized unsaturated fats** (e.g. **rancid tuna**) and/or **deficient in vitamin E**. Rare in cats fed commercial foods.

Biopsy of fat – may be grossly yellow to brown.

Abdominal ultrasound examination may reveal peritoneal fluid. Abdominocentesis may reveal a **sterile exudate high in protein and mature neutrophils**, **similar** to that seen with **feline infectious peritonitis**, or a **chylous effusion**. Associated sclerosing encapsulating peritonitis has also been reported.

INHERITED AND ACQUIRED (ANTICOAGULANT RODENTICIDE POISONING) COAGULATION DEFECTS

Classical signs

- Spontaneous bleeding and re-bleeding after trauma.

Clinical signs

Spontaneous bleeding and re-bleeding may occur at various sites, including within the abdomen, although thoracic hemorrhage tends to be more common.

Signs due to acute anemia and abdominal distention vary with the severity of blood loss.

Diagnosis

Abdominal ultrasonography will demonstrate peritoneal fluid. Abdominocentesis will confirm that the fluid is blood.

Cats bleeding from **hemophilia A or hemophilia B** will have **prolonged activated partial thromboplastin time**. Definitive diagnosis is by quantification of factor VIII or factor IX, respectively.

Devon Rex cats bleeding from **inherited vitamin K responsive coagulopathy** will have **prolonged prothrombin time and activated partial thromboplastin time**, which resolve with vitamin K therapy.

Cats bleeding from **coagulopathy due to vitamin K antagonist rodenticide poisoning** will have **prolonged prothrombin time, activated partial thromboplastin time, and PIVKA clotting time**, which resolve with vitamin K therapy.

Cats bleeding from **coagulopathy due to liver disease** (e.g. hepatic lipidosis or cholangiohepatitis) will have **prolonged prothrombin time and/or activated**

partial thromboplastin time. If the **prothrombin time** is elevated, it may **normalize with vitamin K therapy**.

Differential diagnosis

Hemorrhage due to abdominal neoplasia, trauma, or hepatic necrosis, amyloidosis, or peliosis.

Treatment

Transfusion.

Vitamin K for Devon Rex cats, vitamin K antagonist rodenticide poisoning, and cats with liver disease with prolonged prothrombin times (see main references on page 509 for details, The Bleeding Cat).

Environment that minimizes trauma.

GLOMERULONEPHRITIS

Classical signs

- Chronic depression, anorexia, weight loss.
- Polyuria/polydipsia if chronic renal failure.
- Subcutaneous edema and/or ascites if nephrotic syndrome.

Clinical signs

Signs are those of **chronic renal failure and/or nephrotic syndrome**. Concurrent signs may be present from an underlying disease (FeLV infection, FIP, *Mycoplasma* arthritis and other chronic infections, systemic lupus erythematosus and other immune-mediated disorders, mercury intoxication). Dyspnea may occur due to pleural effusion or pulmonary thromboembolism.

Diagnosis

A serum chemistry profile will reveal **azotemia with chronic renal failure, and severe hypoalbuminemia with nephrotic syndrome**.

Urinalysis will reveal **inappropriately low urine specific gravity with chronic renal failure, and marked proteinuria with nephrotic syndrome** (note that proteinuria will raise specific gravity).

Abdominal imaging may reveal small kidneys, altered renal echogenicity or peritoneal fluid.

Peritoneal fluid is a transudate.

Kidney biopsy will reveal glomerulonephritis.

Potential underlying diseases should be investigated. Littermates should be evaluated for familial disease.

Differential diagnosis

Other causes of chronic weight loss and ascites include FIP, neoplasia, pancreatitis, liver diseases, right heart failure, steatitis and tuberculosis. If the peritoneal fluid is a transudate, the main differential diagnosis is neoplasia.

Treatment

Treat the underlying disorder if possible.

Prednisone (initial dose 2–4 mg/kg/day) has been recommended but is of questionable value.

Treatments that are ineffective in most dogs include cytotoxic drugs and cyclosporine.

Treatments of potential benefit in dogs include **ACE-inhibitors** (e.g. enalapril, benazepril) to **reduce hypoproteinemia, n-3 fatty acids to reduce inflammation and inhibit platelets,** and **low-dose aspirin (0.5 mg/kg PO every other day) to inhibit platelets.**

Plasma transfusions will temporarily ameliorate hypoalbuminemia.

NEOPLASIA OBSTRUCTING OR COMPRESSING THE LOWER URINARY TRACT, GRANULOMATOUS URETHRITIS AND URETHRAL STRICTURE

> **Classical signs**
> - Chronic straining to urinate and incontinence.

Clinical signs

Dysuria characterized by increased time in litter box, straining, and dribbling urine from paradoxical incontinence.

Tumors affecting mucosa may cause hematuria.

Urinary bladder may be markedly enlarged (± atonic), **sufficient to cause abdominal distention**.

Diagnosis

Difficulty in passing urinary catheter.

Abdominal radiography will confirm enlargement of the bladder. Contrast urethrogram or excretory urogram may identify **narrowing of urethra or a mass at the trigone**.

Abdominal ultrasonography will confirm enlargement of the bladder and may identify a mass at the trigone.

Definitive diagnosis requires biopsy, which may require surgery.

INTRAHEPATIC ARTERIOVENOUS FISTULA

> **Classical signs**
> - Ascites.

Clinical signs

A fistula between the hepatic arterial system and portal venous system causes **ascites from pre-sinusoidal portal hypertension**. Other signs could include **poor weight gain**, reduced appetite, and **dyspnea secondary** to ascites. Congestive heart failure and hepatic encephalopathy from secondary porto-systemic shunting are theoretical sequelae.

Usually a congenital lesion, therefore seen in **young animal**, but could occur secondary to trauma or surgery.

Diagnosis

Rare.

Abdominal **ultrasound** examination will confirm peritoneal fluid and may detect a **cavernous lesion**. Doppler ultrasound may detect high-velocity turbulent blood flow through the fistula.

Abdominocentesis reveals a **transudate**.

Angiography may be used to confirm the diagnosis.

Exploratory laparotomy may reveal prominent subcapsular hepatic blood vessels.

PORTAL VEIN ATRESIA OR HYPOPLASIA

Classical signs

- Ascites.
- Hepatic encephalopathy.

Clinical signs

An underdeveloped portal venous system causes **ascites from pre-sinusoidal portal hypertension** in a young animal. Other signs could include **hepatic encephalopathy, poor weight gain,** reduced appetite and **dyspnea** secondary to ascites.

Diagnosis

Rare.

Elevated serum bile acids.

Abdominal **ultrasound** examination will confirm peritoneal fluid and a small liver.

Abdominocentesis reveals a **transudate.**

Angiography or exploratory laparatomy may be used to confirm the diagnosis.

LIGATION OF PORTOSYSTEMIC SHUNT

Classical signs

- Ascites.

Clinical signs

Ligation of a portosystemic shunt may cause ascites from pre-sinusoidal portal hypertension.

Diagnosis

Common for 2 days following surgical ligation of a portosystemic shunt. Ascites is less likely to occur with an ameroid constrictor or cellophane banding.

Abdominal **ultrasound** examination will confirm peritoneal fluid.

Abdominocentesis reveals a **transudate** to **modified transudate.**

HEPATIC AMYLOIDOSIS

Classical signs

- Lethargy, anorexia, weight loss, anemia, hepatomegaly.

Clinical signs

Amyloidosis is a systemic disease with deposition of amyloid protein AA in numerous tissues including the liver.

- In most cases, including familial amyloidosis in Abyssinian cats, **renal failure from renal amyloidosis dominates the clinical presentation**. Nephrotic syndrome causing ascites is rare because **amyloid affects primarily the renal medulla**.
- In some cases, including as a familial disease in some lines of **Siamese cats and Oriental shorthair cats, amyloid deposition in the liver is clinically most important**.
  - Signs are mostly due to **chronic liver disease** (lethargy, anorexia, weight loss), or **acute hemorrhage** (anemia, hemoperitoneum) resulting from spontaneous hepatic rupture. Signs of liver failure (icterus, hepatic encephalopathy) are not common.
  - **Abdominal distention** may occur due to **hepatomegaly, splenomegaly, intestinal dilation** and **hemoperitoneum.**

Diagnosis

Liver enzymes are normal to variably elevated.

Liver biopsy will demonstrate amyloid. If amyloidosis is suspected, biopsy of the intestinal tract may be considered to demonstrate amyloid deposition because there is an increased risk of hemorrhage from liver biopsy.

HEPATIC NECROSIS

Classical signs

- **Acute depression and anorexia.**

Clinical signs

Hepatic necrosis may result from a wide variety of mechanisms (e.g. tissue hypoxia, free radical formation) and specific etiologies (e.g. **feline infectious peritonitis**, virulent systemic feline calicivirus infection, toxoplasmosis, **acetaminophen** and **diazepam toxicosis**).

Clinical signs are due to the specific cause and to acute liver injury, which may range from subclinical to fulminant hepatic failure with hepatic encephalopathy.

Necrotic liver tissue may spontaneously hemorrhage resulting in peritoneal fluid and acute anemia.

Diagnosis

Liver biopsy will demonstrate necrosis.

Abdominal ultrasonography will confirm the presence of peritoneal fluid. Abdominocentesis will confirm that the fluid is blood.

PELIOSIS HEPATIS

Classical signs

- Spontaneous abdominal hemorrhage.

Clinical signs

Variable clinical signs include:

- **Spontaneous abdominal hemorrhage from irregular blood-filled cystic spaces**, which may result in pale mucous membranes, collapse or abdominal distention.
- Signs of liver disease, including hepatomegaly or jaundice. Telangiectasia is often present.
- Weight loss, dyspnea.

Diagnosis

Abdominal radiographs may reveal hepatomegaly or loss of abdominal detail.

Abdominal ultrasound examination will reveal hypoechoic regions in liver ± peritoneal fluid.

Fine-needle aspiration of liver lesions should yield blood. Abdominocentesis may yield blood.

Histology of liver biopsy will confirm the diagnosis.

Peliosis hepatis may be caused by *Bartonella henselae* infection in humans, and the two have been associated

in a dog, so testing for this organism should be considered.

HEPATIC ABSCESS

Classical signs

- Lethargy, anorexia, and weight loss.

Clinical signs

Non-specific signs are most common.

In a case series about a quarter of cats had a fever and about a third were hypothermic. One third of cats had abdominal pain.

Diagnosis

Rare disorder.

Variable neutrophilia, anemia, hypoalbuminemia, hyperbilirubinemia and elevation in liver enzymes.

Ultrasound may demonstrate hypoechoic or mixed hypoechoic/hyperechoic lesions in the liver and abdominal effusion.

Abdominal fluid cytology usually reveals degenerate neutrophils and bacteria. Degenerate neutrophils without bacteria and hemorrhagic effusion have also been seen.

Culture of hepatic lesions.

PERI-RENAL PSEUDOCYSTS

Classical signs

- Abdominal distention.
- Polyuria and polydipsia.
- Inappetence and weight loss.

Clinical signs

Abdominal distention occurs due to the formation of unilateral or bilateral fluid-filled sacs. The sacs lack an epithelial lining and contain either a transudate of serum, urine, or uncommonly, blood.

About 75% of cats have concurrent chronic renal failure, but cause and effect are not known.

Cats are presented for abdominal distention and/or clinical signs of chronic renal failure such as polyuria, polydipsia, inappetence and weight loss.

Diagnosis

Abdominal radiography will demonstrate large kidneys. Ultrasonography will demonstrate small kidneys within fluid-filled structures.

Presence of fluid may be confirmed by abdominocentesis. Analysis of fluid will reveal a transudate, urine or blood.

Routine hematology and serum biochemistry may reveal changes consistent with chronic renal failure.

EXTRA-UTERINE FETUSES

Classical signs

- None.

Clinical signs

Most "ectopic pregnancies" are not associated with clinical signs, and are an incidental finding during ovariohysterectomy.

Because **extra-uterine fetuses usually occur secondary to uterine rupture**, marked hemorrhage at the time of rupture or septic peritonitis may occur, which may result in peritoneal fluid.

Ascites without systemic signs of illness may also occur.

Diagnosis

Abdominal radiography or ultrasonography will demonstrate a mummified fetus ± peritoneal fluid.

BUDD–CHIARI-LIKE SYNDROME

Classical signs

- Marked abdominal distention due to ascites.

Clinical signs

Budd-Chiari-like syndrome is congenital or acquired **obstruction of the venous outflow of the liver,** including the hepatic venules, hepatic veins and caudal vena cava, causing **post-sinusoidal portal hypertension**. It is rare in cats. Cases have included veno-occlusive disease and fibrous webs in the caudal vena cava.

The predominant clinical sign is **progressive abdominal distention due to fluid**.

Diagnosis

Angiography will demonstrate caudal vena caval obstruction.

Liver biopsy will demonstrate veno-occlusive disease.

Abdominocentesis will reveal a modified transudate.

PNEUMOPERITONEUM

Classical signs

- Marked abdominal distention.

Clinical signs

Mild pneumoperitoneum usually occurs following laparotomy and intentional marked pneumoperitoneum occurs during laparascopy.

Marked spontaneous pneumoperitoneum usually results from a **perforating gastric ulcer or neoplasm, rupture of the stomach or large intestine**, or less often as an **extension from pneumothorax or pneumomediastinum**. Small intestinal rupture usually does not cause marked pneumoperitoneum unless it is a complication of endoscopy, which uses insufflation. Gas may also enter from penetrating abdominal wounds or perforation of the bladder during traumatic urinary tract catheterization, or may be produced by intra-abdominal bacteria, but such gas does not usually cause abdominal distention.

The predominant clinical sign of marked pneumoperitoneum is marked **abdominal distention due to air**, and acute onset of depression if associated with gastrointestinal tract rupture.

- Perforating gastric ulcers may result in marked pneumoperitoneum without generalized peritonitis and may be associated with minimal systemic signs.
- Gastrointestinal perforation may occur with minimal-to-absent pneumoperitoneum.

Diagnosis

Radiography will demonstrate free air in the abdomen. This is best seen along **the peritoneal surface of the diaphragm and the fundus of the stomach**. **Lateral views** obtained **in dorsal or sternal recumbency** will demonstrate the air if standard views are inconclusive.

With marked pneumoperitoneum, abdominocentesis will reveal air. Abdominocentesis may also reveal abdominal fluid, the characteristics of which will vary with the cause.

UMBILICAL, INGUINAL, TRAUMATIC ABDOMINAL WALL HERNIA*

Classical signs

- Localized swelling of the abdomen.

Clinical signs

Congenital or acquired hernias are usually evident as localized changes in abdominal contour.
- Owners may misinterpret marked **displacement of abdominal fat or organs into the hernia as abdominal distention**.

With acquired traumatic abdominal hernias there are usually also internal or external signs of motor vehicle trauma or fight wounds.
- Ventral abdominal herniation may be associated with rupture of the cranial pubic ligament.

Diagnosis

The focal nature of the lesion is usually evident on abdominal palpation, especially if the hernia is reducible.

Abdominal imaging or surgical exploration may be necessary to confirm the hernia.

LEPTOSPIROSIS

Classical signs

- Undefined.

Clinical signs

Positive titers and seroconversion to *Leptospira* spp. have been documented in various sick cats.

Clinical signs are variable and many are attributable to concurrent diseases.
- **Abdominal distention due to ascites has been reported.**

Diagnosis

The **disease in cats is rare compared to dogs.**

Most cats with positive titers have had some **evidence of liver disease**, e.g. increased liver enzymes, bilirubin or ascites.

Currently diagnosis in dogs relies on demonstrating a **four-fold rise in acute and convalescent titers**, and arguably the same criteria should be applied to cats.

GASTRIC DILATION-VOLVULUS

Classical signs

- Tympanic cranial abdomen, shock.

Clinical signs

Gastric dilation-volvulus is rare in cats. Clinical signs are similar to dogs.

Abdominal distention occurs because of dilation of the stomach with air.

Diagnosis

Abdominal radiography will demonstrate marked gastric distention with air.

RUPTURED GALL BLADDER OR BILE DUCT

Classical signs

- Progressive icterus and abdominal distention.

Clinical signs

Rupture of the gall bladder or biliary tract is rare in cats. Causes include motor vehicle trauma, falling from heights, penetrating trauma (e.g. bullet wound) or cholelithiasis.

Bile peritonitis causes **mild systemic signs** in dogs unless secondary infection occurs.

Diagnosis

Abdominal ultrasonography will demonstrate **peritoneal fluid. The gall bladder is small with gall bladder rupture and small-to-large with bile duct rupture.**

Abdominocentesis will reveal a **dark bile-stained modified transudate to (usually septic) exudate** containing high levels of bilirubin pigment with or without crystals. It should be noted that ascites in an animal that is icteric from pre-hepatic or hepatic causes also contains some bilirubin, because of diffusion of bilirubin from the blood into the ascitic fluid. If there is question as to whether the source of bile is the blood or the biliary tract, **the bilirubin level in the abdominal fluid may be compared to serum, with a higher level in the fluid indicating biliary tract rupture**. (In one case series of dogs and cats, bilirubin level in the fluid was consistently at least two times the serum level.)

ABDOMINAL FLUKE INFECTION

> **Classical signs**
>
> - Chronic weight loss, anorexia, vomiting, diarrhea, jaundice.

Clinical signs

Platynosomum spp., *Metorchis* spp.,*Opisthorchis* spp., *Clonorchis* spp. and *Amphimerus* spp. are **bile duct parasites** in numerous mammals, including cats.

Infections may be subclinical or may cause chronic weight loss, anorexia, vomiting, diarrhea and jaundice. Some infections may cause hepatic neoplasia or hepatic cysts.

Fluke infection of the peritoneal cavity causing ascites has been reported rarely.

Diagnosis

Infection is usually diagnosed by finding characteristic operculated eggs on fecal floatation.

Abdominal ultrasonography may demonstrate **hepatic tumors or cysts and peritoneal fluid**.

Abdominocentesis may rarely reveal **peritoneal fluid containing single-end operculated eggs**.

SCLEROSING ENCAPSULATING PERITONITIS

> **Classical signs**
>
> - Variable (rare disorder).

Clinical signs

The abdominal mesothelial lining becomes replaced by fibrous tissue resulting in encasement of abdominal organs. Clinical signs reported in dogs and cats due to the peritonitis or underlying disorders include anorexia, vomiting, abdominal pain, abdominal mass and ascites.

Diagnosis

Biopsy of peritoneum reveals fibrous tissue.

IDIOPATHIC CHYLOUS ASCITES

> **Classical signs**
>
> - Ascites.

Clinical signs

Idiopathic chylous ascites is rare compared to idiopathic chylothorax.

Peritoneal effusion with or without concurrent pleural effusion.

Diagnosis

Abdominocentesis reveals chylous effusion.

Neoplasia or other underlying causes of effusion are not identified.

RECOMMENDED READING

Auman M, Worth LT, Drobatz KJ. Uroperitoneum in cats: 26 cases (1986–1995). J Am Anim Hosp Assoc 1998; 34: 315–324.

Bonczynski JJ, Ludwig LL, Barton LJ, Loar A, Peterson ME. Comparison of peritoneal fluid and peripheral blood pH, bicarbonate, glucose, and lactate concentration as a diagnostic tool for septic peritonitis in dogs and cats. Vet Surg 2003; 32: 161–166.

Center SA, Harte J, Watrous D, et al. The clinical and metabolic effects of rapid weight loss in obese pet cats and the influence of supplemental oral L-canitine. J Vet Intern Med 2000; 14: 598–608.

Connallly H. Cytology and fluid analysis of the acute abdomen. Clin Tech Small Anim Pract 2003; 18: 39–44.

Costello MF, Drobatz KJ, Aronson LR, King LG. Underlying cause, pathophysiologic abnormalities, and response to treatment in cats with septic peritonitis: 51 cases (1990–2001). J Am Vet Med Assoc 2004; 225: 897–902.

Fossum TW, Wellman M, Relford RL, Slater MR. Eosinophilic pleural or peritoneal effusions in dogs and cats: 14 cases (1986–1992). J Am Vet Med Assoc 1993; 202: 1873–1876.

Haney DR, Levy JK, Newell SM, Graham JP, Gorman SP. Use of fetal skeletal mineralization for prediction of parturition date in cats. J Am Vet Med Assoc 2003; 223: 1614–1616.

Hartmann K, Binder C, Hirschberger J, et al. Comparison of different tests to diagnose feline infectious peritonitis. J Vet Intern Med 2003; 17: 781–790.

Mandell DC, Drobatz K. Feline hemoperitoneum: 16 cases. Vet Emerg Crit Care 1995; 5: 93–97.

Paltrinieri S, Parodi MC, Cammarata G. In vivo diagnosis of feline infectious peritonitis by comparison of protein content, cytology, and direct immunofluorescence test on peritoneal and pleural effusions. J Vet Diagn Invest 1999; 11: 358–361.

Steyn PF, Wittum TE. Radiographic, epidemiologic, and clinical aspects of simultaneous pleural and peritoneal effusions in dogs and cats: 48 cases (1982–1991). J Am Vet Med Assoc 1993; 202: 301–312.

Tasker S, Gunn-Moore D. Differential diagnosis of ascites in cats. In Practice 2000; 22: 472–479.

Wright KN, Gompf RE, DeNovo RC. Peritoneal effusion in cats: 65 cases (1981–1997). J Am Vet Med Assoc 1999; 214: 375–381.

23. The bleeding cat

Anthony Abrams-Ogg

KEY SIGNS

- Rule out a local lesion.
- Confirm a bleeding tendency.
- Identify a vascular, platelet or clotting disorder.

MECHANISM?

- Bleeding is caused by vascular injury or a disturbance of one or more stages of normal hemostasis.
- The stages of normal hemostasis are: vasoconstriction and formation of a platelet plug (primary hemostasis), formation of a fibrin clot (secondary hemostasis) and clot dissolution (fibrinolysis).

WHERE?

- Bleeding caused by a vascular injury may occur at any site.
- Bleeding caused by a non-traumatic vascular disorder varies with the specific disorder.
- Bleeding due to a platelet disorder tends to be cutaneous and mucosal.
- Bleeding due to a coagulopathy tends to be subcutaneous and internal.

WHAT?

- The **most common causes of bleeding** are **local lesions**. These result from trauma, inflammation or neoplasia.
- The most common causes of **bleeding tendencies** are liver diseases, neoplasia, and infectious diseases. Most of this is subclinical.
- The most common causes of abnormal clinical bleeding are hepatic lipidosis, retroviral-induced megakaryocytic hypoplasia and vitamin K antagonist poisoning.

QUICK REFERENCE SUMMARY

Diseases causing a bleeding cat

VASCULAR DISORDERS

ANOMALY

- Cutaneous asthenia (Ehlers–Danlos syndrome) (p 519)
Inherited fragile skin and/or fragile vessels may lead to vascular trauma.

continued

continued

METABOLIC

● Renal failure*** (p 494)

Uremia causes alimentary tract ulceration, systemic hypertension causes retinal hemorrhages, a platelet function defect may be present, coagulation defects may be present, and hemolytic-uremic syndrome is an uncommon complication of renal transplantation.

● Hyperadrenocorticism (p 520)

Acquired fragile skin may lead to vascular trauma.

● Systemic hypertension** (p 495)

Systemic hypertension may cause retinal hemorrhages and, less often, epistaxis. The most common cause of hypertension is chronic renal failure. Other causes include hyperthyroidism, diabetes mellitus, hyperadrenocorticism and polycythemia vera. Rare disorders that may cause hypertension include multiple myeloma, pheochromocytoma and hyperaldosteronism.

NEOPLASTIC, INFLAMMATION, TRAUMA

● Local lesions causing localized hemorrhage *** (p 492)

Tumors (e.g. cutaneous squamous cell carcinoma), local inflammation (e.g. cat bite abscesses, idiopathic cystitis), and trauma (e.g. lacerations) may cause local bleeding at the site.

● Motor vehicle and other major blunt trauma*** (p 493)

Major trauma can cause mild to severe local bleeding at numerous sites.

● Strangulation (p 519)

External choking injury may cause scleral hemorrhage.

TOXIC

● Snake bite envenomation (p 503)

Snake venom toxins may cause edema and bleeding around the bite.

PLATELET DISORDERS

ANOMALY

● Chediak–Higashi syndrome (p 520)

An inherited platelet function defect causes prolonged bleeding after trauma.

● Idiopathic thrombocytopathia (p 520)

An inherited platelet function defect causes spontaneous mucosal bleeding.

● Von Willebrand's disease (p 521)

An inherited von Willebrand's factor (a platelet adhesion protein) deficiency causes prolonged bleeding after trauma.

METABOLIC

● Megakaryocytic hypoplasia** (p 495)

Reduced platelet production may be due to hematopoietic neoplasms in the bone marrow, retroviral infections, histoplasmosis infecting the bone marrow, idiopathic causes (which are probably immune-mediated) and toxicoses. Severe thrombocytopenia causes spontaneous mucosal bleeding and prolonged bleeding after injury.

- **Disseminated intravascular coagulation* (p 501)**

Acute and chronic DIC are characterized by variable thrombocytopenia, although clinical bleeding is uncommon.

- Splenomegaly (p 521)

Splenic sequestration may contribute to thrombocytopenia when there is marked splenomegaly.

INFLAMMATION (INFECTIOUS)

- **Feline leukemia virus (FeLV) infection** (p 499)**

Bleeding tendencies may be caused by megakaryocytic hypoplasia, immune-mediated platelet destruction, and DIC secondary to infections and neoplasia. Clinical bleeding is uncommon except with severe thrombocytopenia.

- **Feline immunodeficiency virus (FIV) infection** (p 500)**

Bleeding tendencies may be caused by megakaryocytic hypoplasia, prolongation of clotting times due to unknown mechanisms, and DIC secondary to infections and neoplasia. Clinical bleeding is uncommon except with severe thrombocytopenia.

INFLAMMATION (IMMUNE)

- Immune-mediated thrombocytopenia (ITP) (p 506)

ITP may be primary or secondary to neoplasia, infectious diseases or drugs. Transient thrombocytopenia may occur following vaccination in dogs, but has not been documented in cats. Severe thrombocytopenia causes spontaneous mucosal bleeding and prolonged bleeding after injury.

IDIOPATHIC

- Miscellaneous diseases (p 505)

Thrombocytopenias due to unknown mechanisms have been seen with a variety of diseases not typically associated with abnormal bleeding. Clinical bleeding with these abnormalities is uncommon.

TOXIC

- Antibiotics (p 523)

Antibiotics may have various effects on hemostasis including idiosyncratic megakaryocytic hypoplasia, impaired platelet function, and exacerbating vitamin K deficiency and antagonism.

- Antiplatelet cardiac drugs (p 520)

Aspirin and n-3 fatty acids are given to impair platelet function in an attempt to prevent thromboembolism in cardiomyopathy. Effect, if any, is subclinical. Risk for spontaneous bleeding with newer drugs that block specific platelet receptors is probably low.

- Non-steroidal anti-inflammatory drugs (p 524)

Non-steroidal anti-inflammatory drugs given for analgesia may impair platelet function. Effect on risk for bleeding is probably minimal.

- Miscellaneous drugs (p 524)

Sedatives, anesthetic agents and anti-histamines may impair platelet function. Effect on risk for bleeding is probably minimal.

continued

continued

COAGULOPATHIES
ANOMALY

● Hemophilia A (classical hemophilia) (p 510)
Inherited factor VIII deficiency causes spontaneous internal bleeding and re-bleeding after trauma.

● Hemophilia B (Christmas disease) (p 513)
Inherited factor IX deficiency causes spontaneous internal bleeding and re-bleeding after trauma.

● **Hageman trait* (p 504)**
Inherited factor XII deficiency causes markedly prolonged activated clotting time and activated partial thromboplastin time without clinical signs.

● Vitamin K responsive coagulopathy in the Devon Rex (p 515)
An inherited defect in vitamin K metabolism causes spontaneous internal bleeding and re-bleeding after trauma.

● Factor X deficiency (p 522)
Inherited factor X deficiency causes spontaneous internal bleeding and re-bleeding after trauma.

● Hemophilia C (p 514)
Inherited factor XI deficiency causes excessive bleeding after trauma.

METABOLIC

● **Liver disease** (p 498)**
Vitamin K deficiency (several causes), failure of coagulation factor synthesis, and chronic DIC may cause excessive bleeding after venepuncture and liver biopsy. The liver may be friable.

● Pancreatitis (p 518)
Hemostatic abnormalities are usually subclinical. Clinical bleeding is unlikely unless there is severe DIC or concurrent liver disease.

● Exocrine pancreatic insufficiency (EPI) (p 516)
Vitamin K malabsorption may cause spontaneous or excessive bleeding.

● Inflammatory bowel disease (IBD) (p 517)
Vitamin K malabsorption may cause spontaneous or excessive bleeding.

● **Disseminated intravascular coagulation* (p 501)**
Acute and chronic DIC are characterized by variable prolongation of clotting times, although clinical bleeding is uncommon. DIC may be caused by hematopoietic and solid neoplasms, viral infections (panleukopenia, feline infectious peritonitis), bacterial and fungal sepsis, systemic protozoal infections and hyperthermia. Clinical bleeding is uncommon.

NUTRITIONAL

● Vitamin K deficient diet (p 523)
A diet severely deficient in vitamin K1 or containing a vitamin K antagonist may cause spontaneous internal bleeding and re-bleeding after trauma. Anorexia may contribute to vitamin K deficiency in liver disease.

INFLAMMATION (IMMUNE)

● Circulating anti-coagulant (p 522)

Circulating anti-coagulants may be acquired in immune-mediated diseases and cause spontaneous or excessive bleeding.

IDIOPATHIC

● **Miscellaneous diseases* (p 505)**

Prolongation of clotting times due to unknown mechanisms have been seen with a variety of diseases not typically associated with abnormal bleeding. Clinical bleeding with these abnormalities is uncommon.

TOXIC

● Antibiotics (p 523)

Some antibiotics may exacerbate vitamin K deficiency and antagonism.

● Vitamin K antagonist rodenticides and drugs (p 507)

Poisoning with these compounds may cause severe spontaneous internal bleeding and excessive bleeding following trauma.

● Anti-convulsants (p 523)

Phenobarbital may cause a subclinical vitamin K antagonism.

● Anti-thyroid drugs (p 524)

Anti-thyroid drugs may cause a subclinical vitamin K antagonism.

● Anti-coagulants (p 522)

Anti-coagulant drug overdose may cause spontaneous bleeding.

● **Snake bite envenomation* (p 503)**

Snake venom hematoxins may cause subclinical and clinical bleeding tendencies.

INTRODUCTION

MECHANISM?

Hemostasis following injury to a blood vessel is classically divided into primary hemostasis, secondary hemostasis and fibrinolysis, although there is extensive interaction between these parts.

● **Primary hemostasis** consists of:
  – Vasoconstriction.
  – Formation of the initial platelet plug.
● **Secondary hemostasis** consists of a cascade of coagulation proteins that converts the platelet plug into a stable fibrin clot. Calcium (factor IV) is needed for most steps in the cascade.
  – Secondary hemostasis is classically divided into the extrinsic, intrinsic, and common system, although there is extensive interaction between these pathways.
  – The **extrinsic system** (tissue factor pathway) is initiated when tissue factor (factor III) is expressed on the surface of activated subendothelial fibroblasts and monocytes at sites of vascular injury or inflammation. In a simplified view, tissue factor interacts with factor VII to form a tissue factor–activated factor VII complex that amplifies itself and directly activates

factor X (the start of the common system). The extrinsic system is the main pathway for the **initiation** of coagulation in vivo, but it cannot sustain coagulation.

- The **intrinsic system** (contact activation pathway) is activated by exposure to subendothelial tissue following vascular injury. Activation of contact activating factors (factors XII [Hageman], high-molecular-weight kininogen, prekallikrein), XI, IX and VIII occurs. Contact activation by factor XII is probably of minimal importance in initiating normal coagulation in vivo. However, while the extrinsic system is most important for initiating coagulation, the intrinsic system is important in **sustaining** coagulation. In a simplified view, thrombin resulting from extrinsic system activation ultimately results in factors IX and VIII (together with calcium and platelet phospholipid) forming a "tenase complex" on the surface of activated platelets, which activates factor X. The contact activation factors are important in inflammation and fibrinolysis.

- The **common system** is activated by the end-products of the extrinsic and intrinsic systems (i.e. the tissue-factor-activated factor VII and tenase complexes, respectively). In a simplified view, the initial step is activation of factor X, which then activates factor V. Activated factors X and V (together with calcium and platelet phospholipid) form a "prothrombinase complex" on the surface of activated platelets, which activates thrombin (factor II), which in turn converts fibrinogen (factor I) to fibrin. Factor XIII then stabilizes the fibrin clot, converting the fibrin monomer to a fibrin polymer.

- **Fibrinolysis** refers to clot dissolution by the plasminogen-plasmin system.

Bleeding is most often caused by local vascular injury. Normal hemostasis ensues and the degree of bleeding is **appropriate** for the injury. Causes of vascular injury include:

- **Sharp and blunt trauma**. This includes clinical procedures (e.g. venepuncture, dentistry, surgery).
- **Tissue inflammation**. Inflammation disrupts blood vessels and causes vasodilation. The latter increases blood flow to the area and promotes extravasation of red blood cells.

- **Neoplasia**. Neoplasia may disrupt blood vessels, promote inflammation, promote angiogenesis and promote fragile vasculature (e.g. endothelium without a vessel wall).

Bleeding is less often caused by a disorder of primary or secondary hemostasis. Such disorders may cause **subclinical abnormalities** in test results or **abnormal clinical bleeding**.

Abnormal bleeding is spontaneous or excessive.

- **Spontaneous bleeding** occurs as a result of the minor trauma of daily activity.
- Similar to other organ systems, **hemostasis has a large reserve capacity** – a severe deficiency is required for spontaneous bleeding to occur, for example, a platelet count < $10–20 \times 10^9$/L (10 000–20 000/μl), or a factor VIII level < 10% normal is required for spontaneous bleeding to occur.
  - Bleeding diatheses are less common in cats than in dogs.
- **Excessive bleeding** occurs following trauma or development of other local lesions. The degree of bleeding is **inappropriate** for the severity of the lesion.

Bleeding disorders may be **inherited** or **acquired**.

- Inherited disorders are as common in mixed-breed cats as in purebreds.

Multiple mechanisms may contribute to bleeding in an individual patient.

Acute blood loss causes acute anemia and hypovolemia. Signs include lethargy, anorexia, hypothermia, pallor, tachycardia, weak pulses and dyspnea.

Chronic blood loss causes iron-deficiency anemia.

Regardless of cause, acute substantial bleeding may cause signs due to a **space-occupying effect** and/or inflammation incited by the presence of blood. Signs include mucosal and cutaneous swellings (hematomas); neurologic signs from bleeding into or around the central nervous system; lameness, muscle pain, muscle stiffness, joint swelling and joint pain (hemorrhage into muscles and joints); uveitis; dyspnea from pulmonary or pleural hemorrhage, or tracheal compression by a jugular hematoma; acute cardiac tamponade from pericardial hemorrhage (causing tachycardia and hypotension similar to hypovolemia), abdominal **distention** and abdominal pain (presumably due to hemorrhage within organs), dysuria due to a clot within the bladder, and possibly vomiting due to a clot within the stomach.

WHERE?

Bleeding may be the result of a local lesion or a disturbance in primary or secondary hemostasis.

Bleeding from a **local lesion** may occur into or from any tissue and is **appropriate for the severity of the lesion**.

- Bleeding varies with the severity, type and location of lesion. Hemostasis may be insufficient to stop bleeding, and manipulation of the lesion may reactivate bleeding.
- Presence of blood clots in shed blood rules out a typical coagulopathy, but not a platelet disorder, as the cause of bleeding.

Absence of blood clots in shed blood does not rule in a coagulopathy.

- Initial bloodshed may be too rapid to immediately activate coagulation (e.g. laceration of a large vessel).
- Clots may have been removed (e.g. swallowed) and only red blood cells not incorporated into the clot remain.
- Clot lysis may have occurred.
- Blood in body cavities and the intestinal tract may not clot because of defibrination on epithelial surfaces and clots may be digested.

Vascular disorders may result in either spontaneous or excessive bleeding at the site of the disorder.

- Vascular disease secondary to systemic hypertension commonly causes retinal hemorrhages and less commonly epistaxis.
- Other vascular disorders are not common causes of bleeding in cats.

Platelet disorders may result in either spontaneous or excessive bleeding.

- **Spontaneous bleeding** occurs because blood vessel walls are continuously sustaining minute injuries and being plugged by platelets. A platelet disorder permits bleeding at sites of minute injury in small vessels resulting in the following signs:
  - Bleeding at multiple sites.
  - Petechiation and ecchymoses, especially in dependent areas and areas subject to normally high wear and tear (e.g. gums).

- Bleeding from mucosal surfaces – epistaxis, melena and hematuria.
- Intraocular hemorrhage.
- **Risk of spontaneous bleeding is related to the platelet count**, but quantification of the risk is imprecise, in part because of imprecision in platelet counting, especially in cats (see discussion below). The following values are derived from humans and dogs; cats are at less risk of bleeding for a given platelet count. Indeed, signs of clinical bleeding in cats are usually absent or mild until almost no platelets are evident on a blood smear. Bleeding is worse at a given platelet count if there is concurrent vasculopathy, platelet function defect, coagulopathy, fever, or, possibly, anemia.
- Platelets $< 80 \times 10^9$/L ($< 80\,000$/μl) – increased bleeding at surgery.
- Platelets $< 50 \times 10^9$/L ($< 50\,000$/μl) – microscopic spontaneous bleeding.
- Platelets $< 20 \times 10^9$/L ($< 20\,000$/μl) – mild risk of spontaneous clinical bleeding.
- Platelets $< 10 \times 10^9$/L ($< 10\,000$/μl) –moderate risk of spontaneous clinical bleeding.
- Platelets $< 5 \times 10^9$/L ($< 5\,000$/μl) – severe risk of spontaneous clinical bleeding.

- **Excessive bleeding** may be characterized by:
  - Occurrence immediately following injury, because the initial platelet plug does not form.
  - Increased rate of bleeding.
  - Prolonged bleeding.
    - **Prolonged bleeding after venepuncture is one of the most common initial signs of thrombocytopenia.** It should not be dismissed and attributed to the venepuncture technique in a cat at risk for a bleeding disorder.

Coagulopathies may result in either spontaneous or excessive bleeding.

- **Spontaneous bleeding** occurs because vasoconstriction and platelet plugs are insufficient to stop bleeding from larger vessels. Coagulation is necessary, and a coagulopathy permits bleeding from larger vessels into tissues and body cavities resulting in the following signs:
  - More localized bleeding (although widespread hemorrhage may occur).
  - Subcutaneous hematomas and intramuscular hemorrhages.

– Bleeding into body cavities (pleural space, peritoneal cavity, joints).
– Scleral hemorrhage.
● **Excessive bleeding** may be characterized by:
– Delayed bleeding and rebleeding because the initial platelet plug is not stabilized by a fibrin clot.
– **Detection of a bruise following venepuncture is one of the most common initial signs of coagulopathy.** It should not be dismissed as a result of venepuncture technique in a cat at risk for a bleeding disorder.
– Increased rate of bleeding if a larger vessel is injured.

Differences are not absolute between bleeding due to platelet disorders and coagulopathy, and clinical signs overlap. Bleeding patterns seen with both include cutaneous and subcutaneous bleeding at venepuncture sites, gingival bleeding, retinal hemorrhages, cerebral hemorrhages, pulmonary hemorrhages and widespread bleeding.

WHAT?

To diagnose the cause of bleeding:
● Rule out a local lesion.
● Confirm abnormal bleeding with tests of hemostasis.
● Characterize abnormal bleeding as a defect in primary and/or secondary hemostasis based on clinical signs and tests of hemostasis.
● Determine if the hemostatic defect is inherited or acquired.
● Determine the mode of inheritance if inherited.
● Determine an underlying cause if defect is acquired.

The most common causes of bleeding are local lesions – trauma, inflammation and neoplasia.

The most common causes of impaired hemostasis are liver diseases, neoplasia and infectious diseases. Most of the alterations in hemostasis are subclinical.

The most common causes of abnormal clinical bleeding are hepatic lipidosis, retroviral-induced megakaryocytic hypoplasia and vitamin K antagonist poisoning.

TESTS OF HEMOSTASIS

Tests of hemostatic function are necessary to determine what stage of the hemostatic process is abnormal.

If the blood sample is being collected by using a winged-infusion set ("butterfly"), jugular catheter, or vacuum tube draw, then the first 2–5 ml should be discarded or used for serum chemistry determinations. This may reduce platelet clumping and premature activation of coagulation. In most cases a blood sample is obtained by venepuncture using a syringe and needle, in which case the EDTA (platelet count) and citrate tubes (coagulation tests) should be filled first, and the remaining blood used for serum chemistry determinations.

Routine tests of hemostasis include:
● **Platelet count.**
– Used for detecting **thrombocytopenia**.
– Platelet counts may be obtained by estimation from a blood smear, manual counting, or with automated cell counters.
– To **estimate platelet count**, prepare a routinely stained blood smear. Examine the blood smear monolayer where red cells are close together and 50% are touching. Normally there are about 10–30 platelets/oil immersion field (magnification $= \times 1000$); each platelet $\approx 20 \times 10^9$/L (20 000/μl). This requires a properly prepared blood smear. An alternative method that avoids a blood smear uses a disposable counting chamber and supravital stain (ZynoStain, Zynocyte, MA, USA) (Tasker et al, 2001).
– **Manual counting** may be performed using a Unopette microcollection system (Becton Dickinson) and a hemocytometer.
– **Automated cell counters** use impedance (Coulter principle), quantitative buffy coat (QBC) or light scattering properties (flow cytometry).
– Platelet counting in cats has historically been problematic because cats are prone to **artifactual thrombocytopenia** due to **platelet clumping**. Platelet clumping results from difficulties in obtaining blood samples and increased aggregatability of platelets.
– Citrate samples are superior to EDTA samples, although platelet clumping may still occur.
– If a citrated blood sample has been obtained for coagulation testing (see below), consider using this sample for platelet counting.
– A solution containing citrate, theophylline, adenosine and dipyradamole (CTAD) con-

tains platelet inhibitors and reduces platelet clumping. It is commercially available in a vacuum tube (CTAD tube [formerly Diatube-H], Becton Dickinson).
- Manual agitation and vortex mixing of blood samples does not reliably break up platelet clumps.
- The effect of delay in processing the sample on the platelet count is controversial, but the general recommendation is to perform the platelet count as soon after collection as possible.
- Automated cell counters that use light-scattering technology may detect platelet clumps.
- Some clumping may occur without dropping the platelet count below normal range.
- **Examination of a blood smear is always recommended**. This can be used to verify a platelet count obtained by manual or automated methods. This is especially important when platelet counts are obtained in-house using quantitative buffy coat technology.
  - Closely examine the feather edge of the blood smear to identify platelet clumps. Also examine the blood sample to identify a blood clot in the tube.
  - Evaluation of a blood smear in a bleeding cat will rapidly determine whether or not the cat is bleeding due to thrombocytopenia.
    - If there are $\geq$ 1–2 platelets per oil field, it is unlikely the cat is suffering from spontaneous hemorrhage. If there are $\geq$ 3–4 platelets per oil field, it is unlikely that the cat will bleed excessively.
    - If platelet clumps are present, the platelet count is probably adequate and bleeding is not due to thrombocytopenia.
- The most reliable results are obtained with manual counting, estimation from a well-prepared blood smear, and automated cell counters using flow cytometry.
- **Reference ranges** vary with the method of counting – a typical range is 200–600 $\times$ 10^9/L (200 000–600 000/µl).
- **Buccal mucosal bleeding time (BMBT).**
  - BMBT is typically used for detecting disorders of platelet function when platelet numbers are normal.

- The test is used most often for screening cats with uremia prior to kidney biopsy.
- Do not routinely perform if cat has thrombocytopenia. **BMBT is usually prolonged when the platelet count is < 50 $\times$ 10^9/L (50 000/µl)**, and progressive prolongation is expected with worsening thrombocytopenia. A platelet count of 10–15 $\times$ 10^9/L (10 000–15 000/µl) is likely to result in a BMBT of 5–6 minutes. BMBT may be performed in a cat with thrombocytopenia to detect a concurrent platelet function defect, if bleeding is considered to be excessive for the platelet count and clotting tests are normal.
- Ketamine-acepromazine sedation is normally used, but BMBT with other sedatives or anesthetics is similar.
- Place cat in lateral recumbency and fold up the upper lip. Secure the lip with a tightly tied gauze strip passed through the mouth, around the head rostral to the ipsilateral ear, and caudal to the contralateral ear.
- Avoiding obvious blood vessels, make a 5–6 mm long by 1 mm deep incision in the buccal mucosa of the everted lip above the molars or premolars; this is best done using a spring-loaded device (e.g. Triplett Bleeding Time Device, Helena Laboratories). Blot the blood with a filter paper 1–2 mm from the incision. The incision should not be stretched or touched during the test. However, if a fibrin film forms over the incision it should be teased away using the filter paper to touch the blood as it wells up.
- **Normal BMBT is 1–3.25 min**.
- **Prolonged BMBT in an animal with a normal platelet count indicates a vascular defect, platelet function defect or von Willebrand's disease.** Anemia will prolong bleeding time in humans, rabbits, and dogs, but this effect has not been evaluated in cats. A coagulopathy will not immediately affect BMBT, but rebleeding may occur. If the incision is made in an inflamed area, bleeding time will be prolonged.
- In general, the longer the BMBT value, the more likely the risk of bleeding, but there are no precise values defining the risk.
- **Activated clotting (coagulation) time (ACT).**
  - The intrinsic system is initiated by contact activation. In the ACT siliceous (diatomaceous) earth or glass particles are used to provide a very

large surface for contact activation. Blood clots via the intrinsic and common pathways.

– Add 2 ml fresh blood to an ACT tube pre-warmed to 37°C using a heating block or human axilla. Invert the tube rapidly five times and incubate at 37°C for 60 s. Quickly tip the tube gently to observe for clot formation. If no clot is observed, quickly re-incubate for another 10 seconds, and then re-examine for clot formation. Repeat observations every 10 seconds until the very first signs of a clot appear. **Time to first clot formation is the activated clotting time.** After clot formation is first noted, re-incubate and re-examine every 10 seconds. A complete solid clot, which is detected by tipping the tube upside down, normally forms within another 10 s. The formation of an incomplete "soft" clot is indicative of the presence of heparin (in low concentration) or low fibrinogen levels.

– Earlier **reported ranges for ACT in cats** vary from < 65–75 s to 60–125 s. In the author's practice the accepted range is 60–90 s. In a recent study (Bay et al, 2000), normal range was 55–165 s.

  – In that study, blood was collected by direct draw into ACT vacuum tubes. The most common practice is to collect blood with a syringe, and then inject the blood into the ACT tube. It is possible that syringe collection and injection shortens ACT by increasing platelet activation (although this is not important in humans), and by initiating coagulation before the blood enters the ACT tube.

  – Traumatic venepuncture inconsistently prolongs ACT.

– **Prolonged ACT indicates a defect in the intrinsic or common system of coagulation.**

  – The clotting process requires phospholipid from the platelets in the blood, so it has been suggested that **severe thrombocytopenia** ($<10 \times 10^9$/L [< 10 000/μl]) may also prolong ACT. This has not been proven in the cat, and probably a virtual absence of platelets would be necessary.

– ACT is not affected by sedation with ketamine and acepromazine.

– Although ACT depends to some extent on the operator, a defect in the intrinsic or common pathway causing clinical bleeding will usually result in an ACT > 1.5–2 min.

– There is **no direct correlation between the degree of prolongation of ACT and the risk for bleeding.** The risk for bleeding at a given ACT value will vary with the underlying disorder causing the coagulation abnormality. In general, for a given disorder, the longer the ACT value the more likely the risk of bleeding, but there are no precise values defining the risk.

● **Activated partial thromboplastin time (aPTT).**

  – In this test, calcium, a contact activator and a platelet phospholipid substitute are added to plasma, and the time to clot formation is measured. Normal blood clotting via the intrinsic system requires contact activation and the thromboplastin effect of platelet phospholipid. (A thromboplastin is a substance having procoagulant activity.) The various platelet phospholipid substitutes used in the test have only partial thromboplastin activity, hence the name of the test.

  – Most laboratories perform this assay with a fibrometer or photo-optical device, which detects the formation of fibrin strands. The assay should only be performed in a laboratory that has validated its assay for use in cats.

  – Blood is collected into 3.2% citrate anti-coagulant (9 parts blood:1 part citrate). Underfilling, overfilling or a clot in the citrate tube invalidates the results. The margin for error in the blood:citrate ratio in cats is not known. Citrate vacuum tubes are designed to draw the correct amount of blood.

  – The sample should be centrifuged promptly and kept refrigerated or frozen until assayed. If the sample cannot be centrifuged promptly, it should be refrigerated until assayed.

  – Prolonged aPTT > 20–25% of a control sample (prepared from a pool of donors) and/or outside the normal range indicates a defect in the intrinsic or common system of coagulation.

    – It may also be beneficial to submit an additional control sample from a clinically normal cat collected and handled in exactly the same manner as the patient sample in order to detect artifactual prolongation of the aPTT.

    – When comparing serial test results, results from one laboratory cannot be directly compared against results from another laboratory because of differences in methodology, including use of different thromboplastins.

– As with ACT, there is no direct correlation between the degree of prolongation of aPTT and the risk for bleeding. The risk for bleeding at a given aPTT value will vary with the underlying disorder causing the coagulation abnormality. In general, for a given disorder, the longer the aPTT value the more likely the risk of bleeding, but there are no precise values defining the risk.

● **Prothrombin time (PT).**
  – This test is similar to the aPTT, except that a thromboplastin with tissue factor-like activity is added in excess to the test system, thus mimicking the extrinsic system. The assay should only be performed in a laboratory that has validated its assay for use in cats.
  – Collect sample as for aPTT.
  – Prolonged PT > 20–25% of control sample and/or outside the normal range indicates a defect in the extrinsic or common system of coagulation.
    – It may also be beneficial to submit an additional control sample from a clinically normal cat collected and handled in exactly the same manner as the patient sample in order to detect artifactual prolongation of the PT.

      When comparing serial test results, results from one laboratory cannot be directly compared against results from another laboratory because of differences in methodology, including use of different thromboplastins. To facilitate comparison in humans an international normalized ratio (INR) may be calculated as INR = (patient PT/mean normal PT)^{ISI}, where ISI represents the international sensitivity index of the thromboplastin. The validity of using INR in cats has not been extensively evaluated.
    – PT results are typically shorter than aPTT results.
  – As with ACT and aPTT, there is no direct correlation between the degree of prolongation of PT and the risk for bleeding. The risk for bleeding at a given PT value will vary with the underlying disorder causing the coagulation abnormality. In general, for a given disorder, the longer the PT value the more likely the risk of bleeding, but there are no precise values defining the risk.

● **Proteins induced by vitamin K antagonism or absence (PIVKA).**

– PIVKA clotting time is similar to PT, but a **different thromboplastin is used** to activate coagulation, and the **plasma is diluted, resulting in longer clotting times**. The test was introduced as a **more sensitive assay than the standard PT** for monitoring warfarin therapy in humans. The assay is more sensitive both because the thromboplastin is more sensitive to factor X deficiency, and because the longer clotting times facilitate detection of subtle changes. It is also believed, but not proven, that the test is more sensitive than the PT to detect vitamin K deficiency or antagonism because the PIVKAs (uncarboxylated clotting factors, see Vitamin K antagonist poisoning, below) inhibit the thromboplastin and the factor X conversion of prothrombin to thrombin.
  – **PIVKA time is a modified PT, and does not actually measure concentration of PIVKAs.**
  – The test was first introduced as the Thrombotest™, and this name is used interchangeably with PIVKA. The former is recommended to avoid the confusion that arises from the term PIVKA.
– PIVKA time is more sensitive than PT to detect subclinical and clinical coagulopathies in cats due to vitamin K deficiency.
  – Most cats (> 95%) with a bleeding tendency due to vitamin K deficiency will have a prolonged PIVKA time.
  – It is controversial whether or not PIVKA time is more sensitive than the PT for the detection of vitamin K antagonism in dogs. This has not been evaluated in cats. Certainly any cat with clinical hemorrhage due to vitamin K antagonist poisoning will have a prolonged PT. PIVKA time may be more useful than PT for the monitoring of warfarin therapy for prophylaxis of thromboembolism in cats with cardiomyopathy.
– PIVKA time is not specific for vitamin K deficiency or antagonism. Similar to the PT, **it will be prolonged in any disorder affecting factors II, VII, IX and X**, including congenital factor VII deficiency and some cases of DIC.
– Collect sample as for PT and aPTT.
– Although the Thrombotest is a simple test for a reference laboratory to perform, it is not as

widely offered by such laboratories as are PT and aPTT. Point-of-care instruments are available.

- **Thrombin time (TT) and fibrinogen (factor I) level.**
  - Thrombin measures the time required for thrombin to convert fibrinogen to fibrin. The test is performed by adding thrombin to diluted citrated plasma.
  - Collect sample as for aPTT and PT.
  - Prolonged TT is due primarily to hypofibrinogenemia and thus **TT is a precise method to assay fibrinogen level.** Thrombin time is also **prolonged by inhibitors such as heparin and fibrin degradation products.**
  - **Fibrinogen level** can also be measured in a clinic or laboratory by heat precipitation as follows (this method is best for measuring increased levels of fibrinogen and may not be sufficiently sensitive to measure decreased levels):
    - Fill two microhematocrit tubes with EDTA (or citrated) blood.
    - Immerse one of the tubes in a 56–58°C (133–136°F) water bath for 3 minutes to precipitate fibrinogen.
    - Centrifuge both tubes at standard rate and time, and measure microhematocrit and total protein (using a refractometer).
    - [Total Protein in the room temperature sample (albumin + globulin + fibrinogen)] – [Total Protein in the heated sample (albumin + globulin)] = fibrinogen.
    - An alternative, less precise, method is to obtain serum from a separate clot tube and subtract total protein in the serum sample from total protein in the plasma sample.
  - Several other methods for measuring fibrinogen level, including immunologic assays, are in use in reference laboratories.
- **Fibrin-degradation products (FDPs).**
  - FDPs are the breakdown products of fibrinogen and fibrin monomers by plasmin.
  - The latex agglutination test is most commonly used.
    - This was originally exclusively a serum test, where blood is collected in a special tube containing a soybean trypsin inhibitor and fer-de-lance (*Bothrops atrox*) venom to promote rapid and complete clotting of the sample. The rapid clotting facilitates emergency testing, while the complete clotting circumvents

inhibition of clotting in samples from patients treated with heparin.The venom typically causes hemolysis of the sample.
    - Assays that use citrated plasma are now available. This facilitates measurement of FDPs as part of a coagulation screen.
  - **Increased FDPs suggest accelerated fibrinolysis by the plasmin system.**
  - **The test is infrequently positive in cats**.
    - D-dimers, measured by immunologic assays, are another marker of fibrinolysis, and represent breakdown products of cross-linked fibrin. Little is currently known of the utility of d-dimer measurement in cats.
- **Schistocytes and other poikilocytes**.
  - Fragmented and other abnormal red cells may appear with disseminated intravascular coagulation (DIC).
- **Specialized tests of hemostasis.**
  Other tests of hemostasis are used in research laboratories and may be required to investigate a novel bleeding disorder.
  - **Platelet aggregation** is the test most often used to further investigate a defect of primary hemostasis. In the most widely used method, various aggregating agents are added to platelet-rich plasma, and a **change in plasma turbidity** is detected by a spectrophotometer as the platelets aggregate. Whole blood aggregometry is an alternative, but less widely used, technique. Platelet aggregation is very sensitive, and in vitro defects may not result in clinically relevant effects.

DISEASES CAUSING BLEEDING

LOCAL LESIONS CAUSING LOCALIZED HEMORRHAGE***

Classical signs

- Clinically evident localized bleeding.
- Local signs of trauma, inflammation or neoplasia.

Clinical signs

Diseases where clinical bleeding may be the chief complaint or a clinical problem include:

- **Bleeding into or from skin, underlying tissues, ears and footpads** with lacerations, puncture wounds, blunt trauma, ruptured cat bite abscesses and bleeding tumors (see The Cat With Skin Lumps and Bumps, page 1067 and The Cat With Non-Healing Wounds, page 1081). Vasculitis usually results in edema, but may rarely cause local bleeding.
- **Bleeding from oral cavity** due to lacerations and puncture wounds, periodontal disease, and oral neoplasms (see The Cat With Bad Breath or Oral Lesions, page 602).
- **Epistaxis** from nasal trauma, rhinitis and neoplasms (see The Cat With Upper Respiratory Tract Signs of Chronic Nasal Disease, page 19).
- **Ocular hemorrhage** from corneoscleral lacerations, severe uveitis, and ocular neoplasms (see The Cat With Eye Problems, page 1165).
- **Hematuria** from major trauma to the kidney or bladder, idiopathic lower urinary tract disease, neoplasms of the kidney or bladder (see The Cat With Urinary Tract Signs, page 173). Clot formation in the bladder may cause or exacerbate signs of lower urinary tract disease.
- **Vaginal bleeding** from pyometra, spontaneous abortion or lochia (see The Infertile Queen, page 1145).
- **Melena** from intestinal neoplasia, which may cause iron-deficiency anemia (see The Cat With Signs of Gastrointestinal Tract Disease, page 578).
- **Hematochezia** from colitis (and rarely acute enteritis), and colonic and anorectal neoplasms (see The Cat With Signs of Gastrointestinal Tract Disease, page 578).
- **Hemoptysis** from major blunt trauma, acute heart failure and less commonly lung lobe torsion and primary lung neoplasms (see The Dyspneic or Tachypneic Cat, page 47).
- **Hemothorax** from major blunt trauma, penetrating trauma and spontaneous bleeding from the thymus (see The Dyspneic or Tachypneic Cat, page 47).
- **Hemopericardium** from major blunt trauma, penetrating trauma or neoplasia (rare) (see The Dyspneic or Tachypneic Cat, page 47).
- **Hemoperitoneum** from major blunt trauma, penetrating trauma, liver disorders (especially hepatic amyloidosis and peliosis hepatis), and bleeding neoplasms (see The Cat With Abdominal Distention or Abdominal Fluid, page 443).

Diagnosis

See the appropriate chapters listed above.

Tests of hemostasis (platelet count, BMBT, ACT, aPTT, PT) are either normal or not sufficiently abnormal to account for the hemorrhage.

Differential diagnosis

If a local lesion is not apparent, a hemostatic defect is likely.

Local lesions and hemostatic defects may be concurrent.

Systemic hypertension may cause retinal hemorrhages and epistaxis.

Treatment

Treat the local lesion – see the appropriate chapters listed above.

Use fluid therapy and/or whole blood transfusion (10–20 ml/kg) to correct acute hypovolemia and anemia.

MOTOR VEHICLE AND OTHER MAJOR BLUNT TRAUMA***

Classical signs

- Shorn nails, fractured mandible, fractured pelvis, dyspnea.

Clinical signs

External signs of trauma include shorn nails, and bleeding from skin and oral cavity lacerations.

Internal signs of trauma include palpable fractures, non-palpable bladder, hemoperitoneum and dyspnea from pneumothorax, hemothorax, diaphragmatic hernia, pulmonary contusions, neurogenic pulmonary edema, shock and pain.

The cat may be in **shock** with pale mucous membranes and weak pulses.

Diagnosis

Diagnosis is facilitated if the event is witnessed, e.g. hit by motor vehicle, fall from a height, kicked by a horse.

Physical examination findings consistent with trauma are supportive evidence.

Radiographic findings often reveal fractures and thoracic abnormalities. Intra-abdominal bleeding may cause loss of detail on abdominal radiographs, but ultrasound, abdominocentesis and diagnostic peritoneal lavage are superior for its detection.

- Thoracic injuries and resulting dyspnea are more common and clinically important than abdominal injuries following blunt trauma in cats. Abdominal hemorrhage may occur, but is rarely life threatening.

Hemostatic testing is usually normal in traumatized cats, although mild thrombocytopenia may occur secondary to massive bleeding. Trauma does not appear to be an important trigger for DIC in cats.

Differential diagnosis

Differential diagnoses for hemoperitoneum include anti-coagulant rodenticide poisoning, inherited coagulopathy (e.g. hemophilia A and B), ruptured neoplasm (e.g. hemangiosarcoma) and spontaneous bleeding from a diseased liver (e.g. amyloidosis, peliosis hepatis).

Differential diagnoses for hemothorax include anti-coagulant rodenticide poisoning, inherited coagulopathy (e.g. hemophilia A and B), and spontaneous bleeding from the thymus.

Treatment

See the appropriate chapters for treatment of specific traumatic disorders.

RENAL FAILURE***

Classical signs

- Lethargy, inappetence, weight loss, polyuria, polydipsia.
- Pale mucous membranes (anemia).

See main reference, page 235 (The Cat With Polyuria and Polydipsia).

Clinical signs

Cats with chronic renal failure show varying **lethargy, inappetence, weight loss, polyuria, polydipsia,** intermittent vomiting and anemia.

Uremic stomatitis and uremic gastroenteritis may cause bleeding in acute and chronic renal failure, contributing to anemia in the latter.

Hypertension may cause retinal hemorrhages and/or retinal detachment.

Hemolytic-uremic syndrome is an uncommon complication of renal transplantation.

Diagnosis

Hemostatic testing is usually normal.

- Mildly prolonged aPTT and mild thrombocytopenia (mechanisms not known) have been seen in chronic renal failure.
- Uremic thrombocytopathia has not been documented in cats, but probably occurs. Determining BMBT prior to renal biopsy is recommended.
- Hemolytic-uremic syndrome results in thrombocytopenia.

Differential diagnosis

If a cat with chronic renal failure is showing signs of acute bleeding other than retinal hemorrhages, a concurrent local or hemostatic disorder should be pursued.

Treatment

The use of **H2-blockers and/or sulcralfate** may reduce **gastrointestinal bleeding**.

Dental prophylaxis may reduce oral cavity bleeding.

Amlodipine, enalapril or **benazapril** is recommended for treatment of **hypertension** (see The Blind Cat or Cat With Retinal Disease, page 1171).

No specific treatment is recommended for the hemostatic disorders. If BMBT is prolonged and requires correction prior to an invasive procedure, treatments useful in humans and/or dogs include:

- **Whole blood or packed red cell transfusion**, or **recombinant human erythropoietin therapy** to improve anemia, because uremic bleeding is worse at a lower hematocrit.
- **Fresh-frozen plasma or cryoprecipitate transfusion**, or desmopressin to improve von Willebrand's factor level and/or function, because defects in von

Willebrand's factor may contribute to the thrombo-cytopathia (in humans) and augmenting von Willebrand's factor may compensate for non-von Willebrand's factor-dependent defects. Fresh-frozen plasma and cryoprecipitate may also contain functional platelet microparticles. Recombinant factor VIIa is beneficial in humans.

- Peritoneal or hemodialysis, to reduce uremic toxins that contribute to bleeding.

SYSTEMIC HYPERTENSION**

> ### Classical signs
>
> - Retinal hemorrhages.
> - Epistaxis.
> - Signs of the underlying disease.

Clinical signs

Sustained systemic blood pressure leads to vascular damage manifested clinically most often as **retinal hemorrhages** and less frequently as **epistaxis**.

Cats with **chronic renal failure** (the most common cause of hypertension) will have varying lethargy, inappetence, weight loss, polyuria, polydipsia and intermittent vomiting.

Cats with **hyperthyroidism**, **diabetes mellitus** and **hyperadrenocorticism** may have systemic hypertension but bleeding and other signs of organ damage do not commonly occur without concurrent renal failure.

Cats with **multiple myeloma** show non-specific signs of lethargy, inappetence and weight loss.

Cats with **polycythemia vera** have dark mucous membranes and may seizure.

Hyperaldosteronism (may cause weakness and polyuria/polydipsia due to hypokalemia) and **pheochromocytoma** (may cause polyuria/polydipsia) can cause hypertension, but the risk for abnormal bleeding is not known. These disorders are both rare in the cat.

Diagnosis

Routine work-up is required to identify the primary disease.

Hemostatic testing is normal or may identify abnormalities secondary to underlying (e.g. myeloma) or concurrent (e.g. FIV infection) diseases.

Differential diagnosis

Differential diagnoses for retinal hemorrhages include a platelet disorder or coagulopathy.

Differential diagnoses for epistaxis include trauma, rhinitis, neoplasia, a platelet disorder or coagulopathy.

Treatment

Amlodipine, enalapril or benazapril are used most often to treat renovascular hypertension (see The Blind Cat or Cat With Retinal Disease, page 1171).

For other conditions, treatment of the primary disease may be sufficient to resolve hypertension.

MEGAKARYOCYTIC HYPOPLASIA**

> ### Classical signs
>
> - Signs of the primary disease such as leukemia, lymphoma, FeLV/FIV infection, histoplasmosis (e.g. fever, inappetence, weight loss, gingivitis, lymphadenopathy, hepatosplenomegaly, dyspnea, diarrhea).
> - Signs of concurrent cytopenias (e.g. pale mucous membranes from anemia, fever secondary to neutropenic sepsis).
> - History of drug use known to cause myelosuppression.
> - Platelet disorder bleeding (e.g. prolonged bleeding after venepuncture, melena, epistaxis, petechiation).

Pathogenesis

Megakaryocytic hypoplasia reduces platelet production (hypoproliferative thrombocytopenia).

Megakaryocytic hypoplasia occurs most commonly as part of generalized bone marrow failure or dyshematopoiesis resulting in pancytopenia. Causes of bone marrow failure include:

- **Hematopoietic neoplasia** causing myelophthisis. Neoplasms include lymphoid leukemia, myeloid leukemia, myelodysplastic syndrome, multiple myeloma, malignant histiocytosis and mast cell tumor.

- **Infections** causing generalized bone marrow failure or dyshematopoiesis. Infectious agents include feline leukemia virus, feline immunodeficiency virus, *Histoplasma capsulatum*, and, possibly, *Ehrlichia* spp.
  - Feline panleukopenia virus infection causes transient myelosuppression, but acute thrombocytopenia is due to disseminated intravascular coagulation.
- **Cytotoxic anticancer drugs** and large-field radiation therapy produce predictable dose-dependent effects.
  - Cats are more sensitive to azathioprine toxicosis than dogs, probably because of decreased levels of thiopurine methyltransferase, the enzyme responsible for the drug's metabolism.
- Idiosyncratic, immune-mediated, and toxic **drug reactions** have been reported with chloramphenicol, griseofulvin (especially in FIV-infected cats), cephalosporins, ribavirin, albendazole, anti-thyroid drugs (propylthiouracil, methimazole, carbimazole), and phenobarbital.

Occasionally no cause is found and/or megakaryocytic hypoplasia is the only bone marrow abnormality. Some of the idiopathic cases are due to immune-mediated mechanisms. A diagnosis of immune-mediated hypoplasia is usually based on ruling out other causes of megakaryocytic hypoplasia, presence of other disorders that are typically immune-mediated, and response to immunosuppressive therapy.

Clinical signs

In most cases thrombocytopenia is noted during work-up of the primary disease or work-up of other signs, e.g. fever.

Clinical bleeding is occasionally the chief complaint or noted during examination or work-up.

Spontaneous bleeding includes petechiation, ecchymoses, epistaxis, ocular hemorrhages, hematuria and melena.

Excessive bleeding is usually first noted as **bleeding from venepuncture sites**. Biopsy sites, suture lines and other local lesions may also bleed excessively.

Signs due to anemia (e.g. pale mucous membranes, tachycardia) and local effects of hemorrhage (e.g. hematoma formation) vary with severity and acuteness of blood loss.

Signs of underlying hematopoietic neoplasia, FeLV or FIV infection, or histoplasmosis include fever, inappetence, weight loss, lymphadenopathy, hepatosplenomegaly, dyspnea and diarrhea.

- FeLV or FIV infection may cause gingivitis.

Fever may be present due to spontaneous infection secondary to concurrent neutropenia.

Diagnosis

History and physical examination findings are consistent with a primary disease (e.g. drug therapy).

A complete blood count will reveal thrombocytopenia.

- Artifactual thrombocytopenia is common in cats. A platelet count generated by a laboratory instrument or manual count should be verified with a blood smear, and the blood smear should be closely examined for platelet clumps.

Bone marrow biopsy will reveal **megakaryocytic hypoplasia**. Concurrent erythroid hypoplasia, myeloid hypoplasia and neoplasia may also be identified.

- If feline leukemia virus infection is suspected but peripheral blood tests are negative, then obtain a fluorescent antibody (FA) or PCR test on a bone marrow aspirate or ELISA test on a bone marrow core biopsy. **It should be noted that PCR testing has not been standardized and is more likely to give false-positive results than ELISA and FA if the laboratory does not maintain the highest standards of quality control.**

Differential diagnosis

Other causes of thrombocytopenia are usually associated with normal to increased platelet counts on bone marrow biopsy. For many of these causes the primary disease is sufficiently characterized on routine work-up to explain thrombocytopenia without the need for bone marrow biopsy. Other causes of thrombocytopenia include:

- DIC (**platelet consumption**).
- Immune-mediated thrombocytopenia (**platelet destruction**). This is a rare disorder in the cat.
- Marked splenomegaly (**platelet sequestration**). This is an uncommon cause of thrombocytopenia in the cat.
- Severe bleeding (**platelet loss**).
  - **Severe bleeding** may result in mild thrombocytopenia. In a series of cats with anticoagulant rodenticide poisoning, a platelet count as low as 58×10^9/L (58,000/µl) was noted (reference 9). If severe bleeding is associated with mild thrombocytopenia, it is more likely that the low platelet count is a result of, rather than the cause of, the bleeding.

Treatment

Treat the primary disease if possible.

Thrombocytopenia may be transiently improved by **transfusion of fresh whole blood, platelet-rich plasma, or fresh-frozen plasma** (which contains functional platelet particles), 10–20 ml/kg, or platelet concentrate, 1–2 units/cat.

- This is recommended before biopsy of internal organs if the platelet count is < 50×10^9/L (50 000/µl).
- Platelet transfusions may be used prophylactically against spontaneous hemorrhage in humans with platelet counts < 10–20×10^9/L (10 000–20 000/µl). This is not recommended in cats because spontaneous critical hemorrhage is rare in thrombocytopenic cats, and because most practices have a limited donor blood supply.

Augmenting one part of hemostasis compensates to some extent for a deficiency in another part. To this end **inhibitors of fibrinolysis** (e.g. aminocaproic acid), which augment coagulation, have been useful in treating thrombocytopenia in humans but have not been evaluated in cats.

General treatment measures for cats with a bleeding tendency include the following recommendations. These are most important in cats with moderate to marked defects in hemostasis:

- Minimize exuberant exercise and risk for trauma at home (keep indoors).
- Handle gently in the hospital and provide a well-padded cage.
- Feed soft food to minimize gingival trauma.
- Minimize invasive procedures and injections. If injection is required, use 25-G or smaller needles. The intravenous route is preferred (with the exception of vitamin K). Subcutaneous and especially intramuscular injections may cause hematomas that may impair absorption of the drug in addition to causing discomfort.
- Apply moderate manual pressure or pressure bandages to sites of active bleeding when possible.
- Do not drain hematomas unless they are causing a problem (e.g. tracheal compression).
- Avoid over-exuberant intravenous fluid therapy, which dilutes platelet and coagulation factor concentrations. Synthetic colloids may cause platelet dysfunction.
- Avoid drugs that significantly decrease platelet function (e.g. aspirin), antagonize vitamin K, or have direct anti-coagulant effects (e.g. heparin).
  - **Penicillins, some cephalosporins, tetracyclines, gentamicin and sulfa drugs** have been demonstrated **to variably impair platelet function in vitro or in vivo** in humans, rabbits or dogs. Worsening hemorrhage is likely to be seen only in severely thrombocytopenic patients. Effects of these drugs in cats are not known. However, amoxicillin, cefazolin, cephalexin, doxycycline, and enrofloxacin at standard doses do not impair platelet function in normal dogs and are unlikely to have any clinically relevant hemostatic effects in cats.
  - Acepromazine and some antihistamines impair platelet function in humans. Acepromazine does not impair platelet function in dogs and these drugs are unlikely to have any clinically relevant hemostatic effects in cats.

Prognosis

Prognosis is determined by the primary disease.

If megakaryocytic hypoplasia cannot be promptly corrected and if the cat is clinically bleeding from severe thrombocytopenia, the prognosis for long-term transfusion support is poor because of donor exhaustion and possibly platelet alloimmunization.

LIVER DISEASE**

Classical signs

- Lethargy, inappetence, weight loss, vomiting, icterus.
- Spontaneous or excessive bleeding may occur.

See main reference page 421 (The Yellow Cat or Cat With Increased Liver Enzymes).

Pathogenesis

The **most common causes of liver disease in the cat are lipidosis, cholangiohepatitis and lymphoma**. Less common causes include congenital portosystemic shunts, amyloidosis, non-lymphoid neoplasia, feline infectious peritonitis, peliosis hepatis, toxoplasmosis and toxins (e.g. diazepam).

Liver disease may cause bleeding tendencies by several mechanisms including:
- Acquired platelet function defects (not proven in cats).
- Decreased synthesis of coagulation factors.
  - Primary **hepatocellular failure affecting synthesis** of all factors.
  - **Vitamin K deficiency** (contributing to coagulopathy in about 50% of cases).
    - Intrahepatic **cholestasis** and extrahepatic bile duct obstruction prevent release of **bile acids** into the small intestine that are **needed for absorption of vitamin K1 and K2**.
    - Anorexia and antibiotic therapy contribute to vitamin K deficiency.
- Synthesis of abnormal prothrombin (not proven in cats).
- **DIC** causing consumption of platelets and coagulation factors.
- **Decreased clearance of plasminogen activators** thus promoting fibrinolysis (not proven in cats).

In general, **fever decreases the half-life of coagulation factors** and wound healing increases consumption of coagulation factors (e.g. after exploratory laparotomy). Both of these may be present with liver disease.

The **liver may be more fragile** with hepatic lipidosis, amyloidosis and peliosis hepatis increasing the risk of bleeding after liver biopsy. Spontaneous hemoperitoneum may occur with amyloidosis and peliosis hepatis.

Coagulation abnormalities are **more likely** to be present if there is **concurrent pancreatitis.**

Clinical signs

More than 80% of cats with liver disease may have a coagulation abnormality, but **abnormal clinical bleeding is uncommon**.

Excessive bleeding may occur following venepuncture and liver biopsy.

Severity of coagulopathy correlates to some extent to increase in alkaline phosphatase value, likely due to cholestasis.

In other species acute bleeding into the intestinal tract may precipitate hepatic encephalopathy, but this has not been documented in the cat.

Diagnosis

Combining results of several studies, coagulation abnormalities may be categorized as follows:
- **Vitamin K deficiency:** Normal platelet count, prolonged PT, ± prolonged aPTT, normal TT.
- **Synthesis failure:** Normal platelet count, prolonged PT, prolonged aPTT, prolonged TT.
- **Indeterminate:** Normal platelet count, normal PT, prolonged aPTT, normal TT.
- **DIC:** Low platelet count, prolonged PT, prolonged aPTT, prolonged TT; or 3 of the following: low platelet count, prolonged PT or aPTT, prolonged TT or hypofibrinogenemia, decreased antithrombin III (not routinely available), presence of FDPs, red blood cell fragments.

Vitamin K deficiency may also be identified by improvement in coagulation following vitamin K1 therapy.

PIVKA time is more sensitive in identifying abnormal coagulation than are PT and aPTT. Cats may show a bleeding tendency with a prolonged PIVKA time and normal PT and aPTT.

More than one mechanism may contribute to coagulopathy.

Differential diagnosis

In most cases the cat with liver disease is presented for subacute to chronic non-specific signs and coagulopathy is identified in the work-up of liver disease.

A large number of disorders may be associated with subacute non-specific signs and subclinical coagulopathy, including neoplasia, retroviral infections, FIP, heart disease and pancreatitis. Routine work-up will help identify the primary disease.

Treatment

Vitamin K1, 2.5–5 mg/kg SC for 1–2 days, will usually **normalize PT and aPTT in 1–2 days** if vitamin K deficiency is solely responsible for coagulopathy. (**PIVKA values take 3–5 days to normalize.**) The need for further vitamin K1 therapy will depend on success of managing the primary disease.

Prognosis

Prognosis is determined by the primary liver disease.

Prognosis for resolution of a vitamin K deficient state is excellent.

FELINE LEUKEMIA VIRUS (FELV) INFECTION**

Classical signs

- Lethargy, inappetence, weight loss, unkempt haircoat, fever, anemia, gingivitis, recurrent upper respiratory infections, opportunistic infections.
- Cats with megakaryocytic hypoplasia may have platelet disorder type bleeding.

See main reference on page 540 (The Anemic Cat).

Pathogenesis

FeLV infection can cause bleeding tendencies by several mechanisms. These include:

- **Megakaryocytic hypoplasia**.
- Immune-mediated platelet destruction.
- DIC secondary to infections and neoplasia.

Clinical signs

Clinical bleeding is uncommon except with severe thrombocytopenia, in which case bleeding is typical of platelet disorders, e.g. petechiation, epistaxis, melena, prolonged bleeding after venepuncture.

Diagnosis

FeLV antigen test.
- Bleeding tendencies are most likely to **occur during persistent viremia**, in which case ELISA and FA tests are usually both positive.
- If peripheral blood tests are negative and another cause of megakaryocytic hypoplasia has not been determined, obtain a FA or PCR test on a bone marrow aspirate or ELISA test on a bone marrow core biopsy. **It should be noted that PCR testing has not been standardized and is more likely to give false-positive results than ELISA and FA if the laboratory does not maintain the highest standards of quality control.**

Hemostatic testing may reveal thrombocytopenia, and prolonged PT, ACT, and aPTT and hypofibrinogenemia if DIC is present.

Differential diagnosis

The main cause of clinical bleeding in FeLV-infected cats is megakaryocytic hypoplasia. If a FeLV-positive cat is bleeding without severe thrombocytopenia (usually platelets $< 20 \times 10^9$/L, $<200\ 000/\mu l$), another hemostatic disorder should be investigated.

A concurrent disease may be responsible for subclinical hemostatic defects including liver disease, cardiomyopathy, pancreatitis, renal failure, other systemic infections, lymphoma and other neoplasms, and snakebite envenomation and other toxicoses.

Feline immunodeficiency virus (FIV) infection causes similar signs to FeLV infection and may also cause megakaryocytic hypoplasia and other hemostatic defects. An FIV test may be used to rule this out.

Most causes of megakaryocytic hypoplasia, ITP and DIC may be identified by routine work-up.

Treatment

Thrombocytopenia and other hemostatic defects may be transiently improved by transfusion of **fresh** whole blood, **platelet-rich plasma**, or **fresh-frozen plasma (which contains functional platelet particles)**, 10–20 ml/kg. Bleeding due to **thrombocytopenia** may also be treated with platelet concentrate, 1–2 units/cat.

- Transfusion is recommended **before biopsy** of internal organs **if the platelet count is** < 50×10^9/L (50,000/dl).

Treat infections and neoplasia.

Recombinant human **interferon-α,** 1 unit/cat PO q 24 h may ameliorate myelosuppression.

Bone marrow transplantation for megakaryocytic hypoplasia may be considered if available.

Prognosis

Prognosis for severe FeLV-induced megakaryocytic hypoplasia is poor.

Long-term prognosis with other hemostatic defects is determined by the FeLV-associated underlying disease.

FELINE IMMUNODEFICIENCY VIRUS (FIV) INFECTION**

Classical signs

- Lethargy, inappetence, weight loss, unkempt haircoat, fever, generalized lymphadenopathy, gingivitis, diarrhea, dermatitis, recurrent upper respiratory infections, opportunistic infections, neurologic signs, uveitis.
- Various hemostatic abnormalities may occur but are usually subclinical.

See main reference on page 339 (The Thin, Inappetent Cat).

Pathogenesis

The following hemostatic defects may occur with FIV infection:

- **Thrombocytopenia**. This may be due to the primary infection or secondary to other disease processes, e.g. neoplasia, bone marrow failure with griseofulvin therapy.
  - FIV infection in-itself does not commonly cause severe megakaryocytic hypoplasia.
  - FIV infection in-itself does not appear to cause platelet function defects.
- **Prolongation of aPTT**. The mechanism is not known, but it is not due to specific factor deficiencies, DIC, or a circulating inhibitor.
- **Prolongation of TT**. The mechanism is not known, but it is not due to hypofibrinogenemia or dysfibrinogenemia.
- **DIC** secondary to infections and neoplasia.

Clinical signs

Clinical bleeding is uncommon.

Severe thrombocytopenia may cause bleeding typical of platelet disorders, e.g. petechiation, epistaxis, melena, prolonged bleeding after venepuncture.

Prolongation of the aPTT and TT do not result in abnormal bleeding.

Diagnosis

FIV antibody test (ELISA, FA, western blot).

- Antibody is **usually detectable within 2 months** of infection, but may take up to 6 months, therefore a negative test should be repeated if FIV is being considered in the differential diagnoses of a cat with thrombocytopenia.
- PCR test for viral DNA. **It should be noted that PCR testing has not been standardized and is more likely to give false-positive results than antibody tests if the laboratory does not maintain the highest standards of quality control.**

Neutropenia and lymphopenia are common concurrent hematologic abnormalities in symptomatic cats.

Hemostatic testing may reveal the following abnormalities due to FIV infection: low to normal platelet count, normal BMBT unless thrombocytopenic, shortened to normal PT, normal to prolonged ACT and aPTT, normal to prolonged TT and normal to increased fibrinogen. In addition, prolonged PT, ACT and aPTT and hypofibrinogenemia may occur if DIC is present.

Differential diagnosis

FeLV infection causes similar signs to FIV infection. FeLV infection causes severe megakaryocytic hypoplasia more commonly than FIV infection, and other hemostatic defects may also occur. A FeLV antigen test may be used to rule this out.

Most **other causes of megakaryocytic hypoplasia** and **DIC** may be identified by routine work-up.

Concurrent disease may be responsible for the hemostatic defect. Subclinical coagulation abnormalities have been identified with a number of disorders including liver disease, cardiomyopathy, pancreatitis, renal failure, other systemic infections, lymphoma and other neoplasms, and snake bite envenomation and other toxicoses.

Treatment

The **prolonged aPTT and TT** may be corrected by transfusion of **fresh or fresh-frozen plasma**, 10–20 ml/kg.

- This is recommended before biopsy of internal organs, although the need for such transfusion is not known.

Bleeding due to **thrombocytopenia** may be transiently improved by transfusion of **fresh whole blood**, **platelet-rich plasma** or **fresh-frozen plasma** (which contains functional platelet particles), 10–20 ml/kg, or platelet concentrate, 1–2 units/cat.

- This is recommended **before biopsy** of internal organs **if the platelet count is** $< 50 \times 10^9$/L (50 000/dl).

Prognosis

Prognosis for severe FIV-induced megakaryocytic hypoplasia is poor.

Myelosuppression associated with griseofulvin or other drug therapy will usually resolve, but intensive supportive care is required.

There is no specific prognosis associated with the unique FIV-associated coagulation defects.

Long-term prognosis is usually determined by other FIV-associated diseases.

DISSEMINATED INTRAVASCULAR COAGULATION (DIC)*

Classical signs

- Signs of underlying sepsis or non-septic inflammation (e.g. anorexia, depression, fever, hypothermia, tachycardia, abdominal pain).
- Signs of underlying neoplasia (e.g. inappetence, weight loss, lymphadenopathy, hepatosplenomegaly, abdominal mass, dyspnea).
- Signs of underlying FIP (e.g. inappetence, weight loss, fever, abdominal distention, dyspnea).
- Signs of underlying liver disease (e.g. inappetence, weight loss, icterus).
- Signs of other underlying diseases, e.g. hyperthermia (temperature $\geq 42°C$ [107.6°F]), shock, snake bite wound.
- Spontaneous and excessive bleeding at various sites may occur, but is uncommon.

Pathogenesis

Concurrent **intravascular activation of hemostasis and accelerated fibrinolysis** lead to **microvascular thrombosis and embolism**.

Thrombosis and embolism may lead to organ failure.

Bleeding tendencies occur secondary to consumption of platelets and coagulation factors, increased plasmin activity, and circulating anti-coagulants, including fibrin degradation products (FDPs).

Numerous disease processes may trigger DIC, including thromboembolism due to cardiomyopathy, neoplasia (e.g. hemangiosarcoma, hepatic, biliary and pulmonary carcinomas, mesothelioma, lymphoma, myeloid leukemia, malignant histiocytosis), infections (e.g. bacterial sepsis, tuberculosis, histoplasmosis, cytauxzoonosis, toxoplasmosis), non-infectious inflammation (e.g. pancreatitis, immune-mediated diseases), heat stroke, major trauma, penetrating head trauma, shock and snake bite envenomation.

DIC has wide clinical and pathological spectra and may be **acute to chronic, localized to generalized, and subclinical to fulminant**. A broad definition is used here to include most cases of consumptive thrombocytopenia and microangiopathic disorders.

Acute DIC is not as common in cats as in dogs. The most common causes are **panleukopenia virus** infection, other **overwhelming infections** (e.g. cytauxzoonosis), and **neoplasia**.

The most common causes of **subacute to chronic DIC** are **liver diseases, neoplasia and FIP** (due to vasculitis).

Thrombocytopenia has also been noted with several other diseases (see Miscellaneous diseases, page 505), where the thrombocytopenia is likely consumptive in origin.

Clinical signs

Signs of the primary disease.

Most DIC is **subclinical**.

Superficial and deep spontaneous **bleeding may occur**, but it is uncommon.

Venepuncture and biopsy sites, suture lines, and internal and external injuries may bleed excessively.

Signs due to anemia and local effects of hemorrhage vary with severity of blood loss.

Diagnosis

Identification of a primary disease.

Diagnosis is controversial in all species and there is not a single test or combination of tests that rules in or rules out DIC.

Laboratory abnormalities consistent with DIC include:
- Low platelet count, prolonged ACT, prolonged aPTT, prolonged PT, prolonged TT, hypofibrinogenemia, decreased antithrombin III concentration, presence of FDPs, and red blood cell fragments.
- One approach uses **presence of three of the above abnormalities** (counting prolonged PT and/or aPTT as one abnormality) as criteria for diagnosing DIC.
  - Another approach uses low platelet count, prolonged PT, prolonged aPTT, and prolonged TT as diagnostic of DIC in liver disease.

  - In the author's opinion, firm diagnostic criteria should not be used. Rather, the probability of DIC increases with the number of consistent laboratory abnormalities: e.g. it is possible that a cat with only thrombocytopenia has DIC, it is more likely that a cat with thrombocytopenia and prolonged ACT has DIC, while it is highly probable that a cat with thrombocytopenia, prolonged PT and aPTT, hypofibrinogenemia and increased FDPs has DIC. Scoring systems based on this approach have been used in humans.
- Measuring **antithrombin III**, which tends to be consumed in DIC, may add specificity but probably does not increase sensitivity to the diagnosis of DIC.
- Measurements of **D-Dimer** are being used with increasing frequency to support the diagnosis of DIC in dogs. Little is currently known of the utility of D-dimer assay in the diagnosis of DIC in cats. D-dimer is a more specific marker of thrombosis than are FDPs, but D-dimer is not specific for DIC. D-dimer levels will be increased in thromboembolic disorders including arterial and pulmonary thromboembolism.
- There is poor correlation between degrees of coagulation abnormalities, severity of underlying clinical disease and risk for hemorrhage.

Differential diagnosis

Differential diagnoses for the various primary diseases are discussed throughout this book. If a hemostatic defect is identified in the work-up of the primary disease, the possibility of a defect unrelated to the primary disease should be considered, e.g. Hageman trait.

Differential diagnoses for abnormal hemostasis with liver disease include vitamin K deficiency, synthesis failure and undetermined causes (which might be mild DIC).

In cats with neutropenia due to myelosuppression and secondary sepsis, thrombocytopenia may be due to concurrent megakaryocytic hypoplasia rather than DIC.

Treatment

Treat the primary disease.
- This is the most important treatment. If this is not possible, other treatments will ultimately fail.

Adequate **fluid therapy** to promote microvascular circulation, but not excessive fluid therapy, which will promote edema and bleeding.

If clinically bleeding, **transfuse** to replace platelets and/or clotting factors and anti-thrombin III with fresh whole blood, platelet-rich plasma, or fresh/fresh-frozen plasma, 10–20 ml/kg.

Heparin therapy is controversial.
- It is recommended because, although bleeding is clinically more obvious, **thrombosis causes most of the organ damage.**
- The goal is to **block microvascular thrombosis** while not aggravating bleeding.
- In cats with fulminant DIC, doses of 50–200 units/kg SC q 6–8 h have been recommended; 75–100 units SC q 8 h is used most often. The dose may be incubated for 30 minutes in the blood product prior to transfusion to activate antithrombin III, although the value of this practice is unproven. An initial **goal is prolongation of the ACT or aPTT to 1.5–2 times** the mean value of normal range or aPTT control value.
- It should not be used in cats with subclinical, subacute or chronic DIC, unless thromboembolism is present.
  - If thromboembolism is present, an initial dose of 200 units/kg SC q 6–8 h is recommended.

Prognosis

The prognosis is largely determined by the primary disease.

Acute diffuse DIC has a very poor prognosis.

SNAKE BITE ENVENOMATION*

Classical signs

- Bite wound on cranial half of body ± local swelling or bleeding (Viperidae, Crotalidae).
- Paresis/paralysis or bleeding tendency depending upon species of snake.

Clinical signs

Cats are believed to be less likely to be bitten by most snake species than dogs, and to be more resistant to hematoxins.

- Resistance to hematoxins may in part reflect cats playing with, and subsequently being bitten, by smaller snakes (thus receiving less venom), and/or only cats with mild–moderate envenomation surviving long enough to be presented to a veterinarian.

Venoms from **Elapidae** snakes (e.g. Australian tiger snake and brown snake, North American coral snakes, Indian cobras) are predominantly **neurotoxic**, although **procoagulants and myolysins** may cause significant complications.
- Signs include areflexic dilated pupils, dysphagia (salivation), dyspnea (respiratory paralysis), hindlimb ataxia and flaccid quadriplegia.
- Local reaction to the bite wound may be minimal.
- Although neurologic signs predominate, cats with tiger or brown snake bites may have significant disturbances of hemostasis.
  - **Potent procoagulants**, especially in the brown snake venom, act as **prothrombin converters, resulting in consumption of fibrinogen**.
  - 10–30% of cats show evidence of hemostatic abnormalities. Typical signs include **non-clotting blood, prolonged coagulation times** (ACT typically 180–240 s), **continuous bleeding from wounds** and venepuncture sites, hematemesis and hematuria.

Venoms from **Viperidae** (e.g. common adder in Britain and continental Europe, *Vipera palaestina* in the Middle East) are predominantly hematoxic, although some have neurotoxic properties.
- **Edema ± bleeding/bruising around the bite** is typical, but is not predictive of systemic toxicosis.
- Widespread bleeding is uncommon with bites from the common adder and *V. palaestina*, but may occur.

Venoms from **Crotalidae** (e.g. North American rattlesnakes, copperhead, cottonmouth, and South American fer-de-lance and bushmaster) are predominantly **hematoxic**, although some (e.g. Majove rattlesnake, Asian habu snake) are potent neurotoxins.
- **Severe regional swelling** may occur surrounding the bite from massive extravasation of plasma and red cells, but local reaction is not predictive of systemic toxicosis.
- Hypotension may result from pooling of blood in lungs and thoracic vessels.
- **Widespread bleeding may occur.**

– Clinical reports of Massassauga rattlesnake bites to cats are lacking. In dogs envenomation may cause marked prolongation of clotting times but clinical bleeding is rare.

Venoms from most **Colubridae** are mild and clinical reports of bites to cats lacking.
● The boomslang of central and South Africa produces a powerful **hematoxin** that is procoagulant and causes DIC in humans and dogs.

Diagnosis

Diagnosis is based on a history of exposure to the snake (try to identify species) and/or physical examination findings.

CBC may reveal hemoconcentration, hemolysis, echinocytosis, rubricytosis or thrombocytopenia.

Serum chemistry profile may reveal hypoproteinemia, hypokalemia and elevated CK, ALT, urea and creatinine levels.

Urinalysis may reveal myoglobinuria or hemoglobinuria, and glucosuria.

Hemostatic testing may reveal variable thrombocytopenia, prolonged PT and/or ACT, aPTT, and increased FDPs (i.e. DIC).

A Snake Venom Detection Kit (CSL Limited, Australia) can be used for identification of the presence and type of Australian snake venom. Testing is also available from commercial veterinary laboratories. Urine is preferred over blood because of non-specific binding with plasma proteins. A swab of the bite site is most accurate, but is rarely identifiable in cats with bites from Australian snakes.

Differential diagnosis

See The Weak and Ataxic or Paralyzed Cat (page 952) for differential diagnosis of neurologic signs.

Differential diagnoses for the local reaction include angioedema from insect envenomation, animal bite wounds, sharp and blunt trauma.

Differential diagnoses for hemostatic abnormalities include other causes of DIC.

Treatment

Keep animal calm.

If a bite on a limb is witnessed, application of a tourniquet or cold pack by the owner for 10–20 min may be beneficial, but should not delay transport to a veterinarian.

Supportive care.

Specific **antivenom** (antivenin) therapy.
● Observe for allergic reactions.
● Premedication with an anti-histamine, e.g. diphenhydramine, 1 mg/kg IV as a slow bolus over 10–15 min is recommended. This will not potentiate the venom.

If there are signs of hemostatic abnormalities, treat as for DIC (page 502) (see Disseminated intravascular coagulation, above) with transfusions of fresh whole blood, fresh plasma or fresh-frozen plasma.

Antibiotic therapy for secondary wound infection and delayed surgical management of the wound may be necessary.

HAGEMAN TRAIT*

Classical signs
● None.

Pathogenesis

Hageman trait refers to **reduced synthesis, release or function of factor XII** (Hageman factor).

Activation of factor XII to XIIa is the first step in the intrinsic system. As previously noted, this does not appear to be an important mechanism for the initiation of coagulation in vivo.

Factor XII is involved in the **conversion of plasminogen to plasmin**, which is responsible for clot dissolution (fibrinolysis).

Factor XII is also involved in inflammation.

Clinical signs

Spontaneous bleeding does not occur.

Prolonged ACT and aPTT are usually noted incidentally, e.g. when hemostasis is evaluated prior to biopsy.

Concurrent thrombocytopenia or thrombocytopathia was believed to have triggered bleeding in a cat following modified-live virus vaccination. This would appear to be an uncommon event, and is not reported in humans with Hageman trait.

Humans with Hageman deficiency are at increased risk for thromboembolic events as a result of a deficient fibrinolytic system. It is not known if cats with Hageman trait and cardiomyopathy are at increased risk of arterial thromboembolism.

It is not known if cats with Hageman trait have blunted inflammatory responses.

Diagnosis

No signs of abnormal bleeding unless another disease process affecting hemostasis is present.

Hageman trait is the most common inherited coagulation factor deficiency in cats, but prevalence is not known. Although stated to be common, recent large retrospective reviews of hemostatic disorders in sick cats have not identified any cases.

Hemostatic testing reveals normal platelet count and BMBT, normal PT, and markedly **prolonged ACT and aPTT** (e.g. aPTT > 50 s, often > 100 s, where the upper limit of normal range is 25 s).

Definitive diagnosis is based on **quantification of factor XII activity** (FXII:C), similar to the diagnosis of hemophilia A, and ruling-out acquired factor XII deficiency (see Circulating anti-coagulant, below).

Differential diagnosis

Hemophilia A, B (and C) are the main differential diagnoses for markedly prolonged ACT and aPTT as solitary abnormalities.

If a cat is presented with bleeding and a prolonged ACT and aPTT are found, a judgment must be made as to whether the bleeding is appropriate for the injury. For example, a cat with hemothorax and prolonged ACT and aPTT could have hemophilia A or chest trauma and Hageman trait, but in the former case there would be no evidence of injury.

Hemophilia B and Hageman trait have occurred concurrently.

Vitamin K antagonist poisoning – PT is prolonged as well as aPTT.

DIC – thrombocytopenia is often present, in addition to signs of a primary disease.

Acquired factor XII deficiency has been reported in humans but not in cats.

Treatment

None required.

Prognosis

Normal life expectancy.

Transmission

Factor XII deficiency is a heritable single-gene defect that is autosomal recessive.

Prevention

Probably none is required.

MISCELLANEOUS DISEASES*

Classical signs

- Signs of the primary disease.

Clinical signs

Thrombocytopenia, increased ACT/aPTT/PIVKA time, or **decreased antithrombin III** levels have been noted in various diseases not typically associated with bleeding tendencies. Diseases include hypertrophic cardiomyopathy, congenital cardiac disorders, pleural effusions not due to feline infectious peritonitis, diabetes mellitus, hyperthyroidism, hypertension, chronic renal failure, urinary tract infection, urethral obstruction, rhinitis, *Mycoplasma haemofelis* infection (haemobartonellosis), primary neurologic diseases, and non-anti-coagulant toxicoses.

DIC may be the mechanism for at least some of these abnormalities. The close **interaction** between the **intrinsic system and inflammation via factor XII**

may be responsible for some alterations in ACT and aPTT.

Hemostatic abnormalities are subclinical.

Diagnosis

Clinical signs and work-up of the primary disease.

IMMUNE-MEDIATED THROMBOCYTOPENIA (ITP)

Classical signs

- Platelet disorder bleeding (e.g. prolonged bleeding after venepuncture, melena, epistaxis, petechiation).

Pathogenesis

In ITP, **platelets become antigenic** leading to **accelerated platelet destruction** by the macrophage–monocyte system, particularly in the spleen.

In **primary**, **or idiopathic, ITP** an underlying disease is not found and the disease is considered to be auto-immune.

In **secondary** ITP, a primary, or underlying, disease is found, e.g. FeLV infection, where there is immune-complex deposition on the surface of infected platelets.
- **Lymphoma** is another primary disease associated with ITP, and ITP may be the mechanism of thrombocytopenia associated with various other neoplasms.
- Thrombocytopenia caused by **anti-thyroid drugs** (propylthiouracil, methimazole, carbimazole) is presumed to be immune-mediated because affected cats may have antinuclear antibodies.
- **Modified live virus vaccination** has been associated with thrombocytopenia and thrombocytopathia in dogs, typically occurring within 2–4 weeks of vaccination. Thrombocytopenia varies from a sub-clinical, self-limiting fall within normal range to severe thrombocytopenia requiring immunosuppressive therapy. Post-vaccinal thrombocytopenia or thrombocytopathia has been suspected in cats based on post-vaccinal bleeding in cats with other-wise sub-clinical hemostatic defects (see Hageman

trait, page 504 and Vitamin K responsive coagulopathy in the Devon Rex, page 515).

ITP may be concurrent with other autoimmune diseases, e.g. hemolytic anemia, myasthenia gravis, and systemic lupus erythematosus.

Clinical signs

Primary ITP is rare. There is usually marked thrombocytopenia and signs are typical of platelet disorder bleeding, including **petechiation, epistaxis, melena and hematuria**.

Signs of an underlying disease may be present, e.g. lymphadenopathy with lymphoma.

Splenomegaly may be present due to hyperplasia, extra-medullary hematopoiesis and neoplasia.

Thrombocytopenia may be an incidental finding in a work-up.

Anemia and associated signs vary.

Diagnosis

Rule out other causes of thrombocytopenia based on clinical signs and work-up.

Hemostatic testing reveals **thrombocytopenia, normal PT and aPTT**, and normal to increased fibrinogen level. Platelet counts $< 10 \times 10^9$/L (10 000/µl) are stated to mildly prolong ACT, but this effect is poorly documented.

Bone marrow biopsy reveals increased numbers of megakaryocytes.

Demonstration of **platelet or megakaryocyte-associated antibody** by immunofluorescence (test may not be readily available). Platelet and megakaryocyte-associated neutrophils have also been reported.

Response to immunosuppressive therapy.

Differential diagnosis

Megakaryocytic hypoplasia is distinguished from ITP on the basis of identification of a disease that causes decreased platelet production, e.g. myeloid leukemia, on bone marrow biopsy.

- Note that idiopathic megakaryocytic hypoplasia and pancytopenia may be immune-mediated in origin. If there are any megakaryocytes present in the marrow biopsy, testing by immunofluorescence for megakaryocyte-associated antibody should be performed. ITP and immune-mediated megakaryocytic hypoplasia are both uncommon but well-documented causes of thrombocytopenia in cats. Whether or not concurrent immunologic attack on platelets and megakaryocytes is occurring in some cases is not known.
- Note that FeLV infection may cause both megakaryocytic hypoplasia and decreased platelet lifespan.

In **DIC** a primary disease can usually be identified, thrombocytopenia tends to be mild–moderate, and there may be prolongation of PT, aPTT, and TT, hypofibrinogenemia, increased FDPs, and red cell fragments.

Splenomegaly as a cause of thrombocytopenia is probably rare. If it is due to neoplasia it may be identified by splenic biopsy, but this does not rule out that thrombocytopenia is due to secondary ITP. An increase in the platelet count with prednisone treatment of a non-hematopoietic neoplasm, e.g. hemangiosarcoma, gives putative evidence that ITP is present.

Severe bleeding may result in mild thrombocytopenia. In a series of cats with anti-coagulant rodenticide poisoning, a platelet count as low as $58 \times 10^9/L$ (58 000/μl) was noted. If severe bleeding is associated with mild thrombocytopenia, it is more likely that the low platelet count is a result of, rather than the cause of, the bleeding.

Treatment

Prednisone 2–4 mg/kg PO until platelet count is normal or stable (usually within one week). The dose is slowly tapered after 2 weeks with re-measurement of platelet count.

If there is no response, then strategies used in dogs may be tried, e.g. vincristine 0.02 mg/kg IV, cyclophosphamide 50 mg/m^2 PO alternate days, cyclosporine 5 mg/kg PO bid.

If the cat is acutely weak from blood loss, a **transfusion** should be given (10–20 ml/kg whole blood), especially if the PCV < 15.

Prognosis

Based on a limited number of cases, the prognosis is good.

VITAMIN K ANTAGONIST RODENTICIDES AND DRUGS

> **Classical signs**
> - Spontaneous or excessive internal or external bleeding.

Pathogenesis

Vitamin K is normally obtained from the diet and intestinal flora, and absorbed in the intestinal tract.

Vitamin K is essential for carboxylation of clotting factors II, VII, IX and X. The uncarboxylated clotting factors cannot bind calcium, a necessary step in clot formation.

Vitamin K is converted to inactive vitamin K-epoxide during the carboxylation process.

The enzyme, **epoxide reductase**, converts vitamin K-epoxide back to active vitamin K. This cycle conserves vitamin K and precludes the need for daily intake.

Anti-coagulant rodenticides inhibit epoxide reductase preventing the re-cycling of vitamin K, such that hepatic stores become rapidly depleted, leading to coagulopathy.

There are numerous products classified chemically as **hydroxycoumarins** (e.g. warfarin) and **indandiones** (e.g. diphacinone). Second-generation products are those effective against warfarin-resistant rats and are more potent. Potency is related to degree and duration of enzyme inhibition. The half-life of second-generation products is much longer than warfarin.

Most toxicity data are based on other species or limited data. As rules-of-thumb, single-dose oral LD$_{50}$ for warfarin is 5–50 mg/kg, for diphacinone 15 mg/kg, and for bromadialone and brodifacoum 25 mg/kg. Ten percent of the LD$_{50}$ is a rule-of-thumb to determine the minimum toxic dose. The lack of information is not a big concern since ingestion is rarely observed or quantifiable with cats.

Anti-coagulant rodenticide poisoning may occur from either **ingesting the poison** (primary toxicosis) or **a poisoned rodent** (secondary toxicosis). Secondary toxicosis is unlikely with warfarin, but may occur with second-generation products, and indeed may be the most common cause of anti-coagulant rodenticide poisoning in cats. Secondary toxicosis was suspected as the cause of poisoning in a recent case series.

Cats with cardiomyopathy may be treated with vitamin K antagonists as prophylaxis for thromboembolism.

Clinical signs

Signs appear **2–5 days after exposure**.
- Severity and time to onset of signs depends on amount of poison ingested and the animal.
  - The **higher the dose of poison the earlier and more severe the signs**. For a given amount of poison, **exposure over several days is more toxic** than a single large exposure.
  - Because cats put less physical stress on their tissue compared to dogs, signs tend to appear later in cats after exposure than in dogs.
  - Signs appear earlier and are more severe in very young and old animals.
- The newer generation poisons do not necessarily cause earlier onset of signs.

Signs of **acute anemia** and **hypovolemia** are present. Other non-specific signs include **depression** (which may appear before detectable anemia), non-localizable **pain and fever**.

Localizing signs of hemorrhage include scleral hemorrhages, otic hemorrhages, epistaxis, cough, hemoptysis and dyspnea (pulmonary hemorrhage), inspiratory dyspnea or restrictive breathing (hemothorax), abdominal pain (presumably due to hemorrhage within organs), abdominal distention (hemoabdomen), lameness, muscle pain and stiffness (hemorrhage into muscles), lameness and joint swelling (hemarthrosis), neurologic signs (cerebral hemorrhage), ecchymoses, subcutaneous hematomas and excessive bleeding from wounds.
- Pleural hemorrhage, mediastinal hemorrhage, and subcutaneous hematomas appear to be most common.

- Mucosal surface bleeding (petechiation, melena, hematochezia) may also occur.

Sudden death may occur due to cerebral hemorrhage, hemopericardium, pulmonary or mediastinal hemorrhage, or exsanguination into the pleural or abdominal cavities.

Diagnosis

Anti-coagulant poisoning is less common in cats than dogs because of difference in eating habits.

Feces may be colored (e.g. green) from dye in bait with primary toxicosis.

Measuring hematocrit and total protein may help identify blood loss as a cause of lethargy, bearing in mind that in the first few hours of bleeding these parameters may not change appreciably.

Reticulocytes will appear after 4 days of the onset of hemorrhage, but this is late in the disease process and not usually useful to identify blood loss as a cause of acute anemia.

Radiographs and ultrasound examinations may detect fluid accumulation in organs and body cavities.

Maintaining a high index of suspicion when a cat at risk has appropriate signs will lead to hemostatic testing.
- **PT is the most valuable routine test.**
  - Factor VII has the shortest half-life of the vitamin K dependent factors and is in the extrinsic system. The other vitamin K dependent factors have longer half-lives and are in the intrinsic or common system.
  - PT becomes prolonged before aPTT does, but by the time a cat is presented with clinical bleeding, both **PT and aPTT are usually prolonged**.
  - If PT is not prolonged, then a prolongation of aPTT is not due to vitamin K antagonism.
- Platelet count is normal, or may be mild to moderately decreased if there is marked hemorrhage. BMBT should be normal, but rebleeding may occur.
- Response to vitamin K1 (see Treatment, below).
- **PIVKA time is increased** (see Tests of hemostasis, above). PIVKA time is more sensitive than PT to vitamin K antagonism, but is not necessary to make the diagnosis in the bleeding animal, nor, despite its

name, is it specific for a vitamin K dependent coagulopathy.

- Analytic confirmation of the poison in the blood is possible through some diagnostic laboratories.

Differential diagnosis

Trauma, e.g. by a motor vehicle, can result in similar patterns of hemorrhage and systemic signs. This is differentiated on the basis of evidence of injury (e.g. sheared nails, lacerations, fractured pelvis) and hemostatic testing.

Differential diagnoses for bleeding at a specific site include **local lesions at that site**. These are differentiated on the basis of other signs of these processes and normal hemostatic test results.

Liver and gastrointestinal diseases may result in vitamin K deficiency, but the signs of the primary disease are present (e.g. jaundice, diarrhea) and are usually subacute to chronic.

Fulminant DIC causing overt bleeding is not common in cats, and there will be clinical or laboratory signs of an underlying disease. If in doubt, response to vitamin K therapy rules out DIC.

Hemophilia A, B and C are characterized by a normal PT and prolonged aPTT.

Acute heart failure causes dyspnea and the same systemic signs as acute hypovolemia due to hemorrhage, and nasal and oral cavity blood-tinged liquid may be present. A heart murmur and arrhythmia may be present with both. Pulmonary crackles are more likely to be caused by heart failure. Acute heart failure is more common than anti-coagulant poisoning, and, while radiographic pulmonary changes may be the same, cardiomegaly is usually present with heart failure and the heart may be smaller with hemorrhage. Echocardiography and hemostatic testing will definitively distinguish the two.

Treatment

Post-exposure treatment.

- Induce **vomiting** with xylazine, 0.44 mg/kg IM, or with hydrogen peroxide, 2 ml/kg, or syrup of ipecac, 3–6 ml/kg diluted 1:1 with water, PO or preferably by stomach tube, if ingestion of the poi-

son is witnessed or suspected within several hours prior to consultation. (See Acute poisoning in The Cat With Depression, Anorexia or Dehydration, page 285). Examine vomitus for evidence of bait (some are colored green) or a rodent; consider saving vomitus for toxicologic analysis.

- Administer an **adsorbent and cathartic** by stomach tube if the cat is sufficiently cooperative and:
  - Examination of vomitus confirms ingestion and a toxic dose is suspected.
  - Ingestion is known, induced vomiting did not adequately eliminate poison, and it is less than 12 hours post-ingestion.
  - Ingestion is suspected, it is considered to be too late to induce vomiting, and it is **less than 12 hours post-ingestion**.
    - Give a slurry of activated charcoal, 1.0–5.0 g/kg, preferably using a preparation that includes sorbitol as a cathartic. If activated charcoal without cathartic is used, follow with sodium sulfate, 1/2 level teaspoon per kg in 5–10 volumes of tepid water, by stomach tube. If sorbitol or sodium sulfate is not available, use lactulose, 3 ml/kg PO.
- **Measure PT** at 48 and 72 hours and begin vitamin K1 therapy if PT is prolonged. Obtaining a baseline PT may be helpful to facilitate detection of early changes in PT. A less desirable alternative is to measure baseline ACT and then at 72 and 96 hours, and begin vitamin K1 therapy if ACT is > baseline.
- In some cases it may be less expensive or more convenient (e.g. cat is obstreperous in hospital) to empirically treat with vitamin K1 than to monitor coagulation.

Vitamin K1. The synthetic product is phytonadione which has the same activity as natural phylloquinone.

- The purpose of therapy is to provide a **daily source of vitamin K until the toxin is eliminated** and the vitamin K–vitamin K epoxide cycle can resume. Vitamin K1 is expensive but the small size of the doses makes therapy less expensive in cats compared to most dogs and allows empirical use of higher, longer doses.
- **Improvement in the PT is expected within 8–12 hours and normalization by 24–48 hours**.
- Preferred route is PO as it has the best absorption.
  - The **injectable products may be given orally**. Feed canned food as **fat promotes absorption**.

The daily dose may be given in one or two daily treatments. Some prefer the latter to ensure that the cat ingests at least some vitamin K1 each day.

– If animal is vomiting give SC.
– **Avoid IV injection** because of the risk for anaphylactoid reactions associated with vehicles in the preparation (this risk may be less with some newer formulations). If IV injection is necessary (e.g. severe hematoma formation at injection site), pre-treat with diphenhydramine or tripelenamine, or equivalent anti-histamine, 1 mg/kg IV over 20 minutes (rapid injection causes hypotension), or acepromazine, 0.05–0.1 mg/kg IV. Dilute the vitamin K1 product in 5% dextrose or other approved diluents listed in the product circular, give slowly over 60 minutes, and observe closely for anaphylactoid reactions and urticaria.

• Vitamin K1 dose:
  – **Warfarin, fumarin, pindone, valone** – 1 mg/kg for **1–2 weeks**.
  – **Bromadiolone, diphacinone, chlorophacinone, brodifacoum** – 2.5–5 mg/kg for **3–4 weeks.**
  – **If product is not known** – 2.5–5 mg/kg for **3–4 weeks** (assume secondary poisoning with a second-generation product).
  – Do not give higher doses – response is not better and there may be a risk of causing Heinz body hemolytic anemia.
  – **Measure PT 2, 3 and 5 days after discontinuing treatment**, especially if poison is not known, to ensure treatment was sufficiently long. Alternatively measure ACT at 3, 4 and 6 days.

Provide supplemental **oxygen** using an oxygen tent (do not use a nasal catheter) if the cat is dyspneic or tachypneic.

Transfusion is required for the actively bleeding cat with existing or potential hypovolemic shock or other life-threatening hemorrhage.

• **3–8 hours are required for vitamin K to raise coagulation protein levels.**
• Transfusion is preferred for volume support since fluid therapy will dilute remaining clotting factors and platelets.
  – Fresh whole blood (10–20 ml/kg) is the most practical blood product to use and will replace lost red cells, coagulation factors, and provide volume.
  – Plasma (10–20 ml/kg). The vitamin K dependent factors are stable in plasma so fresh-frozen plasma is not necessary. Packed red cells are then given for red cell replacement.
  – If only stored whole blood is available, this will provide some coagulation factor activity in addition to red cells.

Thoracocentesis should be used to relieve life-threatening pleural blood, and pericardiocentesis to relieve life-threatening cardiac tamponade.

Crystalloid or synthetic colloid **fluid therapy** may be necessary for the animal in shock, but minimum required volumes should be used to minimize dilution of clotting factors and platelets.

Avoid drugs that may enhance toxicosis by altering metabolism of poison. Such drugs commonly used in cats include sulfonamides, metronidazole, fluoroquinolones and cimetidine. Ranitidine and famotidine are safe to use.

Prognosis

Prognosis is excellent with prompt treatment.

Prevention

Prevent exposure to anti-coagulant poisons by proper storage of products and confining cats when products are in use.

For weeks to months after the initial episode, animals are more sensitive to toxicosis upon re-exposure to long-acting rodenticides. This is likely because the poison is still present in the liver and stores of vitamin K have not yet fully recovered.

HEMOPHILIA A (CLASSICAL HEMOPHILIA)

Classical signs

• Excessive internal or external bleeding in young male cats.

Pathogenesis

Hemophilia A is caused by reduced synthesis, release or function of **factor VIII** (anti-hemophilic factor).

- It is a heritable single-gene defect that is X-linked recessive (see Transmission).

Factor VIII is probably synthesized in the liver.

Severity of clinical signs correlates with factor VIII level.
- Bleeding tendency is worst if levels < 1%.
- Bleeding tendency is less if levels are 5–30%.
- Carriers are clinically normal with levels ≈ 50%.

The various individual cases and hemophiliac families reported are probably due to new and different mutations in the large factor VIII gene and subsequent inbreeding. Hemophiliac cats may thus vary in the severity of factor VIII deficiency.

Clinical signs

Clinical signs are usually noted in **cats less than a year of age**, but occasionally the diagnosis is made in an older cat.

Most cases are diagnosed as a result of investigation of **persistent or recurrent bleeding after neutering or declawing.**

History may reveal previous excessive bleeding from wounds, hematomas, lameness (hemarthrosis), and unexplained internal bleeding.

Although umbilical bleeding in neonates and bleeding at the time of teething have not been specifically reported, some family histories have reported fatal bleeding diatheses in related kittens.

Hematomas probably form at subcutaneous vaccination sites but go unnoticed. Vaccination does not trigger bleeding at other sites.

Signs due to anemia and **local effects of hemorrhage** vary with severity of blood loss. Signs are acute to subacute in onset.

Males are affected the most. However, because cats may have minimal signs, males may breed, resulting in affected females (see Transmission).

Diagnosis

Hemophilia A is rare.

Hemostatic testing reveals normal platelet count and BMBT (may rebleed), normal PT, and markedly **pro-**

longed ACT and aPTT (typically aPTT is > 1.5–2 times control value, and aPTT > 40 s where the upper limit of normal range is 25 s).
- **Prolonged aPTT is corrected by adding plasma** (which contains factor VIII), but not serum (which does not contain factor VIII), to the sample. This result allows a presumptive diagnosis of hemophilia A as inherited deficiencies of the other coagulation factors consumed during clotting are not known.

Definitive diagnosis is based on quantification of factor VIII activity (FVIII:C) and ruling out acquired factor VIII deficiency (see Circulating anti-coagulant, below). Measuring factor VIII activity quantifies the ability of the patient's plasma to correct the prolonged aPTT of factor VIII deficient plasma. In hemophiliacs FVIII:C is < 25–30% of normal.

Differential diagnosis

Differential diagnoses for bleeding at a specific site include **local lesions at that site**. These are differentiated on the basis of other signs of injury or inflammation and normal hemostatic test results.

Abnormal bleeding due to a **platelet disorder** is ruled out on the basis of a normal platelet count and BMBT.

Hemophilia B and C are characterized by a prolonged ACT and aPTT that is corrected by adding serum to sample, and by a low factor IX or XI quantification.

Cats with coagulopathy secondary to **liver failure** will have clinical and laboratory signs of liver disease, e.g. subacute to chronic inappetence, jaundice, hepatic encephalopathy, and increased liver enzymes, respectively, and may have a prolonged PT.

Cats with **vitamin K antagonist poisoning** and other vitamin K related disorders have a prolonged PT and will respond to vitamin K therapy.

Fulminant DIC causing overt bleeding is not common in cats, and there will be clinical or laboratory signs of an underlying disease.

Acquired factor VIII deficiency has been reported in humans but not in cats.

Treatment

Transfusion with 10–20 ml/kg **fresh whole blood, fresh plasma**, or **fresh-frozen plasma** (frozen within 8 hours of collection and stored for < 1 year), or 2 units cryoprecipitate.

- By definition, **fresh products are those used within 8 hours of collection**. Factor VIII levels begin to decline after 8 hours of refrigeration, and in humans only 50% of factor VIII activity is present after 24 hours, but in dogs 85% of activity remains. Some factor VIII activity is probably present in both up to two weeks. The stability of feline factor VIII is not known. While ideally fresh blood products should be used, blood or plasma that is more than 8 hours old is still likely be beneficial to a hemophiliac.
- If plasma products are used, 25–70 ml packed red cells may also be needed.
- Transfusion may be used during a bleeding episode or prophylactically before a procedure.
- **Collect sufficient blood samples for hemostatic testing prior to transfusion.**
- A single transfusion may stop active bleeding in a cat if there is no underlying injury or inflammatory disorder.
- Half-life of factor VIII post-transfusion is probably only 8–12 hours, so repetitive transfusions every 12–24 hours may be necessary.
- Cats with absolute factor VIII deficiency may theoretically become refractory to transfused factor VIII because of antibody formation.

Treatment with vitamin K1 is of no benefit, except as a diagnostic test to rule out vitamin K antagonist poisoning.

Treatments in dogs and/or humans not evaluated in cats include desmopressin, lyophilized factor VIII, recombinant human factor VIII, recombinant factor VIIa, inhibitors of fibrinolysis (e.g. aminocaproic acid), liver transplantation, and gene therapy.

Prognosis

In most cases **spontaneous bleeding is minimal** or mild.

Prognosis is good for **cats kept in an environment that minimizes trauma and exuberant exercise**.

Bleeding tendency appears to be less in mature cats compared to juveniles. An explanation for this may be factor VIII levels increasing with age, as has been seen in normal cats.

Transmission

Factor VIII deficiency is a heritable single-gene defect that is **X-linked recessive**.

Based on classical mendelian inheritance, where "X" and "Y" are sex-chromosomes, "H" is the normal factor VIII gene, "h" is the abnormal factor VIII gene, and approximately half the litter are males and half females:

- Breeding an unaffected male (X^H,Y) to a normal female (X^H,X^H), will result in all normal males and all normal females, i.e. none in litter are bleeders. This is, of course, the normal situation.
- Breeding an unaffected male (X^H,Y) to a carrier female (X^H,X^h), will result in 50% of the males in the litter being affected, and 50% of the females being carriers, i.e. approximately 25% of the litter (all males) are bleeders. This is the most likely natural scenario in the random appearance of hemophilia.
- Breeding an unaffected male (X^H,Y) to an affected female (X^h,X^h), will result in all males being affected and all females being carriers, i.e. approximately 50% of litter are bleeders (all males).
- Breeding an affected male (X^h,Y) to a normal female (X^H,X^H), will result in all males being normal and all females being carries, i.e. none in litter are bleeders.
- Breeding an affected male (X^h,Y) to a carrier female (X^H,X^h), will result in 50% of the males being affected, and 50% of the females being affected females, i.e. 50% of litter are bleeders (half male, half female).
- Breeding affected male (X^h,Y) to an affected female (X^h,X^h), will result in all males being affected and 50% all females being affected, i.e. 75% in litter are bleeders (all male, half female). This is the least likely naturally occurring situation.

Prevention

Parents and littermates may be tested for factor VIII:C to identify affected cats (males and homozygous females) and carriers (heterozygous females).

- Normal cats have normal factor VIII:C levels.
- In most species, **carrier females have ≈ 40–60% normal factor VIII:C**, but the upper range may overlap with the lower range of normal. One confirmed carrier had a factor VIII:C of 69%. Breeding

studies are the only way to identify carriers with low normal factor VIII:C.

- Clinically **affected cats have < 25–30% factor VIII:C**.

A breeder should be advised not to breed affected and carrier/suspected carrier cats. One strategy would be to only breed cats with factor VIII:C ≥ 100%.

For clients who are not breeders, or if factor VIII testing of related cats is cost-prohibitive, neuter and spay all related cats. Measure ACT first to identify affected cats that will require transfusion prior to surgery.

HEMOPHILIA B (CHRISTMAS DISEASE)

> ### Classical signs
>
> - Spontaneous or excessive internal or external bleeding in young male cats.

Pathogenesis

Hemophilia B is caused by reduced synthesis, release or function of **factor IX** (Christmas factor).

- It is a **heritable single-gene defect** that is **X-linked recessive**. Newly arising cases probably represent new mutations.

Factor IX is produced by vitamin K dependent synthesis in the liver.

Severity of clinical signs correlate with factor IX level similar to hemophilia A.

- Most affected cats have levels < 10%.
- Carriers typically have levels ≈ 40–60%.
  - Carriers may have up to ≈ 80% normal levels, perhaps because factor IX levels increase with stress.

Clinical signs

Clinical signs are usually noted in **cats less than a year of age**, but occasionally the diagnosis is made in an older cat.

Signs of **spontaneous bleeding** are mild to moderate. Signs include **hemothorax** and **hemoabdomen, shifting lameness due to hemarthrosis, subcutaneous swellings, bruises, gingival bleeding**.

Excessive bleeding following injury or procedures, e.g. neutering, declawing, venepuncture.

Family history may reveal fatal bleeding diathesis/unexplained death in related kittens.

Other than bleeding tendencies being more severe, signs are otherwise identical to hemophilia A.

Males are affected the most. Because **signs are more apparent than in hemophilia A**, males are less likely to breed and produce affected female offspring (see Transmission).

Diagnosis

Hemophilia B is rare.

Hemostatic testing reveals normal platelet count and BMBT (may rebleed), normal PT, and markedly **prolonged ACT and aPTT**.

- In contrast to hemophilia A, **prolonged aPTT in hemophilia B is corrected by adding serum** (which contains factor IX but not factor VIII) to the sample. Prolonged aPTT in both hemophilia A and B is corrected by adding plasma. This result is consistent with a deficiency of any of the non-consumable clotting factors, and its main value is to rule out hemophilia A.

Definitive diagnosis is based on quantification of factor IX activity (FIX:C), similar to hemophilia A, and ruling out acquired factor VIII deficiency (see Circulating anti-coagulant, below).

Differential diagnosis

Differential diagnoses and differentiation for bleeding for hemophilia B are similar to those for hemophilia A.

- **Acquired factor IX deficiency** has been reported in humans but not in cats.

Comparing hemophilia B to hemophilia A, with the former:

- Spontaneous bleeding is more common.
- Prolonged ACT and aPTT are corrected by adding serum to sample.

Treatment

Transfusion with 10–20 ml/kg fresh or stored whole blood, fresh, fresh-frozen, refrigerated, or frozen plasma. Factor IX is stable during normal refrigeration time for red cell banking (up to 35 days) and in frozen plasma. If plasma products are used, 1–2 units of packed red cells may also be needed.

- **Collect sufficient blood samples for hemostatic testing prior to transfusion**.
- A single transfusion may stop active bleeding in a cat if there is no underlying injury or inflammatory disorder.
- **Half-life of factor IX post-transfusion is probably only 24 hours**, so repetitive transfusions every 24–48 hours may be necessary.
- Cats with absolute factor IX deficiency may theoretically become refractory to transfused factor IX because of antibody formation.

Treatments in dogs and/or humans not evaluated in cats include lyophilized factor IX, recombinant factor VIIa, inhibitors of fibrinolysis (e.g. aminocaproic acid), and gene therapy.

Prognosis

Prognosis is good for cats kept in an environment that minimizes trauma and exuberant exercise, but bleeding episodes requiring transfusion are likely to occur.

Transmission

Factor IX deficiency is a heritable single-gene defect that is **X-linked recessive**. See Hemophilia A for inheritance patterns.

Prevention

As for hemophilia A, but testing for factor IX.

HEMOPHILIA C

Classical signs

- Excessive bleeding in a young cat (single case).

Pathogenesis

Hemophilia C is caused by reduced synthesis, release or function of **factor XI** (plasma thromboplastin antecedent).

Congenital hemophilia C has recently been described in a young female cat.

Clinical signs

Excessive bleeding following injury or procedures, in this case neutering and declawing.

Diagnosis

Hemophilia C is rare.

Hemostatic testing reveals normal platelet count and BMBT (may rebleed), normal PT, and markedly **prolonged ACT and aPTT**.

- In contrast to hemophilia A, as with hemophilia B, **prolonged aPTT in hemophilia C is corrected by adding serum** (which contains factor XI but not factor VIII) to the sample. Prolonged aPTT in hemophilia A, B and C is corrected by adding plasma. This result is consistent with a deficiency of any of the non-consumable clotting factors, and its main value is to rule out hemophilia A.

Definitive diagnosis is based on quantification of factor IX activity (FXI:C), similar to hemophilia A, and ruling out acquired factor XI deficiency (see Circulating anticoagulant, below).

Differential diagnosis

Differential diagnoses and differentiation for bleeding for hemophilia C are similar to those for hemophilia A.

Acquired factor XI deficiency in a cat has been reported.

Treatment

Transfusion with 10–20 ml/kg fresh or stored whole blood, fresh, fresh-frozen, refrigerated, or frozen plasma should be considered if there is critical hemorrhage. Factor XI is stable during normal refrigeration time for red cell banking (up to 35 days) and in frozen plasma. If plasma products are used, 1–2 units of packed red cells may also be needed.

- **Collect sufficient blood samples for hemostatic testing prior to transfusion.**
- In the case reported, transfusion was not necessary.

- **Half-life of factor XI post-transfusion is probably longer (2–3 days) than factor VIII or IX.**
- Cats with absolute factor XI deficiency may theoretically become refractory to transfused factor IX because of antibody formation.

Treatments in humans not evaluated in cats include lyophilized factor XI, recombinant factor VIIa, and inhibitors of fibrinolysis (e.g. aminocaproic acid).

Prognosis

Prognosis is probably good for cats kept in an environment that minimizes trauma and exuberant exercise.

Transmission

Transmission in cats is unknown. In humans, dogs and cattle transmission is autosomal recessive.

Prevention

As for hemophilia A, but testing for factor XI.

VITAMIN-K RESPONSIVE COAGULOPATHY IN THE DEVON REX

Classical signs

- Spontaneous and excessive bleeding in Devon Rex cats.

Pathogenesis

Vitamin K is essential for carboxylation of clotting factors II, VII, IX and X. The uncarboxylated clotting factors cannot bind calcium, a necessary step in clot formation (see Vitamin K antagonist rodenticides and drugs).

The enzyme responsible for carboxylation has reduced affinity for vitamin K, impairing its function.

Clinical signs

Spontaneous bleeding in Devon Rex cats including hemothorax, intrapulmonary hemorrhage, hemarthrosis and otic hemorrhages. Reported cases range from 5 months to 2 almost years.

Excessive bleeding after venepuncture, neutering and other surgical procedures.

For cases with a defect not sufficiently severe to cause spontaneous hemorrhage, the age of detection will depend on the age when a procedure is performed. Most cats are neutered at a young age, resulting in detection of the defect at that time.

Signs due to anemia and local effects of hemorrhage vary with severity of blood loss.

Some affected cats may not show spontaneous or excessive bleeding, also consistent with **variable severity of the defect.**

In one case a bleeding episode was suspected to have been triggered by concurrent decreased platelet function associated with modified-live virus vaccination.

Diagnosis

Consistent signalment (young Devon Rex cats) and signs of spontaneous or excessive bleeding are highly suggestive.

No evidence of other vitamin K related disorders.
- No history of exposure to vitamin K antagonist poisons.
- No clinical or laboratory evidence of liver disease.
- No diarrhea (exocrine pancreatic insufficiency and inflammatory bowel disease).

Hemostatic testing reveals normal platelet count and BMBT (may rebleed), and **prolonged PT, ACT and aPTT**. PIVKA time has not been reported but is presumably prolonged.

Quantification of vitamin K dependent factor activities, using techniques similar to factor VIII quantification in hemophilia A.

Normalization of PT, ACT, aPTT and factor activities **with vitamin K therapy**.

Differential diagnosis

Vitamin K antagonist rodenticide poisoning may be ruled out in some cases on lack of exposure history.
- **If exposure is possible**, then the cat should be confined in a rodenticide-free environment and **treated with vitamin K for 6 weeks**. After stopping

vitamin K therapy, PT ± aPTT should be monitored. Clotting times will become abnormal again with the genetic defect but remain normal if the cat had been poisoned.

- **Toxicological analysis of blood** can be used to identify presence of a rodenticide.

Other toxins and drugs significantly impairing vitamin K function are rare and may be ruled out by history and improvement with drug withdrawal.

Cats with **coagulopathy secondary to liver failure** will have clinical and laboratory signs of liver disease, e.g. subacute to chronic inappetence, jaundice, hepatic encephalopathy, and increased liver enzymes, respectively.

Exocrine pancreatic insufficiency and inflammatory bowel disease severe enough to cause vitamin K deficiency also cause **diarrhea**.

Differential diagnoses for bleeding at a specific site include **injury or inflammation** at that site. These are differentiated on the basis of other signs of injury or inflammation and normal hemostatic test results.

Abnormal bleeding due to a **platelet disorder** is ruled out on the basis of a normal platelet count and BMBT.

Thrombocytopenia is often present in **DIC**, in addition to signs of a severe illness causing DIC.

Treatment

Vitamin K1 at an initial dose of 5 mg/day PO, and then tapered to a minimum dose required to keep PT normal.

Cats with life-threatening bleeding may require **transfusion** (see Vitamin K antagonist rodenticides and drugs).

- Caution: There is a **high-prevalence of type B blood type** in this breed. Be sure to blood-type or cross-match donor and recipient prior to transfusion.

Prognosis

Excellent with vitamin K1 therapy.

Transmission

Mode of inheritance is not known, but defect is likely to be autosomal.

Prevention

Recommendations are tentative.

Measure PT in parents and littermates to identify affected cats.

- If PT testing is cost-prohibitive, **ACT should be useful for initial screening** (prolonged test result identifying affected cats); but if ACT is normal, PT should be performed.

Do not breed affected cats. Treat with vitamin K and neuter.

Consider not breeding related unaffected cats, in case defect is autosomal recessive.

EXOCRINE PANCREATIC INSUFFICIENCY (EPI)

> ### Classical signs
> - Chronic diarrhea, weight loss, polyphagia.
> - Excessive bleeding may occur.
> - Rare in cats.

Pathogenesis

Dietary triglycerides are normally **digested by pancreatic lipase to monoglycerides and fatty acids**.

This process is needed for solubilization and **subsequent absorption of fat-soluble vitamins**, including vitamin K.

In EPI, **lipase deficiency** can therefore result in **vitamin K deficiency**.

Vitamin K deficiency leads to coagulopathy due to deficiencies of factors II, VII, IX and X (see Vitamin K antagonist rodenticides and drugs).

Vitamin K **deficiency is usually mild** since there is not complete absence of intestinal lipolysis.

Clinical signs

Chronic diarrhea, weight loss, normal to increased appetite (see The Cat With Signs of Chronic Small Bowel Diarrhea, page 751).

Greasy soiling of the haircoat (especially perianal) may occur.

Clinical bleeding is rare and is most likely to be excessive, e.g. following venepuncture, rather than spontaneous.

Prevalence of subclinical clotting factor deficiency is not known.

Diagnosis

See The Cat With Signs of Chronic Small Bowel Diarrhea (page 752) for diagnosis of EPI.

Hemostatic testing in the bleeding cat reveals **normal platelet count and BMBT** (may rebleed), and **prolonged PT, ACT and aPTT**.

Cats with EPI and clinically normal hemostasis may have high normal range values or mild prolongation of PT, ACT and aPTT. A sub-clinical effect may be better documented by measuring **elevated PIVKA** time and quantification of factor VII using a technique similar to factor VIII quantification in hemophilia A.

Differential diagnosis

Differential diagnoses for a cat with chronic diarrhea and coagulopathy include:
- **Inflammatory bowel disease.** This is differentiated from EPI by normal trypsin-like immunoreactivity and intestinal biopsy showing inflammation.
- **Primary intestinal disease** and secondary **cholangiohepatitis** or **hepatic lipidosis**. These are identified by routine laboratory work-up and biopsy. Appetite is usually reduced with liver disease.
- **Feline leukemia virus** and **feline immunodeficiency virus** infections. Both viral diseases may be associated with chronic diarrhea, but appetite is usually reduced. Coagulopathies may occur with retroviral infections, but are usually subclinical. Both viruses may cause thrombocytopenia.
- Unrelated causes of diarrhea and abnormal bleeding.

Treatment

See The Cat With Signs of Chronic Small Bowel Diarrhea (page 752) for treatment of EPI.

Cats with EPI and clinical or laboratory evidence of coagulopathy should be given **vitamin K1**, 5 mg/kg SC daily until normalization of PT. The need for further treatment will depend on response to vitamin K1 treat-

ment and improvement of diarrhea with pancreatic enzyme supplementation.

Concurrent supplementation with vitamin E (tocopherol) may increase vitamin K1 requirements.

Avoid unnecessary antibiotic therapy that may **reduce intestinal bacterial production of vitamin K2**.
- Antibiotic treatment may be necessary to treat small intestinal bacterial overgrowth.

Prognosis

The prognosis for normalization of hemostasis is excellent.

INFLAMMATORY BOWEL DISEASE (IBD)

Classical signs

- Chronic diarrhea, weight loss, variable appetite.
- Spontaneous or excessive bleeding may occur (uncommon).

See main reference, The Cat With Signs of Chronic Small Bowel Diarrhea (page 769) for treatment of IBD.

Pathogenesis

Vitamin K deficiency leads to coagulopathy due to deficiencies of factors II, VII, IX and X (see Vitamin K antagonist rodenticides and drugs).

Vitamin K1 is the main source of vitamin K for mammals.
- It is obtained from the diet (phylloquinone) and absorbed in the proximal small intestine.
- **Severe intestinal malabsorption** may result in **vitamin K1 deficiency**.
- The main causes of **malabsorption** in cats are **IBD, hyperthyroidism and intestinal lymphoma** Vitamin K deficiency has been documented with IBD, and is probably responsible for some of the increased PIVKA times seen occasionally in hyperthyroidism, but has not been investigated in lymphoma.

Vitamin K2 (menaquinone) is also an **important source of vitamin K for mammals**.

- It is produced by **intestinal bacteria** (especially *Escherichia coli* and *Bacteroides* spp.) and absorbed in the ileum and colon.
- If IBD affects predominantly the proximal small intestine, bacterial synthesis provides sufficient vitamin K2 to prevent coagulopathy.

Clinical signs

Chronic diarrhea, chronic intermittent vomiting, weight loss, appetite varying from episodic inappetence to polyphagia (see The Cat With Signs of Chronic Small Bowel Diarrhea, page 768).

Clinical bleeding is uncommon but spontaneous bleeding diathesis has occurred.

Based on prolonged PIVKA time**, prevalence of sub-clinical factor deficiency in severe IBD is approximately 30%.**

Diagnosis

Hemostatic testing in a bleeding cat reveals **normal platelet count and BMBT** (may rebleed), and prolonged PT, ACT and aPTT.

Cats with IBD and clinically normal hemostasis may have high normal range values or mild prolongation of PT, ACT and aPTT. A sub-clinical effect may be better documented by measuring **elevated PIVKA time** and quantification of factor VII using a technique similar to factor VIII quantification in hemophilia A.

Differential diagnosis

As for exocrine pancreatic insufficiency.

Treatment

Cats with IBD and clinical or laboratory evidence of coagulopathy should be given **vitamin K1**, 5 mg/kg SC daily until normalization of PT. The need for further treatment will depend on response to vitamin K1 treatment and improvement of diarrhea with corticosteroid therapy and dietary manipulations.

If intestinal malabsorption is not adequately controlled and ongoing vitamin K supplementation is needed, oral supplementation with vitamin K1 may be tried.

- Concurrent use of **medium-chain triglyceride** supplementation, 1–2 ml/kg/day PO will **promote vitamin K absorption** and promote weight gain, but the product is **unpalatable**.
- If oral vitamin K1 therapy is unsuccessful, vitamin K3 therapy may be considered. Vitamin K3 is a synthetic vitamin K that is less fat-soluble and is **absorbed in the colon**. Unfortunately it causes a **dose-dependent Heinz-body hemolytic anemia** and **methemoglobinemia**, and a safe but effective dose in the cat has not been determined.

Avoid unnecessary antibiotic therapy that may reduce intestinal bacterial production of vitamin K2.

Prognosis

The prognosis for normalization of hemostasis is excellent but ongoing vitamin K1 therapy may be needed until the underlying disorder is resolved.

PANCREATITIS

> **Classical signs**
> - Depression and anorexia.

See main reference on page 272 (The Cat With Depression, Anorexia or Dehydration).

Clinical signs

The most common signs are non-specific.

Hypothermia, vomiting, abdominal pain and occasionally a palpable cranial abdominal mass may be present.

Icterus may be present from concurrent liver disease or extra-hepatic bile duct obstruction.

Hemostatic abnormalities may be present due to DIC of varying severity or due to concurrent liver disease.
- Hemostatic abnormalities are usually subclinical. Clinical bleeding is unlikely unless there is severe DIC or concurrent liver disease.

Cats with concurrent liver disease and pancreatitis are more likely to have hemostatic defects and clinical bleeding than with either disease on its own.

Diagnosis

See The Cat With Depression, Anorexia or Dehydration (page 273).

Hemostatic testing may reveal evidence of DIC (e.g. thrombocytopenia, prolongation of clotting times), evidence of **vitamin K deficiency** (prolonged PT and PIVKA time), and/or evidence of other hemostatic disorders associated with concurrent liver disease (see Liver disease, above).

Differential diagnosis

See The Cat With Depression, Anorexia or Dehydration (page 275). Pancreatitis is difficult to definitively diagnose without biopsy. Many diseases in the cat cause non-specific signs and sub-clinical hemostatic defects. Systematic elimination of diseases by work-up helps narrow the list of differential diagnoses.

Treatment

See The Cat With Depression, Anorexia or Dehydration (page 277).

If there is clinical bleeding, treat with vitamin K as for liver diseases and transfusions as for DIC.

STRANGULATION

Classical signs
- Scleral hemorrhage.

Clinical signs

Non-fatal strangulation may result in scleral edema and hemorrhage, and neurologic signs. Pulmonary edema has also been seen in dogs.

Diagnosis

History is diagnostic. Usually the collar or leash is caught in a tree.

Skin lesions around neck.

Hemostatic testing is normal.

CUTANEOUS ASTHENIA (EHLERS–DANLOS SYNDROME)

Classical signs
- Excessive wounding since birth.
- Subcutaneous hematomas or seromas.

Clinical signs

Signs are present from birth, but may worsen with age.

Skin is hyperextensive and wounds easily with minor trauma, and may feel softer. Scars from previous wounds may be present. Signs result from abnormal collagen synthesis, and will vary in degree with the specific genetic defect.
- The chief complaint may be **bleeding from the skin, but bleeding is appropriate for the wound**.
- Bleeding into the skin without a wound (petechiation, ecchymoses) is not characteristic of the diseases described to date in cats.
- **Subcutaneous hematomas and seromas may occur** because blood and lymphatic vessels are fragile or are injured when the skin stretches.

Concurrent signs include **joint laxity, lens luxation and cataracts**.

Reported in domestic shorthaired, domestic longhaired, Himalayan and Burmese cats.

Diagnosis

Clinical signs are highly suggestive.

Skin extensibility index (SEI) > 19%. SEI = height of fold/body length × 100, where, with the cat standing, a fold of lumbosacral skin is pulled upwards and the height from the top of the spine to the top of the fold is measured, and body length is measured from the occipital crest to the base of the tail.

Skin biopsy for histopathology and/or electron microscopy of skin to document collagen abnormalities, special biochemical analyses, and measurement of tensile strength.

Hemostatic testing is normal.

HYPERADRENOCORTICISM

Classical signs

- Polyuria, polydipsia, polyphagia.
- Abdominal distention, alopecia, fragile skin.

Clinical signs

Polyuria, polydipsia and polyphagia commonly occur because of insulin-resistant diabetes mellitus.

Abdominal distention commonly occurs because of muscle wasting and hepatomegaly.

Cutaneous signs include **patchy alopecia** (most common), symmetrical alopecia and fragile skin.

Fragile skin may bleed when it is torn, but bleeding is typically slight.

Cats, unlike dogs, do not appear to bleed more easily from venepuncture sites.

Diagnosis

See The Cat With Polyuria and Polydipsia (page 251).

Hemostatic testing is normal.

CHEDIAK–HIGASHI SYNDROME

Classical signs

- Persian cats with congenitally dilute smoke-blue hair coat.

Clinical signs

Signs are present from birth and are associated with an autosomal recessive defect.

Affected **Persian cats** have a **dilute smoke-blue hair** coat and yellow-green irises.

Ophthalmologic evaluation reveals epiphora and blepharospasm in bright light and a red fundus.

Prolonged bleeding occurs at venepuncture sites, surgical sites and following minor and major trauma,

because of a **platelet function defect**. Spontaneous bleeding and bleeding diathesis do not occur.

Diagnosis

Clinical signs.

Routine blood smear reveals large pink cytoplasmic inclusions in granulocytes and larger than normal eosinophil granules.

Hemostatic testing reveals prolonged BMBT (9.33 → 20 min) and decreased platelet aggregation.

IDIOPATHIC THROMBOCYTOPATHIA

Classical signs

- Spontaneous epistaxis and gingival bleeding.

Clinical signs

Bleeding results from an **abnormality in platelet function affecting aggregation**.

Presumed to be a congenital defect since signs are apparent at a young age.

Recurrent epistaxis and gingival bleeding have been seen.

Diagnosis

Clinical signs.

Hemostatic testing reveals normal platelet count and prolonged BMBT.

Abnormal platelet aggregation in vitro.

ANTIPLATELET CARDIAC DRUGS

Classical signs

- None.

Clinical signs

β-blockers and calcium-channel blockers inconsistently inhibit platelet aggregation in vivo.

Acepromazine, at one time extensively used in the management of arterial thromboembolism, inhibits platelet aggregation in humans, but does not in dogs and presumably has minimal effect in cats.

Aspirin, n-3 fatty acids, and cyproheptadine variably inhibit platelet aggregation in vitro but have a minimal effect on BMBT when used as single agents.

- These drugs have been given to cats in an attempt to prevent arterial thromboembolism due to cardiomyopathy.
  - Newer classes of **antithrombotic drugs** in humans **inhibit platelet aggregation** by preventing binding of fibrinogen or ADP to specific platelet receptors. These drugs have been shown to impair platelet function in normal cats. Clopidogrel currently shows the most promise for clinical use.

The effect of the older drugs on bleeding in cats with a bleeding disorder is not known, but is unlikely to be marked in most circumstances. Aspirin should probably be avoided in cats with a moderate to marked hemostatic disorder. The effect of the newer platelet receptor blocking drugs on bleeding in cats with a bleeding disorder is not known, but these drugs should likewise probably be avoided in cats with a moderate to marked hemostatic disorder.

Diagnosis

History of drug therapy.

If a cat receiving one of these drugs has abnormal bleeding, another cause of the bleeding should be ruled out.

SPLENOMEGALY

Classical signs

- Enlarged spleen on abdominal palpation.
- Signs of a primary disease.

Clinical signs

Mild to markedly **enlarged spleen on abdominal palpation**.

Other signs of a primary disease causing splenomegaly may be present. Diseases include bacterial, fungal and protozoal infections, non-infectious inflammation and immune-stimulation, and neoplastic infiltration. Splenomegaly may also result from portal hypertension and extra-medullary hematopoiesis. Most causes of lymphadenopathy may also cause splenomegaly (see The Cat With Enlarged Lymph Nodes, page 393).

The most common cause of marked splenomegaly is **neoplasia, especially mast cell tumor and lymphoma**.

Although the spleen of the cat is non-sinusoidal, **splenic sequestration of platelets does normally occur**. Splenomegaly could potentially contribute to thrombocytopenia, but it does not appear to be an important mechanism and a bleeding tendency is unlikely.

Diagnosis

Routine work-up to identify primary disease.

Aspiration or surgical biopsy of spleen.

Hemostatic testing may reveal **thrombocytopenia** and coagulopathy (e.g. DIC) secondary to the primary disease.

VON WILLEBRAND'S DISEASE

Classical signs

- Not known (rare disease).

Clinical signs

There is a report of a 9-year-old male neutered cat with persistent oral bleeding after tooth extraction.

In dogs the most common signs are those of excessive or prolonged bleeding following injury.

Diagnosis

Hemostatic tests reveal **prolonged BMBT**, normal to slightly prolonged ACT and aPTT, and decreased von Willebrand's factor (vWf:Ag).

FACTOR X DEFICIENCY

Classical signs

- Not known (rare disease).

Clinical signs

There is a report of a cat with **mild excessive bleeding after declawing** and **seizures** attributed to intracranial hemorrhage at 3 years of age.

The defect appeared to be inherited. The mother and one sibling were subclinically affected.

Diagnosis

Hemostatic tests reveal normal platelet count and BMBT, markedly prolonged PT, ACT, and aPTT and normal TT.

Russell's viper venom time (RVVT) is prolonged.

Factor X:C is decreased.

Rule out acquired factor X deficiency (reported in humans but not cats). See Circulating anti-coagulant, below.

CIRCULATING ANTI-COAGULANT

Classical signs

- Not known (rare disease).

Clinical signs

Primary or secondary autoimmune diseases may be associated with **acquired circulating anti-coagulants (inhibitors)**, e.g. the lupus anti-coagulant in systemic lupus erythematosus. The anti-coagulant may result in spontaneous or excessive bleeding. Paradoxically, animals and humans with lupus anti-coagulants are **also at risk for thrombosis**.

Inhibitors to most coagulation factors have been reported in humans. There is a report of a 5-year-old cat with persistent **epistaxis** due **to inhibition of factor XI** (plasma thromboplastin antecedent) causing a prolonged aPTT.

Diagnosis

Hemostatic test results will vary with the coagulation factor inhibited and platelet abnormalities.

A circulating inhibitor is demonstrated by mixing equal volumes of patient and normal plasma. If the prolonged coagulation time in the patient plasma is normalized, then it was due to a factor deficiency. (This test works because PT and aPTT do not become prolonged until there is < 25% function, so the normal plasma adds sufficient factors to the deficient plasma to normalize the test). If the **prolonged coagulation time** in the patient plasma is **not normalized** (i.e. the patient plasma prolongs coagulation time in normal plasma), then an inhibitor is present.

- If an inhibitor is demonstrated, more specific mixing studies may be performed using specific factor C assays to identify the specific factor inhibitor.

ANTI-COAGULANTS

Classical signs

- Spontaneous bleeding with excessive anticoagulation.

Clinical signs

Heparin, low-molecular-weight heparin and warfarin may be used as prophylaxis against thromboembolism in cats with cardiomyopathy (see The Cat With Signs of Heart Disease, page 130).

Heparin may be used in the treatment of pulmonary thromboembolism and DIC (see above).

There is a **narrow therapeutic margin** between effective and excessive anti-coagulant therapy. Excessive therapy will result in spontaneous hemorrhage.

Diagnosis

History of anti-coagulant therapy.

Prolongation of ACT, aPTT, PT, PIVKA time and TT with heparin and warfarin therapy. The ACT, aPTT and TT are usually used to monitor heparin therapy, while PIVKA time and PT are used to monitor warfarin therapy. Routine coagulation tests are not affected by low-molecular-weight heparin, where plasma anti-factor Xa activity is used to monitor therapy.

VITAMIN K DEFICIENT DIET

Classical signs

- Spontaneous bleeding with certain fish diets.

Clinical signs

The cat has a **relatively low dietary vitamin K requirement** and it is difficult to experimentally induce vitamin K deficiency.

Some commercial fish-based diets caused a vitamin K responsive bleeding diathesis during feeding trials, possibly due to an anti-vitamin K factor in the diet.

Diagnosis

The main cause of vitamin K deficiency is anorexia.

If no other explanation exists to account for a vitamin K responsive coagulopathy, diet should be investigated.

ANTI-CONVULSANTS

Classical signs

- None (with respect to bleeding).

Clinical signs

Phenobarbital and diphenylhydantoin (rarely used in cats) cause **mild reduction in hepatic synthesis of vitamin K dependent clotting factors**. This is only a problem in a cat with another vitamin K related disorder.

Diagnosis

Sub-clinical effect may be **documented by PIVKA** time and/or quantification of vitamin K dependent factor activities using techniques similar to factor VIII quantification in hemophilia A. If a clinical effect

occurs, hemostatic tests reveal prolonged PT ± prolonged ACT and aPTT.

ANTIBIOTICS

Classical signs

- Abnormal bleeding associated with antibiotic therapy.

Clinical signs

Penicillins and some cephalosporins variably impair platelet function in humans, rabbits and dogs, and may exacerbate thrombocypenic bleeding. This is most important in humans with penicillins, when the platelet count is $< 20 \times 10^9$/L (200,000/μl) or in the presence of other hemostatic defects. Amoxicillin, cefalexin, and cefazolin at standard doses do not impair platelet function in normal dogs and are unlikely to have any clinically relevant hemostatic effects in cats.

Other antibiotics that alter platelet aggregation *in vitro* in humans, rabbits or dogs include **tetracyclines, gentamicin and sulfonamides**. The clinical effect, if any, is less important than with the penicillins. Fluoroquinolones do not appear to impair platelet function. Doxycyline and enrofloxacin at standard doses do not impair platelet function. Doxycycline and enrofloxacin at standard doses do not impair platelet function in normal dogs. These antibiotics are unlikely to have any clinically relevant hemostatic effects in cats.

An idiosyncratic drug reaction may result in thrombocytopenia and platelet-type bleeding.

Antibiotic therapy may reduce bacterial synthesis of **vitamin K2** (menaquinone) by killing intestinal bacteria (especially *Escherichia coli* and *Bacteroides* spp.). Numerous antibiotics have been implicated in humans. This is not usually a concern in the animal with otherwise normal hemostasis, but may promote coagulopathy in animals at risk for vitamin K deficiency.

Moxalactam, cefamandole and cefoperazone may directly **impair vitamin K dependent factor** synthesis. These antibiotics are infrequently used in cats.

Sulfonamides, metronidazole and possibly fluoro-quinolones may **exacerbate vitamim K antagonist rodenticide poisoning**.

Actinomycin D, an anti-tumor antibiotic, may be a vitamin K antagonist, but the clinical relevance of this in cats is not known.

Diagnosis

Abnormal bleeding associated with antibiotic therapy and improvement upon withdrawing therapy.

If vitamin K deficiency or antagonism is causing bleeding, hemostatic testing reveals prolonged PT ± prolonged ACT and aPTT, and improvement in coagulopathy with vitamin K1 injection (assuming normal liver function).
- Sub-clinical effect may be documented by PIVKA time and quantification of vitamin K dependent factor activities using techniques similar to factor VIII quantification in hemophilia A.

ANTI-THYROID DRUGS

> ### Classical signs
>
> - Epistaxis, oral hemorrhages.
> - Prolonged bleeding following procedures.

Clinical signs

Spontaneous bleeding (e.g. epistaxis, oral hemorrhages, melena) and excessive bleeding (e.g. following venepuncture or surgery) due to **anti-thyroid drugs** (propylthiouracil, methimazole, carbimazole) is usually due to **thrombocytopenia** caused by **peripheral destruction or megakaryocytic hypoplasia**.

Methimazole and carbimazole may interfere with **activation of the vitamin K-dependent clotting** factors II, VII, IX and X. This effect in cats is minimal – PIVKA time may be increased, but an increase in PT is unlikely.

Diagnosis

Increased PIVKA time compared to baseline in a hyperthyroid cat being treated with an anti-thyroid drug.

Presumably quantification of vitamin K dependent factor activities could also demonstrate a deficiency.

NON-STEROIDAL ANTI-INFLAMMATORY DRUGS

> ### Classical signs
>
> - None (with respect to bleeding).

Clinical signs

Non-steroidal anti-inflammatory drugs (NSAIDs) are being prescribed with increasing frequency for analgesia in cats.

Similar to aspirin, non-selective NSAIDs impair platelet function by inhibition of cyclooxygenase-1. This may result in prolonged bleeding times and increased surgical hemorrhage in humans and dogs. The effect on bleeding time in cats has not been well investigated, but, given that aspirin has minimal effects on BMBT in the cat, NSAIDs are also **likely to have minimal effects.**

Diagnosis

History of drug therapy.

If a cat receiving one of these drugs has abnormal bleeding, another cause of the bleeding should be ruled out.

MISCELLANEOUS DRUGS

> ### Classical signs
>
> - None (with respect to bleeding).

Clinical signs

Numerous drugs inhibit platelet aggregation in various species in vitro. These include:
- Anesthetic and sedative agents: acepromazine, diazepam, ketamine, propofol and halothane, but not barbiturates or isoflurane. Acepromazine and propofol do not inhibit platelet function in normal dogs.

- Anti-histamines: H1 and H2 blockers. H2 blockers are frequently given to thrombocytopenic animals with gastrointestinal hemorrhage because ulceration cannot be ruled out. Famotidine has less of an effect on platelets than either cimetidine or ranitidine. Sulcralfate will provide local gastrointestinal protection without any effect on platelets.
- The effect of these drugs on platelet function in cats is not known, but they are unlikely to have any clinically relevant hemostatic effects.

- Disturbances of platelet aggregation in vitro may not have any clinical relevance in vivo.

Diagnosis

History of drug therapy.

If a cat receiving one of these drugs has abnormal bleeding, another cause of the bleeding should be ruled out.

RECOMMENDED READING

Bay JD, Scott MA, Hans JE. Reference values for activated coagulation time in cats. Am J Vet Res 2000; 63: 750–753.

Day M, Mackin A, Littlewood J (eds). Manual of Canine and Feline Haematology and Transfusion Medicine. Quedgeley, Gloucester, British Small Animal Veterinary Association, 2000.

Evans RJ. The blood and haemopoietic system. In: Chandler EA, Gaskell CJ, Gaskell RM (eds) Feline Medicine and Therapeutics, 2nd edn. Oxford, Blackwell Scientific Publications, 1994, pp. 192–226.

Jordan HL, Grindem CB, Breitschwert EB. Thrombocytopenia in cats: A retrospective study of 41 cases. J Vet Intern Med 1993; 7: 261–265.

Kohn B, Weigart C, Giger U. Haemorrhage in seven cats with suspected anti-coagulant rodenticide intoxication. J Feline Med Surg 2003; 5: 295–304.

Lisciandro SC, Hohenhaus A, Brooks M. Coagulation abnormalities in 22 cats with naturally occurring liver disease. J Vet Intern Med 1998; 12: 71–75.

Peterson JL, Couto CG, Wellman ML. Hemostatic disorders in cats: A retrospective study and review of the literature. J Vet Intern Med 1995; 9: 298–303.

Tasker S, Cripps PJ, Mackin AJ. Evaluation of methods of platelet counting in the cat. J Small Anim Pract 2001; 42: 326–332.

Thomas JS, Green RA. Clotting times and antithrombin III activity in cats with naturally developing diseases: 85 cases (1984–1994). J Am Vet Med Assoc 1998; 213: 1290–1295.

PART 8

Cat with abnormal laboratory data

24 The anemic cat

Michael R. Lappin

KEY SIGNS

- Pale mucous membranes.
- Weakness, depression, lethargy.
- Increased heart and respiratory rates.
- ± Splenomegaly.
- ± Melena or hematochezia.

MECHANISM?

- Blood loss or red blood cell destruction (hemolysis) produces a regenerative anemia. **Failure of the bone marrow** to produce adequate red blood cells produces a non-regenerative anemia.

WHERE?

- Hemolytic anemia is intravascular or extravascular (liver, spleen), whereas blood loss anemia can be into body spaces (abdomen, thorax) or out of the body (usually GIT).
- Non-regenerative anemia indicates a **bone marrow** problem.

WHAT?

- Hemoplasmosis (previously *Hemobartonella felis*) are the most common cause of regenerative anemia.
- Non-regenerative anemia is most commonly the result of **chronic disease, especially infectious disease**.

QUICK REFERENCE SUMMARY

Diseases causing an anemic cat

REGENERATIVE ANEMIA (> 60 000 RETICULOCYTES/ML) – HEMOLYSIS

ANOMALY

● Hereditary hemolytic anemia (pyruvate kinase deficiency, osmotic fragility, porphyria)
Rarely, diseases like pyruvate kinase deficiency in Abyssinian cats result in hemolysis. Hereditary hemolytic anemias usually result in mild, intermittent regenerative anemia and weight loss. Porphyria produces severe macrocytic, hypochromic anemia and brown discoloration of the teeth.

METABOLIC

● Hypophosphatemia* (p 534)

Extreme hypophosphatemia during treatment of ketoacidotic diabetic cats can result in increased red blood cell fragility. Onset of anemia, muscle weakness or ataxia after intensive treatment of a diabetic cat is suspicious.

● Microangiopathic hemolytic anemia* (p 534)

Red blood cells can be damaged when passing through abnormal vessels resulting in schistocytes. Disseminated intravascular coagulation (fibrin strands), dirofilariasis, and splenic tumors or hematomas can damage red blood cells. Lethargy, anorexia and depression may be present in addition to the signs of the underlying disease. Schistocytes are evident on thin blood smears but are hard to detect in cats.

INFECTIOUS

● Hemoplasmosis*** (p 530)

In most parts of the world, the most common causes of hemolytic anemia are infectious, especially from *Mycoplasma haemofelis*, and *Candidatus* M. haemominutum infection. Typically cats present with pale mucous membranes, anorexia, mild to marked depression and sometimes fever.

● Cytauxzoonosis

Typically cats present with pale mucous membranes, anorexia, depression and fever. Dyspnea, collapse and death occur commonly.

IMMUNE

● Immune-mediated hemolytic anemia** (p 532)

Primary immune-mediated hemolytic anemia in cats is unusual when compared to dogs but secondary immune-mediated red cell destruction can occur secondary to drugs, vaccines and infectious agents. Anemia is usually regenerative but may be non-regenerative. Depression, and variable fever, splenomegaly and icterus occur. Agglutination or a positive Coomb's test are indicative of an immune-mediated process.

TOXINS

● Drugs and toxins** (p 533)

Some drugs like acetaminophen and benzocaines and other toxins result in Heinz body anemia in cats which is usually regenerative. Other drugs and toxins induce non-regenerative anemia (see below). Lethargy, anorexia, weakness, pale mucous membranes and elevated heart and respiratory rates are often present.

continued

continued

BLOOD LOSS

● Local diseases of blood vessels** (p 536)

Blood loss anemia can occur when blood vessels are damaged by trauma, erosive diseases like tumors or fungal infections, and vasculitis-like systemic lupus erythrematosus. Signs include anemia, and evidence of internal or external bleeding such as melena, hematochezia, hematuria, dyspnea, hemothorax or hemoabdomen.

● Platelet abnormalities (primary hemostatic defects)** (p 537)

Diseases of platelets including those resulting in thrombocytopenia or those resulting in decreased platelet function. Anemia together with petechiae and ecchymoses at more than one site are typical signs. Hemorrhage may involve the fundus of the eye, mucous membranes of the mouth, vulva, and penis, and skin including ears.

● Factor abnormalities (secondary hemostatic defects)** (p 538)

Decreased amounts or function of coagulation factors. Typically there is anemia together with evidence of hemorrhage at more than one site involving fundus of the eye, mucous membranes of the mouth, vulva, and penis, and skin including ears. Dyspnea, coughing, hemothorax or hemoabdomen may also be evident.

● Hypertension* (p 539)

Systemic arterial hypertension rarely results in significant blood loss and anemia, except if epistaxis is involved. Retinal hemorrhage and epistaxis are most common sites of visible hemorrhage.

NON-REGENERATIVE ANEMIA (< 60 000 RETICULOCYTES/µL)

DEGENERATIVE

● Renal failure** (p 540)

Anemia occurs in many cats with chronic renal failure, but presenting complaints are usually those of renal disease not anemia. Polyuria, polydipsia, inappetance and weight loss are typical.

METABOLIC

● Hypoadrenocorticism

While rare in cats, hypoadrenocorticism does occur and results in anemia. Depression, lethargy, vomiting, diarrhea, anorexia and weakness occur.

● Hypothyroidism

Rarely, anemia may result from hypothyroidism following treatment of hyperthyroidism. Lethargy, weight gain, seborrhea and delayed hair regrowth are typical.

● Iron deficiency

While rare in cats, chronic blood loss can result in microcytic anemia. Lethargy, anorexia, weight loss and signs of chronic gastrointestinal disease resulting in chronic blood loss may be present. Severe flea infestation in young kittens may result in anemia.

● Folic acid antagonism/deficiency

Chronic administration of pyrimethamine or sulfa drugs can result in macrocytic anemia. Dietary insufficiency (tuna diet), malabsorption, and congenital defects may also cause folic acid deficiency.

● **Anemia of chronic disease*** (p 539)**

Diseases associated with chronic inflammation, usually infectious or neoplastic, can result in anemia of chronic disease. Chronic anorexia, lethargy and weight loss, with or without fever, are typically present.

NEOPLASTIC

● **Myelophthitic diseases* (p 546)**

Neoplasms of the bone marrow can crowd out red blood cell precursors. Lethargy, anorexia, weight loss and pale mucous membranes are often present.

INFECTIOUS

● **Feline leukemia virus** (p 540)**

Lethargy, anorexia and weight loss are typical. Anemia may be a main presenting sign. Signs may be referable to secondary infections or neoplasia.

● **Feline infectious peritonitis (FIP), feline immunodeficiency virus (FIV)** (p 545)**

Other classic viral diseases associated with non-regenerative anemia in cats include feline infectious peritonitis and feline immunodeficiency virus. Lethargy, anorexia, weight loss and fever are typical. Signs are referable to secondary infections (FIV) or effusion into body cavities and pyogranulomatous inflammation of the liver, kidney, eye or CNS (FIP).

● **Ehrlichiosis and anaplasmosis**

Uncommon diseases in cats compared to dogs. Lethargy, anorexia, depression and fever are the most common signs. Other signs reported include hyperesthesia, lameness or joint pain, pale mucous membranes, splenomegaly, dyspnea, diarrhea and uveitis.

IMMUNE

● **Immune-mediated (pure red cell aplasia)**

Immune-mediated reactions can be directed at precursor cells resulting in non-regenerative anemia. Lethargy, anorexia, weight loss and pale mucous membranes are often present. Heart and respiratory rates may be elevated once anemia is severe.

TOXINS

● **Drugs/toxins* (p 546)**

Usually a history of exposure to substances like chloramphenicol, which damage the bone marrow. Typically there is lethargy, anorexia and depression together with a history of administration of drugs known to cause bone marrow damage. Vomiting and diarrhea may be evident.

INTRODUCTION

MECHANISM?

Anemia is defined as a packed cell volume of less than 27%.

Anemia is either **regenerative or non-regenerative**.

● **Regenerative anemia** is characterized by reticulocyte counts greater than 60 000/µl; **non-regenerative anemia** has less than 60 000/µl.
● By definition, it takes from 3–5 days after acute development of anemia to have maximal reticulocytosis, and so acute anemia may initially appear as non-regenerative.

- If the anemia has been present for 3–5 days and the reticulocyte count is < 60 000 the anemia is non-regenerative.

The two primary differential diagnoses for **regenerative anemia are hemolysis** (destruction of red blood cells) and **blood loss.**

Loss can occur out of the body through wounds, the gastrointestinal tract, or the nose. Bleeding into body cavities and parenchymal organs also occurs.

- If the **blood loss is out of the body, total protein** concentrations are usually **decreased,** whereas blood loss into a body cavity and hemolytic anemias usually has normal total protein concentrations.

Blood loss can result from local diseases of vessels like **trauma or erosion of the vessel** due to diseases like neoplasia. **Vasculitis, hypertension, factor abnormalities and platelet** abnormalities also can result in blood loss anemia.

There are multiple mechanisms for **hemolytic anemia** including **infectious diseases, primary immune-mediated diseases, microangiopathic diseases, toxins, congenital diseases and metabolic diseases.**

Non-regenerative anemias generally imply **bone marrow dysfunction**, which can be caused by many things including infectious diseases, toxicities, neoplasia, chronic inflammation and metabolic diseases.

WHERE?

Hemolytic anemia is intravascular or extravascular, but is usually extravascular **(liver, spleen)** in cats.

Blood loss in regenerative anemia can be into body spaces **(abdomen, thorax)** or out of the body **(usually GIT)** as a result of **local vascular damage**, or **systemic coagulation or platelet problems.**

Non-regenerative anemia indicates a **bone marrow problem.**

WHAT?

Hemotropic mycoplasmas (previously hemobartonellosis) are the most common causes of regenerative anemia. Less common causes are immune-mediated, drug- or toxin-associated, vascular damage from

trauma, tumors or fungal infection, coagulopathies and thrombocytopenia.

Non-regenerative anemia is most commonly the result of **chronic disease** (infectious, neoplastic or renal failure). Infectious diseases include **feline leukemia virus, feline infectious peritonitis, feline immunodeficiency virus and ehrlichiosis.**

DISEASES CAUSING ANEMIA: REGENERATIVE ANEMIA DUE TO HEMOLYSIS

HEMOPLASMOSIS***

Classical signs

- Previous history or presence of fleas.
- Pale mucous membranes.
- +/− splenomegaly or icterus.
- Lethargy, anorexia, depression.
- +/− fever.

Transmission

Mycoplasma haemofelis and *Candidatus* M. haemominutum and the causes of feline infectious anemia (previously hemobartonellosis).

Experimentally the organisms can be transmitted by intramuscular, intraperitoneal or intravenous administration of infected blood and transplacentally.

Transmission by the cat flea *Ctenocephalides felis* has been shown for *M. haemofelis*, but not *Candidatus* Mycoplasma haemomintum.

Cats with hemobartonellosis may have a history of fighting.

Pathogenesis

The organisms are epicellular parasites of red blood cells (RBC).

M. haemofelis (previously known as the large form) **is most pathogenic.**

Anemia is from immune-mediated reactions that are organism specific or directed at RBC membrane proteins that have been modified by the parasitism.

Antibody-coated red blood cells are removed by the reticuloendothelial system, and intravascular lysis is unusual; Coomb's positive test results are common.

Level of parasitemia fluctuates rapidly making diagnosis difficult based on cytology.

The **acute phase** of disease usually **develops within 3 weeks**; spontaneous recovery followed by recurrence from the chronic carrier state can occur.

Anemia associated with *Candidatus* Mycoplasma haemomintum is often detected in cats with current feline leukemia virus infection.

In locations where feline leukemia virus is common, approximately 50% of infected cats are co-infected with the virus; co-infection with feline immunodeficiency virus is rare.

Clinical signs

Infection is most common in **male cats** less than 3 years of age, and occurs most often in the spring.

Cats are usually presented for **depression, lethargy and anorexia.**

Pale mucous membranes are a common physical examination abnormality. **Fever and icterus** are also common.

Splenomegaly occurs in some from extramedullary hematopoiesis and immune stimulation.

Fleas or flea dirt may or may not be noted.

Chronic infection may lead to recurrent hemolytic anemia or intermittent fever, depression and anorexia without hemolytic anemia.

Diagnosis

Diagnosis is based on cytological demonstration of the organism on the surface of RBC. However, the organism may be difficult to find even though clinical signs are present, and at least 50% of cats are falsely negative on cytological examination.

The organism may dislodge from the surface of RBCs placed in EDTA in cytologically negative suspect cats. In suspect cats, repeat cytological assessment using smears made from blood without anti-coagulants.

Polymerase chain reaction (PCR) is available commercially. PCR is positive in some cytologically nega-

tive cats suggesting it is more sensitive. Some healthy cats are PCR positive and so the predictive value for presence of disease is not 100%.

Macroscopic or microscopic agglutination, spherocytosis, or Coomb's positive test results are suggestive.

Differential diagnosis

Any infectious, immune-mediated, or neoplastic cause of hemolytic anemia can look similar as a result of signs associated with fever and anemia. Demonstration of the organism by cytological assessment or PCR differentiates mycoplasma-associated hemolytic anemia from other causes.

Treatment

Doxycycline at 10 mg/kg, PO, q 24 hours for the first week and then continued q 24 hours for 2 weeks. If the cat will tolerate treatment, a total of 4 weeks of treatment may result in more cats becoming PCR negative.

While tetracycline at 22 mg/kg, PO q 8 hours can be effective it is no longer recommended since doxycycline is superior.

Enrofloxacin at 5–10 mg/kg, PO, q 12–24 hours for 2–3 weeks may be effective in cats that are intolerant of tetracyclines. Doses over 5.5 mg/kg may be associated with retinal toxicity and blindness in a small percentage of cats.

For cats that do not tolerate or are resistant to tetracyclines and enrofloxacin, **imidocarb diproprionate** at 5 mg/kg, IM or SQ, q 2 weeks, for 2–4 injections can be used.

Chloramphenicol at 15 mg/kg, PO, q 12 hours for 3 weeks has been used but not studied experimentally; this drug also has been associated with bone marrow suppression.

Prednisolone at 1–2 mg/kg, PO, q 12 hours should be used for at least the first week of therapy because of the immune-mediated pathogenesis.

Treatment lessens clinical signs of disease but does not resolve infection in many cats.

While there is no PCV that alone indicates when to transfuse, **whole blood transfusions** are generally indicated if the PCV is dropping rapidly and heart and respiration rates are elevated at rest.

Blood typing should be performed if possible in breeds prone to the B type (British short hair, Devon Rex, Cornish Rex, Japanese bobtail, Scottish fold, Sphinx, Somoli).

Cross-match results may be hard to interpret due to spontaneous agglutination.

Since *M. haemofelis* is the most common cause of hemolytic anemia in cats, **treatment should be considered for all suspect cats**, even if the organism cannot be found.

Prognosis

Most treated cats survive. The prognosis is worse for those with concurrent immunodeficiency-inducing diseases.

Because treated cats are usually not cured, exacerbations are common.

Prevention

Flea control and housing cats indoors lessen potential for exposure.

Cats used as **blood donors should be tested** for both *Mycoplasma haemofelis* and *Candidatus* Mycoplasma haemomintum using PCR techniques. Donor cats exposed to fleas should be regularly retested.

IMMUNE-MEDIATED HEMOLYTIC ANEMIA**

Classical signs

- Lethargy, anorexia, depression, +/– fever.
- Pale mucous membranes.
- +/– splenomegaly or icterus.

Pathogenesis

Primary immune-mediated hemolytic anemia (IMHA) is rare and the cause unknown.

Secondary IMHA occurs from hypersensitivity reactions against drugs (like beta-lactam antibiotics), modified-live vaccines, neoplasms, and infectious agents like *M. haemofelis* and feline leukemia virus.

RBC can be lysed in the bloodstream (**intravascular**) or removed by the reticuloendothelial system (**extravascular**), with the latter being most common.

Large concentrations of anti-RBC antibodies result in cross-linking and macroscopic or **microscopic agglutination**.

Spherocytes are formed when fixed reticuloendothelial cells remove part of the antibody or complement-coated RBC membrane.

The immune reaction can be directed at RBC precursors resulting in non-regenerative anemia.

Clinical signs

Depression, lethargy and anorexia are common presenting complaints.

History of recent vaccination (within 1 month) or antibiotic administration may be present.

History of fleas is common in cats with hemotropic mycoplasmosis.

Fading kitten syndrome occurs in kittens with a history of a type B queen mated to a type A tom (neonatal iso-erythrolysis; see page 1134).

Pale mucous membranes, tachycardia and tachypnea are common.

Splenomegaly and lymphadenopathy occur in some cats.

Icterus is dependent on rapidity of anemia development. White blood cells are activated commonly resulting in fever.

Diagnosis

Presence of spherocytes is classic but difficult to document in cats compared to dogs since normal RBC of cats is relatively small, and they do not have central pallor.

Macroscopic or microscopic agglutination. If agglutinating cells are noted, mix 1 drop of blood in EDTA with 1 drop 0.9% NaCl and repeat the thin blood smear. If cells are no longer clumped, massive roulette formation was occurring and not agglutination.

Direct Coomb's testing can be used in cases without spherocytes or autoagglutination to confirm presence of IgG, IgM or complement on the surface of RBC. EDTA blood is submitted to the laboratory for reaction with Coomb's reagent (anti-IgG, anti-IgM, anti-complement). Optimally, the laboratory should provide a titer, not the result of a single dilution. Feline-specific Coomb's reagent must be used.

Antinuclear antibody testing can be performed. Some cats with systemic lupus erythematosus will be positive and have primary immune-mediated hemolytic anemia.

Erythrophagocytosis can be noted on **bone marrow examination**; maturation arrest of RBC development may be detected if immune response is directed at precursor cells.

Differential diagnosis

Any infectious or neoplastic cause of hemolytic or blood loss anemia can look similar because the signs of fever and anemia are not specific, and immune destruction of RBC may be partly involved in the pathogenesis of the anemia. Diagnosis is often based on exclusion of infectious and neoplastic causes, and demonstration of agglutination or a positive Coomb's test.

Treatment

Dexamethasone at 1 mg/kg, IV, once on day 1.

Prednisolone at 2–4 mg/kg, PO, q 12 hours initially followed by decreasing doses every other week provided anemia is resolving. If maintenance treatment is required, the target dose is approximately 0.5 mg/kg, PO, q 48 h.

Doxycycline at 5–10 mg/kg, PO, q 12 hours for at least 14 days in all cats with hemolytic anemia due to possible hemobartonellosis.

Dexamethasone administered at 0.1–0.2 mg/kg, PO, q 12 hours in cats resistant to prednisolone.

Cyclosporine at 1–5 mg/kg, PO, q 12–24 hours, for 7–14 days is indicated for acute treatment of **cats that are autoagglutinating** or undergoing **intravascular hemolysis**.

Cyclophosphamide at 6.25–12 mg/cat, PO, 4 days weekly for 1–2 weeks has been used in some cats acutely but is not currently used by the author.

Chlorambucil at 0.2 mg/kg, PO, q 24 hours may be needed in some cats with glucocorticoid-induced side effects or incomplete control, and should be used in place of cyclophosphamide for long-term management.

Azathioprine at 0.3 mg/kg, PO, q 72 hours may be needed in some cats with glucocorticoid-induced side effects or incomplete control, but extreme bone marrow suppression can occur and chlorambucil is preferred.

Whole blood transfusion may be indicated if the **PCV is dropping rapidly**, the cat is depressed, and if heart and respiration rates are elevated at rest.

Prognosis

Prognosis with primary IMHA is unknown since it is rare.

Theoretically, secondary IMHA should have a good prognosis since the initiating antigen (*M. haemofelis*, vaccines, antibiotics) can be removed.

Prevention

Avoid over-stimulating cat immune systems with antibiotics and vaccines.

Cats with primary or secondary IMHA should be housed indoors and no longer vaccinated.

Lessen exposure to fleas to potentially avoid infection by *M. haemofelis*.

DRUGS/TOXINS**

> **Classical signs**
>
> - Lethargy, anorexia, depression.
> - Pale mucous membranes and elevated heart and respiratory rate.
> - History of exposure to oxidative toxin.

Pathogenesis

Oxidation of the globin in hemoglobin leads to formation of **Heinz bodies** (precipitated hemoglobin).

Anemia results from cell lysis or framentation in capillaries because of fragility, **or removal** by the fixed reticuloendothelial system of the spleen and liver.

Clinical signs

Lethargy, anorexia, weakness, pale mucous membranes and elevated heart and respiratory rates occur.

History of exposure to oxidative toxins like acetaminophen (iatrogenic), onions (foodstuffs like babyfood), zinc (United States pennies, airline carrier hardware), propothiouracil (iatrogenic), methylene blue (iatrogenic), phenazopyridine (iatrogenic), vitamin K1 (iatrogenic), propylene glycol (food stuffs; carrier in some medications), and benzocaine derivatives (iatrogenic).

Diagnosis

Heinz bodies (intracytoplasmic irregular retractile granules) are seen cytologically on thin blood smears.

Methemoglobin levels can be elevated; blood has a brown color.

Treatment

Remove the source of the oxidant injury.

N-acetylcysteine at 140 mg/kg, PO, once followed by 70 mg/kg, PO every 4–6 hours if severe methemoglobinemia is present.

Supportive care including whole blood transfusion if needed.

HYPOPHOSPHATEMIA*

> **Classical signs**
> - Anemia, muscle weakness in diabetic cat.
> - Ataxia, seizures.

Clinical signs

Extreme hypophosphatemia may occur during **initial treatment of ketoacidotic diabetes mellitus**, and result in muscle weakness, ataxia, seizures and **pale mucous membranes**.

Liver disease may result in red blood cell fragility.

Diagnosis

Measurement of serum phosphorus concentrations.

Treatment

Administer potassium phosphates at 0.03–0.12 mmol/kg/h until normophosphatemic.

Alternately, prevent hypophosphatemia (and hypokalemia) by giving calculated potassium requirements as 30% potassium chloride and 50% potassium dihydrophosphate.

Phosphate concentrations are usually maintained within normal concentrations by diet alone after resolution of the ketoacidotic crisis.

MICROANGIOPATHIC HEMOLYTIC ANEMIA*

> **Classical signs**
> - Lethargy, anorexia, depression.
> - Clinical signs of the primary disease.

Clinical signs

Diseases that involve small vessels like **disseminated intravascular coagulation** (fibrin strands), **dirofilariasis**, and **splenic tumors or hematomas damage RBC** resulting in formation of schistocytes or fragments.

History, physical examination, and laboratory assessment support the primary disease.

Lethargy, depression, weakness and pale mucous membranes may result if anemia is severe.

Diagnosis

Schistocytes are seen cytologically on thin blood smears.

Diagnostic work-up for the suspected primary cause should be performed.

CYTAUXZOONOSIS

> **Classical signs**
> - Fever, depression, shock and death.
> - Indoor/outdoor cats in the Gulf Coast states.
> - History of tick exposure.

Transmission

Bobcats are subclinically infected by *Cytauxzoon felis* and so are probably the natural host.

Transmission occurs from infected bobcats to domestic cats by *Dermacentor variabilis*.

Pathogenesis

Transmission of the organism results in clinical illness in 5–20 days.

Schizonts and macroschizonts form in **mononuclear phagocytes**, line the lumen of veins, and **obstruct blood flow through tissues** (tissue phase).

Merozoites released from infected macrophages **infect erythrocytes causing hemolytic anemia** (erythrocyte phase).

Clinical signs

Most infected cats are presented for **depression.**

Physical examination usually reveals **fever, anorexia, dyspnea, depression, collapse, icterus**, and **pale mucous membranes.**

Hypothermia develops in some cats preceeding death.

Death is a common sequel, but strains of *C. felis* that spontaneously resolve have now been recognized.

Most cases of cytauxzoonosis are in **outdoor cats**, but ticks are generally not identified

The **course of disease is generally 1 week or less** in cats infected with pathogenic strains.

Cats infected with non-pathogenic strains may live for years.

Diagnosis

Regenerative anemia, neutrophilic leukocytosis or leukopenia, thrombocytopenia or thrombocytosis, **hemoglobinemia, hemoglobinuria**, bilirubinemia and bilirubinuria are the most common laboratory abnormalities, but vary between patients.

Antemortem diagnosis is based on demonstrating the **ring-shaped erythrocytic phase on thin blood smears** which occurs in most cats with acute illness.

The organism can be detected in infected macrophages in bone marrow, spleen, liver, or lymph node aspirates stained with Wright's or Giemsa stains.

Serologic testing can be used to confirm exposure, but is usually not needed clinically

PCR assay has been studied experimentally and may be available in the future.

Differential diagnosis

Any infectious, immune-mediated, or neoplastic cause of hemolytic anemia can look similar due to the signs associated with fever and anemia. Identification of the organism is diagnostic.

Treatment

Fluid therapy and blood transfusion should be administered as indicated (see hemobartonellosis).

Imidocarb administered at 5.0 mg/kg, IM, every 14 days for two doses or **diminazene** at 2.0 mg/kg, IM, every 7 days for two doses are the drugs of choice but no treatment is known to be effective.

Parvaquone, buparvaquone, thiacetarsamide and tetracycline therapy have also been attempted.

Zoonotic potential and prevention

Cytauxzoon felis is not known to infect people.

Tick control should be maintained, and cats in endemic areas should be housed indoors.

HEREDITARY HEMOLYTIC ANEMIA (PYRUVATE KINASE DEFICIENCY, OSMOTIC FRAGILITY, PORPHYRIA)

> ### Classical signs
> - Lethargy, anorexia, weight loss.
> - Pale mucous membranes.
> - Young Abyssinian, Somalis, Siamese or DSH cat.

Clinical signs

Congenital diseases resulting in hemolysis are **rare in cats**.

Pyruvate kinase deficiency has been described in Abyssinian cats, Somalis and DSH with **intermittent, regenerative anemias**.

Increased osmotic fragility of erythrocytes causing **hemolytic crises** with macrocytic regenerative anemia and splenomegaly has also been documented in Abyssinians and Somalis.

Cats with hereditary hemolytic anemias exhibit **intermittent anemia and weight loss**, and the clinical signs appear to be **ameliorated by splenectomy**.

Porphyria in a family of Siamese cats was associated with **severe macrocytic, hypochromic anemia** with poikilocytosis, Howell–Jolly bodies, and nucleated red blood cells.

Porphyria in domestic shorthair cats is inherited as an autosomal dominant trait, and is characterized by only a **mild anemia**.

Porphyrins produce a **brownish discoloration of teeth**, bones (at necropsy), and urine, all of which fluoresce bright pink-red with ultraviolet light.

Diagnosis

Measure pyruvate kinase activities.

Measure blood porphyria concentrations. Demonstrate fluorescence of porphyrins in teeth or urine.

Treatment

Supportive care including transfusion if indicated.

Splenectomy for anemias caused by pyruvate kinase deficiency and increased osmotic fragility.

REGENERATIVE ANEMIA DUE TO BLOOD LOSS

LOCAL DISEASES OF BLOOD VESSELS**

Classical signs

- Anemia.
- Bleeding internally or externally.

Classical signs—Cont'd

- Evidence of trauma, neoplasia, inflammatory or erosive disease.
- Melena, hematochezia, hematuria, dyspnea, hemothorax or hemoabdomen.

Pathogenesis

Blood vessels are damaged by trauma (blunt trauma, foreign bodies, etc.), erosive diseases resulting from tumors, chronic infections (fungal in particular), toxicities (mainly gastrointestinal), or vasculitis like systemic lupus erythematosus.

Clinical signs

Weakness and lethargy are common presenting complaints.

Blood usually is lost into tissues, spaces like the **pleural space and peritoneal cavity**, the **gastrointestinal tract** (including palate of the cat), or any external damaged tissue like the nose.

Bleeding may or may not be evident, depending on where the blood is lost.

Melena or hematochezia may be present in cases with gastrointestinal blood loss; exceptions include small volume, chronic bleeding and acute loss.

Acute dyspnea or weakness associated with pale mucous membranes and evidence of **hemothorax or hemoabdomen** on centesis are typical findings.

In contrast to blood loss from coagulopathies or hypertension, local diseases usually do not result in evidence of bleeding at distant sites. The exception is vasculitis.

Fungal and neoplastic diseases of the nose that result in epistaxis usually have mucopurulent discharge prior to development of epistaxis.

Other clinical signs are associated with the primary disease.

Diagnosis

Diagnostic work-up and findings are dependent on the individual primary disease and site of bleeding.

PLATELET ABNORMALITIES (PRIMARY HEMOSTATIC DEFECTS)**

Classical signs

- Anemia.
- Petechiae and ecchymoses at more than one site.
- Hemorrhage involving fundus of the eye, mucous membranes of the mouth, vulva, and penis, and skin including ears.

Pathogenesis

Platelet diseases can be divided into those inducing **thrombocytopenia** and those inducing **platelet dysfunction**.

The differential categories for thrombocytopenia include consumption, destruction, decreased production and sequestration.

The most common causes of platelet consumption are **disseminated intravascular coagulation** and consumption at sites of inflammation.

The most common cause of platelet destruction is **immune-mediated** which can be either primary or secondary to drugs and vaccines.

Platelets are produced by the bone marrow and so any bone marrow disease can potentially result in thrombocytopenia. **Neoplasia and feline leukemia** virus are common examples.

Sequestration of platelets usually occurs in the spleen or liver but is not a primary disease.

Platelet function abnormalities can be iatrogenic (aspirin), congenital (rare in cats), or acquired (hyperglobulinemia).

Clinical signs

Diseases of platelets usually result in **petechiae and ecchymoses**.

Ingestion of aspirin may be known.

Clinical signs are usually consistent with where the primary bleeding is occurring and the primary disease resulting in hemorrhage.

Most bleeding disorders will have evidence of **hemorrhage in more than one site**. The fundus of the **eye, mucous membranes of the mouth, vulva, and penis**, and the skin especially ear and ventral abdomen are good places to evaluate for evidence of hemorrhage.

Diagnosis

Platelet count should be made; **spontaneous hemorrhage** generally occurs with **platelet counts of < 50 000 platelets/µl**.

Platelet estimates can be made; under oil immersion (1000×), every **one platelet per field** equates to approximately **20 000** platelets/µl.

When thrombocytopenia is suspected, scan the blood smear evaluating for clumps which may falsely lower the count.

If giant platelets are present, decreased production of platelets is unlikely.

If persistent thrombocytopenia is present, a **bone marrow** examination is indicated to evaluate for **myelophthitic disease** and **latent feline leukemia virus infection** (IFA or PCR; see FeLV section).

Platelet function deficits in cats are rare, however **von Willebrand's disease** does occur.

Bleeding time assesses platelet function and should be less than 5 minutes.

Bleeding time should only be performed in cats with normal platelet counts and factor tests (ACT, etc.).

Treatment

Treatment varies with the primary disease (see appropriate section) but frequently includes administration of **fresh whole blood transfusion** if life-threatening hemorrhage is occurring.

Fresh plasma can be used if red blood cells are not needed.

For suspected secondary immune-mediated thrombocytopenia, remove the potential source if possible (antibiotic or vaccine).

Primary immune-mediated thrombocytopenia is rare in cats, but treatment is as discussed for hemolytic anemia (see appropriate section).

FACTOR ABNORMALITIES (SECONDARY HEMOSTATIC DEFECTS)**

Classical signs

- Anemia.
- Evidence of hemorrhage at more than one site involving fundus of the eye, mucous membranes of the mouth, vulva, and penis, and skin including ears.
- Dyspnea, coughing, hemothorax or hemoabdomen.

Pathogenesis

Factor abnormalities can be divided into **decreased amounts** (liver disease, DIC, hemophilia, cholestasis, warfarin toxicity) or **decreased function of coagulation factors** (circulating anti-coagulants like heparin).

Hepatic insufficiency leads to **decreased production** of procoagulants.

Hepatic cholestasis results in **absence of vitamin K** and **failure to convert factors II, VII, IX and X** to active coagulants.

DIC results in factor consumption

Hemophilia is the congenital lack of a factor or factors.

Warfarin toxicity results in vitamin K antagonism and the resultant failure to convert factors II, VII, IX and X to active coagulants.

Increased amounts of **circulating anticoagulants** are most common with **mast cell tumors (heparin) or DIC (fibrinogen degradation products)**.

Clinical signs

Most bleeding disorders will have evidence of **hemorrhage in more than one site**.

Decreased amounts or function of coagulation factors usually results in **bleeding into body cavities** like the chest and peritoneal cavity.

The **fundus of the eye** and **mucous membranes of the mouth, vulva and penis** are good places to evaluate for evidence of hemorrhage.

Clinical signs are usually consistent with where the primary bleeding is occurring and the primary disease resulting in hemorrhage.

Ingestion of vitamin K antagonistic rodenticides may be known.

Cats with **hepatic insufficiency** usually have other clinical signs like weight loss, anorexia, polyuria/polydipsia.

Cats with **cholestasis** commonly have other clinical findings like weight loss, anorexia and icterus.

DIC is a syndrome induced by other diseases; clinical findings are consistent with the primary disease.

If severe enough to cause spontaneous hemorrhage, **hemophilia** usually presents in **younger cats**.

Diagnosis

Activated clotting time (ACT; normal < 65 seconds) can be used in clinical settings to assess the intrinsic and common coagulation pathways. Factor VII is the only factor deficiency not screened by the activated clotting time (extrinsic pathway), but factor VII hemophilia is rare and so the **ACT is an excellent clinical screening test for factor deficiencies**. Thrombocytopenia < 50 000 platelets/µl can **prolong the ACT by up to 10–15** seconds due to **lack of platelet phospholipid**.

The **activated partial thromoplastin time** and **prothrombin time** as well as specific assessment of different factors or **proteins induced by vitamin K absence** or antagonism are performed on **citrated plasma**; samples should be collected and stored prior to starting treatment.

Treatment

Treatment varies with the disease, but frequently includes administration of **fresh whole blood** transfusion if life-threatening hemorrhage is occurring.

Frozen plasma can be used to supply coagulation factors if red blood cells or platelets are not needed.

If vitamin K antagonists are the cause of the hemorrhage, **vitamin K1** should be given **subcutaneously at 1–5 mg/kg, q 12 hour for 24 hours**. Dose is dependent on the type of anti-coagulant ingested. Warfarin can be treated with 1–3 mg/kg and long-acting products should be treated with 3–5 mg/kg. Oral administration of vitamin K1 is initiated on day 2 at 1–5 mg/kg, q 12 hours for 2 weeks (warfarin) to 6 weeks (long-acting anti-coagulant) depending on the type of anti-coagulant ingested.

Vitamin K1 given intravenously can result in an anaphylactoid reaction.

When vitamin K1 therapy is discontinued, the cat should be **returned in 72 hours for assessment** of an ACT or prothrombin time. If increased at that time, two more weeks of therapy should be prescribed prior to the next evaluation.

HYPERTENSION*

Classical signs

- Sudden onset of blindness with dilated pupils from retinal hemorrhage.
- Epistaxis.
- Evidence of diseases causing hypertension, especially renal disease or hyperthyroidism.

Pathogenesis

Systemic arterial hypertension in cats is usually from **renal disease, hyperthyroidism, hyperadrenocorticism** and **idiopathic** (essential).

Clinical signs

Systemic arterial hypertension can result in hemorrhage; **retinal hemorrhage and epistaxis** are most common.

With the exception of epistaxis, volume of blood loss is usually small and so anemia is rare.

Diagnosis

Systolic blood pressure > 175 mmHg using a Doppler system is abnormal.

- Some normal cats will appear hypertensive due to epinephrine release from the stress of measuring the blood pressure.

Renal and endocrine causes of hypertension should be excluded by bloodwork and urinalysis.

Treatment

ACE-inhibitors, calcium channel blockers, beta-blockers, and sodium restriction are used to manage systemic arterial hypertension in cats.

See appropriate sections for specific treatment recommendations (page 134).

NON-REGENERATIVE ANEMIA (< 60 000 RETICULOCYTES/μL)

ANEMIA OF CHRONIC DISEASE***

Classical signs

- Chronic lethargy, anorexia and depression.

Pathogenesis

Activation of leukocytes by the primary disease results in the **production of cytokines like interleukin 1**.

In the face of inflammatory cytokines, **macrophages fail to release iron** to be used for red blood cell production.

Red blood cell life span is slightly shortened.

Response of the bone marrow to erythropoietin may be blunted.

Clinical signs

Diseases associated with chronic inflammation, usually infectious or neoplastic, can result in anemia of chronic disease.

Clinical signs are those usually related to the primary disease with minimal clinical findings associated with the anemia.

The **anemia is generally mild** compared to those associated with FeLV or immune-mediated diseases.

Diagnosis

Diagnosis is usually based on exclusion of other causes of non-regenerative anemia combined with documentation of a chronic neoplastic or inflammatory disease.

Mild normocytic-normochromic, non-regenerative anemia (**PCV is generally 18–27%**).

Platelet counts are generally normal.

Neutrophilia and monocytosis may be present due to chronic inflammation induced by the primary disease.

Bone marrow cytology shows **increased iron stores in bone marrow macrophages**.

Differential diagnosis

FeLV, myelophthtic disease, ehrlichiosis, anemia of renal failure, hypoadrenocorticism.

Treatment

Remove the source of the chronic disease.

Whole blood transfusion if indicated.

Erythropoietin and other bone marrow stimulants are unlikely to be effective.

RENAL FAILURE**

> ### Classical signs
>
> - Weight loss, inappetence.
> - Polyuria, polydipsia.
> - ± Intermittent vomiting.
> - Pale mucous membranes.

Clinical signs

Polydipsia, polyuria, inappetence, weight loss, intermittent vomiting, "rubber jaw", small kidneys, and other findings consistent with chronic renal failure (see page 234).

The **non-regenerative anemia** is generally **mild to moderate (PCV ≥ 18) from erythropoietin lack**, unless accompanied by blood loss anemia from gastrointestinal hemorrhage or hemolysis from hypophosphatemia. Other factors contributing to anemia in renal

failure include shortened red cell survival, and the effects of uremic toxins such as parathyroid hormone on erythropoiesis.

Diagnosis

Documentation of **azotemia with suboptimal urine-concentrating ability** (see page 645).

Exclude other causes of non-regenerative anemia.

Mild to moderate **normocytic, normochromic, non-regenerative anemia** (PCV = 15–27%).

Neutrophil and platelet numbers are generally normal.

Differential diagnosis

Any cause of non-regenerative anemia.

Treatment

Human recombinant erythropoietin.
- 100 U/kg, SC, 3 days weekly for induction.
- Adjust dose and frequency to maintain PCV > 20 for maintenance.
- Antibodies may be generated against the human recombinant product inactivating it, which occurs in 20–30% of treated cats.
- Severe immune-mediated reactions rarely occur.
- Some clinicians use erythropoietin to induce remission of anemia and attempt to use anabolic steroids to maintain remission.
- If iron deficiency is present, response to erythropoietin can be blunted.

If clinically indicated, administer a blood transfusion while waiting for an erythropoietin response. Indication is inappetence, and increased heart and respiratory rates at rest.

Anabolic steroids (see page 1339).

FELINE LEUKEMIA VIRUS**

> ### Classical signs
>
> - Lethargy, anorexia, weight loss; usually in cats < 6 years.
> - +/− clinical findings consistent with lymphoma; masses, etc.
> - +/− secondary infections of any organ system.

Pathogenesis

Feline leukemia virus (FeLV) is a single-stranded **RNA virus** that produces reverse transcriptase enzyme.

The envelope protein **p15e** is associated with the development of **immunosuppression**.

The core protein **p27** is present in the cytoplasm of infected cells as well as in the peripheral blood, saliva and tears of infected cats; detection of p27 is the **basis of the immunofluorescence and ELISA tests** for FeLV.

The envelope **glycoprotein 70** (gp70) contains **subgroup antigens** A, B or C; these subgroups are associated with the infectivity, virulence and disease caused by individual strains of the virus.

All cats carry subgroup A either alone or in combination with B or C.

Subgroup A may cause malignancy by itself, but co-infection with B or C may have a synergistic effect on oncogenicity.

Exposure to gp70 results in the production of neutralizing antibodies in some cats.

Feline coronavirus-associated cell membrane antigen is a FeLV-induced antigen expressed on the surface of cells with virus-induced **malignant transformation**. Antibodies formed against this antigen can be detected in some cats.

Stages of infection after oral exposure and resultant immunofluorescent antibody (IFA) and enzyme-linked immunosorbent assay (ELISA) test results:

- Stage I. **Replication in local lymphoid tissues**; 2–12 days post-inoculation (PI); IFA negative; ELISA negative.
- Stage II. **Dissemination in circulating lymphocytes and monocytes**; 2–12 days PI; IFA negative; ELISA positive.
- Stage III. **Replication in the spleen, distant lymph nodes and gut** associated lymphoid tissue; 2–12 days PI, IFA negative, ELISA positive.
- Stage IV. **Replication in bone marrow cells and intestinal epithelial crypts**; 2–6 weeks PI; IFA negative; ELISA positive.
- Stage V. **Peripheral viremia**, dissemination via infected bone marrow derived neutrophils and platelets; 4–6 weeks PI; IFA positive; ELISA positive.
- Stage VI. **Disseminated epithelial cell infection** with virus secretion in saliva and tears; 4–6 weeks PI; IFA positive; ELISA positive.

Following exposure, cats either become persistently infected, develop latent or sequestered infection, **become immune carriers** or **have self-limiting infection**.

Whether or not infection occurs following natural exposure to FeLV is determined by the virus subtype or strain, the virus dose, the age of the cat when exposed, and the cat's immune responses.

Approximately **30% of the cats with self-limiting infection** will have **provirus present (latent infection)** which can be **associated with p27-negative lymphoma** and possible reactivation to persistent viremia.

Some cats with latent infection also have evidence of immunosuppression.

Latent infection can be activated by the administration of glucocorticoids or other immunosuppressive drugs or pregnancy.

Atypical or sequestered (localized) infection occurs in up to 26% of cats exposed to FeLV; the **bone marrow, spleen, lymph node** and small intestine are the tissues most commonly involved. It is unknown what percentage of these cats develops clinical disease but some cats will transmit the virus to offspring.

In experimental studies, 100% of neonatal kittens, 70–85% of weanling kittens, and **15–30% of cats > 4 months old were infected** when exposed; adults may be more difficult to infect than kittens due to the maturation of macrophage function.

Subgroup C induces aplastic anemia from tropism for macrophages resulting in increased secretion of tumor necrosis factor-alpha.

Immunodeficiency syndromes are likely to occur secondary to **T lymphocyte depletion** (both CD4+ and CD8+ lymphocytes) **or dysfunction**, and either neutropenia or neutrophil function deficits.

Myeloproliferative diseases likely develop from viral induction of **bone marrow growth-promoting substances**.

Transmission

The **principal route of infection** is **prolonged contact with infected cat saliva and nasal secretions**; biting is not required but can transmit infection.

Fomite transmission and aerosol transmission are unlikely due to **poor survival of the organism in the environment**.

Transplacental infection and transmission by milk occur but more kittens are probably infected when **licked and groomed by the infected queen**.

FeLV has been detected in semen and vaginal epithelium and so venereal transmission is possible.

The role of blood-sucking arthropods in the transmission of FeLV is largely unknown but considered of minimal importance.

Clinical signs

Any age, gender or breed of cat can develop signs of FeLV infection but the **majority are male** and **between 1–6 years of age**.

Most FeLV-infected cats are evaluated for **non-specific signs** such as **anorexia, weight loss and depression** or for evaluation of abnormalities associated with specific organ systems.

Of FeLV-infected cats evaluated at necropsy, **23% have evidence of neoplasia** (96% – lymphoma/leukemia complex) and the remainder die from non-neoplastic diseases including those from **secondary infections due to immunosuppression**.

Gastrointestinal abnormalities.
- **Stomatitis and halitosis** may be secondary to **overgrowth of normal bacterial flora** or **persistent calicivirus** infection from immunosuppression.
- **Vomiting and diarrhea** occur in some FeLV-infected cats and may be due to opportunistic infections such as **salmonellosis, giardiasis or cryptosporidiosis or lymphoma**.
- A form of enteritis clinically and histopathologically resembling panleukopenia but apparently related to FeLV infection has been described, and is possibly secondary to enteric coronavirus infection.

Icterus.
- **Pre-hepatic icterus** is related to immune-mediated destruction of red blood cells induced by FeLV or secondary infection by *M. haemofelis* or *Candidatus* Mycoplasma haemomintum (*Haemobartonella felis*).
- **Hepatic icterus** is related to **hepatic lymphoma**, hepatic lipidosis and focal liver necrosis.
- **Post-hepatic icterus** may occur due to **alimenteric lymphoma**.

Respiratory abnormalities.
- Sneezing, nasal discharge, pneumonia, bronchitis and pyothorax occur in some FeLV-infected cats from immunosuppression and secondary infections.
- Dyspnea and restrictive breathing pattern with muffled heart or lung sounds are common in cats with **thymic lymphoma**; these **cats are generally < 3 years** of age and may have decreased cranial chest compliance on palpation.

Lymphadenopathy due to lymphoma or hyperplasia of lymphoid tissues occurs in FeLV-infected cats.

Neoplasia.
- **Mediastinal (thymic), multicentric** and **alimenteric** lymphoma are common neoplasms associated with FeLV.
- Fibrosarcomas occasionally develop in young cats co-infected with FeLV and feline sarcoma virus.
- Lymphocytic, myelogenous, erythroid and megakaryocytic leukemia all are reported secondary to FeLV infection; **myelodysplasia and myelofibrosis** also occur.

Urinary tract abnormalities.
- Urinary tract problems most frequently associated with FeLV-infected cats are urinary incontinence and renal failure.
- **Renal failure** is generally secondary to renal lymphoma or glomerulonephritis.
- **Urinary incontinence** has been predominantly a small bladder, nocturnal incontinence that appears to be caused by either sphincter incompetence or detrusor hyperactivity.

Ocular abnormalities.
- Intraocular lymphoma induces uveitis and glaucoma in some cats; cats are generally presented for miosis, blepharospasm or cloudy eyes.

- Aqueous flare, mass lesions, keratic precipitates, lens luxations and glaucoma are often found on ocular examination.
- If anterior uveitis is present, the abnormality is usually because of co-infection with FIP, *T. gondii*, *C. neoformans* or FIV.

Reproductive abnormalities.
- FeLV-infected queens may be presented for abortion, stillbirth or infertility.
- Kittens that are infected in utero but survive to parturition generally develop accelerated FeLV syndromes or die as a part of the kitten mortality complex.

Neurologic abnormalities.
- Nervous system disease is likely to develop due to **polyneuropathy** or **lymphoma**.
- Neurologic abnormalities are occasionally secondary to other infectious agents like FIP or *T. gondii*.
- Anisocoria, ataxia, weakness, behavioral change and urinary incontinence are the most common neurologic signs.
- Neurologic examination commonly reveals **tetraparesis or paraparesis** and **decreased conscious proprioception**.
- Leukemic cells were detected in the bone marrow of 69% of a group of cats with spinal lymphoma.

Secondary infections.
- **Concurrent infections by viral, bacterial, fungal, rickettsial and parasitic agents** are commonly detected in FeLV seropositive cats; it is difficult clinically to determine which are primary and which are secondary to FeLV-induced immunosuppression.
- A strong association exists between FeLV and infections with **feline infectious peritonitis** virus and hemotropic mycoplasmas (previously *Haemobartonella felis*).
- Secondary infections may be more difficult to treat in FeLV-infected cats that are immunosuppressed.

Musculoskeletal abnormalities.
- **Multiple cartilaginous exostosis** occur in some cats.
- **Polyarthritis with resultant stiffness** and lameness with or without swollen, hot and painful joints occurs in some cats and has been attributed to immune complex deposition.

Laboratory abnormalities.
- **Anemia is common; non-regenerative** anemia occurs alone or in combination with decreases in lymphocytes, neutrophils and platelets.
- Evidence of abnormal red blood cell release from the bone marrow characterized by **increased numbers of circulating nucleated red blood cells without an appropriate reticulocytosis** is common.
- Examination of bone marrow often documents a **maturation arrest in the erythroid line**.
- **Regenerative anemia** is detected in some cats with immune-mediated destruction of erythrocytes induced by FeLV or in some cats co-infected with *M. haemofelis*.
- Microagglutination of erythrocytes or positive direct Coomb's testing occurs in some cats.
- **Neutropenia** occurs in some due to bone marrow suppression or immune-mediated destruction.
- **Renal azotemia** occurs in cats with renal lymphoma.
- **Hyperbilirubinemia** occurs due to pre-hepatic hemolytic anemia or hepatic disease associated with lymphosarcoma.
- Increased activities of liver enzymes develop secondary to hepatic lipidosis or hepatic lymphosarcoma.
- **Proteinuria** occurs in some FeLV-infected cats secondary to glomerulonephritis.
- **Malignant lymphocytes** characteristic of FeLV-induced lymphosarcoma are easily identified cytologically, and occasionally are identified in peripheral blood smears and in cerebrospinal fluid.
- Leukemias can be detected in peripheral blood smears and on bone marrow aspirates.

Diagnosis

Detection of FeLV antigens in neutrophils and platelets by IFA or in whole blood, plasma, serum, saliva or tears by ELISA are most commonly used clinically to document infection by FeLV.

Antibody titers to FeLV envelope antigens (neutralizing antibody) and against virus-transformed tumor cells (FOCMA antibody) are available in some research laboratories but clinical use is limited due to poor prognostic value.

Results of IFA and ELISA testing during the dissemination of FeLV are listed under Pathogenesis.

- The **ELISA can detect p27 antigen prior to infection of bone marrow** and release of infected neutrophils and platelets and so can be positive in some cats during early stages of infection or during self-limiting infection even though IFA results are negative.
- **Positive serum test results** occur anywhere between **2 and 30 weeks** (generally 2–8 weeks) after infection.
- Systemic epithelial tissue (including salivary glands and tear glands) infection occurs after bone marrow infection.
- There is generally a delay of 1–2 weeks after the onset of viremia before ELISA tear and saliva tests become positive.
- Since p27 can be detected by ELISA in cats that are developing self-limiting infection, **all cats positive by serum ELISA should have the results confirmed immediately by IFA** or should be **isolated and retested by ELISA in 4–6 weeks.**
- Some ELISA-positive cats that revert to negative have become latently infected; the majority of latently infected cats are negative by ELISA and IFA but the virus can be isolated from the bone marrow.
- **False-positive ELISA** results can develop secondary to poor laboratory technique and are more common with whole blood, tears or saliva than with serum or plasma.
- **False-negative ELISA** using tears or saliva occur during early stages of infection.
- Results of the IFA test are accurate 98% of the time.
- **False-negative IFA** results may occur when leukopenia or thrombocytopenia prevents evaluation of an adequate number of cells.
- **False-positive IFA** results can occur if the blood smears submitted for evaluation are too thick.
- A positive IFA indicates that the cat is viremic and contagious; **viremia will be sustained for life in 90–97% of cats with positive IFA results**.
- Virtually all IFA-positive cats will also be ELISA positive.
- The rare combination of IFA-positive and ELISA-negative results suggests technique-related artifact.
- Negative ELISA results correlate well with negative IFA results and an inability to isolate FeLV.
- Cats that are ELISA-positive and IFA-negative are termed discordant; discordant results are usually due to false-positive ELISA results, false-negative IFA results, or self-limiting infection.
- **Cats that are ELISA-positive and IFA-negative** are probably not contagious at that time, but should be **isolated until retested 4–6 weeks later** since progression to persistent viremia and epithelial cell infection may be occurring.
- There is no reliable means of **identifying local or latent FeLV infections** other than **virus isolation and polymerase chain reaction on bone marrow cells**.
- Positive ELISA or IFA results do not document immunodeficiency or disease induced by FeLV; many seropositive cats have disease manifestations induced by secondary invaders.

Treatment

Antiviral drugs.
- Use of antiviral drugs is controversial.
- Numbers of reported cats is minimal and so definitive statements cannot be made for predicted response. The **primary goal of treatment is to improve quality of life** evidenced by attitude, appetite and physical appearance.
- If used, **zidovudine (AZT)** should be administered at 5 mg/kg bid. Cats should be monitored for development of anemia.
- 9-(2-phosphonoyl-methoxyethyl) adenine **(PMEA)** treated cats have greater therapeutic responses but more adverse effects than AZT-treated cats.

While nothing has been able to consistently clear viremia, immunotherapy may benefit some clinically ill, persistently viremic cats. The practitioner should realize that controlled studies for most are lacking and the following should be considered primarily anecdotal.
- **Interferon-alpha.** Prevents release of budding virons. 30 units (1 ml) PO, once daily or once daily, every other week. 10 000 units/kg, SQ daily for several weeks if life threatened.
- *Staphylococcus* **A.** B lymphocyte and T lymphocyte activation, immune-complex binding, interferon induction, and immunoglobulin Fc binding. 1 ml/kg intraperitoneally, twice weekly for 10 weeks followed by 1 ml/kg intraperitoneally, twice weekly every fourth week for life.

- *Propionibacterium acnes*. Activation of macrophages and natural killer cells. Increased production of interferon, tumor necrosis factor, and interleukin 1. 0.5 ml IV, twice weekly for 2 weeks followed by 0.5 ml IV, weekly for 20 weeks.
- **Acemannan.** Enhanced release of tumor necrosis factor, prostaglandin E_2, and interleukin 1-alpha by macrophages. 2 mg/kg, IP, once weekly for 6 weeks.
- **Pind-orf.** Inactivated parapox ovis virus.

Antibiotics are often indicated **for secondary infections** and should be used at the high end of the dose range for an extended duration.

Supportive care including fluid therapy, appetite stimulants and enteral nutrition supplied via force feeding or nasogastric, pharyngostomy, gastrostomy or jejunostomy tube placement may be indicated.

Blood transfusions, erythropoietin, hematinic agents, vitamin B12, folic acid and anabolic steroids generally have been unsuccessful in the management of the non-regenerative anemia.

Immunosuppressive therapy may be required in the management of hemolytic anemia but has the potential for virus activation.

Prognosis

The **majority of cats (> 80%)** with persistent viremia will **die** of an FeLV-related illness **within 2–3 years**.

Most cats with self-limiting infection will be subclinically affected.

Prevention

Avoid exposure; house cats indoors.

Test and removal of seropositive cats can result in virus-free catteries and multiple-cat households.

Multiple FeLV vaccines have been developed and licensed in the last several years.
- Due to variation in challenge study methodology and the difficulty of assessing preventable fraction of a disease with a relatively low infection rate, long subclinical phase, and multiple field strains, efficacy of individual vaccines continues to be in question.

- Vaccination of cats not previously exposed to FeLV should be considered in cats at high risk (i.e. particularly kittens less than 1 year old in contact with potentially infected cats).
- Owners should be warned of the potential efficacy of less than 100%.
- Cats should be tested for FeLV prior to vaccination.
- Vaccination is not indicated in seropositive cats.
- Vaccination does not induce seropositivity.
- Soft tissue sarcomas develop at the vaccination site in 1:1000 to 1:10 000 cats given adjuvanted vaccines.

Zoonotic aspects

While FeLV will grow in some human cell cultures (with the exception of subgroup A), antigens of FeLV have never been documented in the serum of humans suggesting that this virus is species specific.

Human complement lyses FeLV.

FELINE INFECTIOUS PERITONITIS VIRUS (FIP), FELINE IMMUNODEFICIENCY VIRUS (FIV)**

Classical signs

- Lethargy, anorexia, weight loss.
- +/– fever, pleural or abdominal effusion (FIP).
- +/– CNS, hepatic, renal disease (FIP).
- +/– secondary infections of any organ system (FIV).

See main references page 339, The Thin, Inappetant Cat (FIV), and page 372, The Pyrexic Cat (FIP).

Clinical signs

Anemia is not usually a main presenting sign, and occurs as a consequence of chronic disease. Signs of the agent predominate.

Typically FIP presents as fever, weight loss, anorexia and lethargy. Highly proteinaceous pleural or abdominal effusions may be present, or there may be evidence of hepatic, renal, ocular or CNS disease.

Cats with signs from FIV often have lethargy, anorexia and weight loss associated with secondary infections of the skin, and gastrointestinal or respiratory tracts.

Diagnosis

Diagnosis of FIV is based on the appropriate antibody test, whereas pre-mortem diagnosis of FIP is usually presumptive, unless biopsy samples are available for histological examination.

DRUGS/TOXINS*

Classical signs

- Lethargy, anorexia and depression.
- Other specific signs of the toxin.
- Vomiting and diarrhea are common.

Clinical signs

Usually there is a **history of exposure to the drug or toxin**; grizeofulvin, azathioprine, estrogens, chloramphenicol, some chemotherapeutic agents and non-steroidal anti-inflammatory agents are most common.

Mechanism varies with the toxin. **Bone marrow suppression** (azathioprine, estrogens, chloramphenicol, chemotherapeutic agents) is the mechanism for non-regenerative anemia. Any drug can be protein bound and serve as a hapten for **secondary immune-mediated hemolytic** anemia (see Regenerative anemia). Other drugs and toxins result in bleeding (see Regenerative anemia). **Idiosyncratic reactions** can occur with most drugs or toxins, but each one listed here also is an intrinsic toxin damaging the bone marrow if the toxic dose is exceeded.

Weakness, lethargy, pale mucous membranes, tachycardia and tachypnea may be present due to anemia.

Other clinical findings from the toxin inducing non-regenerative anemia may be present.

Hemorrhage (thrombocytopenia) or **evidence of infections (neutropenia)** may be evident.

Non-steroidal anti-inflammatory agents can cause clinical findings consistent with gastrointestinal bleeding or renal disease.

Diagnosis

Severe normocytic-normochromic, non-regenerative anemia.

Most drugs and toxins damage the bone marrow and so **have concurrent thrombocytopenia** and **neutropenia**.

Since bone marrow damage is present, anemia may be severe.

Bone marrow hypoplasia can be documented by cytologic examination of bone marrow aspirates or histology of core biopsies but these techniques do not prove the cause of damage.

Historical evidence of exposure to a drug or toxin is the best way to determine cause of anemia.

Differential diagnosis

FeLV, myelophthitic disease, ehrlichiosis.

Treatment

Whole blood transfusions are given as needed.

Recombinant erythropoietin can be administered as described for renal failure-associated non-regenerative anemia, but is unlikely to be effective since maximal erythropoietin responses are likely occurring.

Antibiotics may be indicated if fever due to neutropenia is occurring.

MYELOPHTHITIC DISEASES*

Classical signs

- Lethargy, anorexia and depression.

Clinical signs

Abnormalities result from neoplastic infiltration (lymphoma and myeloproliferative neoplasms most common) into the bone marrow inducing loss of normal bone marrow cells.

Findings may be consistent with the primary neoplasia; i.e. masses.

Weakness, tachycardia and pale mucous membranes result from anemia.

Fever or other evidence of secondary infections develop if neutropenia is present

Bleeding results from thrombocytopenia.

Diagnosis

Pancytopenia (aplastic anemia) is most common; pure red cell aplasia is unusual.

Lymphoma, myeloproliferative disease or multiple myeloma are often detected on bone marrow cytology or biopsy.

Circulating malignant cells may be detected.

Differential diagnosis

FeLV, drugs or toxins, ehrlichiosis.

Treatment

Treat the neoplasm primarily.

Supportive care.

EHRLICHIOSIS AND ANAPLASMOSIS

Classical signs

- Lethargy, anorexia, depression and fever.
- Lameness from polyarthritis.
- Pale mucous membranes.

Transmission

It is unknown how clinically ill, naturally exposed cats are infected with an *Ehrlichia canis*-like organism.

Ixodes spp. ticks have been associated with several cases with *Anaplasma phagocytophilum* (previously *E. equi*) infection.

Exposure to arthropods has been reported in about 30% of the cases in the literature.

Pathogenesis

Pathogenesis is unknown, but it is likely similar to dogs based on clinical and laboratory findings.

In dogs, infection may result in either a regenerative or non-regenerative anemia.

Early in infection, acute aplastic anemia occurs because of destruction of progenitor and proliferative cells in the bone marrow. The resulting anemia is usually mild or absent because of the long erythrocyte lifespan.

Secondary immune-mediated anemia may occur.

In the chronic phase of the disease, hemopoietic stem cell injury results in moderate to severe non-regenerative anemia.

Cats experimentally infected with *Neorickettsia risticii* develop **morulae in mononuclear cells** and occasionally develop **fever, depression, lymphadenopathy**, anorexia and diarrhea.

Cats experimentally infected with *A. phagocytophilum* develop **morulae in neutrophils and eosinophils**.

Cases proven by genetic sequencing were *E. canis* (North America and France) or *A. phagocytophilum* (Sweden, Ireland, Denmark and North America).

Ehrlichia-like morula have been detected in mononuclear cells or neutrophils of naturally exposed cats in the United States, Kenya, France, Sweden, Brazil and Thailand.

Other cases have been diagnosed based on the combination of positive *E. canis* or *A. phagocytophilum* serology, clinical or laboratory findings consistent with ehrlichial infection, exclusion of other causes, and response to an anti-rickettsial drug. However, it is unknown whether these cats were ill from the *Ehrlichia* spp. infection.

Clinical signs

Cats are usually **young** and both males and females have been affected.

Cats infected by *A. phagocytophilum* have only been diagnosed in areas with *Ixodes* ticks.

Fever, inappetence, lethargy, **weight loss, hyperesthesia or joint pain**, and **pale mucous membranes** are the most common abnormalities. **Splenomegaly, dyspnea**, uveitis, diarrhea and lymphadenomegaly are also detected in some.

Concurrent diseases are rarely reported but included hemotropic *Mycoplasma* infection and lymphosarcoma.

Anemia was reported for some cats; most are non-regenerative and both cats with known regenerative anemia were infected with a hemotropic *Mycoplasma* spp.

Leukopenia, leukocytosis characterized neutrophilia, lymphocytosis, monocytosis, and intermittent thrombocytopenia can occur.

Thromobocytopenia is the most common abnormality in cats infected by *A. phagocytophilum*.

Hyperglobulinemia was reported for some cats; protein electrophoresis documented polyclonal gammopathy in the cat assayed.

Epidemiologic associations have been made with ocular discharge, **monoclonal gammopathy** or **polyarthritis** in *E. canis* seropositive cats and with outdoor exposure and vomiting in *N. risticii* seropositive cats.

Diagnosis

Morulae appear as clusters of short rods in the cytoplasm of leukocytes.

Determination of species by PCR or culture and electron microscopy.

Presumptive diagnosis based on the combination of positive serologic test results, clinical signs of disease consistent with *Ehrlichia* infection, exclusion of other causes of the disease syndrome, and response to anti-rickettsial drugs.

Some cats with suspected clinical ehrlichiosis had antibodies against *E. canis* and *N. risticii* and some had antibodies against *E. risticii* alone or *E. canis* alone.

Positive serologic test results occur in healthy cats as well as clinically ill cats, and so a diagnosis of clinical ehrlichiosis should not be based on serologic test results alone.

Some cats proven by PCR assay to be infected by an *E. canis* like organism were negative for *E. canis* antibodies.

All cats proven by PCR assay to be infected by *A. phagocytophilum* have also been seropositive.

Differential diagnosis

Infectious, neoplastic, or immune-mediated diseases resulting in fever, polyarthritis and anemia.

Treatment

Clinical improvement after therapy with tetracycline, doxycycline, or imidocarb dipropionate was reported for most cats.

Doxycycline at 10 mg/kg, PO, q 24 h, for a minimum of 4 weeks.

Imidocarb at 5 mg/kg, IM, q 14 days for 2 doses.

Prognosis

Good.

Prevention and zoonotic aspects

Avoid exposure, house cats indoors.

Ehrlichia canis and *A. phagocytophilum* infect people as well as cats. However, transmission is from tick exposure not contact with cats.

If indicated, use tick control on high-risk cats.

IMMUNE-MEDIATED (PURE RED CELL APLASIA)

Classical signs

- Lethargy, anorexia and depression.

Clinical signs

Most cases of pure red cell aplasia are thought to be due to **primary or secondary immune-mediated destruction of red blood cell precursors**.

Lethargy or weakness, pale mucous membranes, and elevated heart and respiration rates occur at rest.

Clinical course may be protracted due to the slow development of anemia.

Diagnosis

Feline leukemia virus infection, drugs and toxins should be excluded.

CBC generally reveals **severe normocytic-normochromic, non-regenerative anemia** with normal neutrophil and platelet numbers.

Bone marrow examination reveals either **maturation arrest or lack of erythroblasts**.

IFA or polymerase chain reaction for FeLV should be performed on bone marrow cells.

Spherocytes, positive direct Coomb's test results and autoagglutination might be present in some affected animals.

Differential diagnosis

FeLV, myelophthitic disease, ehrlichiosis, anemia of chronic disease.

Treatment

Immunosuppressive therapy as described for regenerative hemolytic anemia (see page 533) should be prescribed.

Several blood transfusions may be required; since the bone marrow is involved, response to therapy is more delayed.

Recombinant erythropoietin can be administered as described for renal failure-associated non-regenerative anemia (see page 540), but is unlikely to be effective since maximal erythropoietin responses are likely occurring.

FOLIC ACID ANTAGONISM/DEFICIENCY

> ### Classical signs
> - Lethargy, anorexia and depression.

Clinical signs

Folic acid is required for DNA synthesis, which is important in red blood cell production; **insufficient folic acid** results in **macrocytic anemia as a matura-tion defect**. Mechanisms include folic acid antagonist administration, dietary insufficiency, malabsorption and congenital defect.

History of chronic (> 2 weeks) **administration of folic acid antagonists** including **pyrimethamine** and **sulfa drugs.**

Clinical signs are associated with anemia and those of the disease the antibiotic was being used to treat.

Diarrhea and weight loss may be associated with **malabsorption syndromes**.

The cat may have been fed a **folic acid deficient diet** like **tuna**.

Diagnosis

Macrocytic-hypochromic, or macrocytic-normochromic non-regenerative anemia with nuclear remnants.

Mean corpuscular volume >55 fl.

Neutropenia with hypersegmented neutrophils may be present

History of drug administration.

Bone marrow cytology shows **erythroid hyperplasia** and **megaloblastic changes**.

Serum folate concentrations decreased (normal = 13–38 µg/L) with normal cobalamin concentrations.

Treatment

Stop drug treatment.

Folic acid supplementation at 0.004–0.01 mg/kg/day, PO.

Signs resolve within 3 weeks of supplementation.

IRON DEFICIENCY

> ### Classical signs
> - Lethargy, anorexia and depression.

Clinical signs

Most commonly develops from **chronic loss of blood from the body**.

The most common site of loss is the **gastrointestinal tract**.

Iron is required for the production of hemoglobin; lack of iron leads to **microcytic, hypochromic anemia**.

Melena or hematochezia may or may not be present.

Clinical signs including **vomiting, diarrhea and weight loss** that are associated with gastrointestinal diseases resulting in chronic blood loss.

Gastrointestinal parasites (hookworms) and **fleas** can result in iron deficiency anemia in **kittens**.

Clinical signs of end-stage liver disease or portosystemic shunts including failure to thrive and central nervous system disease.

Melena or hematochezia may or may not be present.

The primary disease generally is chronic and low grade; acute blood loss usually does not result in iron deficiency and thus is usually regenerative.

Diagnosis

Mild to severe microcytic-hypochromic, non-regenerative anemia.

Mean corpuscular volume is generally < 39 fl.

Bone marrow iron stores subjectively are decreased.

Decreased serum iron concentrations and **increased total iron binding capacity**.

Thrombocytosis and occasionally neutrophilia are present from non-specific bone marrow stimulation.

Serum bile acids, ultrasound, contrast studies, scintigraphy and hepatic biopsy can be used to document portosystemic shunts or end-stage liver disease.

Differential diagnosis

Any cause of non-regenerative anemia.

Treatment

Control underlying disease.

Ferrous sulfate 50–100 mg/cat, PO, q 24 hours.

It requires weeks to months to correct iron deficiency since the gastrointestinal transferrin system can only absorb small concentrations of iron daily.

HYPOADRENOCORTICISM

Classical signs
- Weakness, lethargy, anorexia.
- Vomiting or diarrhea.

Clinical signs

Very rare in cats.

Cats are usually presented for evaluation of **depression, lethargy, vomiting, diarrhea and anorexia** (see page 253).

Bradycardia in the face of shock may be present due to hyperkalemia.

Clinical signs of anemia are unusual, because the anemia is mild.

Diagnosis

Normocytic-normochromic, non-regenerative anemia usually with a PCV of 15–27.

ACTH stimulation to document hypoadrenocorticism.

Treatment

Treatment of shock and hyperkalemia acutely.

Glucocorticoid and mineralocorticoid supplementation (see page 254).

HYPOTHYROIDISM

Classical signs
- Lethargy, weight gain.
- Poor coat, seborrhea sicca, slow hair regrowth after clipping.

Clinical signs

Extremely rare cause of anemia post-thyroidectomy or I[131] treatment.

Most cats maintain enough thyroid function and never become anemic.

Obesity, lethargy and pale mucous membranes.

Poor coat, seborrhea sicca, slow hair regrowth after clipping and thick skin.

Decreased total and free T4 concentrations after treatment for hyperthyroidism.

Diagnosis

Normocytic-normochromic, non-regenerative anemia usually with a PCV of 15–27.

Treatment

Levothyroxine supplementation (see page 1354).

RECOMMENDED READING

Breitschwert EB, Abrams-Ogg AC, Lappin MR, et al. Molecular evidence supporting *Ehrlichia canis*-like infection in cats. J Vet Intern Med 2002; 16: 642–649.

Couto CG. Disorders of hemostatis. In: Couto G, Nelson R (eds) Small Animal Internal Medicine. Mosby, St. Louis, MO, 1998, pp. 1192–1206.

Foley JE, Harrus S, Poland A, et al. Molecular, clinical, and pathologic comparison of two distinct strains of *Haemobartonella felis* in domestic cats. Am J Vet Res 1998; 59: 1581–1588.

Jensen WA, Lappin MR, Kamkar S, Reagan, W. Use of a polymerase chain reaction assay to detect and differentiate two strains of *Haemobartonella felis* in naturally infected cats. Am J Vet Res 2001; 62: 604–608.

Lappin MR. Infectious diseases section. In: Couto G, Nelson R (eds) Small Animal Internal Medicine. Mosby, St. Louis, MO, 1998, pp. 1239–1337.

Neer TM, Breitschwerdt EB, Greene RT, et al. Consensus statement of ehrlichial disease of small animals from the infectious disease study group of the ACVIM. J Vet Int Med 2002; 16: 309–315.

Stubbs CJ, Holland CJ, Reif JS, et al. Feline ehrlichiosis; literature review and serologic survey. Comp Cont Ed Pract Vet 2000; 22: 307–317.

Tasker S, Lappin MR. *Haemobartonella felis*: recent developments in diagnosis and treatment. J Fel Med Surg 2002; 4: 3–11.

Tasker S, Binns SH, Day M J, et al. Use of a PCR assay to assess prevalence and risk factors for *Mycoplasma haemofelis* and *Candidatus* Mycoplasma haemominutum in cats in the United Kingdom. Vet Record 2003; 152: 193–198.

25. The cat with polycythemia

Jacquie Rand and Annette Litster

KEY SIGNS

- Increased red cell concentration in peripheral blood.
- Injected mucous membranes.

MECHANISM?

- Dehydration resulting from disease of many organs may produce relative polycythemia. Polycythemia may be an appropriate physiological response to hypoxia caused by pulmonary or cardiac disease. Alternatively, inappropriate polycythemia may be associated with renal space-occupying masses or other visceral tumors. Inappropriate primary polycythemia results from a rare myeloproliferative disorder, polycythemia vera.

WHERE?

- Gastrointestinal tract, renal or skin (burns) disease causing excessive fluid loss.
- Cardiac or respiratory disease causing chronic hypoxia.
- Renal (space-occupying masses) or visceral (neoplastic conditions) conditions associated with inappropriate erythropoietin secretion.
  Bone marrow associated with myeloproliferative disease.

WHAT?

- The most common cause of polycythemia is dehydration. Hyperthyroidism produces mild polycythemia in many cats. Appropriate polycythemia associated with hypoxia from chronic respiratory or cardiac disease is less common. Primary or secondary inappropriate polycythemia is very rare.

QUICK REFERENCE SUMMARY

Diseases causing polycythemia

DEGENERATIVE

- **Cardiac disease* (p 561)**
  Cardiac conditions such as cardiomyopathy which result in tissue hypoxia or cyanosis from cardiac failure may stimulate increased erythropoietin production, resulting in increased red

blood cell mass. Clinical signs may include dyspnea, lethargy, weakness, a gallop rhythm, heart murmur and arrhythmia. Mucous membranes may be pale or cyanotic with prolonged capillary refill time.

ANOMALY

● Congenital heart disease* (p 561)

Congenital cardiac anomalies associated with right to left shunting, e.g. tetralogy of Fallot, reverse patent ductus arteriosus, and atrial or ventricular septal defects may cause secondary polycythemia in young cats. There may be a history of lethargy and stunted growth, and on clinical examination, dyspnea, cyanosis and a heart murmur may be noted. PCV is often markedly elevated (> 60%).

● Renal space-occupying mass

Renal conditions such as renal cysts and hydronephrosis have been associated with inappropriate erythrocytosis secondary to increased erythropoietin production, but these are very rare. Kidneys are unilaterally or bilaterally enlarged on abdominal palpation, and there may be associated clinical signs of renal disease such as polyuria and polydipsia.

NEOPLASTIC

● Polycythemia vera*(p 563)

Primary polycythemia is caused by a myeloproliferative disorder, similar to polycythemia vera in humans. There may be a history of bleeding, seizures, polydipsia and polyuria, and physical examination reveals dark pink mucosa with a PCV often exceeding 60%. Circulating erythropoietin levels are normal or low. This condition is very rare in cats.

● Neoplasia (p 565)

Neoplasia of a wide variety of organs including the kidneys, liver, adrenal gland, female reproductive tract and central nervous system have been associated with inappropriate polycythemia. The condition is characterized by increased circulating erythropoietin levels without a hypoxic stimulus. Impaired renal blood flow secondary to a space-occupying mass, or tumor secretion of erythropoietin or erythropoietin-like substances have been hypothesized as possible causes of erythrocytosis. Clinical signs relate to the type of tumor involved and its anatomical location.

METABOLIC

● Dehydration*** (p 557)

Derangement of fluid balance from a variety of causes is the most common cause of polycythemia in cats. Polycythemia occurs most commonly when **excessive fluid loss** through the gastrointestinal tract **(vomiting or diarrhea)** or kidney **(diabetes mellitus or renal failure)** is coupled with **inadequate fluid intake**. Typically there is depression and anorexia, and signs that relate to the underlying condition such as polyuria, polydipsia, vomiting or diarrhea. Skin tents on pinching, mucous membranes are dry, and may have delayed refill. Accompanying laboratory abnormalities include increased total protein, increased urine specific gravity and pre-renal azotemia.

continued

continued

● **Hyperthyroidism** (p 560)**

Hyperthyroidism may be associated with a mild increase in PCV, possibly from a direct effect of thyroxine on erythrocyte precursors. Affected cats are usually older (> 8 years), with a history of weight loss despite a robust appetite. Associated clinical signs include irritable behavior, tachycardia, sometimes with a gallop rhythm, polyuria, polydipsia and often chronic vomiting.

● **Severe obesity (Pickwickian syndrome) (p 568)**

Morbid obesity may predispose to tissue hypoxia from inadequate alveolar ventilation because of fat accumulation in the thorax and compression of upper airways. Blood O_2 saturation levels are low (<92%) and there are slightly to markedly increased circulating levels of erythropoietin.

PHYSICAL

● High altitude (p 568)

Decreased O_2 levels in the atmosphere at high altitudes may stimulate increased renal erythropoietin production in response to tissue hypoxia. The cat is otherwise clinically normal, although there may be mild dyspnea with a fast, shallow respiratory pattern. Circulating erythropoietin levels are elevated.

PSYCHOLOGIC

● Stress-induced splenic contraction (p 567)

The stress response in cats may include splenic contraction, with a resultant infusion of stored splenic erythrocytes into the circulation. Affected cats usually have an appropriate history and may have other accompanying signs such as dilated pupils and behavioral changes. Hemoconcentration caused by stress is usually mild and transient.

IATROGENIC

● Excessive blood transfusion or overdose of exogenous erythropoietin (p 564)

This is a potential, although previously unreported, cause of polycythemia. The diagnosis is made with an appropriate history and clinical signs of erythrocytosis such as weakness, injected mucous membranes and neurological signs.

IMMUNE

● Acute systemic anaphylaxis (p 566)

Acute systemic anaphylaxis results from an extremely rapid and overwhelming immune reaction to a foreign antigen. It may cause hemoconcentration, most likely from a combination of fluid loss caused by increased vascular permeability, and splenic contraction in response to acute shock. There should be a history of exposure to a foreign antigen, usually protein. Anaphylaxis may occur on the first exposure to the inciting antigen. Clinical signs include acute dyspnea, collapse, pale mucus membranes and other signs of hypotensive shock.

INFLAMMATION

● **Chronic pulmonary disease* (p 562)**

Chronic pulmonary disease such as feline asthma/bronchitis complex may cause tissue hypoxia, resulting in increased erythropoietin production and erythrocytosis. There is usually a history of chronic coughing, with dyspnea and lethargy in more severe cases. Clinical signs include crackles and wheezes on thoracic auscultation.

INTRODUCTION

MECHANISM?

Increased red cell concentration may result from a **relative or absolute** increase in erythrocytes.

A relative increase in red blood cells is caused by **dehydration.** In dehydration, a reduction in plasma volume causes hemoconcentration, resulting in erythrocytosis and increased total plasma protein concentration. Blood oxygen saturation levels are normal.

Transient absolute polycythemia may occur with excitement when **splenic contraction** releases red cells into circulation.

Absolute polycythemia may be an appropriate physiological response to **chronic hypoxia** from cardiac or pulmonary disease, and is mediated by increased serum erythropoietin levels.

- Signs relate to the **underlying cardiac cause** and include a cardiac murmur and cyanosis consistent with right to left shunting of blood causing hypoxia, e.g. tetralogy of Fallot, atrial or ventriclar septal defect (ASD or VSD).
- Clinical signs of **chronic primary lung pathology** include coughing, dyspnea, wheezes and crackles, which accompany generalized hypoxia in more severe cases.

Alternatively, **absolute polycythemia** may be caused by **increased, but physiologically inappropriate, erythropoietin secretion**, associated with a variety of **neoplastic conditions or space-occupying renal masses**. In these cases, blood oxygen saturation levels are normal.

- **Secondary causes of inappropriate polycythemia** include **visceral tumors** involving the kidneys, liver, adrenal gland, female reproductive tract and central nervous system. These occasionally secrete erythropoietin or an erythropoietin-like substance **without a hypoxic stimulus.** While these tumors have been reported to cause polycythemia in humans and dogs, they are yet to be reported as a cause of polycythemia in the cat.
  - Clinical signs are expected to relate to the type of tumor involved, its anatomical location, and the polycythemia.

- **Space-occupying renal masses** including neoplasia, cysts or hydronephrosis may impair renal blood flow and stimulate secretion of inappropriate concentrations of erythropoietin.
  - Polycythemia from a **renal space-occupying mass** is sometimes accompanied by signs of renal failure, such as polydipsia/polyuria, reduced urine specific gravity and azotemia.

Primary inappropriate polycythemia is called polycythemia vera, and is a neoplastic proliferation of erythroid cells, associated with low or **undetectable erythropoietin concentrations**. Typically **PCV is greater than 60–65%.**

Once the PCV exceeds 65%, the ensuing **hyperviscosity increases peripheral resistance, decreases cardiac output and decreases oxygen transport to the tissues**. Increased blood volume distends vessels and together with sluggish flow, **predisposes to thrombosis and vessel rupture**. It is hypothesized that erythrocytosis impairs renal tubular concentrating mechanisms, resulting in polyuria and polydipsia.

Clinically, polycythemia causes **injected mucous membranes, torturous retinal blood vessels**, and there may be a history of **intermittent bleeding diatheses**.

Insufficient vascular perfusion of the central nervous system may result in **neurological signs such as seizures, ataxia, abnormal behavior and/or blindness**.

WHERE?

Relative polycythemia may result from **gastrointestinal or renal disease,** and rarely from extensive **skin burns** which cause excessive fluid loss, or **severe disease of any organ** sufficient to cause marked lethargy and inadequate fluid intake.

Absolute polycythemia from a physiological increase in erythropoietin concentration may result from **cardiac or pulmonary disease.**

Absolute polycythemia from a pathological increase in erythropoietin concentration may result from space-occupying **renal disease or neoplasia of a wide variety of organs.**

Primary absolute polycythemia is the result of a myelodysplastic condition of the **bone marrow.**

WHAT?

The **most common cause** of polycythemia is **dehydration. Hyperthyroidism,** acquired cardiac disease such as **cardiomyopathy,** and respiratory disease including **feline asthma/bronchitis complex** are less common causes of polycythemia. Renal cysts and hydronephrosis are rare causes of polycythemia in cats. All other causes of polycythemia are uncommon, with **congenital cardiac disease** the most common cause of severe polycythemia. **Polycythemia vera** and neoplasia secreting erythropoietin-like products are very rare causes of severe polycythemia in cats.

DIAGNOSIS

Relative polycythemia from dehydration should be suspected if **plasma protein is elevated** and there is **clinical evidence of dehydration.**
- **PCV is usually ≤ 60%.**
- Treatment with fluids normalizes PCV and plasma protein concentration.

Cats that are very stressed at the time blood is collected may have **transient polycythemia.**
- **PCV** is usually ≤ 60 and polycythemia is **mild and transient.**

Absolute polycythemia should be suspected **if plasma protein is normal** and there is **no evidence of dehydration,** in an **unstressed** cat.

Appropriate polycythemia (in response to hypoxia) is differentiated from inappropriate polycythemia by measurement of **oxygen saturation** of arterial blood.
- **Appropriate polycythemia** is likely **if arterial oxygen saturation is less than 92%** (normal ≥ 97%).
- **Cardiac and pulmonary systems should be examined** initially using auscultation and thoracic radiographs, and if indicated, by echocardiography and electrocardiography.

Inappropriate polycythemia should be suspected if **arterial oxygen saturation is normal.**

Secondary causes of inappropriate polycythemia include visceral tumors or a space-occupying renal mass such as neoplasia, cyst or hydronephrosis. These should be investigated using renal palpation, abdominal radiographs, abdominal ultrasonography and/or intravenous pyelogram.

Serum erythropoietin assay helps differentiate secondary from primary inappropriate polycythemia. However, accurate measurement of feline erythropoietin is compromised by the **lack of an assay technique validated for use in cats**. A human ELISA assay technique has been successfully used to detect erythropoietin in cat serum and is available through Dr Urs Giger at the University of Pennsylvania.

Serum erythropoietin concentrations are normal or increased in most cases of **secondary inappropriate polycythemia.**

Primary polycythemia (polycythemia vera) is likely if **PCV > 60–65%** and there is **no evidence of dehydration, hypoxia, cardiac or pulmonary disease, neoplasia or a space-occupying renal lesion**.
- **Erythropoietin** is low or **undetectable** in **primary polycythemia**.
- Primary polycythemia may be accompanied by **leukocytosis and thrombocytosis**.
- Bone marrow typically has increased cellularity, with erythroid hyperplasia or panhyperplasia, normal maturation within the erythroid line, and **normal morphology of cells**.

TREATMENT

In relative polycythemia, intravenous or subcutaneous balanced electrolyte solutions should be administered to correct dehydration.

Primary polycythemia vera can be treated by a combination of regular, intermittent phlebotomy and fluid therapy. More severe cases may require **adjunct chemotherapy with hydroxyurea.**

In secondary polycythemia (appropriate or inappropriate), the underlying disease must be diagnosed and treated, and symptomatic therapy with phlebotomy and fluid therapy should be provided to manage the erythrocytosis.

DISEASES CAUSING POLYCYTHEMIA

DEHYDRATION***

> **Classical signs**
>
> - Skin tenting.
> - Tacky mucus membranes.
> - Combination of increased PCV and plasma protein concentration.
> - Signs attributable to underlying disease.

Pathogenesis

A relative increase in red cells occurs as a result of **dehydration**. The increase in red cell concentration is secondary to decreased plasma volume from dehydration. **Total red cell mass is normal,** although red cell mass can only be determined using radio-isotope-tagged autologous red blood cells, a technique not generally available in practice.

Relative polycythemia occurs most commonly when **excessive fluid loss** through the gastrointestinal tract (**vomiting or diarrhoea**) or kidney (**diabetes mellitus or renal failure**) is coupled with **inadequate fluid intake**.

Clinical signs

Clinical signs of dehydration include **skin tenting, tacky mucus membranes and high plasma protein levels**.

- Dehydration is assessed initially by examining **skin turgor,** usually by drawing the skin at the back of the neck upward.
  - It is not until there is **5% dehydration** that there is **subtle loss of skin elasticity**.
  - At **6–8% dehydration**, there is a **delay in return of the skin to its normal position**, the capillary refill time may be slightly prolonged, and mucous membranes may be dry to touch.
  - At **10–12% dehydration**, tented skin stands in place; mucus membranes are dry; the eyes are sunken in the orbits; there is prolonged capillary refill time; and there may be signs of shock.
  - By **12–15% dehydration**, signs of shock are present and death is imminent.

Accompanying clinical signs are attributable to the **cause of the dehydration. Renal and gastrointestinal tract fluid losses** are common causes of dehydration, and present with **polyuria and polydipsia,** or **vomiting and diarrhea**, respectively, coupled with inadequate fluid intake.

Massive fluid deficits can occur after **burns** because of fluid losses from the skin.

Acute viral respiratory disease can cause dehydration because of **losses from ocular and nasal discharges and hypersalivation.**

Diagnosis

Characteristic clinical signs of dehydration are accompanied by **hemoconcentration, normal blood oxygen saturation and increased total plasma protein concentration**.

Differential diagnosis

Since clinical signs of dehydration are characteristic, **differential diagnoses mainly refer to the condition causing the dehydration**, rather than to dehydration itself.

Treatment

Fluid and electrolyte therapy is initially required to **restore intravascular volume** because this is most critical for survival, and then to **replace fluid and electrolytes in the extravascular compartments** including both intracellular and interstitial fluid. Many patients that are dehydrated have adequate circulating blood volume to maintain tissue perfusion, and do not need rapid volume expansion.

Of total body water, **2/3 is intracellular** and **1/3 is extracellular**. Only about **1/6 of body water is intravascular.**

- **Sodium and chloride** are the major electrolytes in the **extracellular fluid**.
- **Potassium and phosphates** are the major electrolytes in **intracellular fluid**.

Type of fluid selected should be based on the **electrolyte and acid–base status** of the cat, and whether it is being used for replacement or maintenance.

Crystalloids are the most common types of fluids used, and have sodium as their major osmotically active particle. Sodium and water rapidly traverse semipermeable membranes such as the endothelium, and **only 20–33% remains in the vascular space 30 min after administration.**

- **Crystalloids** may be **balanced** and have a similar electrolyte composition and osmolality to normal plasma (e.g. lactated Ringer's solution, Plasma-lyte A or Normisol-R), or **unbalanced**. Unbalanced fluids (eg. 0.9% NaCl, 5% dextrose in water) are used to correct specific deficits in plasma electrolyte concentrations or water, and should be chosen only after serum electrolyte concentrations have been determined.

- Fluids may also be classified as **replacement fluids**, provided to correct electrolyte or pH imbalances, or **maintenance fluids**, which are restricted in sodium, contain additional potassium and are **hypotonic** when administered or after metabolism of dextrose, e.g. Plasma-Lyte 56, Normosol M, 0.45% NaCl with added potassium, or 0.45% NaCl with 2.5% dextrose and added potassium, Plasma-Lyte 56 with 5% dextrose, and Normisol-M with 5% dextrose.

Metabolic acidosis is the most common acid–base disorder, and is usually corrected with volume expansion, correcting the underlying disease, and using fluids with an alkalizing effect. Where there is **severe metabolic acidosis or hepatic failure**, $NaHCO_3$ may need to be added to the IV fluid infusion.

- **Fluids containing lactate or buffers metabolized to lactate** (acetate and gluconate) are alkalizing, because lactate is metabolized to bicarbonate by the liver, which makes it suitable for the treatment of metabolic acidosis.
  - **Lactated Ringer's solution** is buffered by lactate.
  - **Plasma-Lyte and Normosol** are buffered by acetate and gluconate.

Metabolic alkalosis is usually corrected once chloride deficits are corrected. Metabolic alkalosis occurs as a result of **chloride depletion and dehydration**, because to maintain intravascular volume, the renal tubules reabsorb bicarbonate along with sodium instead of the depleted chloride.

- **Normal saline** is unbuffered and has an acidifying effect.

Hypotonic fluids should be used when there are free water deficits or when serum sodium is elevated.

- **Hypotonic fluids** include 5% dextrose in water and 0.45% sodium chloride with 2.5% dextrose. These fluids have similar osmolalities to plasma prior to administration, but once administered the dextrose is metabolized and the remaining fluid becomes hypotonic.

- Five percent dextrose in water is useful as a carrier fluid for administration of drugs and does not add extra electrolytes to the cat. For example, it can be used as a constant rate infusion (CRI). Drugs such as metoclopramide or morphine may be administered as a constant rate infusion (CRI) in 5% dextrose in water.

Hypertonic fluids result in rapid volume expansion because the high sodium concentration (e.g. 7.5% NaCl) or dextrose (**10% dextrose**) attracts water from the extravascular compartments, and small volumes (3–5 ml/kg) can be administered. However, the effect is short term (~30 min), and they should be administered with additional crystalloids, with or without colloids. Administer the dose slowly IV over 5–10 minutes. Hypertonic saline is most useful in cats that require small volume resuscitation, for example after head trauma or pulmonary contusions. It can be combined with colloids such as Hetastarch.

- **Hypertonic saline** causes volume expansion equivalent to colloids, but at 1/4 the volume administered.

- **Dose is** 3–5 ml/kg of 7.5% NaCl administered slowly IV over 5–10 minutes.

Colloids contain osmotically active particles that are too large to cross vessel walls, and most of the infused volume remains in circulation. **Colloids** are indicated for **rapid restoration of circulating fluid volume** and to **slow loss of fluid from the intravascular space**.

- The addition of **colloids** to the fluid therapy regimen may also be appropriate where losses are ongoing from the intravascular space, such as with burns, acute shock, systemic inflammatory response syndrome (SIRS), sepsis or acute systemic anaphylaxis. Commercially available hetastarch solution may be used for up to 30% of the maintenance IV fluid requirements in severe cases while losses are ongoing.

- In general, when administering **colloids, divide the dose into four aliquots and administer slowly IV over 10–15 minutes. Recheck the cat** after each aliquot, carefully evaluating the lungs for signs of

pulmonary edema. Use a **syringe pump or infusion pump** because cats are very sensitive to the volume expansion effects of colloids, and manual administration increases the risk of adverse effects such as pulmonary edema. Hypothermic cats are particularly sensitive to colloids, and administering hypertonic saline or colloids to cats with undiagnosed and asymptomatic hypertrophic cardiomyopathy may precipitate pulmonary edema.

Colloid solutions include **dextran, hydroxyethyl starch** (HES) and hemoglobin-based oxygen-carrying solutions such as **Oxyglobin®**. They are contraindicated for use in very dehydrated, oligouric patients because the possibility of renal damage is increased. The fluid attracted intravascularly comes from within cells, exacerbating intracellular dehydration.

- **Colloid osmostic pressure** (COP) and volume-expanding capacity varies with the colloid as follows:
- 6% hetastarch has a COP of 30 mmHg, and expands the volume by 1–1.3 ml per ml of colloid infused, and stays in the vascular space for 12–48 h.
- 10% dextran 40 has a COP of 40 and expands the volume by 1–1.5 ml per ml of colloid infused, and stays in the vascular space for 4–8 h.
- 6% dextran 70 has a COP of 40 and expands the volume by 0.8 ml per ml of colloid infused, and stays in the vascular space for 4–8 h.
- **Dextran** is made from high-molecular-weight linear glucose polymers produced by bacteria, and is available as Dextran 40 and 70, but Dextran 40 is rarely used in veterinary medicine because of its association with acute renal failure. The dose rate is 5–10 ml/kg, beginning with the lower dose.
- **Hydroxyethyl starch** is composed primarily of amylopectin, and is a branched polysaccharide closely resembling glycogen. It is available as Hetastarch and Pentastarch. The standard dose rate is 10–15 ml/kg/day, but administer 2–5 ml/kg initially and re-evaluate the cat.
- **Oxyglobin®** is used primarily for its oxygen-carrying capacity, but can be used for its colloidal effect. However it is expensive to use solely for volume expansion. The COP of Oxyglobin is 37 mmHg, thus, it has slightly more colloidal pull than Hetastarch, and retains oxygen-carrying capacity for up to 40 h. The dose rate in cats is 1–2 ml/kg/h with a total dose of 15 ml/kg.

- **Haemaccel®** is a colloid solution available in Europe and Australasia that is comprised of 3.5% polygeline, a gelatin-based colloid.

To achieve a very rapid increase in intravascular volume using low volumes of infused fluids, **colloids and hypertonic saline** can be combined. Replacement or maintenance crystalloids are administered concurrently to maintain or replenish interstitial and intracellular fluid levels, and are administered at 50% of the volume that would be required if they were used alone. Examples of combinations used are:

- Combine 1.3 ml/kg of 23.4% NaCl with 2.7 ml/kg of 6% hetastarch, and administer slowly over 10–15 minutes. Mixing the solutions together results in a 7.5% NaCl solution.
- 20% NaCl at 1.5 ml/kg combined with Dextran 70 at 3 ml/kg and administer slowly over 10–15 minutes. Mixing results in approximately 7% NaCl.

Plasma can be used as a colloid, but it is best used when there is a specific indication such as pancreatitis or a coagulation disturbance. It is not the preferred method of replacing albumin or improving the oncotic pressure, because the volume of plasma required to measurably increase serum albumin concentration is very large. However, it can be used as a component of fluid therapy to help increase plasma oncotic pressure in a hypoproteinemic cat, and to decrease the tendency for loss of intravascular fluid. Plasma can be administered at 20 ml/kg over 4 h in place of 1/3 of the calculated crystalloid fluid volume to be administered.

The **intravenous route of fluid administration** is preferred for correction of severe dehydration, major electrolyte and acid–base imbalances, and shock. While the jugular, cephalic, femoral and saphenous veins are available for IV catheter placement, the cephalic vein is the site of choice as the catheter is most readily secured at that site and less commonly soiled with urine and feces than in caudal limb sites.

Fluid rates administered depend on the requirement of the animal.

If the cat has insufficient plasma volume to maintain tissue perfusion, intravascular volume must be restored rapidly.

- **Inadequate tissue perfusion is indicated by**:
  - Tachycardia and tachypnea, and sometimes bradycardia.

- Pale mucus membranes and increased capillary refill time (> 2 s).
- Cold extremities.
- Anuria or oliguria (<1 ml/kg/h urine produced).
- Decreased central venous pressure (< 5 cmH$_2$O).
- **Inadequate interstitial hydration** is evident as tacky mucus membranes, skin tenting and sunken eyes.

Crystalloids can be used alone, but colloids and hypertonic saline result in much more rapid restoration of normal perfusion, because only small volumes need to be administered (3–5 ml/kg), and they act immediately to attract water into the vascular space.

- When **tissue perfusion is inadequate**, for example from **severe dehydration or shock**, crytalloids administered alone can be infused at **40–55 ml/kg/h** for a total dose of 45–60 ml/kg to **restore circulating intravascular volume**. This volume should be reduced by 40–60% if colloids are administered together with crytalloids.
  - In general, the patient should be reassessed after 1/4 to 1/3 is administered or after 15 min, because IV fluids administered too rapidly can cause pulmonary edema. Intravascular volume is usually restored over the first 2 hours.
- If the electrolyte status of the patient is unknown, use a crystalloid most like plasma in sodium and potassium content, pH and osmolality, such as **lactated Ringer's**, **Normosol-R or Plasma-Lyte A**. These have an alkalizing effect which is useful because patients with reduced circulating blood volume are usually acidotic. 0.9% NaCl can also be used.

For hemodynamically stable patients with dehydration, fluid deficits are corrected over the first 12–24 hours, followed by maintenance fluid rates. Maintenance rates of **70 ml/kg/day (3 ml/kg/h)** are calculated, and the dehydration fluid deficit is added to the maintenance figure. Dehydration fluid deficit is calculated by the following formula: % dehydration × body weight (kg) = fluid deficit (liters).

- For example, a 5 kg cat that is 10% dehydrated requires 500 ml (0.1 × 5 L) to correct the fluid deficit and 350 ml (70 × 5 ml) for maintenance, which is 850 ml in the first 24 h, or 35 ml/h or 0.59 ml/min. Using a microdrip set with 60 drops per ml, the infusion rate is 35 drops per minute (0.59 ml × 60 drops/ml), or just over one every 2 seconds. This rate may be increased in the first 4–6 h to correct the fluid deficit more rapidly.

- Replacement fluids include **lactated Ringer's, Normosol-R or Plasma-Lyte A.**

If ongoing maintenance fluids are required over several days because fluid intake is inadequate or there are continuing fluid losses, change to a **maintenance fluid** that resembles the amount of free water and electrolytes that would be consumed daily and are being lost. Maintenance solutions are hypotonic crystalloids that are lower in sodium and chloride but higher in potassium concentration than plasma, such as Plasma-Lyte 56, Normosol M, 0.45% NaCl with added potassium, or 0.45% NaCl with 2.5% dextrose and added potassium.

- Maintenance fluid rates are **70 ml/kg/day,** but if there are **ongoing fluid losses from polyuria, diarrhea or vomiting,** then calculate an additional **5%/kg requirement** (or 50 ml/kg/day), which is nearly equivalent to doubling the daily maintenance rate. **Fever** can increase fluid requirements by 15–20 ml/kg/day.

Potassium is usually added to fluids at the following rates, and the infusion rate of the fluid is adjusted so the rate does not exceed 0.5 mmol (mEq)/kg/h.

Serum potassium concentration (mmol or mEq/L)	Potassium supplementation to 1 L of IV fluids
>3.5	20 mEq
30 mEq	3.0–3.5
40 mEq	2.5–3.0
60 mEq	2.0–2.5
80 mEq	< 2.0

Prognosis

The prognosis ultimately depends on the **inciting condition**, but acute dehydration treated with prompt and vigorous fluid therapy has an excellent prognosis.

HYPERTHYROIDISM**

Classical signs

- Weight loss despite polyphagia.
- Polyuria/polydipsia.
- Tachycardia, sometimes with a gallop rhythm.
- Mild erythrocytosis in some cases.

See main reference The thin cat (or cat with weight loss) and a good appetite on page 304 for details.

Pathogenesis

Many hyperthyroid cats have **mild increases in PCV**, which are thought to be a **direct effect of thyroid hormone stimulating red cell precursors. Erythropoietin production** may also be increased in hyperthyroidism, because of the increased metabolic rate.

Clinical signs

There is usually a history of **weight loss despite polyphagia**.

Cats are often **hyperexcitable** and the **coat is often unkempt** from poor grooming.

Vomiting and polyuria/polydipsia occur in about one third of cats.

On physical examination, there may be **palpable thyroid nodules, and tachycardia or a heart murmur** on cardiac auscultation.

Diagnosis

Serum total thyroxine (T$_4$) is usually increased, unless there is an accompanying medical condition that may suppress total T$_4$ to the upper half of the reference range (**"sick euthyroid syndrome"**). In these cases, a diagnosis of hyperthyroidism can be made by detection of **increased serum free T$_4$** or by a triiodothyroxinine (T$_3$) suppression test.

Differential diagnosis

Other causes of **mild absolute erythrocytosis with normal blood O$_2$ saturation**, such as **stress-induced splenic contraction**, must be differentiated from erythrocytosis associated with hyperthyroidism.
- Demonstration of increased thyroxine is diagnostic for hyperthyroidism, although stress-induced splenic contraction could occur concurrently and compound the mild polycythemia.

Treatment

The treatment of choice for hyperthyroidism is **radioactive I^{131} therapy** where available.

Hyperthyroidism is commonly treated with oral daily **methimazole**, which is generally continued for the life of the cat.

Surgical treatment by unilateral or bilateral thyroidectomy may be recommended if the cat has acceptable anesthetic risk factors. Careful surgical technique is necessary to avoid **post-operative hypoparathyroidism** and life threatening hypocalcemia.

Adjunctive treatment with beta-blockers or other hypotensive agents may be necessary to manage the **cardiovascular complications** of hyperthyroidism.

Prognosis

The prognosis for successful management of hyperthyroidism is generally **very good provided associated complicating factors such as thyrotoxic heart disease are well controlled**.

CARDIAC DISEASE INCLUDING CONGENITAL DISEASE*

> ### Classical signs
>
> - Abnormal cardiac rhythm or rate, often accompanied by a cardiac murmur.
> - Blood O$_2$ saturation is reduced (<92%).
> - Advanced cases may present with acute dyspnea.
> - Usually cardiomegaly on thoracic radiography.

See main references The Cat With Abnormal Heart Sounds and/or an Enlarged Heart and The Cat With Tachycardia, Bradycardia, or an Irregular Rhythm on pages 140, 157 for details.

Pathogenesis

Cardiac failure causes **chronic hypoxia, stimulating increased secretion of erythropoietin, resulting in polycythemia**.

The most dramatic increases in PCV occur in young cats with **congenital heart disease with right to left shunting** (e.g. tetralogy of Fallot, reverse patent ductus arteriosus, atrial or ventricular septal defects), but appropriate secondary polycythemia may also occur with **left-sided or biventricular congestive heart failure**, as occurs with cardiomyopathy.

Clinical signs

Feline cardiac disease **usually presents at an advanced stage**, with dyspnea and hypoxia (oxygen saturation <92%).

There may be **open-mouth breathing and cyanosis**.

Mucosae are dark pink, or purple if the polycythemia is caused by hypoxia from right to left shunting of blood in the heart or lungs.

Tachycardia and arrhythmia may be detected on cardiac auscultation, with accompanying **crackles and wheezes** on thoracic auscultation from pleural effusion and/or pulmonary edema.

Congenital cardiac disease often causes **stunted growth** in comparison with littermates.

Diagnosis

Initial diagnosis may be made on **auscultatory abnormalities**, together with other signs of cardiac failure such as **dyspnea and hypertension**.

Thoracic radiology reveals **cardiomegaly** with or without **pulmonary edema** and/or **pleural effusion**.

Cardiac chamber abnormalities, abnormal wall thicknesses and/or pressure or flow irregularities may be detected using **echocardiology**.

ECG abnormalities may be detected, although this is not as common in cats as in dogs.

Differential diagnosis

Other causes of chronic hypoxia, such as **pulmonary disease**, should be differentiated from hypoxia from congenital or degenerative cardiac disease.

Treatment

Treatment of cardiac conditions is dependent on **correct diagnosis of the cause of cardiac failure**.

Medical therapy is instituted to treat the **physiological effects of cardiac failure**. This may include treatment for hypertension, cardiac rate disturbances, arrhythmia, pulmonary edema and/or pleural effusion. See The Cat With Abnormal Heart Sounds and/or an Enlarged Heart and The Cat With Tachycardia, Bradycardia, or an Irregular Rhythm on pages 124, 157 for treatment details.

Hypoxia in tetralogy of Fallot is decreased when the condition is treated by **aortic banding**, which reduces right-to-left blood flow.

Hematocrit should be reduced to 45% before surgery is performed to treat any underlying conditions, to decrease the risk of thromboembolism during surgery. This is achieved by performing phlebotomy and administering intravenous fluids.

Prognosis

The prognosis for feline cardiac disease is guarded and may be poor if the disease is initially diagnosed at an advanced stage.

CHRONIC PULMONARY DISEASE*

Classical signs

- ± History of chronic coughing.
- Dyspnea may be acute, chronic or intermittent.
- Cyanosis and open-mouth breathing in severe cases.
- Crackles, wheezes and sometimes muffled cardiac sounds.

See main references The Cat With Stridor (page 32), The Dyspneic or Tachypneic Cat (page 47), The Cat With Hydrothorax (page 71) and The Coughing Cat (page 90) for details.

Pathogenesis

Respiratory disease causes **chronic hypoxia**, stimulating increased **secretion of erythropoietin** and resulting in **polycythemia**.

The most common cause of chronic pulmonary disease in cats is feline asthma/feline bronchitis complex, which is an idiopathic inflammatory condition causing a combination of bronchoconstriction, chronic airway inflammation and excessive mucus production. Parasitic pulmonary disease such as lungworm or heartworm may also cause chronic respiratory signs with intermittent hypoxia.

Clinical signs

Coughing, intermittent dyspnea and hypoxia (oxygen saturation <92%) are the most common clinical signs of chronic feline respiratory disease. Dyspnea may be acute, chronic or intermittent.

There may be **open-mouth breathing and cyanosis** in severely affected cats.

Crackles and wheezes from **bronchial disease and/or pleural effusion** may be heard on thoracic auscultation.

Diagnosis

Chronic pulmonary disease presents with **auscultatory abnormalities**, together with a **history of intermittent or continuous dyspnea and often chronic coughing**.

Thoracic radiology reveals **characteristic lung patterns** associated with **bronchial, pleural or pulmonary disease**.

Bronchoalveolar lavage cytology and microbiology is useful in the diagnosis of inflammatory or bacterial (e.g. *Mycoplasma felis*) lung disease.

Fecal flotation and examination should be performed to check for **parasites such as lungworm** (*Aleurostrongylus abstrusus*).

Serology should also be performed to detect **heartworm** (*Dirofilaria immitis*) infection in endemic areas, as clinical signs of feline heartworm disease are generally respiratory in nature.

Toxoplasma **serology** may be performed as the lungs are a common site for the extra-intestinal (tissue) phase of the disease.

Differential diagnosis

Other causes of chronic hypoxia, such as congenital or degenerative cardiac disease, should be differentiated from hypoxia caused by chronic pulmonary disease.

Treatment

Treatment of respiratory conditions is dependent on the **correct diagnosis of the cause of the respiratory condition,** using a **thorough diagnostic work-up procedure**.

Specific therapies are needed to treat **respiratory infections**.

Symptomatic medical therapy is recommended for **chronic inflammatory pulmonary disease** such as **feline asthma/bronchitis complex. Oral corticosteroid therapy** at anti-inflammatory dose rates and bronchodilators such as terbutaline or aminophylline may reduce the severity and frequency of dyspneic episodes. **Inhaled corticosteroid and/or bronchodilator therapy** can be administered using pediatric asthma inhalers.

Prognosis

The prognosis for feline respiratory disease is **good for most respiratory infections**, although **chronic infections may result in chronic inflammatory disease** even after successful treatment of the infection.

POLYCYTHEMIA VERA*

> ### Classical signs
>
> - Injected dark pink mucous membranes.
> - ± History of intermittent bleeding diatheses.
> - ± Systolic ejection (hemic) murmur.
> - ± Central nervous system signs, such as seizures.
> - PCV > 60% with low serum erythropoietin concentration and normal blood O_2 saturation.

Pathogenesis

Polycythemia vera results from an **absolute increase** in red cell mass because of a **clonal proliferation of neoplastic erythroid stem cells** in the bone marrow associated with myeloproliferative disease.

- Erythroid precursors proliferate independent of erythropoietin in a normal orderly pattern of maturation.

Because normal feedback inhibition of erythrocytosis does not occur, **circulating erythropoietin levels are usually very low**.

Polycythemia vera is **very rare in cats.**

There is often **leukocytosis and thrombocythemia**.

The erythrocytes produced in polycythemia vera are **morphologically normal**.

Clinical signs

Mucosae are dark pink.

Bleeding may occur from numerous sites, e.g. nose, gums, skin, gastrointestinal tract, urinary tract or in the eye.

Central nervous system signs such as seizures, abnormal behavior, ataxia and blindness often occur because of reduced vascular perfusion of the central nervous system.

There may be a history of **polydipsia and polyuria**.

Dilated tortuous retinal vessels and retinal hemorrhage may be observed on ophthalmic examination.

A systolic ejection murmur (hemic murmur) may be present over the base of the heart secondary to abnormal viscosity.

Diagnosis

Polycythemia vera is diagnosed when there is a **combination of marked erythrocytosis (PCV > 60), low or undetectable serum erythropoietin levels, normal plasma protein concentration and normal blood O_2 saturation levels**.

The **bone marrow** has **increased cellularity with erythroid hyperplasia or panhyperplasia**. There is relatively normal maturation of erythroid precursors and cells have **normal morphology**, with no evidence of neoplasic features. Myeloid to erythroid ratio may be normal, or reflect erythroid hyperplasia.

Differential diagnosis

Polycythemia vera needs to be differentiated from other more common causes of erythrocytosis, such as **dehydration, hyperthyroidism and chronic hypoxic cardiac or pulmonary disease**.

Treatment

Primary polycythemia should be treated with **phlebotomy and intravenous fluids** to reduce PCV to below 60%.

Ten ml/kg/day of blood should be removed, and replaced with an equivalent volume of fluid (0.9% NaCl or balanced electrolyte solution) or the cat's own plasma.

- Regular phlebotomies may be adequate to maintain PCV. If phlebotomies are required more than once a month to maintain PCV < 60%, hydroxyurea therapy should be tried.

Bone marrow can be suppressed using **hydroxyurea** indefinitely (15–30 mg/kg q 24 h with food, reduce dose to 15 mg/kg q 24–48 h after 7–14 days).

- Complete blood counts should be performed every 7–14 days until PCV is normal, then every 3–4 months.
- When using hydroxyurea, serious bone marrow depression resulting in anemia, thrombocytopenia and leukopenia may occur, so cats receiving the drug need to be monitored carefully. If leukopenia, thrombocytopenia or anemia develops, stop the drug until blood counts are normal, and then resume at a lower dose.

Prognosis

The prognosis for polycythemia vera is **guarded**, depending on the response to treatment and the incidence of side effects of the therapies used.

EXCESSIVE BLOOD TRANSFUSION OR OVERDOSE OF EXOGENOUS ERYTHROPOIETIN

> ### Classical signs
>
> - Injected mucus membranes.
> - Weakness.
> - CNS signs including seizures.

Clinical signs

This is a potential, although previously unreported, cause of polycythemia.

Expected clinical signs are those of erythrocytosis, i.e. weakness, injected mucus membranes and neurological signs.

Diagnosis

The diagnosis is made using a combination of an appropriate history and clinical signs.

NEOPLASIA

> ### Classical signs
>
> - Signs are referable to the causative space-occupying mass.
> - Mucosae may be dark pink.
> - Signs of hyperviscosity, e.g. tortuous retinal vessels, seizures, bleeding diatheses, polyuria, polydipisia.

Pathogenesis

It is hypothesized that **renal** and other **visceral tumors** may **secrete erythropoietin or an erythropoietin-like substance**, resulting in erythrocytosis. While these tumors have been reported to cause polycythemia in humans and dogs, they are yet to be reported as a cause of polycythemia in the cat.

This kind of polycythemia is **secondary to another pathological condition and inappropriate,** since blood O_2 saturation levels are normal.

Clinical signs

Clinical signs are **referable** to the underlying neoplasia and polycythemia.

Mucus membranes are dark pink.

Signs of hyperviscosity include tortuous retinal vessels, seizures and other CNS signs, and intermittent bleeding diathesis.

Diagnosis

Erythrocytosis associated with neoplasia is diagnosed when there is a **combination of marked erythrocytosis (PCV > 60)**, normal or **increased serum erythropoietin** levels, **normal plasma protein** concentration, and normal **blood O_2 saturation levels**.

Visceral tumors are diagnosed ideally by **abdominal ultrasound**, although **intravenous pyelography** may also be a valuable imaging technique for renal masses.

Serum erythropoietin levels are normal or elevated, and blood O_2 saturation levels are normal.

Differential diagnosis

Secondary inappropriate polycythemia **must be differentiated from relative polycythemia** in dehydration, **secondary polycythemia** due to hypoxia, and from **primary polycythemia**.

- In neoplastic conditions, there is a **normal plasma protein** concentration, normal **blood O_2 saturation and normal or increased serum erythropoietin** concentration. This differentiates secondary inappropriate polycythemia associated with neoplasia from other conditions causing polycythemia.

Treatment

Treatment should be directed at the tumor, which is the **underlying cause of the polycythemia**.

Polycythemia may reoccur if metastatic foci secrete erythropoietin or an erythropoietin-like substance.

Prognosis

The prognosis **depends on the underlying cause of the polycythemia**. The prognosis with neoplasia varies according to the tumor type.

RENAL SPACE-OCCUPYING MASS

> ### Classical signs
>
> - Signs are referable to the causative space-occupying mass.
> - Dark pink mucosae.
> - Signs of hyperviscosity, e.g. tortuous retinal vessels, seizures, bleeding diatheses, polyuria, polydipisia.
> - ±Signs of renal insufficiency, such as azotemia, reduced urine specific gravity, polydipsia and polyuria.

Pathogenesis

A **space-occupying renal mass** such as a cyst, hydronephrotic disease or tumor may induce local tissue **hypoxia, stimulating renal oxygen sensors**, resulting in increased erythropoietin production. These sensors are thought to be located in the juxtaglomerular complex.

Some renal tumors may secrete erythropoietin or an erythropoietin-like substance, resulting in erythrocytosis.

This kind of polycythemia is **secondary to another pathological condition and inappropriate,** since blood O_2 saturation levels are normal.

Clinical signs

Clinical signs are **referable to the inciting condition**, whether renal or neoplastic. Lethargy, weight loss and inappetence are common.

Mucus membranes are **dark pink.**

Signs of hyperviscosity may be present including tortuous retinal vessels, seizures and other CNS signs, and intermittent bleeding diathesis.

Signs of renal insufficiency, such as azotemia, reduced urine specific gravity, polydipsia and polyuria may be present. However, not all cases of polycythemia from renal space-occupying masses will be accompanied by signs of renal insufficiency, due to the relatively large functional reserve of the kidneys.

Diagnosis

Renal space-occupying masses are best visualized using **abdominal ultrasound**, although **intravenous pyelography** may also be a valuable imaging technique.

Serum erythropoietin levels are normal or **elevated, and blood O_2 saturation levels are normal.**

Differential diagnosis

Secondary inappropriate polycythemia **must be differentiated from relative polycythemia** caused by dehydration, **secondary polycythemia** from hypoxia and **primary polycythemia**.
- When a renal space-occupying mass is causing polycythemia, **plasma protein** concentration and **blood O_2 saturation levels should be normal,** while serum **erythropoietin** concentration is often inappropriately high. These factors differentiate secondary inappropriate polycythemia due to a renal space-occupying mass from other conditions causing polycythemia.

Treatment

Treatment should be directed at the space-occupying mass, which is the **underlying cause of the polycythemia**.

Nephrectomy may be considered in cases of secondary inappropriate polycythemia from a renal space-occupying mass, but nephrectomy is considered a last-resort treatment as the resultant reduction in functional renal mass may precipitate renal insufficiency or failure. Also, polycythemia may reoccur if metastatic foci secrete erythropoietin or a functionally similar substance.

Prognosis

The prognosis **depends on the underlying cause of the polycythemia. Polycystic renal disease is a degenerative condition with a poor prognosis,** and most **renal tumors have a guarded prognosis,** at best. The prognosis with other kinds of neoplasia varies according to the tumor type.

ACUTE SYSTEMIC ANAPHYLAXIS

> ### Classical signs
> - Acute dyspnea.
> - Hypotensive shock.
> - Collapse.
> - Pale mucous membranes.

Pathogenesis

Acute systemic anaphylaxis is caused by **exposure to a foreign antigen**, usually protein, and generally by the intravenous route.

While prior exposure to the antigen is usually necessary for sensitization to occur, **anaphylaxis may occur on first exposure to the antigen**. This is termed an anaphylactoid reaction.

Anaphylaxis causes **increased vascular permeability**, allowing potentially large amounts of plasma to escape from the intravascular space, resulting in hemoconcentration.

It is also hypothesized that epinephrine is released during acute shock, causing splenic contraction and the infusion of large numbers of stored erythrocytes into the circulation.

Clinical signs

Clinical signs of acute systemic anaphylaxis vary between species, as **the major organs affected in the reaction are species-specific.**

Since **the "shock organ" in the cat is the lung**, pulmonary signs such as severe acute dyspnea predominate.

Signs of **hypotensive shock**, such as pallor and collapse, accompany the pulmonary signs.

The onset of clinical signs occurs in seconds to minutes after exposure to the inciting antigen.

Occasionally, **cutaneous swelling** may be noted around the face and paws.

Diagnosis

Polycythemia may be evident on hematological examination. Typically, mucus membranes are pale and signs are peracute. This is in contrast to other causes of polycythemia where mucous membranes are dark pink and there are often signs suggesting chronic disease such as weight loss. Diagnosis is made by a **combination of appropriate history and characteristic clinical signs**.

No laboratory tests are currently available to make a definitive diagnosis of acute systemic anaphylaxis.

Blood O_2 saturation is acutely and severely reduced.

Differential diagnosis

Polycythemia associated with anaphylaxis is usually readily distinguishable from all other causes of polycythemia due to its peracute onset. Accompanying clinical signs differentiate it from dehydration, which is associated with more chronic signs including anorexia and depression.

Acute systemic anaphylaxis must be differentiated from **other causes of acute shock** such as major trauma.

Treatment

Acute shock caused by anaphylaxis should be treated by a combination of **intravenous fluid therapy at shock dose rates** (perhaps including colloids in the protocol), **supplemental O_2** and intravenous high-dose **prednisolone** sodium succinate (100 mg/cat IV). The rate of fluid administration should be as rapid as possible to restore circulating blood volume. In cats, 150 ml can be given rapidly in the first hour but additional fluids should be administered more slowly to prevent pulmonary edema. Fluid therapy may be evaluated by monitoring blood pressure, packed cell volume and urine output.

Adjunctive therapy with bronchodilating agents (epinephrine 0.2 ml/cat of a 1:1000 dilution IV; terbutaline 0.1 mg/kg SC or IV) and antihistamines (chlorpheniramine maleate 1 mg/kg SC) may also be used.

Prognosis

Since acute systemic anaphylaxis is such an acute, overwhelming and life-threatening condition, the prognosis is guarded to poor, depending on how promptly and aggressively therapy is initiated, and perhaps on the amount of inciting antigen to which the cat was exposed and the rapidity of exposure.

STRESS-INDUCED SPLENIC CONTRACTION

> **Classical signs**
>
> - The stress response in cats may include splenic contraction, with a resultant infusion of stored splenic erythrocytes into the circulation.
> - Hemoconcentration caused by stress is usually mild and transient.

Diagnosis

Affected cats often have an appropriate history of acute stress. This may be stress associated with surgery or other treatment, as well as the flight-or-fight response to acute stress.

There may be associated signs of acute stress such as dilated pupils and behavioral changes.

Erythrocytosis should resolve promptly after the inciting incident.

SEVERE OBESITY (PICKWICKIAN SYNDROME)

Classical signs

- Cats are morbidly obese (body condition score 9/9), have chronic dyspnea and difficulty with normal ambulation.

Diagnosis

While the Pickwickian syndrome causing chronic hypoxia and resultant erythrocytosis has not been reported in cats, it is logical to assume that this may occur.

Morbid obesity may predispose to tissue hypoxia from inadequate alveolar ventilation because of fat accumulation in the thorax and compression of upper airways.

Blood O_2 saturation levels are expected to be low (<92%), and there should be slightly to markedly increased circulating levels of erythropoietin.

HIGH ALTITUDE

Classical signs

- Mild polycythemia in an otherwise healthy cat living at altitude.
- Decreased O_2 levels in the atmosphere at high altitudes stimulate increased renal erythropoietin production in response to tissue hypoxia.

Diagnosis

Expected signs include mild polycythemia in an otherwise healthy cat.

A presumptive diagnosis is based on finding mild polycythemia in a cat living at high altitude (e.g. > 5000 feet/1500 m).

RECOMMENDED READING

Giger U. Polycythemia: Is it p. vera? Proc 21st ACVIM Forum 2003: 742–744.

Nitchke EK. Erythrocytosis in dogs and cats: Diagnosis and management. Compend Contin Educ Pract Vet 2004; 26: 104–118.

Veterinary Information Network (VIN) at www.vin.com has many excellent board discussions and conference proceedings on use of fluids for dehydration and resuscitation including several by J Wohl, L Barton and TM Rieser.

26. The cat with hyperlipidemia

Boyd Robert Jones

> **KEY SIGNS**
>
> - Lipemia (lactescent appearance of plasma).
> - Lipemia retinalis (lipemic appearance of retinal vessels with a pink or salmon color).
> - Cloudy cornea or anterior chamber.
> - Cutaneous xanthomata (yellowish subcutaneous nodules or plaques).

MECHANISM?

- Hyperlipidemia is an increase in the **plasma triglyceride and/or cholesterol** concentrations.
- Hyperlipidemia may result from a **primary defect** in triglyceride or cholesterol metabolism.
- Hyperlipidemia may also occur when lipoprotein metabolism is altered by **systemic disease**.

WHERE?

- Abnormalities occur in blood/plasma, eye, skin, peripheral nerves, spleen, kidney and liver.
- Hyperlipidemia should be suspected when there is a persistent fasting hyperlipidemia (> 12 hours after feeding) or when a cat has any of the following signs:
- Lipemia retinalis.
- Cloudy cornea or anterior chamber.
- Cutaneous xanthomata.
- Peripheral neuropathy.
- Splenomegaly.

WHAT?

- The most common causes of hyperlipidemia are **idiopathic** and **secondary systemic diseases**, such as **diabetes mellitus**.

QUICK REFERENCE SUMMARY

Diseases causing hyperlipidemia

ANOMALY

● Inherited hyperchylomicronemia (p 575)

Domestic shorthair cats. May have no clinical signs, or signs of hyperlipidemia such as lipemia retinalis, xanthomata or peripheral neuropathy. Caused by a breed-related defect in lipoprotein lipase (LPL) activation due to a point mutation in the gene for LPL.

● Cholesterol ester storage disease (p 576)

Siamese < 1 year old, corneal clouding, intermittent diarrhea and vomiting, hepatomegaly. Lysosomal acid lipase (cholesterol ester hydrolase) deficiency results in accumulation of cholesterol esters in lysosomes.

METABOLIC

● Nephrotic syndrome (p 576)

Hypercholesterolemia occurs in the nephrotic syndrome as a sequel to protein-losing nephropathy. Proteinuria with hypoalbuminemia are classical findings.

● **Diabetes mellitus**(p 574)**

Hypertrigylceridemia occurs in some cats with diabetes. LPL activity is reduced, but the cause of the hypertriglyceridemia is likely multifactorial. Hypercholesterolemia may also occur and results from increased hepatic synthesis of cholesterol.

● **Idiopathic hyperlipidemia*** (p 573)**

May have no clinical signs, or have signs of hyperlipidemia. Any breed may be affected but Burmese kittens are over-represented and may present with severe anemia, lethargy and dyspnea. The cause of many cases of hyperlipidemia will be unconfirmed. The cause in most of these cases is due to a so far unidentified defect in lipid metabolism.

INTRODUCTION

MECHANISM

Definition of terms

Hyperlipidemia is an **increase** in the **plasma triglyceride and/or cholesterol concentrations**.

Hyperlipidemia may result from a primary defect in lipoprotein metabolism or from lipoprotein metabolism being altered by systemic disease.

Lipemia is the **lactescent appearance of plasma** and indicates an increase in the plasma triglyceride concentration in chylomicrons and/or low-density lipoproteins.

Lipid metabolism

Medium- and short-chain fatty acids are bound to albumin and transferred from the intestine directly to the liver via the portal vein.

Cholesterol and triglycerides are insoluble in plasma and their transport through the bloodstream relies upon their incorporation into specialized lipid–protein complexes called lipoproteins.

There are **four classes of lipoproteins (chylomicrons, VLDL, LDL and HDL),** each with separate physical and chemical characteristics.

Each of the four lipoprotein classes have discrete roles in plasma lipid transport.

- Chylomicrons and VLDL are the primary transporters of triglycerides.
- LDL and HDL are the cholesterol transporters (LDL are the cholesterol suppliers; HDL are the cholesterol scavengers).

All lipoproteins share a **common structure.**
- The hydrophobic components (triglycerides and cholesteryl esters) are carried in the core of the particle.
- These are surrounded by a polar coat of phospholipids, special proteins called **apolipoproteins**, and a small amount of free cholesterol.

Chylomicrons are **formed in the intestinal mucosa.** They transport dietary triglycerides from the small intestine to adipose tissue for storage, to skeletal muscle for use as energy substrate, and to lactating mammary tissue for milk fat synthesis.
- Chylomicrons are the largest and lightest of the lipoproteins, and remain at the **origin on gel** electrophoresis.
- Triglycerides are removed from chylomicrons through the action of the enzyme **lipoprotein lipase.**
  - **Lipoprotein lipase** is located on the luminal surface of **capillary endothelium** in adipose tissue, skeletal and cardiac muscle, and lactating mammary tissue.
  - Lipoprotein lipase is **activated by apolipoprotein C-II** (apoC-II) on the surface of the chylomicron, and releases the triglycerides as fatty acids.
  - Chylomicrons are **cleared** from the blood **within 12 hours after eating**, and therefore, are not normally present in the fasted cat.
  - Removal of triglycerides from the chylomicron leaves a smaller remnant particle that is rich in cholesterol.
  - The remnant particle is removed from the circulation by specific cell surface receptors in the liver that recognize apolipoprotein E (apoE) present on the surface of these particles.

Very-low-density lipoproteins (VLDL) export triglycerides and cholesterol from the major site of endogenous synthesis in the liver, and deliver triglycerides to peripheral tissues.
- VLDL are also known as **pre-β lipoprotein** because of the electrophoretic mobility.

- Triglycerides are released to adipose tissue, skeletal and cardiac muscle, and lactating mammary tissue by lipoprotein lipase.
- The cholesterol-rich remnant particles are processed by a second lipase, called **hepatic lipase**, to form LDL.

Low-density lipoproteins (LDL) are formed from VLDL and deliver cholesterol to peripheral tissues such as the adrenal and reproductive glands.
- These lipoproteins migrate in the **β-position** on electrophoresis.
- Cholesterol delivery is facilitated by the interaction of the structural protein of LDL (apolipoprotein B-100) with specific receptors, called the LDL receptors.
- LDL receptors are also found in high concentrations in the liver where they remove excess LDL.

High-density lipoproteins (HDL) scavenge cholesterol that is excess to tissue needs and transport it to the liver. The HDL are the major carriers of cholesterol.
- HDL are the smallest and most dense lipoproteins and migrate in the **α-position** on electrophoresis.
- In the liver, cholesterol is excreted as bile salts, stored, or redistributed to other body tissues as VLDL and LDL.
- HDL are secreted into the circulation **from the liver and intestine** as small immature discoidal particles.
- The free cholesterol picked up from peripheral tissues is esterified by the enzyme lecithin:cholesterol acyl transferase (**LCAT**) to form cholesteryl esters, which enter the core of the particles.
  - In humans, the cholesteryl esters are transferred from HDL to chylomicrons, VLDL and LDL and hence back to the liver.
  - Cats lack the enzyme responsible for this, cholesteryl ester transfer protein (**CETP**), so that the HDL continue to pick up free cholesterol and expand under the action of LCAT.
  - These large HDL particles then acquire apoE and are subsequently removed from the circulation by the remnant and LDL receptors in the liver.

Hyperlipidemia

Diagnosis of hyperlipidemia is based on history, physical examination, examination of plasma and special laboratory tests.

Understanding the metabolic origins of hyperlipidemia provides the basis for the investigation of patients and for therapeutic management.

Fasting hypertriglyceridemia results from defects in **metabolism of chylomicrons and/or VLDL.**

Hypercholesterolaemia results from defects in the metabolism of **LDL and HDL.**

Compositional changes in certain lipoproteins, for example cholesterol-enrichment of VLDL or triglyceride-enrichment of LDL, may also occur in certain disorders.

Hypertriglyceridemia

Plasma concentrations of triglycerides are raised when the amounts of chylomicrons and/or VLDL increase in the circulation.
- **Chylomicrons and VLDL** are both catabolized by the enzyme **lipoprotein lipase**, which removes the triglycerides from these particles.
- Defects in the activity of lipoprotein lipase, either genetic or acquired, result in reduced clearance of chylomicrons and VLDL and hypertriglyceridemia.

Persistence of chylomicrons in the circulation for > 12 hours after ingestion of a fat-containing meal and in fasting plasma are abnormal and suggest **impaired lipoprotein lipase activity.**

Chylomicrons rise to the surface and form a **creamy layer** when plasma is **refrigerated** for 12–14 hours. VLDL remain in suspension and produce a turbid or lactescent sample.

Hypercholesterolemia

Raised plasma cholesterol concentrations generally result from **deranged metabolism of LDL and HDL.**

Raised HDL concentrations have been found in certain types of **secondary hyperlipidemia** in cats, but the precise metabolic origins of this change is unclear.

Hypercholesterolemia does not produce visible lipemia (opalescence) as HDL and LDL are too small to refract light.

WHERE?

Signs of hyperlipidemia cause problems in the following organs: blood/plasma, eye, skin, peripheral nerves, spleen, kidney, liver.

The most common signs include:
- **Lipemia retinalis** (lipemic appearance of retinal vessels with a pink or salmon-colored appearance rather than red).
- **Cloudy cornea or lipemic aqueous** (cloudy anterior chamber of eye).
- **Cutaneous xanthomata** (well-circumscribed soft, smooth, alopecic subcutaneous nodules or plaques, which may have a yellowish appearance and may ulcerate in locations prone to trauma, often multiple over the trunk and head, less frequently involve the limbs).
- **Peripheral neuropathy** resulting in paresis or paralysis of cranial or spinal nerves (e.g. 3rd sympathetic producing Horner's syndrome, trigeminal, tibial or radial nerves).
- **Splenomegaly.**

WHAT?

The **most common cause of hyperlipidemia is idiopathic.** The abnormality in lipid metabolism is unidentified.

The most common metabolic cause is **diabetes mellitus.**

The inherited diseases are uncommon but occur most frequently in **young kittens** (weaning to 6 months age).

Diagnosis is based on history and physical examination, blood examination, special diagnostic tests and histopathology.

LABORATORY REFERENCE RANGES

Reference values (adult cats):
- Cholesterol 1–4.5 mmol/L (40–170 mg/dl)
- Triglyceride 0.2–1.1 mmol/L (20–100 mg/dl)

Clinical pathology laboratories have their own reference ranges for both cholesterol and triglycerides. Always compare your results with your own laboratory's reference ranges.

There are no significant breed or gender differences which affect plasma lipid values in cats.

Pregnancy is not a cause of secondary hyperlipidemia.

During **lactation**, the concentration of cholesterol decreases owing to a reduction in VLDL cholesterol and LDL cholesterol concentrations and suppression of HDL cholesterol production.

The plasma cholesterol concentration in suckling kittens up to 8–12 weeks of age is significantly higher than the adult reference range reflecting the fat content of the queen's milk.

The cat with hyperlipidemia – what to do

Is the hyperlipidemia from a recent meal?
- Fast overnight and resample. Plasma should be cleared of lipid in 7–8 hours in a healthy cat.
- The presence of hypercholesterolemia in the absence of triglyceridemia does not give visibly lipemic plasma.
- If hyperlipidemic, measure the **plasma cholesterol and triglyceride**. If **triglyceride** is elevated there is a defect in **chylomicron or VLDL** metabolism. If the **cholesterol** is elevated there is more likely a defect in **LDL and/or HDL** metabolism.
- Is the hyperlipidemia **secondary to other diseases**? Eliminate other diseases including:
  - Diabetes mellitus (polyuria, polydipsia, weight loss, persistent hyperglycemia, glycosuria).
  - Nephrotic syndrome (proteinuria, hypoalbuminemia, hypercholesterolemia).

If no secondary disease is identified, the problem is probably a primary disorder of lipid metabolism.

Specialized tests are available and can be applied in the investigation. They are useful in lipidemic cats to determine the metabolic basis for the hyperlipidemia, which helps determine therapy.

These tests include:
- **Chylomicron refrigeration test:** Harvest serum or plasma and refrigerate at −4°C overnight. Chylomicrons, if present will rise to form a "cream" layer (the supranatant). If the infranatant is lactescent this indicates elevated triglyceride in VLDL.
- **Tests of chylomicron clearance:** Fast for 24 hours. Collect a basal blood sample. Feed a small meal of a high-fat tinned cat food (4–5 g per cat). Collect

blood at 7, 12 and 24 hours post-prandially. Measure triglyceride in each sample. Triglyceride values should return to baseline by 7 hours and remain stable for 24 hours. Cats with altered triglyceride metabolism will show elevated triglyceride values which fail to return to baseline by 24 hours.
- **Quantification of the individual lipoprotein classes** by qualitative methods (gel electrophoresis). Electrophoresis confirms the relative abundance of a lipoprotein class: chylomicrons (origin), VLDL (pre-Beta), LDL (beta) and HDL (alpha 1).
- **Lipoprotein separation** and quantification[#].
- **Assay of lipoprotein lipase activity.** The Heparin response test. Collect a basal blood sample. Administer 100 IU heparin intravenously and collect a second blood sample after 10 minutes. Measure triglyceride in each sample. A reduction in triglyceride indicates LPL activity. Special lipid laboratories can complete more specialized LPL assays[#] on each sample. This procedure is advised.
- **Assay of LCAT activity[#].**
- **PCR analysis** for a specific genetic disease[#].
  - The tests marked [#] are available in a small number of research laboratories and are not available to most veterinarians.

DISEASES CAUSING HYPERLIPIDEMIA

IDIOPATHIC HYPERLIPIDEMIA***

Classical signs

- None.
- Lipemia retinalis.
- Cutaneous xanthomata.
- Anemia.
- Lipemic aqueous or cornea.
- Hypertriglyceridemia and/or hypercholesterolemia.

Pathogenesis

Idiopathic hyperlipidemia includes all cats with hypertriglyceridemia and/or hypercholesterolemia for which the defect in lipid metabolism is unidentified. Currently most cats with hyperlipidemia are classified as idiopathic.

Burmese kittens are over-represented, but any breed may be involved.

Pathogenesis is unknown, but it is probably due to a primary defect of lipid metabolism, if secondary causes (diabetes nephrotic syndrome) have been eliminated.

There is probably one phenotypic expression for **many different genetic mutations**, which may involve the enzyme lipoprotein lipase or other essential molecules in lipoprotein metabolism, e.g. apolipoproteins.

The pathogenesis of the concurrent clinical signs and anemia is unknown.

Clinical signs

There may be no clinical signs, just hyperlipidemia.

Alternatively, a variety of clinical signs may occur including:
- **Lipemia retinalis**.
- **Cutaneous xanthomata**.
- **Lipemic aqueous**.
- Frequently associated with severe anemia (PCV < 11%) in kittens around the time of weaning. Kittens may present with acute lethargy, dyspnea and death within 48 h. Usually the entire litter has severe fasting hypertriglyceridemia. Reported in purebred (including Siamese, Persian, Burmese, Oriental) and domestic shorthair breeds.

Diagnosis

Confirmation of hypertriglyceridemia and/or hyper-cholesterolemia.

Other diagnostic tests may indicate where the abnormality of lipid metabolism is located by the relative distribution of the lipoproteins.

Treatment

Severely anemic kittens need emergency treatment with **supplemental oxygen and a blood transfusion** to survive.

The plasma **triglyceride** should be **reduced to less than 5.5 mmol/L** (500 mg/dl), which minimizes the risk of hyperlipidemia-associated signs.

Feed either a homemade or commercial **diet low in saturated fats**, calorie restricted, and high in fiber to reduce lipid values. Wean kittens onto a low-fat diet.

Once hypertriglyceridemia resolves, many kittens can tolerate normal cat food.

Gemfibrozil (Lopid, Parke Davis, 7.5–10 mg/kg daily) may help reduce triglyceride values if dietary therapy alone fails.

Marine (fish) oils which are rich in n-3 fatty acids may reduce plasma triglycerides by decreasing the synthesis of VLDL. Dose at 10–30 mg/kg PO daily for cats that are unresponsive to dietary fat restriction.

Always check body weight at regular intervals if cats are on a calorie-restricted or reducing diet to ensure normal weight is maintained.

DIABETES MELLITUS**

> **Classical signs**
> - Polyuria, polydipsia.
> - Polyphagia or inappetance.
> - Weight loss.
> - Persistent hyperglycemia, glycosuria.

See main references on page 236 for details (The Cat With Polyuria and Polydipsia).

Pathogenesis

Hyperlipidemia occurs in **some cats with diabetes mellitus**.

Rarely, cats with diabetes have concurrent hyper-adrenocorticism or acromegaly, conditions which result in insulin-resistant diabetes mellitus.

The hypertriglyceridemia results from a combination of **reduced lipoprotein lipase activity** as insulin is required for normal activity of this enzyme, **increased synthesis of VLDL** due to poor regulation of hormone-sensitive lipase, **increased flux of non-esterified fatty acids** to the liver and **increased triglyceride synthesis**.

The raised cholesterol concentrations reflect **increased hepatic synthesis**, which leads to down-regulation of LDL receptor activity and increased LDL.

Clinical signs

Signs of diabetes mellitus (polyuria, polydipsia, weight loss).

Lipemic plasma.

Lipemia retinalis.

Cutaneous xanthomata (very rare finding in diabetic cats).

Diagnosis

Increased plasma or serum glucose and glycosuria, together with signs of diabetes (see Diabetes mellitus in The Cat With Polyuria and Polydipsia, page 237).

Treatment

Insulin or oral hypoglycemic drugs. See Diabetes mellitus for treatment details, page 237.

Feeding a low-fat diet is essential.

INHERITED HYPERCHYLOMICRONEMIA

Classical signs

- Domestic short-haired cats.
- Hyperchylomicronemia and hypertriglyceridemia.
- Lipemia retinalis (if triglyceride > 15 mmol/L).
- Cutaneous xanthomata.
- Peripheral neuropathies.
- Reduced appetite and lethargy.
- or NO CLINICAL SIGNS other than hyperlipidemia.

Pathogenesis

Absent lipoprotein lipase (LPL) activity.

Inherited as an **autosomal recessive** mode of inheritance.

Heterozygotes have intermediate LPL activity consistent with an autosomal recessive trait.

Molecular basis for the LPL deficiency is a single base-pair change in the lipoprotein lipase gene. An arginine for glycine transposition is present at amino acid residue 412 in exon 8.

This mutation results in the expression of **catalytically inactive enzyme**, which fails to be activated or to bind appropriately.

Clinical signs

No clinical signs other than hyperlipidemia may be evident.

Alternatively, a variety of clinical signs may occur including:
- Lipemia retinalis.
- **Cutaneous xanthomata.**
- **Peripheral nerve paralysis involving**:
  - 3rd sympathetic cranial nerve (Horner's syndrome with protrusion of 3rd eyelid, miosis, narrowed palpebral fissure).
  - Tibial nerve.
  - Radial nerve.
  - Trigeminal nerve.
- Splenomegaly.
- Xanthomata in other organs including:
  - Intestine.
  - Heart.
  - Liver.

In kittens there is increased still-birth rate, reduced body mass and reduced growth rates.

Diagnosis

Gross lipemia of fasting blood samples. Blood looks like **"cream of tomato soup"**.

Massive **hyperchylomicronemia** and **elevated VLDL**. Cream layer and lactescent serum or plasma are present after refrigeration.

Raised triglycerides (15–150 mmol/L, 1300–13 000 mg/dl).

Raised triglyceride and cholesterol in chylomicrons and VLDL.

Lowered LDL cholesterol.

Reduced fat tolerance. Post-prandial plasma lipid values are significantly elevated for > 48 hours after fat ingestion in homozygous cats.

There is no difference in lipoprotein composition between normal and affected genotypes except for an increase in the ratio of apoC to apoE in chylomicrons and VLDL.

Pre- and post-heparin plasma contains increased LPL mass, but no enzymic activity, that is, triglyceride does not decrease after heparin.

PCR mismatch analysis can detect normal cats, homozygotes and heterozygotes for this genetic defect.

Treatment

A **low-fat diet** either homemade or commercial will reduce blood lipid values and clinical signs will regress after 4–12 weeks.

Siblings and parents should be tested, and affected homozygotes and heterozygotes neutered and not bred.

The prevalence of this mutation in cat populations is very low.

CHOLESTEROL ESTER STORAGE DISEASE

Classical signs

- Siamese cats.
- Corneal clouding.
- Hepatomegaly.
- Intermittent vomiting and diarrhea.

Pathogenesis

Lysosomal lipase (cholesterol ester hydrolase) hydrolyzes cholesterol esters in various lipoproteins as they are removed from plasma and enter the cellular compartment.

Deficiency of this enzyme results in **cholesterol ester accumulation within lysosomes** which may result in organ failure and death.

The condition is transmitted as an **autosomal recessive** mode of inheritance in the **Siamese**.

Homozygous recessive cats are more severely affected than the heterozygotes.

Clinical signs

Siamese breed.

Onset of signs **before 1 year of age.**

Corneal clouding.

Intermittent vomiting and diarrhea.

Hepatomegaly.

Diagnosis

History of **vomiting and diarrhea with corneal clouding**.

Plasma cholesterol values are in the reference ranges.

Plasma triglyceride and low-density lipoprotein are **increased**.

Plasma and serum are grossly normal.

Heparin response test indicates normal lipoprotein lipase activity.

Cytoplasmic vacuolation containing cholesterol esters is present in a proportion of neutrophils (16%), **lymphocytes (56%), and monocytes (60%),** stained by Wright-Giemsa.

Acid lipase activity in cultivated fibroblasts and hepatocytes is markedly decreased compared with controls.

Differential diagnosis

Other inherited metabolic and lysosomal storage diseases.

Treatment

In theory, a **reduced-fat diet** and treatment with one of the **HMG CoA-reductase inhibitors** (statins) should reduce cholesterol synthesis, and up-regulate LDL-receptor activity thus reducing plasma cholesterol, triglyceride and the LDL cholesterol concentrations. This treatment was not attempted in the reported cases.

NEPHROTIC SYNDROME

Classical signs

- Proteinuria.
- Hypoalbuminemia.
- Peripheral edema.
- Ascites.
- ± polydipsia, polyuria.

Pathogenesis

Rare disease in cats.

Hypercholesterolemia is a common **sequel to protein-losing glomerulopathy.**

LDL and HDL cholesterol concentrations are both increased.

The exact **pathogenesis** of the cholesterol elevation is **unknown.**

Clinical signs

Peripheral edema.

Ascites.

± polydipsia and polyuria.

Diagnosis

Proteinuria.

Hypoalbuminemia.

Concurrent hypercholesterolemia.

RECOMMENDED READING

Ginzinger DE, Lewis MES, Yuanhong MA, et al. A mutation in the lipoprotein lipase gene is the molecular basics of Chylomicronemia in a colony of domestic cats. J Clin Invest 1997; 97: 1257–1266.

PART 9

Cat with signs of gastrointestinal tract disease

27. The cat with salivation

Victor Hans Menrath

KEY SIGNS

- Drooling.
- Excessive salivation.

MECHANISM?

- Ptyalism (**drooling**) occurs as a result of either: **excessive saliva production** or **normal production of saliva** but inability to swallow or retain saliva in the mouth.

WHERE?

- Oral causes – mouth (including pharynx) and tongue.
- Extra-oral causes – includes **central nervous system** and **gastrointestinal tract** causes.

WHAT?

- **Fear** or **stress** is the most common cause of **non-pathological** ptyalism in the clinic situation. Careful **examination of the oral cavity** is essential to distinguish **oral** from **extra-oral causes.**
- Recurrent, **intermittent**, non-stress-induced ptyalism in **young** cats (usually less than 1 year) is likely to be caused by **portosystemic shunt.**
- Other causes of recurrent, **intermittent** ptyalism (usually in cats more than 1 year old) include **hiatal hernia, gastroesophageal intussusception** and **diaphragmatic hernia.**
- Most other causes of ptyalism are likely to be **acute in onset** and produce **continuous drooling. Pain** is a major cause of ptyalism in cats.

QUICK REFERENCE SUMMARY
Diseases causing salivation

ANOMALY

● **Portosystemic shunt (PSS)* (p 588)**

Congenital liver abnormality causing intermittent central nervous system (CNS) signs with ptyalism. Usually in young cats (< 1 year). Often associated with eating. Affected cats are often very stunted in size.

MECHANICAL

● **Esophageal foreign body* (p 590)**

Repeated swallowing attempts with neck outstretched/retching, regurgitating white or blood stained foam.

● **Oral foreign body** (p 586)**

Acute onset of salivation, gagging and pawing at the mouth. Dysphagia, halitosis and inappetence may be evident. Most commonly associated with a bone lodged laterally between the 4th upper premolars.

NEOPLASTIC

● **Oral neoplasia* (p 587)**

Squamous cell carcinoma most common. Often under tongue or associated with a canine tooth or in tonsillar region. Ulcerated and/or proliferative.

PSYCHOLOGICAL

● **Psychogenic causes*** (p 582)**

Ptyalism can be caused by stress, fear, pleasure and pain.

INFECTIOUS

● Rabies (p 599)

Progressive central nervous system signs of muscle fasciculation, weakness, ataxia combined with behavioral changes, low-grade fever and ptyalism in unvaccinated cats. Serious zoonosis.

● **Feline herpes virus** (p 583)**

Pronounced ptyalism can occur in the very early stage of the disease. Invariably followed by the normal classical signs of viral upper respiratory disease – i.e. sneezing, naso-ocular discharge, etc.

● **Feline calicivirus** (p 582)**

Ptyalism as a result of tongue laceration due to virus, usually in young kittens. Often associated with other upper respiratory signs – e.g. chemosis, sneezing, coughing.

● Feline spongioform encephalopathy (FSE) (p 600)

Progressive central nervous signs including hindlimb ataxia, behavioral changes, hyperesthesia, head tremor and muscle fasciculation. Ptyalism.

continued

continued

● Feline panleukopenia (parvo virus) (p 600)

Continuous ptyalism has been recorded in a 3-month-old kitten suffering from feline panleukopenia caused by feline parvovirus.

INFLAMMATORY

● Esophagitis* (p 591)

Characterized by repeated attempts at swallowing, ptyalism, "neck stretching" and regurgitation of ingested food, often with mucoid foam. Early treatment essential to prevent secondary esophageal stricture.

● Periodontal disease/periodontitis*** (p 582)

Saliva-stained perilabial fur, often reluctance to pick up food, quidding and pawing at mouth.

IMMUNE

● Feline oral inflammatory disease (plasmacytic-lymphocytic stomatitis)** (p 585)

Mild to severe granulomatous inflammation in fauces. Often extremely painful and refractory to treatment. Cats resent mouth examination.

● Eosinophilic granuloma complex (EGC)** (p 586)

Orange-white lesions on tongue surface, soft and hard palate. Usually associated excessive grooming due to skin allergy. Lesions often painful.

TOXIC

● Household cleaners and disinfectants* (p 587)

Common cause of chemical burns on tongue. Especially shower recess cleaners.

● Acetaminophen (paracetamol) toxicity (p 595)

Facial edema, cyanosis and chocolate urine. Prompt treatment is essential.

● Organophosphate and carbamate toxicity (p 594)

Carbamate toxicity is most common. Miosis, muscular twitching and hypersalivation.

● Pyrethrin and pyrethroid toxicity (p 595)

Salivation, tremors, seizures. No definitive test for diagnosis.

● Spider envenomation (p 597)

Severe pain, vocalization, hyperexcitability and ataxia early, progressing to muscular weakness and collapse. Severe, prolonged ptyalism, possibly due to pain.

● Dieffenbachia (dumb cane) poisoning (p 598)

Sudden onset of salivation immediately after chewing plant. Tongue paralysis is characteristic.

● D-limonene, linalool and crude citrus oil extracts (p 598)

Used in insecticidal sprays and shampoos. Ptyalism may be the only clinical sign. Muscular tremors and ataxia can occur in more severely affected cases.

● Lead poisoning (p 596)

Gastrointestinal signs (inappetance, diarrhea) and/or CNS signs (behavioral changes, seizures, blindness).

- **Oral medication** (p 584)

Can be unpleasant tasting or irritant to the oral mucous membranes. Some drugs can cause a delayed hypersalivation (e.g. trimethoprim-sulfa combinations).

TRAUMA

- **Tongue laceration** (p 584)

Sudden onset, inability to eat, rapid secondary bacterial infection.

- **Jaw fracture/dislocation** (p 584)

Inability to chew, slack jaw, asymmetry of jaw.

- Hiatal hernia/gastroesophageal intussusception (p 592)

Uncommon, intermittent salivation, age of cats. Intussusception can be rapidly fatal.

- Diaphragmatic hernia with incarcerated stomach (p 598)

Very uncommon, intermittent salivation, often associated with feeding and dyspnea.

INTRODUCTION

MECHANISM?

Ptyalism (hypersalivation, drooling, hypersialosis) occurs as a result of

Either: excessive saliva production due to stimulation of the salivary nuclei located in the brainstem via **local receptors** (taste and tactile) in **the mouth** and on **the tongue**, or via **higher centers** in the central nervous system (CNS).

Or: **normal** or **increased** saliva production but with an inability to swallow or retain the excessive saliva in the mouth due to an **anatomical** problem.

WHERE?

Oral causes mouth (including pharynx) and tongue.

Extra-oral causes including CNS and gastrointestinal tract (especially esophagus and stomach).

WHAT?

The most common non-pathological cause of ptyalism in **the clinic situation** is **fear** or **stress** and occurs especially in very nervous cats. These cats do not have ptyalism at home.

Medication or attempted medication with **unpleasant-tasting oral medication.**

Pleasure is a common **non-pathological** cause of ptyalism **at home**. This often occurs in older cats and is usually associated with other signs of pleasure, e.g. purring and kneading of paws.

Ptyalism **at home** unassociated with pleasure and ptyalism **in the clinic,** unassociated with fear or stress **suggests a pathological cause**.

Careful history-taking will help differentiate **pathological** from **non-pathological** causes of ptyalism.

Careful examination of the oral cavity will help differentiate **oral** from **extra-oral** causes of ptyalism.

Recurrent, intermittent (non-stress-induced) ptyalism **in young cats** (<1 year old) is likely to be caused by **portosystemic shunt**.

Other causes of recurrent, intermittent ptyalism include **hiatal hernia**, **gastroesophageal intussusception** and **diaphragmatic hernia.**

Most other causes are likely to be **acute in onset** and produce **continuous drooling.**

Pain is a major cause of ptyalism in the cat – usually combined with **dilated pupils.**

DISEASES CAUSING SALIVATION

PSYCHOGENIC CAUSES***

> **Classical signs**
>
> - Ptyalism.
> - Dilated pupils.

Pathogenesis

Fear, anxiety, pleasure, nausea.

May be exacerbated by underlying or concomitant **hyperthyroidism**.

Anticipation of unpleasant experience (e.g. tableting or painful injection).

Especially in "**highly-strung**" cats, e.g. Siamese.

Makes oral medication virtually impossible.

Probably the most common cause of ptyalism in the cat in the clinic situation.

Clinical signs

Drooling, ptyalism.

Usually **during traveling** or **at veterinary clinic**.

Often triggered by cat **recognizing unpleasant event to come**.

Pupils dilated when due to stress or fear.

Repeated lip smacking and swallowing

Treatment

0.01 mg/kg PO or SC **atropine** 1/2 hour **before traveling/-event**.

Diazepam 0.5 mg/kg PO or SC 1/2 hour **before traveling/-event**.

Above drugs can be **combined**.

PERIDONTAL DISEASE/PERIODONTITIS***

> **Classical signs**
>
> - Dysphagia.
> - Pawing at mouth.
> - Halitosis.
> - Ptyalism.

See main reference on page 604 for details (The Cat With Bad Breath or Oral Lesions).

Clinical signs

Severe peridontal disease will result in tooth loss, deep pockets with heavy anaerobic infections and strong halitosis.

Cat may show signs of attempting to pick up food, dropping it and pawing at mouth.

Peri-labial fur may be saliva stained.

Feline odontoclastic resorptive lesions ("neck lesions") can also be very painful and show similar signs.

Diagnosis

Probing to identify periodontal pockets. Tapping affected teeth will cause jaw "chattering".

FELINE CALICIVIRUS**

> **Classical signs**
>
> - Sneezing, coughing, oculonasal discharge.
> - Oral ulceration, especially tongue.
> - Ptyalism.

See main reference on page 11 for details.

Clinical signs

Sudden onset of **acute conjunctivitis (usually one eye first).**

Rapidly followed by sneezing, coughing, pyrexia.

Tongue ulceration is common – ulcer is usually large, in the **central tongue** it is often butterfly-shaped. Ulceration of the nose philtrum, dorsal surface hard palate, footpads can also occur.

Most commonly in **kittens 8–12 weeks of age**.

Salivation due to **ulceration** and **pain in the tongue**.

Occasional **viral pneumonia, lameness ("limping kitten syndrome")**.

Growth rate of kittens is often temporarily delayed.

Diarrhea can occur and be protracted.

Diagnosis

Clinical signs.

Response to antibiotics.

PCR, viral isolation.

Treatment

Supportive nursing and broad-spectrum antibiotics, e.g. doxycycline (2.5 mg/kg PO q 24 h), cephalexin (30 mg/kg PO q 12 h).

Maintain hydration.

FELINE HERPES VIRUS**

> ### Classical signs
>
> - Sudden onset of severe ptyalism.
> - Depression, inanition, dehydration.
> - Pyrexia followed by sneezing, coughing naso-ocular discharge.

See main reference on page 7 for details (The Cat With Acute Sneezing or Nasal Discharge).

Pathogenesis

Caused by **feline herpes virus I.**

Viral replication in oral mucosa and/or perhaps salivary glands causes massive production of saliva in the **very early stages of the course of the disease**. Viral parotiditis could be involved in the cause of salivation.

Severe clinical signs are usually associated with a **very short incubation period** (1–4 days) (i.e. severity of signs is **virus dose-responsive**).

Salivation is followed by varying degrees of **pharyngitis, laryngitis, tracheitis and esophagitis** and classical signs of viral upper respiratory tract infection, i.e. coughing, sneezing, runny eyes and nose.

May have concurrent FeLV, FIV, calicivirus, bordetella or mycoplasma infection.

Clinical signs

Hypersalivation syndrome usually occurs in adult unvaccinated or poorly vaccinated cats, with **novel exposure**.

Severe **drooling salivation** with **depression** and **rapid dehydration** precedes classical signs of viral upper respiratory tract disease.

Pyrexia usually lasts for period of hypersalivation (24–48 h).

Often followed by severe pharyngitis, laryngitis, tracheitis, esophagitis (retching, choking cough, vomiting) and requires long periods of intensive care if signs are severe.

Diagnosis

PCR, viral isolation.

Classical signs of viral upper respiratory tract infection (i.e. sneezing, coughing etc.) follow salivation within 24–48 h.

Treatment

Rapid **dehydration** can occur – IV fluid support, steam inhalation therapy.

Place **feeding tube** (esophagostomy, gastrostomy).

Be prepared for **2–4 weeks intensive nursing** if signs are severe.

Prevent secondary bacterial rhinitis and sinusitis with **broad-spectrum antibiotics**, e.g. cephalexin (30 mg/kg PO; 15 mg/kg q 12 h) or amoxycillin/clavulanic acid (12.5 mg/kg PO q 12 h) which should be continued for **4 weeks minimum**.

Prognosis

Good with good intensive care.

Cat will almost always become a **herpes virus carrier**.

ORAL MEDICATION**

> **Classical signs**
>
> - Ptyalism, excessive salivation.
> - Usually immediately following oral medication.
> - Sometimes ptyalism delayed.

Clinical signs

Acute ptyalism following attempted or successful oral medication.

Often associated with rapid tongue movements in an attempt to remove drug or taste from mouth.

Ptyalism is often delayed for 5–10 minutes after the successful administration of trimethoprim-sulfa tablets.

Ptyalism is self-limiting and usually short duration (e.g. 5–10 minutes).

Treatment

Treatment is not necessary.

Reassure owner that it is self-limiting.

TONGUE LACERATION**

> **Classical signs**
>
> - Ptyalism.
> - Dysphagia.
> - Halitosis.

Pathogenesis

Trauma from cat's **own teeth biting on tongue** (e.g. car accident, falling from height).

Trauma from cat fight – claw slicing tongue.

Clinical signs

Hemorrhage may be significant if acute.

Reluctance to groom.

Paws and chest are sticky with foul-smelling saliva.

Rapid secondary bacterial infection.

Diagnosis

Obviously lacerated tongue.

Treatment

Surgical debridement and repair with absorbable sutures (e.g. 4/0 plain gut).

Antibiotics. Parenteral or paste-form best, e.g. cephalexin (15 mg/kg IM q 12 h), amoxycillin/clavulanic acid (8.5 mg/kg SC or IM q 24 h).

JAW FRACTURE/DISLOCATION**

> **Classical signs**
>
> - Ptyalism.
> - Mouth held open ("slack-jawed").
> - Jaw asymmetry.

Clinical signs

Excessive salivation.

Unable to close jaw.

Jaw dislocation without fracture is uncommon – temporo-mandibular dislocation can be **rostrodorsal (most common)** or **caudo-ventral**. **Dislocation** is almost invariably **bilateral**.

Mandibular symphyseal separation is most common and is often associated with temporo-mandibular dislocation and/or fracture of the mandible, causing jaw asymmetry.

Diagnosis

Symphyseal separation is usually obvious on examination.

Careful palpation of both horizontal and vertical sections of mandibles from inside mouth under anesthesia will help to identify fractures.

Careful radiography.

Treatment

Rostral tempero-mandibular joint (TMJ) dislocation can be reduced by placing a ballpoint pen or pencil horizontally across the mouth **behind** the lower molars and forcibly closing mouth until joints relocated.

Caudal TMJ dislocations are reduced in a similar fashion but the mandible is forced rostrally.

Surgical repair of symphyseal separation by using circlage stainless steel wire.

FELINE ORAL INFLAMMATORY DISEASE** (PLASMACYTIC-LYMPHOCYTIC STOMATITIS/FAUCITIS) (PLASMA CELL GINGIVITIS AND PHARYNGITIS)

Classical signs

- Ptyalism.
- Difficult prehension.
- Halitosis.
- Pain, reluctance to open mouth.
- Severe faucitis, gingivitis.

Pathogenesis

Etiology unknown. Suggested causes are **viral** (especially **calicivirus**), **bacterial** and **immunological** (possibly hypersensitivity to plaque proteins).

The condition appears to be the result of a **chronic-immune-mediated process** because lymphocytes and plasma cells predominate, and lesions respond to immunosuppressive drugs.

Moderate to severe **calicivirus-induced gingivitis** occurs commonly in young (8–12 weeks) kittens with or without concomitant tongue ulceration. Gingivitis often persists as chronic **gingival hyperplasia** through adulthood, predisposing to excessive plaque, periodontal disease and early loss of teeth. A small percentage of these cats develop plasmacytic-lymphocytic faucitis later in life, usually middle age.

Clinical signs

Intense oral pain and resentment to oral examination occurs with **severe faucitis**. Bright red proliferate granulomatous tissue **may partially occlude pharynx** in severe cases.

Dysphagia, excessive salivation and **weight loss** occur in severe cases.

Severe faucitis is often associated **with FIV or FeLV** infection.

Treatment

Thorough dental prophylaxis and **complete** extraction of all teeth showing resorptive lesions. Severe faucitis often responds to extraction of all molars and premolars and any **retained root tips**.

Antibiotic therapy using amoxycillin (10 mg/kg PO q 12 h), metronidazole (10 mg/kg PO q 12 h) or clindamycin (5.5 mg/kg PO q 12 h) often results in improvement, but rarely complete resolution of inflammation. Doxycycline (25 mg/kg PO q 24h) has anti infammatory effects.

In most cases, antibiotic therapy will need to be combined with **immunosuppresive therapy**. Many cases will not be able to be medicated orally and will require **parenteral therapy,** e.g. methylprednisolone acetate (2–4 mg/kg IM).

If the cat can be medicated orally, prednisolone (2 mg/kg PO q 12 h) for 10 days, then taper.

For very refractive cases, may have to use **azathioprine** (0.3 mg/kg PO q 72 h), or **cyclophosphamide** (6.25–12.5 mg/cat once daily, 4 days PO per week) or **chlorambucil** (0.1–0.2 mg/kg q 24 h PO initially, then q 48 h) or **aurothioglucose** (0.5–1 mg IM every 7 days). Cyclosporine (5 mg/kg PO q 12–24h) can be very effective.

A topical gel (Bonjela ®, choline salicylate, cetalkonium chloride, Reckitt & Coleman Pharmaceuticals, UK) applied with or without sedation/anesthetic has been reported to ameliorate the faucitis and gingivitis in affected cats. The gel is rubbed into the lesions in the mouth over a period of about 2 minutes once a week until signs regress. Note that this is an off-label use of this product designed as an oral analgesic gel in humans and contains salicylate. To date there have been no reported adverse reactions with its use in cats.

Prognosis

This condition, in its severe form remains **one of the most difficult and frustrating to treat in feline practice.** Thorough oral debridement is essential.

Most cases eventually end up requiring chronic medication with immunosuppressants for the rest of their lives.

ORAL FOREIGN BODY**

> **Classical signs**
>
> - Ptyalism, acute onset.
> - Gagging, pawing at mouth.
> - Halitosis.
> - Dysphagia.

Pathogenesis

Usually **sliver of bone** jammed laterally between 4th upper premolars.

Linear foreign body (string, cotton) around base of tongue.

Clinical signs

Salivating, **pawing at mouth** – sometimes bleeding laceration around mouth from self-trauma.

Dysphagia, **halitosis**.

Diagnosis

Self evident on oral examination.

Examine roof of mouth and under tongue.

Treatment

Remove foreign body.

Antibiotics if secondary infection from self-trauma or foreign body damage.

EOSINOPHILIC GRANULOMA COMPLEX (EGC)**

> **Classical signs**
>
> - Ptyalism.
> - Dysphagia.

Pathogenesis

Immune-mediated process resulting in granuloma formation (eosinophilic granuloma) in the oral cavity, especially the **dorsum of the tongue** and **hard palate**, but can occur in other areas, e.g. soft palate.

Histopathology shows typical **granuloma formation with collagen degeneration**.

Usually associated with a concurrent pruritic **skin disease** and **excessive grooming**.

The **cause of this association is unknown**. Oral mucous membrane trauma from excessive grooming could cause the lesions, or both the oral and skin lesions may be a reaction to antigens, such as flea antigen, on the coat.

Clinical signs

Salivation and **dysphagia** usually only occurs in severe cases of eosinophilic granuloma complex with associated glossitis.

Oral exam reveals single or multiple raised, firm 1–2 mm white-yellow nodules, scattered throughout mouth, but especially on dorsum tongue surface causing the surface of the tongue to have **"cobble-stone" appearance.** Associated glossitis may occur **causing** difficulty in prehension and swallowing.

Evidence of **over-grooming** and **itchy skin disease** is usually present.

Halitosis may occur with secondary bacterial infection.

Diagnosis

Lesions have a very characteristic appearance.

Histopathology confirms diagnosis.

Differential diagnosis

Oral neoplasia. Squamous cell carcinoma usually occurs on the **ventral surface** of the tongue in the region of frenulum and has an ulcerated, red appearance.

Treatment

Treatment can be difficult and frustrating.

Treat concurrent **skin allergy** and **ectoparasites** to achieve control.

Change to a **novel protein diet**.

Regular **manual grooming** and **bathing**.

Prednisolone (2 mg/kg PO q 12 h for 5–10 days, then taper).

Megestrol acetate (2.5–5 mg/cat PO for 4 days, then 2.5–5 mg q 5–7 days until lesions regress).
NB This drug, although very effective, has numerous side effects **especially in the Burmese breed** (diabetes mellitus, pyometra, obesity, iatrogenic Cushings disease).

Cyclosporine (5 mg/kg PO q 12–24h).

Doxycycline (2.5 mg/kg PO q 24h).

ORAL NEOPLASIA *

Classical signs

- Ptyalism, often blood stained.
- Halitosis.
- Dysphagia.

Pathogenesis

Squamous cell carcinoma is the most common neoplasm. Usually on the ventral surface of the tongue causing immobility of the tongue but sometimes tonsillar crypt or under the canine tooth.

Usually in older cats (> 10 years).

Other tumors include **epulis**, **fibroscarcoma** and **lymphoscarcoma**.

Clinical signs

Excessive salivation, often blood stained. Signs usually present longer than 1 week.

Dysphagia, difficulty in prehension.

Facial distortion, halitosis.

Weight loss due to inability to eat or metastatic disease.

Diagnosis

Biopsy and histologic examination.

Radiography to assess extent of tumor invasion.

Differential diagnosis

Inflammatory polyps – usually have stalk.

Intra-oral abscess and granulation tissue can have a similar appearance – differentiate by **biopsy** or trial **antibiotics**.

Eosinophilic granuloma complex (linear granuloma) has characteristic white-yellow nodules – differentiate by **biopsy** or trial corticosteroids.

Treatment

Treatment of lingual squamous cell carcinoma in the cat **has not proved successful,** however some of the newer chemotherapic agents may be more effective combined with tumor excision.

Mandibular masses can be treated by **partial mandibulectomy**.

Prognosis

Grave for squamous cell carcinoma of the tongue.

For other tumors, the prognosis will depend on the tumor type and suitability for treatment.

HOUSEHOLD CLEANERS AND DISINFECTANTS*

Classical signs

- Ptyalism, acute onset.
- Dysphagia.
- Depression, saliva-stained front feet.

Pathogenesis

Most common household cleaning products and disinfectants are **extremely toxic to cats**.

These include **chlorine** (sodium hypochlorite), **strong alkalis**, **strong acids**, **pine oils**, **phenolic compounds**, **hydrocarbons** and **quaternary ammonium compounds**.

Most cause **contact necrosis** of **skin** and **mucous membranes** especially if undiluted or incorrectly diluted.

Most toxicities occur when the cat **licks water containing cleaner residues** (e.g. shower recess cleaners) or by licking paws after walking through the chemical.

This causes corrosive damage of the tongue surface, mucous membranes of the mouth and occasionally, esophagus.

Clinical signs

Acute onset of **hypersalivation, depression, dysphagia**.

Front legs are often wet and stained with saliva.

Rapid secondary bacterial infection occurs in the mouth causing halitosis.

Tongue slightly swollen, partially immobile, and the **dorsal surface initially appears very pale and dull (early necrosis).**

Sloughing may occur to variable extent of the surface of the tongue leaving **raw, ulcerated surface** – usually within 36–48 hours.

There is rapid onset of **dehydration** due to saliva loss and inability to lap water.

Neurological signs (muscle weakness, fasciculations, seizures) may occur with **quaternary ammonium** and **pine oil/phenolic compound toxicities.**

Esophageal corrosion may occur with choking, gagging and retching and regurgitation of white foam.

Other areas of body may be affected, e.g. pads of feet.

Diagnosis

History of exposure.

Occasionally characteristic **smell of toxic agent,** e.g. chlorine.

Methemoglobinemia indicates toxicity involves phenolic compound.

Treatment

Wash corrosive material off cat.

Supportive fluids, nutrition, and **broad-spectrum antibiotics,** e.g. cephalexin (15 mg/kg IM q 12 h).

Corticosteroids in the early stages, especially if **esophagitis is suspected,** e.g. dexamethasone (0.1–0.2 mg/kg IV, IM q 12–24 h).

Pain control in the early stages, e.g. buprenorphine (0.005–0.01 mg/kg IV, IM q 4–8 h).

PORTOSYSTEMIC SHUNT*

Classical signs

- Ptyalism, excessive salivation.
- Repeated swallowing and lip smacking.
- Behavioral and neurological signs including seizures.
- Signs are intermittent, progressive and often associated with eating.
- Usually in young cats (< 1 year).

Pathogenesis

Portosystemic shunts (portocaval shunt, portovascular anastomosis) are **vascular communications** between portal and systemic venous systems.

Clinical signs are the result of **gut-produced neurotoxins** bypassing normal detoxification in the liver, entering the systemic circulation and affecting the CNS.

These gut-produced neurotoxins include ammonia, mercaptans, GABA agonists, benzodiazepam ligands and tryptophan.

Portosystemic shunts can be **congenital or acquired, intrahepatic or extrahepatic.**

Most **feline** portosystemic shunts are **congenital**, single and **extrahepatic**.

Reduced blood supply to the liver often results in a **small liver**.

High urinary excretion of ammonia and uric acid may result in **urate urolithasis** and/or **ammonium biurate crystals** in urine.

Clinical signs

CNS disturbances associated with hepatic encephalopathy are most frequent, occurring in 95% of cases of feline portosystemic shunting.

Neurological signs vary considerably and include mild behavioral changes (aggressive behavior, staring into space, head-pressing), **ataxia**, **weakness**, **stupor**, blindness, dilated pupils, tremors, seizures, coma and **death**.

The hallmark of the CNS signs is that they are **intermittent, progressive in severity** and **often precipitated by a high-protein meal**.

Hypersalivation is an especially prominent clinical sign (78%).

Signs wax and wane with episodes lasting minutes to hours and may or may not be associated with feeding.

Signs related to **hepatic dysfunction** include **stunted growth, delayed anesthesia recovery, diarrhea, polydipsia/polyuria and lethargy**.

Signs of urinary tract disease as a result of **urate urolithiasis** include **hematuria, dysuria and pollakiuria**.

Signs often abate with **antibiotic administration** (i.e. reduced production of toxic metabolites by enteric bacteria).

In cats, clinical signs of hepatic encephalopathy most commonly **become apparent at about 6 months of age**.

Diagnosis

Serum bile acids – 2 hours post-prandial **always** elevated with portosystemic shunts (>100 µmol/L).
- Serum bile acids are specific indicators of hepatobiliary disease in the cat. Fasting bile acids are normally less than 5 µmol/L and 2 hour post-feeding bile acids usually less than 20 µmol/L. Cats with portosystemic shunt usually have elevated (>100 µmol/L) bile acids 2 hours after feeding. Serum bile acids concentration cannot however differentiate between hepatocellular, vascular or cholestatic liver disease.

Ammonia tolerance test: more specific than bile acids, but not practical unless in-house ammonia testing available as ammonia is very labile. Cats with portosystemic shunt may have normal fasting blood ammonia levels. Blood is taken 30 minutes after a challenge with 100 mg/kg ammonium chloride. This ammonia-loading test, although very specific, has a propensity for inducing vomiting and excessively high serum ammonia levels causing severe CNS signs.

Hematology – RBC **microcytosis** may occur (MCV < 39 fl).

Biochemistry – normal to decreased BUN, hypocholesterolemia, mild increase in ALT and AST.

Ultrasonography – can be useful to visualize shunt vessel especially with **intrahepatic shunts**.

Portography – contrast portogram via mesenteric vein provides definitive diagnosis and location of shunt vessel.

Urinalysis – may reveal ammonium biurate crystals or urate uroliths.

Liver biopsy – histology shows periportal fibrosis, bile duct hyperplasia.

Transcolonic portal scintigraphy – availability likely to be restricted.

Differential diagnosis

The combination of intermittent, **recurrent ptyalism** and **neurological signs** associated **with eating** in a **young cat** is **almost pathognomonic** for portosystemic shunt.

Viral encephalitides such as **rabies and feline spongioform encephalopathy** can present with severe CNS disturbances combined with ptyalism but these diseases are always **progressive** and signs are **continuous.**

Lead poisoning can occasionally present with clinical signs of intermittent neurological disturbances and hypersalivation in the cat. Blood lead levels will confirm or rule out diagnosis.

Pyrethrin and **pyrethroid toxicity** produces signs of hypersalivation and neurological signs. Signs are continuous and history of recent exposure generally confirms diagnosis.

Organochlorine (chlorinated hydrocarbon) and **organophosphate toxicity** is characterized by hypersalivation and neuromuscular disturbances including muscular disturbances such as muscular twitching, weakness and seizures. History of exposure and serum cholinesterase levels (OP) will confirm diagnosis.

Treatment

The medical management of portosystemic shunt encephalopathy plays a vital role in **both pre-** and **post-surgical treatment.**

Medical management on its own, however, is **palliative at best**.

Medical management consists of:

- Minimize formation and absorption of **ammonia** and other toxic substances by the administration of **oral antibiotics** (**ampicillin** (20–40 mg/kg PO q 8 h), **metronidazole** (10–25 mg/kg PO 24 h), and **oral lactulose** 2.5–5 ml q 8 h). The dose of lactulose (a palatable syrup) should be increased or reduced to produce soft stools 2–3 times daily.
- **Retention enemas** can be used to treat **hepatic coma**. The enema consists of **neomycin** (15 mg/kg) plus **lactulose** (diluted 1:2 with warm water) and is given in doses of 40–200 ml and repeated until colon is completely empty and then given every 6–8 hours as long as the coma persists.
- Determine **blood glucose**, **fluid**, **electrolyte** and **acid–base** status of patient and normalize balances using **lactated Ringers** solution supplemented with **2.5–5% dextrose** and **potassium chloride** depending on laboratory results.

Control seizures with diazepam (0.25–0.5 mg/kg IV q 6–8 h).

Dietary therapy – the ideal diet should contain the **minimum amount of high-biological-value protein**, highly available **carbohydrates** as the primary source of energy, adequate levels of **arginine** and **minerals,** and be **palatable.** Diets designed for renal-failure cats generally meet these requirements although, in severe cases, even more protein restriction may be required.

Surgery is ultimately the treatment of choice as it offers the possibility of cure.

- Surgery involves isolating the shunting vessels and **partial** (using ameroid constrictor band) or **complete ligation** depending on measured portal venous pressure.
- Rapidly fatal **portal hypertension** and gastrointestinal venous stasis may occur with complete ligation of the shunting vessel and **close observation is required for 48 hours** in case repeat surgery is required to relax the ligature.
- Clinical signs of hepatic encephalopathy may recur months after surgery, necessitating repeat surgery to re-ligate the shunting vessel.

Prognosis

Good if surgery successful.

Often difficult to manage medically without surgery.

ESOPHAGEAL FOREIGN BODY*

Classical signs

- Hypersalivation, dysphagia.
- Gagging, retching, swallowing, outstretched neck.
- Regurgitating white or blood-tinged foam.

Pathogenesis

Caudal-pointing papillary spines on the tongue and the playful nature of cats make **linear foreign body** (string, cotton thread) ingestion common. These are **often wrapped around the base of the tongue**.

Other foreign bodies include sewing needles, fish hooks, hair balls, V-shaped cooked avian bones (e.g. wish-bone) and string attached to the end of continental sausages. These usually lodge at **thoracic inlet, base of the heart** or **at diaphragm hiatus**.

Complications include secondary aspiration pneumonia, esophageal perforations, regional esophagitis with or without secondary stricture and bronchoesophageal fistula.

Clinical signs

Acute onset of gagging, retching, ptyalism, often with **neck stretched forward**.

Regurgitation of **white foam** often stained with **fresh blood.**

Signs of depression, anorexia, fever, cough and dyspnea can suggest **esophageal perforation** or **aspiration pneumonia**.

Signs are generally continuous and persistent.

Diagnosis

History of playing with or eating a **potential foreign body**.

Plain and/or contrast **radiography** to demonstrate foreign body.

Endoscopy is useful to confirm the presence of a foreign body and to assess damage to the esophagus.

Check under tongue for linear foreign body (e.g. cotton or string).

Differential diagnosis

Pharyngeal **foreign body** or **acute pharyngitis**. Examine pharynx under general anesthetic.

Acute **viral** esophagitis/pharyngitis/laryngitis. Usually other viral signs predominate (i.e. sneezing, running eyes, etc.). Both calici and herpes virus possible.

Acute **gastroesophageal intussusception** or **hiatal hernia** – usually **intermittent** signs.

Caustic chemical pharyngitis/esophagitis (rare) is always associated with chemical burning of the **dorsum of the tongue**.

Treatment

Retrieval of the foreign body by **endoscopy**.

Perforating foreign bodies require **thoracotomy and esophagotomy**.

Sewing needles and fish hooks on string can often by retrieved by passing a plastic tube down the string to dislodge and guard the foreign body during retrieval.

Broad-spectrum **antibiotics** (amoxicillin 20 mg/kg SC or IM q 12 h).

Withhold food and water for 24–48 hours.

Intravenous or **subcutaneous fluid** support will be required first 24–48 hours.

Some foreign bodies can be pushed into the stomach and retrieved by gastrotomy.

Prognosis

Good **unless esophageal perforation has occurred.**

ESOPHAGITIS*

Classical signs

- Excessive salivation.
- Repeated attempts at swallowing.
- Anorexia, dysphagia.
- Regurgitation.

Pathogenesis

Most commonly due to **gastric reflux** during and after **anesthesia**.

Pre-anesthetic and anesthetic agents suppress normal esophageal motility and can cause the lower esophageal sphincter to relax allowing **gastric reflux**.

Refluxed in **hydrochloric acid** can reduce esophageal pH to 2.0 and cause protein denaturation of the esophageal mucosa.

Once esophagitis exists, the **lower esophageal sphincter becomes incompetent, perpetuating reflux**.

Tilting of the surgery table and **poor patient preparation** (food-filled stomach) before surgery **predisposes cats to reflux esophagitis.**

Esophagitis can occur secondary to **esophageal foreign bodies** or **persistent vomiting**.

Rarely, esophagitis can result from **ingestion of caustic agents**.

Pooling of gastric fluids and resultant esophagitis characteristically occurs in the region of the **base of the heart**.

Young animals with **congenital esophageal hernia** are likely to have a higher risk for reflux esophagitis.

Occasionally, esophagitis associated with **severe feline herpes virus or calicivirus** infection occurs.

Pain and **inability to swallow** probably plays a major role in pathogenesis of ptyalism.

If untreated, esophagitis often leads to **secondary esophageal stricture**.

Clinical signs

Dysphagia, excessive salivation, repeated swallowing attempts with out-stretched neck occurs in the **early, acute phase** of the disease syndrome.

Regurgitation of white froth, often blood stained occurs in the early stages of acute, severe esophagitis.

Signs generally occur **within 24–48 hours of anesthetic** if post-anesthetic esophagitis.

Intense pain associated with swallowing attempts may cause the cat to cry out.

Concomitant oral ulceration and stomatitis may indicate caustic **chemical ingestion.**

Regurgitation of food and/or vomiting can occur in milder cases of esophagitis, hiatal hernia or healing/stricture phase of severe acute esophagitis.

Diagnosis

History of **chemical exposure**, ingestion of a **foreign body** or a **recent anesthetic**.

Survey radiographs of the esophagus are often unremarkable.

Endoscopy reveals variable hyperemia, bleeding, ulceration and pseudomembranes of the esophageal mucosa, or a foreign body.

Post-anesthetic reflux esophagitis lesions are characteristically in the region over the **base of the heart.**

Reflux **due to severe vomiting or hiatal hernia** characteristically causes esophagitis in the **distal esophagus**.

Endoscopy can differentiate a **functional** esophageal stricture due to severe mucosal and sub-mucosal inflammation and edema from a **fibrous stricture** (forming subsequent to severe esophagitis).

Differential diagnosis

Hiatal hernia usually causes **intermittent** signs of vomiting, ptyalism, regurgitation and dyspnea. Plain radiography shows a soft tissue density dorsal to the vena cava in the caudal thorax. Contrast radiography reveals the gastric fundus in the region of the terminal esophagus.

Gastroesophageal intussusception – may cause intermittent signs but often causes persistent and severe clinical signs of vomiting and salivation leading to rapid onset of vascular shock and death. Plain or contrast radiography or endoscopy to confirm.

Diaphragmatic hernia involving the stomach – rapid expansion of incarcerated stomach after eating due to accumulating gases causes rapid onset of dyspnea, salivation and attempts to vomit. Plain or contrast radiography to confirm presence of stomach in the chest. **Often history of feeding immediately prior to onset of signs.**

Treatment

Acute reflux or chemical esophagitis must be treated aggressively in the early stage in an attempt to prevent fibrous esophageal stricture.

Preferably, all medication should be given **parenterally for the first 5–6 days.**

Broad-spectrum antibiotics to control secondary bacterial infections (amoxicillin/clavulanic acid).

Corticosteroids to prevent stricture (dexamethasone 0.2 mg/kg IM or IV q 12–24 h).

Sucralfate suspension to protect mucosa per os if not vomiting (0.25 g PO q 8–12 h).

Cimetidine (10 mg/kg IV, IM PO q 6–8 h) or **ranitidine** (2.5 mg/kg IV q 12 h; 3.5 mg/kg PO q 12 h) to **reduce gastric acidity**.

Metoclopramide (0.2 mg/kg IV, IM, PO q 6–8 h) or **cisapride** (5 mg/cat q 8–12 h) to promote gastric emptying.

Narcotics for pain control e.g. methadone 0.1–0.5 mg/kg IV or IM q 4–6 h

Placement of **gastrotomy** or **esophagotomy** tube for nutrition while "resting esophagus" – leave in place 5–7 days.

Surgical repair of hiatal hernia, gastroesophageal hernia or diaphragmatic hernia.

Prognosis

Esophageal stricture due to fibrosis and scarring secondary to esophagitis is common and is characterized by repeated regurgitation after eating.

This can be treated with gradual dilatation of stricture by balloon dilation catheter or bouginage. Often requires repeated dilation over weeks or months to achieve resolution of signs.

HIATAL HERNIA/GASTROESOPHAGEAL INTUSSUSCEPTION

Classical signs

- Ptyalism.
- Vomiting/regurgitation.

Classical signs—Cont'd

- May or may not be related to eating.
- Dyspnea, hematemesis, collapse, shock, death with large intussusceptions.
- Signs often intermittent

Pathogenesis

Hiatal hernia denotes herniation of the distal esophagus and proximal stomach into the thoracic cavity.

Hiatal hernias tend to be **intermittent** in nature but can be persistent.

Gastroesophageal intussusception occurs when the stomach (and occasionally duodenum, spleen, etc.) prolapses (invaginates) into the distal esophagus with resultant compromise of blood supply to the prolapsed segment. **Gastroesophageal intussusception** is **usually acute** and **persistent** but can be chronic with intermittent signs.

Congenital or acquired laxity of the hiatus is suspected to predispose to both hiatal hernias and gastroesophageal intussusception.

Diaphragmatic hernia may predispose to post-surgical gastroesophageal intussusception.

Reflux esophagitis occurs with both gastroesophageal intussusception and hiatal hernias.

Clinical signs

Although uncommon, both gastroesophageal intussusception and hiatal hernias are a significant **rule-out in ptyalism**.

Chronic intermittent vomiting is characteristic for both **hiatal hernia** and **chronic gastroesophageal intussusception**.

Chronic, intermittent ptyalism can occur **with or without vomiting** and weight loss.

Acute bouts of **respiratory distress** may occur.

Large, acute gastroesophageal intussusception can cause rapid onset of shock associated with hematemesis, dyspnea, collapse and sudden death.

Diagnosis

Gastroesophageal intussusception:

- **Plain thoracic radiographs** show the presence of a **soft tissue mass** in the esophagus cranial to the diaphragm. The gastric gas bubble in the cranial abdomen is often missing indicating that the stomach has prolapsed into the esophagus.
- The diagnosis can be confirmed with a **barium swallow** in which the barium will not pass beyond the intussusception.
- Endoscopy will reveal.

Hiatial hernia:

- The hernial sac is formed by the stretched phreno-esophageal ligament and **sliding hernias** are frequently associated with **gastric reflux** and **esophagitis**.
- **Plain radiographs** may or may not reveal herniation of the stomach and diagnosis is usually confirmed by **barium swallow under fluoroscopy** or by **endoscopy**.
- Applying **abdominal pressure during radiography** may help induce hernia.
- **Endoscopy** is also valuable in assessing the degree of esophagitis due to gastroesophageal reflux.

Differential diagnosis

Megaesophagus is often associated with hiatal hernia and gastroesophageal intussusception. **Regurgitation** is a predominant sign. Confirm that the megaesophagus is unassociated with hiatal hernia or gastroesophageal intussusception by esophagram.

Esophageal foreign body. Signs of gagging, retching, salivation, repeated attempts at swallowing generally acute onset and continuous. History of eating or playing with **foreign body**. LOOK UNDER TONGUE! Confirm with plain and/or contrast radiographs or endoscopy.

Porto-systemic shunt. Severe pain associated with gastroesophageal intussusception may induce signs that may be confused with portosystemic shunt. Portosystemic shunt can be confirmed with serum bile acids.

Diaphragmatic hernia with incarcerated stomach. Confirm with X-rays/contrast.

Treatment

Medical treatment:

- Control of **esophagitis** and clinical signs with **ranitidine** (3.5 mg/kg PO q 12 h) or **cimetidine** (5–10 mg/kg PO q12 h).
- Feed **low-fat diet**. Fat delays gastric emptying time and it is therefore desirable to feed **low-fat diets. Elevated feedings** may help some cats and should be trialled especially if megaesophagus is present.
- If no response to medical therapy **surgical repair** is warranted.

Surgical repair involves anatomical replacement of herniated organs, reduction in size of esophageal hiatus, phrenicoesophageal plexy and left-sided fundic gastropexy.

ORGANOPHOSPHATE AND CARBAMATE TOXICITY

Classical signs

- Ptyalism, lacrimation, vomiting, diarrhea, pollakiuria.
- Miosis, muscular tremors, seizures.
- Dyspnea, respiratory failure.
- Bradycardia, depression, death.
- Rapid onset of clinical signs.

Pathogenesis

Organophosphates (OPs) and carbamates cause **inhibition of acetylcholinesterase** (AChE) and pseudo-cholinesterase, which allows **accumulation of acetylcholine** (ACh) in RBCs and the post-synaptic receptors of nervous tissue and muscle.

Accumulation of ACh results in **marked excitation of all effector organs**.

OPs are generally considered **irreversible** inhibitors of AChE activity, while **carbamates are slowly reversible** inhibitors.

OPs are **stored in fat** and slowly released into the circulation. **Lean, long-haired breeds** of cats are **more severely affected**.

Cats are more susceptible to OP toxicity than **dogs**. Poisoning often occurs following use of **canine flea products on cats**.

Most cat poison cases are due to **carbamates**.

Clinical signs

Early signs include **apprehension, increased swallowing, ptyalism, muscular twitching around the face and eyes. Miosis** and **bradycardia** occur.

Muscular twitching progresses to **whole-body muscle fasciculations** and **generalized tetany** causing a stiff-legged gait progressing to a **sawhorse stance** (i.e. all four legs stiff and apart).

Abdominal pain, cramping **diarrhea, vomiting** and **frequent urination** occurs commonly and eventually progresses to **muscular weakness** and **paralysis**.

Death can occur due to **respiratory failure**.

Delayed neuropathy: certain OPs (e.g. fenthion) can cause a delayed (usually 7–10 days) neuropathy causing **hindlimb weakness** and **characteristic ventroflexion of the neck**. All the other signs of acute OP poisoning are **absent** when delayed signs occur. Delayed neuropathy may occur after minimal exposure and there may be no history of acute signs in the preceding 7–10 days.

Diagnosis

History of recent application of OP or carbamate and characteristic signs.

Cholinesterase assay – whole blood, serum or plasma. Results should be interpreted in light of clinical signs and time of onset of signs.

Differential diagnosis

Pyrethrin toxicity – history of exposure.

Quaternary ammonium toxicity – history of exposure and ptyalism with **mouth ulcers** rather than generalized parasympathetic signs as occur with OPs.

Treatment

Establish **IV fluid line** and (oxygen/ventilation if needed).

Atropine IV (0.25–0.5 mg/kg) repeated to effect can be given S/C once stabilized. **Do not over-atropinize**.

Diazepam (1 mg/kg IV) **repeated to effect** to control **seizures**.

Muscle fasciculations can be controlled with **diphenhydramine** (2–4 mg/kg PO q 8 h).

2-PAM (20 mg/kg IM or IV) is effective against confirmed OP toxicity **if given in the first 24 hours**. **Repeat 8 hourly until stable**. Can be given with atropine. **Do not use in carbamate toxicity**.

Prevent further absorption – **wash cat with hair shampoo**, and give **activated charcoal** PO.

Diphenhydramine is used to treat delayed neuropathy (2–4 mg/kg PO q 8 h).

Prognosis

Generally good with treatment.

PYRETHRIN AND PYRETHROID TOXICITY

Classical signs

- Ptyalism.
- Tremors, ataxia, seizures.
- Depression or hyperexcitability.
- Vomiting, diarrhea.

Pathogenesis

Popular insecticide for use on cats.

Slows the closing of the sodium ion gate in nerve cells resulting in repetitive discharges or membrane depolarization.

Extremely bitter taste of topically-applied pyrethroids.

Clinical signs

Ptyalism, tremors, ataxia, seizures.

Occasionally **dyspnea** and **coma** occurs.

Hyperthermia, vomiting and **diarrhea** can occur.

Rapid onset of signs post exposure (within a few hours).

Diagnosis

History of exposure, clinical signs.

No definitive diagnostic clinical test available to date.

Differential diagnosis

Organophosphate/carbamate toxicity – blood cholinesterase level low.

Treatment

Diazepam (0.2 mg/kg IV) **to effect** to control **tremors** or **seizures**.

Phenobarbital IV if not controlled with phenobarbital add pentobarbital IV. NB **Phenobarbital** is an **anticonvulsant** where **pentobarbital stops muscular activity**. Pentobarbital is associated with paddling on recovery, which can be difficult to distinguish from seizure activity, and makes it less suitable for acute seizure control.

Wash cat to reduce further absorption.

Recovery usually in 1–4 days.

Small doses of **atropine** (0.01–0.02 mg/kg IV, IM, SC q 6–8 h) can be used to control salivation. (**Do not over-atropinise.**)

IV fluids, O_2, ventilation in severely affected cases.

ACETAMINOPHEN (PARACETAMOL) TOXICITY

Classical signs

- Ptyalism.
- Pale, blue-tinged mucous membranes.
- Facial edema, respiratory distress.
- Anorexia, vomiting.
- Hemoglobinuria.

Pathogenesis

Acetaminophen is widely used as an **antipyretic** and **analgesic in human medicine**.

Most common drug-induced toxicosis in the cat.

Metabolized in the liver to **glucuronide** and **sulfate conjugates**.

Cats are **deficient in glucuronyltransferase** and the glucuronidation and sulfation biotransformation routes are **rapidly saturated**, causing acute toxicity.

Hepatic necrosis and **methemoglobinemia** results.

Fatal methemoglobinemia usually occurs before signs of hepatic necrosis develops.

Cats are poisoned by as little as 50–60 mg/kg: that is, one adult tablet.

Clinical signs

Cyanosis and **tachypnea**.

Salivation and **abdominal pain**.

Facial edema and **often edema of the paws**.

Heinz body anemia.

Chocolate-colored urine (hemaglobinuria, hematuria).

Jaundice.

Rapid onset of clinical signs (within a few hours of ingestion).

Death ensues 18–36 hours after ingestion, if untreated.

Diagnosis

History of drug administration.

Characteristic combination of **facial edema** and **chocolate-colored urine**.

Heinz bodies on RBCs.

Methemoglobinemia.

Progressive rise in **liver enzymes**.

Low blood glutathione levels.

Serum acetaminophen concentration maximally elevated within 1–3 h after ingestion.

Differential diagnosis

Phenolic and **phenolic compound toxicity**.

Nitrite poisoning.

Treatment

Prompt and **early treatment** is essential.

Gastric lavage within 4–6 hours of ingestion.

Activated charcoal per os.

N-acetylcysteine (Mucomyst) 140 mg/kg as a 5% solution PO or IV as a loading dose, then 70 mg/kg PO or IV q 4 h for 3–5 additional treatments.

Ascorbic acid 125 mg PO q 6 h.

Electrolyte and fluid therapy.

Handle patient with **least stress**.

A rough estimate of the methemoglobin content of blood can be made by comparing the color of the patient's drop of blood against that of a drop of blood from a normal cat against a white background (e.g. white absorbent paper). A noticeable brown coloration compared with normal blood indicates a methemoglobin content of more than 10%. This subjective test can be used to monitor the effectiveness of treatment and should be performed every 2–3 hours.

Good nursing and **maintain body temperature.**

Whole blood transfusion if necessary to treat **hemolytic anemia**.

Recovery usually within 48 h.

Prognosis

Guarded to poor if severe methemaglobinuria (>50%) or hemolysis.

Good with very early and aggressive treatment.

LEAD POISONING

Classical signs

- Gastrointestinal – diarrhea, vomiting, inappetance.
- CNS signs – behavioral changes, depression, seizures.
- Occasionally, intermittent ptyalism.

Clinical signs

Usually in **young cats**.

Vague, **chronic gastrointestinal signs** most common – e.g. inanition, **inappetance**, poor growth, occasionally diarrhea and vomiting.

CNS signs can occur in more severe cases and include behavioral changes (depression, aggression, lethargy) seizures and blindness.

Occasionally, intermittent ptyalism.

Diagnosis

History of access to lead, e.g. old house renovation (lead-based paint, dust from sanding).

Blood lead greater than 0.4 ppm.

Treatment

Chelation of lead with calcium disodium ethylene diamine tetra-acetate (CaEDTA) 100 mg/kg SC daily in four divided doses. Dilute CaEDTA to a concentration of about 10 mg CaEDTA/ml with 5% dextrose solution for 5 days. In severe cases, a further 5-day course can be given after a rest period of 5 days.

Relapses of clinical signs of lead poisoning are common and are treated as they arise.

SPIDER ENVENOMATION

Classical signs

- Ptyalism.
- Hyperexcitability.
- Ataxia, paralysis.

Pathogenesis

Latrodectus spp. spiders include **black widow** (USA), **red back spider** (Australia) and **katipo** (New Zealand).

Venom contains **alpha-latroxin**, a **potent neuro-toxin**. The toxin opens cation-selective channels at the presynaptic nerve terminals, causing **release of large amount** of acetylcholine and **norepinephrine resulting in sustained muscle spasm**.

The mechanism of **severe pain** at the bite site and regions remote from the actual bitten area is not well understood.

Clinical signs

Initially, **severe pain** characterized by **crying out**.

Hyperexcitability, **ataxia**, **muscle rigidity** and spasm, progressing to **muscle weakness** and collapse.

Prolonged, **severe ptyalism**, possibly due to pain.

Death can occur from **respiratory failure**.

Diagnosis

Clinical signs.

History of contact with latrodectus spider.

Laboratory evaluation not helpful.

Treatment

Latrodectus antivenine results in dramatic improvement of clinical signs if given in the acute phase of the disease and good results can be achieved even if given 24 hours after envenomation.
- **Premedicate** with **antihistamine** (chlorpheniramine 2.5–5 mg IM or SC) and have epinephrine (2.5–5 µg/kg IV) on hand. Latrodectus antivenine is prepared from the hyperimmune serum of horses.
- Dose of antivenine is 1 vial (500 units) given by **intramuscular** injection.
- In life-threatening situations the **intravenous route** can be used but the risk of **anaphylaxis** is greater.

Muscle spasm can be controlled with small doses of **intravenous diazepam** (0.2–0.5 mg/kg q 6 h), but **avoid respiratory depression**.

Supportive care includes **intravenous fluids, cortisone** and **atropine** (to control salivation).

Prognosis

Good with use of antivenine; guarded without.

DIEFFENBACHIA ("DUMB CANE") POISONING

Classical signs

- Ptyalism.
- Tongue paralysis.
- Dysphagia.

Pathophysiology

Dieffenbachia is a popular decorative indoor plant. The leaves contain **irritant calcium oxalate crystals**, which the plant can propel into the tissues of the mouth of cats chewing on the plant by means of special contractile cells.

Plant extract also contains **protealytic enzymes**, which trigger the release of histamines and kinins and contribute to clinical signs.

Plant is also known as "**dumb cane**" because it produces **paralysis of the tongue**.

Clinical signs

Sudden onset of signs. There is **immediate pain on chewing plant**.

Immediate **salivation**. Often **head shaking**.

Sometimes **change in voice**.

Examination of mouth reveals mild to moderate mucosal edema and **tongue paralysis** and **swelling.**

Diagnosis

History of plant chewing.

Treatment

Symptomatic – rinse mouth with water or **milk** to precipitate soluble oxalates.

Antihistamines (diphenhydramine 2–4 mg/kg IV, IM, PO q 6–8 h), and **corticosteroids** (dexamethasone 0.1–0.2 mg/kg IV, IM, PO q 12–24 h) to relieve pain and swelling.

Prognosis

Prognosis is very good as clinical signs regress after 24–48 hours.

DIAPHRAGMATIC HERNIA WITH INCARCERATED STOMACH

Classical signs

- Uncommon.
- Intermittent bouts of ptyalism often associated with dyspnea.
- Anxious expression, often after eating.

Pathogenesis

Stomach, with or without other abdominal organs, is chronically incarcerated in pleural cavity by constricting diaphragm subsequent to **traumatic diaphragmatic hernia**.

Sudden expansion of the stomach due to a large meal, with or without associated gas production causes **acute onset of hypersalivation with anxious expression**.

Rapid expansion of stomach volume after eating causes **sudden onset nausea,** which in turn, causes ptyalism.

Clinical signs

Sudden onset of salivation with **intent, anxious expression** and varying degrees of **dyspnea**.

Usually signs occur **immediately after eating.**

Differential diagnosis

Portosystemic shunt is associated with elevated postprandial bile acids and CNS signs.

Diagnosis

Plain and/or contrast radiography.

Treatment

Surgical repair of hernia.

D-LIMONENE, LINAPOOL, AND CRUDE CITRUS OIL EXTRACTS

Classical signs

- Moderate to severe ptyalism.
- Muscular tremors (shivering).
- Ataxia.

Clinical signs

Used as insecticidal sprays or shampoos.

Immediate sign of toxicosis is hypersalivation which lasts 15 minutes to 1 hour.

More severely affected cats develop muscular tremors and ataxia. Hypothermia occurs.

Clinical signs generally abate within 4 hours.

Treatment

Wash cat in unmedicated shampoo.

Maintain body temperature.

DIBUTYL PHTHALATE

> **Classical Signs**
>
> - Profuse salivation and foaming.
> - Occasional retching and/or vomiting.

Clinical Signs

Used luminescent agent in "Glo-Jewellary" and as insect repellent

Has extremely bitter taste and causes immediate hypersalivation when cat bites into toy.

Signs of hypersalivation generally self limiting once taste removed from mouth.

RABIES

> **Classical signs**
>
> - CNS signs, behavioral changes.
> - Ptyalism, frothing.
> - Fever.

Pathogenesis

Single-stranded RNA Lyssavirus.

Virus inoculation via **bite wound** from rabid animal or **via mucous membrane** contact with infected body fluids, e.g. saliva.

Viral replication occurs in myocytes and spreads to neuromuscular junctions and neurotendinal spindles.

Virus spreads to CNS via intra-axonal fluid within peripheral nerves, then to peripheral sensory and motor neurons.

Salivary glands contain **large amounts of virus which is shed in saliva.**

Infection through contact with infected reservoir animals (bats, skunks, raccoons and foxes) or **infected dogs** and **cats.**

Clinical signs

Initial clinical signs are present for **only 24 hours** and include **low-grade fever** and **behavioral changes** (e.g. irritability, hiding or increased affection).

The **excitatory stage** ("**furious rabies**") may last 2–4 days and is not always exhibited.

Signs include **muscle fasciculations**, **ptyalism**, **weakness**, **ataxia** and **increased aggressiveness** and **irritability**.

The **final stage ("dumb" rabies)** lasts 1–4 days and **general paralysis and convulsions precede death.**

Diagnosis

History of **no vaccination** with approved killed vaccine.

History of **exposure to bite** or **scratch wounds from infected dogs or cats.**

History of exposure to reservoir animals including foxes, skunks, raccoons and bats.

Typical clinical signs with progression almost invariably to **death within 7–10 days**.

EXTREME ZOONOTIC POTENTIAL.

Immediately notify authorities when rabies is suspected. Follow official policy for handling suspected rabies cases, including tissue or fluid samples.

Minimal changes in CSF analysis and **routine blood** analysis.

Histological confirmation with finding **Negri bodies** within the CNS on post-mortem.

Immunofluorescent antibody test on CNS tissue.

Differential diagnosis

Portosystemic shunt – intermittent, often associated with eating. Lack of rapid progression of signs over 7–10 days resulting in death. Confirm with post-prandial serum bile acids.

Pyrethrin and pyrethroid toxicity – no behavior changes and history of exposure and serum cholinesterase levels (OP) will confirm diagnosis.

Feline spongiform encephalopathy also has combination of neurological signs and hypersalivation. Histopathology differentiates.

Treatment

No treatment should be attempted. Almost uniformly fatal.

Follow official guides for management of suspected rabies case.

Prognosis

Always grave.

FELINE SPONGIFORM ENCEPHALOPATHY (FSE)

Classical signs

- CNS signs, progressive.
- Hypersalivation.

Clinical signs

Progressive neurological signs including ataxia (especially pelvic limbs), behavioral changes, hyperesthesia, head tremor, muscle fasciculations.

Ptyalism.

Diagnosis

Histopathology shows discrete **vacuolation** of gray matter throughout CNS.

Treatment

Supportive only.

Prognosis

Grave.

FELINE PANLEUKOPENIA (PARVO VIRUS, FELINE ENTERITIS, FELINE DISTEMPER)

Classical signs

- Vomiting, diarrhea.
- Lethargy.
- Severe dehydration.
- High mortality.

Clinical signs

Usually in young (2–6 months) kittens.

Acute-onset vomiting, often severe diarrhea.

Fever in early stages of disease.

Rapid dehydration.

Severe depression.

Although not generally a feature of feline panleukopenia, continuous ptyalism has been recorded as the predominate clinical sign in kitten with confirmed panleukopenia at post-mortem examination.

Diagnosis

No vaccination history, recent exposure to virus.

Panleukopenia is the most consistent clinical finding. Complete blood counts show leukocyte counts between 500 and 3000 cells per microliter during the acute phase of the disease.

Canine parvovirus antigen fecal immunoassay will detect feline parvovirus antigen in feces of affected cats.

Viral isolation from feces or affected tissues.

Histopathology.

Treatment

Rehydration, intravenous fluids.

Re-establishment of electrolyte balance.

Broad-spectrum antibiotics (amoxicillin/clavulonic acid 62.5 mg/cat PO q 12 h).

Whole blood transfusion in severely affected cats.

Prognosis

Guarded to poor in young kittens.

If cat survives 5 days, prognosis improved markedly.

RECOMMENDED READING

Sherding RD (ed). The Cat: Diseases and Clinical Management, 2nd edn. WB Saunders Company, Philadelphia, 1994.

The Veterinary Clinics of North America, Small Animal Practice, Toxicology for the Small Animal Practitioner 1975; 5: 4623–4652.

The Veterinary Clinics of North America, Small Animal Practice, Non-cardiac Surgical Diseases of the Thorax 1987; 17: 2333–2358.

The Veterinary Clinics of North America, Small Animal Practice, Liver Disease 1995; 25: 2337–2355.

Tilley, Smith. The 5 Minute Veterinary Consult – Canine and Feline, 3rd edn. Lippincott, Williams and Wilkins, 1997.

28. The cat with bad breath or oral lesions

Gary John Wilson

> **KEY SIGNS**
> - Bad breath.
> - Oral mass, ulceration or inflammation.
> - Calculus.

MECHANISM?

- Bad breath occurs from the production of volatile sulfur-containing compounds. Hydrogen sulfide and methyl mercaptan account for approximately 90% of these. Gram-negative bacteria are primarily responsible for malodor production.

WHERE?

- Oral cavity, nasal cavity, nasopharynx and respiratory tract.

WHAT?

- Most cats with bad breath have periodontal disease.

QUICK REFERENCE SUMMARY

Diseases causing bad breath or oral lesions

ORAL CAVITY

ANOMALY

- Congenital anomaly of hard palate (cleft palate) (p 610)

Cleft palate results in rhinitis and secondary bacterial infection and nasal discharge in young kittens.

MECHANICAL

- **Oral foreign body* (p 609)**

Foreign bodies include grass seed, bone fragments and hair. They are usually acute onset associated with sneezing, rubbing the face, pawing at the mouth, coughing or gagging.

NEOPLASTIC

- **Oral neoplasia** (p 607)**

Visible tumors often with secondary bacterial infection and periodontal disease. Signs may include rubbing face, pawing at mouth or facial distortion.

INFECTIOUS (BACTERIAL)

- **Periodontal disease*** (p 604)**

Chronic disease with halitosis, inflamed gums and calculus on teeth.

- Oronasal fistula (p 610)

Chronic occasional sneezing and nasal discharge associated with dental disease or trauma.

- **Bacterial infection of tongue lacerations* (p 609)**

Halitosis with purulent open wound on or under tongue.

- **Oral ulcerations associated with viral causes (herpesvirus and calicivirus)* (p 607)**

Oral lesions are more common with calicivirus infection and the vesicles rupture to form oral ulcers, which allows secondary bacterial invasion.

IMMUNE/IDIOPATHIC

- **Feline oral inflammatory disease (plasmacytic-lymphocytic gingivopharyngitis complex, plasmacytic-lymphocytic stomatitis/faucitis)** (p 606)**

Chronic severe inflammation of gingiva and fauces.

- Eosinophilic granuloma complex (p 611)

Lip ulcer or raised firm lesions especially on the tongue or hard palate. Oral lesions postulated to be secondary to chronic licking.

TRAUMA

- Mandibular and maxillary fractures (p 610)

Inability to chew, salivation and rapid secondary infection of traumatized tissue.

- Tooth fracture with periapical abscessation (p 610)

Fractured teeth often go unnoticed in cats and will progress to pulp death and periapical abscessation and possible external discharge.

TOXIC

- Oral ulcerations associated with uremic or toxic causes (p 607)

Oral ulceration may occur with uremia or associated with concentrated cleaning agents, allowing secondary bacterial invasion.

EXTRA-ORAL CAUSES OF BAD BREATH (NASAL CAVITY, ESOPHAGUS, LOWER AIRWAY)

INFECTIOUS

Bacterial:

- **Bacterial rhinitis secondary to viral upper respiratory tract disease* (p 608)**

Chronic mucopurulent or hemorrhagic nasal discharge and sneezing.

continued

continued

● Infections associated with esophageal or lower airway disease (p 609)
Infections secondary to primary disease of the esophagus or lower respiratory tract.

Fungal:

● Cryptococcosis (p 611)
Chronic mucopurulent or hemorrhagic nasal discharge, sneezing and occasional facial distortion with associated halitosis.

INTRODUCTION

MECHANISM?

Volatile sulfur-containing compounds are the major contributors to malodor (bad breath).

Hydrogen sulfide and methyl mercaptan account for approximately 90% of the total sulfur content of mouth air.

Anaerobic Gram-negative bacteria utilize sulfur-containing amino acids for the generation of volatile sulfur-containing compounds.

WHERE?

Diseases of the oral cavity, nasal cavity, nasopharynx and the respiratory tract may cause bad breath and oral lesions.

Any malodor from the oral cavity indicates disease.

History and detailed physical examination (often under anesthesia) are essential for diagnosis.

Oral lesions should be expected if the cat is reluctant to allow oral examination (or shows any other signs of oral pain).

WHAT?

The most common diseases causing bad breath and oral lesions are:
● **Periodontal disease.**
● **Feline oral inflammatory disease** (plasmacytic-lymphocytic gingivopharyngitis complex).

Diagnosis is made after examination under general anesthesia, radiography, laboratory tests or a combination of these.

DISEASES CAUSING BAD BREATH OR ORAL LESIONS

PERIODONTAL DISEASE***

Classical signs

● Halitosis (bad breath).
● Calculus on teeth.
● Inflamed gums.

Pathogenesis

Plaque is a matrix of bacteria, salivary glycoproteins, food particles, epithelial cells and leukocytes, which adheres to the tooth surface.

Plaque can only be **removed mechanically**; it cannot be rinsed off.

Supragingival plaque occurs above the gum line and subgingival plaque below.

Subgingival plaque bacteria are responsible for the pathology found in periodontal disease.

Initially **edema and inflammation** of the gum margins (gingivitis) is seen, which is followed by **loss of epithelial attachment** at the base of the gingival sulcus with subsequent periodontal pocket formation.

Destructive processes continue with eventual **loss of the periodontal ligament and alveolar bone** (periodontitis).

If allowed to progress untreated, eventually the **tooth will be lost**.

As periodontal disease progresses, the bacteria change initially from anaerobic Gram-positive bacteria to Gram negative to anaerobes, and finally to fusiforms and spirochetes.

The halitosis is due to the **production of volatile sulfur compounds by the plaque bacteria** (especially by the anaerobes).

Chronic low-grade **bacteremia** from periodontal disease can have **systemic effects** on other organs (especially kidney, myocardium and liver).

Clinical signs

Healthy gingiva is **shiny with a sharp margin**, which appears almost transparent under magnification and has a sulcus depth which is less than 0.5 mm.

With gingivitis the margins are **edematous and inflamed** (red line around edge of marginal gingiva) and may **bleed on probing**. Halitosis will be present and supragingival calculus may be present.

As disease progresses, **pocket formation begins** with associated subgingival plaque. Halitosis and **supragingival calculus** will be present and subgingival calculus may also be present.

Further deterioration leads to bone loss, deep pocket formation, furcation exposure (loss of bone between tooth roots of multi-rooted teeth) and **tooth mobility.**

Severe periodontal disease will result in tooth loss, deep pockets with heavy anaerobic infections and strong halitosis. The cat may show signs of systemic disease and refuse to eat or **attempt to swallow food without chewing.**

Diagnosis

History of halitosis and, in severe cases, there may be a reluctance to chew food and occasional pawing at mouth.

Clinical signs are diagnostic.

In the anesthetized cat, determine **the severity of disease** by a thorough oral examination. This will include palpation of loose teeth and the **use of a periodontal probe** to check for the presence of periodontal pockets.

Evaluate radiographically to assess loss of **crestal bone** (bone between teeth) and loss of bone around the tooth roots.

Differential diagnosis

Feline oral inflammatory disease (or plasmacytic-lymphocytic gingivopharyngitis complex) has similar signs in the early stages to early periodontal disease but cats rapidly **develop a severe inflammation of the whole gingiva** and often a concurrent faucitis (compared to inflammation of the gum margin only with periodontal disease). The tissues are grossly inflamed and are friable, bleed easily and are extremely painful.

Feline odontoclastic resorptive lesions may appear similar to localized areas of periodontal disease with **gingival hyperplasia** covering the resorptive lesion. **Probing under general anesthesia** will reveal the lesion. These lesions are also extremely painful and cats will often avoid using these teeth.

Treatment

Dental prophylaxis to eliminate the bacteria causing odor and to remove diseased tissue so as to allow the reattachment of the gingiva.
- This is done under general anesthesia to ensure that subgingival plaque is removed.
- The steps involved are **supragingival scaling, subgingival scaling, polishing** and flushing (**irrigation**) of the sulcus.

For the more severe cases treatment may also involve **periodontal surgery** to expose affected tissue and to allow complete subgingival cleaning and extraction.

Antibiotics are usually not required.

Prognosis

Good if secondary organ damage has not occurred.

Prevention

Daily brushing is recommended but does require owner and cat compliance.

Chewing raw meaty bones such as chicken wings will help to mechanically remove the plaque.

Calculus control diets, which are designed to remove the adhered plaque as they are chewed, due to their abrasive nature or to compete with plaque for salivary calcium ions.

Dental chews will help in mechanically removing plaque.

FELINE ORAL INFLAMMATORY DISEASE** (OR PLASMACYTIC-LYMPHOCYTIC GINGIVOPHARYNGITIS COMPLEX, PLAMACYTIC-LYMPHOCYTIC STOMATITIS/FAUCITIS)

Classical signs

- Halitosis.
- Grossly inflamed gums especially in premolar and molar areas.
- Gums bleed easily.
- Very painful and cats often bad tempered.

Pathogenesis

The etiology of this condition is **unknown**. Suggested causes have been bacterial, viral (especially calicivirus) and immunological (possible hypersensitivity to plaque proteins).

The condition may be the result of chronic immune-mediated processes.

Lymphocytes, plasma cells and neutrophils are the predominate cells found at biopsy.

Clinical signs

Intense oral pain (and often bad-tempered cats which resent oral examination).

When eating, affected cats often attempt to **swallow the food without chewing** due to the oral pain. The appetite appears reduced due to the cat's reluctance to prehend food.

Halitosis.

Dysphagia, **excess salivation** and weight loss in severe cases.

Proliferation of gingiva with extensive inflammation. The tissue is friable and bleeds readily on palpation.

Most frequently involves the **gingiva caudal to the canine teeth** and **the fauces** but can occur associated with the incisors as well.

In severe cases the **entire gingiva** (not just the gingival margin) as well as the fauces becomes grossly inflamed.

More prevalent in **purebred cats**.

Diagnosis

Clinical signs are diagnostic in severe cases.

In early cases, the severe inflammatory reaction of the gingival margin (which bleeds easily on palpation) is suggestive.

The diagnosis can be confirmed by **biopsy** if necessary.

Differential diagnosis

Periodontal disease. The inflammation is less acute, less severe and restricted to the gingival margin.

Chronic calicivirus faucitis and gingivitis. The inflammatory response is less severe with calicivirus.

Acute herpesvirus and calicivirus infections. This is associated with lingual and palatal ulcerations and other signs of respiratory tract infection such as sneezing and oculonasal discharge.

Treatment

Initially, a careful and thorough **dental prophylaxis** and appropriate antibiotic therapy (must be effective against anaerobes such as *Actinomyces* sp., *Peptostreptococcus* sp. and the black pigmented bacteroides) will give relief although only temporary in most instances.

Corticosteroid therapy will produce improvement whilst used.

Permanent resolution is common following **extraction of all teeth** caudal to the canines (but these teeth must be extracted completely including all of the roots).

In cases that suffer recurrence following extraction (less than 5%), **acupuncture** may result in resolution.

Acupuncture alone will produce short-term relief.

Prognosis

The **prognosis is guarded** for those treated **without extraction**.

With complete extraction, the prognosis is fair to good.

Prevention

Until the etiology is understood, no prevention is possible.

ORAL NEOPLASIA**

Classical signs

- Presence of oral mass.
- Dysphagia, excessive salivation, hemorrhage.
- Halitosis.

Pathogenesis

Neoplasia may involve gingiva, tongue, oral mucosa or tonsils.

Squamous cell carcinoma is the most common neoplasm in cats and is most often found on the **ventral tongue**.

Other types of oral tumor are infrequent in the cat.

Neoplasia usually occurs in older cats (> 10 years).

Clinical signs

Oral mass.

Excessive **salivation, dysphagia** or **oral hemorrhage**.

Facial distortion.

Halitosis.

Poor body condition due to inability to eat or metastatic disease.

Diagnosis

Biopsy and histologic examination.

Radiography to assess the extent of hard tissue tumors.

Differential diagnosis

Intra-oral abscess and granulation tissue can have a similar appearance to neoplasia but will be differentiated by biopsy.

Eosinophilic granuloma complex is often smaller and can be differentiated by biopsy.

Treatment

Treatment of lingual squamous cell carcinoma in the cat has not proved successful.

Mandibular masses can be treated by **partial mandibulectomy** (the complete hemimandible can be removed if necessary).

Prognosis

The prognosis for squamous cell carcinoma of the tongue is **grave**.

For other tumors, the prognosis will depend on the tumor type and suitability for treatment.

ORAL ULCERATIONS FROM VIRAL, UREMIC OR TOXIC CAUSES*

Classical signs

- Excessive salivation.
- Tongue and pharyngeal ulceration.
- Anorexia.

See main reference on page 578 for details (The Cat With Salivation).

Pathogenesis

Feline herpesvirus and feline calicivirus can cause an **ulcerative stomatitis** in association with upper respiratory tract disease.
- **Calicivirus infection most commonly** causes oral lesions especially on the tongue and hard palate.
- The lesions begin as vesicles, which coalesce and rupture, forming ulcers.
- Lesions caused by herpesvirus occur less frequently but are usually more severe.

Cats with uremia produce increased ammonia in the saliva. Uremia also causes damage to blood vessels resulting in vasculitis. Ulceration of the oral mucosa may be caused by the combination.

Toxic causes of oral ulceration in the cat are most frequently associated with household cleaning agents.

- These toxic agents include **sodium hypochlorite** and **sodium hydroxide** that are used for cleaning showers and bathrooms, and **quaternary ammonium compounds.**
- The cat damages the oral mucosa whilst **licking the walls or floor** or from licking it **off their feet.**
- These cats may also have lesions on their feet if exposure was from walking in the chemical.

Clinical signs

Excessive salivation and oral pain.

Oral ulceration associated with concurrent upper respiratory tract disease.

Fever is often present associated with herpesvirus and calicivirus ulceration but not with uremic or toxic ulcers.

Sudden onset of salivation, dysphagia and depression with toxic ulceration.

Loss of sense of smell, fever and oral pain results in anorexia.

Halitosis.

Diagnosis

Presence of oral ulcers.

Virus identification using PCR if ulcers are associated with upper respiratory tract disease.

Blood tests for uremia.

History of exposure to toxins liable to produce oral ulceration.

Differential diagnosis

Electrical or heat burns to the tongue and oral mucosa are rare in the cat. Lack **of fever** and history of potential for exposure help to differentiate these from infectious causes.

Treatment

Antibiotics to control secondary bacterial infections.

Fluid therapy, soft foods and adjunct therapy (for the primary disease) until lesions are healed.

Pain control.

BACTERIAL RHINITIS SECONDARY TO VIRAL UPPER RESPIRATORY TRACT DISEASE*

Classical signs

- Chronic sneezing and snuffling.
- Mucopurulent nasal discharge.
- Stertorous respiration.

See main reference on page 21 for details (The Cat With Signs of Chronic Nasal Disease).

Clinical signs

Chronic mucopurulent nasal discharge.

Chronic sneezing and snuffling.

Stertorous respiration.

Halitosis may be present.

Diagnosis

History of clinical signs after an acute upper respiratory tract infection.

Radiography demonstrating **fluid densities in nasal cavity and sinuses** with loss of turbinates.

Cytology showing many neutrophils with intra- and extracellular bacteria and no evidence of *Cryptococcus* sp. or neoplastic cells.

Differential diagnosis

Neoplasia. Usually older cats and radiographic signs are more often unilateral. Biopsy will differentiate.

Cryptococcosis. Often has nasal distortion or visible polyp protruding through nares. Differentiate with cytology or serology.

Treatment

Long-term broad-spectrum antibiotic therapy.

Surgery (rhinotomy) to curette sinuses may be tried as a salvage procedure.

ORAL FOREIGN BODY*

Classical signs

- Gagging, pawing at mouth.
- Halitosis.
- Dysphagia.

Clinical signs

Sudden onset of gagging and pawing at the mouth.

Dysphagia. The cat will often **appear very hungry** but has **difficulty swallowing.**

Rapid jaw and tongue movements.

Diagnosis

Evidence of foreign body or trauma caused by the foreign body in the oral cavity or pharynx.

Most commonly the tongue or pharynx are involved especially with **string or cotton.**

Differential diagnosis

Oral tumors. These can be differentiated visually from a foreign body.

Traumatic lacerations. These are usually associated with hemorrhage and no foreign body will be found on examination.

Treatment

Removal of the foreign body.

BACTERIAL INFECTION OF TONGUE LACERATIONS*

Classical signs

- Hemorrhage.
- Reluctance to groom and excessive salivation.

Clinical signs

Hemorrhage may be significant if acute.

Sudden onset of reluctance to groom, excessive salivation and reluctance to eat.

Halitosis develops as tissue becomes infected.

Laceration may be on the dorsal surface or **sublingual (more often).**

Diagnosis

Visualize the laceration.

Differential diagnosis

Foreign bodies can usually be seen.

Ulcerations secondary to trauma.

Treatment

Surgical debridement and repair.

INFECTIONS ASSOCIATED WITH ESOPHAGEAL AND LOWER AIRWAY DISEASE

Classical signs

- Dysphagia, regurgitation (esophageal disease).
- Dyspnea, coughing (lower airway disease).

Clinical signs

Halitosis.

Dysphagia, regurgitation and possible reluctance to eat with esophageal disease. **Esophageal tumors and foreign bodies** are most often associated with halitosis.

Dyspnea, coughing with lower airway disease. **Foreign bodies, airway tumors** and **purulent bacterial infections** are most frequently associated with halitosis.

Diagnosis

Radiography to demonstrate lesions.

Auscultation and ultrasonography.

ORONASAL FISTULA

Classical signs

- Occasional sneezing.
- Unilateral nasal discharge.
- Excessive licking of nose.

See main reference on page 27 for details (The Cat With Signs of Chronic Nasal Disease).

Clinical signs

Most often **associated with dental disease**; occasionally occurs after **trauma**, with formation of a fistula in the hard palate.

Occasional sneezing.

Unilateral nasal discharge (usually mucopurulent but may be hemorrhagic). If associated with dental disease or unilateral traumatic fistula.

Excessive licking of nose.

Oronasal fistula visible if tooth is absent.

Advanced periodontal disease.

Halitosis.

Diagnosis

Presence of oronasal fistula on periodontal probing (vigorous movement of probe results in blood from nostril).

MANDIBULAR AND MAXILLARY FRACTURES

Classical signs

- Mouth held open (often with tongue protruding).
- Jaw asymmetry.
- Excessive salivation.

Clinical signs

Unwilling (or unable) to close mouth and tongue protruding.

Asymmetry of jaw.

Hemorrhage in acute stages.

Excessive salivation.

Halitosis associated with secondary bacterial infection of traumatized tissue.

Diagnosis

Palpation and radiographic demonstration of fracture.

TOOTH FRACTURE WITH PERIAPICAL ABSCESSATION

Classical signs

- Presence of fractured tooth.

Clinical signs

Fractured tooth.

Oral pain in acute phase (< 48 hours) then no pain until periapical abscess forms.

Calculus build-up on teeth on affected side of mouth due to reluctance to chew with affected tooth.

Halitosis may be present if the periapical abscess is draining intra-orally.

Diagnosis

Presence of **fractured crown**.

CONGENITAL ANOMALY OF THE HARD PALATE (CLEFT PALATE)

Classical signs

- Snuffling and nasal discharge.
- Visible evidence of cleft.

Clinical signs

Snuffling and nasal discharge, which is usually bilateral.

In **young kitten** with congenital cleft, milk is visible coming from the nose during feeding.

In **traumatic cleft**, dried blood around the nose and mouth and facial injuries.

Halitosis is associated with rhinitis and secondary infection from food in the nasal passages.

Diagnosis

Evidence of cleft.

CRYPTOCOCCOSIS

Classical signs

- Chronic nasal discharge.
- Facial distortion (nasal bones).

See main reference on page 25 for details (The Cat With Signs of Chronic Nasal Disease).

Clinical signs

Chronic nasal discharge and snuffling.

Distortion of bridge of nose or nasal polyp is present in most cases.

Depression and anorexia.

Other organs may be affected.

Diagnosis

Serology for cryptococcus antibody.

Cytology for identification of the organism.

EOSINOPHILIC GRANULOMA COMPLEX

Classical signs

- Ulcerated lesion near the midline of the upper lip.
- Raised firm lesions in the oral cavity (especially tongue and hard palate).

See main reference on page 1088 for details (The Cat With Non-Healing Wounds).

Clinical signs

Ulcerated lesion on **the upper lip** near the midline.

Raised firm lesions (with yellow-white spots throughout) **in the oral cavity** especially on the **tongue and hard palate**.

Diagnosis

Biopsy.

RECOMMENDED READING

DeBowes LJ, Mosier D, Logan E et al. Association of periodontal disease and histologic lesions in multiple organs from 45 dogs. J Vet Dent 1996; 13: 57–60.

Harvey CE, Emily PP. Small Animal Dentistry. St. Louis, Mosby, 1993, pp. 89–143, 150–155.

Hennet P. Chronic gingivo-stomatitis in cats: long-term follow-up of 30 cases treated by dental extractions. J Vet Dent 1997; 14: 15–21.

Tonzetich J. Production and origin of oral malodor: a review of mechanisms and methods of analysis. J Periodontol 1977; 48: 13–20.

Wilson GJ. Feline Dentistry and Oral Cavity Diseases. Sydney, University of Sydney Post Graduate Foundation in Veterinary Science, 2002.

29. The cat with signs of regurgitation (acute or chronic)

Debra L Zoran

KEY SIGNS

- Passive elimination via the mouth of swallowed food.
- Food is typically undigested.
- Gagging or retching may occur concurrently.

MECHANISM?

- Regurgitation is a **passive** act that may involve several anatomic regions of the alimentary tract: oral cavity, oropharynx, esophagus or occasionally the stomach.
- Oral or pharyngeal disease is more often associated with dysphagia (difficulty swallowing).
- Regurgitation is a more typical presenting sign of **esophageal disease.**
- Regurgitation is **not associated with prodromal signs** (no anxiety, nausea or hypersalivation), there will be **no abdominal muscular activity,** and is often composed of recently swallowed food (undigested, whole).
- In cases of chronic megaesophagus, where food may sit undisturbed for hours in the distal esophagus, the food may have a more liquid, unformed character.
- The pH of the material may be **neutral, slightly basic (oral) or slightly acidic** (stomach), but is typically in a range of pH 4–7.

WHERE?

- Regurgitation is usually associated with **disease of the esophagus**:
- **Megaesophagus** (acquired or congenital).
- Associated with esophageal anomalies, e.g. diverticular structures, vascular ring anomalies.
- **Esophagitis**, esophageal strictures or foreign bodies.
- Associated with oropharyngeal disease, e.g. stomatitis-pharyngitis complex.
- Parasitic diseases of the esophagus.
  Signs of **gagging or retching** are often associated with regurgitation (or vomiting) in cats and include many oral, dental and pharyngeal infectious, inflammatory, neoplastic or toxic disorders.

WHAT?

- The most common causes of regurgitation in cats are esophagitis (due to a variety of infectious or inflammatory causes), esophageal stricture, esophageal foreign bodies, and more rarely pharyngeal or esophageal neoplasia.

QUICK REFERENCE SUMMARY
Diseases causing signs of regurgitation
ANOMALY

● Vascular ring anomalies (persistent right aortic arch – PRAA) (p 623)

Vascular ring anomalies cause regurgitation soon after the kitten is weaned onto solid food.

● Esophageal diverticular structures (p 624)

These may be clinically silent or associated with regurgitation, painful swallowing, lethargy and decreased appetite, depending on the size of the diverticular structure.

MECHANICAL

● **Esophageal foreign body** (p 616)**

Foreign bodies may cause gagging, retching or regurgitation, depending on what they are, how long they have been present in the esophagus, and whether or not they are caustic.

● **Esophageal stricture* (p 618)**

This is a complication of esophagitis that results in regurgitation due to narrowing or nearly complete obstruction of the esophageal lumen.

● Eating too fast (food gulping) (p 628)

Regurgitation of undigested food may be caused by eating too fast or food gulping.

● Hiatal hernia (gastroesophageal intussusception) (p 625)

This is a rare disorder associated with intermittent regurgitation or vomiting due to herniation of the stomach through the esophageal hiatus.

● Esophageal fistula (p 625)

This is an abnormal communication between the esophagus and respiratory system that usually results from foreign body penetration or a ruptured diverticulum. Clinical signs will include regurgitation as well as respiratory signs (e.g. coughing, dyspnea, etc.).

IDIOPATHIC

● **Esophageal hypomotility/idiopathic megaesophagus (acquired or congenital)* (p 621)**

Regurgitation may or may not be associated with eating. Aspiration pneumonia is a common complication resulting from the frequent regurgitation.

● Dysautonomia (p 627)

Regurgitation occurs due to the development of megaesophagus secondary to abnormal functioning of the autonomic nervous system. This rare disorder is also associated with abnormal colonic and ocular muscle functions, among other things.

IMMUNOLOGIC

● **Myasthenia gravis (acquired or congenital)* (p 622)**

Myasthenia gravis can be acquired or congenital and results in megaesophagus (regurgitation) secondary to the presence of antibodies to the acetylcholine receptor in the neuro-muscular junction, with the end result being smooth muscle dysfunction.

continued

continued

INFLAMMATORY

- **Esophagitis*** (p 615)**

Esophagitis is an inflammatory disease of the esophagus that has multiple causes such as reflux disease, post-anesthesia, chronic vomiting, caustic or irritant ingestion and results in regurgitation and may progress to esophageal strictures if left untreated or if severe.

INHERITED

- **Hereditary myopathy of Devon Rex cats (p 626)**

This is an inherited myopathy in young Devon cats that presents as generalized appendicular weakness. Ventroflexion of the head and neck, dorsal protrusion of the scapulae and megaesophagus with regurgitation are the main clinical features of hereditary myopathy.

NEOPLASTIC

- **Esophageal neoplasia (squamous cell carcinoma, metastatic neoplasia)* (p 619)**

This is a rare tumor in cats, but is the most common tumor of the esophagus. The tumor creates an obstructive lesion that results in regurgitation, weight loss and anorexia.

- **Mediastinal neoplasia* (p 628)**

Thymic lymphoma and thymoma commonly result in extraesophageal obstruction and regurgitation.

TOXIC

- **Lead poisoning* (p 619)**

Lead poisoning is usually marked in the early phases with vomiting and GI signs. Neurologic signs develop late or with chronic exposure and may lead to the development of smooth muscle dysfunction (megaesophagus) and regurgitation.

- **Plant ingestion* (p 620)**

Regurgitation secondary to plant consumption is usually due to their irritant or caustic properties that result in the development of esophagitis.

INTRODUCTION

MECHANISM?

Regurgitation is the passive removal of ingesta, saliva, and other material from the upper GI tract (oral cavity, oropharynx and esophagus).

Regurgitation of stomach contents can occur but is much **less common than vomiting.**

Regurgitation is **not associated with abdominal muscle contraction**, has no **prodromal signs** (no anxiety, nausea or hypersalivation preceeding it), and the material is typically composed of recently swallowed food (undigested, may still be whole) with saliva.

In cases of **chronic megaesophagus,** where food may sit undisturbed for hours in the distal esophagus, the food may have a **more liquid, unformed character.**

The pH of the material may be neutral, slightly basic (oral) or slightly acidic (stomach), but is typically in a range of **pH 4–7.**

Diseases of the esophagus rarely cause hematologic or biochemical abnormalities, and their **diagnosis often requires contrast radiography, endoscopy** or other sophisticated imaging techniques.

WHERE?

Classically, regurgitation is considered to be the hallmark of esophageal disease.

Gagging or retching, painful swallowing or dysphagia can all be signs of esophageal disease, however, most of the time these signs are associated with oral or oropharyngeal disease (see page 602, The Cat With Bad Breath or Oral Lesions).

WHAT?

Esophageal diseases that may be associated with regurgitation include esophagitis, cardiac anomalies (e.g. persistent right aortic arch), mechanical problems (e.g. strictures, foreign bodies or fistula), metabolic disorders (megaesophagus – acquired, congenital or idiopathic), or toxic (plant ingestion, etc.).

Many diseases of the esophagus may be difficult, if not impossible **to treat**.

Megaesophagus, strictures, diverticuli, hiatal hernias, fistulae and esophageal neoplasia are all very difficult to manage or cure.

Esophagitis is the most common and potentially most treatable esophageal disease of cats other than foreign bodies and ingestion of plant material.

DISEASES CAUSING SIGNS OF REGURGITATION

ESOPHAGITIS***

Classical signs

- Regurgitation is the most common sign.
- Vomiting, gagging, retching, anorexia, weight loss and lethargy.

Pathogenesis

Esophagitis can be caused by a wide variety of insults, including **infectious** (e.g. calicivirus).
- **Gastroesophageal reflux disease** (persistent vomiting, **anesthesia,** lower esophageal sphincter abnormalities, hiatal hernias).
- **Chemical** (caustic agents) or **thermal injury**.

- **Drugs** (primarily due to direct injury if retained in the esophagus, e.g. doxycycline, potassium gluconate, propranolol).
- Secondary to **trauma from esophageal foreign bodies.**

Other than traumatically induced esophagitis, the most common cause of esophageal inflammation in cats is **reflux of acid, pepsin and stomach contents into esophagus as a result of anesthesia or chronic vomiting**.

The esophagus does not have the mucosal protection mechanisms that are present in the stomach, and thus, acid and chemical mucosal injury from reflux will set into motion **a localized inflammatory response** that, if uncorrected, can result in esophageal stricture formation or perforation.

Clinical signs

Regurgitation following eating is the predominant clinical sign in cats with esophagitis, but vomiting, anorexia, weight loss, lethargy and gagging may also be observed.

Onset of regurgitation following an anesthetic procedure or foreign body retrieval is highly suspicious of esophagitis.

Diagnosis

A history of a recent **onset of regurgitation after an anesthetic procedure** should immediately suggest esophagitis.

Concurrent oral ulceration suggests chemical, thermal, calicivirus or uremic ulceration.

History (chemical, thermal, anaesthesia, drugs, foreign bodies) usually identifies the problem.

Esophagitis in cats due to consumption of **a chemical or thermal agent** may be associated with **completely normal baseline blood work.**

Survey radiography may be helpful **if the esophageal inflammatory process is also causing motility disturbances** that can be seen as **esophageal dilatation** radiographically. Rarely, contrast radiography may be useful in identifying areas of **mucosal irregularity** suggestive of esophagitis. **Contrast radiographs are**

most helpful in identification of **esophageal stricture** formation.

Definitive diagnosis of esophagitis, and any complications associated with it, is achieved by **endoscopic examination of the esophagus and biopsy**.

Note: a normal-appearing mucosa does not rule out esophagitis. However, in most cases, **mucosal erythema, hemorrhage and increased friability** are common findings.

Differential diagnosis

Essentially any cause of regurgitation or chronic vomiting should be considered as a differential because the signs are so non-specific and many overlap with other diseases.

Treatment

Treatment of esophagitis is first aimed at **correcting the underlying cause**. If the cause cannot be identified and corrected, management of the esophagitis will be extremely difficult.

Symptomatic therapy then is used to **control the inflammatory process** that is ongoing in the esophageal mucosa. This type of approach will require both **"resting" the esophagus** and **pharmacologic therapy**.

In cats with **mild esophagitis**, simply **withdrawing food for 24–48 hours is often sufficient** to allow mucosal healing. Upon re-feeding, the diet should be **a soft, low-fat, non-abrasive food** that will not re-injure the tissue.

When **severe esophagitis** is present, **feeding should be administered via alternative feeding methods.**

Provide enteral nutrition via a gastrostomy or jejunostomy tube (pharyngostomy or nasogastric tubes will continue to irritate the esophagus and may allow continued gastroesophageal reflux) **or use total parenteral nutrition if the cat is also vomiting.**

Corticosteroids (0.5–1.0 mg/kg PO q 12 h) **are indicated if stricture formation is expected** to occur, but **will not help in cases where a stricture has already occurred** and may reduce healing in severe cases, so must be used with **caution.**

Prophylactic antibiotics that are effective against pathogens present in the oral mucosa are **only indicated** (amoxicillin, clavamox, cephalexin, clindamycin) **in severe esophagitis cases** where mucosal damage is so severe that normal mucosal defenses are compromised.

Reduction of gastric acidity with histamine-2 blockers (famotidine 0.5–1.0 mg/kg PO q 24 h) or protein pump inhibitors (omeprazole 1 mg/kg PO q 24 h) is also indicated, especially if gastroesophageal reflux disease is suspected.

Mucosal cytoprotectants, such as sucralfate (250–500 mg PO q 8–12 h made into a slurry) have also been recommended to reduce further mucosal injury, however their effectiveness is questioned.

Drugs that **increase lower esophageal sphincter tone**, metoclopramide (0.1–0.2 mg/kg PO q 12 h) and cisapride (5 mg/kg PO q 12 h), **are indicated when acid reflux is suspected** and may be required long-term to prevent disease recurrence in cats with this disease.

In all cases, the **treatment should be continued for at least 2–3 weeks beyond the resolution** of clinical signs to prevent recurrence and allow complete healing of the tissue.

Prognosis

The prognosis is **good in cats with mild esophagitis or when severe esophagitis is managed aggressively** and does not result in stricture formation.

In cases of esophagitis that develop **strictures**, the prognosis is **guarded to fair**. See section on stricture management for details.

ESOPHAGEAL FOREIGN BODY**

Classical signs

- Acute onset of regurgitation is the most common sign.
- Gagging or retching are also observed, especially when the object is in the cranial esophagus.
- Rarely, acute respiratory distress may also occur.

Pathogenesis

Esophageal foreign bodies are relatively common in cats because of their curious nature, propensity to chew on or ingest string or like objects, and their consumption of hair (or bones) from prey or grooming.

String foreign bodies will usually pass through the GI tract if they are not anchored.

Common reasons for string foreign bodies to become anchored include, attachment around the **base of the tongue** or if the string is attached to a needle that becomes lodged in the wall of the esophagus or GI tract.

The **greatest dangers from esophageal foreign bodies are perforation and esophagitis.**

Esophageal perforation is a life-threatening condition because it **leads to fulminant (tension) pneumothorax and pneumomediastinum. Extremely small perforations** (needle punctures) may not result in tension pneumothorax but instead cause **mediastinitis and pleuritis or even fistula formation**.

Esophagitis is important because it **can lead to esophageal stricture if the inflammatory response is severe** or chronic.

Clinical signs

An acute **onset of regurgitation or anorexia are the most common presenting signs**, and these may be associated with **hypersalivation, gagging, retching or anxiety**.

If the foreign body causes an **esophageal perforation**, the cat may present in **extreme respiratory distress**.

The severity of the signs observed often relate to what the object is (e.g. string, hair, bones, needles, wire), whether the object is causing a **partial or complete obstruction**, and the **duration** that it has been present (e.g. presence of esophagitis, stricture, etc.).

Diagnosis

The **acute onset of hypersalivation and regurgitation is often suggestive of an esophageal foreign body**, and the diagnosis is frequently confirmed by visualizing string entrapped around the base of the tongue.

Survey radiographs will often reveal a radio-opaque foreign object.

Endoscopy may be required in some cases **to identify small or radiolucent objects**, and is very useful in retrieving some objects.

In some cases, **contrast radiographs may be required to identify radiolucent objects or fistula.**

Because of the **acute onset of clinical signs** in cats with esophageal foreign bodies, **a routine database is usually completely normal.**

Cats that develop a **small esophageal perforation** may have an **inflammatory leukogram.**

Differential diagnosis

Primary differentials include ingestion of a caustic, irritating or noxious substance that causes acute **esophagitis.**

Oral ulceration is usually present **following ingestion of caustic or irritating substances.**

Other causes of regurgitation are typically associated with **clinical signs of a chronic nature** (esophageal hypomotility, gastroesophageal reflux esophagitis, neoplasia) and thus are less likely.

Treatment

The initial goal is the **immediate removal of the foreign object** from the esophagus. This must be **done carefully to minimize further esophageal damage and complications** (e.g. vagal tone induced bradyarrhythmias, further mucosal trauma or development of a perforation).

Endoscopic retrieval should be attempted first because of the difficulties associated with esophageal surgery, **unless there is radiographic evidence of a perforation.**

Use of both a rigid proctoscope and a flexible endoscope has been very successful. The flexible scope is used to manipulate the object free with grasping tools, and the proctoscope to protect the esophagus from further damage as the object is moved orad.

If the object cannot be safely removed in an oral direction, but can be propelled into the stomach, this is the next best option. The object may be allowed to pass (bony material) through the GI tract on its own or can be removed by gastrostomy.

Thoracotomy to remove an esophageal foreign body is only used as a last resort, when all other efforts have failed, or when an esophageal perforation is eminent or has occurred.

Following removal of the object by endoscopy, close inspection of the esophagus to determine the extent of injury is important.

If there is severe esophagitis or a small perforation (needle), medical management of these conditions should include placement of a nasogastric or gastrostomy tube for feeding and medical management of esophagitis (gastric acid blockers, motility modifiers, mucosal protectants, and possibly antibiotics will be required). Therapy should be continued for 2–3 weeks beyond cessation of clinical signs.

Prognosis and prevention

Prevention is clearly aimed at reducing the opportunity for cats to ingest these objects by "cat-proofing" the home and preventing prey-catching and consumption. However, it is impossible to foresee all possible problems, so early recognition is also important to a successful outcome.

The prognosis is good to excellent if the object can be immediately retrieved and the damage to the esophagus is minimal.

In cases of a chronic esophageal foreign body, presence of severe esophagitis, perforation or great difficulty in removing the object, the prognosis is guarded to poor.

Cats that develop esophageal strictures resulting from severe esophagitis may require repeated bouginage to allow passage of ingesta.

Cats requiring thoracotomy and esophageal surgery to remove a foreign object will have a very guarded prognosis to survive the procedure, let alone return to normal function.

ESOPHAGEAL STRICTURE*

Classical signs

- Regurgitation is most common sign.
- Vomiting, anorexia, weight loss and lethargy.

Pathogenesis

Esophageal strictures are a complication of severe esophagitis, and are most commonly associated with gastroesophageal reflux esophagitis which occurs most commonly as a complication of persistent vomiting or can occur as a result of reflux during general anesthesia. There is usually a lag of 2–3 weeks between anesthesia and stricture formation.

Less frequent causes of esophageal strictures are reflux esophagitis as a result of gastroesophageal reflux or hiatal hernia.

Strictures form when the esophageal mucosa is severely damaged and the inflammatory process extends down into the submucosa and muscular layers.

Clinical signs

Regurgitation following eating is the most common presenting complaint. Liquid may be able to pass depending on the severity of the strictured area.

If the stricture is caused by severe esophagitis secondary to chronic vomiting, other signs may include weight loss, lethargy and anorexia.

Diagnosis

The diagnosis may be suspected on survey radiography, but can be confirmed with contrast films or endoscopy.

Endoscopy should be used to evaluate esophageal strictures and to obtain biopsies to rule out esophageal neoplasia, if indicated.

Routine blood work will typically be normal, unless the cat is also chronically vomiting, or the regurgitation has been present long enough to affect serum protein levels or hydration status.

Differential diagnosis

All causes of regurgitation should be considered in the initial approach, but the finding of a narrowed lumen on contrast radiographs narrows the primary differentials to neoplasia, peri-esophageal masses, foreign bodies and stricture.

Treatment

Esophageal strictures can be corrected one of two ways: by **balloon or bougie dilation or surgical removal**.

Every effort to correct the problem by stretching the strictured area with balloon catheterization or bougienage should be made, because of the difficulty of the surgical procedure and the numerous complications associated with it.

In most cases, **multiple dilation procedures are required** to slowly stretch out the stricture site to an approximately normal size.

Balloon catheters dilate the stricture site with radial forces and can be used endoscopically or fluoroscopically, thus providing better visualization of the site and better control over the force exerted.

Bougies dilate with longitudinal shearing and may require multiple procedures. Bougies are associated with a greater risk of tearing or perforation and thus balloon dilation is preferred.

Corticosteroid therapy (1.0–2.0 mg/kg/day) **to prevent further fibrosis** has been recommended but is controversial and **has not been proven effective in this regard.**

In many cases of stricture, the inciting cause is long resolved, but if **esophagitis is ongoing due to gastric reflux, this should be managed as well** (see section under esophagitis).

Prognosis

The prognosis is **guarded** for cats with esophageal strictures. Many cats can be helped temporarily with dilation procedures, but the stricture recurs or requires repeated procedures to maintain an open esophageal passageway.

LEAD POISONING*

> ### Classical signs
>
> - Inappetance, weight loss.
> - Behavior changes (irritable, aggressive).
> - Regurgitation secondary to megaesophagus is rare.
> - Vomiting or diarrhea.
> - Seizures or other central nervous system signs.

See main reference on page 596 for details.

Clinical signs

Early clinical signs include gastrointestinal tract signs such as **inappetance, salivation, vomiting and weight loss**.

Other **less common signs** of lead toxicity include **diarrhea**, and abnormalities of the hemogram are less common in cats than dogs (basophilic stippling, nucleated RBCs).

In the **late stages**, other **central nervous system signs** such as ataxia and seizures may occur.

Regurgitation secondary to megaesophagus is **very rare** in cats.

Diagnosis

Serum blood lead levels are the definitive means of diagnosis of lead poisoning.

The diagnosis is helped by a **history of exposure** to lead-containing paints usually associated with home renovation or other objects such as batteries.

Signs of **inappetence, weight loss and behavioral changes** should prompt consideration of lead poisoning as a differential.

Hematologic findings are often absent.

Survey radiographs in cats that have a history of regurgitation will reveal **esophageal dilation or megaesophagus,** and in long-standing cases, may reveal **aspiration pneumonia** as well.

ESOPHAGEAL NEOPLASIA* (SQUAMOUS CELL CARCINOMA, METASTATIC NEOPLASIA)

> ### Classical signs
>
> - Regurgitation secondary to obstruction, esophagitis or motility disturbances.
> - Weight loss, inappetance and respiratory signs are also common.

Clinical signs

Esophageal neoplasia creates an **obstructive lesion** that is associated with regurgitation, **especially after ingestion of food,** and is typically seen in **older cats.**

Other signs may include **weight loss, anorexia and respiratory signs** if aspiration pneumonia occurs.

The most common neoplasm is squamous cell carcinoma, although esophageal tumors in general are rare in cats, and the tumor will metastasize early to regional lymph nodes and lung.

Diagnosis

The presence of **regurgitation as the predominant clinical sign** will lead the clinician to suspect esophageal disease.

Because many of these cats are older, a variety of hematological and biochemical abnormalities may be present, but **there are no typical changes associated with esophageal disease on the blood work.**

The diagnosis may be suggested by finding an **intraluminal or mass lesion obstructing the esophageal lumen on contrast radiography.**

Endoscopic evaluation and biopsy are the least invasive and most efficient means of obtaining a definitive diagnosis of esophageal neoplasia, although **surgical approaches** will also give diagnostic information as well.

Surgical resection of most esophageal neoplasms is difficult if not impossible due to the fact that most tumors are well advanced at the time of diagnosis. **Surgical excision of thymomas is often rewarding** as the mass is usually **benign and discrete.**

PLANT INGESTION*

Classical signs

- Intermittent or persistent regurgitation or vomiting of plant material.

See main reference on page 646 for details.

Clinical signs

Regurgitation or vomiting after ingestion of **plants containing materials that are irritating, caustic or abrasive**.

Signs may be intermittent or chronic in nature depending on the availability of the plants.

Other signs include **dysphagia, gagging or repeated swallowing efforts**.

Diagnosis

Plants that are associated with esophageal or gastric irritation include: Poinsettia (*Euphorbia* spp.), Mistletoe (*Phoradendron* spp.), Aloe vera, Crown of Thorns (*Euphorbia* spp.), Snow on the Mountain (*Euphorbia* spp.), Azalea (*Rhododenderon*), Castor bean (*Ricinus* spp), Rosary pea (*Abrus*), English ivy (*Hedera*), Daphne (*Daphne*), Christmas rose (*Helleborus*), Holly (*Ilex*), Privet (*Ligustrum*), Iris (*Iris*), Narcissus (*Narcissus*), Phildendron (*Philodendron*), Wisteria (*Wisteria*).

Diagnosis is based upon historical exposure or evidence of exposure in the regurgitated material.

In some cats, **endoscopy should be performed to rule out esophagitis due to other causes** and **determine the extent of the lesions**.

Differential diagnosis

Other causes of esophagitis, especially gastroesophageal reflux disease and other causes of chronic vomiting should be considered.

Treatment

Most cases are not associated with severe esophagitis that requires alternative alimentation routes or aggressive medical therapy.

Reduction of hyperacidity with **histamine-2 blockers** (famotidine 0.5–1.0 mg/kg PO q 24 h), administration of **anti-emetics** (primarily for the prokinetic action of metoclopramide) as needed and feeding a **bland diet** is all that will be required in most cats.

In cats with severe esophagitis, more aggressive therapy will be required to prevent formation of strictures or fistula. See section on esophagitis.

ESOPHAGEAL HYPOMOTILITY/IDIOPATHIC MEGAESOPHAGUS (ACQUIRED OR CONGENITAL)*

Classical signs

- Regurgitation, often not associated directly with eating.
- Cats may develop aspiration pneumonia resulting in:
  respiratory distress, coughing, wheezing, lethargy, anorexia.

Pathogenesis

Esophageal hypomotility disorders may be **idiopathic** in origin or occur secondary to a known disease entity (**acquired or secondary megaesophagus**).

Idiopathic megaesophagus appears to be caused by a **defect in peristalsis** due to abnormal neural signal pathways and increasing evidence suggests that the disease is inherited (Siamese cats have the greatest prevalence).

The secondary causes of megaesophagus are numerous and include:

- **Neuromuscular disorders** (dysautonomia, myasthenia gravis, polymyopathies and polyneuropathies, e.g. tetanus may cause regurgitation secondary to hiatal hernia).
- **Inflammatory disorders** (e.g. esophagitis).
- **Obstructive disorders** (foreign objects, peri- or intra-esophageal masses, ring structures, hiatal hernia).
- **Stomach or pyloric dysfunction** resulting in chronic regurgitation or reflux.
- **Toxicity** (e.g. lead).

The secondary causes of megaesophagus that have major importance clinically are **discussed separately** in this chapter.

Diagnosis

The history and signalment of chronic regurgitation will be suggestive of esophageal disease.

Survey radiographs are usually all that is required to confirm the presence of megaesophagus. Survey radiographs also are important in determining the presence of **aspiration pneumonia**, the most common complication of megaesophagus.

Cats with aspiration pneumonia may **have hematologic or biochemical profile abnormalities**, but these will be **non-specific.**

- **Contrast radiographs are rarely indicated but will confirm the diagnosis** in cases with minimal dilation.

Other diagnostics are used to determine if the disease is congenital, acquired or idiopathic.

- **Fluoroscopy** (to evaluate motility).
- **Endoscopy** (for esophagitis or obstructive disorders).
- **Neuromuscular examination** (muscle or nerve biopsies, electrodiagnostics, e.g. EMG, nerve conduction testing).
- Measurement of **antibodies to acetylcholine receptors** (myasthenia gravis).
- **Blood lead levels.**
- Creatine kinase measurement is of little value as the polymyopathies in cats that cause megaoesophagus, i.e. Devon Rex myopathy and myasthenia, are not associated with increased creatine kinase levels.
- **Testing of endocrine and autonomic** (e.g. dysautonomia) **function.**

Idiopathic megaesophagus is a diagnosis made by exclusion of all other possible causes.

Differential diagnosis

There are numerous differentials for regurgitation (esophageal hypomotility, inflammatory, obstructive, neoplastic, toxic or chemical irritants, or due to gastro-esophageal reflux), but once megaesophagus is found on survey radiographs, the list of differentials is reduced to the idiopathic, congenital or acquired forms of megaesophagus.

Treatment

Treatment of esophageal hypomotility disorders in cats is **symptomatic, unless a reversible cause** for the megaesophagus **is identified and corrected** before the esophagus is permanently damaged.

Other **supportive measures** include managing dehydration with **fluid therapy** as needed, **elevated feeding of multiple, small, liquid meals** (note: although **some cats will respond better to foods that are solid or semi-solid**) to facilitate gravitation of food into the stomach, and **management of aspiration pneumonia** if it occurs (bronchodilators, antibiotics if needed, oxygen supplementation, and coupage).

If oral feeding is unsuccessful, despite trying different food types and consistencies, **gastrostomy tube feeding** may be required for long-term management. Nasogastric and esophagostomy tubes are generally not good long-term options for feeding management.

Prognosis

The **prognosis depends upon several factors but especially upon the cause.** If an underlying disorder can be identified and corrected (e.g. dilation due to PRAA), the prognosis may be favorable.

Idiopathic megaesophagus and megaesophagus due to neuromuscular function disorders (dysautonomia or myasthenia gravis) is **guarded to poor.**

MYASTHENIA GRAVIS* (CONGENITAL OR ACQUIRED)

> ### Classical signs
>
> - Regurgitation due to megaesophagus, and generalized muscle weakness.
> - Dysphonia and cervial ventroflexion are more common in cats.

See main reference on page 896 for details.

Clinical signs

Regurgitation is reported due to megaesophagus. **Generalized muscle weakness** is seen in the generalized and acute fulminating forms of the condition, but not in focal myasthenia.

Dysphonia and cervial ventroflexion are more common in cats than in dogs.

Congenital myasthenia is more common in **Siamese and DSH cats**, while **acquired myasthenia** appears to be more common in **Somalis and Abbysinians** and occurs in slightly older kittens (4–6 months).

Acquired myasthenia has a **bimodal age distribution,** with most affected cats being young adults (2–3 years) or older (9–10 years).

Diagnosis

The definitive diagnosis is made by the demonstration of **antibodies (Ab) to the acetylcholine receptor (AchR), either in serum or neuromuscular junction biopsies**.

The **EMG** in cats with myasthenia will show the **classic decremental response** (each successive spike will have a lower magnitude, corresponding to the fatigue of the muscle.

Acquired myasthenia gravis is believed to be an **immunologic disease resulting in the destruction of AchR by immunoglobin produced against the receptor**, but **thymoma** and other diseases are also seen in conjunction with acquired myasthenia.

Congenital myasthenia is due to **lack of AchR**, rather than immune-mediated destruction of receptors. This form of myasthenia is **rare in cats**.

An **intravenous ednophonium chloride test** may be performed on cats with generalized muscle weakness. This short-acting cholinesterase-inhibiting drug results in alleviation of weakness in about half of affected cats.

Muscle biopsy may show histopathologic signs of myositis.

Differential diagnosis

Other causes of megaesophagus, including idiopathic ME, PRAA, chronic esophagitis, metabolic or toxic causes.

Treatment

Supportive care for acquired myasthenia and associated megaesophagus includes:

Elevated feedings.

Tube (NG, gastrostomy) **feeding.**

Management of aspiration pneumonia as required with antibiotics and bronchodilators.

Immunosuppressive therapy (prednisolone 2–6 mg/kg/day or azathioprine).

Acetycholinesterase antagonists (pyridostigmine bromide 0.2–2.0 mg/kg q 8–12 h PO).

If available, **plasmapheresis** may be used in some cats with acquired megaesophagus.

Thymectomy is indicated in cats with a thymoma and associated megaesophagus.

Congenital myasthenia does not respond well to immunosuppressive therapy and thus supportive care is essential.

Some cats with severe megaesophagus succumb to aspiration pneumonia.

VASCULAR RING ANOMALIES (PERSISTENT RIGHT AORTIC ARCH – PRAA)

Classical signs

- Regurgitation when kitten is weaned onto solid foods.

Pathogenesis

The vascular ring anomalies are **congenital malformations of the aortic arches** which result in a ring around the esophagus that results in an esophageal obstruction.

In cats, a **persistent right aortic arch is the most common anomaly** causing esophageal obstruction and regurgitation.

Other rare, but reported anomalies include the double aortic arch and the left aortic arch with right ligamentum arteriosum.

The obstruction of the esophagus with persistent right aortic arch anomaly is created because the esophagus is trapped by the aorta on the right, the heart base ventrally, and the ligamentum arteriosum dorsolaterally on the left.

Clinical signs

The classical sign associated with a vascular ring anomaly is the **acute onset of regurgitation in a kitten** that has just been **weaned onto solid food**.

In most kittens, regurgitation will occur immediately after eating, but **later in the course of the disease,** as the esophagus becomes more dilated and non-functional, **regurgitation may occur at any time** with no relationship to food intake.

Other signs include respiratory distress, coughing or lethargy associated with aspiration pneumonia that occurs secondary to regurgitation.

Diagnosis

A presumptive diagnosis is often made based on the history and signalment, however, **survey radiographs** followed by introduction of **contrast media** are required to make the definitive diagnosis and **differentiate megaesophagus due to a vascular ring structure** from other causes.

Routine hematology and serum biochemistry values will be normal unless the kitten has developed an aspiration pneumonia or secondary bacterial pneumonia as sequelae to the anomaly.

Echocardiography can be used to determine which type of vascular ring structure is involved, but is not necessary to make the diagnosis.

Differential diagnosis

The primary differential for this disease is congenital megaesophagus, but the presence of the **constricted area at the base of the heart,** along with onset of signs at the time that the kitten begins to consume solid food will help differentiate the two diseases.

Other causes of regurgitation will be readily ruled out by the survey radiographs.

Treatment

The only treatment is surgical removal of the constricting band to release the entrapped esophagus.

In kittens with long-standing esophageal dilatation due to the vascular ring, **esophageal hypomotility cranial to the stricture may be permanent** and require life-long management (see Management of megaesophagus).

Treatment of aspiration pneumonia is supportive: oxygen supplementation, fluids, antibiotics if a bacterial component is present, and respiratory therapy (bronchodilators, expectorants, coupage) as needed.

Prognosis

The prognosis is **guarded to good.** If esophageal function returns after the removal of the constricting band, the prognosis is very good, but in those kittens with residual esophageal dilatation and hypomotility, the long-term prognosis is guarded to poor.

ESOPHAGEAL DIVERTICULAR STRUCTURES

Classical signs

- Regurgitation, pain when swallowing, lethargy, and decreased appetite.

Pathogenesis

Esophageal diverticula are **sac-like dilations of the esophageal wall** that can be **congenital or acquired.**

Acquired diverticula are secondary to one of two scenarios:

Trauma or an obstruction (e.g. foreign body) **that causes increased intraluminal pressure** resulting in a dilation or diverticulum developing **cranial to the injury site.**

Esophageal fibrosis secondary to an inflammatory process (either in the esophagus or in the surrounding tissues) that **causes a contraction of esophageal tissue** and the formation of a diverticular sac.

Congenital diverticula are rare in cats.

Clinical signs

Clinical signs are usually **only observed with a large diverticula.**

Signs that may occur include:
- **Regurgitation.**
- **Inappetence and weight loss.**
- **Pain when swallowing** or thoracic pain.
- Respiratory signs.
- Fever.

Respiratory signs can be secondary to aspiration pneumonia or can be associated with an **inflammatory process in the lungs that is the cause of esophageal fibrosis** and diverticulum formation.

Diagnosis

There is no classic history or signalment that will lead to a presumptive diagnosis, however, **the signs will be suggestive of esophageal disease** in most cases.

Hematologic and serum biochemical profiles are typically **normal.**

Survey radiographs may be suggestive if there is a large diverticulum, but in most cases **contrast studies are necessary to confirm the presence of the sac-like structure**.

Endoscopic examination of the esophagus is also diagnostic and also may provide information about the cause or any associated complications. In cats that have **very small diverticula, endoscopy will be a more helpful diagnostic procedure than contrast radiographs** which could miss the lesion.

Differential diagnosis

Any cause of regurgitation should initially be considered a differential. But blood work and radiographs (survey and contrast) will help to rule out some of the more common causes of regurgitation, which include megaesophagus, esophageal foreign bodies, esophageal masses and peri-esophageal masses.

Endoscopic examination will be required to rule out esophagitis and other inflammatory causes of regurgitation.

Treatment

Diverticula should be managed as conservatively as possible, due to the difficulties and complications associated with esophageal surgery.

If an **underlying cause can be identified and corrected,** this greatly improves the chances for treatment success.

Conservative management of diverticula includes **preventing food accumulation in the sac,** either by **elevated feedings of gruel or liquid diets or by placement of a gastromy tube to by-pass the esophagus.**

If the conservative management fails, either due to the cause or size of the diverticulum, **surgical excision and reconstruction are options,** but esophageal dysfunction and stricture are common sequelae to surgery.

Prognosis

The prognosis for cats with an esophageal diverticulum **depends on its cause and size.**

In cats that have a small diverticulum for which the cause has been identified and removed, the prognosis is **guarded to good.**

If the diverticulum is large, the **cause is uncorrectable,** or there is **no response to conservative management,** the prognosis is **poor.**

HIATAL HERNIA/GASTROESOPHAGEAL INTUSSUSCEPTION

> **Classical signs**
>
> - Intermittent or persistent regurgitation or vomiting.

Pathogenesis

Hiatal hernia is the **protrusion of any abdominal contents through the esophageal hiatus** of the diaphragm into the thorax. With gastroesophageal intussusception, the stomach is prolapsed into the lumen of the distal esophagus.

Hiatal hernia is **an uncommon problem in cats,** but occurs due to **enlargement of the hiatal membrane** (may occur from trauma) or as a result of **laxity in the phrenoesophageal membrane.** Hiatal hernias have been reported in association with generalized tetanus.

Cats more commonly have **sliding hiatal hernias**, with cranial displacement of the abdominal esophagus and part of the stomach through the esophageal hiatus.

Gastroesophageal intussusception can cause both esophagitis and esophageal obstruction.

Clinical signs

Intermittent or persistent regurgitation or vomiting are the most common signs.

Some cats may show **abdominal pain on palpation** of the anterior abdomen.

Respiratory distress may be seen with large hiatal hernias or gastroesophageal intussusceptions.

Diagnosis

Survey radiographs of the thorax may reveal a **soft tissue density and gas in the region of the caudal dorsal mediastinum,** but **contrast radiography** will confirm the presence of the hernia (unless it is a sliding hernia that is in the normal position at the time of radiographs) or untussusception.

In some cases **fluoroscopy** will assist in identifying a sliding hernia.

Differential diagnosis

Diagnosis may be difficult if the hernia is sliding or the intussusception is intermittent and the signs are intermittent in nature. All the major esophageal disorders (esophagitis, hypomotility, stricture, etc) should be considered and ruled out by appropriate testing.

Treatment

If the cat is symptomatic, treatment is as for **reflux esophagitis** (histamine-2 blockers, metoclopramide and sucralfate as needed).

In cats with persistent clinical signs that do not improve with conservative medical therapy, **surgical intervention is indicated.**

Prognosis

Fair to good, especially since cats with hiatal hernias or gastroesophageal intussusceptions tend to have intermittent clinical signs.

ESOPHAGEAL FISTULA

> **Classical signs**
>
> - Regurgitation or dysphagia occurring in conjunction with coughing or respiratory distress.

Pathogenesis

Fistula development is the result of esophageal ischemia and necrosis that ultimately leads to a small perforation. The process of healing leads to development of a **fibrous tract** and a **communication develops** between the esophagus and the respiratory system.

The most common pathway in cats is between the left caudal lung lobe or the accessory lung lobe and the esophagus.

The **most common cause** of fistula development is an **esophageal foreign body** that penetrates (e.g. needle) but other causes include **diverticular structures** and **neoplasia**.

Clinical signs

Signs are referrable to **both the esophagus and lower respiratory tract**.

Signs of esophageal disease include **regurgitation, painful swallowing or repeated swallowing attempts**.

The majority of signs are **respiratory, and include dyspnea, coughing, tachypnea, anorexia, fever and weight loss**, associated with the accumulation of esophageal contents in the affected lung lobe.

The smaller the fistula, the fewer the clinical signs and the more difficult it is to diagnose.

Diagnosis

A large fistula may be visualized on survey radiographs, as well as the **pulmonary changes associated with pneumonia** (increased alveolar and interstitial pattern).

In cats with a very small fistula, contrast radiographs may be required to identify the structure. In some cases, these may be so small that endoscopy is not a means of definitive diagnosis either.

Endoscopic examination should be performed **to obtain biopsies to determine if the lesion is neoplastic** or not.

If there is significant pulmonary disease, the cat may have an **inflammatory leukogram**.

Differential diagnosis

Diverticular structures, esophageal strictures, radiolucent esophageal foreign objects, and aspiration pneumonia secondary to esophageal hypomotility, should all be considered when a differential list is being formulated.

Treatment

The only treatment is surgical closure of the fistula and correction of the underlying cause if it is still present (e.g. diverticulum, neoplasia).

In some cats, **lobectomy** may be necessary as well.

Symptomatic therapy for the pneumonia and esophageal disease includes: esophageal rest (nasogastric or gastrostomy tube), **antibiotic and bronchodilator therapy** as needed, and drugs to control esophagitis if it is present (e.g. ranitidine, metoclopramide, sucralfate, etc).

Prognosis

Guarded. Any esophageal disease that requires surgical correction must be regarded as having a guarded prognosis because of the high rate of complications that occur following surgery (e.g. stricture).

Prevention

Rapid identification and correction (removal) of esophageal foreign bodies, diverticular structures or neoplasia (if possible).

HEREDITARY MYOPATHY OF DEVON REX CATS

Classical signs

- Young Devon Rex cats.
- Appendicular weakness and fatigability.
- Passive ventroflexion of the head and neck.
- Dorsal protrusion of the scapulae.
- Megaesophagus is common, and choking and laryngospasm may occur when eating.

See main reference on page 900 (The Cat With Neck Ventroflexion) for details.

Pathogenesis

The disease is inherited in an **autosomal recessive** fashion. The pathological defect causing the **muscle weakness** has **not been determined.**

Clinical signs

Affected cats have **ventroflexion of the head and neck** because weakness of the dorsal cervical muscles leads to an inability to support the head. Ventroflexion is **accentuated during locomotion, micturition and defecation.**

A **high-stepping forelimb gait, head bobbing and progressive dorsal protrusion of the scapulae** may also be seen, particularly following exertion, stress or excitement.

Cats often have problems **prehending and swallowing food,** partly because of their abnormal head position and partly because of oropharyngeal weakness.

Acute upper airway obstruction may develop due to accumulation of ingesta in the vicinity of the larynx, and this may lead to fatal laryngospasm.

Diagnosis

Diagnosis is made on a combination of **history, breed and clinical signs.**

Routine bloodwork including serum K+, creatine kinase and aspartate transaminase shows **no abnormalities.**

Muscle tone, and spinal reflexes are all within normal limits.

Sparse fibrillation potentials and positive sharp waves are present on EMG.

Muscle biopsy reveals highly variable muscle fiber sizes, with increased numbers of nuclei, internal nucleation and split or degenerating fibers.

Survey or contrast radiographs may reveal megaesophagus with a U-shaped diverticulum at the thoracic inlet.

Differential diagnosis

Other myopathies such as X-linked muscular dystrophy, nemaline myopathy and hypokalaemic polymyopathy should be considered, as well as **myasthenia gravis.**

Treatment

Symptomatic treatment for reflux esophagitis may be given, including histamine-2 blockers (famotidine 0.5–1.0 mg/kg PO q 24 h), drugs that increase esophageal sphincter tone (cisapride 5 mg/kg PO q 12 h), and mucosal cytoprotectants (sucralfate 250–500 mg PO q 8–12 h).

Other supportive measures include elevated feeding of small, liquid meals, or even gastrostomy tube feeding.

Prognosis

Guarded to poor. Most of these cats suffer from chronic reflux esophagitis with megaesophagus and many die suddenly of laryngospasm after choking on food.

Prevention

Because the condition is associated with an autosomal recessive gene, the **parents of any affected kittens should no longer be used for breeding.**

DYSAUTONOMIA

> **Classical signs**
>
> - Regurgitation secondary to megaesophagus.
> - Constipation.
> - Mydriasis.
> - Dry mucous membranes of mouth and eye.

See main reference on page 792 for details.

Pathogenesis

Generalized degeneration of the autonomic ganglia results in loss of GI tract motility, and loss of autonomic control to the eye and heart.

Clinical signs

Clinical signs usually develop over **48 hours** and **depression and anorexia** are present in nearly all cats.

Regurgitation occurs secondary to megaesophagus. Vomiting often occurs and regurgitation may be reported as vomiting.

Constipation is commonly reported.

Mydriasis is present with **normal vision** and third eyelids are commonly prolapsed.

Keratoconjunctivitis sicca and dry oral mucous membranes may be present.

Other signs include **bradycardia** (60–120 bpm) and **hypotension**

Anal areflexia has been reported.

Dysuria in association with a distended urinary bladder also occurs.

The disease is **rare in the US** (some regional areas especially in the central mid-west have more cases) but was more common in Europe in the 1980s.

It is usually seen in **young (< 3 years) cats.**

Diagnosis

The constellation of clinical signs is suggestive of **autonomic nervous system dysfunction.**

There is **no definitive diagnostic test for dysautonomia,** but the following tests of autonomic function are supportive:
- Intraocular **physostigmine** fails to provoke a response, but **pilocarpine** causes immediate miosis.
- Intradermal skin testing – There is no response to histamine (no wheal or flare).
- **Epinephrine should not be given to cats with dysautonomia because fatal arrhythmias may develop.**
- **Cats will respond to atropine** (increased heart rate), which proves that the **post-ganglionic receptors are still able to appropriately respond to stimulus.**

EATING TOO FAST (FOOD GULPING)

Classical signs

- Intermittent regurgitation of food immediately after ingestion, often in tubular form.

Clinical signs

Intermittent regurgitation of whole food, often in tubular form, immediately after it is consumed.

There are **no other abnormal clinical findings** other than the cat appears to gulp or swallow its food without chewing it.

Diagnosis

All clinical, biochemical, radiographic and endoscopic studies (if performed) **will be normal.**

This is a **diagnosis of clinical presumption** based on history, physical exam and the ability to control the signs by feeding smaller meals more frequently or reducing the competition for food that may create food gulping.

Differential diagnosis

Hiatal hernia, mild gastroesophageal reflux, mild esophageal hypomotility or lower esophageal sphincter disease.

Food intolerance and food allergy may cause vomiting very soon after eating which could be mistaken for regurgitation.

Treatment

Feed the cat **smaller meals more frequently** or change feeding location or time to **reduce competition for food** or the tendency to eat rapidly.

MEDIASTINAL NEOPLASIA

Classical signs

- Anorexia.
- Regurgitation.
- Other systemic signs if paraneoplastic disease occurs.
- Thymic lymphoma/thymoma is a mostly benign anterior mediastinal mass, usually found in older cats. Most affected cats are **FeLV negative** and the tumor may be associated with **paraneoplastic syndromes,** such as myasthenia gravis, polymyositis, myocarditis or dermatitis.

See main reference on page 56 for details.

RECOMMENDED READING

August JR (ed). Consultations in Feline Internal Medicine. WB Saunders, Philadelphia, PA. 2001; 4.

Mears EA, Jenkins CC. Canine and feline megaesophagus. Comp Cont Ed 1997; 19(3): 313–326.

Sellon RK, Willard MD. Esophagitis and strictures. Vet Clin North Am Small Anim Pract 2003; 33: 945–967.

Guilford WG, Center SA, Strombeck DR, Williams DA (eds). Strombeck's Small Animal Gastroenterology, 3rd edn. WB Saunders, Philadelphia, PA. 2000.

Tams TR. Esophagoscopy. Small Animal Endoscopy. WB Saunders, Philadelphia, PA. 1999; 2.

30. The cat with signs of acute vomiting

Debra L Zoran

KEY SIGNS

- Active elimination of stomach contents through the mouth.
- ± Preceded by nausea, pacing, and salivation.
- Usually digested food or liquid with acidic or neutral pH.
- ±1 week's duration.

MECHANISM?

- Vomiting is an active process that must be distinguished from regurgitation.
- Vomiting in cats is associated with abdominal muscle contraction, and signs of considerable muscular effort and anxiety prior to the event.
- Vomitus may consist of undigested food material (if swallowed whole), partly digested or even liquid, and may be clear, yellow (bile stained) or brown (food colored).

WHERE?

- Vomiting may result from gastrointestinal disease or extra-intestinal tract diseases.
- Vomiting is rarely associated with colonic disease, except when toxins associated with fecal retention affect the vomiting center and chemoreceptor trigger zone.

WHAT?

- The most common causes of acute vomiting are:
- Mechanical obstructions (including foreign bodies).
- Extra-intestinal tract diseases such as hepatitis.
- Renal failure or pancreatitis, dietary (indiscretion).
- Inflammatory diseases (e.g. IBD).

QUICK REFERENCE SUMMARY

Diseases causing signs of acute vomiting

DEGENERATIVE

- Dysautonomia (p 661)

Dysfunction of the autonomic nervous system resulting in dilated pupils, dry mucous membranes, regurgitation, vomiting, constipation, bradycardia and dysuria.

MECHANICAL

● Gastrointestinal foreign bodies (obstruction)** (p 636)

Acute onset of vomiting that may be projectile if the obstruction is at the pylorus. Vomiting may be intermittent if object is not causing a complete obstruction. Linear foreign bodies (e.g. string) may be evident wrapped around the base of the tongue.

● Intussusception* (p 643)

Acute onset of vomiting, anorexia and lethargy and occurs more often in kittens. The obstruction may be palpated in some cats.

● Motility disturbances (ileus, gastroesophageal reflux)* (p 647)

Vomiting is not associated with eating and usually is bile stained due to presence of duodenal content.

● Antral pyloric hypertrophy/stenosis (p 660)

Vomiting of partially or completely digested food usually several hours after eating, and may be projectile in nature. Siamese cats may be predisposed. Vomiting may appear to be acute in onset in the congenital form, as the vomiting occurs when the kitten begins to eat solid food.

METABOLIC

● Hepatopathies (hepatic lipidosis, cholangitis, drug-induced hepatopathy)** (p 638)

Anorexia, lethargy and vomiting are persistent. Cat may or may not be icteric.

● Diabetes mellitus* (p 643)

Acute onset of vomiting, lethargy, anorexia associated with uncontrolled diabetes mellitus. Cats are usually older, in poor body condition and may be severely dehydrated or in shock if owner does not recognize the condition until late.

● Acute renal failure/pyelonephritis* (p 645)

Acute renal failure is associated with an acute onset of vomiting and depression (may be primary, e.g. ischemic, hypovolemic, or secondary, e.g. post renal obstruction). Other signs include tachypnea, oliguria or anuria, hypothermia. Pyelonephritis causes intermittent vomiting, pain over the sublumbar region, decreased appetite, occasionally fever and polyuria.

● Hypercalcemia (p 652)

There are many causes of hypercalcemia, but the clinical signs most commonly seen are anorexia, vomiting, weight loss and lethargy or weakness.

NEOPLASTIC

● Gastric or small intestinal neoplasia* (p 641)

The most common tumor of the feline digestive system is alimentary lymphoma. Other tumors that occur in the stomach and small intestine are adenocarcinomas (second), and mast cell tumors (third), with fibrosarcomas, leiomyosarcomas and carcinoids occurring rarely. The primary site of gastric tumors is the pylorus. With the exception of lymphoma, which can occur at any age, most tumors occur in old cats. The clinical signs most often observed are anorexia, weight loss and vomiting, which may occur as acute vomiting when the tumor causes a GI obstruction.

continued

continued

NUTRITIONAL

● Food intolerance or dietary indiscretion** (p 635)

Indiscretion is associated with an acute vomiting due to over-eating, eating too quickly or ingesting a foreign substance (food or non-food), e.g. lizards, beetles, plants. Food intolerance causes intermittent vomiting or loose stools, with no pattern or association with eating, and resolves when food source is changed to omit offending substance from diet.

INFLAMMATORY

● Acute pancreatitis** (p 639)

Anorexia and lethargy are the most common signs, with abdominal pain and vomiting being observed much less frequently.

● Gastritis/gastric ulcer disease** (p 637)

Acute onset of vomiting, anorexia and lethargy. May be associated with hematemesis if there are deep erosions or ulcers.

● Septicemia/bacteremia/endotoxemic shock (p 655)

Vomiting is only one of the signs that may occur, others include hypothermia, weakness or collapse, depression, weak or thready pulses, tachypnea and pale to gray mucous membrane color.

● Peritonitis (p 655)

Abdominal pain, distention, fever, decreased appetite and lethargy are the most common presenting signs. Vomiting may occur, but is not a consistent problem.

● Encephalitis/meningitis (p 659)

Vomiting, when it occurs, is due to inflammatory effects on the CRTZ or results from systemic effects of the disease that is causing the encephalitis, e.g. histoplasmosis, toxoplasmosis, cryptococcosis, etc. Most cats with inflammatory CNS disease either have seizures, neurologic deficits, ataxia or dysmetria, or cervical pain.

● Vestibular disease (p 656)

Vomiting is more commonly associated with peripheral vestibular disease. In addition to vomiting, other clinical signs may include head tilt, ataxia, nystagmus and circling.

INFECTIOUS

Viral:

● Feline panleukopenia virus* (p 650)

Infectious viral enteritis of young cats that is often fatal in unvaccinated populations due to the severity of the clinical signs and systemic septicemia. Clinical signs include an acute onset of anorexia and depression, followed by vomiting. Diarrhea may not occur, or is delayed for 24–48 hours. The disease is a relatively rare problem in well, vaccinated cats due to the efficacy of the vaccine.

Bacterial:

● *Helicobacter* spp.* (p 646)

The true importance of *Helicobacter* in feline gastritis is still unknown, but increasing evidence points to them having a role in inflammatory diseases of the stomach, liver and pancreas.

● Salmonellosis* (p 648)

Primarily a problem in young or debilitated cats, as most cats are asymptomatic carriers. In adult cats, vomiting, diarrhea, anorexia and weight loss are more common, while in kittens, systemic signs of infection, including fever or hypothermia, weakness or collapse due to septicemia and endotoxemia.

PARASITIC

● Physaloptera (p 653)

Intermittent vomiting episodes in young, outdoor cats that hunt. Occasionally the small worms are observed in the vomitus.

● *Ollulanus tricuspis* (p 654)

Acute onset of vomiting in free-roaming or colony cats associated with infection with this gastric nematode, which has a direct life cycle.

● Ascarids (p 654)

Intermittent vomiting in young kittens is sometimes observed with large worm burdens due to the mass of worms obstructing normal passage of ingesta. More common signs include unthriftiness, diarrhea and pot-bellied appearance.

TOXIC

● Plant ingestion/toxicity* (p 646)

Many plants do not produce severe toxicity (*Philodendron, Diffenbachia, Euphorbia, Caladium*, etc,), but a few are nephrotoxic (*Lilium* e.g. lilies, *rheum*, e.g. rhubarb, *oxalis* e.g. sorrel) and cause vomiting in addition to signs of renal failure. Other plants that cause vomiting are *ricinus* (castor bean), *robinia* (black locust), and *solanum* (nightshade) to name a few of the more common species.

● Pharmacologic/antibiotic induced* (p 642)

Acute onset of vomiting after initiating antibiotic therapy. Antibiotics associated with vomiting: ampicillin, cephalosporins, tetracycline, erythromycin.

● Ethylene glycol* (p 648)

Vomiting occurs in two stages, one is associated with the initial ingestion of the toxin and is due to alcohol intoxication and metabolic acidosis. Other signs that occur during this time are salivation, depression, ataxia and polydipsia. The second stage occurs 2–3 days later and vomiting, depression and oral ulcers develop secondary to the acute, anuric renal failure, which is the end stage of this toxicity.

● Pyrethrins\pyrethroids\permethrins\organophosphates* (p 644)

Vomiting, diarrhea, hypersalivation, contact dermatitis, ataxia, excitation, seizures and dyspnea are all reported signs of toxicity to these insecticides.

● Anesthetic agents (Xylazine) (p 658)

Xylazine-induced emesis is a well-known side effect of its administration and is often used therapeutically.

● Chemotherapy drug-induced vomiting (p 658)

Those drugs associated with vomiting include: actinomycin-D, cyclophosphamide, cytosine arabinoside, dacarbazine, doxyrubricin, methotrexate, mitoxantrone, vinblastine.

continued

continued

● Non-steroidal anti-inflammatory drug (NSAID) toxicity (p 656)

Vomiting associated with non-steroidal anti-inflammatory drugs (aspirin, ibuprofen) is usually associated with acute gastritis and erosions that occur secondary to the anti-prostaglandin effects on the stomach. Ibuprofen will also cause acute renal failure. Acetaminophen does not induce gastritis but vomiting has been observed in cats due to the hepatotoxicity. Other clinical signs that occur more frequently and are more important include facial edema, pruritus, salivation, tachypnea, depression and cyanosis (due to methemoglobinemia).

● Arsenic poisoning (p 659)

Arsenic is found in herbicides, insecticides, wood preservatives and blood parasiticides. Initial clinical signs include vomiting, diarrhea, anorexia and depression. This is followed by hepatic and renal failure.

INTRODUCTION

MECHANISM?

Vomiting occurs when the **vomiting center in the medulla is stimulated**, which can occur by **several mechanisms**:
● Effect of **blood-borne toxins or drugs**.
● **Afferent impulses from the cerebral cortex, chemoreceptor trigger zone (CRTZ), the vestibular apparatus, or receptors in the pharynx or abdominal viscera**.

The chemoreceptor trigger zone **(CRTZ) is stimulated by:**
● **Blood-borne toxins**, including uremic toxins or drugs.

Vomiting is an **active process** that must be distinguished from regurgitation.

Vomiting in cats is associated with **abdominal muscle contraction**, and signs of **considerable muscular effort and anxiety** prior to the event.

Vomitus may consist of undigested food material (if swallowed whole), partly digested or even liquid, and may be clear, yellow (bile stained) or brown (food colored).

Vomitus is **not typically tubular in form**, nor does it contain large amounts of white frothy material.

The **pH of vomitus is usually acidic** (pH < 4), but **may be neutral (pH 7) if duodenal content is present** (bile reflux).

WHERE?

Vomiting may result from **gastrointestinal disease or extra-intestinal tract diseases**.

Acute vomiting associated with **extra-intestinal diseases** may be due to:
● **CNS disease** (e.g. encephalitis or vestibular disease).
● **Pancreatitis.**
● **Hepatobiliary disease.**
● **Renal disease** causing acute or chronic renal failure.
● **Metabolic or endocrine diseases** including ketoacidotic diabetes mellitus and hypercalcemia.
● **Systemic illness or infection**, e.g. septicemia, pyometra.

Primary gastrointestinal diseases that cause acute vomiting involve the stomach or small intestine:
● **Parasites,** e.g. *Physaloptera, Ollulanus*, etc.
● **Infectious diseases,** e.g. *Salmonella, Helicobacter*.
● **Inflammatory diseases,** e.g. IBD.
● **Neoplasia.**
● **Mechanical,** e.g. foreign body obstruction, intussusception, motility disturbances.
● **Dietary disturbances,** e.g. indiscretion or food intolerance.

Vomiting is **rarely associated with colonic disease**, except when toxins associated with **fecal retention** affect the vomiting center and chemoreceptor trigger zone.

WHAT?

The **most common causes** of acute vomiting are: **mechanical obstructions** (including foreign bodies), extra-intestinal tract diseases (such as hepatitis, renal failure or pancreatitis, dietary indiscretion), and inflammatory diseases (e.g. IBD).

Many cats vomit intermittently, and these episodes are attributed to trichobezoars (hairballs). However, some of these cats may be vomiting due to dietary indiscretion or food intolerance, gastric parasites, motility disturbances, pancreatitis or other acute inflammatory disorders.

Acute, persistent vomiting episodes that occur along with other clinical signs such as lethargy, anorexia or diarrhea, usually signal a more serious problem that should be investigated more thoroughly. Examples of problems fitting this category include intussusception, erosions/ulcers, acute renal failure, neoplasia or inflammatory bowel disease.

DISEASES CAUSING SIGNS OF ACUTE VOMITING

FOOD INTOLERANCE OR DIETARY INDISCRETION**

Classical signs

- Intermittent vomiting.
- Large bowel diarrhea or soft, mucoid feces.

Pathogenesis

Food intolerance is a non-immunologic, adverse reaction to a substance(s) present in food. This reaction may be to a food component such as the type of protein or carbohydrate, or it may be to the colorings, preservatives, flavorings, etc. that are present in pet foods. Natural chemicals in foods such as amines, salicylates and monosodium glutamate may stimulate nerve endings and have also been associated with food intolerance. Highly flavored or "rich" food has more of these chemicals. Cats may be sensitive to more than one food. Signs may require a "binge" or several days of exposure before they are evident.

The actual mechanism associated with vomiting or diarrhea due to food intolerance is unknown.

Food intolerance is usually a cause of chronic, intermittent vomiting, but kittens may present acutely with diarrhea when they are first introduced to new foods. Diarrhea may result when a rapid change in food overwhelms the digestive capacity. Changes in food composition require changes in digestive enzymes.

Ingesting a foreign substance (dietary indiscretion) such as lizards, beetles, moths or plants may cause acute vomiting. Over-eating or eating too quickly is poorly documented as a cause of vomiting in cats.

Clinical signs

Intermittent but persistent vomiting or mucoid, soft feces are common signs. Poor hair coat or failure to thrive may also be noted but this is less common.

Diagnosis

There is no definitive diagnostic test for this problem other than to observe a response to changing the diet.

Differential diagnosis

Intermittent but unrelenting vomiting in an otherwise healthy cat suggests possible motility disturbances, antral pyloric hypertrophy, gastric parasites or early IBD.

Treatment

Changing the diet to a diet that does not contain the offending substance. This may be as simple as changing from a grocery store brand to a premium brand food (or vice versa), but also may require changing to a hypoallergenic food product (IVD's Limited diets, Hill's d/d, Eukanuba Response formula, Waltham, etc.). Kittens often respond to being fed exactly the same food as a sole diet for at least 3 days.

Prognosis

Good if the appropriate food can be found, which is usually not a difficult problem. However, the cat may have to remain on the diet indefinitely.

GASTROINTESTINAL FOREIGN BODIES (OBSTRUCTION)**

Classical signs

- Frequent, severe vomiting episodes with upper GI obstruction.
- Intermittent vomiting with lower intestinal obstruction.
- Anorexia.
- Dehydration.
- Diarrhea is more prevalent with lower intestinal obstructions.
- Abdominal pain.

Pathogenesis

GI foreign bodies occur **more commonly in young cats,** because of their curious nature, tendency to ingest non-food substances (string, rubber bands) and prey (hair, fur, bones).

Linear foreign bodies (e.g. string, yarn, thread, etc.) are the most common foreign body in cats and create problems from the motility disturbances that are created resulting in **intestinal plication** or intussusception, and from the **intestinal perforation** due to string migration through the intestinal wall. Thread, with or without a needle, and string are the most common causes, and in some countries, the string from the end of a sausage is a common culprit.

Linear foreign bodies may first be caught under the **base of the tongue,** creating not only an oral lesion, but also preventing the possible passage of the string through the GI tract. Alternatively, they may become **trapped at the pylorus,** with the rest of the string passing into the small intestine.

Many foreign objects (especially hair, but including string) will pass through the GI tract, so if an obstruction occurs, it may be due to a **disturbance in motility, narrowing of lumen or other pathology** that prevents the normal passage of the object.

Clinical signs

The signs **depend upon the location** of the foreign object and will help in many cases to localize the lesion.

With **gastric or upper small intestinal obstructions, acute onset of frequent vomiting** or gagging is common.

Dehydration, lethargy and anorexia are common in these cats, and they may show evidence of abdominal discomfort (either on palpation or by posture).

In cats with a **lower intestinal obstruction, diarrhea will probably be more likely, vomiting less frequent and severe,** and dehydration and abdominal pain more variable.

If the foreign body is of significant size or if intestinal plication from a linear foreign body is present, these **abnormalities may be palpable**.

Cats that develop an **intestinal perforation** as a result of the foreign body deteriorate rapidly and develop **depression and fever, hypovolemia/shock**.

Diagnosis

History and physical examination findings are very important in pointing to the diagnosis (always **examine under the tongue of vomiting cats**).

Hemogram and serum biochemistry profile findings will likely be normal if the condition is acute.

Long-standing or severe linear foreign bodies or GI perforation will show an **inflammatory response,** evidence of dehydration (hemoconcentration or elevated proteins) and **electrolyte abnormalities** consistent with vomiting (hypokalemia is most common).

The diagnosis is obtained by **imaging studies,** including radiography (plain or contrast), ultrasonography or upper GI endoscopy. Radiographs may reveal evidence of intestinal plication (wash board appearance) which is the classic presentation for string foreign bodies. In some cases, endoscopy will allow retrieval of the foreign object, and is a useful means of assessing other damage (e.g. erosions, ulcers, or tears in the mucosa).

Differential diagnosis

The **acute onset, age of occurrence and history or physical examination findings** usually point to a foreign body.

However, some cats with linear foreign bodies have a **waxing/waning course of vomiting and anorexia** that may not suggest the diagnosis immediately.

Other differentials in those cases would include infectious, dietary or inflammatory gastrointestinal diseases.

Treatment

In cases where the object is still in the stomach, it is sometimes possible to safely **retrieve the object** (needle, small toy, etc.) via an **endoscopic** procedure.

Most GI foreign bodies however, will require **surgical removal**, and some may be a surgical emergency when GI perforation has occurred.

Cats that are severely dehydrated from persistent vomiting, or have suspected intestinal perforation and leakage should be stabilized as much as possible with **aggressive fluid therapy** and **broad-spectrum antibiotics** prior to surgery (e.g. combination of ampicillin/amoxicillin or cefazolin and enrofloxacin, amikacin or cefoxitin). Some cats with a protracted history of vomiting will benefit from **histamine-2 blockers** or GI protectants if gastritis or gastric erosions are suspected.

Motility-modifying agents, such as metoclopramide, should not be used until the obstruction is relieved.

Prognosis

The prognosis is good unless large portions of bowel must be resected which potentially leads to short bowel syndrome.

Prevention

The key is to prevent ingestion of string, rubber bands, needle and thread, string, etc., to not allow cats to ingest prey, and to use caution in the type of pet toys that the cat is allowed to play with.

GASTRITIS/GASTRIC ULCER DISEASE**

> ### Classical signs
> - Acute or chronic vomiting, with or without hemoptysis.
> - Anorexia or reduced appetite.
> - Lethargy.
> - Anterior abdominal pain.

Pathogenesis

Gastritis results from hyperacidity, loss of mucosal protection (mucus, bicarbonate), reduced mucosal blood flow, or mucosal damage from direct trauma, irritation or chemical erosion.

Continued damage leads to development of a **gastric erosion** (lesion in mucosa only) or **ulcer** (lesion affecting the deeper tissue layers of the stomach wall).

Non-steroidal anti-inflammatory drugs **(NSAIDs) reduce the synthesis of prostaglandins** which are necessary for **gastric mucus secretion**. Gastric mucus is the primary means of surface protection against acid, irritants and trauma.

Hyperacidity can occur secondary to liver failure (hypersecretion of gastrin and reduced mucosal blood flow), renal failure (hypergastrinemia) or mastocytosis (increased release of histamine), or can result from long-term use of gastric acid-suppressing drugs (e.g. proton pump inhibitors), or a gastrinoma (gastrin-secreting tumor) which is a very rare endocrine tumor in cats.

A decrease in **bicarbonate** delivery to the gastric mucosa occurs in metabolic acidosis (e.g. renal failure) and in states of reduced blood flow (e.g. shock), thus resulting in mucosal injury.

Clinical signs

Vomiting occurs with or without hematemesis.

Vomiting may be **acute in onset with drug-induced gastritis or ulcers, but for most other causes is chronic** due to the development of hyperacidity from metabolic or inflammatory diseases.

Anorexia or decreased appetite and lethargy occur in cats with severe erosions or ulcers.

Anterior abdominal pain is more common with ulcer disease.

Diagnosis

History of acute onset, exposure to NSAIDs, ingestion of chemical or toxin irritating to gastric mucosa, or episode of ischemia (shock).

Radiographic findings are usually non-diagnostic, but may identify a deep erosion/ulcer with contrast.

A deep erosion or ulcer may be identified via **ultrasound**, but simple gastritis or superficial mucosal erosions will only be diagnosed by endoscopy examination or biopsy.

Endoscopy is the **definitive** way to diagnose **mucosal erosions and ulcers,** and also may help identify a cause via histopathologic examination of the tissue.

Differential diagnosis

Acute gastritis due to erosions/ulcers will mimic many causes of acute vomiting, including dietary indiscretion, **mechanical or obstructive disorders**, infectious causes, toxin-induced (especially plant ingestion), pancreatitis, and metabolic or endocrine diseases such as hepatitis, renal failure or neoplasia.

Treatment

Treatment is aimed at **identification and correction of the underlying cause** of the primary lesion, **reduction of acid secretion** and **protection of the gastric mucosa** to allow it to heal. This is accomplished by:

- Administration of **histamine-2 receptor antagonist (H$_2$RA)** (e.g. cimetidine 5 mg/kg PO q 8 h, ranitidine 0.5–1.0 mg/kg PO q 12 h, or famotidine 0.5–1.0 mg/kg PO q 12–24 h).
  - Famotidine is the most potent and only H$_2$RA to effectively reduce acid in dogs. No studies have been completed in cats.
  - **Proton pump inhibiting drugs** (omeprazole 1 mg/kg PO q 24 h) are the most effective in reducing acid secretion but can be difficult to dose.
  - **Sucralfate** (250–500 mg PO q 8–12 h) is also a useful adjunct therapy for cats with significant gastric erosions or ulcers, as it will act as a surface protectant. Sucralfate must be given in an acidic environment to be effective, so it should be administered at least 1 hour prior to giving histamine-blocking or proton pump-inhibiting drugs.
  - Feeding **nothing per os for the first 24 hours**, then feeding a highly digestible, bland, low-residue diet, either commercial or homemade (e.g. small amounts of low-fat beef, chicken or turkey), will be beneficial.

In cases where treatment of the underlying cause is not possible or where management is the only option (e.g.

chronic renal failure), long-term therapy with histamine blockade will be necessary to help reduce the development of new erosions or ulcers.

In **severe or deep ulcers**, **surgical intervention** may be necessary but this is unusual. Emergency surgical intervention will be necessary in cats that have perforating ulcers. Many deep or perforating ulcers are caused by an invasive neoplasm, or by fungal disease in geographic areas where systemic fungal infections are prevalent.

Cats with severe disease that are unable or unwilling to eat for **more than 3 days** should have **nutritional support** provided, either through placement of a feeding tube for enteral feeding, or by parenteral nutrition.

Prognosis

The majority of cats will recover completely from the insult if the cause can be identified and corrected, and in most other cases the disease can be successfully managed. In cats with ulcers due to neoplasia, the prognosis is guarded to poor.

Prevention

Reduce opportunities for ingestion of toxic or irritating substances.

Management of diseases causing **hypergastrinemia** (renal failure, hepatic disease) should **always include therapy for gastritis.**

Prevent ischemia and shock-induced gastric erosions by rapid replacement of **fluids** following shock, and maintenance of hydration during surgical procedures, etc.

HAPATOPATHIES** (HEPATIC LIPIDOSIS, CHOLANGITIS, DRUG-INDUCED HEPATOPATHY)

> **Classical signs**
>
> - Weight loss, anorexia, vomiting, icterus and depression are the most common signs.

See main reference on page 421 for details.

Clinical signs

Weight loss (often dramatic), anorexia, vomiting, icterus and depression are the most common signs. Other signs may include ascites (this is rare with hepatic lipidosis, but may occur with end-stage hepatopathies or cholangitis).

Most hepatopathies are associated with chronic vomiting, but drug-induced hepatopathies (e.g. glipizide) are associated with acute vomiting.

Diagnosis

The presence of icterus helps to narrow the differentials list to hepatic, pre-hepatic and post-hepatic diseases.

The **hemogram** in cats with hepatic disease is **often abnormal** (e.g. mild, non-regenerative anemia, with RBC morphology having schistocytes, leptocytes or target cells present), but the changes are **not specific** for liver disease. However, it does help **rule out pre-hepatic causes of icterus**.

Serum chemistry abnormalities may include **elevated liver enzyme activities** (mild to marked increases), **hyperbilirubinemia, hypocholesterolemia, hypoalbuminemia**, decreased BUN, and electrolyte alterations (consistent with vomiting or dehydration, e.g. hypokalemia, hypernatremia).

The urinalysis will have **bilirubinuria,** and occasionally may have urate crystalluria if the liver failure is severe or end-stage.

Ultrasonography is the most useful imaging modality, because it can also be used to obtain fine-needle aspirates or biopsies (note: check for a possible coagulopathy before performing a blind biopsy). In cats with hepatic lipidosis the liver is enlarged and hepatocytes are crowded out by lipid, but cats with cholangitis may have a normal, large or small liver.

Liver biopsies taken via surgical exploratory laparotomy have greater accuracy, and will also **allow placement of a gastrostomy or jejunostomy tube** (which is essential for cats with hepatic lipidosis and important for any cat that doesn't eat for longer than 3–5 days). Again, the cat should be checked for a possible coagulopathy before surgery is performed.

ACUTE PANCREATITIS**

Classical signs

- Anorexia, lethargy and depression are the most common signs.
- Vomiting is seen in less than 50% of cats with pancreatitis.

Pathogenesis

The **cause of acute pancreatitis in cats is unknown,** but it has been associated with trauma, some infectious diseases (herpes virus, toxoplasmosis, feline infectious peritonitis, etc.), hepatic lipidosis, drugs, and extension of inflammation from the small intestine. Recently pancreatitis has been **observed to occur in association with inflammatory bowel disease and cholangitis,** but whether it is due to a common inflammatory reaction or innocent bystander situation is unknown.

The destructive process in the pancreas is initiated by **activation of trypsinogen**, which leads to the activation of other proteases, lipases and inflammatory mediators such as kininogens and free radical species. Activation of these processes leads to activation of complement, induction of coagulation disorders such as DIC and hypovolemic shock.

Acute necrotizing pancreatitis is a common finding in cats with diabetes mellitus that die within the first week of diagnosis despite treatment. Histologic evidence of pancreatitis is found in approximately 50% of cats with diabetes mellitus.

In dogs, hyperlipoproteinemia, high-fat/low-protein diets, obesity, some drugs (furosemide, azathioprine, L-asparaginase, sulfonamides, tetracyclines, corticosteroids) and metabolic states (hypercalcemia, uremia) are implicated as risk factors for pancreatitis, but no such association has been reported for cats.

Clinical signs

Anorexia, lethargy and dehydration are the most common presenting signs in cats, unlike the classic signs of vomiting and abdominal pain that are exhibited in dogs.

Fewer than a third of cats with pancreatitis will present with vomiting, abdominal pain, diarrhea, tachypnea or dyspnea, or a palpable anterior abdominal mass.

Cats tend to have a **more variable clinical course** than the disease in dogs, with some cats having a course of anorexia, lethargy and weight loss that does not suggest acute illness, while other cats will present with acute deterioration, severe shock and collapse.

A critically ill diabetic cat that does not respond to appropriate therapy within the first 24–48 hours of therapy should be suspected of having acute necrotizing pancreatitis.

Diagnosis

Diagnosis of pancreatitis in cats is very difficult, primarily because of the vague clinical presentation.

Hematologic changes, if they occur, are non-specific: neutrophilia, hemoconcentration, thrombocytopenia (late), and anemia (late).

Serum **biochemical abnormalities are common, but also non-specific**: hyper- or hypoglycemia, elevated alanine aminotransferase, elevated serum alkaline phosphatase, hyperbilirubinemia, hypercholesterolemia, hypokalemia, hypophosphatemia, hypocalcemia. **Serum amylase and lipase values are unreliable and uninterpretable** (pancreatitis in cats has been associated with elevations, decreases and normal values of both enzymes).

Hypocalcemia, when present, is suggestive of acute necrotizing pancreatitis and a poorer prognosis.

Radiographic abnormalities are highly variable but those that may be observed include decreased contrast in the right, cranial abdomen; dilated and gas-filled small intestines; or a mass effect in the area of the pancreas with transposition of duodenum, stomach and transverse colon.

Ultrasonography is a very useful diagnostic tool for evaluating pancreatic pathology. Changes in pancreas size, echogenicity and the presence of masses can often be detected. **However, pancreatic abnormalities found via ultrasound may persist for months** after the condition has resolved.

An elevated serum trypsin-like immunoreactivity (TLI) assay (the feline-specific assay must be used) cannot accurately predict pancreatitis in cats, however, a value of greater than 100 µg/L has been reported to have an 80% specificity and 33% sensitivity for pancreatitis.

A feline pancreatic lipase immunoreactivity (fPLI) assay has been recently developed and validated. This assay is very specific (90%), and highly sensitive (100%), for acute pancreatitis but only 65% specific for chronic pancreatitis.

A recent study showed that the combined use of fPLI and abdominal ultrasound was nearly 100% specific and sensitive for acute pancreatitis.

Differential diagnosis

The vague and non-specific clinical signs make it impossible to rule out other causes of extra-intestinal and intestinal disease until a complete work-up has been performed.

In very ill cats, the other major differentials include peritonitis, septicemia and endotoxic shock.

Treatment

Oral alimentation should be withheld for 1–3 days if vomiting is present in cats with pancreatitis to reduce pancreatic secretions. Return to full feed gradually and feed cats a highly palatable, but highly digestible, diet (Hills feline i/d, Iam's low residue diet, etc.). In cats that are not vomiting, and especially those that have been anorectic for more than 3 days, oral alimentation should not be withheld and feeding tubes should be placed, if needed.

Eliminate, if possible, any predisposing factors that are present.

Aggressive fluid therapy is the cornerstone of treatment, not only to correct the dehydration that occurs from vomiting, but also to reduce the effects of microvascular stasis on the pancreas and other vascular beds (pulmonary, renal, hepatic). In some cases colloid therapy in addition to crystalloids is very beneficial. Attention to the need for **potassium supplementation**, phosphorus, and other electrolytes, such as magnesium, sodium and chloride are essential.

In cats with concurrent hepatic lipidosis or those that must be held off food for greater than 5 days, **enteral nutrition via a jejunostomy tube or total parenteral nutrition will be a necessary** component of the treatment plan. J-tubes must be surgically placed, which may increase the risk of complications due to pancreatitis. Total parenteral nutrition requires strict attention to sterility and close monitoring of electrolytes and is more suited to referral institutions than general practice.

Vomiting should be controlled with **antiemetic therapy**. Either **metoclopramide** (0.1–0.2 mg/kg IV q 8 h) or chlorpromazine (0.01–0.025 mg/kg IV) are effective, but it is important when using any phenothiazine antiemetics that you ensure adequate volume expansion so that hypotension is avoided. If gastritis is suspected histamine-2 blockers such as ranitidine or famotidine should also be considered.

Corticosteroids are indicated **in cats that are in shock** and may be helpful in cats with chronic pancreatitis from concurrent IBD or cholangitis.

Abdominal pain should be controlled with butorphanol (0.1–0.8 mg/kg IV q 4–6 h), buprenorphine (0.03 mg/kg q 6–8 h) or meperidine (2–4 mg/kg IM q 6–8 h).

Antibiotics should not be routinely used in pancreatitis. **Indications for use of antibiotics include evidence of toxic changes in the neutrophils, the cat is febrile, or other signs of sepsis or septicemia** are present. In cases where a pancreatic abscess is suspected or a concern, parenteral cephalosporins (cefazolin, 20–30 mg/kg IV, cephalothin 20–35 mg/kg IV) combined with fluorinated quinolones are recommended.

The **major complications** of pancreatitis include: development of pancreatic abscesses, pancreatic fibrosis resulting in obstruction of the common bile duct or development of diabetes mellitus, peritonitis, pulmonary thromboembolism, acute renal failure, and disseminated intravascular coagulation. In those cases, surgical intervention may be required (abscess, peritonitis, stricture), but in cases where respiratory, cardiovascular, renal or coagulation abnormalities develop the prognosis is guarded to poor.

Prognosis

Cats with **concurrent hepatic lipidosis or cholangitis and acute necrotizing pancreatitis have a worse prognosis.** These cases are more difficult to manage (require TPN or jejunostomy feeding) and have more complications (coagulation abnormalities and tendency toward development of pulmonary thromboembolism).

GASTRIC OR SMALL INTESTINAL NEOPLASIA*

Classical signs

- Chronic, progressive vomiting that may include hematemesis.
- Weight loss.
- Anorexia.
- Lethargy or depression.
- Diarrhea may occur if the location of the lesion is in the small intestine.

See main reference on page 675 for details (The Cat With Chronic Vomiting).

Clinical signs

Acute vomiting may occur occasionally or the signs occur acutely, while the disease itself is chronic.

Typically chronic, progressive vomiting that may include hematemesis is observed.

Weight loss, anorexia, lethargy or depression are also common.

Diarrhea may occur if the location of the lesion is in the small intestine.

Signs occur in **older cats**, however, **lymphoma** occurs in cats of **all ages** and may be associated with FeLV infection.

Diagnosis

Palpation of the abdomen may reveal a **mass or thickened intestinal loops** in some cases.

Hematology and serum chemistry profiles are usually **non-specific,** but help to rule out other causes of vomiting. The most frequent hematologic abnormality is **anemia of chronic disease** (normocytic, normochromic), but blood loss anemia is also observed. The abnormalities found in the chemistry profile depend on the extent of the disease and severity of vomiting, and are non-specific.

The most helpful diagnostic procedures are imaging techniques: radiography, ultrasonography or possibly endoscopy. Depending on the location and size of the mass, **ultrasonography** will not only allow visualization of the lesion, but may also allow diagnosis via **fine-needle aspiration or biopsy**.

Ultimately, **histopathologic examination of the tissue is necessary for a definitive diagnosis**, and in many cases, surgical exploratory for both biopsy and resection is the best approach.

Differential diagnosis

Inflammatory bowel disease – This is usually not associated with hematemesis or severe weight loss, and occurs in young to middle-aged cats.

Metabolic diseases, e.g. hyperthyroidism, chronic renal or liver diseases.

Chronic pancreatitis.

Treatment

For **adenocarcinoma, mast cell tumors** and other tumors that tend to occur as **solitary mass lesions**, surgical removal via intestinal resection is the primary approach. **Biopsies should be obtained of liver, regional lymph nodes and mesenteric tissues** to determine if metastasis has occurred or its extent. Chemotherapy has not been proven effective for adenocarcinoma or intestinal mast cell tumors.

Lymphoma is generally an infiltrative neoplasm and **chemotherapy** using the COP protocol is the treatment of choice. See main reference on page 676 for details.

PHARMACOLOGIC (ANTIBIOTIC-INDUCED)

Classical signs

- Anorexia.
- Vomiting.
- Diarrhea.

Pathogenesis

Vomiting associated with antibiotics is a common occurrence and can occur with almost all of the popular antibiotics, including: **amoxicillin, cephalexin,** **erythromycin**, lincomycin, sulfasoxazole, **tetracycline**, trimethoprim-sulfadiazine.

The **mechanism for induction of nausea or vomiting varies** for each drug. For example, erythromycin is a prokinetic and is highly acidic, causing a direct irritant effect on the gastric epithelium.

Some drugs can be given without inducing vomiting if they are given with food, while others may induce vomiting whether or not food is present because the effect is not directly on the stomach.

Clinical signs

Anorexia or a decrease in appetite is the most common sign of drug-associated discomfort, followed by **vomiting** or regurgitation.

Diarrhea may occur following antibiotic use, but is usually associated with a disruption in microflora of the colon resulting in colitis or large bowel diarrhea.

Diagnosis

The diagnosis may be straightforward if the cat was previously not vomiting and started vomiting after the drug was administered. However, if drugs are being given to treat a disease for which vomiting or diarrhea are already present, differentiating the drug effect from the disease will be quite difficult.

An especially important example of this is in **cats with cholangitis** that have **signs of vomiting due to their disease, and have to be on long-term antibiotic therapy** to treat their disease. It is sometimes very difficult to determine whether a worsening of clinical signs is due to the therapy or a worsening of the disease. In those cases, careful assessment of the physical findings and blood work changes will be necessary to separate the two problems.

Treatment

The best approach is to stop use of the antibiotic in question, and if antibiotic therapy is still required, switch to an appropriate antibiotic of another class.

Prognosis and prevention

Some antibiotics are best given with food (e.g. beta lactams), and in those cases, adverse effects are sometimes avoided by using the drug as it is recommended.

The vomiting is easily controlled by changing to another antibiotic, so the prognosis is excellent.

KETOACIDOTIC DIABETES MELLITUS*

Classical signs

- Vomiting.
- Lethargy or depression.
- Anorexia and weight loss.
- Polyuria/polydipsia.

See main reference on page 236 for details (The Cat With Polyuria and Polydipsia).

Clinical signs

At the time of diagnosis, one third of diabetic cats have a history of vomiting, and with ketoacidosis, an acute onset of vomiting may occur.

Vomiting, lethargy or depression, anorexia, polyuria/polydipsia and weight loss are the classical signs of ketoacidotic diabetes mellitus in cats.

Diabetic cats may also present without weight loss or depression, and polyphagia and polydipsia are still prominent signs.

Cats with **severe, long-standing ketoacidotic diabetes mellitus** may have **neurologic signs** such as stupor, obtundation and coma.

Diagnosis

Typical hemogram and serum chemistry abnormalities include mild non-regenerative anemia (chronic disease), leukocytosis, lymphopenia, hyperglycemia, elevated liver enzyme activities, hypokalemia, hypo-magnesemia, hypophosphatemia, and metabolic acidosis.

The **urinalysis, in conjunction with the presence of hyperglycemia, is diagnostic** and shows **glucosuria and ketonuria.** Cats may be ketonemic and have acetone breath before ketonuria is detected on the dipstick.

Many cats will also have **concurrent bacteriuria**, with elevated protein, blood or white cells.

INTUSSUSCEPTION*

Classical signs

- Acute vomiting, anorexia and lethargy, usually in kittens.
- Abdominal discomfort.
- Endotoxemia or shock may ensue if the intussusception is complete.

Pathogenesis

The exact pathophysiology of the development of intussusception is unknown.

Uncoordinated peristalsis resulting in vigorous contraction of a segment of bowel into an adjacent quiescent segment that occurs due to any variety of causes is involved, and a common predisposing cause in cats is a string foreign body.

The end result is that a segment of intestine telescopes or invaginates into the adjoining, distal segment of bowel, causing an intraluminal obstruction, vascular compromise of the affected bowel segments and ultimately the development of entoxemia and shock.

Bowel **regions that undergo changes in diameter** (gastroesophageal junction and iliocolic junction) seem to be **at the greatest risk,** but intussusceptions occur at any location, and are classified according to their location within the gastrointestinal tract.

Intussusceptions cranial to the jejunum are termed **high intussusceptions** and generally are **more severe** (signs are more acute and have more rapid clinical deterioration) than distal intussusceptions.

Siamese and Burmese cats appear to have a predilection for development of intussusceptions.

Most intussusceptions occur in **young animals** (< 1 year of age).

Intussusceptions are rare in cats compared to dogs.

Clinical signs

An acute onset of vomiting and lethargy, with diarrhea occurring occasionally, is typical in kittens.

With **high intussusceptions,** vomiting, abdominal discomfort, anorexia, lethargy, dehydration and hypovolemia leading to shock are the most common clinical signs.

Low intussusceptions (at the iliocolic junction) typically present with bloody, mucoid diarrhea, tenesmus, intermittent vomiting and weight loss. In many of these cases, the intussusception can be **palpated.**

Diagnosis

Hemogram and serum biochemistry profiles will be variable depending on the severity and location of the intussusception, however, dehydration, electrolyte abnormalities, anemia and leukocyte changes have all been observed depending on the cause of the intussusception.

Radiographs and/or ultrasound examination of the gastrointestinal tract are the best means of confirming the diagnosis. A gas- or fluid-filled, dilated loop of bowel is present immediately cranial to the intussusception, which may not be visualized without using a contrast agent. If there is not too much gas to obstruct adequate images, intestinal intussusceptions are usually readily identified using ultrasound, and are characterized by visualizing the folds of intestine layered on top of one another.

Contrast studies may be used but should not be done at the expense of delaying treatment in severely ill cases.

Endoscopic examination or colonoscopy can also be used to obtain a diagnosis, especially with low intussusceptions, but this is rarely needed and may be very difficult in kittens.

Differential diagnosis

Many **diseases that can precipitate an intussusception** (viral enteritis, foreign bodies, gastroenteritis, intestinal parasitism, etc.) also have clinical signs that **mimic it.**

A thorough physical examination, diagnostic evaluation, and close patient monitoring are essential.

Treatment

Intussusception must be considered a **surgical emergency**. Cats with signs of shock or endotoxemia should be prepared for surgery by **correcting fluid and electrolyte imbalances, administration of broad-spectrum, parenteral antibiotics** (combinations such as ampicillin/amoxicillin or cefazolin and enrofloxain, amikacin, cefoxitin or imipenam), **and use of histamine-2 blockers** (ranitidine or famotidine) or protectants (e.g. sucralfate) if gastric erosions or ulceration is suspected.

Motility-enhancing drugs, such as metoclopramide, **are contraindicated in patients with GI obstruction** and should not be used.

After surgical correction, which is most commonly surgical resection and anastomosis, **if gastric ulceration is not a complicating factor, oral alimentation should be instituted in the first 24 hours**, to enhance the return of normal motility and reduce the possibility of post-operative ileus.

Prognosis and prevention

The key point is that correction of the intussusception does not necessarily alleviate the problem unless the **underlying cause can be identified and corrected.** Otherwise **recurrences are possible** and even likely.

Surgical procedures, such as multiple enteroplexy, are recommended to reduce the risk of recurrence.

Prognosis is **guarded to good if** the anesthesia and surgical procedure is **uncomplicated.**

PYRETHRINS/PYRETHROIDS/-PERMETHRINS /ORGANOPHOSPHATES*

Classical signs

- Vomiting, diarrhea.
- Hypersalivation, agitation.
- Contact dermatitis.
- Tremors, ataxia, and possibly seizures.

See main reference on page 594 for details (The Cat With Salivation).

Clinical signs

Signs associated with contact exposure or ingestion of pyrethrin/pyrethroid-containing pesticides are **generally mild.**

Vomiting, diarrhea, hypersalivation and agitation are the most common signs seen with exposure to permethrins in cats. This is currently the most commonly reported toxicity in cats in the United States due to the accidental or inadvertent exposure of cats to the over-the-counter flea products available for dogs.

Severely affected cats may develop **muscle tremors, ataxia, excitation or seizures.**

Organophosphate insecticides cause a combination of signs that include **salivation, lacrimation, increased defecation and urination due to the stimulation of the parasympathetic nervous system**. Other clinical signs that may occur are vomiting, tremors, ataxia, hyperthermia, dyspnea and seizures. Severely poisoned cats may die from the systemic effects of the toxin.

Diagnosis

History of exposure to or ingestion of products containing permethrin (most common) or pyrethroids.

There is generally no need for further diagnostic testing since signs will abate with removal of pyrethrins or permethrins from the skin or GI tract and supportive care.

With **organophosphates,** if there is no known exposure, but the toxicity is suspected based on clinical signs, measurement of **serum cholinesterase activity levels** may aid diagnosis. Levels less than 25% of normal are highly suggestive of OP toxicity.

ACUTE RENAL FAILURE/PYELONEPHRITIS*

Classical signs

- Anorexia or decreased appetite.
- Polyuria/polydipsia, and weight loss. Occasional chronic vomiting, in advanced cats.
- Cats with pyelonephritis may only have vague signs of inappetence, fever or abdominal discomfort.

See main reference on page 278 for details.

Clinical signs

Anorexia or decreased appetite, polyuria/polydipsia, and weight loss are the classic signs of renal disease.

Renal failure is a rare cause of acute vomiting in the cat.

In cats that do vomit, the signs are generally chronic and associated with the effects of increased uremic toxins causing nausea by their effects on the CRTZ and also by associated hypergastrinemia and the direct effects on the stomach.

Cats with pyelonephritis may only have vague signs of **inappetence, fever or abdominal discomfort**.

Diagnosis

Palpation of the abdomen may reveal **enlarged or painful kidneys** (acute renal disease, pyelonephritis, FIP, renal neoplasia or polycystic kidney disease), or **small, misshapen kidneys** (chronic renal disease).

Marked azotemia (elevated BUN and creatinine), hyperphosphatemia, hyperkalemia and metabolic acidosis in conjunction with isosthenuria (or impaired urine-concentrating ability, e.g. urine specific gravity < 1.030) and oliguria/anuria are classically associated with acute renal failure, while mild azotemia, hypokalemia, hyperphosphatemia, and metabolic acidosis with isosthenuria and polyuria/polydipsia are found with chronic renal diseases.

Pyelonephritis and other inflammatory diseases of the kidneys have fewer hematologic or biochemical changes. Some cats may have an inflammatory leukogram (neutrophilia with or without a left shift), but azotemia does not occur until late (renal failure develops).

Urinalysis is very helpful in distinguishing infectious, or inflammatory, renal diseases from other problems.

Pyelonephritis is difficult to diagnose definitively and is only confirmed by culture of organisms directly from the kidney, either via ultrasound-guided **pyelocentesis or during a surgical exploratory**.

Other tests of renal function include intravenous pyelograms or scintigraphic assessment of GFR, but these are not universally available.

Ultrasound is also a useful tool for assessing renal size and infrastructure, and is helping to assess the patency of the ureters, presence of calculi, neoplasms, cysts or other abnormalities.

Differential diagnosis

The wide range of clinical signs resulting from various renal diseases can mimic many different diseases, and so the initial history and physical examination are extremely important.

Most of the more common extra-intestinal, systemic diseases that can cause vomiting should be considered in the initial differentials, but the history, physical exam, minimum database, and urinalysis (with culture if bacteria or WBC are present) will rule out most of the diseases of concern (e.g. diabetes mellitus, hepatopathies, hyperthyroidism, etc.).

Imaging studies will help rule in or out the other major differentials: neoplasia, pancreatitis and mechanical disturbances.

Inflammatory bowel disease requires histopathologic confirmation, which can be obtained by endoscopic biopsies or via a surgical exploratory.

Treatment

The treatment of each individual renal disease is different, and the reader is referred to the primary reference for details.

HELICOBACTER SPP.*

Classical signs

- Anorexia.
- Vomiting.
- Usually associated with chronic vomiting, but may have acute onset of signs.

See main reference on page 682 for details

Clinical signs

The predominant clinical sign continues to be **chronic, intermittent vomiting**.

Diagnosis

The disease mimics so many other causes of vomiting that a thorough diagnostic evaluation is required to make the diagnosis.

Typically, the **hemogram and serum chemistry profile is completely normal,** especially since the vomiting episodes are not frequent enough to cause electrolyte imbalances or dehydration.

The most useful diagnostic test is **endoscopic examination and biopsy. The organisms will be visualized best via histopathologic examination,** but cytology or culture of the gastric contents has also yielded the organisms in some cases. However, **culture of *Helicobacter pylori* requires special media and culture conditions** to be successful, but is the best means of finding this pathogenic species.

Clo-tests, which are enzymatic tests of the presence of urease used in humans to screen for *Helicobacter* spp. organisms in gastric content, have not been adequately evaluated in cats; however, because cats have some *Helicobacter* spp. as normal flora, this test is not likely to be helpful.

PLANT INGESTION/TOXICITY*

Classical signs

- Most plants do not cause severe toxicity, but may cause drooling, vomiting or diarrhea due to their irritant effects on mucous membranes.
- Severe toxicity may result in hepatic or renal failure, with vomiting, diarrhea, depression, anorexia occurring secondary to these effects.

Pathogenesis

Most plants do not cause severe toxicity, but may cause **drooling, vomiting or diarrhea** due to their irritant effects on mucous membranes.

Severe toxicity may result in hepatic or renal failure, with vomiting, diarrhea, depression, anorexia occurring secondary to these effects.

Plants associated with an **acute onset of vomiting following ingestion** include mistletoe, azalea, black nightshade, Christmas cherry, Christmas rose, daffodil, glory lily, jessamines, lantana, larkspur, poinsettia, rhododendron, tulip, wild rosemary, youpon holly (to name a few).

The **specific cause of vomiting or other signs of toxicity is very plant-dependent** and quite variable in severity.

Clinical signs

Vomiting is the most common sign following ingestion of plant material, whether or not it is poisonous/toxic to the gastrointestinal tract or not. Other signs may include **anorexia, drooling, dysphagia or diarrhea.**

Diagnosis

History of exposure or ingestion is essential in many cases, because there is so much variability in presentation.

Plants that cause vomiting due to **irritation or direct GI upset**: *Philodendron* (sweetheart vine), *Diffenbachia* (dumb cane), *Euphorbia* (poinsettia), *Caladium* (elephants ear), *Ricinus* (castor bean), *Robinia* (false acacia) and *Solanum* (potato, Christmas cherry) spp. to name a few of the more common plants.

Plants that cause vomiting secondary to **nephrotoxicity**: *Lilium* (lily), *Rheum* (rhubarb) and *oxalis* spp.

Differential diagnosis

Acute onset of vomiting in an otherwise healthy cat: consider dietary indiscretion, foreign body or ingestion of other toxins.

Cats ingesting plants that are **nephrotoxic** will have signs that are indistinguishable from other causes of vomiting due to systemic metabolic, infectious or inflammatory diseases.

Treatment

In most cases, the vomiting is **self-limiting** after the offending plant is removed from the GI tract.

Gastric protectants or histamine-2 antagonists may be indicated if severe gastritis develops.

Gastric lavage may be helpful if large amounts of irritant plants are consumed and will reduce further absorption of more toxic metabolites from other plants.

Other treatments that may be necessary **include fluid therapy, antiemetics and offering food that is bland or highly digestible.**

Once signs of nephrotoxicity are observed following lily plant ingestion, progression to anuric renal failure and death is unavoidable. Supportive care with fluid therapy may slow the onset of signs, but there is no effective treatment.

MOTILITY DISTURBANCES* (GASTROESOPHAGEAL REFLUX, ILEUS)

Classical signs

- Vomiting or regurgitation (esophagitis).
- Abdominal distention or abdominal pain due to accumulation of gas in the bowel.
- Anorexia.

See main reference on page 615 for details.

Clinical signs

Vomiting or regurgitation (due to esophagitis) or diarrhea may all be observed, depending on the segment of bowel affected.

Anorexia and dysphagia are more common with esophagitis.

Mild abdominal distention or abdominal pain due to accumulation of gas in the bowel can occur.

Epigastric pain and hypersalivation are due to esophagitis.

Diagnosis

Ileus may be suspected by **palpation of flaccid, dilated loops of bowel. Gut sounds are decreased or absent**.

Survey abdominal radiographs may show dilated, gas- and fluid-filled loops of bowel.

Adynamic ileus can be confirmed by a contrast study using barium-impregnated polyethylene spheres (BIPS), scinitigraphy or fluoroscopy to assess motility. Contrast radiographs or endoscopy will be required to identify esophagitis.

Esophagitis may be clinically silent but if regurgitation, hypersalivation and anorexia are present should be considered.

SALMONELLOSIS*

Classical signs

- Most cats have asymptomatic infections.
- In young kittens watery or hemorrhagic diarrhea is the most common sign.
- Vomiting, lethargy and anorexia may also occur, but are uncommon and usually associated with septicemia.

See main reference on page 719 for details (The Cat With Signs of Acute Small Bowel Diarrhea).

Clinical signs

Cats may develop one of **three possible clinical syndromes**: (1) asymptomatic carrier state, (2) gastroenteritis, or (3) fulminant septicemia/bacteremia.

Gastroenteritis is typically characterized by diarrhea that may be watery, mucoid, bloody or all three. Typically, **fever, depression and anorexia are first observed**, followed by vomiting, abdominal pain and diarrhea.

Cats with septicemia or bacteremia may not have any GI signs, and instead are febrile, lethargic, anorectic and may show signs of septic shock (e.g. hypovolemia, weakness, poor capillary refill time, acute renal failure).

The disease may persist for 3–4 weeks in severely ill cats, and shedding may occur for up to 6 weeks.

Diagnosis

History and physical examination will be important suggestive factors but there are numerous causes of acute diarrhea in young cats.

Routine hematology and serum biochemistry profiles are typically unremarkable in the early phases, but will show evidence of dehydration, electrolyte imbalance and leukocyte abnormalities in the later stages. **Cats with bacteremia/septicemia will have a left shift** (greater than 500 band neutrophils found on hemogram) or **degenerative neutropenia** (neutropenia in the presence of toxic changes and without evidence of band cells) and may have hepatic or renal compromise as a result of the endotoxemia.

Definitive diagnosis depends on the isolation of *Salmonella* **spp.** from properly cultured fecal samples or from blood cultures in cats with bacteremia.

ETHYLENE GLYCOL*

Classical signs

- Vomiting occurs after ingestion due to the direct toxicity of ethylene glycol to the GI tract.
- 24–36 h later, lethargy, vomiting, anorexia and depression occur secondary to renal failure.

Pathogenesis

Automobile antifreeze is the most common source of this toxin for small animal poisoning.

Other sources of ethylene glycol include household cleaning products, lacquers and cosmetics.

Ethylene glycol itself is not nephrotoxic, but is an alcohol that results in **signs of stupor, vomiting and weakness**. It is the **metabolism of ethylene glycol to glycoaldehyde, glyoxylic acid, glycolate and oxalic acid that result in the development of acute, oliguric to anuric renal failure** and ultimately death due to direct toxic effects on the nephron.

Renal injury is also a result of deposition of calcium oxalate crystals in the tubular lumen that lead to tubular obstruction and back leak, however, this is less a cause of death than the other mechanisms.

Clinical signs

Initial signs occur within the first few hours following ingestion and include **vomiting, hypersalivation, ataxia and depression**, which are associated with alcohol intoxication.

If the cat is not treated at this stage, metabolism of the ethylene glycol leads to formation of severe metabolic acidosis, oxalate crystalluria and renal shutdown (acute anuric renal failure) within 24–48 hours.

Signs of ethylene glycol poisoning at this stage mimic those of all causes of acute, anuric renal failure and include vomiting, depression to obtundation, severe dehydration and hypovolemia due to vomiting, and lack of urine production once dehydration is corrected.

In the end stage of anuric renal failure, cats often become over-hydrated, with the development of pulmonary edema, peripheral edema and ascites.

Once the development of anuric renal failure has begun, the prognosis is grave, and only dialysis and renal transplantation will save the cat.

Diagnosis

The diagnosis is often made based upon a **history of known or suspected exposure** to/ingestion of ethylene glycol (antifreeze). In cats, amounts of less than a teaspoon can be potentially fatal.

When there is no known exposure to ethylene glycol and the animal is presented in acute renal failure, an index of suspicion is required to make the diagnosis. **Presence of oxalate or hippurate crystals** in the urine of a cat in acute renal failure is highly suggestive of ethylene glycol ingestion.

Definitive diagnosis can be made by **toxicologic analysis of serum** for presence of metabolites of ethylene glycol in the blood or by using a commercially available blood test kit for use in clinical practice settings that detects the presence of ethylene glycol in blood. This test is most effective when used within 12–24 hours of ingestion.

Cats with ethylene glycol toxicity will have markedly increased serum osmolality, a profound metabolic acidosis (with increased anion gap) and calcium oxalate crystalluria to support the diagnosis.

Differential diagnosis

Exposure to **poisonous plants**, especially the lily family which cause acute renal failure.

Ketoacidotic diabetes mellitus, acute renal failure due to infectious or other causes, hepatic disease/failure are important extra-intestinal differentials.

In older cats, neoplasia should be considered.

Intussusception or foreign body obstruction should be considered **in young cats.**

Treatment

Immediately **evacuate the stomach** by inducing emesis to prevent further absorption of the toxin.

If the ingestion just occurred, administer activated charcoal to reduce additional absorption of the ingested material from the GI tract. However, absorption of ethylene glycol is within minutes, so once clinical signs are present, this is not indicated.

If the cat has signs of acute toxicity and exposure is > 2–3 hours prior to presentation, administration of 20% ethanol (5 ml/kg IV q 4 h) is recommended to compete with the alcohol dehydrogenase and slow metabolism of the ethylene glycol to its nephrotoxic metabolites.

In acute toxicity, give 4-methypyrazole (4-MP), an ethylene glycol antagonist, which, if administered within 4 hours of ingestion, will prevent metabolism of the drug to its toxic metabolites. Between 4–12 hours after ingestion, 4-MP will be less effective, but still may help reduce the severity. After 12 hours, the prognosis is grave. In general, 4-MP is less effective in cats than in dogs.

Management of acute renal failure is essential, and includes correction of fluid deficits using isotonic fluids, correction of electrolyte disturbances and correction of metabolic acidosis with cautious use of sodium bicarbonate therapy.

Close assessment of urine output is essential to prevent fluid overload. An indwelling urinary catheter should be placed to measure output, and furosemide and mannitol should be administered to promote increased diuresis and urine flow.

In cats with oliguric or anuric renal failure, hemodialysis may ultimately be required to manage the renal failure.

Prognosis

The prognosis is **guarded** if the intoxication is immediately discovered, the material removed from the GI tract and preventative measures instituted to control metabolism of the poison.

In cats **that are presented greater than 4–6 hours after ingestion** the prognosis is **very guarded to poor**, and in cats already **showing signs of anuric renal failure the prognosis is grave.**

FELINE PANLEUKOPENIA VIRUS*

> ### Classical signs
>
> - Anorexia, vomiting, depression, weakness and dehydration are commonly observed signs.
> - Disease is most severe in kittens, and has a high mortality rate.
> - Diarrhea is less frequent and occurs later in the course.

Pathogenesis

The disease is caused by a **feline parvovirus which only infects rapidly replicating cells** (e.g. intestinal epithelium, granulocytes, and if infected early in life, granular cells of the cerebellum and developing retina).

In **rapidly dividing cells**, the virus causes cell cytolysis thus destroying the affected cell populations.

- In the **bone marrow**, cells of the white cell series are affected, and lymphoid tissue throughout the body undergoes necrosis, resulting in a rapid and severe decrease in white cell numbers that eventually results in **panleukopenia.**
- In the **GI tract**, the **crypt cells are destroyed** resulting ultimately in the destruction of the intestinal epithelium. This leads to **malabsorption, vomiting and diarrhea, and secondary bacteremia.** The colon is less affected because of the slower mitotic rate of colonocytes.

If the **queen is infected while the kittens are in utero, the kittens will be stillborn, aborted, or fetal death will result in resorption**, depending upon the stage of the pregnancy. **Young kittens infected during the neonatal period (< 10 days after birth) will have cerebellar hypoplasia (ataxia, hypermetria) and retinal dysplasia (blindness).**

In **unvaccinated feline populations**, the disease is associated with **very high morbidity and mortality**, and is highly infectious. However, **vaccination is extremely effective in preventing the disease**, and

cats properly vaccinated against panleukopenia virus are probably immune for life.

Clinical signs

Anorexia, depression and extreme lethargy are very common clinical signs initially. These are followed by **vomiting, diarrhea and dehyration** that can be quite severe. Typically, persistent vomiting, which may be bile-stained, occurs as an early sign in most cats, and can be associated with acute dehydration.

Diarrhea occurs later in the course of the disease and is not present in all cats.

In the **acute form**, most kittens are **febrile**, and may become **septicemic**. In the late stages of the disease, the cat will almost always become hypothermic.

Kittens affected with **cerebellar hypoplasia** will be **ataxic, hypermetric, dysmetric, incoordinated and have a base-wide stance.** These kittens will be otherwise normal both neurologically and physically at birth, and clinical signs will not be apparent until 3–4 weeks post-partum when they begin to walk.

Most affected animals will be kittens that have come from an unvaccinated queen or from a premise with many unvaccinated cats in close proximity. The highest morbidity and mortality is in kittens 3–5 months of age.

Sudden death may be observed in kittens anywhere from 4 weeks to 12 months of age.

Diagnosis

The **history, signalment and physical examination findings** are all suggestive of the disease.

However, in its milder forms, the disease can be difficult to differentiate from many gastrointestinal diseases, including salmonellosis.

The **most consistent hematologic abnormality is panleukopenia**, with leukocyte counts typically ranging between 500–3000 cells/μl. The **nadir in the white cell count occurs 4–6 days after infection**. Because the disease is so acute, serum biochemistry values are usually within normal limits. There is a correlation between the degree of leukopenia and severity of the illness.

There is no licensed ELISA test kit for the feline parvovirus, however, the **canine test kit will detect the**

feline parvovirus in feces as well. The test is very sensitive and specific (> 90%) for parvoviruses. **False positives may occur following vaccination with modified live virus vaccines, and false negatives may occur early in the course of disease** (days 1–3 post-infection) before viral shedding is actively occurring.

Serologic testing is still an important diagnostic test for feline panleukopenia, but it **requires paired samples (acute and convalescent) that show a rise in titer to be definitive**, and therefore is the most useful in cattery situations to help plan preventative management programs.

Other tests that can be performed include virus isolation on feces or tissues and electron microscopy for detection of virus particles in the feces.

Differential diagnosis

In its severe form, few diseases mimic feline panleukopenia. However, milder clinical forms of the disease must be differentiated from all other infectious causes of gastrointestinal disease.

In particular, **feline leukemia virus** can present in some cats with a **panleukopenia-like syndrome**. The diagnosis is made when the cat is tested for feline leukemia virus and found to be positive. Most FeLV cats are also anemic, which helps in differentiation of the two viruses.

Salmonella infections in cats are **usually subclinical**, but when they are severe, can present with a fulminant gastroenteritis. Non-regenerative hypochromic anemia, lymphopenia, thrombocytopenia, neutropenia with a left shift, and toxic leukocytes are found in cats with systemic disease and endotoxemia. A mature neutrophilic leukocytosis is more characteristic of chronic or localized disease.

Rarely, cats with **griseofulvin toxicity** develop a severe leukopenia and GI signs that resemble panleukopenia. In contrast to the viral disease, the leukopenia caused by griseofulvin toxicity is persistent. Griseofulvin toxicity is more likely to occur in FIV-positive cats.

Treatment

Treatment is supportive, but must be **aggressively administered** if it is to be successful. The key is maintenance of **fluid and electrolyte balance and prevention of secondary bacterial infection** until the body is able to neutralize the virus with antibody.

Aggressive fluid therapy is the cornerstone of treatment, to correct the dehydration that occurs from vomiting. Attention to the need for **potassium supplementation**, phophorus, and other electrolytes, such as magnesium, sodium and chloride are essential.

In cats that are unable to eat for 3–5 days, enteral nutrition via a feeding tube or total parenteral nutrition may be a necessary component of the treatment plan. Once the vomiting is controlled, oral alimentation (via nasoesophageal, esophageal or gastrostomy tubes) can be instituted. It is important to **begin nutritional support as soon as possible**, as the GI tract requires this protein to repair the injured epithelium. In addition, further immunosuppression will occur if protein malnutrition occurs in addition to the leukopenia resulting from the viral attack.

Vomiting should be controlled with **antiemetic therapy**. Either **metoclopramide** (0.1–0.2 mg/kg IV q 8 h) or chlorpromazine (0.01–0.025 mg/kg IV) are effective, but it is important when using any phenothiazine antiemetics that you ensure adequate volume expansion so that hypotension is avoided. If gastritis is suspected histamine-2 blockers should also be considered.

Antibiotic therapy is very important in these kittens, as they are at great risk of development of systemic septicemia due to the loss of intestinal epithelium and leukopenia that ensues as a result of the viral infection. **Four-quadrant therapy** (Gram positive, Gram negative, anaerobes and aerobes) is important. Combination therapy using ampicillin (10–20 mg/kg q 8 h)/amoxicillin (5–10 mg/kg q 12 h) and either amikacin (6–8 mg/kg q 24 h) or enrofloxacin (2.5 mg/kg q 12 h) are good choices.

Prognosis

Guarded. The older the kitten is when it is infected, the more likely it is to survive the disease. However, in young kittens, mortality will be very high, despite aggressive therapy.

The more severe the leukopenia, the poorer the prognosis, with white cell counts below 500 cells/μl having a grave prognosis.

Kittens with mild cerebellar hypoplasia may make suitable pets, as the condition is not progressive.

Prevention

Vaccination is the key to prevention. Current vaccines are very effective in preventing the disease and have been responsible for reducing the incidence of the disease in cats to a very low level. Further, once a cat has been appropriately vaccinated for this disease, the immunity is likely to be life-long.

Maternal antibodies derived from the queen will be protective, but by 12 weeks of age are waning. Kittens should be vaccinated every 2–3 weeks from 6–7 weeks of age until they are 12 weeks of age.

The virus is extremely hardy, and will persist in the environment for years, unless it is killed by appropriate disinfectants (clorox). Before presenting any new cats to a household that has had a cat with panleukopenia in it, the new cat should be vaccinated appropriately (kittens > 12 weeks should have had two vaccinations 2–3 weeks apart).

In catteries where there are panleukopenia outbreaks, control is achieved by vaccination, isolation of susceptible cats from infected cats, and good hygiene measures to prevent further spread.

HYPERCALCEMIA (HYPERCALCEMIA OF MALIGNANCY, HYPERPARATHYROIDISM/ CHOLECALCIFEROL POISONING, IDIOPATHIC)

Classical signs

- Anorexia, vomiting, lethargy or muscle weakness and weight loss may be the only outward signs.
- Other signs include polyuria/polydipsia, muscle wasting and shivering/tremors.

See main references on page 245 (The Cat With Polyuria and Polydipsia for details).

Clinical signs

Cholecalciferol poisoning (e.g. Rampage, Quintox) **results in vomiting, lethargy and depression within 3 hours of ingestion**. Within 2–3 days of ingestion, diarrhea and acute renal failure occur.

Hypercalcemia occurs in a minority of cats with chronic renal failure. Acute decompensation of renal function may lead to acute onset of vomiting.

Hypercalcemia of malignancy, hypercalcemia secondary to hyperparathyroidism and idiopathic hypocalcemia cause **vague clinical signs of greater than 1 week duration**. These signs include anorexia, vomiting, lethargy or muscle weakness and weight loss as the most common signs observed.

Idiopathic hypercalcemia has been reported in cats where acidifying diets were implicated. Idiopathic hypercalcemia was associated with chronic vomiting, weight loss, dysuria, inappropriate urination, anoxeria, pollakiuria and lethargy.

Diagnosis

Primary hyperparathyroidism (HPT) is much rarer in cats than hypercalcemia of malignancy and hypercalcemia of malignancy is rare in cats compared to dogs.

A history of potential exposure to rodenticides containing cholecalciferol is valuable if hypercalcemia is associated with acute vomiting and depression.

The most common neoplasms associated with hypercalcemia are hematopoietic (lymphoma, multiple myeloma), solid tumors with bony metastasis, e.g. squamous cell carcinoma, and apocrine cell adenocarcinoma of the anal sac, which is rare in cats.

Hematologic abnormalities in HPT and cholecalciferol poisoning are **uncommon,** but non-regenerative anemia is commonly associated with chronic renal failure.

The **serum chemistry abnormalities include hypercalcemia** (serum total and ionized), **hyperphosphatemia (cholecalciferol), renal failure and elevated liver enzyme activities** (hypercalcemia of malignancy, cholecalciferol).

Phosphorus is elevated in renal failure and cholecalciferol toxicity but normal or decreased for all other causes of hypercalcemia.

Azotemia is also common with hypercalcemia due to the development of nephrocalcinosis or other renal damage.

Imaging studies are very important in **ruling out occult neoplastic disease** as the source of the hypercalcemia.

Serum PTH is elevated with HPT and chronic renal failure, but low with neoplastic diseases, idiopathic hypercalcaemia and cholecalciferol toxicosis.

PTH-related protein (PTHrP) is decreased with HPT and cholecalciferol toxicity, but increased with neoplasia and chronic renal failure. PTHrP is usually undetectable in idiopathic hypercalcemia.

Ionized calcium levels may be helpful in ruling out renal failure as a cause of hypercalcemia (e.g. ionized calcium is low in renal failure and elevated in all other hypercalcemic diseases).

Idiopathic hypercalcemia is associated with an increased serum total calcium or serum ionized calcium concentration, or both. Serum phosphorus, albumin and 25-hydroxycholecalciferol (vitamin D3) concentrations are normal in cats with idiopathic hypercalcaemia.

PHYSALOPTERA

Classical signs

- Vomiting.
- Worms may be present in vomitus.

Pathogenesis

Physaloptera spp. are spirurid worms that **are transmitted to cats by ingestion of infective larvae present in coprophagous beetles, bugs or in transport hosts such as birds, rodents or frogs**. They are **most prevalent in the southern United States**, where conditions are favorable for the intermediate/transport hosts of these parasites to persist.

Physaloptera spp. **are small (2.5–5.0 cm)** worms with cuticular collars and spiraled tails that **cause acute gastritis even when they are present in very small numbers**.

Clinical signs

Vomiting is typically the only clinical sign, and worms may be present in vomitus. In most cases, **cats are otherwise completely healthy,** vomiting is inter-mittent, and rarely associated with severe bouts of vomiting, dehydration or illness.

Diagnosis

Hematology and serum biochemistry profile are within normal limits.

Fecal examination may expose the ovoid to ellipsoidal, thick-shelled, **larvated eggs** ($30–40 \times 20$ μm), but **this is not a reliable means of making the diagnosis.**

Radiographs will be unremarkable, but **endoscopic examination will allow visualization of the worms.**

Oftentimes, the diagnosis, if not confirmed by direct visualization of worms in stomach via endoscopy, is made by **response to appropriate treatment**.

Differential diagnosis

Other infections with spirurid worms, e.g. *Spiroceri*, will produce similar eggs and occasionally cause vomiting.

Gastritis, gastric trichobezoars and dietary indiscretion or food intolerance should all be considered, because the signs are similar (mild, intermittent).

Treatment

Anthelmintics such as **fenbendazole** (25–50 mg/kg PO q 24 h for 3–5 days) or **pyrantel** which are effective in the stomach will be curative.

Cats that are on **monthly heartworm preventative-containing** ivermectin plus pyrantel (Heartguard) will have effective control of any infection or re-infection. It is not known whether selemectin or milbemycin are effective (at the heartworm-preventative dose) in preventing or treating physaloptera.

Consider **histamine-2 blockers** (e.g. ranitidine or famotidine) or **sucralfate to reduce gastritis,** if the signs are severe.

Prognosis

Good. **Response to treatment is excellent** and because there is no migration of parasites beyond the stomach wall, re-treatment is unnecessary unless the cat is re-infected.

Prevention

Prevent ingestion of the carrier beetles, bugs or transport hosts (birds, rodents).

ASCARIDS

Classical signs

- Abdominal distention, colicky abdominal pain.
- Poor body condition, not nursing or eating.
- Diarrhea or abnormal feces.

See main reference on page 717 for details (The Cat With Signs of Acute Small Bowel Diarrhea).

Clinical signs

The most common signs of roundworm infection in kittens are **abdominal distention, colicky abdominal pain, poor body condition/hair coat and diarrhea or soft feces.**

Vomiting worms or vomiting due to masses of worms obstructing passage of ingesta is **very uncommon** in cats (compared to dogs), as is the clinical sign of coughing due to larval migration.

Adult cats develop innate immunity and thus, unless they are immunocompromised, rarely have clinical signs of intestinal roundworm infection.

Diagnosis

Fecal flotation will reveal spherical egg (*Toxocara cati*) with pitted outer shell membrane containing a single zygote, and approximately 75 μm in size. Toxascaris is also an ovoid egg of similar size but has a smooth shell.

Some cats may have a **peripheral eosinophilia,** suggestive of parasite infestation, but **this is not a consistent finding** nor one that is specific for roundworm infection.

Treatment

Anthelmintics such as **pyrantel** (5–10 mg/kg PO once) or **fenbendazole** (25–50 mg/kg PO q 24 h for 3 days)

must be given to all cats/kittens that are housed together.

Pyrantel is not absorbed from the GI tract to any appreciable amount and thus is **the safest to use in kittens under 4–6 weeks of age.**

Repeat treatment in 3–4 weeks to effectively kill prepatent stages.

Reinfection is prevented by **good sanitation.**

Roundworms have **zoonotic potential** (visceral or ocular larval migrans), although this is not as great a problem as the canine roundworm.

OLLULANUS TRICUSPIS

Classical signs

- Vomiting.

Pathogenesis

Ollulanus tricuspis is a nematode parasite infecting the **gastric glands of cats** resulting in **acute gastritis and vomiting.** The life cycle of the parasite is direct.

The life cycle is completed in the cat with **infection of other cats occurring via ingestion of parasite-containing vomitus.**

The parasite is **found worldwide**, but there have only been sporadic reports of infection in the United States. **Free-roaming and colony cats are more likely to be exposed and infected than are household cats.**

Clinical signs

Vomiting is the most common clinical sign, and occasionally the worms may be found in the vomitus.

Anorexia and weight loss may be observed in severely parasitized cats.

Infection occurs **primarily in adult cats in colonies or high-density environments** (catteries, shelters or homes with many cats living together) that have the opportunity for close intimate contact necessary for parasite transmission.

Diagnosis

Detection of the parasites can be difficult because **no ova are released** and the **larvae and adults are digested during normal passage through the gastrointestinal tract. Gastric lavage, examination of vomitus or endoscopic examination** are the recommended procedures for diagnosis of these parasites.

Differential diagnosis

The major differentials are *Physaloptera* spp. and larval forms of *Aelurostrongylus* spp. (the lung worm), which may be coughed up and swallowed.

Treatment and prognosis.

Little is reported about treatment regimes for *Ollulanus* spp. but it is likely that **fenbendazole (25–50 mg/kg PO q 24 h for 3–5 days)** would be effective against these nematodes.

Prevention

Keeping cats from contacting/ingesting infected vomitus by housing cats indoors, or by isolating cats that are known to be infected, is an effective means of prevention.

PERITONITIS

> **Classical signs**
>
> - Abdominal pain, lethargy, ascites, anorexia and fever are common signs.
> - Vomiting or diarrhea are less frequent, but often observed in more severe cases.

See main reference on page 467 for details.

Clinical signs

Abdominal discomfort/pain, lethargy and anorexia are common signs and must be differentiated from FIP or other causes of abdominal effusion.

This is a **rare clinical problem in cats,** and occurs **most often secondary to intestinal perforation** (e.g. string foreign body).

Vomiting or diarrhea are not common signs, but when they occur they are often associated with severe disease.

Fever and abdominal distention/effusion may also be present.

Diagnosis

Abdominal radiographs (plain, contrast) and ultrasonography will suggest peritonitis and may pinpoint location or cause (ruptured gallbladder, pancreatitis, bowel rupture). **Radiographic findings** consistent with peritonitis **include loss of abdominal detail** that is often focal, but may include the entire abdomen. **Ultrasound can readily detect any fluid accumulation in the peritoneal space** that is occurring as a result of the inflammatory process.

Definitive diagnosis confirming the presence of peritonitis can be obtained by **abdominocentesis or diagnostic peritoneal lavage and cytologic/bacteriologic examination of fluid.**

Cytology of periotoneal fluids consistent with peritonitis is characterized by **increased cellularity** (primarily neutrophils, with or without intracellular bacteria if the process is septic), and protein and is often described as an exudate. **The key to differentiating peritonitis from FIP or neoplastic causes of abdominal effusion is examination of cell types,** as FIP is typically pyogranulomatous, but with a low to moderate cell count, and neoplastic infiltrates will most commonly be lymphocytes or carcinomatous.

Hematology is non-specific, and usually shows **an inflammatory leukogram**, stress leukogram or sequestration of neutrophils (neutropenia).

SEPTICEMIA/BACTEREMIA/ENDOTOXIC SHOCK

> **Classical signs**
>
> - Generalized depression, fever or hypothermia.
> - Tachycardia/tachypnea and signs of shock.
> - Vomiting is not consistently present but does occur.

Clinical signs

This is a **rare clinical problem in cats**.

Cats with septicemia are severely depressed, may be febrile or hypothermic (although this is often a poor prognostic sign), and will have **systemic signs of shock** (tachycardia, tachypnea, decreased capillary refill).

Other signs, especially in cats with septic shock, may include **vomiting or bloody diarrhea and anorexia.**

There is **no particular age, breed or sex predilection to development of septicemia or endotoxemia**, but cats with severe infections, immunocompromise (e.g. FeLV or FIV+) or stress may be prediposed.

Diagnosis

Hemogram may reveal neutrophilia progressing to neutropenia and thrombocytopenia. There may be hyperglycemia early, progressing to hypoglycemia later. Hyperkalemia, elevated liver enzymes and azotemia are common, and bacteriuria may be present.

Blood culture is indicated in patients with suspected bacteremia to confirm the infection exists. Blood cultures should be obtained in a sterile manner from multiple venipuncture sites (if possible), and, ideally, samples should be obtained over several hours (every 2–4 hours collect a new sample) to maximize the opportunity to obtain a positive sample. **Urine culture** is also helpful in cases with renal seeding of the infection.

Imaging studies are important in further evaluating the extent of illness and may help identify a focus of infection (radiographs of chest, abdominal ultrasound).

VESTIBULAR DISEASE

Classical signs

- Head tilt, circling, falling.
- Infrequent vomiting and anorexia may occur.

See main reference on page 933 for details.

Clinical signs

Occasionally cats with an acute onset of vestibular disease vomit, but signs of **head tilt** (away from the affected side with peripheral vestibular disease and towards the affected side with central vestibular disease), circling, falling, ataxia, and horizontal (more typical for peripheral disease) or rotary (more typical of central disease) **nystagmus** are much more prominent than GI signs.

Vomiting or anorexia occur due to disequilibrium effects, **but are not common clinical signs of cats with vestibular disease.** Vomiting is usually only seen in the first 1–2 days after onset and is infrequent (1–2 single episodes in the first 48 hours).

Vomiting is more common with peripheral vestibular disease or idiopathic vestibular syndrome, and is rarely associated with central vestibular disease.

Altered consciousness, postural deficits or other cranial nerve deficits are not typically seen.

Diagnosis

History and physical examination findings are highly suggestive of vestibular disease.

Evaluation of cats with vestibular disease should include a **minimum data base** (hematology, serum chemistry profile and urinalysis), otoscopic examination, radiographs of the tympanic bulla. **CT of the bulla and area of the 8th nerve are also important diagnostic tests.**

Major causes of vestibular signs include: idiopathic vestibular syndrome (diagnosis of exclusion), otitis media/interna (diagnosis by myingotomy, culture, radiographs or CT), middle ear polyps (CT), trauma, neoplasia (radiographs or CT), endocrine diseases causing neuropathies (diabetes mellitus and hyperadrenocorticism) and toxic insults (aminoglycoside antibiotics, topical chlorhexidine or iodophor compounds).

A minor cause of vomiting is **motion sickness** from the vestibular dysfunction during car rides.

PHARMACOLOGIC TOXICITY (NON-STEROIDAL ANTI-INFLAMMATORY DRUG (NSAID) TOXICITY)

Classical signs

- Anorexia.
- Vomiting, with or without hematemesis.
- Abdominal pain.
- Diarrhea, with or without melena.

Pathogenesis

Cats are much more sensitive to the effects of NSAIDs because they have a reduced capacity to metabolize these drugs in their liver (**poor glucuronyl transferase activity**).

The adverse consequences of NSAID ingestion on the gastrointestinal tract are due to multifactorial effects on the tissue, including direct toxicity to the epithelium, increased back diffusion of acid, decreased synthesis of prostaglandins, mucus and bicarbonate, decreased mucosal blood flow and microvascular injury.

Acetaminophen (paracetamol), which is an analgesic, antipyretic drug sometimes included in the NSAID group, does not have the same toxic effects on the gastrointestinal tract. In fact, the **toxicity of acetaminophen in cats is very high**, but the toxic effect is **due to the oxidant effects on red cells causing methemoglobinemia, hemolysis, Heinz body anemia and hepatotoxicity.**

Clinical signs

Cats that have **ingested aspirin, ibuprofen or related NSAIDs** are likely to show **acute signs of GI upset** which may include anorexia, vomiting (with or without hematemesis), or abdominal pain.

Chronic ingestion of these drugs may result in **inappetence, vomiting or diarrhea** (with or without melena).

Acute overdoses of NSAIDs, especially ibuprofen, naproxen, etc., may result in acute oliguric or anuric renal failure.

Cats that have ingested **acetaminophen** (paracetamol) will have **hypersalivation and vomiting early**, followed by development of **cyanosis** (methemoglobinemia) and **facial pruritus** within a few hours. Later, untreated cats may develop **edema of the face and paws**, and will ultimately develop liver failure if they survive the initial toxicity.

Diagnosis

History of ingestion and appropriate clinical signs are usually enough to support NSAID-induced gastritis or ulceration as the cause of the GI signs.

Typically, the **hematology and serum chemistry profile will be normal with NSAIDs other than acetaminophen,** unless the cat has severe erosions or ulcers that have been bleeding. In those cases, **anemia of blood loss** will be present, and in some cases can be quite dramatic.

Cats may present in **acute, oliguric or anuric renal failure,** and in these cats, severe azotemia, hyperphosphatemia, hyperkalemia and severe metabolic acidosis may be present.

Confirmation of gastritis, gastric erosions or ulcers requires imaging studies. The most definitive means of diagnosis is via **endoscopy** whereby through both visualization and histopathology the diagnosis can be confirmed. **Severe ulcers** can also be visualized on **contrast radiographs or via ultrasound.**

Differential diagnosis

Other differentials to consider are acute pancreatitis, mechanical obstructions, infectious agents such as *Helicobacter* that cause acute gastritis and acute gastritis/gastric disease of other causes.

Treatment

Stop further ingestion of NSAIDs, and **remove as much of the drug from the GI tract as possible** (lavage, induce vomiting, administer activated charcoal). This is especially important if the ingestion was an accidental overdose and has occurred within the past 2–4 hours, although gastric lavage is most useful if performed within 1 hour of ingestion.

In cases where the signs of acute gastritis or gastric ulceration are associated with **blood loss, a transfusion may be necessary.** This is especially true if perforation has occurred and immediate surgical intervention is necessary.

Treatment is non-specific, as with any gastritis or ulcer patient: administer **histamine-2 blockers** (ranitidine or famotidine), **mucosal cytoprotectants** (sucralfate), and antiemetics (metoclopramide) if indicated. If the cat is dehydrated from the vomiting episodes, **fluid therapy** and possibly potassium supplementation will also be indicated.

Prognosis

Good with appropriate therapy and aggressive management unless there is gastric or duodenal perforation, or acute renal failure has developed before the cat presents to the hospital.

Prevention

NSAIDs should be used cautiously in cats and cats that receive these drugs require frequent careful evaluation.

Accidental exposure to medications not intended for cats should be prevented.

Misoprostil (a prostaglandin agonist) has not been evaluated in cats as a gastric protectant.

TOXICITY (CHEMOTHERAPY DRUG-INDUCED VOMITING)

Classical signs

- Anorexia.
- Vomiting, with or without hematemesis.
- Abdominal pain.
- Diarrhea, with or without melena.

Pathogenesis

Nausea and vomiting are **frequent complications of cancer chemotherapy** drugs. There are many different chemotherapeutic agents and they all vary in their effects; however, **cisplatin, doxorubicin, vincristine and methotrexate commonly cause gastrointestinal side effects.**

The cause of the vomiting may be due to **direct stimulation of the CRTZ or toxicity to the gastrointestinal tract** by inhibiting the rapidly dividing stem cells that populate the GI epithelium. **Vincristine** does not have direct cellular toxicity, but may induce **ileus**, which can result in vomiting, diarrhea or both.

Clinical signs

The **most common GI signs observed with cancer chemotherapy drugs are non-specific**, and include anorexia, vomiting, with or without hematemesis, abdominal pain due to bloating from ileus, diarrhea, pyrexia due to development of secondary infections, or lethargy.

Diagnosis

A history of cancer chemotherapy and appropriate clinical signs are often sufficient to make a presumptive diagnosis. However, it is always important to bear in mind that the **vomiting could be unrelated to the drugs**, and represent an additional problem associated with the disease or a new problem that is unrelated to the disease.

Differential diagnosis

Vomiting may be due to the neoplastic disease itself.

Treatment

Vomiting associated with cancer chemotherapy can be difficult to manage in some situations. The **most effective anti-emetic drugs** for this purpose are the drugs that block the effects on the CRTZ, such as **metoclopramide**. In very severe cases, ondansetron or dolasetron are other alternatives.

In animals that have uncontrollable vomiting, the treatment regimen may have to be altered to allow the cat to have reasonable quality of life.

Prognosis

Guarded, primarily because of the presence of cancer requiring chemotherapy for treatment or control.

ANESTHETIC AGENT (XYLAZINE)

Classical signs

- Lethargy, sedation.
- Vomiting.
- Bradycardia.
- Hypotension.

Pathogenesis

Xylazine is an **alpha-2 adrenergic antagonist** sedative-anesthetic that will induce emesis in cats within minutes of administration due to direct effects on the CRTZ.

Clinical signs

Clinical signs associated with xylazine administration are either associated with the **sedation effects** (which also include some profound cardiovascular effects such as bradycardia and hypotension) or **vomiting**.

Diagnosis

Vomiting is such a common side effect following administration of xylazine that the **drug is used frequently to induce vomiting.**

Treatment

There is no need to treat vomiting associated with xylazine administration since it is self-limiting.

ENCEPHALITIS/MENINGITIS

Classical signs

- Neurologic signs predominate and depend on the location.
- Ataxia, dementia, nerve deficits, or cervical pain may be evident.
- Vomiting is often associated secondary to the systemic illness (fungal, bacterial, protozoal or viral) that is causing the disease.

See main reference on pages 829, 859 for details (The Cat With Seizures, Circling and/or Changed Behavior and The Cat With Tremor or Twitching).

Clinical signs

Neurologic signs predominate and depend on the location in the brain that is affected. If the rostral fossa is affected, seizures, circling, pacing, personality change, and decreased responsiveness are common. If the caudal fossa is affected, depression, head tilt, facial paralysis, incoordination and other brainstem abnormalities are noted.

Vomiting is uncommon, but is often associated with the presence of systemic illness (fungal, bacterial, protozoal or viral) that has also affected the CNS.

Other clinical signs, such as fever, depression, weakness, hypotension or shock may be observed with cats that are systemically ill.

Some cats with only central nervous system disease will have a normal physical examination, with only neurologic deficits or abnormalities found with careful assessment.

Diagnosis

Hematology and serum biochemistry profiles help define **systemic or infectious causes** (e.g. viral, bacterial or fungal causes).

Radiographs of cervical, thoracic and lumbar spine are used to **rule out diskospondylitis** or evidence of **neoplasia**.

Cerebrospinal spinal fluid analysis (cytology and culture) may be essential for the diagnosis, but caution should be exercised during CSF collection due to possible elevated intracranial pressure which could cause tentorial herniation.

Imaging studies (**MRI and CT scanning**) are important means of lesion localization and identification, but are not universally available.

ARSENIC POISONING

Classical signs

- Vomiting, diarrhea, anorexia and depression occur early.
- Arsenic toxicity eventually results in hepatic and renal failure (depression, anorexia, vomiting and diarrhea along with oliguria or anuria, or icterus and ascites.

Pathogenesis

Arsenic may be present in herbicides, insecticides, wood preservatives and treatments used for blood parasites (including heartworm).

Cats appear to be more commonly poisoned than dogs, possibly due to consumption of prey or insects killed by the toxin.

Toxicity may be acute, resulting in immediate and life-threatening illness, **or chronic**, and more insidious.

Clinical signs

Acute arsenic toxicity is **associated with vomiting**, diarrhea or hematochezia, abdominal pain, weakness and shock-like signs (e.g. rapid, weak pulses, prostration, subnormal body temperature and collapse).

Chronic, low-grade exposure to arsenic may be impossible to detect clinically, **as anorexia is the only consistent sign.**

Diagnosis

Historical information of exposure to heavy metals is a very important means of getting the diagnosis, however, such information is not always known.

The **hemogram and serum chemistry profile** will be **unremarkable** when the cat presents with signs of gastrointestinal disturbance.

Arsenic poisoning also causes **hepatocellular necrosis**, which will be evidenced by elevations in serum alanine aminotransferase and alkaline phosphatase enzymes. Other abnormalities may include elevations in bilirubin, bile acid values and decreases in albumin (end stage).

Nephrotoxicity associated with arsenic poisoning is also associated with isosthenuria, azotemia and eventually oliguria/anuria.

Definitive diagnosis is made by measurement of **arsenic concentrations in urine (acute), kidney, liver, vomitus or hair (chronic).**

Differential diagnosis

Other heavy metal toxicoses (e.g. lead), ingestion of caustic agents, or ingestion of poisonous plants should be considered.

Acute renal failure due to other infectious or metabolic causes may mimic arsenical nephrotoxicity.

Treatment

The first step is to **remove the source of arsenic** if possible. If the toxin has been ingested, **lavage the stomach and administer activated charcoal** to minimize further absorption of the agent from the GI tract.

Promote excretion of the toxin from the body **by starting fluid diuresis and administration of BAL** (British anti-Lewisite, dimercaptol) at a dose of 2.5–5 mg/kg in oil, IM, q 4 h for 2 days, then q 12 h up to 10

days. BAL toxicity may occur (e.g. vomiting, tremors or convulsions), which will require cessation of the drug.

DMSA (dimercepto succinic acid) is often used in children, because it is less toxic than BAL, but its effectiveness in cats has not been evaluated.

If the cat is in acute, oliguric or anuric renal failure, dialysis may be necessary.

ANTRAL PYLORIC HYPERTROPHY/STENOSIS

> **Classical signs**
>
> - Vomiting is the primary sign, and usually is observed several hours after eating.
> - Projectile vomiting will be observed if the pylorus is obstructed.

See main reference on page 694 for details of The Cat With Signs of Chronic Vomiting.

Clinical signs

Vomiting is the most common sign. In adult cats, the vomiting occurs as a chronic problem, but in kittens may occur as acute vomiting in a kitten that is just beginning to consume solid foods.

In **congenital pyloric stenosis**, the kittens begin to vomit shortly after they are started on solid food.

Acquired pyloric hypertrophy in adult cats has a more variable presentation, but is usually associated with intermittent vomiting of digested food several hours after consumption.

If the pylorus is completely obstructed the **vomiting may be projectile**.

Chronic intermittent vomiting and gastric distention may lead to **gastroesophageal reflux or esophagitis** which may be associated with regurgitation or inappetence and the resulting weight loss.

Diagnosis

History and signalment are suggestive of a gastric emptying disturbance.

Hemogram, serum chemistries and urinalysis are **typically unremarkable.**

Survey radiographs of the abdomen may be **normal or show gastric distension**. Contrast radiographs may identify **hypertrophic gastric mucosa or a narrow gastric outflow pathway ("beak sign")**.

Ultrasonography may be able to detect a thickened pyloric antrum.

Fluoroscopy or scintigraphy can be used to evaluate gastric peristalsis and emptying, but are not universally available.

Gastric endoscopy may be normal or may reveal thickened folds of mucosa, the pyloric antrum may not insufflate normally, or the pylorus may be too stenotic to allow passage of the endoscope through the orifice.

Definitive diagnosis requires an exploratory laparotomy and histopathologic examination of tissue.

DYSAUTONOMIA

Classical signs

- Vomiting or regurgitation, diarrhea, anorexia and constipation are the primary GI signs.
- Dry eyes, mucous membranes and nose may be observed.
- Bradycardia.
- Dilated pupils.

See main reference on page 792 for details (The Constipated or Straining Cat).

Clinical signs

Dysautonomia is generally seen as an **acute onset of depression, anorexia, constipation, dry external nares and mouth, reduced tear production or dry eye, bradycardia, regurgitation** (due to megaesophagus) and **dilated pupils**.

Other clinical signs that may be present, but are less common, include anal areflexia, fecal incontinence, and dysuria or urinary incontinence.

The disease occurs **primarily in Great Britain**, but sporadic cases have been reported in the United States and elsewhere.

Most affected cats are young (< 3 years old) and have no breed or sex predisposition.

Diagnosis

In general, routine **hemogram, biochemistry tests and urinalysis are within normal limits**.

Megaesophagus may be observed on routine thoracic radiographs.

Constipation or obstipation may also be detected on abdominal radiographs.

Schirmer tear tests will be abnormal (< 5 mm) in most animals.

Ophthalmic pharmacology testing may be helpful, but is not 100% reliable in detecting dysautonomia. However, in dysautonomic cats phospholine iodide will have no miotic effect, and pilocarpine will have an exaggerated miotic effect.

Low plasma or urinary catecholamine concentrations also confirms sympathetic insufficiency.

RECOMMENDED READING

August JR. Consultations in Feline Internal Medicine. WB Saunders, Philadelphia, PA. 2001, 4.
Ettinger SW, Feldman EC. Textbook of Veterinary Internal Medicine, 5th edn. WB Saunders, Philadelphia, PA. 2005.
Greene's Infectious Diseases of Dogs and Cats, 2nd edn. WB Saunders, Philadelphia, PA. 2005.
Kirk's Current Veterinary Therapy, XIII, 2000.

31. The cat with signs of chronic vomiting

Debra L Zoran

> ## KEY SIGNS
>
> - Active elimination of stomach contents through the mouth.
> - ± Preceded by nausea, pacing, and salivation.
> - Usually digested food or liquid with acidic or neutral pH.
> - ≥ 2 weeks duration.

MECHANISM?

- Vomiting occurs when the vomiting center in the medulla or when afferent impulses from the cerebral cortex, chemoreceptor trigger zone (CRTZ), or receptors in the pharynx or abdominal viscera is stimulated.
- Vomiting is an **active process** that must be distinguished from regurgitation.
- Vomitus may consist of undigested food material (if swallowed whole), partly digested or even liquid, and may be clear, yellow (bile stained) or brown (food colored).
- The **pH of vomitus is usually acidic** (pH < 4), but may be neutral (pH 7) if duodenal content is present (bile reflux).

WHERE?

- Chronic vomiting can be caused by **primary gastrointestinal diseases** or by **extra-intestinal diseases** or disorders that may have no apparent association with the GI tract.
- Vomiting is **rarely associated with primary colonic disease**.
- Extra-intestinal causes of vomiting include:
- Hepatobiliary disease.
- Pancreatic disease (e.g. pancreatitis, neoplasia).
- Renal disease causing acute or chronic renal failure.
- CNS disease (e.g. vestibular disease, encephalitis, seizure disorders, neoplasia).
- Metabolic diseases (e.g. hyperthyroidism, ketoacidotic diabetes mellitus or Addison's disease).
- Cardiomyopathy or congestive heart failure.
- Systemic illness or infection affecting the CRTZ or cortex (e.g. septicemia).

WHAT?

- Primary gastrointestinal diseases that cause chronic vomiting include:
- Parasites (e.g. *Physaloptera*).
- Infectious diseases (e.g. *Helicobacter*).
- Inflammatory diseases (e.g. IBD, gastritis or gastric ulcer disease).
- Neoplasia.

- Mechanical (e.g. antral pyloric hypertrophy/stenosis, obstruction, intussusception).
- Dietary disturbances (e.g. food intolerance or food allergy).

    The **most common causes of chronic vomiting** are: **inflammatory diseases** (e.g. food allergy or IBD), **dietary** (dietary indiscretion or food intolerance), **neoplastic** diseases and **metabolic or extra-intestinal disturbances** (e.g. renal, hepatic or pancreatic disease).

QUICK REFERENCE SUMMARY

Diseases causing signs of chronic vomiting

ANOMALY

- Dysautonomia (p 695)

This is a disorder of the autonomic nervous system resulting in GI signs due to motility disturbances in the esophagus, stomach, small and large intestine. The esophagus and colon are most dramatically affected and thus regurgitation and constipation are more prevalent than other signs. Chronic vomiting may occur or regurgitation may be reported as vomiting. Acute onset of anorexia, depression, dilated pupils without blindness, prolapsed third eyelids and bradycardia are common.

MECHANICAL

- **Foreign bodies* (p 688)**

Foreign bodies are often associated with an acute onset of vomiting, but string ingestion may cause chronic intermittent vomiting when the obstruction is incomplete or motility disturbances are intermittent.

- Antral pyloric hypertrophy/stenosis (p 694)

Acquired or congenital thickening of the pyloric tissue may result in vomiting due to motility disturbances, obstruction of outflow or both. Vomiting usually occurs several hours after eating and may be projectile. Rarely   stenosis is functional with no evidence of thickening.

- Intussusception (p 692)

Intussusception is usually associated with acute onset of severe vomiting, but sliding, intermittent or incomplete intussusception may have chronic, intermittent vomiting.

METABOLIC

- **Hyperthyroidism** (p 670)**

Intermittent vomiting occurs in conjunction with weight loss, polyphagia and polyuria. Other signs include hyperactivity, irritability, poor grooming habits and large, bulky or mucoid feces.

- **Hepatic diseases (hepatic ipidosis, cholangitis, hepatic cirrhosis, portosystemic anomalies, etc.)** (p 674)**

Vomiting is often associated with hepatic diseases or failure (of any cause). Other signs of hepatic disease include fever, weight loss, icterus, anorexia and lethargy. Cats in severe hepatic failure may show signs of hepatoencephalopathy, including drooling, apparent blindness, stupor, pica or altered behavior.

continued

continued

● Chronic renal failure* (p 680)

Intermittent vomiting is due to the effects of azotemia and hypergastrinemia on the gastric mucosa. The most common signs are polyuria, polydipsia, weight loss and decreased appetite.

● Congestive heart failure* (p 689)

Intermittent vomiting often occurs in the late stages of the disease, in addition to the signs of cardiovascular and respiratory distress or failure.

● Diabetes mellitus* (p 681)

One third of cats with diabetes have a history of vomiting. Cats with severe ketoacidosis secondary to unregulated diabetes mellitus often present with signs of anorexia, weight loss and a sudden onset of vomiting and depression. Polyuria and polydipsia are also present and may have been ongoing for several months prior to the development of the severe signs of illness.

● Hypercalcemia* (p 683)

Vomiting often occurs secondary to hypercalcemia. Other clinical signs associated with hypercalcemia include polyuria/polydipsia, anorexia and lethargy. Severe hypercalcemia may cause muscle weakness and dystrophic calcification of tissues (e.g. skin, kidneys, stomach, etc.).

● CNS diseases (encephalitis, seizure disorders, vestibular disease, neoplasia)* (p 690)

Vomiting is an uncommon sign of neurologic disease, but chronic intermittent vomiting may be associated with many different diseases of the CNS, and should be considered whenever signs of neurologic disease coexist with vomiting, especially vestibular signs (e.g. head tilt, nystagmus, rolling) or signs suggesting hepatoencephalopathy (e.g. drooling, behavior changes or apparent blindness).

● Hypoadrenocorticism (Addison's disease) (p 691)

This is an uncommon endocrine disease in cats that often presents with only vague clinical signs of lethargy, anorexia and weight loss. Vomiting and diarrhea are less common signs in cats, as are changes in the electrocardiogram associated with hyperkalemia.

NEOPLASTIC

● Intestinal adenocarcinoma** (p 677)

Anorexia, weight loss and lethargy are the most common signs, but vomiting often occurs when the tumor reaches a size that causes motility disturbances or bowel obstruction. The most common location is the distal small intestine.

● GI lymphosarcoma** (p 675)

This tumor tends to be more infiltrative and may involve large segments of small bowel, stomach or colon. Signs range from anorexia and weight loss to vomiting or diarrhea, depending on the location of the tumor.

● Intestinal mast cell tumor* (p 687)

These tumors are often solitary and primarily affect the distal small intestine, and may cause no signs, other than weight loss and anorexia, until late in the disease when vomiting develops either secondary to tumor size or presence of metastatic foci.

● Systemic neoplasia (generalized lymphoma, systemic mast cell tumor)* (p 689)

Vomiting may occur due to neoplasia involving abdominal organs resulting in direct effects, organ dysfunction or the release of vasoactive substances (e.g. mast cell tumor) that cause gastritis. The most common clinical signs associated with neoplasia include anorexia, weight loss or lethargy and usually occur in older cats.

- Other intestinal neoplasia (fibrosarcoma, carcinoids, plasmacytoma, leiomyosarcoma, etc.) (p 693)

The presence of vomiting as a clinical sign depends on the location and size of the tumor(s) and its effects on the local (abdominal) environment.

- Gastrinoma (p 696)

Gastrinoma may cause chronic vomiting due to gastritis or gastric ulcer disease that is unresponsive to routine therapy.

NUTRITIONAL

• Food intolerance* (p 669)

Food intolerance is a non-immune-mediated condition associated with intermittent diarrhea or vomiting, with no pattern or association with eating, and it resolves when the food source is changed to omit the offending substance from diet. The clinical significance of food intolerance is unknown relative to other causes of vomiting because of the difficulty in obtaining a definitive diagnosis.

IMMUNOLOGIC

• Food allergy (dietary hypersensitivity)* (p 667)

Chronic vomiting is a common clinical presentation in cats with food allergy, and cutaneous signs may also be present.

• Idiopathic inflammatory bowel disease (IBD)* (p 671)

IBD causes chronic, intermittent or recurrent vomiting, anorexia, weight loss and diarrhea in cats. It is a diagnosis of exclusion and requires histopathologic confirmation.

INFLAMMATORY

• Chronic pancreatitis** (p 673)

Pancreatitis in cats is often **not** associated with vomiting, especially chronic pancreatitis. The most common signs are anorexia, lethargy and weight loss.

• Gastritis/gastric ulcer disease (p 679)

This is usually associated with an acute onset of vomiting, but low-grade gastritis may result in intermittent signs that do not prompt immediate attention.

INFECTIOUS:

Viral:

• Feline viral diseases (FeLV, FIV, FIP) (p 684)

Vomiting is not a common presenting sign for any of the primary feline viral diseases, but is associated with FeLV or FIV primarily secondary to the systemic disease that is occurring as a result of the infection. In cats with FIP, vomiting may be associated with focal granuloma formation in the GI tract or abdomen or may occur secondary to systemic disease (hepatic, CNS, renal). Other common clinical signs are anorexia, lethargy, fever or dyspnea.

Bacterial:

• Helicobacter spp.* (p 682)

The true importance of *Helicobacter* organisms in cats as a cause of chronic gastritis and vomiting is still not known, but there have been increasing numbers of cats with chronic gastritis and presence of these organisms that respond to appropriate therapy.

continued

continued

Protozoal:

- **Toxoplasmosis* (p 686)**

  Intermittent vomiting is a common sign in infected cats, but will occur in conjunction with other signs of systemic disease (respiratory, CNS, ocular).

Fungal:

- **Histoplasmosis* (p 685)**

  GI histoplasmosis is less common than respiratory or disseminated disease, but vomiting will still often be observed, especially when there is hepatic involvement. The most common signs are respiratory (e.g. coughing or signs of respiratory distress) or lethargy, anorexia and weight loss associated with disseminated disease.

Parasitic:

- Physaloptera (p 690)

  Chronic intermittent vomiting may be associated with undiagnosed infection with the stomach worm *Physaloptera*.

- Heartworm disease *(Dirofilaria immitus)* (p 691)

  Dirofilariosis is a disease with primarily regional importance. Cats with heartworm disease may not have signs of respiratory or cardiovascular disease (e.g. coughing or changes in breathing pattern), but instead present with intermittent vomiting, anorexia or weight loss.

Toxin/drug:

- **Pharmacologic (drug-associated vomiting)** (p 678)**

  Drugs are a common cause of acute vomiting in cats. However, chronic vomiting may occur in cats that are on long-term drug therapy (e.g. chemotherapy, theophylline, etc.).

- Lead poisoning (p 692)

  Lead poisoning is an uncommon cause of vomiting in cats, as they are generally more fastidious in their eating habits. In cats ingesting lead-containing materials, both gastrointestinal (vomiting, diarrhea, anorexia) and neurologic (seizures, ataxia, megaesophagus, tremors) signs are typical.

INTRODUCTION

MECHANISM?

Vomiting occurs when the **vomiting center** in the medulla is stimulated, which can occur by several mechanisms:

- Effect of blood-borne toxins or drugs.
- Afferent impulses from the cerebral cortex, chemoreceptor trigger zone (CRTZ), or receptors in the pharynx or abdominal viscera.

The **CRTZ** is stimulated by:

- Blood-borne toxins or drugs.
- Impulses from the vestibular apparatus.

Vomiting is an active process that must be distinguished from regurgitation.

Vomiting in cats is associated with **abdominal muscle contraction, considerable muscular effort and anxiety** prior to the event.

Vomitus may consist of undigested food material (if swallowed whole), partly digested or even liquid, and may be clear, yellow (bile stained) or brown (food colored).

Vomitus is not typically tubular in form, nor does it contain large amounts of white frothy material.

The pH of vomitus is usually acidic (pH < 4), **but may be neutral** (pH 7) if duodenal content is present (bile reflux).

WHERE?

Vomiting may be associated with **gastrointestinal disease or extra-intestinal tract diseases**.

Gastrointestinal **disease involving the stomach and/or small intestine** causes vomiting.

Vomiting is **rarely associated with primary colonic disease**.

Extra-intestinal causes of vomiting include:
- **Hepatobiliary disease**.
- **Pancreatic disease** (e.g. pancreatitis, neoplasia).
- Renal disease causing acute or chronic **renal failure**.
- CNS disease (e.g. vestibular disease, encephalitis, seizure disorders, neoplasia).
- Metabolic diseases (e.g. **hyperthyroidism**, ketoacidotic diabetes mellitus or Addison's disease).
- Cardiomyopathy or congestive heart failure.
- Systemic illness or infection affecting the CRTZ or cortex (e.g. septicemia).

WHAT?

Primary gastrointestinal diseases that cause chronic vomiting include:
- Parasites (e.g. physaloptera, etc.).
- Infectious diseases (e.g. *Helicobacter*).
- Inflammatory diseases (e.g. IBD, gastritis or gastric ulcer disease).
- Neoplasia.
- Mechanical (e.g. antral pyloric hypertrophy/stenosis, obstruction, intussusception).
- Dietary disturbances (e.g. food intolerance or food allergy).

The most common causes of chronic vomiting are: dietary (indiscretion or food intolerance), **neoplastic diseases, metabolic or extra-intestinal disturbances** (e.g. renal, hepatic or pancreatic disease) and **inflammatory diseases** (e.g. IBD).

Diagnosis is based on the minimum data base, multiple fecal examinations, survey or contrast radiography, radionucleotide or scintigraphic studies (e.g. thyroid disease, motility studies, evaluation for portosystemic shunts, vascular diseases, etc.), ultrasound examination, endocrine testing, evaluation of serum TLI, cobalamin/folate assays, titers for various infectious agents, neurologic examination and diagnostics (e.g. CSF,

computed tomography, etc.), endoscopic examination and biopsy or surgical exploratory with biopsy.

Many diseases that cause chronic vomiting are diseases from which complete recovery is not possible (e.g. IBD, food allergy, motility disturbances, chronic renal disease, etc.) and thus, **long-term therapy including dietary or pharmacologic treatment will be necessary**.

In some cases, the prognosis will be very guarded to poor for long-term survival (e.g. neoplasia, cardiomyopathy), and this should be discussed with the owner.

Occasional vomiting is considered a normal phenomenon in cats, both for removal of ingested hair, but also as a protective mechanism following consumption of new or unusual foods. This should be taken into consideration when evaluating a cat for chronic vomiting.

DISEASES CAUSING SIGNS OF CHRONIC VOMITING (>3 WEEKS DURATION)

FOOD ALLERGY (DIETARY HYPERSENSITIVITY)***

Classical signs

- Chronic vomiting, usually < once per day, immediately to > 12 h after eating.
- Diarrhea is less frequent and more often large bowel in character.
- Weight loss.
- Dermatological signs in some cats (miliary dermatitis, pruritus).

Pathogenesis

Food allergy is an immunologic reaction usually to the protein (or glycoprotein) component of food.

Food allergy may also be associated with dermatological signs.

Approximately 25% of cats with GI signs from food allergy also have dermatologic signs consisting of pruritus, miliary dermatitis and alopecia.

The pathogenesis of food allergy is poorly understood, but is thought to be a combination of two main mechanisms. Firstly, direct toxicity caused by the ingestion of the food causing **release of histamine and other vasoactive amines**. Secondly, indirect effects are mediated via an amplification system, which responds to the food by releasing mast cell products, the production of **eicosanoids** and other inflammatory mediators, initiation of the kinin cascade, and other events that result in the clinical syndrome.

Clinical signs

Signs associated with food allergy are non-seasonal, affect a wide range of ages, breeds and both sexes, and are present in one or all three of these systems: the gastrointestinal tract, the skin or the respiratory tract.

Cats with food allergy may have vomiting/diarrhea, anorexia and weight loss, but may also have **dermatologic signs**, which may include rodent ulcers, eosinophilic plaques, miliary dermatitis, otitis externa or generalized pruritus, alopecia and erythema. A combination of GI and dermatologic signs should raise the index of suspicion of a food-related problem.

Head and neck pruritus appears to be especially **common in cats with food allergy**.

In some cats, food allergy may be associated with systemic signs such as feline asthma, rhinitis, stomatitis or other respiratory tract signs. However, this is poorly documented.

In a study of cats with documented food sensitivity (food intolerance and food allergy), there was a history of vomiting (56%), diarrhea (25%), or vomiting and diarrhea (19%).

Vomiting usually occurred less than once daily, a few minutes to > 12 h after eating and most commonly consisted of bile.

Large bowel signs (mucus and fresh blood in feces or excessive straining to defecate) were slightly (57%) more common than small bowel signs. Flatulence occurred in 38% of cats.

Weight loss occurred in 70% of cats.

Appetite was variably affected and either normal, increased or decreased.

Some cats were reported as irritable (38%) or lethargic (25%).

Dermatologic signs occurred in 25% of cats and consisted of miliary dermatitis, pruritis and alopecia.

Diagnosis

The **diagnosis of food allergy** is confirmed by performing **elimination/challenge trials.** However, **the diagnosis of food allergy** may require a **more specific approach to the elimination/challenge trials than is possible with commercially available diets** because of the difficulty in removing all sources of allergy from commercial diets.

The best **elimination diet** for making a definitive diagnosis **in these cases is a home-prepared diet containing novel protein and carbohydrate source,** e.g. lamb, venison, duck, kangaroo, crocodile or ostrich with potato or rice (and added vitamin and mineral supplementation).

Gastrointestinal signs usually resolve within 1–3 weeks but dermatologic signs may require that these diets be **fed a minimum of 6–8 weeks or 2 weeks after all symptoms resolve**.

The cat should then be changed to a **hypoallergenic commercial cat food** (e.g. IVD Limited diets, Hill's d/d diet or z/d diet, Royal Canin's Selected protein diets, or Eukanuba's Response Formula feline) containing food ingredients the cat has been successfully tested with or never exposed to.

Skin tests are inadequate for diagnosis of food allergies because they have a high incidence of false positives and negatives, and are only useful in determining which adverse reactions to foods have an IgE-mediated pathogenesis.

Serum radioallergosorbent (RAST), ELISA, or tests that are variations on the theme, are all available commercially to **test for the presence of antigen-specific IgE in the serum.** However, the difficulties present with skin testing still exist, i.e. non-IgE-mediated and delayed hypersensitivity reactions will also be missed. Not all food allergies cause systemic effects or cause increased systemic levels of IgE and so will be negative using serum IgE testing. Findings of a recent study suggest that type I hypersensitivities account for only 25% of gastrointestinal food sensitivities in cats. Gastroscopic food sensitivity testing has been tested in humans and dogs, but not in cats, and its utility remains to be established for the routine diagnosis of food hypersensitivity.

Differential diagnosis

The main differential diagnosis for food allergy is food intolerance and they are usually clinically indistinguishable.

Cats with food allergy causing **dermatologic signs** must be differentiated from cats with atopy, flea allergy dermatitis, psychogenic alopecia or insect bite hypersensitivity.

The **gastrointestinal signs** of either syndrome can mimic many other causes of chronic GI disease, including gastritis, pancreatitis, and small bowel diseases such as IBD or colitis. The severity and duration of each event depends on the amount of antigen ingested, the immune response and the sensitivity of the patient. The more severe the presentation, the more differentials that must be included, e.g. neoplasia, extra-intestinal disease, etc.

Treatment

Treatment is initiated during the diagnostic phase by **feeding the elimination diet**. The key to effective therapy is to **find the offending agent(s) and remove them from the diet**.

Corticosteroids may provide partial relief, especially where type I hypersensitivity reactions are involved, but in general are not effective in maintaining remission or symptomatic relief for cats with food allergies.

Antihistamines have not been proved effective in preventing the gastrointestinal symptoms associated with food allergy.

Some animals will eventually develop allergies to components in the elimination diet. In these cases, feeding diets containing protein hydrolysates will be most effective. Unlike regular protein molecules, the molecular size of these hydrolysates is too small to crosslink IgE bound to mast cells.

Prognosis

The prognosis for control of food allergy is excellent if the offending agent(s) can be identified and eliminated from the diet. However, in some cases, that is not possible and affected animals will have recurrent or persistent clinical signs.

FOOD INTOLERANCE***

> ### Classical signs
>
> - Chronic vomiting, usually < once per day, immediately to >12 h after eating.
> - Diarrhea is less frequent and more often large bowel in character.
> - Weight loss.
> - Dermatological signs in some cats (miliary dermatitis, pruritus).

Pathogenesis

Food intolerance is a non-immunologic reaction to a substance or multiple substances in food. This reaction can occur to proteins or other food components, but it can also be associated with food coloring, additives, preservatives or flavorings. Naturally occurring chemicals such as amines, salicylates and monosodium glutamate are present in food, especially highly flavored rich food.

These distinctions are **difficult to distinguish clinically**.

Food sensitivity may also be associated with dermatological signs.

Approximately 25% of cats with GI signs from food sensitivity also have dermatologic signs consisting of pruritus, miliary dermatitis and alopecia.

The pathogenic mechanisms of food intolerance are poorly understood, but a combination of direct toxicity caused by the ingestion of the food causing **release of histamine and other vasoactive amines**, and indirect effects that are mediated via an amplification system which responds to the food by releasing mast cell products, production of **eicosanoids** and other inflammatory mediators, initiation of the kinin cascade, and other events that result in the clinical syndrome.

Clinical signs

Cats with **food intolerance** traditionally have been thought to have **gastrointestinal tract signs only**, because the syndrome is not an immunologic reaction.

However, humans with food intolerance may have dermatologic signs, mouth ulcers and other systemic signs. In cats, **vomiting, diarrhea, weight loss, poor coat condition and lethargy** are the most frequently observed clinical signs. It is unknown whether dermatologic signs also occur with food intolerance in cats.

The most common clinical signs of food intolerance are the same as food allergy, i.e. vomiting and/or diarrhea. The vomiting is often intermittent and may not necessarily follow any particular pattern in relation to eating. If diarrhea occurs, it is probably more likely to be large bowel in character (mucus and fresh blood in feces or excessive straining to defecate) than small bowel (low frequency, loose to watery feces passed without straining or mucus).

Weight loss may occur, along with a change in appetite.

Diagnosis

The diagnosis of food intolerance is confirmed by performing elimination/challenge dietary trials.

An elimination trial (either using commercial hypoallergenic diets or premium diets that have reduced food colorings, preservatives, additives, etc.) of 4–6 days should be embarked upon first before proceeding to a more specific food elimination trial requiring controlled food preparation (single novel protein and carbohydrate source). Gastrointestinal signs usually resolve quickly. Vomiting may cease immediately and diarrhea usually within 3 days. Recrudescence of GI signs with challenge usually occurs within 4 days but may take up to 10 days with dermatologic signs.

Differential diagnosis

Food intolerance and food allergy are clinically indistinguishable as they both present with the same clinical signs and are usually highly diet responsive.

Other chronic causes of GI signs include gastritis, pancreatitis and small bowel diseases such as IBD or colitis. As a general rule, more severe clinical presentations require a more thorough clinical workup to eliminate a wider range of differential diagnoses, e.g. neoplasia and extra-intestinal disease.

Treatment

Food intolerance is highly diet-responsive once the offending agent(s) has been identified. This is usually done by using an elimination diet.

Since the condition is not immunologically mediated, drugs that modify or suppress the immune response are unlikely to be beneficial.

Prognosis

Once the inciting food(s) has been eliminated from the diet, food intolerance has an excellent prognosis.

HYPERTHYROIDISM**

> ### Classical signs
>
> - Weight loss.
> - Polyphagia.
> - Vomiting and/or diarrhea.
> - Hyperactivity.
> - Poor grooming habits.

See main reference on page 304 for details.

Clinical signs

Weight loss despite a voracious appetite (polyphagia) is the most common owner complaint.

Vomiting and polyuria/polydipsia occur in a third of cats.

Other signs that occur less commonly are restlessness or irritability, poor grooming habits, decreased appetite, lethargy, panting or dyspnea and large bowel diarrhea.

The most prevalent physical exam findings are a palpable thyroid nodule, thin body condition, tachycardia or heart murmur and hyperactivity or irritability.

There is **no breed or sex predilection** for hyperthyroidism, but **most (90%) are old cats (> 10 years)**. Cats < 6 years of age are rarely affected.

Diagnosis

Presumptive diagnosis is often suggested by the **age, history and clinical presentation**.

Hematology changes include **erythrocytosis, and a stress leukogram (leukocytosis, neutrophilia, lymphopenia).**

Serum biochemistry profile changes: **increases in liver enzyme activities (ALT, SAP, GGT, LDH, AST) occur in greater than 50% of cases**, hyperglycemia and pre-renal azotemia are less common. Hyperphosphatemia and hyperbilirubinemia are uncommon (< 10% of cats).

The **urine specific gravity will usually be > 1.035 (>50%),** but cats with polydipsia/polyuria or underlying renal disease will have unconcentrated urine (urine SG < 1.035).

Definitive diagnosis is made by finding **elevated serum thyroxine (total T$_4$) levels** in most cats (98%).

In a few cats the total T$_4$ is in the upper half of the normal range and measurements of **free T$_4$, a T$_3$ suppression test** (useful for diagnosis of mild hyperthyroidism, but takes 3 days), **TRH stimulation test** (preformed over 4 hours, side effects common from TRH administration) or **radionuclide (^{99}Tc, pertechnate) imaging** examination (requires special equipment and isolation for 24 hours) **may be required to make the diagnosis**.

Differential diagnosis

Diabetes mellitus, chronic renal failure, liver disease are common extra-intestinal causes of vomiting, weight loss and polyuria/polydipsia that must be differentiated from hyperthyroidism.

Primary GI diseases that may cause similar signs are food intolerance/food allergy, IBD and gastrointestinal neoplasia.

Treatment

Medical therapy with anti-thyroid drugs that inhibit the synthesis of thyroid hormones, such as methimazole or carbimazole (2.5–5 mg/kg q 8–12 h, PO) are commonly used treatments. However, these drugs must be administered daily and have side effects which are potentially problematic. Vomiting and anorexia are relatively common side effects, while hematologic abnormalities are rare.

Calcium ipodate (15 mg/kg PO q 12 h) decreases serum T$_3$ (but not T$_4$) concentrations acutely, but the effect is only short term. Thus, it is not useful in long-term management of the disease.

Adjunctive therapy for hyperthyroid heart disease: beta-adrenergic receptor-blocking agents (propranolol, atenolol for heart rate control, and furosemide, calcium channel antagonists and ACE-inhibitors as needed for heart failure (see page 132).

Surgical thyroidectomy is a highly effective treatment, especially for unilateral disease, but requires an anesthetic procedure and careful technique to preserve the parathyroid glands. If bilateral thyroidectomy is required, the patient will require oral thyroid hormone supplementation. Recurrence of hyperthyroidism in the remaining gland or tissue is common.

Radioiodine therapy is the simplest, safest and most effective therapy for the majority of cats, except cats with chronic progressive renal disease/failure and cats that will not eat in confinement. The major disadvantage is the requirement for special facilities for use of radioisotopes and the cat cannot be handled for 7–21days. This makes fluid therapy difficult if the cat goes into renal decompensation during that time, or requires other medication.

IDIOPATHIC INFLAMMATORY BOWEL DISEASE (IBD)*

Classical signs

- Vomiting with or without diarrhea.
- Weight loss and anorexia or decreased appetite.

Pathogenesis

Inflammatory bowel disease (IBD) is an **idiopathic inflammatory disease** of the feline GI tract characterized by **infiltration of the lamina propria and mucosa with inflammatory cells** of various types (lymphocytic, plasmacytic, granulocytic, granulomatous, eosinophilic or combinations of these).

A **lymphocytic/plasmacytic infiltration is the most common lesion in cats**.

The **etiology is unknown** but believed to involve genetic, immunologic, dietary, bacterial and mucosal factors.

Lymphocytes and plasma cells are normal components of the feline GI tract, and increased numbers in the GIT occur in response to many infectious agents. **Differentiation of feline IBD from other diseases requires a complete examination to rule-out other causes for the infiltration**. In IBD, there should also be evidence of **mucosal disease** (e.g. erosion, villous blunting, loss of normal structure in other ways, loss of normal function).

Eosinophilic IBD is rare in cats, and in some cases it is found in association with **hypereosinophilic syndrome** (infiltration of eosinophils in many body tissues including liver, spleen, lymph nodes, etc.).

Other forms of IBD, such as granulomatous and neutrophilic IBD are also rare in cats.

Most forms of IBD involve the small intestine, sparing the stomach and colon, however, enterocolitis and gastritis may also occur.

Recently **an association has been observed between cats with idiopathic IBD and concurrent cholangitis and pancreatitis.** The true relationship between these observations and clinical IBD is not known.

Clinical signs

Vomiting and weight loss are the most common signs, but diarrhea and anorexia are also frequently observed signs.

Middle-aged (> 4 years) cats are most frequently affected, but all ages have been reported to have IBD.

There is **no breed or sex predilection,** but purebred cats may be at increased risk compared to DSH cats.

If there is concurrent cholangitis or pancreatitis, cats may also present with icterus, abdominal pain or fever.

Diagnosis

The diagnosis is based upon several factors: (1) **histologic infiltration** of inflammatory cells, usually lymphocytes and plasma cells in the GI tract; (2) the presence of inflammatory cells is associated with **mucosal abnormalities and functional disturbances;** (3) there are **no other identifiable causes for the infiltration** identified; and (4) the signs of the disease are **chronic** (> 3 weeks in duration).

It is especially important to rule out parasitic, infectious, dietary and extra-intestinal (e.g. hepatic, renal or pancreatic) causes of disease, as these may cause similar lesions to IBD.

The only means of ruling out dietary causes of vomiting is via an elimination trial, which must be conducted using an elimination diet prior to making a diagnosis of IBD.

Endoscopic examination and biopsy is the **most common procedure** used to obtain the diagnosis. **Multiple (6–8), good-quality** (containing submucosa and properly oriented) **biopsies should be obtained from the small intestine and stomach**. Biopsies should be taken from all regions of the stomach and lymphoid follicles should be avoided when obtaining biopsies from the duodenum. **Full-thickness biopsies obtained surgically are also acceptable** if endoscopy is unavailable, and equal care should be taken to assure biopsy quality (proper handling to minimize artifact and orientation on the biopsy sponge to prevent curling and crush artifacts).

The major difficulty associated with endoscopic diagnosis of IBD is differentiation of IBD from lymphoma, which will not be possible if the biopsy samples are not deep enough (contain submucosa) or if they have significant mucosal artifacts that prevent adequate assessment of mucosal abnormalities. In some cases where histologic differentiation is impossible, immunocytochemistry techniques may have to be employed to distinguish the cell origin (c.g. lymphoma cells tend to be monoclonal, while lymphocytes from cats with IBD will be polyclonal).

Non-specific laboratory abnormalities that may be found in cats with IBD include: hypoproteinemia, hyperglycemia (stress induced), **hypokalemia, elevated liver enzyme activities and a stress leukogram.**

Serum cobalamin and folate levels may be decreased in cats with IBD due to malabsorption.

Radiography and ultrasonography generally do not assist with the diagnosis, but are important in ruling out other causes of the clinical signs, e.g. neoplasia.

Differential diagnosis

Neoplasia (lymphoma is of special mention because it may have a similar histologic appearance to IBD).

Food intolerance or hypersensitivity (food allergy).

Parasitic infections of the GI tract, especially giardia, which are difficult to diagnose.

Infectious diseases such as *Campylobacter*, salmonellosis, *Clostridium*, etc.

Extra-intestinal causes of vomiting such as hyperthyroidism, uncontrolled diabetes, renal failure and pancreatitis.

Treatment

In most cats, a **combination of dietary modification and pharmacologic therapy** (anti-inflammatory, immunosuppressive) is successful in controlling the clinical signs.

Dietary therapy involves three main strategies: (1) low-residue, highly digestible diets; (2) hypoallergenic, elimination diets aimed at controlling food allergies; or (3) high-fiber diets for cats with IBD that primarily involves the large bowel.

The mainstay of **pharmacologic therapy** in cats with IBD is **prednisone (2–4 mg/kg PO q 12–24 h)**. This dose is tapered after the first 2 weeks to the lowest dose that will maintain remission. Some cats can be weaned off prednisone after 3–6 months and maintained on a controlled diet (or diet with metronidazole), while others will require life-long steroid therapy.

In refractory cases, dexamethasome (0.25 mg/kg PO q 12–24 h) may be used as well, but is not suitable for alternate day therapy because of the long half life.

Metronidazole is often added (10–15 mg/kg PO q 12 h) to the treatment plan because of the anaerobic, antiprotozoal and immunomodulating effects of the drug.

Other antibiotics that may be useful include tetracycline (20 mg/kg PO q 8 h), doxycycline (5–10 mg/kg PO q 12 h) or **tylosin powder** (10–20 mg/kg PO q 12 h).

In cats that do not completely respond to corticosteroids or that become refractory to standard treatment approach, **chlorambucil** (1 mg PO q 3 days) **or azathioprine** (0.3–0.5 mg/kg PO q 2–3 days) can be added to the regimen. Toxicity (leukopenia) is a major risk with azathioprine use, and should be monitored by hemograms every 2–3 weeks.

Prognosis

Guarded. Cats will frequently respond well to dietary and pharmacologic therapy, but relapses are common and long-term management is required. There is no known cure for IBD and owners should be educated about the nature of the disease to encourage compliance and understanding.

CHRONIC PANCREATITIS*

> **Classical signs**
> - Lethargy.
> - Anorexia.
> - Vomiting is observed in less than 30% of cases.

See main reference on page 639 for details (The Cat With Signs of Acute Vomiting).

Clinical signs

Lethargy and anorexia have been the most commonly observed clinical signs.

In general, **vomiting and anterior abdominal pain occur less frequently.**

Signs may be protracted, with low-grade vomiting occurring in some cats, while others have acute signs.

Diagnosis

A certain **degree of clinical suspicion** is required to make the diagnosis of pancreatitis in cats because the signs are so vague.

Cats with chronic pancreatitis may develop **secondary complications** such as exocrine pancreatic insufficiency, diabetes mellitus, obstruction of the common bile duct or cholangitis.

Hematology and serum chemistry profiles are non-diagnostic, but may show dehydration, electrolyte imbalances, elevated liver enzymes, mild hyperbilirubinemia or a leukocytosis.

Serum lipase and amylase values are not helpful, as they may be elevated, normal or low in normal cats or cats with pancreatic disease.

Imaging studies are the most useful way to obtain a presumptive diagnosis of pancreatitis. **Radiographs of the anterior abdomen** may reveal evidence of local peritonitis, gas in the duodenum or anterior jejunum, or a mass. **Ultrasound examination remains the most reliable technique to evaluate the pancreas** and determine the presence of swelling, abscess or fibrosis. It is important to note that **ultrasonographic changes in chronic pancreatitis persist for months**.

Elevations in serum **trypsin-like immunoreactivity (TLI) assay** have been suggested as a means of detecting pancreatitis, but this **has not be shown to be consistently accurate** either, and is of less use in chronic pancreatitis.

The assay for feline pancreatic lipase (fPLI) has been developed and is a sensitive and highly specific test for acute pancreatitis. However, in cats with chronic pancreatitis, the fPLI may be normal, or mildly increased but below levels diagnostic for pancreatitis, which can make test interpretation difficult.

Differential diagnosis

The list of problems causing anorexia and lethargy in cats is lengthy and includes multiple organ systems and abnormalities.

Treatment

Nothing should be fed for 1–2 days if the cat is vomiting until the vomiting can be controlled. However, a fast of longer than 3 days is to be avoided if at all possible in most cats.

Intravenous fluid therapy should be administered, using a balanced electrolyte solution (either replacement or maintenance fluids) to maintain hydration, correct pancreatic ischemia and reduce the risk of complications of pancreatitis.

Anti-emetics (e.g. metoclopramide 0.1–0.2 mg/kg) may be used if the cat is vomiting.

Cats with severe pancreatitis may be unable to eat for several days (3–5), thus, **parenteral or partial enteral nutrition** will be necessary to prevent development of malnutrition, feline hepatic lipidosis and impaired immunity.

Steroid therapy may be indicated in cats with concurrent IBD or cholangitis.

HEPATIC DISEASES (HEPATIC LIPIDOSIS, CHOLANGITIS, HEPATIC CIRRHOSIS, PORTOSYSTEMIC ANOMALIES)

Classical signs

- Lethargy or depression, vomiting, anorexia and weight loss are common signs.
- Icterus, ascites, hepatomegaly or microhepatica are variable.

See main references on page 421 for details (The Yellow Cat or Cat With Elevated Liver Enzymes).

Clinical signs

Vomiting occurs primarily because of the gastritis that occurs secondary to changes in blood flow and release of GI hormones, and because of mediator release (stimulation of the vomiting center) secondary to presence of toxins from decreased hepatic clearance or function.

Liver diseases often present with the relatively non-specific signs of **anorexia, weight loss, vomiting, and lethargy or depression with or without icterus.**

Other signs include **ascites, edema formation, bleeding disorders due to deficiency of coagulation factors or DIC,** and in cases with severe hepatic failure, signs of **hepatoencephalopathy** (dementia, personality changes, seizures, stupor or coma). Prolongation of clotting times is quite common in cats with hepatopathy.

Diagnosis

Icterus (hyperbilirubinemia) may be caused by **prehepatic (hemolysis), hepatic or post-hepatic (bile duct obstruction)** diseases which all must be considered.

The **hemogram** is important in **differentiating hemolysis from hepatic causes of icterus. Anemia is a common problem** and may be either regenerative (secondary to blood loss or hemolysis) or non-regenerative (e.g. anemia of chronic disease, bone marrow suppression). Typically the anemia of chronic disease is less severe (PCV > 20), than that seen with hemolysis or severe blood loss.

Target cells (leptocytes) on the blood smear are also suggestive of liver disease.

Serum biochemical profile results will be supportive of the diagnosis, with the most common findings being **elevated liver enzymes, hyperbilirubinemia**, decreased BUN, decreased albumin and total protein, hypocholesterolemia, and electrolyte disturbances consistent with vomiting (hypokalemia, hypochloridemia, hypernatremia).

A **serum bile acid assay** is the most reliable, easiest to perform and most readily available liver function test. **A pre- and 2-hour post-prandial assay should be submitted** to evaluate liver function. Other function tests include blood ammonia and bromosulfophthalein (BSP) retention.

Measurement of sulfated bile acids in urine is a newly developed test to diagnose liver disease. In many cats that will not eat, obtaining a serum post-prandial bile acid sample is difficult, and this test may provide additional information about the status of liver function in inappetent cats.

Imaging studies (radiographs, **ultrasound**) are used to assess liver size, morphology and structure, and may be used to obtain **aspirates or biopsies** of liver via ultrasound-guided techniques.

In all cases of suspected liver failure, **evaluation of coagulation function is essential**, not only for therapeutic purposes (e.g. determining the presence of DIC, coagulopathies), but also prior to obtaining tissue for biopsy.

The **definitive diagnosis** typically requires **histopathologic examination** of liver tissue, however, in cases of suspected vascular anomalies, a venous portogram or portal scintigraphy is necessary to define the abnormal vascular structures.

Differential diagnosis

Icteric cats: Immune-mediated hemolytic anemia, pancreatic or gastric abscess or tumor obstructing common bile duct, hemolytic anemia secondary to red cell parasites, primary liver diseases (hepatic lipidosis, cholangitis, and hepatic lymphoma or carcinoma) are the most common diseases.

Cats with ascites: Ascites may be caused by prehepatic (cardiac), hepatic or post-hepatic (GI lymphatic obstruction, protein-losing enteropathy, severe protein-losing nephropathy or mesenteric hypertension (torsion) or venous thrombosis or vasculitis), and these must be separated. **Ascites due to cardiac failure is very rare in the cat.** Hepatic disease, vasculitis from feline infectious peritonitis or lymphatic obstruction associated with neoplasia are the most common causes of ascites in cats.

Treatment

Treatment is based upon **identifying the primary problem**. The reader is referred to the main reference (page 421) for details.

GI LYMPHOSARCOMA**

Classical signs

- Weight loss.
- Intermittent or persistent vomiting.
- Small or large bowel diarrhea.
- Lethargy or depression.

Pathogenesis

In the United States and other countries where **feline leukemia virus (FeLV) is prevalent, FeLV infection is the most common cause of all types of lymphoma except the alimentary form**, which is only associated with viremia 25–30% of the time. In areas **where FeLV infection is rare** (e.g. east coast of Australia), **most cats with lymphoma are FeLV negative**.

Some evidence suggests that the alimentary form of lymphoma arises from transformed multipotent lymphoid or monocyte precursors or from FeLV-transformed B-lymphocytes, and thus may still be associated with FeLV.

Alimentary lymphoma is the **second most common GI tumor** (adenocarcinoma is first), and occurs in **older cats** (> 8 years).

The **most common site** for lymphoma is the **jejunum or ileum**, with the duodenum being a rare site of occurrence. Lymphoma is the most common tumor found in the feline stomach (although it is still a rare disease), but is found unfrequently in the colon compared to adenocarcinoma.

Lymphoma can occur as a **solitary mass causing an obstructive lesion, or as diffuse disease** affecting many sections of the GI tract and occurring throughout all layers of the bowel wall.

Clinical signs

The **most common clinical signs** associated with intestinal lymphoma in cats are **anorexia, lethargy and weight loss**.

Vomiting and diarrhea are variably observed, depending on the location of the lesion, the nature of disease (diffuse vs. a solitary mass) and duration of disease e.g. fever, hematemesis, icterus, ascites and melena.

Cats that are FeLV positive may also have clinical signs consistent with the disease in other locations (e.g. anemia, leukemia, etc.).

Diagnosis

Hematology may be normal or there may be an anemia of chronic disease (that may be masked by dehydration) in cats that are FeLV negative. **FeLV-positive cats may have a wide variety of hematologic changes**, which should be further investigated with a bone marrow examination.

Serum biochemistry profile values also may be within normal limits, or there may be **increases in liver enyzmes, hypercalcemia or hypoproteinemia**. Pre-renal azotemia and electrolyte disturbances may occur in cats with severe vomiting.

The **majority of cats (70–75%) are FeLV antigen negative**.

Radiographs may be normal or may reveal thickened bowel loops or a solitary mass lesion.

Ultrasonography is useful for localizing solitary masses, evaluating mesenteric lymph nodes (which are also typically involved), and for identifying thickened intestinal loops.

The **definitive diagnosis** is made by **histopathologic evaluation** of affected segments of bowel. **Ultrasound-guided aspirates** often will provide sufficient tissue sample for the diagnosis (intestinal wall, mass or lymph nodes).

If the lesion is in a location accessible by **endoscopy, biopsies** can be obtained by this method. However, **endoscopic biopsy samples can be easily misread as IBD or visa versa**, and the diagnosis can be missed if the lesion is present only in the submucosa.

If these diagnostic modalities are not available or provide inconclusive results, full-thickness biopsies obtained by surgical exploratory are usually definitive.

Staging the disease requires histologic evaluation of regional (mesenteric) lymph nodes, liver and spleen, radiographic evaluation of lungs and examination of bone marrow aspirates (if indicated) for evidence of metastasis.

Differential diagnosis

The major differential is **lymphocytic plasmacytic IBD**.

Intestinal adenocarcinoma, foreign body, FIP, fungal or algal infections of the GIT, other intestinal tumors (e.g. mast cell tumor) and hyperthyroidism must all be considered.

Treatment

Chemotherapy is provided in stages: induction of remission, intensification, maintenance and rescue. In general, **cats are more difficult to rescue** (compared to dogs) **once the cancer is out of remission**, which is why their survival times are shorter than dogs.

A typical protocol used to induce remission is the COAP protocol: cyclophosphamide (200–300 mg/m^2 PO q 3 weeks), vincristine (0.5 mg/m^2 IV q 1 week), cytosine arabinoside (100 mg/m^2 IV or SC for 2 days only), and prednisolone (50 mg/m^2 PO q 24 h for 7 days, then EOD). If remission is only partially achieved, intensification with doxorubicin (25 mg/m^2 IV q 3 weeks) or mitoxantrone (4–6 mg/m^2 IV q 3 weeks) can be tried.

Maintenance chemotherapy protocols may include continuation of the COAP protocol or use of the LMP protocol (chlorambucil, methotrexate, prednisone).

In **cats with small cell (highly differentiated) lymphoma of the GIT**, the combination of chlorambucil (20 mg/m² PO every other week) and prednisolone (20 mg/m² PO EOD), with or without methotrexate (2.5 mg/m² PO EOD) is often successfully used.

Other protocols that have been successfully used to treat feline lymphoma include COP (cyclophosphamide, vincristine and prednisone), VCM (vincristine, cyclophosphamide and methotrexate), or VCM plus L-asparaginase.

Nutritional support should be used as needed (especially in cats that are vomiting or not eating enough to maintain normal function).

Control of secondary infections is also sometimes necessary and should be implemented as required. In cats with alimentary lymphosarcoma, metronidazole is often used as the antibiotic choice.

Prognosis

FeLV status does not influence whether or not remission occurs, but is a significant predictor of survival, with FeLV-negative cats having much longer survival times. FeLV-positive cats in stages III–V had no differences in survival than FeLV-negative cats, but in stage I–II, survival is 18 months versus 4 months, respectively, for negative cats and cats with the virus.

The **overall prognosis is guarded to poor** in cats with alimentary lymphoma. Most cats with alimentary lymphoma respond poorly to chemotherapy, but those that do respond may have a survival time of more than one year. Cats with a solitary mass in the GIT that can be resected have a better prognosis.

Most cats with lymphoma treated with multiple agent chemotherapy protocols are expected to live **3–9 months**, with 20% living longer than 1 year. **Untreated cats can only be expected to survive 4–8 weeks**. Cats that are **FeLV positive also have shorter survival times.**

Survival does not appear to be influenced by the extent of the disease, anatomic location or clinical stage, which is an important predictor in some types of lymphoma.

INTESTINAL ADENOCARCINOMA**

Classical signs

- Weight loss and lethargy or depression are the most prevalent signs.
- Intermittent to persistent vomiting or hematochezia develop as the tumor obstructs or ulcerates the epithelial surface.

Pathogenesis

The **most common non-hematopoietic tumor** of the feline GI tract is the adenocarcinoma.

Most intestinal adenocarcinomas occur in the **jejunum and ileum**, with the duodenum rarely affected. Colonic adenocarcinoma is uncommon and usually occurs in **very old cats (e.g. 16 years)**.

Siamese cats represented 70% of 225 reported cases of **intestinal adenocarcinoma** and had a mean age of 10–11 years.

Domestic shorthair cats had the most reported cases of **colonic adenocarcinoma**.

Feline leukemia virus appears to have no role in the pathogenesis of this disease, since all 28 cats in one study that were tested were found to be FeLV negative.

Adenocarcinomas occur either as **annular or intraluminal tumors**.

Metastasis of adenocarcinomas is typically **within the abdominal cavity and not to the lungs.**

Clinical signs

The most commonly observed clinical signs are **anorexia, lethargy, weight loss and vomiting**.

Hematochezia, melena or diarrhea are primarily observed in cats with **colonic disease**.

In cats that are not eating and are vomiting persistently, dehydration may also occur. Fever and abdominal effusion are also late-stage findings associated with metastasis of the tumor.

Diagnosis

Hematologic and serum biochemical profiles are often normal.

Abnormalities may include: hemoconcentration, non-regenerative anemia of chronic disease, electrolyte imbalances or pre-renal azotemia, hypoproteinemia or hypoalbuminemia due to GI protein loss, or elevated liver enzyme activities (metastatic disease).

Radiographs of the thorax rarely reveal metastatic lesions.

Abdominal radiographs may show a mass, enlarged lymph nodes or signs of an intestinal obstruction (e.g. dilated, air-filled bowel segment, abnormal gas patterns, or differences in bowel size or location relative to neighboring bowel). Some cats will have tumors with osseous **metaplasia** (**mineralization**) or **ascites** that will imply neoplasia. Contrast studies may be very useful in delineating intraluminal or annular lesions.

Ultrasonography is also very helpful in identifying mass lesions and their extent for staging, and can be used to direct **fine-needle aspirates or biopsies** for diagnosis.

In cats with colonic disease, **colonoscopic evaluation and biopsy may also be useful**.

Surgical exploratory is the best way to obtain the definitive diagnosis, get **accurate staging information**, and will also allow **resection of the affected segment** of bowel if that is indicated.

Differential diagnosis

Intestinal foreign body or obstruction, other intestinal neoplasia, inflammatory bowel disease, vomiting and weight loss due to extra-intestinal disease (chronic renal failure, etc.), fungal or algal diseases of the intestine, and FIP granuloma should all be included in the differential list.

Treatment

The **only reported and effective treatment** for intestinal adenocarcinoma in cats is **surgical resection**.

The **role of adjuvant chemotherapy** for feline intestinal adenocarcinoma has not been explored.

Nutritional support may be necessary in cats that do not eat enough to meet at least resting energy requirements (RER = 30 × BW (kg) + 70) and cats with cancer may require additional calories (RER × 1.5).

Cats with large colonic resections may require very highly digestible diets to reduce the fecal volume and load on the colon.

Prognosis

The **presence of metastatic disease is not necessarily a poor prognostic sign** in cats with adenocarcinoma, and should not be a disincentive for performing a surgical resection and anastomosis.

The **average survival for cats with the disease is 4–15 months** (with or without metastatic disease), but some cats live several more years following aggressive surgical resection.

PHARMACOLOGIC (DRUG-ASSOCIATED VOMITING) **

> ### Classical signs
>
> - Vomiting observed after administration or ingestion of a drug.

See main reference on page 642 for details.

Clinical signs

In some cases, vomiting is expected following drug administration (e.g. chemotherapy, xylazine), while in others it is not usual (e.g. tetracycline, erythromycin), and in others it represents toxicity or accidental exposure (NSAIDs, narcotics, digitalis).

The **signs observed will depend on the drug that is administered,** e.g. chemotherapy drugs may cause vomiting, anorexia, lethargy, hair loss, etc., while vomiting caused by chloramphenicol or erythromycin may be the only clinical sign.

Diagnosis

Diagnosis is largely dependent upon obtaining an **extensive, accurate history** that includes a complete history of drugs the cat is taking or has taken, toxins it has been exposed to and the potential for accidental or malicious poisoning.

Some **commonly used drugs known to cause vomiting in cats include** many, if not most, **antibiotics** (e.g. amoxicillin, cephalexin, enrofloxacin, tetracycline, erythromycin, metronidazole, clindamycin), **chemotherapy drugs** (dacarbazine, cisplatin, doxorubicin, methotrexate, cyclophosphamide), **methimazole, potassium bromide, glipizide, and antifungal drugs** (e.g. itraconazole, amphotericin).

In some cases, **determination of blood levels of a specific drug** will confirm the presence of a drug or toxin that was unknown or unexpected. Alternatively, hair and urine samples can also be used in some cases to determine the presence of metabolites of various drugs or chemicals.

If the suspected exposure is recent, evacuation of the stomach and analysis of its contents will also provide a means of determining the presence of drugs or chemicals.

Differential diagnosis

Other acute causes of vomiting such as food intolerance/dietary indiscretion, parasitic diseases, infectious diseases, foreign bodies or gastritis due to other causes should be considered when the history is not helpful in identifying exposure.

Treatment

Choice of treatment depends on whether the vomiting is expected (e.g. chemotherapy) and can be controlled with anti-emetics (e.g. metoclopramide or chlorpromazine), or is due to unexpected toxicity or accidental ingestion.

Supportive care for toxicity or accidental ingestion includes removal of stomach contents and gastric lavage, administration of activated charcoal to reduce absorption of contents, administration of gastric protectants as indicated (NSAID ingestion will cause gastritis), anti-emetics (metoclopramide or chlorpromazine), and fluid support to prevent or treat dehydration.

In cats with vomiting due to intolerance (e.g. tetracycline), changing the drug protocol to another that will be effective is generally all that is indicated.

GASTRITIS/GASTRIC ULCER DISEASE

> ## Classical signs
>
> - Frequent vomiting is typical, but intermittent vomiting will occur in some cats.
> - Hematemesis or melena occurs with severe gastritis or bleeding ulcers.

See main reference on page 637 for details (The Cat With Signs of Acute Vomiting).

Clinical signs

Vomiting, either frequently or intermittently, is the primary clinical sign. Severe gastritis and ulcer disease will result in **anorexia, abdominal discomfort, lethargy or weight loss**.

Cats with severe gastritis or ulcer disease may also have **hematemesis or melena** from mucosal bleeding.

Diagnosis

Endoscopic examination of the gastric mucosa will often reveal the surface erosions or ulcers, however, **histologic examination** of the tissue is required to make a diagnosis of gastritis. Mild or chronic gastritis lesions may not have an abnormal mucosal appearance.

Gastric or duodenal ulcers can also be identified by **contrast radiography and by ultrasonography** in some cases, but these techniques are not as useful as endoscopy.

Most cats with gastritis will have a **normal hemogram and chemistry profile**. Cats with bleeding ulcers may have evidence of **acute** (non-regenerative if peracute, regenerative if recent) **or chronic blood loss** (may be either regenerative or non-regenerative depending on amount of hemorrhage).

Differential diagnosis

Helicobacter spp. infection, parasites (*Physaloptera, Ollanus* spp.), IBD, neoplasia, gastritis due to other extra-intestinal diseases.

In cats with ulcers that do not respond to standard therapy, ulcer disease due to a **gastrinoma should be**

ruled out. Diagnosis of a gastrinoma is made histologically by finding a neuroendocrine tumor, usually in the abdomen, and by confirming the presence of **hypergastrinemia** (serum gastrin levels that are extremely elevated) not due to secondary causes.

Treatment

Specific treatment is aimed at identifying and correcting the underlying cause.

Non-specific treatment for gastritis or gastric ulcers involves **reduction of gastric acid secretion, protection of the mucosa** to allow healing and **reduction of gastric retention or vomiting**. This is accomplished by:

Histamine-2 blockers: ranitidine (0.5–1.0 mg/kg PO q 12 h), famotidine (0.5–1.0 mg/kg PO q 12–24 h).

Proton pump inhibition: omeprazole (0.5–1.0 mg/kg PO q 24 h), note: this drug is difficult to dose in cats as it must be recompounded, but is the most effective acid suppression drug.

Mucosal protection: sucralfate (250–500 mg PO q 8–12 h) note: give at least 2 hours before giving H$_2$ blockers.

Anti-emetics: metoclopramide (0.1–0.2 mg/kg PO q 8–12 h) as needed to control vomiting, promote gastric emptying and reduce gastroesophageal reflux.

Feed only highly digestible, low-fat foods (e.g. Hill's i/d diet, Purina EN, Iams low-residue diet, etc.) **in small amounts.** In some cats, it is best to give them nothing per os until the gastritis/ulcer healing has begun and the vomiting is under control (1–3 days).

Hydration should be maintained with **IV or SQ fluids as needed**, if the cat is unable to eat or has severe vomiting.

CHRONIC RENAL FAILURE*

Classical signs

- Polyuria/polydipsia.
- Weight loss.
- Anorexia.
- Lethargy.
- Poor/hair coat/unkempt appearance.
- Vomiting.

See main reference on page 235 for details (The Cat With Polyuria/Polydipsia).

Clinical signs

Polyuria/polydipsia, anorexia or decreased appetite, and **weight loss** are the most common clinical signs of chronic renal failure.

An unkempt hair coat, decreased grooming and reduced overall activity level are also often observed.

Intermittent vomiting or diarrhea due to hypergastrinemia and uremia and uremic ulcers or stomatitis occur in severe cases.

Polyuria is profound until the late stages of the disease, when oliguria gradually develops with the progression to end-stage kidney disease.

Diagnosis

History and physical examination findings are suggestive of the diagnosis in a geriatric cat.

Hematology, serum biochemistry profile and urinalysis will confirm the presence of **azotemia, isosthenuria** or poorly concentrated urine (1.015–1.035), **mild to moderate non-regenerative anemia,** dehydration may also be present, along with **hypokalemia, hyperphosphatemia,** and evidence of chronic metabolic acidosis (low total CO$_2$).

Differential diagnosis

Hyperthyroidism, diabetes mellitus, hepatic disease (hepatic lipidosis if cat is/was obese) and neoplasia (lymphoma, adenocarcinoma, etc.) are important differentials in an old cat with polyuria/polydipsia and weight loss.

Treatment

Supportive. Fluid therapy as needed. **Sub-cutaneous fluids may be very important adjunctive therapy** in cats that do not drink enough or are vomiting, and have severe polyuria that results in dehydration and worsening azotemia.

Dietary manipulation. Feeding a diet that has a **moderate or low quantity of high-quality protein, reduced phosphorus, and relatively high in calories**, to maintain weight, decrease azotemia and reduce the effects of renal secondary hyperparathyroidism.

Phosphorus binders (e.g. amphogel) may be needed when dietary manipulation no longer is effective in reducing serum phosphorus levels.

Potassium supplementation (potassium gluconate) is needed in most cats with chronic renal failure due to potassium wasting and total body potassium depletion that occurs.

In cats with frequent vomiting, histamine-2 blockers (famotidine 0.5–1.0 mg/kg PO q 24 h, ranitidine 0.5–1.0 mg/kg) may be helpful in reducing hyperacidity and gastritis that occurs secondary to azotemia and hypergastrinemia.

Cats in more advanced stages of renal disease may have a significant **non-regenerative anemia (PCV < 20)** due to the lack of erythropoietin production from the failing kidney, which may respond, for a limited period of time, to treatment with **recombinant human erythropoietin.**

DIABETES MELLITUS*

Classical signs

- Polyuria/polydipsia.
- Weight loss.
- Polyphagia or anorexia.
- Lethargy, weakness and/or depression.
- Vomiting.

See main reference on page 236 for details (The Cat With Polyuria and Polydipsia).

Clinical signs

Signs of **polydipsia, polyuria, polyphagia and weight loss** may be **present for months prior to diagnosis**.

Approximately **one-third of cats with diabetes mellitus have a history of vomiting**. An **acute onset of vomiting** may occur with **ketoacidosis**.

The **classical signs of ketoacidosis** include **polyuria, polydipsia, anorexia, weight loss, dehydration, vomiting, weakness and depression**.

In some cats, other clinical signs may include **peripheral nerve dysfunction (plantegrade stance), dementia or stupor/coma**.

Diagnosis

The **clinical signs and history** of polyuria/polydipsia suggest that diabetes mellitus should be considered.

The **hemogram is non-specific,** hemoconcentration and a stress leukogram are common, however, some cats have an inflammatory leukogram secondary to infection (a common sequelae of unregulated diabetes mellitus).

A **serum biochemistry profile and urinalysis** will be **diagnostic.** The finding of **hyperglycemia with glucosuria with or without ketonuria, and in some cases bactiuria/pyuria is typical**. Other abnormalities likely to be observed include elevated liver enzymes, hypokalemia (may be severe), hypophosphatemia (may be severe), hypomagnesemia, low total CO_2 values (supportive of acidosis), and azotemia (may be pre-renal or renal in origin).

Other studies, such as imaging, blood gas analysis, etc. are used to further characterize the disease relative to severity and cause (e.g. pancreatitis, etc.), but **should not be done at the expense of initiating appropriate and immediate therapy.**

Differential diagnosis

The **differentials are numerous, based upon the history and clinical signs** (e.g. renal failure, hepatic disease, poisoning, neoplasia and inflammatory bowel disease) but a minimum data base will serve to confirm the presence of diabetes mellitus.

Treatment

Ketoacidotic diabetes mellitus can be a medical emergency, as many cats will have severe metabolic acidosis, dehydration and electrolyte disturbances that are life threatening unless addressed.

Fluid therapy (0.9% NaCl or Normosol) is the essential, but must be used judiciously in conjunction with **replacement of potassium, phosphorus and magnesium**, which are often severely depleted. Serum potassium may rapidly decrease during initial therapy and should be monitored very closely (q 2–4 h).

Insulin replacement is instituted with a short-acting insulin (e.g. regular insulin, 0.1–0.2 U/kg, IV or IM q

2–6 h or as a constant rate infusion). **Frequent monitoring (q 1–2 h) of blood glucose concentrations is necessary** so that when the blood glucose level drops below 16.8 mmol/L SI (300 mg/dl), 5% dextrose is added to the fluids.

In cats that are not severely acidotic, and are still eating and not vomiting, insulin treatment may be instituted with NPH insulin (0.25–0.5 U/kg, SQ q 12 h), or where available PZI or glargine, with monitoring of blood glucose levels (q 2–3 h).

Cats that have urinary tract or other infections should be treated with appropriate **antibiotics**.

Vomiting is controlled with metoclopramide (0.1–0.2 mg/kg q 12 h) as needed.

Cats that are able to eat without vomiting should be fed a **highly palatable diet** (see page 238). **High-protein, reduced-carbohydrate diets** are advantageous in both thin and obese diabetic cats unless they have concurrent renal disease and need to eat a lower-protein diet.

HELICOBACTER SPP.*

> ### Classical signs
>
> - The classical sign is vomiting.

Pathogenesis

Helicobacter organisms known to **colonize the feline stomach** include: *H. pylori*, *H. felis*, and *H. bizzozeronii*. Other *Helicobacter* spp. that have been identified in the small intestine and liver of cats include *H. cinaedi* and *H. fennelliae*. The significance of these organisms and their ability to cause clinical disease is unknown.

H. felis is commonly found in the stomach of cats and may not be a feline pathogen, but **H. pylori**, which causes peptic disease in humans, is believed to also be associated with **gastritis in cats**, especially cats in **colonies or catteries**. *H. bizzozeronii* is the most common gastric colonizer in cats, and has experimentally produced chronic gastritis in kittens.

Infection is primarily transmitted via the **oral–oral route. Organisms are present in vomitus, oral secretions and saliva**, and may be transmitted via improperly disinfected dental equipment, endoscopes and other instruments, or via contact with oral secretions directly.

Infection with *Helicobacter* organisms results in **increased infiltration of the mucosa with polymorphonuclear cells and mononuclear cells**, and is classified as **chronic gastritis**.

Persistent infection is associated with increased development of gastric lymphoid follicles, especially in the antrum, the location of heaviest concentration of organisms in most cats.

At this time, there does not appear to be a breed or sex predilection for infection or development of signs.

The classical sign is chronic vomiting due to gastritis, but the incidence and true importance of *Helicobacter* spp. in gastritis in cats is not known.

Clinical signs

Chronic vomiting, weight loss and in some cases, pica are reported in clinically affected cats.

However, **these organisms will be present in clinically healthy animals**, so a direct cause-and-effect relationship cannot be established.

Diagnosis

The diagnosis **is made by histologic examination of gastric mucosal tissue (usually obtained** via endoscopy). Either a **special silver stain or modified Giemsa stain** must be used to identify the organisms.

Culture and organism identification is also required to make a definitive diagnosis, since not all spiral organisms are pathogens or *Helicobacter* spp. *Helicobacter* spp. require **special media and handling for** successful culture in vitro.

Helicobacter **spp. produce urease** that can be used to provisionally diagnose their presence, by placing biopsy samples in urea broth or by using the **commercially available test** (CloTest). However, **this test is neither sensitive nor specific for *Helicobacter* infection**.

Serologic assays used in humans are not reliable for testing in cats because of the cross-reactivity between other spiral organisms (commonly present in normal cats) and *H. pylori* (the suspected pathogen).

Differential diagnosis

Chronic gastritis due to other causes such as hepatic disease, pancreatitis, chronic renal failure or IBD may result in a similar clinical presentation.

Treatment

There have been various treatment regimens recommended for cats with *Helicobacter* infection, but none have been well substantiated.

The triple therapy regimen has been the mainstay of treatment for *Helicobacter* infection. This is bismuth (0.5–2 ml/kg PO q 4–6 h), metronidazole (62.5 mg PO q 24 h), and amoxicillin (15–20 mg/kg PO q 12 h). This regimen with the addition of famotidine (0.5–1.0 mg/kg PO q 24 h) has been recommended in refractory or severe cases.

Famotidine (0.5–1 mg/kg PO q 24 h), ranitidine (1–2 mg/kg PO q 12 h), or omeprazole (0.5–1.0 mg/kg PO q 24 h), in addition to antibiotic therapy have more recently been recommended.

Other antibiotics that may be used include tetracycline (22 mg/kg PO q 8 h), clarithromycin (7.5 mg/kg PO q 12 h), or azithromycin (5 mg/kg PO q 24–48 h).

Pepto-bismol can be used (1 ml/kg PO q 24 h) to control gastritis due to *Helicobacter* infection, but salicylate toxicity has occasionally been observed in individual cats.

The **duration of treatment for infected cats** has also not been well substantiated, but **14–28 days** has been the standard recommendation.

Prevention

Unknown, but careful attention to cleanliness of endoscopes and dental equipment is advised.

Public health

H. felis and *H. heilmannii* both are capable of colonization of humans and cats, but are not particularly pathogenic. *H. pylori* has not been isolated reliably from pet cats, so the zoonotic potential of *Helicobacter* in pet cats as a cause of human gastritis (a significant problem) has not been shown.

Most epidemiologic studies do not incriminate pet contact with human infection, and only contact with commercially reared cats has been shown to have any potential for risk, suggesting the possibility of a reverse zoonotic infection.

HYPERCALCEMIA* (MALIGNANCY, CHOLECALCIFEROL TOXICITY, CHRONIC RENAL FAILURE, HYPERPARATHYROIDISM, IDIOPATHIC HYPERCALCEMIA)

Classical signs

- Signs vary with the cause of hypercalcemia.
- Anorexia, vomiting and weight loss are typical.
- Polyuria and polydipsia are late signs, due to renal failure.
- Muscle weakness or tremors may occur acutely.

See main reference on page 245 (The Cat With Polyuria and Polydipsia) for details.

Clinical signs

Vomiting may be due to the disease causing the increased serum calcium or to the direct effects of elevated calcium stimulating vomiting receptors both peripherally or centrally.

The signs are dependent upon the cause of hypercalcemia, which can be due to the presence of malignancy, ingestion of cholecalciferol-containing rodenticides, endocrinopathies (primarily primary hyperparathyroidism) or idiopathic.

Signs associated with large elevations in serum calcium include **anorexia, vomiting, muscle weakness, polyuria and polydipsia**, **shaking/tremors and weight loss**.

Hypercalcemia has also been associated with the **development of calcium-containing nephroliths or uroliths**, which may cause signs of renal or bladder dysfunction.

Generally, **in cats, hypercalcemia is rare,** but if present is most commonly caused by renal failure or is secondary to malignancy. In some cats, the cause cannot be identified. Other rarer causes include vitamin D toxicosis, primary hyperparathyroidism, hyperthyroidism, hypoadrenocorticoism and granulomalous disease.

Diagnosis

Hypercalcemia of malignancy is most often secondary to lymphoma, but may be due to multiple myeloma, adenocarcinoma and squamous cell carcinoma. Diagnosis of this disorder is based upon finding the primary tumor, an elevation of PTH-rP but not of iPTH in serum, and a response to therapy.

Primary hyperparathyroidism is rare in cats, but will be associated with an increased iPTH assay, a decrease in serum phosphorus and lack of other primary abnormalities.

Cholecalciferol poisoning is associated with a decrease in both the iPTH assay and PTH-rP assay, hyperphosphatemia and often evidence of mineralization of abdominal and other soft tissues.

Chronic renal failure (renal secondary hyperparathyroidism) is associated with an elevated iPTH and PTH-rP assay, but normal or decreased ionized calcium. Ionized calcium will be elevated with all other causes of hypercalcemia.

Recently, idiopathic hypercalcemia has been reported in cats and acidifying diets were implicated. This is associated with an increased serum total calcium or serum ionized calcium concentration, or both. Serum iPTH concentrations are low or in the low–normal range, while serum PTHrP is usually undetectable. Serum 25-hydroxycholecalciferol (vitamin D3) concentrations are normal in affected cats, as are serum phosphorus and albumin levels.

Phosphorous concentrations are normal or low–normal in all causes of hypercalcemia except cholecalciferol toxicity or renal failure, unless renal failure develops secondary to hypercalcemia.

Treatment

Specific treatment of hypercalcemia is directed at correcting the underlying cause if possible.

Supportive therapy measures to control or reduce hypercalcemia include **correction of fluid deficits and fluid diuresis** with physiologic saline (60–180 ml/kg/day) and **administration of drugs that induce calciuresis** (furosemide 2–4 mg/kg PO q 12 h, or prednisolone 1–2 mg/kg PO q 12 h).

In severe, life-threatening hypercalcemia, where the above measures are inadequate, **sodium bicarbonate** (0.5–2 mEq/kg in IV fluids over 6 hours), **salmon calcitonin** (4 U/kg IV q 12–24 h) **and dialysis** (peritoneal or hemodialysis) **may be necessary.**

Other long-term therapeutic measures include feeding **a low-calcium diet** (Hill's k/d, u/d).

FELINE VIRAL DISEASES (FeLV, FIV, FIP)

> ## Classical signs
>
> - Weight loss, anorexia and lethargy are the most common signs.
> - Vomiting is less common.
> - ± Fever

See main reference on pages 540, 339, 372 for details.

Clinical signs

Specific signs depend upon the effect of the infection on the individual cat, e.g. development of neoplastic disease, bone marrow involvement, secondary infections and local (granuloma formation in FIP) or systemic disease (CNS, respiratory, hepatic, effusions).

The **most common signs** are **weight loss, anorexia and lethargy or depression**.

Feline leukemia virus (FeLV) is often associated with **neoplastic disease** (lymphoma, bone marrow infiltration) or **bone marrow dyscrasias** (cytopenias, myelodysplasias, etc.). Vomiting may occur associated with lymphoma.

Feline immunodeficiency virus (FIV) results in immunodeficiency disease that often results in **secondary infections** being the cause of significant morbidity and mortality. The skin, respiratory system and the gastrointestinal tract are most often affected.

The **classical presentation of effusive feline infections peritonitis (FIP)** is anorexia, lethargy, fever, weight loss, abdominal enlargement and dyspnea due to the **pleural and peritoneal effusion** of fluid.

Non-effusive FIP may present with a **wide variety of clinical signs depending on the system involved,** including chorioretinitis, fever, vomiting and/or diarrhea, abdominal pain (renal, liver), anorexia, lethargy and weight loss.

Diagnosis

Diagnosis of FeLV is by **ELISA antigen testing** and confirmation with serum or bone marrow IFA if the diagnosis is in doubt. PCR testing can also be performed in FeLV-suspect cats for confirmation.

FIV infection is detected by an **antibody test** and confirmed either via western blot analysis or **PCR testing** for the presence of viral proteins. (Note: vaccinated cats will test positive on the antibody test.)

Diagnosis of FIP is a very difficult process because of the lack of a definitive test that is sensitive and specific enough to differentiate enteric corona viral infections from FIP (a mutant of enteric corona virus).

Antibody titers are available, but detect the presence of any corona virus (feline enteric, canine enteric, FIP, etc.). Most cats from catteries, shelter situations or large, multi-cat populations will be exposed to enteric corona virus because of the ubiquitous nature of the virus in these settings (up to 85–90%). Thus, antibody testing of cats from these environments will be quite difficult to interpret. **Specific ELISA tests for the 7B protein** in FIP have **not proved to be reliable** in the field.

Serum PCR testing for FIP shows great promise for becoming a definitive diagnostic test, but the currently available serum tests still are not reliable tests for distinguishing FIP versus enteric corona virus. **The PCR test is an excellent means of ruling out FIP (negative test means the cat does not have FIP).** However, **a positive serum PCR test does not prove the cat has FIP.**

The **definitive diagnosis of FIP** still requires **histologic examination of tissues** for the classical changes or virus isolation. This is not usually necessary in cats with effusive FIP, but non-effusive FIP has such variable clinical signs and progression that the diagnosis is quite challenging.

PCR on tissue samples which have classic changes is also a good diagnostic test for FIP.

HISTOPLASMOSIS*

> ### Classical signs
>
> - Dyspnea, wheezing or coughing are classical signs.
> - Signs of gastrointestinal, CNS, or hemolymphatic system disturbances occur with systemic involvement.

See main reference on page 755 for details.

Clinical signs

The **classical presenting signs are respiratory: dyspnea, wheezing or coughing**.

In cats with systemic histoplasmosis, the gastrointestinal tract, CNS or the skeletal system may be involved. The **GI tract signs are typically associated with diarrhea**, but in some cases, vomiting is observed, along with anorexia, weight loss and lethargy.

In generalized histoplasmosis, more non-specific signs may occur, such as anorexia, weight loss, fever, lymphadenopathy and lethargy.

Nervous system signs are rare and typically associated with seizures, changes in mentation or meningitis (neck or back pain, other neurologic signs such as ataxia, cranial nerve signs or weakness).

The **hemolymphatic system** involvement is manifest primarily as **bone marrow infiltration** with the fungus, which crowds out the red cell, white cell and/or platelet precursors, so the clinical signs are variable depending on the extent of marrow destruction.

Diagnosis

This disease has a **regional occurrence**, so a supportive history in a cat from an endemic area is suggestive.

In cats with **pulmonary histoplasmosis**, there may be very few hematologic or serum biochemical changes (e.g. leukocytosis, mild anemia, hyperproteinemia due to increased gamma globulins).

Disseminated histoplasmosis will often be associated with increases in liver enzyme activities, abnormal hemogram (bone marrow involvement causing anemia, thrombocytopenia, etc.), or changes associated with protein losing enteropathy (hypoproteinemia, hypo-albuminemia, hypocholesterolemia, altered serum electrolytes).

Radiographs will be useful in cats with pulmonary disease, but less helpful with evaluation of other organs. Cats with intestinal histoplasmosis often have thickened loops of bowel that can be seen radiographically or via ultrasound imaging. **Ultrasound** may be useful in assessing liver and GI tract involvement.

Serology is available for detection of systemic fungal infections, including histoplasmosis, but the tests have a **high percentage of false negatives** in cats.

The **definitive diagnosis is obtained by finding organisms** in the affected tissues.

Endoscopic or surgical biopsy, fine-needle aspirates by ultrasound guidance, bone marrow examination or bronchial washing are necessary to obtain the diagnosis. In cats with signs of GI disease, especially diarrhea, rectal scrapings may also reveal the organism.

TOXOPLASMOSIS*

Classical signs

- Toxoplasmosis is a systemic disease involving multiple organs systems.
- Respiratory tract signs (dyspnea, coughing, rhinitis).
- CNS signs (ataxia, behavioral changes, seizures, circling).
- Hepatic disease signs (vomiting, diarrhea, icterus, anorexia, lethargy, weight loss, abdominal effusion, or discomfort).
- Cardiac signs (arrhythmias, sudden death).
- Ocular signs (chorioretinitis, anterior uveitis, optic neuritis, blindness, anisocoria, glaucoma or retinal detachment).
- Rarely GIT granuloma causing vomiting.

See main reference on page 375 for details.

Clinical signs

Toxoplasmosis is a systemic, multi-organ disease that often affects young kittens, but adult cats are also infected, especially those with FIV or feline leukemia virus infection.

Infected cats most frequently have respiratory tract disease (dyspnea, coughing, rhinitis), **CNS disease** (ataxia, behavioral changes, seizures, circling), **hepatic disease** (vomiting, diarrhea, icterus, anorexia, lethargy, weight loss, abdominal effusion or discomfort), **cardiac disease** (arrhythmias, sudden death) **or ocular disease** (chorioretinitis, anterior uveitis, optic neuritis, blindness, anisocoria, glaucoma or retinal detachment).

Adult cats with FIV have more multi-systemic signs, while cats without FIV often have ocular or neurologic signs only.

Occasionally, toxoplasma granulomas (tissue cysts) form in the GIT or pancreas, rather than encysting in muscle, and result in chronic vomiting. The encysted organisms cause immune complex formation that is responsible for the granuloma formation and the chronic, but sublethal clinical disease.

Diagnosis

Hemogram abnormalities: **non-regenerative anemia, neutrophilic leukocytosis, lymphocytosis and eosinophilia** are most commonly observed.

Lymphopenia may be present in cats with FIV or end-stage disease.

Biochemical abnormalities are common with systemic disease and include: hypoproteinemia, hypoalbuminemia, hyperglobulinemia, elevated liver enzyme activities (hepatic involvement), increased creatine kinase (muscle involvement), hyperbilirubinemia (cats with cholangitis), proteinuria is also relatively common.

In focal GIT *Toxoplasma* granuloma, biochemical abnormalities may be minimal.

Diagnosis is based on finding the organism in tissues (cytology or histopathology) or by serologic testing.

Thoracic radiographs in cats with acute disease will reveal a diffuse interstitial pattern with a mottled lobar distribution.

Fecal examination for oocysts in cats is usually not helpful since less than 1% of infected cats shed the oocysts on any given day.

Serologic testing is currently the best method of detection, but because of the presence of antibodies in both healthy and diseased cats, titers must be used cautiously. **No single serologic test can definitively confirm toxoplasmosis.**

Serum ELISA tests for IgM, IgG and IgA are readily available and have been used to try to distinguish acute from chronic infections in cats. Finding of a **high IgM titer, along with a four-fold increase over 2–3 weeks (or decrease) in IgG titer** (in the presence of appropriate clinical signs, and response to anti-toxoplasma drugs, e.g. clindamycin) is suggestive of recent or active toxoplasmosis.

Other tests of serum IgG supportive of toxoplasma infection are the **modified agglutination test (MAT)** and the latex agglutination test (LAT). The MAT is the most sensitive test of IgG antibody, but is not uniformly available. The LAT cannot distinguish antibody classes, thus is less useful.

Aqueous humor and CSF titers are also useful, but should be compared with serum titers to determine if local immunoglobulin production is occurring.

INTESTINAL MAST CELL TUMOR*

> ### Classical signs
>
> - Weight loss and anorexia are the most common early signs.
> - Intermittent or persistent vomiting, diarrhea and lethargy or depression become more prevalent with advancing disease.

Pathogenesis

Mast cell tumors of the intestine are the **third most common GI tract neoplasm** in cats behind lymphoma and intestinal adenocarcinoma.

These are tumors of **old (mean age = 13 years) cats**, with **no breed or sex predilection**. They occur with about the same frequency as mast cell tumors of the lymphoreticular system (e.g. spleen, lymph nodes and bone marrow), but **cats with intestinal mast cell tumors typically do not have circulating mast cells.**

Intestinal mast cell tumors are usually solitary, and affect the **distal small intestine**, but multiple masses can occur. Typically, they appear as a **segmented nodular thickening in the small intestine**.

Mast cell tumors of the GI tract are usually **poorly differentiated** (thus cytologic examination is difficult) and **highly malignant,** with metastasis to the mesenteric lymph nodes, liver and spleen. They are generally not functional tumors and are **not typically associated with gastrointestinal ulcer disease**. However, there may be chronic bleeding from the tumor into the GIT.

No association with FeLV, FIV or FIP has been reported.

Clinical signs

The **most common clinical signs** in cats with an intestinal mast cell tumor are **weight loss, lethargy and anorexia.**

Intermittent or persistent **vomiting, diarrhea and lethargy** or depression become **more prevalent with advancing disease**.

Vomiting and/or diarrhea may also be observed, but often not until late in the disease.

Other signs include ascites, splenic enlargement (metastasis), and rarely, mast cells in circulation (bone marrow involvement).

Diagnosis

Palpation of an intestinal mass in an older cat is suggestive of neoplasia, but **these tumors may be very small.**

Abnormalities of the hemogram or serum chemistry profile are uncommon, but may include anemia (non-regenerative), hypoproteinemia and elevated liver enzyme activities.

Survey radiographs may identify a mass, evidence of intestinal obstruction, or mild peritoneal effusion, but contrast radiography will be required to identify the location and extent of many of these tumors.

Ultrasonography is a useful tool in identifying the location, extent and presence of metastatic lesions. **Fine-needle aspiration or biopsy** of these masses by ultrasound guidance may be useful, but because of the poorly differentiated nature of the tumor they may also be non-diagnostic.

Analysis of peritoneal effusion fluid may be helpful if mast cells are present, but as with fine-needle aspirates, the effusion may be suggestive of neoplasia, but not necessarily give a definitive diagnosis.

Definitive diagnosis requires histopathologic examination of the tissue, which is usually best achieved by wide surgical resection and anastomosis.

Staging of the tumor is achieved by biopsy of mesenteric lymph nodes, spleen, liver and bone marrow aspiration (if indicated). **The tumor rarely metastasizes out of the abdomen**.

Differential diagnosis

Other intestinal neoplasia, foreign body, fungal or algal disease, inflammatory bowel disease, and extra-intestinal causes of anorexia, weight loss and vomiting (chronic renal failure, hyperthyroidism, etc.) are all differentials that should be considered.

Treatment

Surgical resection is the only known treatment. Surgical margins must be > 5 cm beyond the visible edge of the lesion because of the cellular invasion that occurs along the tumor mass.

Metastasis occurs early in the course of the disease to the spleen, liver and regional lymph nodes.

Other forms of therapy (**chemotherapy, radiation, etc.) have either been ineffective or not evaluated. Adjunct therapy with cimetidine, anti-histamines and prednisone** may be tried to control signs associated with mast cell degranulation, but are **often not helpful** because these tumors are typically poorly differentiated and **do not produce granules or GI ulcer disease**.

Nutritional support (enteral or parenteral nutrition) may be required for cats that do not want to eat or are vomiting.

Prognosis

The **prognosis is poor** for cats with this disease.

Despite surgical removal, **cats with intestinal mast cell tumors rarely live longer than 4 months**.

FOREIGN BODIES*

> ## Classical signs
>
> - The classical sign is an acute onset of frequent vomiting.
> - Intermittent vomiting will occur in some cats with foreign bodies that are causing an intermittent or incomplete obstruction (e.g. string).

See main reference on page 636 for details.

Clinical signs

The **classical sign is an acute onset of frequent vomiting**, but intermittent vomiting will occur in some cats with foreign bodies that are causing an **intermittent or incomplete obstruction** (e.g. string).

There may or may not be palpable abnormalities in the intestinal tract, and most cats will be clinically normal otherwise.

Diagnosis

The **definitive diagnosis** is usually made by **contrast radiography**, however, survey radiographs or **ultrasound examination** may also reveal abnormalities that are consistent with a GI foreign body.

String foreign bodies often are found attached to the base of the tongue, thus a **thorough oral exam is always essential in cats with a suspected GI foreign body.**

Some foreign bodies can be found and retrieved by **gastrointestinal or colonic endoscopy**. In many cases, these foreign objects are metallic and will be visible on survey radiographs.

Differential diagnosis

Gastric parasites, heartworm disease, *Helicobacter* spp. gastritis, food intolerance, food allergy, and antral pyloric hypertrophy or stenosis are primary differentials because they all may cause vomiting in the absence of other signs of disease.

Treatment

Surgical removal of the foreign body is required if it is not able to be retrieved and removed via an endoscopic procedure.

CONGESTIVE HEART FAILURE*

> **Classical signs**
>
> - Coughing or dyspnea.
> - Lethargy.
> - Anorexia.
> - Exercise intolerance.
> - Weight loss.

See main reference on page 124 for details (The Cat With Abnormal Heart Sounds and/or an Enlarged Heart).

Clinical signs

Classical signs of congestive heart failure include **dyspnea, coughing, cyanosis, pale mucous membranes**, poor pulse quality, inappetence, exercise intolerance/weakness and lethargy. Cats are usually presented with acute dyspnea and cyanosis.

The **signs may be quite variable** depending on the cause of heart failure. **Valvular disease** is often associated with an **audible murmur**, while **heart muscle diseases** often are associated with **tachycardia, gallop rhythm and weak pulses**.

Other signs that may be observed in cats with heart failure include collapse, vomiting, weight loss, limb paresis/paralysis due to thromboembolic disease, and rarely, abdominal distention.

Other cats may develop pleural effusion that increases respiratory effort but is not associated with coughing or increased lung sounds (decreased or absent lung sounds are present).

Vomiting episodes are typically chronic, but infrequent and more commonly associated with heart muscle disease (myopathy) rather than valvular disease.

Diagnosis

History and physical examination findings will be suggestive of congestive heart failure, especially if the cat has a murmur, gallop rhythm or other signs referable to primary heart disease.

Hematology and serum biochemical profile data may reveal **mild, non-specific changes,** such as anemia of chronic disease, prerenal azotemia, elevations in liver enzyme activities secondary to congestion, and changes in electrolytes and proteins consistent with dehydration. If myositis is a differential for the cause of heart failure, elevated creatine kinase values may be useful additional information.

Imaging studies are necessary to make a **definitive diagnosis**. In particular, **thoracic radiographs** will be helpful in assessing **cardiac size and pulmonary involvement** (edema vs. pleural effusion, etc.). **Cardiac ultrasound examination** is the best diagnostic test for evaluating cardiac muscle function, size and presence of valvular or other defects.

Electrocardiography may also be useful to detect or document any **arrhythmias.**

SYSTEMIC NEOPLASIA*(GENERALIZED LYMPHOMA, SYSTEMIC MASTOCYTOSIS)

> **Classical signs**
>
> - Weight loss.
> - Lethargy or depression.
> - Anorexia.
> - Enlarged spleen or liver, lymph nodes or bone marrow involvement.

Clinical signs

The **most common clinical finding** is marked **hepatomegaly or splenomegaly** along with **enlarged lymph nodes** (mesenteric).

Other common signs are **vomiting and anorexia**.

In some cases, **peritoneal effusion** will be present, which along with the hepatomegaly or splenomegaly will be observed as **profound abdominal enlargement**.

Diagnosis

Definitive diagnosis is obtained by **fine-needle aspiration of the enlarged liver, spleen or lymph nodes.**

Mast cells or lymphoblasts/cytes may also be found in the systemic circulation on routine hematology, and will also be found on examination of **bone marrow aspirates**. In addition, **anemia and cytopenias are also common findings** on hematologic exams.

Ultrasound or radiographic evaluation will reveal the extreme size of the liver and spleen and ultrasound guidance can be used in obtaining fine-needle aspirates (especially of lymph nodes or sections of the liver that have obvious structural abnormalities).

CNS DISEASES* (ENCEPHALITIS, VESTIBULAR DISEASE, SEIZURE DISORDERS, NEOPLASIA)

Classical signs

- Neurologic signs localized to the region of the CNS that is affected (e.g. vestibular disease is associated with loss of balance, ataxia, falling to one side, head tilt, nystagmus, etc.).
- Vomiting is infrequent.

Clinical signs

The predominant clinical signs will be **neurologic signs that are localized to the region of the CNS that is affected.** Vestibular disease can be associated with vomiting, but typical signs include loss of balance, ataxia, falling to one side, head tilt and nystagmus. **Most neurologic diseases that cause vomiting affect the CNS,** not the spinal cord or peripheral nervous system, except for the peripheral parts of cranial nerve VIII located in the inner ear.

Vomiting is an infrequent but still important sign of CNS disturbance most often associated with involvement of the **peripheral vestibular system.**

Cats with signs of **hepatoencephalopathy** (changes in behavior, stupor, drooling or ataxia) may vomit from the effects on the CNS or the GIT.

Diagnosis

A thorough **neurologic examination** is the first step in determining if neurologic disease is present and in attempting to determine if the disease is affecting the central, spinal or peripheral nervous system.

Other important diagnostic tests for diseases in the CNS include CSF analysis, including culture and serology (FIP, toxoplasmosis, fungal disease), computed tomography or MRI imaging, electroencephalogram, and brainstem auditory-evoked response (middle/inner ear).

Radiographs of the middle/inner ear areas are non-specific and very difficult to evaluate, and have **largely been replaced by CT** as a means of assessing this region. However, **middle and inner ear infections** can also be diagnosed via **myringotomy and culture of fluid** from the middle ear.

Unless a systemic disease process is the cause of the CNS signs, the **minimum data base is likely to be normal.**

PHYSALOPTERA

Classical signs

- The classical sign is frequent vomiting, but intermittent vomiting will occur in some cats.

See main reference on page 653 for details (The Cat With Signs of Acute Vomiting).

Clinical signs

The **predominant clinical sign is vomiting**. Most cats will present with an acute onset of vomiting, but others may have intermittent, chronic vomiting.

Diagnosis

Fecal floatation and finding of the **larvated eggs** in the feces (**shedding is intermittent**, so multiple feces are required) is diagnostic, but unrewarding.

Finding of **small worms in vomitus or on endoscopic examination.**

Response to a **therapeutic trial with fenbendazole** (25 mg/kg PO q 24 h for 3–5 days).

HEARTWORM DISEASE (*DIROFILARIA IMMITIS*)

Classical signs

- Signs are variable.
- No signs may be present.
- Signs of respiratory disease (tachypnea, dyspnea).
- Intermittent vomiting.
- Signs of cardiovascular disease (lethargy, anorexia, coughing, weakness).
- Sudden death.

See main reference on page 139 for details.

Clinical signs

Anorexia and weight loss are the **most common signs** observed in cats with dirofilariasis.

Respiratory signs such as wheezing, dyspnea, and occasionally coughing are less common than in dogs, and often **mimic feline asthma**.

Intermittent vomiting is a relatively frequent sign associated with feline heartworm disease that may occur in the absence of other clinical signs.

Sudden death is a complication of heartworm disease in cats, and may occur in 20–30% of infected cats.

Diagnosis

A history of **living in a heartworm endemic area** along with the **appropriate clinical signs** in the absence of heartworm preventative use should arouse clinical suspicion.

Hematology may reveal an **eosinophilia or basophilia**.

Unless cats have developed heart failure, the chemistry profile and urinalysis are usually normal. Cats that are in right congestive heart failure may have elevated liver enyzme activities or azotemia.

Radiographs of the thorax will reveal the **classic changes associated with heartworm disease**, which are enlarged pulmonary arteries, arterial tortuosity or blunting, pulmonary interstitial pattern and right-sided cardiac enlargement.

Ultrasound can also be used to identify worms in the main pulmonary artery or right ventricle, but the sensitivity of this test is highly dependent on operator experience.

A **heartworm antibody test** is the recommended **screening test** for cats, and while it does not confirm infection, it is an accurate means of confirming exposure. However, **it may remain positive for 18 months or more after resolution of infection, and also may be positive if arrested larval infection has occurred.**

Because cats generally have only 1–2 worms present, the **standard heartworm antigen tests used in dogs are often not sensitive enough to detect the disease in cats.**

A feline antigen test has been developed, and detects the presence of a single male worm, but false-negative tests still occur. Antigen tests should not be the sole means of evaluating cats for heartworm infection.

HYPOADRENOCORTICISM (ADDISON'S DISEASE)

Classical signs

- Lethargy, anorexia and weight loss are most common.
- Vomiting.
- Polyuria, polydipsia.
- Clinical signs may wax and wane.

See main reference on page 252 for details.

Clinical signs

This is a very rare disease in cats.

The classical signs are **lethargy, anorexia and weight loss**. Other signs that may be seen are vomiting, polyuria/polydipsia, weakness and waxing/waning signs.

Most cats (> 50%) will be **hypothermic, dehydrated or depressed on physical examination**, but other signs such as weak pulses, bradycardia and collapse are less common.

Diagnosis

The **history and clinical signs will be vague in early cases**, so that a degree of clinical suspicion is required to make the diagnosis.

Anemia, lymphocytosis and eosinophilia are relatively uncommon (< 20%) findings in cats.

Serum biochemistries and urinalysis show **hyponatremia, azotemia (pre-renal or renal), and hyperphosphatemia** in the majority of cats. Hyperkalemia and hypochloridemia are also common, but not seen in every case.

Other less common (< 30% cases reported) abnormalities include metabolic acidosis, increased liver enzyme activities, hypercalcemia and hyperbilirubinemia.

Slightly more than 50% of affected cats will have an **unconcentrated urine sample (SG < 1.030)**, supporting renal azotemia.

The **definitive diagnostic test** for hypoadrenocorticism is an **ACTH stimulation test**, which will reveal a low resting cortisol concentration, and no response (no increase in cortisol levels) following administration of ACTH (Cosyntropin 0.125 mg/cat, IM), at either the 30 or 60 min post-administration sampling times. Administration of steroids by any route (oral, parenteral or topically) or progestins (e.g. megestrol acetate) will suppress cortisol response to ACTH. This suppression may persist for weeks after the last time of administration, especially if administration was chronic.

Radiographic changes include microcardia and hypoperfusion of the lungs due to hypovolemia. **ECG changes classically observed in dogs,** such as peaked T waves, reduced or absent P waves, or atrial standstill are not seen in cats.

If serum electrolyte concentrations are normal, but a subnormal response to ACTH administration is observed, the cat may have: (1) residual mineralocorticoid secretion; (2) secondary hypoadrenocorticism from pituitary or hypothalamic disease causing only glucocorticoid deficiency but this has not yet been reported in cats; or (3) **secondary hypoadrenocorticism due to exogenous administration of glucocorticoids or progestogens.** Although this is the most common cause of secondary hypoadrenocorticism and suppressed adrenal response to ACTH, it rarely causes sufficient lethargy for veterinary attention to be sought. If clinical signs consistent with hypoadrenocorticism are present in a cat with a suppressed ACTH stimulation test secondary to steroid administration, the signs are most likely caused by another disease.

To differentiate pituitary or hypothalamic disease from exogenous drug administration as the cause of secondary hypoadrenocorticism, **plasma ACTH concentration** is measured.

INTUSSUSCEPTION

Classical signs

- The classical sign is an acute onset of frequent vomiting.
- Intermittent vomiting will occur in some cats.

See main reference on page 643 for details.

Clinical signs

An **acute onset of vomiting, abdominal pain or anorexia is the most common sign**. However, in some cats with **sliding, intermittent or incomplete intussusception**, the signs may be intermittent. **Weight loss and vomiting** will be more prevalent in these cats.

Diagnosis

A palpable abdominal mass may help direct the diagnostic approach if it is present.

Contrast radiographs or ultrasound examination of the GI tract are the most definitive means of making the diagnosis.

Intussusception rarely presents as a chronic problem, so in these cases, abnormalities associated with chronic GI dysfunction (e.g. hypoproteinemia, hypoalbuminemia) may be present.

LEAD POISONING

Classical signs

- Gastrointestinal signs include anorexia, vomiting, diarrhea and abdominal pain.
- Neurologic signs include aggression, nervousness, tremors, seizures, blindness and dementia.

See main reference on page 596 for details.

Clinical signs

Gastrointestinal signs include anorexia, vomiting, diarrhea and abdominal pain. Weight loss is common.

Neurologic signs include aggression, nervousness, tremors, seizures, blindness and dementia.

GI signs tend to occur **acutely** and **before neurologic signs**. **CNS signs** are associated with **severe toxicity or chronicity.**

Diagnosis

There may be a history of exposure to lead-containing materials in the environment (paints, roofing materials, batteries, used motor oil, lead shot, etc.).

Characteristic clinical signs (the **combination of gastrointestinal and neurologic signs**) are suggestive.

There are **typical hemogram changes** including basophilic stippling of RBCs, and increased numbers of nucleated RBCs, although these are not as common in the cat as in the dog.

Radiographs may reveal radiopaque material in the GIT.

The **definitive diagnosis** is made by measurement of a **blood lead level** (> 0.5 ppm is diagnostic).

Treatment

Gastric lavage or **induction of emesis** should be performed to remove the offending materials from the stomach, **if ingestion was recent**. If the material can be retrieved by endoscopy or surgical removal (e.g. it is a large object) it should be done.

Oral activated charcoal should be administered to reduce the absorption of the material from the GIT.

An IV catheter should be placed and **supportive fluid therapy** (Normosol or LRS, 40–60 ml/kg IV) should be commenced.

Calcium EDTA to chelate lead and hasten excretion can also be used (25 mg/kg q 6 h IV as 10 mg Ca EDTA/ml in dextrose, maximum 2–5 days).

If seizures or other severe neurologic signs are present, **appropriate seizure control** (e.g. IV valium 2.5–5 mg or phenobarbital 1–4 mg/kg IM) should be used.

If the cat is debilitated and anorectic, **nutritional support** may also have to be instituted.

OTHER INTESTINAL NEOPLASIA (FIBROSARCOMA, CARCINOIDS, PLASMACYTOMA, LEIOMYOSARCOMA, ETC.)

Classical signs

- Weight loss.
- Lethargy or depression.
- Anorexia.
- Vomiting and/or diarrhea.

Clinical signs

The **clinical signs observed will depend upon the tumor location** in the GI tract.

In cats, **anorexia, weight loss and lethargy are the most common clinical signs** of any gastrointestinal neoplastic disease.

Vomiting and/or diarrhea may be observed, but will be variable depending on whether the tumor is in the small intestine or colon, and whether it is diffuse or solitary in extent.

Diagnosis

Palpation of an intestinal mass is an important diagnostic tool, since many of these tumors are solitary and produce strictures or obstructions.

Hematology and serum biochemistry profiles may be **within normal limits** in cats with intestinal neoplasia.

Abnormalities associated with secondary effects of the tumor include dehydration, electrolyte imbalances, anemia of chronic disease, etc.

Radiographs of both the thorax and abdomen are an important, but sometimes non-diagnostic, tool. Radiographs are best for assessment of **pulmonary metastasis**.

Ultrasound is an invaluable tool for **lesion localization**, determination of **lesion extent** and in some cases, obtaining a **fine-needle aspirate** or biopsy of the lesion.

Definitive diagnosis is by **histopathologic evaluation of a biopsy** or tissue obtained after surgical resection.

ANTRAL PYLORIC HYPERTROPHY/STENOSIS

> ### Classical signs
>
> - Vomiting several hours after eating.
> - Projectile vomiting will be observed if the pylorus is obstructed.
> - Abdominal distention or pain may be observed due to gastric distention.

Pathogenesis

Antral pyloric hypertrophy is a condition that involves **hyperplasia of the pyloric musculature**, **pyloric mucosa or both**, which results in narrowing or complete obstruction of the gastric outflow tract.

The condition can be **congenital or acquired**, but in either case, the exact cause is unknown.

Both **neural dysfunction and endocrinopathies (hypergastrinemia)** have been proposed to be involved in the disease.

The obstruction of gastric outflow results in **gastric retention and subsequent gastric distention. Gastric distention stimulates gastrin secretion** which is trophic to antral tissues and may further contribute to mucosal hypertrophy.

In some cases of **congenital pyloric stenosis** there is no antral hypertrophy. The gastric retention is believed to be due to a **motility disturbance** that results in a functional obstruction.

For reasons that are yet unknown, the disorder has been observed primarily in **Siamese cats**.

Clinical signs

Vomiting is the most common sign.

In **congenital pyloric stenosis**, kittens begin to vomit shortly after they commence solid food.

Acquired pyloric hypertrophy has a more variable presentation, but is usually associated with **intermittent vomiting of digested food several hours after consumption**. If the pylorus is completely obstructed the vomiting may be projectile.

Chronic intermittent vomiting and gastric distention may lead to **gastroesophageal reflux or esophagitis** which may be associated with **regurgitation or inappetence and weight loss**.

Diagnosis

History and signalment will be suggestive of a gastric emptying disturbance.

Hemogram, serum chemistries and urinalysis are typically **unremarkable**.

Survey radiographs of the abdomen may be normal, show gastric distention, or pyloric abnormalities. **Contrast radiographs** may identify hypertrophic gastric mucosa or a narrow gastric outflow pathway ("beak sign").

Ultrasonography may detect a thickened pyloric antrum if it is present.

Fluoroscopy or scintigraphy can be used to evaluate **gastric peristalsis and emptying**, but are not universally available.

Gastric endoscopy may be normal or may reveal thickened folds of mucosa, the pyloric antrum may not insufflate normally, or the pylorus may be too stenotic to allow passage of the endoscope through the orifice.

Definitive diagnosis requires an **exploratory laparotomy and histopathologic examination of tissue** for antral pyloric hypertrophy, but motility disturbances can only be diagnosed via fluoroscopy/scintigraphy, and hypergastrinemia can be detected by measurement of serum gastrin levels.

Differential diagnosis

Neoplasia (gastric adenocarcinoma, leiomyosarcoma, lymphosarcoma) of the gastric, pancreatic or duodenal tissues resulting in pyloric thickening and obstruction should be considered, especially in older cats.

Neoplasia of surrounding tissues resulting in gastric outflow obstruction from an external source, or a gastric foreign body resulting in obstruction or decreased out-flow may also result in similar clinical signs.

Gastric ulcer disease may result in chronic vomiting and abnormal motility.

Extra-gastrointestinal causes of vomiting include hepatic, renal, metabolic, inflammatory (pancreatitis) or endocrine causes.

Treatment

Definitive treatment for pyloric antral hypertrophy/stenosis is **surgical correction of the outflow obstruction.**

In cats with **motility disturbances**, **gastric prokinetic therapy** (metoclopramide 0.1–0.2 mg/kg PO q 12 h, or cisapride 5 mg/cat PO q 8–12 h) may improve movement of ingesta and reduce clinical signs.

However, **in early cases**, medical management with **feeding of small meals consisting of highly digestible foods** (low residue, low fat, low fiber) may also be helpful.

Following surgical correction of the outflow obstruction, some animals will still require medical therapy with gastric prokinetics because of residual motility disturbances.

Prognosis

The prognosis is **guarded to good with surgical management**, as some animals may still require life-long medical management following surgery to control the clinical signs.

Cats that develop **esophagitis due to reflux disease** may have a **more guarded prognosis** because of the problems associated with esophagitis (stricture development).

DYSAUTONOMIA

Classical signs

- Depression and anorexia.
- Mydriasis, reduced pupillary light reflex, protruding nictitans, normal vision.
- Xerostomia (dry mouth and mucous membranes) and keratoconjunctivitis sicca.
- Retching, regurgitation or vomiting.
- Fecal incontinence or constipation.

See main reference on page 792 for details (The Constipated or Straining Cat).

Clinical signs

Lethargy and anorexia are present in almost all cats and usually develop over a **48-hour period.**

The classical signs are associated with **the dysfunction of both sympathetic and parasympathetic nervous system. Ocular signs include** dilated pupils, decreased or absent pupillary light reflex and protruding nictitans, but have **normal vision**.

Gastrointestinal signs are present in about 95% of cats and include constipation, regurgitation (secondary to megaesophagus) and dry mouth. Vomiting may occur or regurgitation may be reported as vomiting.

Less commonly observed signs are bradycardia, hypotension, urinary incontinence or a distended, easily compressed bladder, proprioceptive deficits and transient syncopal episodes.

Diagnosis

There is **no definitive, antemortem diagnostic test for dysautonomia**.

Diagnosis is made by using the **clinical presentation** along with **radiographic evidence of megaesophagus** and its associated complications, and use of **pharmacologic testing** to evaluate the function of the sympathetic and parasympathetic nervous system.

Direct-acting parasympathomimetic and sympathomimetics produce an effect in diseased cats but not in normal cats because of post-ganglionic denervation hypersensitivity in affected cats. **Indirect (preganglionic) acting agents** produce an **ocular effect in normal cats but not diseased cats.**

Ocular testing with sympathomimetic agents, e.g. 1% hydroxyamphetamine (indirect acting) produces no mydriasis, and 1% phenylephrine (direct acting) produces rapid mydriasis in affected cats.

Ocular testing with parasympathomimetic agents, e.g. 0.5% physostigmine (indirect acting) produces no miosis, and 0.1% pilocarpine (direct acting) produces rapid miosis in affected cats.

Systemic testing using 0.04 mg/kg atropine, subcutaneously, will increase the heart rate if the sympathetic nervous system is normal. Note: Do not use ephedrine, epinephrine or other sympathomimetics, because fatal arrhythmias can be induced.

Failure to demonstrate a wheal and flare response following intradermal injection of histamine (1:1000) indicates a defect in the sympathetic innervation of cutaneous blood vessels.

GASTRINOMA

Classical signs

- Chronic vomiting unresponsive to routine therapy for gastritis and gastric ulcer disease.

Pathogenesis

Chronic gastritis and gastric ulcer disease are produced secondary to a **gastrin-secreting tumor** that arises from the **pancreatic islet cells** (called Zollinger–Ellison syndrome).

This is a **rare disease** that has only been described in three older cats.

The pancreatic tumor may occur as a solitary lesion, or there may be multiple lesions on the liver due to metastasis.

Clinical signs

Typical signs include **chronic vomiting, weight loss and anorexia** in a cat previously diagnosed with gastritis or gastric ulcers on histopathologic examination of the stomach, but **unresponsive to routine therapy.**

Diagnosis

The gastritis and gastric ulcer disease are diagnosed by **endoscopy and histologic examination of the stomach and duodenum.**

However, to make a definitive diagnosis of Zollinger–Ellison syndrome, a **serum gastrin level** must be obtained along with the finding of a **discrete tumor on the pancreatic islets. Very high levels of serum gastrin** are obtained in cats with gastrinoma.

Differential diagnosis

These are rare tumors of the GI tract, so **even finding elevated serum gastrin levels is not sufficient**, since there are other causes for elevations in serum gastrin levels (e.g. chronic renal failure, etc.).

Other causes of chronic gastritis, including *Helicobacter* spp., liver disease and pancreatitis should be explored.

Treatment

Surgical removal of the tumor, if possible, is the treatment of choice. Management of the gastritis and gastric ulcer disease is as for other primary causes of this problem (see section on gastritis for details, page 680).

RECOMMENDED READING

August JR. Consultations in Feline Internal Medicine, 2001.
Rosser J. In: August J (ed) Food Hypersensitivity: New Recommendations for Diagnosis and Management. WB Saunders Company, Consultations in Feline Internal Medicine, 1997, pp. 209–214.
Guilford WG, Jones BR, Markwell PR, et al. Food sensitivity in cats with chronic idiopathic gastrointestinal problems. J Vet Intern Med 2001; 15: 7–13.
Kirk's Current Veterinary Therapy XIII, 2000.
Krecic MR. Comp. Cont. Ed., 2003; 23 (11): pp. 951–973.

32. The cat with signs of acute small bowel diarrhea

Debra L Zoran

KEY SIGNS

- Loose to watery feces.
- ± Melena.
- No mucus or fresh blood.
- < 3 weeks duration.

MECHANISM?

- There are four recognized pathophysiologic mechanisms of diarrhea include osmotic, secretory, increased permeability and altered motility.

Small bowel diarrhea is characterized by:

- Loose to watery feces.
- Increased volume of feces.
- Normal to increased frequency of defecation.
- No straining or tenesmus associated with defecation.
- If blood is present in feces it occurs as melena.
- Increased mucus is not present in the feces.
- Weight loss and vomiting are commonly observed concurrently.

WHERE?

- Small intestinal tract (duodenum, jejunum and ileum).

WHAT?

- Mild, acute small bowel diarrhea is a common problem that may be caused by a variety of self-limiting factors, including dietary, infectious, parasitic or toxic agents. However, severe small bowel diarrhea may be life-threatening and associated with severe systemic or GI disease. Some diseases typically produce chronic diarrhea, but in the early stages are perceived as producing acute diarrhea.

QUICK REFERENCE SUMMARY

Diseases causing signs of acute small bowel diarrhea

MECHANICAL

● Foreign bodies* (p 713)

Diarrhea commonly occurs either due to motility disturbances or irritating effects of the foreign object that may cause increased secretion.

● Intussusception* (p 712)

Acute onset of diarrhea may occur due to alterations in gut motility, however, vomiting is a more prominent clinical sign.

● Motility disturbances

Primary motility disturbances are rare, but secondary causes of abnormal GI motility such as postoperative ileus, post-obstructive disease or metabolic or endocrine causes of ileus are more important causes of diarrhea.

● Short bowel syndrome (p 730)

Spontaneous short bowel syndrome occurs acutely with intussusception, bowel strangulation and intestinal volvulus. Iatrogenic syndrome associated with resection of 75–90% of the small intestine results in severe diarrhea and weight loss. Congenital forms of short bowel syndrome are reported, but are rare.

METABOLIC

● Hyperthyroidism* (p 711)

Intermittent diarrhea, vomiting or voluminous stools in an older cat with a good to ravenous appetite, obvious weight loss and poorly groomed coat are characteristic of this disease.

● Inflammatory hepatobiliary disease (cholangitis)* (p 710)

The clinical presentation of cholangitis is non-specific: anorexia, lethargy, weight loss, vomiting, diarrhea, dehydration, hepatomegaly and icterus. The disease primarily affects male cats greater than 4 years of age.

● Shock (hypovolemic, septic, endotoxic)* (p 722)

Acute diarrhea occurs secondary to gastrointestinal ischemia from severe hypovolemia or sepsis and may contribute to patient morbidity.

● Exocrine pancreatic insufficiency (p 730)

A rare disease in cats, but is typically associated with small bowel diarrhea, weight loss and a ravenous appetite. Diarrhea is typically chronic but may be perceived as acute onset.

NUTRITIONAL

● Food intolerance*** (p 704)

Indiscretion is associated with an acute onset of diarrhea due to overeating, eating too quickly or ingesting a foreign substance (food or non-food). Intolerance presents with intermittent diarrhea or vomiting, with no pattern or association with eating, and resolves when the food source is changed to omit offending substance from diet.

● Food allergy (dietary hypersensitivity)* (p 709)

Vomiting appears to be more common than diarrhea in cats with food allergy, but it is more likely to occur when the disturbance affects more distal aspects of the GI tract.

NEOPLASTIC

- **Tumors of the small intestine* (p 715)**

The most common tumor of the feline digestive system is alimentary lymphoma. Other tumors that occur in the small intestine are adenocarcinomas (second), and mast cell tumors (third), with fibrosarcomas, leiomyosarcomas and carcinoids occurring rarely. With the exception of lymphoma, which can occur at any age, most tumors occur in old cats. The clinical signs most often observed are anorexia and weight loss, with vomiting or diarrhea less common. The diarrhea is often chronic, but the onset may be acute.

IMMUNOLOGIC

- **Idiopathic inflammatory bowel disease (IBD) (p 714)**

Generally considered to be a disorder associated with chronic, intermittent vomiting, diarrhea or weight loss, but acute exacerbations of diarrhea may occur. IBD is described primarily by the predominant inflammatory cell type infiltrating the mucosa. Lymphocytic plasmacytic enteritis is the most common form of IBD, but eosinophilic and suppurative forms of the disease occur as well.

INFECTIOUS

- **Coccidiosis (isosporosis, cryptosporidiosis, toxoplasmosis)** (p 705)**

Infections that result in mild to moderate diarrhea are most common in neonates and immunosuppressed adults. Most adults have asymptomatic infestations. The species of coccidia most commonly associated with disease in cats are *Isospora* spp., *Cryptospordium parvum* and occasionally *Toxoplasma gondii*.

- **Giardiasis** (p 707)**

Acute or chronic small bowel diarrhea is the most common clinical presentation, however in some cats large bowel diarrhea also may occur.

- **Nematode parasites (roundworms, hookworms)* (p 717)**

Common signs occurring in kittens with roundworms (*Toxocara cati, Toxascaris leonina*) include unthriftiness, diarrhea and pot-bellied appearance, however, vomiting may also occur.

- **Salmonellosis* (p 719)**

Diarrhea, weight loss and systemic illness are primarily problems in young or debilitated cats, as most cats are asymptomatic carriers. The disease is most important clinically in young kittens or geriatric cats that develop septicemia due to *Salmonella* spp., and may die acutely. Salmonellosis is a zoonotic disease.

- **_Clostridium perfringens_ enterocolitis* (p 721)**

Diarrhea occurs due to sporulation of clostridial organisms and release of enterotoxin resulting in a secretory diarrhea that is usually small bowel in character, but can also have a large bowel component.

- **Feline coronavirus infections (feline enteric coronavirus/feline infectious peritonitis* (p 718)**

Feline enteric coronavirus causes mild, transient diarrhea in young kittens, and is the source of feline infectious peritonitis virus (FIPV). Systemic infectious disease by FIPV is characterized by vasculitis and granulomatous lesions in affected organs. Since FIPV rarely affects the GI tract singularly, vomiting is often associated with the disease effects on the liver, kidneys or other organs. Rarely FIPV causes intestinal granulomas that obstruct the GI tract and cause vomiting or diarrhea that is usually chronic, but may have an acute onset.

continued

continued

● Feline panleukopenia virus (p 722)

Infectious viral enteritis of young cats that is often fatal in unvaccinated populations. Typically, there is a sudden onset of depression and anorexia. Vomiting is followed by diarrhea, varying from mild to severe. Panleukopenia may result in systemic septicemia and rapid death. A relatively rare problem in vaccinated cats due to the vaccine efficacy.

● Peritonitis (p 729)

Abdominal pain, distention, fever, decreased appetite and lethargy are the most common presenting signs. Vomiting or diarrhea may occur, but is not a consistent problem.

● Feline leukemia virus (p 725)

Systemic retroviral disease associated with neoplasia and bone marrow disease in cats. Diarrhea occurs most commonly secondary to development of GI lymphoma.

● Feline immunodeficiency virus (p 726)

Diarrhea is not a common presenting sign of cats with FIV, but diarrhea can occur secondary to the immunodeficiency disease or result from a purulent form of colitis that can occur in a small number of cats that are infected with FIV.

● Campylobacteriosis (p 726)

An uncommon cause of diarrhea in cats, but will cause mucoid, bloody diarrhea, weight loss, anorexia and fever in affected kittens or young cats. Most affected cats are from shelters or catteries that have crowded conditions and poor hygiene. In adult cats, the disease is usually self-limiting, but it is an important zoonosis.

● *Bacillus piliformis* (Tyzzer's disease) (p 732)

Produces clinical signs that are identical to panleukopenia.

IDIOPATHIC

● **Acute gastroenteritis*** (p 702)**

This acute, mild small bowel diarrhea may be caused by a number of dietary, bacterial, parasitic or toxic agents that are usually self-limiting.

● Hypereosinophilic syndrome (p 729)

Rare disorder that is associated with eosinophilic IBD and systemic eosinophilia (increased circulating eosinophils and increased eosinophils in lymph nodes, etc.). It is usually associated with chronic vomiting, diarrhea and weight loss, and is poorly responsive to treatment.

● Idiopathic juvenile diarrhea (p 727)

This is a condition of kittens and young cats less than one year of age. It causes chronic small bowel diarrhea, which is self-limiting once the kitten reaches adulthood.

Toxic:

● **Pharmacologic (antibiotic-induced diarrhea)** (p 705)**

Acute onset of diarrhea or vomiting after initiating antibiotic therapy. Antibiotics often associated with inducing diarrhea: ampicillin, cephalosporins, clindamycin, metronidazole, tetracycline, etc.

● **Pyrethrins/pyrethroids/permethrins/organophosphates* (p 718)**

Vomiting, diarrhea, hypersalivation, contact dermatitis, ataxia, excitation, seizures and dyspnea are all reported signs of toxicity to these insecticides.

- Heavy metals (lead, arsenic) (p 724)
The two most common heavy metal intoxications are ingestion of lead and arsenic. Both cause severe GI signs: vomiting, diarrhea, anorexia, and depression, but lead poisoning will progress to neurologic signs (e.g. ataxia, tremors and seizures), while arsenic is nephrotoxic and hepatotoxic.

- Plant ingestion/toxicity (p 728)
Plants may irritate mucous membranes and cause acute drooling, vomiting or diarrhea. Plant toxins that result in renal or hepatic failure may cause more severe and prolonged vomiting, diarrhea, depression and anorexia.

INTRODUCTION

MECHANISM?

Acute small intestinal diarrhea is a common clinical problem that is often **mild or self-limiting**.

In general, small bowel diarrhea tends to be **milder in cats than in dogs** because of the **capacity of the feline GI tract to absorb water**.

Some diseases which typically produce chronic diarrhea may present as acute diarrhea.

In some cats, **life-threatening illness** develops due to the severity of fluid loss or as a result of the primary problem causing the small bowel diarrhea (endotoxemia, neoplasia, etc.).

There are **many different causes** of diarrhea, which literally is the presence of increased water in the feces.

The increase in fecal water may be due to a physical, functional or physiologic disturbance in the small intestine, the colon, or both.

Characteristics of small bowel diarrhea include:
- **A large volume of watery or very soft feces**.
- **No mucus or hematochezia**, if blood is present it occurs as **melena**.
- There is little or **no straining or tenesmus**.
- **Weight loss and vomiting** are commonly observed.
- The **frequency** of defecation is **normal to increased**.

Diarrhea may be due to increased **osmotically active substances** present in the lumen. The **most common causes of this type of diarrhea** are **dietary overload/indiscretion** and **malabsorption**, which can be due to deficiency of pancreatic (e.g. EPI) or intestinal brush border enzymes, or upper small bowel diseases (e.g. mucosal or intramural), such as IBD or lymphoma.

Increased secretion of water and electrolytes is another cause of diarrhea which occurs primarily as a result of activation of cellular second messenger pathways (cAMP, cGMP, etc). The **causes of secretory diarrhea in cats** include *Salmonella*, *Clostridium*, *Campylobacter*, *E. coli*, and *Staphylococcus*. Diarrhea due to hyperthryoidism may also be due to a secretory mechanism, but this is unproven.

The presence of **increased intestinal permeability due to inflammation, erosion/ulceration or necrosis** is also an important cause of diarrhea. A major cause of increased permeability diarrhea in cats is IBD, but lymphoma or other causes of intestinal inflammation, such as the enteroinvasive bacteria (e.g. *E. coli*) can also cause diarrhea by this mechanism.

Altered intestinal motility, either increased or decreased segmentation or propulsion movements will cause diarrhea. While it is difficult to prove that altered motility is the primary cause of diarrhea in many cases, it may occur in hyperthyroidism, dysautonomia, some infectious enteropathies and in GI neoplasia.

The **main consequences of acute small bowel diarrhea are dehydration and development of metabolic acidosis** as a result of **fluid and electrolyte losses**.

Infectious and parasitic causes of small intestinal diarrhea may be either **self-limiting or severe**, depending on the pathogenicity of the organism.

Inflammatory bowel disease, neoplasia and other more severe diseases that cause small bowel diarrhea are often associated with other signs of systemic or GI disease, such as **weight loss, anorexia, vomiting or depression**.

WHERE?

Small bowel diarrhea can be the result of **disease in the small intestine** (duodenum, jejunum, ileum) or occur secondary to **systemic illness** (peritonitis, septicemia), **organ failure** (hepatic, renal or pancreatic disease) or **other miscellaneous causes** such as hyperthyroidism.

A careful **history and physical examination** will determine whether the problem is likely related to the GI tract or a systemic problem.

In **otherwise healthy cats with acute diarrhea** that is likely due to dietary indiscretion, mild infectious enteritis or exposure to a self-limiting toxin, a **minimal diagnostic approach is needed**.

In **cats that are dehydrated, clinically depressed, anorectic or vomiting**, a more aggressive approach that includes a **hemogram, chemistry profile, fecal analysis, and radiographs or ultrasound** is indicated.

WHAT?

The **most common causes of mild, self-limiting small bowel diarrhea include food intolerance or dietary indiscretion, and some infectious or parasitic agents**.

Cats with **small bowel diarrhea of a more serious nature** often have **systemic illness/organ failure** (e.g. hepatitis, renal failure, or pancreatic disease such as pancreatitis), **or severe intestinal disease** such as neoplasia or inflammatory bowel disease, which must be carefully evaluated.

Diagnosis is based upon history and physical examination findings, radiography, hematology and serum chemistry profiles, serology if indicated for FeLV/FIV, serum TLI, fecal analysis, fecal cytology or alpha-1 protease inhibitor testing, serum cobalamin/folate assays and histopathology.

DISEASES CAUSING SIGNS OF ACUTE SMALL BOWEL DIARRHEA (<3 WEEKS DURATION)

ACUTE GASTROENTERITIS***

Classical signs

- Vomiting, anorexia or reduced appetite are common.
- Acute gastroenteritis is more common in young cats or kittens, but can occur in any age, breed or sex.
- Mild to severe small bowel diarrhea may also be observed.

Pathogenesis

Mild, acute small bowel diarrhea is a **common presenting complaint**, and may be **caused by a variety of self-limiting disturbances**, including dietary, parasitic, infectious or toxic agents.

Small bowel diarrhea can be caused by **osmotic** (increased unabsorbed substances present in the lumen, such as occurs in overeating or malabsorption), **secretory** (increased secretion of ions and water into the lumen, which is mediated by second messengers such as cAMP or cGMP and often stimulated by bacterial or viral agents), **increased permeability** (increased intestinal permeability occurs from diseases that cause increased inflammation, erosion, ulceration or necrosis), and **altered intestinal motility** (increased or decreased intestinal motility can result in diarrhea, especially when it affects segmentation contractions in the colon).

Cats with self-limiting gastroenteritis require **minimal diagnostic testing** and will respond to **symptomatic treatment.**

Certain strains of *E. coli* may behave as gastrointestinal pathogens. Very little is known about diarrheagenic *E. coli* in cats and further epidemiological investigations on this subject are needed. One recent study showed no difference in the strains of *E. coli* isolated from a group of cats with diarrhea and a control group of cats that did not have diarrhea.

Clinical signs

Acute onset of **vomiting, diarrhea, anorexia** or **lethargy** in an **otherwise healthy cat**.

Dehydration may occur if the signs are severe.

Rarely associated with hematemesis, hematochezia or melena.

Diagnosis

Acute idiopathic gastroenteritis is a pathological description and not a diagnosis. One of the many etiologies listed in this chapter is the likely cause. However in cats that are otherwise healthy, but have mild signs of gastroenteritis and no clinical evidence of dehydration, an extensive diagnostic work-up is rarely indicated or performed so the cause of the signs remains unknown.

A **PCV, TP** and **fecal examination** are simple, inexpensive tests that should be used in cats that seem lethargic or dehydrated.

In cats with **more persistent or severe clinical signs, a dietary change,** more extensive **fecal analysis** (zinc sulfate flotations, culture or cytology) and additional evaluation of the **hemogram or chemistry profile** is indicated.

Differential diagnosis

Food intolerance (ingestion of substances that cause an adverse response that is not immunologically mediated, e.g. not food allergy) or **dietary indiscretion** (ingestion of foreign or usual foods or non-food substances that cause GI disturbance) is a common cause of acute gastroenteritis.

Bacterial or viral infections of the GI tract may be mild and self-limiting, or severe and life-threatening, so the clinical presentation must be carefully evaluated.

Other causes of acute, mild gastroenteritis are ingestion of **toxic substances** (plant material, oil or other materials attached to hair coat, etc.).

Treatment

Fluid therapy is indicated if there are clinical signs of dehydration, or if the cat is unable to drink.

Balanced isotonic replacement electrolyte solutions are the best fluid choices for cats with mild to moderate metabolic acidosis and dehydration secondary to acute diarrhea.

Fluids may be given **subcutaneously** in cats that are only mildly dehydrated.

In cats with severe dehydration or who are intolerant of subcutaneous fluid administration, **intravenous** replacement of fluid deficits is necessary.

Oral rehydration therapy is effective in patients that are mildly dehydrated and can ingest oral fluids.

The maintenance rate for fluid therapy is **40–60 ml/kg/day**, and replacement of fluid deficits is calculated by:

$$BW\ (kg) \times \%\ dehydration = fluid\ deficit\ (liters)$$

Deficits should be replaced over 4–6 hours or more, and ongoing losses estimated and additional fluid amounts added to the maintenance fluid rate calculated.

Potassium supplementation of intravenous fluids should be initiated once the cat is rehydrated and should be **monitored and adjusted based upon serum potassium levels.**

Antimicrobial therapy is not routinely indicated for treatment of acute, mild forms of gastroenteritis.

The **choice of antibiotic** should be **based on the suspected or known causative organism** (*Campylobacter, Clostridium* spp., etc.).

Cats with severe mucosal injury as evidenced by blood loss or hypoproteinemia have the potential to develop septicemia, or signs of systemic sepsis (fever, depression, leukocytosis, hypoglycemia, etc.). These cats should receive **broad-spectrum, parenteral antibiotics** effective against enteral pathogens (e.g. either alone or in combination: ampicillin, enrofloxacin, trimethoprim-sulfadimethoxine, metronidazole or cephalexin).

The **most effective motility-modifying drugs** for treatment of diarrhea are the **opioids** (loperamide 0.08–0.16 mg/kg q 12 h or diphenoxylate 0.05–0.1 mg/kg q 12 h). **Opioids should be used with care** in cats because safe, effective dosages have not been established.

Anticholinergic drugs have no useful role in the symptomatic treatment of diarrhea in cats with gastroenteritis, because they reduce both peristaltic and segmental intestinal motility contractions.

Intestinal protectants and absorbent agents (kaolin, pectin, activated charcoal, barium, bismuth subsalicylate) may or may not be clinically effective, but are not harmful and are likely most beneficial when used in acute, non-specific enteritis.

Bismuth subsalicylate, 0.25 ml/kg q 4–6 h, has been shown to be most effective in acute small-intestinal diarrhea, but should be used cautiously in cats to decrease the **possibility of salicylate toxicity.**

If **vomiting** is a concurrent problem, **anti-emetic therapy** should also be initiated. Metoclopramide, 0.2–0.5 mg/kg q 6–8 h, or prochlorperazine, 0.1–0.5 mg/kg q 8 h, are two commonly used anti-emetics. **Anti-emetic therapy should not be used if a gastric outflow obstruction is suspected.**

Withhold food for 24–48 hours in cats with acute small bowel diarrhea, and only offer water or oral isotonic glucose, amino acid and electrolyte solutions.

Because **most diarrheas in cats are osmotic rather than secretory,** feeding through an acute diarrhea will worsen the signs and may exacerbate the condition. This is in contrast to humans with secretory diarrhea, where feeding is advantageous.

Prognosis

In general, for the majority of cats with acute, non-specific gastroenteritis, the prognosis is excellent.

The prognosis is guarded for cats with severe diarrhea or diarrhea occurring secondary to problems in other body systems.

Prevention

Reduce opportunities for ingestion of toxic or irritating substances.

FOOD INTOLERANCE***

Classical signs

- Intermittent vomiting or diarrhea.
- Inappetence.

Pathogenesis

Food intolerance is a non-immunologic, adverse reaction to a substance(s) present in food. This reaction may be to a food component such as the type of protein or carbohydrate, a particular component (e.g. wheat gluten) or it may be to food colorings, preservatives, flavorings, etc.

Food intolerances may result from an **inability to adequately digest a dietary constituent** (e.g. lactose) or from **metabolic, toxic or pharmacological responses to food components** such as histamine in foods, lectins or from the metabolism of dietary residues by the large intestinal microflora.

The precise **mechanism** associated with vomiting or diarrhea due to food intolerance is **unknown**.

The **mucosa (formerly gut) associated lymphoid tissue is believed to be a major component in the devel-** opment of food intolerance, as it is this tissue that is responsible for promoting tolerance and hyporesponsiveness to harmless dietary antigens.

Intolerance may develop as a result of **abnormal mucosal barrier function,** disturbances in immunoregulation **(decreased tolerance)** or simply an **abnormal recognition or response to certain dietary antigens.**

Clinical signs

Intermittent but persistent vomiting or diarrhea are the most common signs.

Poor hair coat, pruritus, inappetence or failure to thrive may also be noted but these are less common.

Presence of concurrent dermatologic and gastrointestinal signs should prompt consideration of a food allergy.

Diagnosis

There is **no diagnostic test** for this problem other than to **observe a beneficial response to an appropriate dietary trial**. This should be carried out for a minimum of 3 weeks.

Use a highly digestible diet or an elimination diet, either a commercial diet containing a single novel protein source, or a homemade diet of **boiled white rice and a novel meat source** such as duck, venison, rabbit, kangaroo, tofu, horsemeat, etc.

Differential diagnosis

Acute, intermittent diarrhea in an otherwise healthy cat suggests early inflammatory bowel disease, GI parasites, dietary indiscretion, or acute gastroenteritis due to infectious causes.

In some cats, this may be a sign of early renal or liver disease, hyperthyroidism and other primary GI abnormalities such as neoplasia.

Treatment

The **diet should be changed so that it does not contain the offending substance.** This may be as simple as changing from a grocery store brand to a premium brand food (or vice versa), but also may require changing to a hypoallergenic food product (e.g. IVD's Limited diets, Hill's d/d, Eukanuba Response formula, Royal Canin, etc.) or in unresponsive cases, formulating a novel homemade diet that is complete and nutritionally balanced.

In food intolerance, the abnormal gastrointestinal response is non-immunologic, thus the **use of oral prednisolone is not indicated and is unlikely to be beneficial.**

Prognosis

Good if the appropriate diet can be found, which is usually not a difficult problem. However, the cat may have to remain on the diet indefinitely.

Prevention

There is no known method to predict which cats are susceptible to food intolerance, and further, no way to prevent the development of food intolerance.

PHARMACOLOGIC** (ANTIBIOTIC-INDUCED DIARRHEA)

Classical signs

- Anorexia, vomiting or diarrhea may all occur following administration of antibiotics.

Pathogenesis

Vomiting or diarrhea associated with antibiotics is a common occurrence and can occur with almost all of the popular antibiotics, including: **amoxicillin, cephalexin, erythromycin**, lincomycin, sulfasoxazole, **tetracycline**, trimethoprim-sulfadiazine, metronidazole and clindamycin.

The **mechanism for induction of nausea, vomiting or diarrhea varies** for each drug.

Diarrhea often occurs due to a disruption of the enteric microflora that results in overgrowth of pathogenic species or sporulation of normal flora resulting in release of toxins that cause diarrhea.

Clinical signs

Anorexia or a decrease in appetite and vomiting are common occurrences following antibiotic use.

Diarrhea may be liquid and explosive (consistent with **small bowel diarrhea**) or unformed, soft feces with increased mucus (**large bowel character**).

There are **no age, breed or sex predispositions to adverse effects**, but in many cats, once an adverse effect occurs due to one antibiotic, **other closely related antibiotics may cause similar problems.**

Diagnosis

The diagnosis is not difficult because it is **based upon an appropriate history and physical examination findings** (e.g. no other abnormalities are found). A fecal exam and appropriate dietary history will rule out the other potential causes of acute diarrhea.

Treatment

The best approach is to **stop the use of the antibiotic in question**, and if antibiotic therapy is still required, **switch to an appropriate antibiotic of another class**.

Prevention

There is no known way to predict a cat's response to antibiotic therapy, but certain antibiotics (e.g. **clindamycin, cephalosporins, and amoxicillin**) are the **most common culprits.**

COCCIDIOSIS** (ISOSPOROSIS, CRYPTOSPORIDIOSIS, TOXOPLASMOSIS)

Classical signs

- Acute small bowel diarrhea is most common in young cats or kittens.
- In severely infected kittens, weight loss, anorexia and dehydration may also occur.
- Most adult cats will be asymptomatic or have subclinical infections.

Pathogenesis

Coccidian parasites (*Isospora*, *Cryptosporidia*, etc.) are **common intestinal inhabitants** that may occur as commensals or pathogens, depending on the circumstances.

Isospora felis* and *I. rivolta are the two *Isospora* species (also called *Cystoisospora*) that infect cats.

Cryptosporidium parvum is generally accepted to be the **cause of feline cryptosporidiosis.**

Immunocompetent cats will only develop *Cryptosporidia* infections in the GI tract, but immunocompromised cats can have infections of the liver, pancreas, gall bladder and respiratory tract in addition to the GI disease.

Cryptosporidiosis has been **primarily reported in cats with immunosuppressive or immune-mediated diseases** such as FeLV, IBD and intestinal lymphosarcoma.

Unlike most coccidian parasites, the life cycle of *Cryptosporidium* occurs **entirely within one host.**

In other coccidian parasites infection occurs by **ingestion of infective (sporulated) oocysts or tissues from an infected paratenic host (wildlife, large animals, etc.).**

Concurrent disease, malnutrition, stress and immunosuppression appear to be important contributing factors in the development of clinical disease.

Clinical disease is most common in **young kittens from crowded, unsanitary, high-stress conditions.**

Natural infections of **healthy kittens and cats** result in **asymptomatic infections** in almost all cases.

Diarrhea is present in about 10% of cats with the enteroepithelial form of toxoplasmosis but is more common in kittens infected before weaning. Acute diarrhea is most common in neonatal kittens.

Clinical signs

The principal clinical sign of coccidiosis is diarrhea, which may be bloody, mucoid or watery.

Other signs that may be observed include **vomiting, weight loss, lethargy and dehydration**.

Adult cats that are infected with coccidian parasites (including cryptosporidia) are typically **asymptomatic**.

Young or immunocompromised cats with cryptosporidiosis will have profuse, watery diarrhea and mesenteric lymphadenopathy due to intestinal hypersecretion and malabsorption.

Diagnosis

Diagnosis is made by identification of isosporoid oocysts in fresh feces.

The **oocysts of cryptosporidia are smaller than RBCs**, 1/10th the size of isospora, and 1/16th the size of a *Toxocara* oocyst.
- **Special flotation media** (Sheather's sugar or zinc sulfate flotation) is required along with **special staining** (Kinyoun's carbolfuchsin negative) or **phase contrast microscopy, to identify *Cryptosporidia*.**
- Because of their small size, the operator needs to focus up and down on the sample to be able to identify the oocysts.

Other methods of identification of **fecal *Cryptosporidia*** include an **ELISA test**, however, its effectiveness in identifying feline species of *Cryptosporidia* is unknown, a **PCR test for *Cryptosporidium* DNA** in the feces, or **electron microscopy of intestinal biopsy** samples.

Fecal samples submitted to the laboratory should be **preserved in formalin** to minimize the risk of human infection.

Differential diagnosis

The primary differentials are other intestinal parasites or protozoa (giardiasis), infectious diarrhea, toxin-induced diarrhea or dietary disturbances, which are common in young cats adjusting to new foods.

Treatment

Sulfonamides are the drugs of choice for *Isospora*, however they are **coccidiostatic**, not curative. Sulfadimethoxine (15 mg/kg q 12 h × 14 days) alone, or in combination with trimethoprim, is the drug of first **choice.**

Other drugs that may be considered if treatment failure occurs are nitrofurazone, tetracycline, quinacrine, spiramycin or roxithroromycin.

Treatment of subclinical infections of isospora or cryptosporidiosis is **not indicated or necessary,** as full recovery will occur.

Cats or kittens with clinically significant cryptosporidiosis may be treated with **tylosin, clindamycin or azithromycin,** however, the clinical effectiveness of these drugs is not well tested.

Cats or kittens that are **dehydrated and anorectic** will require supportive care in the form of **fluid replacement therapy** or **nutritional support** or both.

Prognosis

The prognosis for complete recovery in immunocompetent cats and kittens is excellent.

Any adult cat with coccidiosis or cryptosporidiosis should be carefully evaluated for the presence of other immunodeficiency (e.g. FIV) or immune-compromising diseases (e.g. neoplasia, IBD, etc.).

Prevention

Coccidiosis is primarily a problem of **poor sanitation, and over-crowded, high-stress conditions** that occur in catteries, shelters and other **population-dense situations**.

Because the **oocysts** (both *Isospora* and *Cryptosporidia*) are **environmentally resistant**, only **aggressive sanitation measures** (daily fecal removal, disinfection of cages, runs and food utensils with steam cleaning or 10% ammonia solutions) will prevent contamination.

Public health

Cryptosporidiosis is a significant zoonosis, and thus, careful precautions must be taken in handling infected animals, their feces and their environments.

Even though the association between human infection and feline cryptosporidiosis is weak, this problem should not be taken lightly, especially in cases of cats owned by **immunocompromised humans.**

GIARDIASIS**

> ### Classical signs
>
> - The most common sign is liquid, to semiformed, diarrhea with increased frequency and urgency.
> - Some animals are asymptomatic, and most remain bright, alert and afebrile.

Pathogenesis

Giardia intestinalis is a commonly encountered **flagellate protozoan parasite,** with a **direct life cycle.**

Giardia cysts are ingested from contaminated water, or directly from **animal to animal** (e.g. in kennels or catteries).

Excystation of the ingested cysts releases two motile trophozoites in the small intestine.

Cysts are approximately 9–13 microns in size but are not routinely identified in flotation solutions because they are **not shed consistently and are small.**

Sugar flotation solutions will cause the cysts to shrivel.

Trophozoites are slightly **larger, tear-drop-shaped, have four pairs of flagella and are binucleated**. The trophozoites attach to the mucosal brush border to absorb nutrients. Little is known about encystation and what triggers it.

Cysts are susceptible to desiccation, but **can exist for months in a cool, moist environment**.

The **pathogenesis** of *Giardia* infection is not well understood but is believed to involve **malabsorption, disturbances in brush border enzyme function and possible enterotoxin production.**

Severe clinical disease is **more common in young cats**, but adults can become infected and symptomatic.

Protective immunity appears to protect cats from the development of clinical signs, but may not protect from shedding, since **some animals will continue to shed organisms despite treatment.**

Clinical signs

Most adult cats infected with *Giardia* spp. remain **asymptomatic**.

The **most common sign observed is the presence of liquid to semiformed diarrhea**, associated with increased frequency and quantity of defecation, in an otherwise healthy cat.

Vomiting, dehydration, lethargy and anorexia may be observed in severe cases, but are uncommon.

Occasionally, chronic small bowel diarrhea with weight loss and poor body condition are observed.

Cats are more likely to also have evidence of acute or chronic large bowel diarrhea (with hematochezia, increased mucus and tenesmus) than are other species affected.

Diagnosis

The diagnosis is made by appropriate fecal examination techniques. **Zinc sulfate flotation is considered to be the most accurate** and practical test. **Three consecutive zinc sulfate flotations will identify 95% of infected animals.**

Other methods include **examination of fresh fecal saline smears** (1 drop saline with a small amount of feces that is spread thin enough to read a newspaper through) for trophozoites (only 40% of infected animals will be identified), **duodenal aspiration** (e.g. instill 10 ml of saline into the duodenum, either through the accessory channel of the endoscope or injected directly during laparotomy, and then aspirate the fluid for examination) **of fluid looking for trophozoites** (requires endoscopy or laparotomy, but is 88% effective), **or fecal ELISA testing for *Giardia* specific antigens** (95% sensitivity, but low specificity).

At this time, the zinc sulfate flotation test appears to be the easiest, most reliable and most accurate method of identifying *Giardia* infections.

Because of the **small size of the cysts (1/8 the size of a *Toxocara* oocyst)**, the operator needs to scan the slide carefully and focus up and down through the different planes to identify the cysts in the preparation.

Differential diagnosis

Other infectious, parasitic, dietary, toxic and idiopathic causes of small bowel diarrhea must be considered since many cats have only mild signs.

Treament

Metronidazole (50 mg/kg/day PO for 5 days) continues to be recommended for treatment of giardiasis in cats. However, **resistant strains of the protozoan are increasingly being reported,** and thus this therapy may not be effective in all cases.

Side effects associated with metronidazole therapy include gastrointestinal upset and neurologic signs,

such as seizures, coma and behavioral changes. All of these are less common in cats than in dogs and are reversible with discontinuation of treatment.

Other drugs that have been recommended for treatment of giardiasis are **quinacrine and furazolidine**, but **these drugs may not eliminate the infection,** only improve the clinical signs.

Albendazole and fenbendazole have been recently shown to be effective in treatment of dogs and cats with giardiasis. Albendazole (25 mg/kg q 12 h × 2 days) is **not approved** for use in cats in the United States and is teratogenic, hepatotoxic and causes bone marrow suppression, and thus is **not recommended. Fenbendazole (50 mg/kg/day × 3 days) has been recommended for treatment of giardiasis in cats.**

Proper disposal of feces and good sanitation is essential to remove any environmental contamination.

Prognosis

With proper diagnosis, treatment and sanitation procedures, *Giardia* infections can be completely controlled.

Prevention

Since the cysts are susceptible to drying and many common disinfectants, **good sanitation** can prevent a once contaminated area from being a source of additional infections.

Avoid allowing cats access to drinking water that may have fecal contamination.

A **vaccine** is now available that purports to reduce shedding of *Giardia* cysts, however, immune system activation has been shown to decrease shedding without having an effect on the infection itself. The vaccine does not prevent infection or reduce severity, and in a study in cats made no significant difference overall.

Public health

Giardia cysts should be considered **potentially zoonotic**.

The infectivity of different strains of *Giardia* for different species is quite variable, but this fact should not preclude the need to take adequate precautions when handling feces.

FOOD ALLERGY (DIETARY HYPERSENSITIVITY)*

Classical signs

- Gastrointestinal signs are variable, but can include vomiting, diarrhea, weight loss or anorexia.
- Food allergy may also produce dermatologic signs usually in the absence of GI signs.

See main reference on page 667 for details.

Clinical signs

Gastrointestinal signs are more variable, but can include vomiting, diarrhea, weight loss or anorexia.

- In cats, vomiting is more common than diarrhea.
- Generally, signs of hypersensitivity involve either the GI tract or skin.
- Clinical signs can occur at any age.

Most common signs are **dermatologic in origin** (pruritus, alopecia, miliary dermatitis, seborrhea), affect the **head, face, ears and inner thigh** especially, and are **non-seasonal** in occurrence.

There are no known breed or sex predispositions for food allergy.

Diagnosis

The **definitive diagnosis of food allergy** is only obtained by **feeding an elimination diet**. The signs usually start to resolve after 4–7 days but may require 6–8 weeks for complete resolution, then reintroduction of the offending diet results in the reappearance of signs.

- The elimination diet chosen depends on the cat's preferences for food, the owner's willingness to make homemade foods, and the clinical situation; however, the **best elimination diet is a diet containing a single, novel protein source** (turkey, venison, duck, kangaroo, etc.) **and a single**, **novel carbohydrate source** (rice, potato, etc.), **with no other additives except a pet vitamin**.
- A **homemade diet** (1/3 cup protein, 2/3 cup carbohydrate) can be used as a diagnostic trial, but is **not a balanced diet for long-term maintenance**. In

most cats, choosing a commercial diet that contains a single, novel protein source will work best for long-term management of these cats.

- Diets that contain **protein hydrolysates** are less antigenic than intact proteins because their molecular structure is too short to bridge IgE receptors on the cell membrane. The usefulness of these diets in cats with food allergy is unknown. Type I (IgE-mediated) hypersensitivity is thought to be involved in only about 25% of food allergy cases. However, these diets give another option for both diagnosis and treatment of cats with food allergy.

Other diagnostic tests, including intradermal skin testing, ELISA testing, RAST testing, and gastroscopic food testing have all been tried in an attempt to find easier methods of making the diagnosis. However, the **only reliable test currently available is the food elimination trial** (which is also what is used in humans).

In most cats, the **hemogram and chemistry profile will be completely normal** or have mild non-specific changes associated with inflammation.

Differential diagnosis

Other differentials such as food intolerance, parasites, and metabolic or neoplastic diseases should be considered. **Inflammatory bowel disease** is also a disease that mimics food allergy and is very difficult to differentiate from it.

Flea allergy is the most common cause of dermatologic signs of allergy, but atopy and food allergy must be considered.

Treatment

Once an elimination diet has been identified that successfully relieves the clinical signs, the cat should remain on that diet indefinitely. However, it is best in most cases to try to **identify a commercial diet that most closely resembles the elimination diet** so that the cat receives a nutritionally complete and balanced diet.

After a period on one diet, **cats may develop hypersensitivity to that new diet**, so new (even more novel) diets will be necessary.

Most cats with food allergy respond only partially or not at all to prednisolone.

INFLAMMATORY HEPATOBILIARY DISEASE (CHOLANGITIS)*

Classical signs

- Weight loss, anorexia and depression.
- Vomiting.
- Icterus.

See main reference on page 427 for details.

Clinical signs

Weight loss (often dramatic), anorexia, vomiting, icterus and depression are the most common signs.

Other signs may include ascites, diarrhea or fever.

Most affected cats are middle-aged or older.

Diagnosis

The presence of **icterus** helps to narrow the differentials list to **hepatic, pre-hepatic and post-hepatic diseases.**

The **hemogram** in cats with hepatic disease is **often abnormal** (e.g. mild, non-regenerative anemia, with abnormal RBC morphology including schistocytes, leptocytes or target cells), but the changes are **not specific** for liver disease. However, it does help **rule out pre-hepatic causes of icterus** which are **rare in cats.**

Serum chemistry abnormalities may include **elevated liver enzyme activities** (sometimes dramatically), **hyperbilirubinemia, hypocholesterolemia, hypoalbuminemia, decreased BUN and electrolyte alterations** (consistent with vomiting or dehydration, e.g. hypokalemia, hypernatremia).

Bilirubinuria is common, but some cats may have urate crystalluria if the liver failure is severe.

Bile acid assay (pre- and 2 hours post-prandial) will show mild to moderate elevations.

Urine sulfated bile acids are a new test of liver function that may be useful in situations where obtaining post-prandial bile acids is impossible, for example in inappetent cats.

Coagulation function (platelet numbers and function, and coagulation factors) should be evaluated since liver disease often adversely affects these functions.

Ultrasonography is the most **useful imaging modality**, and it can also be used to obtain **fine needle aspirates or biopsies**. In cats with cholangitis the liver may be normal, decreased or increased in size, but typically will have a **hyperechoic pattern due to the presence of inflammatory infiltrates.**

The results of tru-cut biopsies do not always reflect the histopathologic diagnosis of surgically obtained wedge biopsies. This was illustrated in a recent study of 189 biopsies, where > 60% of the cats had tru-cut biopsies that failed to confirm the presence of cholangitis, which was confirmed by wedge biopsies.

Liver biopsies taken via surgical exploratory are more diagnostic, and will also allow **placement of a feeding tube** (gastrostomy or jejunostomy tube) during the procedure, which is **essential for any cat that has not eaten for 3–5 days**.

In addition to liver histopathology, samples of hepatic tissue should also be submitted for **aerobic and anaerobic culture.**

Differential diagnosis

Cats that have vomiting, diarrhea, and weight loss in addition to icterus, the list of differentials is narrowed to **pre-hepatic** causes (hemolysis), **hepatic causes** (hepatic lipidosis, hepatic necrosis, hepatic failure, etc.), and **post-hepatic** causes (pancreatitis, neoplasia of stomach, pancreas, duodenum or bile duct, and common bile duct obstruction).

In **cats that are not icteric,** the list of potential causes broadens extensively to include the spectrum of metabolic, neoplastic, toxic and infectious causes of both systemic and primary gastrointestinal origin.

Treatment

Therapy for cats with cholangitis is **largely supportive**, but the histopathologic findings are crucial in **determining severity, the type of inflammatory infiltrate** (which is essential to choosing appropriate therapy), and the overall **prognosis** for the disease.

Most cats with severe liver disease will require fluid therapy to replace deficits, provide maintenance fluid support during the recovery period, and induce diuresis to assist removal of hepatotoxins and prevent tubular sludging from bilirubinuria and casts.

The fluids should be **isotonic, balanced electrolyte solutions**, but **preferably not containing lactate**, which is not converted to bicarbonate in cats with liver failure and thus serves as an additional source of acid. Ringers solution and Normosol-R are replacement electrolyte solutions without lactate.

Vomiting should be controlled with a combination of **anti-emetic therapy** (e.g. metoclopramide or dolasetron) and **acid-blocking therapy (H_2 antagonists** such as famotidine), since **cats with liver disease are prone to development of hypergastrinemic gastritis.**

Diarrhea is rarely severe enough to require therapy and often resolves as the anorexia worsens.

Cholerectic agents (Actigall) should be used to **reduce bile sludging and improve bile salt flow.**

Cats with neutrophilic cholangitis should be given **broad-spectrum parenteral antibiotics**. A penicillin combined with a fluorinated quinolone provides a good spectrum of activity for enteric pathogens. Ideally, the **antibiotic choice should be based upon culture results**, but if the culture is negative or the cat is systemically ill, broad-spectrum antimicrobial chemotherapy should be initiated.

Lymphoplasmacytic cholangitis is believed to be an **immune-mediated** disease and has recently been shown to occur in association with inflammatory bowel disease and pancreatitis. **Prednisolone therapy** (2–4 mg/kg/day) is indicated in cats with lymphocytic plasmacytic hepatic infiltrates.

Nutritional support is often overlooked in cats that do not have hepatic lipidosis, but is crucial for all sick cats due to their requirement for essential amino acids and fatty acids to be provided in the daily diet. Nutrition can be provided in the **short term (1–3 days) via naso-esophageal feeding tubes**, but for longer periods, **esophageal feeding tubes** or a **percutaneous endoscopic gastrostomy (PEG) tube** should be placed to allow larger amounts of food per feeding as well as feeding a blenderized cat food rather than liquid enteral diets.

When initiating enteral feeding in sick cats, **the volume of food must be gradually increased over 3–5 days**, to reduce vomiting and gastric retention of food. A con-stant rate infusion of food over 24 hours is less labor intensive than using initial 1–2 hour feedings of small volumes of food. After the initial introductory period, **the goal is to achieve a daily caloric intake near the resting energy requirement (RER),** calculated as BER = [70 + body wt (kg) × 30].

Most anorectic or ill cats will benefit from addition of **B vitamins** to the fluids, however, **fat-soluble vitamin deficiency may also develop** in cats that are anorectic or have malabsorption. **Supplementation with vitamin K and in some cases, vitamin E** should be considered in those cats. Supplementation with **L-carnitine** may also be beneficial.

Potassium and phosphorus should be supplemented in cats with low serum levels using potassium chloride and potassium phosphate.

Antioxidant therapy with S-adenosylmethionine (SAMe) (20 mg/kg/day PO) is indicated in all cats with cholangitis.

HYPERTHYROIDISM*

Classical signs
● **Weight loss despite a good to ravenous appetite.**
● **Polyuria/polydipsia.**
● **Vomiting, diarrhea or voluminous feces.**
● **Hyperactivity or irritability.**
● **Poor coat condition.**

See main reference on page 304 for details.

Clinical signs

Typical signs include weight loss despite a good to **ravenous appetite, hyperactivity, polyuria/polydipsia**, and a poor coat condition.

Vomiting, diarrhea or voluminous feces are common, and may be observed as an acute problem.

Most cats will have **tachycardia, a gallop rhythm** or other signs associated with congestive heart failure (coughing, increased respiratory rate, weakness) secondary to **thyrotoxic heart disease**.

Gastrointestinal signs associated with hyperthyroidism are often intermittent or relatively mild, with the exception of weight loss and appetite changes.

Diagnosis

The **definitive diagnosis** is an **elevated serum total thyroxine concentration** (T_4).

Other **non-specific abnormalities of the hemogram or chemistry profile** may include hemoconcentration, mild anemia, increased liver enzyme concentrations, including elevated serum alanine aminotransferase activity, or hyperglycemia.

A **thorough assessment of renal function** should be undertaken (BUN, creatinine, UA) before initiating treatment of hyperthyroidism in cats since the **increased renal blood flow associated with hyperthyroidism may result in acute renal decompensation when the thyroid disease is treated** (especially with surgical or radioactive iodine therapy).

Most cats will have a **palpable thyroid nodule.**

Cats with signs of hyperthyroidism but serum total T_4 in the upper half of the normal range should be tested using **free T_4 levels**, as false lowering of the T_4 level may occur due to non-thyroidal illness.

In cats with suspected hyperthyroidism, but normal serum total or free T_4 levels, a T_3 suppression test or radioactive thyroid scan can be performed to confirm the diagnosis.

Cats with signs of cardiovascular disease should also have **thoracic radiographs and an echocardiogram** performed to determine the extent of thyrotoxic heart disease and need for therapy.

Differential diagnosis

The major differentials for an older cat with weight loss, vomiting or diarrhea include neoplasia, exocrine pancreatic insufficiency, hepatic or renal disease and inflammatory bowel disease. However, the presence of cardiovascular signs, a ravenous appetite or hyperactive behavior with the GI signs should point to hyperthyroidism first.

Treatment

Treatment for hyperthyroidism includes **both control of the over-secretion of thyroid hormone as well as its effects on the remainder of the body** (e.g. thyrotoxic heart disease).

There are **three commonly used therapeutic approaches** to treatment of the hyperthyroid condition in cats: (1) **medical management** with methimazole; (2) **surgical removal** of the adenomatous thyroid; and (3) **radioactive iodine treatment** of the cat to obliterate the hyperactive gland(s).

The **treatment method chosen depends on several factors**: (1) the **condition of the cat** (requires assessment of anesthetic and surgical risks, renal function, cardiovascular function; (2) the **availability of radioactive therapy**; (3) the **owner's wishes** (financial and other considerations), and the clinical **judgment of the attending veterinarian**.

Prior to surgical or radioiodine therapy, evaluation of renal function and cardiovascular status is extremely important. **Cats with marginal renal function may not be good candidates for thyroidectomy or radioiodine therapy** which will reduce renal blood flow and metabolism dramatically and may induce an acute exacerbation of renal failure.

Some cats with thyrotoxic heart disease may require calcium channel or beta-blocker therapy, furosemide if they are in heart failure, or aspirin (efficacy unproven) to reduce the risk of thromboembolism. **Many cats with thyrotoxic heart disease respond to treatment of hyperthyroidism alone.**

INTUSSUSCEPTION*

Classical signs

- Anorexia, inappetence or normal appetite are all possible, depending on the location and severity of the obstruction.
- Weight loss.

Clinical signs

Intussusceptions are **rare in cats compared to dogs**. When they occur, they tend to be in the jejunum.

With **high intussusceptions**, vomiting, abdominal discomfort, anorexia, lethargy, dehydration and hypovolemia leading to shock are the most common clinical signs.

Low intussusceptions (at the ileocolic junction) typically present with bloody, mucoid diarrhea, tenesmus, intermittent vomiting and weight loss. In many of these cases, the intussusception can be palpated.

Depending on the location and severity of the obstruction, there may be **anorexia or inappetence and vomiting.**

Diagnosis

Hemogram and serum biochemistry profiles are variable depending on the severity and location of the intussusception, however, **dehydration, electrolyte abnormalities, anemia and leukocyte changes** have all been observed depending on the cause of the intussusception.

Radiographs and/or ultrasound examination of the gastrointestinal tract are the **best means of confirming the diagnosis**. Contrast studies may be used but should not be done at the expense of delaying treatment in severely ill cases.

Endoscopic examination or colonoscopy can also be used to obtain a diagnosis, especially with low intussusceptions.

Differential diagnosis

Many **diseases that can precipitate an intussusception** (viral enteritis, foreign bodies, gastroenteritis, intestinal parasitism, etc.) also have clinical signs that **mimic it.** Therefore, a thorough physical examination, diagnostic evaluation, and close patient monitoring are essential. **Mesenteric volvulus** is a very difficult condition to differentiate from intussusception both clinically and radiographically, but fortunately is very rare in the cat.

Treatment

Intussusception must be considered a **surgical emergency. Cats with signs of shock or endotoxemia** should be prepared for surgery by **correcting fluid and electrolyte imbalances**, administration of **broad-spectrum, parenteral antibiotics** (combinations such as ampicillin/amoxicillin or cefazolin and enrofloxain, amikacin, cefoxitin or imipenam), and use of **histamine-2 blockers** (ranitidine or famotidine) or **protectants** if gastric erosions or ulceration is suspected.

Motility-enhancing drugs, such as metoclopramide, are contraindicated in patients with GI obstruction and should not be used.

After surgical correction, if **gastric ulceration is not a complicating factor, oral alimentation should be instituted in the first 24 hours**, to enhance the return of normal motility and reduce the possibility of postoperative ileus.

FOREIGN BODIES*

Classical signs
- Weight loss, anorexia or inappetence
- Acute onset of vomiting or gagging, occasionally diarrhea is observed.

See main reference on page 636 for details.

Clinical signs

The signs **depend upon the location** of the foreign object.

With gastric or upper small intestinal obstructions, acute onset of frequent vomiting or gagging is common.

Dehydration, lethargy and anorexia are common in these cats, and they may show evidence of **abdominal discomfort** (either on palpation or by posture).

In cats **with a lower intestinal obstruction, diarrhea will be more prevalent** and vomiting less frequent.

If the foreign body is of significant size or if intestinal plication from a linear foreign body is present, these **abnormalities may be palpable**.

Cats that develop an **intestinal perforation** as a result of the foreign body may be quite ill (**depression, fever, hypovolemia/shock**).

Depending on the location and severity of the obstruction, there may be an **acute onset of anorexia or inappetence.**

Diagnosis

History and physical examination findings are very important. Always examine under the tongue of vomiting cats for evidence of a string or thread foreign body.

Hemogram and serum biochemistry profile findings will likely be **normal if the condition is acute**.

Long-standing or severe linear foreign bodies or GI perforation will show an **inflammatory response**, evidence of dehydration (hemoconcentration or elevated proteins) and **electrolyte abnormalities** consistent with vomiting (hypokalemia is most common).

The **diagnosis is obtained by imaging studies**, including **radiography** (plain or contrast studies looking for evidence of an obstructive gas pattern), **ultrasonography or upper GI endoscopy**. In some cases, endoscopy will allow retrieval of the foreign object, and is a useful means of assessing other damage (e.g. erosions, ulcers, or tears in the mucosa).

Differential diagnosis

Acute diarrhea is not the classic clinical sign of a foreign body, but may occur **in combination with vomiting or anorexia**, and can occur without these signs if the obstruction is more distal.

Some cats with linear foreign bodies have a waxing\waning course of vomiting, diarrhea or anorexia that may not suggest the diagnosis immediately.

Other differentials in those cases would include infectious, dietary or inflammatory gastrointestinal diseases.

Treatment

In cases where the object is still in the stomach, it is sometimes possible to safely **retrieve the object** (needle, small toy, etc.) via an **endoscopic** procedure.

Most GI foreign bodies however, will require **surgical removal**, and some may be a **surgical emergency when GI perforation has occurred.**

Cats that are severely dehydrated from persistent vomiting, or have suspected intestinal perforation and leakage should be stabilized as much as possible with **aggressive fluid therapy** and **broad-spectrum antibiotics** prior to surgery (e.g. combination of ampicillin/amoxicillin or cefazolin and enrofloxacin, amikacin or cefoxitin). Some cats with a protracted history of vomiting will benefit from **histamine-2 blockers** or **GI protectants** if gastritis or gastric erosions are suspected.

Motility-modifying agents, such as metoclopramide, should not be used until the obstruction is relieved.

IDIOPATHIC INFLAMMATORY BOWEL DISEASE (IBD) (LYMPHOPLASMACYTIC ENTERITIS, EOSINOPHILIC ENTEROCOLITIS)

Classical signs

- Vomiting, anorexia and weight loss are the most common signs of upper GI IBD.
- Diarrhea can occur.
- Affected cats are usually middle aged or older, with no particular sex or breed predisposition.

See main reference on page 768 for details.

Clinical signs

Typically, IBD is associated with upper GI signs of chronic intermittent **vomiting, weight loss and anorexia**.

Diarrhea is also observed in some cats, when the disease affects the colon or distal small intestine. This occurs less often in cats than in dogs. Acute exacerbation of diarrhea may occur.

Most cats with IBD have chronic signs of GI disease.

The disease is most prevalent in **middle-aged to older cats**, but the range is from **6 months to 17 years.**

There appears to be **no breed or sex predisposition** to IBD in most studies, but purebred cats and males appear to be over-represented in some studies.

Diagnosis

IBD is a diagnosis of exclusion, that requires two steps: (1) the **histopathologic confirmation** of an excessive inflammatory response, and (2) the **elimination of the multitude of potential causes** for GI inflammation.

The majority of cats with IBD will have a **normal hemogram and serum chemistry profile**, however, a few **abnormalities are not uncommon, but they are not specific for IBD**. These include leukocytosis, mild non-regenerative anemia, increases in liver enzyme concentrations, mild hypoalbuminemia and mild hyperglycemia.

Fecal examination (flotation, direct exam, cytology) is **essential** to rule out parasitism.

Ultrasound examination is very important, not only in evaluation of the abdomen for structural abnormalities, but especially for **assessing bowel wall thickness and lymph node enlargement**, which have been shown to correlate well with the severity of IBD. Ultrasound is also important, as it may allow **fine-needle aspiration** of abnormalities which facilitate diagnosis, but also will help determine the best approach to take when obtaining the biopsies (**full thickness vs. endoscopic**).

Radiography, including contrast studies, **has not been shown to be helpful** in differentiating cats with IBD and those with other diseases.

Ultimately, endoscopic examination or **a surgical exploratory** will be necessary to obtain biopsies of the GI tract. Endoscopy is less invasive and allows visualization of the mucosal surface, which may assist in the evaluation of the cat. **Multiple (6–8) biopsies should be taken from multiple sites** (stomach, duodenum, ileum and colon), even if there is no visible evidence of disease.

Since there are no simple, easy tests for food intolerance or food allergy, **dietary elimination trials** should be conducted in all cats with signs of IBD or that have inflammatory infiltrates of the GI tract.

Differential diagnosis

The list of diseases that may mimic, cause or complicate IBD (e.g. cause GI inflammation and similar clinical signs) is extensive: systemic diseases (**hyperthyroidism, pancreatic disease, liver disease**, feline viral diseases, **toxoplasmosis**), parasitic diseases (nematodes, *Giardia, Cryptosporidia*, other parasites such as coccidia, entamoeba), **bacterial infection** (*Helicobacter, Campylobacter, Salmonella, Clostridia*, etc.), metabolic diseases (exocrine pancreatic insufficiency, serum cobalamin or folate deficiency), nutritional disorders (**food intolerance**), immunological conditions (food allergy) and **neoplasia** (**lymphoma**, adenocarcinoma, mast cell tumor).

Treatment

The key to successful treatment of IBD is to have a **correct diagnosis** (and that **is a real challenge**).

Even if food allergy/intolerance has been ruled out, a **highly digestible, hypoallergenic or elimination diet** is important in the treatment of IBD. Cats with IBD have an abnormal gut immune system, **thus the presence of additional dietary antigens will only serve to exacerbate the inflammatory response.**

The mainstay of treatment of IBD in cats is **immunosuppressive doses of prednisolone (2–4 mg/kg/day PO).**

Metronidazole (10–15 mg/kg q 12 h PO) is also very effective, and in some cats, may be as effective as steroid therapy. Many clinicians start with metronidazole and dietary therapy, and then add prednisolone if the response to treatment is incomplete.

In cats with **severe IBD** that is not responsive to metronidazole, prednisolone and dietary therapy, **cytotoxic drugs may be considered**. However, **most cats with IBD do not require additional cytotoxic drug therapy**, to manage their disease. Drugs have may be considered include chlorambucil (2 mg/m^2), azathioprine (0.3 mg/kg EOD) and cyclosporine (5 mg/cat/day). **CBCs should be monitored every 2–3 weeks** to detect myelosuppression early.

Cats with a poor response to treatment or recurrent disease should be carefully re-evaluated (including multiple GI biopsies) to be sure that the diagnosis is correct. Lymphoplasmacytic enteritis can be mistaken for intestinal lymphoma in the early stages or a new problem may have developed.

TUMORS OF THE SMALL INTESTINE*

Classical signs

- Chronic, progressive vomiting that may include hematemesis.
- Weight loss and anorexia may be the earliest, and most consistent signs.
- Lethargy or depression are also common, especially later in the course.
- Diarrhea is more common with infiltrative neoplasms.

See main reference on page 675 for details.

Clinical signs

Weight loss and **anorexia** are the earliest and most common clinical signs.

Lethargy or depression are also common.

Diarrhea is most common with infiltrative neoplasms, such as alimentary lymphoma, which is the most common neoplasm in the feline small intestine.

Vomiting is a common presenting complaint and may be associated with hematemesis.

In the USA there is **no breed predilection** for lymphoma, but **Siamese cats appear to be predisposed to adenocarcinoma.**

Signs typically occur in **older cats**, however, **alimentary lymphoma occurs in cats of all ages.**

Intestinal forms of lymphoma are usually found in FeLV-negative cats, however, the **multicentric form of lymphoma can involve the GI tract and is often associated with FeLV-positive antigenemia** where FeLV is frequent in the feline population.

Both **adenocarcinoma and mast cell tumors of the GI tract** are often associated more with **vomiting and weight loss due to their mass-like, obstructive behavior**.

Diagnosis

Palpation of the abdomen may reveal a **mass or thickened intestinal loops**.

Hematology and serum chemistry profiles are usually non-specific, but help to rule out other causes of vomiting. **The most frequent hematologic abnormality is anemia of chronic disease** (normocytic, normochromic), but blood loss anemia is also observed. The **abnormalities found in the chemistry profile** depend on the extent of the disease and severity of vomiting, and are **non-specific** as well.

The most helpful diagnostic procedures are imaging techniques: radiography, ultrasonography or possibly endoscopy. There are no specific radiographic features of neoplasia, since it may be infiltrative or obstructive in nature. Ultrasound may be more helpful in identification of thickened loops of bowel or mass lesions.

Depending on the location and size of the mass, **ultrasonography will allow visualization of the lesion**, and may also facilitate diagnosis via **fine-needle aspiration or biopsy**.

Ultimately, **histopathologic examination of the tissue is necessary for a definitive diagnosis**.

In **cats with obstructive or mass lesions**, lesions unreachable by the endoscope, or when ultrasound-guided fine-needle aspirates are non-diagnostic, **surgically obtained biopsies and resection** are the best approach.

Differential diagnosis

Alimentary lymphoma is easily (and often) mistaken, especially in the early stages of disease, **for lymphoplasmacytic enteritis (inflammatory bowel disease)**.

Many other severe GI or systemic diseases may resemble intestinal neoplasia, including hyperthyroidism, chronic renal failure or liver disease, pancreatitis, severe food intolerance or sensitivity, and severe forms of infectious enteritis. Differentiation of these diseases is based on **blood testing, exploratory laparotomy and intestinal biopsy**.

In cats with **mass-like or obstructive lesions**, other diseases to consider are **intussusception or foreign bodies, FIP or fungal granulomas, and focal abscesses**. Differentiation often requires exploratory laparotomy or biopsy.

Treatment

For **adenocarcinoma, mast cell tumors** and other tumors that tend to occur as solitary mass lesions, **surgical removal via intestinal resection is the primary approach. Biopsies should be obtained of liver, regional lymph nodes and mesenteric tissues** to determine if metastasis has occurred and its extent.

Chemotherapy has not been proven effective for adenocarcinoma or intestinal mast cell tumors.

Lymphoma of the alimentary tract is generally an infiltrative neoplasm and chemotherapy using combination protocols (COAP, etc.) are the treatments of choice. See main reference on page 676 for details.

NEMATODE PARASITES* (ROUNDWORMS, HOOKWORMS)

Classical signs

- Abdominal distention, colicky abdominal pain.
- Poor body condition, not nursing or eating.
- Diarrhea or abnormal feces.

Pathogenesis

Toxocara cati and *Toxascaris leonina* are the **primary roundworms of cats.** *T. cati* can be transmitted via milk, and by ingestion of the ova or hosts (e.g. rodents) containing the ova. Adult roundworms live in the small intestine.

Ancylostoma tubaeforme is the **most common hookworm of cats**, but is **less pathogenic than the primary hookworm of dogs** (*A. caninum)*. Infections occur by ingestion of larvae, migration of larvae through the skin, via paratenic hosts, or prenatally. However, **hookworms are much less of a problem in cats than in dogs.**

Clinical signs

Kittens are most likely to have clinical signs associated with infestation with helminths.

The clinical signs may include **abdominal distention**, colicky abdominal pain, **poor body condition/hair coat, poor or reduced appetite, diarrhea or abnormal feces**, and **vomiting worms or vomiting due to masses of worms obstructing passage of ingesta.**

Ascarids of cats do not pass through the placenta, so kittens will not develop prenatal infections like puppies do.

Diagnosis

Fecal flotation will reveal **spherical egg (*Toxocara cati*) with pitted outer shell membrane** containing a single zygote, and approximately 75 × 45 μm in size. *Toxascaris* **is also an ovoid egg of similar size** but has **a smooth shell.**

Ancylostoma tubaeforme (60 × 40 μm) is the most common hookworm of cats, and is most prevalent in tropical regions. The eggs are elliptical and slightly smaller than roundworm eggs, but still readily identified on saline fecal flotation.

Infection may be associated with **peripheral eosinophilia, hypoproteinemia**, and mild to severe regenerative anemia (blood loss).

Kittens with severe intestinal parasitism may develop a bowel obstruction or intussusception resulting from the motility disturbance, in these kittens, **radiography, contrast studies or ultrasound examination** will be necessary to identify the problem.

Differential diagnosis

The age and clinical signs are usually supportive of the diagnosis, but other protozoal, infectious or dietary causes of gastroenteritis should be considered.

Treatment

Anthelmintics such as pyrantel (5–10 mg/kg PO once) or fenbendazole (25–50 mg/kg PO q 24 h for 3 days) are effective and can be used for treatment of both kittens and adult cats.

Selemectin (oral monthly heartworm preventative, flea adulticide and nematocide) **may be used to treat or prevent intestinal parasites.**

Repeat treatment in 2–3 weeks (hookworms) and 4–6 weeks (roundworms) to effectively **kill prepatent stages.**

Re-infection is prevented by good sanitation. Feces must be removed from the litter box or collected if outside, and incinerated.

Prognosis

Excellent, except in cats with intestinal obstruction, etc., which have a more guarded prognosis until the problem is surgically corrected.

Public health

Both roundworms (visceral larval migrans) and hookworms (cutaneous larval migrans) have

zoonotic potential, but are not as prone to cause larval migrans as canine parasites.

PYRETRINS/PYRETHROIDS/PERMETHRINS/ORGANOPHOSPHATES*

> **Classical signs**
>
> - Acute onset of vomiting, diarrhea, hypersalivation and agitation.
> - Contact dermatitis.
> - Ataxia and possibly seizures.

See main reference on page 644 for details.

CLINICAL SIGNS

Signs associated with contact exposure or ingestion of pyrethrin/pyrethroid-containing pesticides is **generally mild.**

Vomiting, diarrhea, hypersalivation and agitation are the most common signs of organophosphate toxicity.

Permethrins are very toxic to cats, resulting in central nervous system signs, which include muscle tremors, ataxia, excitation or seizures. Cats may also become **hyperthermic secondary to prolonged muscle activity** or seizures.

Contact dermatitis is not common, but may be observed in cats with the topical preparations.

Diagnosis

History of exposure to or ingestion of products containing permethrin (most common) or pyrethroids.

There is generally no need for further diagnostic testing since **signs will abate with removal of the product** from the skin or GI tract and supportive care.

Differential diagnosis

The history of recent application of a product containing these chemicals is usually definitive.

Treatment

The first and most important step, if the cat is not seizuring, is to **bath the cat to remove any remaining chemical.**

Cats that have **muscle tremors, seizures or other neurologic dysfunction** may need specific therapy such as phenobarbital or valium for seizure control. **Methocarbamol** (a muscle relaxant) may be helpful in decreasing excessive muscle activity.

Organophosphate toxicity is treated with **2-PAM and/or atropine** (0.2–0.4 mg/kg) to control the excessive salivation and defecation.

The signs will be self-limiting once the chemical is removed from the body, so **supportive care** is all that is required. However, some cats may require **1–3 days to recover.**

Since cats will not drink or eat, **fluid therapy may be needed.** In some cats, muscle tremors may be so severe to increase body temperature, **so monitoring (and controlling) body temperature is important.**

FELINE CORONAVIRUS INFECTIONS* (FELINE ENTERIC CORONAVIRUS/FELINE INFECTIONS PERITONITIS)

> **Classical signs**
>
> - Mild to moderately severe diarrhea for 2–5 days, usually in kittens (enteric form).
> - Signs of FIP are vague and variable and include weight loss, fever and anorexia.
> - Occasionally vomiting and chronic diarrhea are observed in cats with FIP.

Clinical signs

Enteric coronavirus infection causes a mild to moderate, self-limiting diarrhea, usually seen in kittens.

Diarrhea is uncommon in adults, but occasionally can be a peracute, severe hemorrhagic diarrhea.
- **Feline enteric coronavirus is important because this virus is the source** of feline infectious peritonitis (FIP). **This occurs by mutation of the enteric virus to the pathogenic, virulent FIP coronavirus that infects and replicates in macrophages.**

The clinical signs associated with feline infectious peritonitis (**FIP**) **virus** infection are quite **variable** and depend a great deal upon the stage when the cat presents to the veterinarian for evaluation.

Cats with **fulminant FIP** will likely be **severely depressed, anorectic and have significant weight loss.** Respiratory distress from **pleural effusion** is also common, as is the presence of **ascites.** Some of these cats will have **gastrointestinal tract signs**, such as vomiting or diarrhea, if there is significant **intestinal, liver or renal dysfunction.**

Cats with the so-called **non-effusive or "dry" FIP**, will have much more **vague clinical signs**, including reduced appetite, fever, mild weight loss and general malaise. Some cats will have mild abdominal **discomfort, respiratory signs, neurological signs and granulomatous retinal lesions.**

In some cats, **FIP granulomas** will cause more **focal signs associated with the body system that is affected.** Vomiting and/or chronic diarrhea from granulomas in the GI tract have been reported, as have central nervous system signs ranging from ataxia to seizures.

Diagnosis

The definitive diagnosis of FIP in cats antemortem is quite difficult, especially in cases of focal or non-fulminant FIP.

Interpretation of serologic tests can be difficult, because most test for antibodies to FECV, rather than for the FIPV form of the virus. While the **negative predictive index is relatively good**, false-negative tests can occur in cats with FIP. **Polymerase chain reaction (PCR) testing** is the best current test, but at present is only definitive for confirmation that a cat **does not have FIP.** The PCR test still has false positives that prevent it from being a good screening/diagnostic test. The 7B ELISA test detects antibody to 7B protein, but both false-positive and false-negative results are common with this test.

Currently, **the definitive test for FIP remains histopathologic examination or immunohistochemistry** and virus isolation.

SALMONELLOSIS*

Classical signs

- Abdominal distention, colicky abdominal pain.
- Poor body condition, not nursing or eating.
- Diarrhea or abnormal feces.

Pathogenesis

Salmonella are motile, **Gram-negative bacilli that are ubiquitous pathogens** able to infect many mammals, birds and reptiles.

Virulence of different strains varies and this is determined by the ability to invade tissues.

Salmonella localize in the lymph nodes and intestinal tract, and **shedding of organisms occurs for 3–6 weeks. Reactivation of shedding or clinical illness may occur after stress**, immunosuppression, other viral infections or crowded environmental conditions.

Salmonella produce enterotoxins which **increase secretions and fluid loss** in addition to the **entero-invasive** effects.

Endotoxemia or bacteremia may occur concurrently with intestinal infection or in the absence of GI signs.

Endotoxemia due to *Salmonella* is believed to only occur in cats with severe immunocompromise.

Clinical signs

There are **several clinical syndromes** that occur: **gastroenteritis, bacteremia/septicemia, organ localization and the persistent asymptomatic carrier state.**

Acute episodes occur 3–5 days after exposure, with the most severe signs in kittens or old cats.

Cats will present with **fever, malaise, vomiting, abdominal pain and diarrhea.**

The **diarrhea** varies from watery to mucoid and may have hematochezia.

Weight loss, dehydration, shock and death will ensue if the cat is not treated aggressively.

Other organ systems may be affected with the systemic illness, including the CNS (seizures) and respiratory tract (pneumonia).

Cats that are presented with endotoxemia or bacteremia often have a subclinical gastrointestinal infection.

Very young kittens, less than 7 weeks old, **will not have fever despite bacteremia. Hypothermia**, weakness and collapse may occur without the onset of GI signs.

Organ localization occurs after clinical or subclinical bacteremia and is less common in cats than it is in humans.

The most common sites of organ localization include pyothorax, meningitis, osteomyelitis and focal abscesses of organs or skin.

Songbird fever is a clinical syndrome of **acute febrile illness** in cats associated with seasonal migrations of birds in the **northeastern United States.** The disease is characterized by **fever, depression, diarrhea** and **anorexia** in young, roaming (outdoor) cats that lasts for 2–7 days and may be self-limiting or very severe.

The vast **majority of cats with salmonellosis (>90%) have transient or no clinical illness.** Occasionally chronic diarrhea will occur for up to 8 weeks. **Recovered cats will shed for up to 6 weeks.**

Diagnosis

History (acute onset) and **physical examination (fever, depression, diarrhea)** will be important suggestive factors but there are numerous causes of acute diarrhea in young cats.

Routine **hematology and serum biochemistry profiles are typically unremarkable in the early phases**, but will show evidence of **dehydration, electrolyte imbalance and leukocyte abnormalities in the later stages.** Cats with bacteremia/septicemia will have a left shift or degenerative neutropenia, hypoglycemia, and may have hepatic or renal compromise as a result of the endotoxemia.

Definitive diagnosis depends on the culture of *Salmonella* spp. from fecal samples, or from urine, CSF, synovial fluid or blood in cats with bacteremia.

Serology can be used, but **many subclinically infected cats will have titers**, thus this method is **not an accurate means of diagnosis.** It is also not useful in acutely ill cats to aid treatment decisions because of the **time delay in seroconversion.**

Fecal cytologic exam will reveal **large number of fecal leukocytes**, thus suggesting an **infectious organism that disrupts the mucosal barrier.**

Differential diagnosis

Other acute, GI infectious diseases, such as feline panleukopenia virus, *Campylobacter* and *Clostridium* should be considered, in addition to *Giardia*, *Cryptosporidia*, dietary indiscretion and toxicity.

Treatment

Acute gastroenteritis, without systemic septicemia, is best treated with **parenteral isotonic replacement fluids.** Maintenance fluid therapy is 40–60 ml/kg/day and replacement includes maintenance plus correction of dehydration, i.e. BW × % dehydration plus additional fluids to replace any ongoing losses. The **replacement fluids are to be given over 12–24 hours**, then the fluid rates can be adjusted to meet the patient's needs for maintenance and ongoing losses.

Cats with **severe hypoproteinemia** due to GI protein loss or septicemia and endotoxemia may benefit from **plasma transfusions or colloid (Hetastarch) therapy.**

Antibiotic therapy is not indicated in treating cats with uncomplicated gastroenteritis, but is **recommended in cats with sepsis or endotoxemia.** Antibiotics that may be effective against salmonellosis include the fluorinated quinolones, aminoglycosides **and trimethoprim-sulfonamide** combinations.

Antibiotic therapy may prolong the period of shedding, and is associated with **development of resistant populations** of *Salmonella* spp.

The presence of neutrophils on a rectal cytology swab justifies antibiotic therapy.

Prognosis

Excellent for cats with mild or subclinical infections, which comprise the majority of the cases.

In cats with septicemia or endotoxemia, the mortality rate is high due to cardiovascular collapse, renal failure and DIC.

Prevention

Enforcement of **strict hygiene** (litter box) and **proper cleaning of cages** (phenolic compounds or bleach) will reduce the risk of subclinical carriers creating disease problems in large population groups or hospitals.

Public health

Salmonellosis should be considered a zoonotic disease.

CLOSTRIDIUM PERFRINGENS ENTEROCOLITIS*

Classical signs

- Acute small bowel diarrhea with or without anorexia or lethargy.

Pathogenesis

Clostridium perfringens is an **anaerobic, Gram-positive, spore-forming rod** that is a **normal inhabitant of the colon** in animals and people.

Enterotoxin formation by *Clostridium* spp. causes **increased membrane permeability** and results in fluid and ion loss. Eventually, the epithelial cells will die and slough.

Most clostridia **exist in the GI tract in their vegetative state**, but under certain conditions (alkaline environment, other concurrent infections, antibiotic therapy or stress) the bacterium will undergo **sporulation and release of enterotoxin**.

Following an infection, the organism can be shed for weeks to months, and because of its stability in the environment, has the potential to infect many other susceptible animals.

Clinical signs

The most common clinical sign is **severe, watery to mucohemorrhagic diarrhea.**

In most cats, the diarrhea only lasts a few days, but in some, it may persist and become chronic. Animals that have severe diarrhea will become dehydrated, lethargic and may be anorexic.

There is **no breed, sex or age predisposition**, but cats from **catteries or in stressed environments** are at increased risk.

Diagnosis

The **history (acute onset, predisposing conditions)** and **physical examination findings (character of the diarrhea)** help to focus the diagnostic approach toward infectious, parasitic and dietary causes of diarrhea.

The presence of the organism can be confirmed by **culture of fresh fecal specimens**, however, **because this is part of the normal flora, this approach is not definitive.**

Similar to the dog, there appears to be a **poor correlation between the presence of fecal endospores and the presence of enterotoxin.**

Reverse passive latex agglutination (RPLA) tests for clostridial enterotoxin are available and have been used in dogs and humans, but have **not been evaluated in cats.** In dogs, the test does not differentiate dogs with clostridial diarrhea from normal dogs, as **> 25% of normal dogs are positive.** An enzyme immunoassay (Techlab, Inc., Blacksburg, VA) appears to be more specific in dogs. **A positive enterotoxin assay determined by ELISA** (regardless of endospore numbers) in the context of clinical signs consistent with clostridial infection is **strongly supportive of clostridial-associated diarrhea.**

PCR tests are also utilized for testing feces for enterotoxin, but are not universally available.

Differential diagnosis

Other enteric bacterial infections, parasitic and protozoal infections, dietary disturbances and toxin exposure should all be ruled out first.

Because this disease can occur in any age of cat, other considerations are **metabolic disease (hyperthyroidism), liver disease and neoplasia.**

Treatment

In severely ill cats, parenteral fluid therapy and introduction of a **bland, highly digestible diet** is necessary.

The primary treatment is the use of **antimicrobial drugs that have a good spectrum against anaerobic bacteria**: metronidazole, tylosin, ampicillin/amoxicillin and clindamycin have all been successfully used.

Addition of dietary fiber (1 tbsp psyllium/cat), or changing to a diet with increased dietary fiber may greatly **reduce the proliferation of clostridial organisms in the large bowel.**

Prognosis

Good with appropriate antibiotic therapy in most cats.

Some cats will have recurrent bouts of diarrhea that require **repeated treatment with antibiotics** or may benefit from **lactulose, which reduces the luminal pH and thus will decrease sporulation.**

SHOCK (HYPOVOLEMIC, SEPTIC, ENDOTOXIC)*

Classical signs

- Acute onset of generalized depression, fever or hypothermia.
- Tachycardia/tachypnea and signs of shock.
- Vomiting is not consistently present but does occur, and bloody diarrhea is also occasionally observed.

See main reference on page 269 for details.

Clinical signs

Cats with endotoxemia or sepsis are **depressed, usually febrile** (**but may be hypothermic**), and show signs of **shock.**

Vomiting or bloody diarrhea may occur in the **later stages** of illness.

Other signs include respiratory distress, weakness, obtundation and seizures.

Diagnosis

Hemogram, serum chemistry and urinalysis show neutrophilia if there has been time for neutrophilia to develop, or neutropenia, thrombocytopenia, hyperglycemia early, progressing to hypoglycemia later. Hyperkalemia, and elevated liver enzymes and BUN are common, as is bacteriuria.

Blood culture is indicated in patients with suspected bacteremia to confirm the infection exists. **Urine culture** is also helpful in cases with **renal seeding of the infection.**

Imaging studies are important in further evaluating the extent of illness and **may help identify a focus of** infection (e.g. radiographs of chest, abdominal ultrasound).

FELINE PANLEUKOPENIA VIRUS

Classical signs

- Acute onset of anorexia, vomiting, pyrexia, depression, weakness and dehydration.
- The disease is most severe in kittens, and has a high mortality rate.
- Diarrhea occurs late in the course of the disease.

Pathogenesis

Feline panleukopenia is a **parvovirus** that requires **rapidly dividing cells** for successful infection (lymphoid tissue, bone marrow and intestinal mucosal crypts).

Infections of kittens in utero, or in the immediate postnatal period, results **in infection of the cerebellum, cerebrum, retina and optic nerves** which may result in seizures, behavioral changes, cerebellar dysfunction and retinal degeneration.

Damage to the intestinal crypt cells results in shortening and eventually loss of the villous (absorptive) cells. Diarrhea is caused by malabsorption and increased permeability.

Kittens infected with panleukopenia are **highly susceptible to secondary bacterial infections** with enteric microflora.

Gram-negative endotoxemia is a common complication and cause of death in kittens.

Infection of the queen early in the pregnancy can result in a wide variety of **reproductive disorders**, including early fetal death, infertility, abortions or fetal mummification. **Late-stage gestation infections** result in the birth of **live kittens with varying degrees of neurologic dysfunction.**

As with canine parvovirus, the feline virus is **highly contagious, and is very persistent** in the environment.

Panleukopenia is **transmitted by direct contact** of susceptible animals with infected cats or their secretions (feces contains the largest amount of virus). However, **fomites** are an important aspect of transmission because of the prolonged survival of the virus in the environment.

Feline panleukopenia can be **inactivated by bleach and formaldehyde,** but is **resistant to other common disinfectants.**

Clinical signs

The majority of cases of clinical panleukopenia are observed in **kittens or young cats under 1 year age.**

Clinical signs vary from **mild to very severe.**

Anorexia, depression and extreme lethargy are very common clinical signs in the early stages.

Vomiting usually occurs but varies in severity and is associated with dehydration.

Diarrhea occurs 24–48 hours after the onset of depression, and may be mild or marked with severe blood-streaked or hemorrhagic diarrhea.

In the **peracute form,** death may occur before diarrhea develops.
- The cat often sits sternally with its head down (flexed).
- **Abdominal palpation** may reveal evidence of pain, enlarged abdominal (mesenteric) lymph nodes and increased gas or fluid in the intestines.

The cat **may or may not be febrile,** but may become febrile if there is sepsis. In the late stages of fatal disease, the cat will almost always become hypothermic. **Hypothermia indicates a grave prognosis.**

Kittens affected in late gestation, or in the first 9 days after birth, are often **ataxic, hypermetric, dysmetric, incoordinated** and have a base-wide stance when they begin to walk at 2–3 weeks of age.

Other neurologic abnormalities include **seizures, behavioral changes and retinal degeneration.**

Prenatally infected kittens may be stillborn or die as fading kittens in the first few days of life.

Many susceptible cats will be infected, but have **sub-clinical or mild GI signs** associated with depression and anorexia for 1–3 days.

Secondary upper respiratory tract infections may occur, especially calici- or herpesvirus infections.

Diagnosis

The **history (acute onset of depression and vomiting), signalment (cat less than 1 year of age) and physical examination findings (fluid- and gas-filled intestines)** are all suggestive of the disease.

The milder forms of the disease that occur in adult cats can be difficult to differentiate from many other gastrointestinal diseases.

The most consistent hematologic abnormality is panleukopenia, with leukocyte counts typically ranging between 500 and 3000 cell/µl. **Because the disease is so acute, serum biochemistry values are usually within normal limits.** Hypoglycemia and elevated liver enzyme concentrations may be detected in cats with endotoxemia.

There is no licensed ELISA test kit for the feline parvovirus, however, the **canine test kit will detect the feline parvovirus in feces** as well. False-positive and false-negative test results can occur.
- **False-positive test results can occur following recent vaccination** with a modified live panleukopenia vaccine, and **false-negative results occur if the kitten is tested before shedding starts,** if there is **low virus burden or late in the course** when shedding becomes more intermittent.

Serologic testing is still an important diagnostic test for feline panleukopenia, but it **requires paired samples (acute and convalescent)** that show a rise in titer to be definitive. **Serology is usually only indicated in a multi-cat facility** so appropriate preventative vaccination programs can be implemented.

Other tests that can be performed include virus isolation on feces or tissues and electron microscopy for detection of virus particles in the feces.

Differential diagnosis

In its severe form, which is typically present in kittens, **few diseases mimic feline panleukopenia.**

Milder clinical forms of the disease in adult cats must be differentiated from **all other infectious causes of gastrointestinal disease** (e.g. campylobacterosis, giardiasis, etc.).

Feline leukemia virus can present in some cats with a panleukopenia-like syndrome, but is easily distinguished from feline panleukopenia by the presence of FeLV antigenemia, persistent leukopenia and anemia in a well, vaccinated cat.

Salmonella **infections** in cats are **usually subclinical,** but can present with a **fulminant gastroenteritis similar to panleukopenia.** In acute salmonellosis, leukopenia may be present.

Treatment

Treatment is supportive, but must be **aggressively administered** if it is to be successful.

The key is **maintenance of fluid** (40–60 ml/kg/day plus correction of dehydration and treatment of ongoing losses) **and electrolyte balance** (add potassium chloride to fluids) and **prevention of secondary bacterial infection** until the body is able to neutralize the virus with antibody.

Antibiotics effective against enteric pathogens (Gram-negative and anaerobic bacteria) must be given to control secondary bacterial infections. Combination therapy with ampicillin (10–20 mg/kg q 8 h) or cephalexin (20–30 mg/kg q 8 h) and amikacin (8 mg/kg q 24 h) or enrofloxacin (5 mg/kg q 24 h) is necessary for broad-spectrum coverage.

Control of vomiting can usually be achieved with metoclopramide (0.2–0.5 mg/kg q 6–8 h) or prochlorperazine (0.1–0.5 mg/kg q 6–8 h) therapy.

Plasma or blood transfusion therapy (up to 20 ml/kg for plasma therapy, or calculate transfusion to increase the PCV to approximately 20%) are indicated in kittens with severe anemia, hypoproteinemia or hypotension.

Young kittens also need nutritional support to prevent the development of hypoglycemia and assist the immune response. **B vitamin supplementation** is also especially important.

- **Nutritional support may include tube feeding** (orogastric, nasogastric) with liquid enteral supplements, **force feeding** of canned or blenderized foods, or **intraosseous/intravenous feeding** (total or partial parenteral nutrition). **If the kitten is not vomiting, the enteral route is preferred,** but **in vomiting patients, parenteral routes of feeding will be necessary.** The most important nutrients to

include are **amino acids and glucose,** which can be given via a peripheral vein or intraosseously.

As with other parvovirus infections, **aggressive supportive care** (fluids, antibiotics, warmth, control of emesis, and nutrition, including gamma globulins if available) is the key to success.

Treatment of adult cats is supportive, but depends on the severity of the clinical signs.

There is **no treatment for the neurological signs.**

Prognosis

The **prognosis for kittens or very young cats** with severe signs of feline panleukopenia is **guarded to grave,** as many die. **Kittens infected before 10 days of age** that survive have **life-long neurologic dysfunction,** which is **not progressive,** and may be acceptable to the owners.

Adult cats are likely to survive without significant disability, and will have **life-long immunity.**

Prevention

The currently **available vaccines for feline panleukopenia are excellent.** Kittens should be vaccinated at 8–9 weeks and then boostered at 12–14 weeks.

Adults have traditionally been revaccinated annually, but this is not necessary. In a recent study, **protective immunity from a killed feline panleukopenia vaccine was found to persist for at least 7 years,** and modified live vaccines are believed to impart life-long immunity.

In young kittens, it is also important to **reduce their risk of exposure by isolation from unvaccinated or ill cats.**

HEAVY METALS (LEAD, ARSENIC)

Classical signs

- Vomiting, diarrhea, anorexia and depression occur early.
- Chronic signs of lead toxicity involve the central nervous system, e.g. seizures, tremors and ataxia are most common.

(continued)

Classical signs—Cont'd

- Arsenic toxicity eventually results in hepatic and renal failure presenting as depression, anorexia, vomiting and diarrhea, along with oliguria or anuria, or icterus and ascites.

See main reference on pages 596, 659 for details.

Clinical signs

There are **two major categories of clinical signs with lead poisoning**: (1) **gastrointestinal signs**, which occur **early in the course of the disease**, and (2) **central nervous system** signs, which are manifest **late in the disease.**

GI tract signs occur early with lead toxicity and may include **vomiting, diarrhea, salivation, inappetence and lethargy.**

Chronic signs of lead toxicity involve the central nervous system, and include **seizures, tremors and ataxia.**

Arsenic causes GI signs early, but is **hepatotoxic and nephrotoxic**, resulting in depression, anorexia, vomiting and diarrhea along with oliguria or anuria, or icterus and ascites.

Lead is commonly found in older paints, while **arsenic is primarily obtained from snail baits.**

Diagnosis

Historical information of exposure to heavy metals is a very important means of getting the diagnosis, however, such information is not always known.

The **hemogram and serum chemistry profile will be unremarkable** when the cat presents with signs of **gastrointestinal disturbance.**

The most **common hematologic abnormality associated with lead poisoning is basophilic stippling** of red cells, which occurs in 30% of cats with lead exposure, and the presence of **nucleated red blood cells** (also 30%). However, these tests are **not pathognomonic for lead poisoning.**

Heavy metals also cause hepatocellular necrosis, which will be evidenced by **elevations in serum ala-**nine aminotransferase and alkaline phosphatase enzymes. Other abnormalities may include elevations in bilirubin, bile acid values and decreases in albumin (in end stage hepatic failure).

Nephrotoxicity associated with arsenic poisoning is also associated with **isosthenuria, azotemia and eventually oliguria/anuria.**

FELINE LEUKEMIA VIRUS

Classical signs

- Clinical signs are incredibly variable and depend on which organ(s) are affected.
- Weight loss, inappetence.
- Occasionally vomiting or chronic diarrhea.
- Diarrhea is rarely observed as an acute onset.
- Anemia may be observed.

See main reference on page 540 for details.

Clinical signs

Inappetence, weight loss, and lethargy are typical non-specific signs.

The **clinical signs** observed in cats infected with feline leukemia virus will be quite **variable and depend upon which body system(s) is affected.**

Neoplasia, immunosuppression and bone marrow disease (especially of the red cell series causing anemia) **are the most common clinical manifestations** of the disease.

Generalized lymphosarcoma is a manifestation of FeLV in cats, and **involvement of liver and mesenteric lymph nodes results in gastrointestinal tract signs**, such as vomiting, anorexia, chronic diarrhea and weight loss. While the diarrhea is generally chronic in nature, the owner may perceive that it is acute in onset. Occasionally, the diarrhea occurs in cats with a good to increased appetite.

Diagnosis

Any ill cat should be tested for infection with feline leukemia virus, due to its many **clinical manifestations**

and the **poor prognosis** that exists for cats that are infected with the virus.

The **hemogram and serum chemistry profile** will likely be **abnormal, especially in cats with systemic illness.** The changes may be mild or subtle (**mild anemia of chronic disease, mild changes in white blood count, liver enzymes, etc.**) in the early stages of the disease, and dramatic (**severe non-regenerative anemia, leukopenia, elevation of liver enzymes, etc.**) when the disease finally progresses to end-stage.

Radiographs and ultrasound examination are useful in detecting lymphosarcoma involving the GI tract.

Biopsy of the GI lesions via fine-needle, tru-cut or wedge resection of tissue will be necessary to **confirm the diagnosis of lymphosarcoma.**

The **definitive diagnostic test** for detection of feline leukemia virus infection in cats is a **serum ELISA test which detects viral antigen.** A positive test should be confirmed using a follow-up ELISA test 8–12 weeks later, or by using an immunofluorescent antibody (IFA) test on whole blood or bone marrow, as the sensitivity and specificity of serological tests such as these are affected by the incidence of disease in the local population and the individual cat's risk factors for infection.

FELINE IMMUNODEFICIENCY VIRUS

Classical signs

- Chronic disease of middle-aged to older cats.
- Most common clinical signs are weight loss, chronic infections and development of neoplastic disease.
- Acute or chronic diarrhea is an uncommon problem but occasionally occurs as the only sign.

See main reference on page 339 for details.

Clinical signs

Clinical signs may be **due to direct effects of the virus or occur secondary to the development of immunodeficiency**, but in either case, occur in **middle-aged to older, male cats that are outdoor or occasionally fight.**

Acute signs include **fever, lymphadenopathy and inappetence.** Other signs include weight loss and non-specific lethargy.

Chronic small bowel diarrhea is one clinical syndrome associated with FIV infection. Other syndromes include non-regenerative anemia, neutropenia, anterior uveitis, glomerulonephritis and central nervous system signs ranging from behavioral changes to seizures.

Diagnosis

History (middle-aged, male, outdoor cat) and **physical examination** (non-specific signs of weight loss, with possible multi-system involvement) findings are suggestive.

Antibodies to FIV are detected in serum by an ELISA test commercially available.

Cats vaccinated for FIV will be positive to the antibody test and cannot be distinguished from infected cats.

Confirmation of the test is not usually necessary in ill cats, but **in healthy cats, confirmation of the positive antibody test by western blot or PCR analysis is suggested.**

Kittens may obtain antibody from milk and not be infected, so **a positive antibody test in kittens under 16 weeks of age should be re-evaluated in 1–2 months** to determine whether the antibody was maternal or infectious.

CAMPYLOBACTERIOSIS

Classical signs

- Abdominal distention, colicky abdominal pain, and diarrhea are the most common signs.
- Kittens are generally in poor body condition, or have other concurrent infections.

Pathogenesis

Campylobacter spp. are **Gram-negative, motile rods** associated with diarrheal disease in many species.

The disease is spread by **fecal–oral mechanisms**, with food and water being primary sources of infection.

The disease is **most prevalent, and clinically significant, in kittens from catteries, shelters or laboratories.**

Most adult cats have asymptomatic infections, and those with diarrhea often have other **concurrent enteric pathogens** present that exacerbate the severity of the disease.

Exposure to *Campylobacter* **results in the development of protective immunity** which may explain why kittens are more prone than adults to the development of clinical disease.

Clinical signs

In cats, **clinical signs of campylobacteriosis are uncommon in the absence of other pathogens.** Most infections are asymptomatic.

Affected cats are usually **less than 6 months** of age.

The primary clinical sign of infection is diarrhea, which may be watery, bloody, mucoid or a combination.

Some kittens will become systemically ill with lethargy, dehydration and anorexia observed.

Diagnosis

History and physical examination findings are important, but **may be unremarkable.**

Routine hematology, chemistry profiles and imaging studies are typically unremarkable.

Diagnosis can be confirmed by culturing freshly obtained fecal samples. Samples can be **transported at room temperature without special handling,** but must be **cultured in a microaerophilic atmosphere.**

Campylobacter **are often cultured from the feces of normal cats** (up to 40%), so it is important to correlate the presence of the organism with the history and clinical signs.

Dark-field or phase contrast microscopy can also be used to identify the motile, curved bacteria on fresh fecal samples. **Gram-stained samples** can also be used to identify the **gull wing-shaped rods in the feces.** However, these approaches are less sensitive and require more technical skill.

Differential diagnosis

Infectious (*Salmonella*, *Clostridium*), parasitic (*Giardia*, *Cryptosporidia*, etc.), and dietary (intolerance or discretion) agents should all be considered.

Treatment

Since most cats with *Campylobacter* infections are asymptomatic or associated with other infections, the **effectiveness of antibiotics for treatment of this disease is unknown.**

Several antibiotics appear to be effective in eliminating the organism, including erythromycin (10 mg/kg q 8 h PO), metronidazole (5–10 mg/kg q 12 h, PO), cephalosporins (20 mg/kg q 12 h PO), and fluorinated quinolones (5 mg/kg q 24 h PO).

Prognosis

Excellent, especially in adult cats.

Public health

Enteric campylobacters are known to be human pathogens, and kittens can be a source of human infection.

Usually kittens with diarrhea are incriminated as causes of human infection, however, because humans can be infected with extremely small amounts of the bacteria, **asymptomatic cats and kittens that are shedding can also be a source of infection.**

The best way to prevent human zoonosis is to stress the importance of exercising appropriate personal **hygiene when handling pet feces or litter boxes.**

IDIOPATHIC JUVENILE DIARRHEA

Classical signs

- The only presenting sign is chronic diarrhea.

Pathogenesis

The **pathogenesis** of idiopathic juvenile diarrhea is **unknown.**

Clinical signs

The disorder occurs **in kittens and young cats under a year of age.**

The only clinical sign is presence of **chronic small bowel diarrhea.**

Kittens are otherwise healthy, active and gain weight

Diagnosis

The diagnosis is one of exclusion. Thus, infectious, parasitic, dietary and mechanical disorders must all be ruled out.

Cats with this syndrome are **often purebred cats**, and the **diarrhea is self-limiting once they reach adulthood.**

Differential diagnosis

Because this is a disease of kittens, bacterial, viral, parasitic, protozoal, dietary and toxic causes of diarrhea must all be carefully considered.

Treatment

There is **no known effective treatment** for this condition. But, since it is self-limiting, owners should be instructed not to give up prematurely.

Prognosis

The prognosis is good once the kitten reaches adulthood.

PLANT INGESTION/TOXICITY

Classical signs

- Acute onset of drooling, vomiting or diarrhea due to the irritant effects on mucous membranes.
- More severe and prolonged vomiting, diarrhea, depression or anorexia may occur if hepatic or renal failure occurs as a result of the toxicity.

See main references on page 646 for details.

Clinical signs

Vomiting is the most common sign following ingestion of plant material, whether or not it is poisonous/toxic to the gastrointestinal tract or not.

Other signs may include anorexia, **drooling, dysphagia or diarrhea.**

Diagnosis

History of exposure or ingestion is essential in many cases, because **there is so much variability in presentation.**

Plants that cause vomiting due to irritation or direct GI upset include *Philodendron, Diffenbachia* (dumb cane), *Euphorbia* (poinsettia), *Caladium, Ricinus* (castor bean), *Robinia and Solanum* (tomato, eggplant or nightshade) spp. to name a few of the more common plants.

Plants that cause vomiting secondary to nephrotoxicity include *Lilium* (lily), *Rheum* (rhubarb) *and Oxalis* spp.

Differential diagnosis

Consider dietary indiscretion, foreign body or ingestion of other toxins if there is an **acute onset of vomiting or diarrhea in an otherwise healthy cat.**

Cats ingesting plants that are **nephrotoxic** will have signs that are indistinguishable from other causes of vomiting due to systemic metabolic, infectious or inflammatory diseases.

Treatment

In most cases, the vomiting is self-limiting after the offending plant is removed from the GI tract.

Gastric protectants (e.g. sucralfate 0.5–1 g/cat PO) **or histamine-2 antagonists** (e.g. famotidine, 0.5 mg/kg PO or SQ q 24 h) may be indicated if severe gastritis develops.

Gastric lavage may be helpful if large amounts of irritant plants are consumed and is important following ingestion of toxic plants to reduce further absorption of toxic substrates.

Other treatments that may be necessary include **fluid therapy, anti-emetics** such as metoclopramide (0.2–0.5 mg/kg PO or SQ q 8 h), and **offering food that is bland or highly digestible.**

Once signs of nephrotoxicity are observed following lily plant ingestion, progression to anuric renal failure and death is unavoidable. Supportive care with fluid therapy may slow the onset of signs, but there is no effective treatment.

HYPEREOSINOPHILIC SYNDROME

> **Classical signs**
>
> - Severe, small bowel diarrhea that may be unresponsive to treatment.
> - The hemogram is characterized by peripheral eosinophilia and there is infiltration of eosinophils in the bone marrow, spleen, liver, lymph nodes and other organs.

See main reference on page 758 for details.

Clinical signs

The **clinical signs** are similar to those of cats with IBD except the **intestinal wall thickening** is more pronounced, **hepatosplenomegaly** is common, and **bloody diarrhea is common.** The diarrhea is usually chronic rather than acute.

Some cats will **cough**, have **skin lesions** (miliary dermatitis) and have **peripheral lymphadenopathy**, but these clinical signs are less common.

Diagnosis

Histopathologic examination of liver, spleen, lymph node or intestinal biopsies provides the definitive diagnosis. There is infiltration of these organs by large numbers of normal eosinophils.

Treatment

The cornerstone of treatment is **high-dose prednisolone therapy** (3–6 mg/kg/day PO), but **relapses are common,** even if the high doses of steroids are maintained.

Hydroxyurea (7.5 mg/kg q 12 h PO) may also be used to reduce eosinophil production. It is administered for 3–14-day courses, as required to maintain the cat in remission.

Nutritional or fluid support is often required until the disease is brought under control.

Prognosis

The prognosis is guarded to poor.

PERITONITIS

> **Classical signs**
>
> - Abdominal pain, lethargy, ascites, anorexia and fever are common signs.
> - Vomiting or diarrhea are less frequent, but often observed in more severe cases.

See main reference on page 467 for details.

Clinical signs

Intestinal perforation secondary to string or other foreign bodies, is the **most common cause of peritonitis. Other causes** include penetrating wounds and chemical peritonitis (due to bile duct rupture).

Abdominal discomfort/pain, lethargy and anorexia are common signs.

Vomiting or diarrhea are not common signs, but when they occur are often associated with severe disease.

Fever and abdominal distention/effusion may also be present.

Diagnosis

Abdominal radiographs (plain, contrast) and ultrasonography will suggest peritonitis and **may pinpoint location or cause** (ruptured gallbladder, pancreatitis, bowel rupture).

Definitive diagnosis confirming the presence of peritonitis is with **abdominocentesis or diagnostic peritoneal lavage and cytologic/bacteriologic examination of fluid.**

Hematology is non-specific: inflammatory leukogram, stress leukogram or sequestration of neutrophils.

SHORT BOWEL SYNDROME

Classical signs

- Severe, and in some cases intractable, small bowel diarrhea.
- Peracute onset of vomiting, depression and anorexia if associated with ischemic intestinal disease.

Pathogenesis

Short bowel syndrome is classically **due to surgical resection of a large segment (75–90%) of the small intestine** that results in **fluid overload to the colon** and resultant diarrhea.

Other causes include ischemic intestinal diseases such as intussusception, bowel strangulation and intestinal volvulus, which are **very rare** in the cat.

Intestinal adaptation occurs in the large bowel, which ultimately results in a return to a soft or semi-formed fecal specimen.

If greater than 85% of the small intestine has been removed the chance for adaptation is poor.

Congenital forms of short bowel syndrome are also rare, and will be seen in kittens with intractable diarrhea.

Clinical signs

Diarrhea, dehydration and weight loss all occur as a result of short bowel syndrome.

Other signs are related to **intestinal malabsorption: deficiency of proteins, vitamins or clotting factors.**

Small intestinal bacterial overgrowth may also occur resulting in **vomiting or anorexia** as well.

If associated with ischemic intestinal diseases, evidence of **endotoxemia and shock** may be present.

Depression, anorexia and vomiting are the most common signs. The **acuteness and severity of the signs** depend on the **extent of the bowel compromise.**

Diagnosis

The diagnosis is **presumptive if surgical resection is the cause.**

Cats are often **hypoproteinemic**, may be **hypocholesterolemic**, and have other **non-specific hemogram or chemistry abnormalities.**

Imaging studies can be used to confirm the diagnosis.

Differential diagnosis

Other diseases that may cause similar signs include severe infectious enteropathies, inflammatory bowel disease or alimentary neoplasia.

Treatment

If the disease is spontaneous in the adult cat, stabilization and prompt surgery is required.

Tincture of **thyme will allow the bowel to adapt when the syndrome is iatrogenic** in origin.

Broad-spectrum antibiotics may be needed.

Low-fat, highly digestible diets are necessary to maximize absorption of nutrients.

Fat-soluble vitamins should be administered as needed. Cobalamin 125–250 µg SQ once per week until serum concentrations are normalized, then every 1–2 months to maintain levels. **Folate** 0.5 mg PO daily until serum levels normalized then as required. **Vitamin E** supplementation may also be needed.

Parenteral nutrition may be required in some cats in the early stages to support them until bowel function returns.

Prognosis

Guarded; in cats where diarrhea persists for longer than 2 months after the resection, the prognosis for a return to function is poor.

EXOCRINE PANCREATIC INSUFFICIENCY

Classical signs

- Weight loss despite a vigorous appetite, which may include pica and coprophagy.

Classical signs—Cont'd

- Fecal characteristics may be normal, soft and voluminous or watery diarrhea.
- Poor haircoat and greasy, flaky seborrhea are also common.

Pathogenesis

Exocrine pancreatic insufficiency (EPI) is **very rare in the cat compared to the dog.**

The **most common cause of EPI** in the cat is **chronic pancreatitis.**

A **less common cause of EPI** is infestation with the **feline pancreatic fluke**, *Eurytrema procyonis*.

Other, possible causes of EPI in cats include **pancreatic adenocarcinoma** and congenital pancreatic acinar hypoplasia or aplasia.

Idiopathic pancreatic acinar atrophy, the most common cause of EPI in dogs, has **not been reported in cats.**

In humans with EPI caused by chronic pancreatitis, diabetes mellitus occurs concurrently. It is **unknown whether cats with chronic pancreatitis and EPI will also progress to develop diabetes mellitus** as well.

EPI is believed to develop when **> 90% of the enzymes of the exocrine pancreas are destroyed.** These enzymes play an integral role in assimilating the major food components: proteins, lipids and carbohydrates.

Pancreatic enzymes increase the efficiency of breakdown of macromolecules in the digestive tract and enhance the transport mechanisms for sugars, amino acids and fatty acids. Thus, **food substances are inefficiently broken down and cannot be readily transported across the intestinal lumen without pancreatic enzymes.**

Diarrhea occurs due to the presence of **large quantities of fats, protein and carbohydrates,** which are **osmotic.**

Maldigestion of these important nutrients leads to **weight loss** and may also cause **deficiencies of vitamins, fatty acids or other essential nutrients.**

Clinical signs

The **most common clinical signs are polyphagia, diarrhea and weight loss.**

Vomiting and anorexia are also **occasionally reported.**

The feces are typically **pale, loose, voluminous**, and they may be quite **malodorous.**

Cats often have a **greasy, flaky haircoat** due to the **fat malabsorption.**

Deficiencies of fat-soluble vitamins can result in a bleeding disorder (**vitamin K-responsive coagulopathy**), which may present as **excessive bleeding from venepuncture sites or spontaneous hemorrhage** (nose bleeds, hematuria, melena, etc.).

Diagnosis

Results from routine **hematology and chemistry profiles** will be **normal in most cats. Occasionally, elevations in hepatic enzymes or neutrophilia** will be observed.

Routine **abdominal radiography and ultrasonography** is usually normal, and is **not diagnostic.**

Fecal proteolytic activity testing will reveal **undetectable levels of enzymes**, which is diagnostic for EPI, but **the test is very labile, so false-positive tests occur to improper sample handling.**

A recently validated radioimmunoassay for **feline trypin-like immunoreactivity (fTLI)** is available, much like the TLI test available for use in dogs.

Severely decreased fTLI concentrations are diagnostic for EPI in cats.

All cats with EPI should have a serum cobalamin and folate assay, since many cats with EPI are cobalamin deficient or have concurrent small bowel disease, causing folate levels to be low.

Differential diagnosis

The **clinical signs are so non-specific** that many other diseases that cause polyphagia, weight loss and diarrhea must be considered: **hyperthyroidism**, diabetes mellitus, corticosteroid treatment or hyperadrenocorticism, **chronic renal failure**, heart failure, liver disease, dental disease, neoplasia, **and chronic intestinal diseases such as inflammatory bowel disease and alimentary lymphoma.**

Treatment

Most cats with EPI can be successfully treated by **dietary supplementation with pancreatic enzymes.** The **powder products** (1 tsp per meal) appear to be **more clinically effective than tablets.**

If the cat refuses to eat the food with pancreatic extract, **raw pancreas can be offered, but it is essential to use bovine pancreas to prevent transmission of Aujeszky's disease in porcine pancreas** in areas where the disease occurs.

A diet that contains low amounts of insoluble fiber should be fed, since insoluble fibers may interfere with pancreatic enzyme activity.

Some cats will not respond to enzyme supplementation alone, and this may be due to **concurrent cobalamin deficiency or small intestinal disease.** Cobalamin supplementation should be given **parenterally** (**100–250 µg SC once weekly** for 6–8 weeks, then monthly or bimonthly as needed).

In cats with suspected vitamin K deficiency, supplementation should also be initiated (vitamin K$_1$ 1 mg/kg/day PO).

Other supplements that should be given include: **tocopherol** (30 IU orally, once daily with food for the first month until levels are normalized), and **folate** (0.5 mg orally, once daily).

It is **unknown whether or not cats develop small intestinal bacterial overgrowth as a complication of EPI** as is common in dogs. However, **in cats that do not respond as anticipated** to pancreatic enzyme supplementation, **addition of metronidazole or tetracycline to the treatment regime** is indicated.

Prognosis

Because EPI is associated with the **irreversible loss of pancreatic acinar tissue, complete recovery is not possible.**

However, with appropriate management, cats with EPI will gain weight, pass normal feces and can live a normal life.

Prevention

There is no known way to prevent the development of EPI, however, if cats with chronic pancreatitis can be recognized and appropriately managed, it may be possible to prevent the consequences of chronic pancreatitis-EPI.

TYZZER'S DISEASE (*BACILLUS PILIFORMIS*)

Classical signs

- The disease occurs primarily in kittens at weaning age, but is rare.
- Rapid onset of depression, abdominal discomfort.
- Death within 24–48 hours is common, but some may have signs several days before death.

Pathogenesis

Disease is caused by *Bacillus piliformis*, a spore-forming, Gram-negative, intracellular bacillus.

This is primarily a disease of laboratory rodents, and is very rare in cats and dogs, but may be seen in kittens and especially weanlings.

The source of the infection is believed to be rodent feces.

The organism proliferates in the intestinal epithelium producing enterocolitis and then **spreads to the liver and systemic circulation.**

Clinical signs

The most common signs are an **acute onset of depression and abdominal discomfort.**

Death usually occurs within 24–48 hours, although **weight loss and recurrent or chronic diarrhea can occur in older cats.**

The **diarrhea is typically infrequent, scant and pasty.**

Diagnosis

There is **no ante-mortem test for Tyzzer's disease,** and most frequently, the diagnosis is made by necropsy.

The lesions are most severe in the ileum, colon and liver, with the ileum and colon being severely thickened.

Special stains **(Giemsa) will reveal the filamentous organisms in the histopathologic specimens.**

The organism is difficult to culture because of its intracellular, microaerophilic nature.

Differential diagnosis

The disease is so peracute that panleukopenia must be considered, as well as other infectious agents that cause severe enteritis and systemic disease.

Treatment

There is no known effective therapy.

Supportive care with antibiotics, fluids and maintenance of body functions (temperature, nutrition) are essential.

Prognosis

Poor.

RECOMMENDED READING

August JR (ed). Consultations in Feline Internal Medicine II. Philadelphia, PA, WB Saunders, 2001.

Ettinger S. Textbook of Veterinary Internal Medicine, Vol. 5. 2000.

Greene CG (ed). Infectious Diseases of Small Animals, 3rd edn. Philadelphia, PA, WB Saunders; 2005.

Guilford WG, Center SA, Strombeck DR, et al (eds). Strombeck's Small Animal Gastroenterology, 3rd edn. Philadelphia, PA, WB Saunders, 1996.

Marks SL, Kather EJ. Bacterial-associated diarrhea in the dog: a critical appraisal. Vet Clin North Am Small Anim Pract 2003; 33: 1029–1060.

Suchodolski JS, Steiner JS. Laboratory assessment of gastrointestinal function. Clin. Tech. Small. Anim. Pract., 2003; 18: 203–210.

33. The cat with signs of chronic small bowel diarrhea

Debra L Zoran

> ### KEY SIGNS
> - Loose to watery feces.
> - ± Melena.
> - No mucus or fresh blood.
> - > 3 weeks duration.

MECHANISM?

- Diarrhea may be defined as a **change in the frequency, consistency or volume** of bowel movements.
- The **four recognized pathophysiologic mechanisms** that cause diarrhea include osmotic, secretory, increased permeability and altered motility.
- **Osmotic diarrhea** and conditions causing **increased permeability** are believed to be the **most common causes of diarrhea**.
- **Classification of diarrhea** by characteristics that tend to be more prevalent in **small vs. large intestinal disease** is a helpful way to develop an appropriate diagnostic and treatment regimen. **Small bowel diarrhea is characterized by:**
- Loose to **watery feces**.
- **Increased volume** of feces.
- **Normal to increased frequency** of defecation.
- **No or little straining or tenesmus** associated with defecation.
- If blood is present in feces it occurs as **melena**.
- No increase in mucus on the feces.
- **Weight loss and vomiting** are commonly observed concurrently.

WHERE?

- The **small intestinal tract** (duodenum, jejunum and ileum) is the site of origin of the diarrhea. However, **diseases in other body systems may cause diarrhea** in an otherwise normal intestinal tract (e.g. liver disease, hyperthyroidism, etc.).

WHAT?

- Chronic small bowel diarrhea is a clinical sign that should be **aggressively evaluated** to determine its cause.
- Cats with chronic diarrhea of small intestinal origin may have any of a number of GI or systemic diseases or disorders, but **metabolic** (hyperthyroidism, renal or liver disease, etc.), **idiopathic** (inflammatory bowel disease), **neoplastic** (lymphoma), and **nutritional** (food allergy or intolerance) are **common causes.**

Diseases causing signs of chronic small bowel diarrhea

ANOMALY

- Intestinal diverticulosis (p 759)

These are rare disorders that are most commonly found in the jejunum, and may be subclinical or associated with vomiting, diarrhea or abdominal pain.

MECHANICAL

- Intussusception (p 756)

Acute onset of diarrhea may occur due to alterations in gut motility, however, vomiting is a more prominent clinical sign.

- Short bowel syndrome (p 760)

This iatrogenic syndrome is associated with resection of 75–90% of the small intestine and results in severe diarrhea and weight loss. Congenital forms of short bowel syndrome are reported, but are rare.

METABOLIC

- **Hyperthyroidism* (p 743)**

Intermittent diarrhea, vomiting or voluminous stools in an older cat with a good to ravenous appetite, obvious weight loss and a poorly groomed coat are characteristic of this disease.

- Exocrine pancreatic insufficiency (EPI) (p 751)

This is a rare disease in cats, but is typically associated with small bowel diarrhea, weight loss and a ravenous appetite.

- Hypoadrenocorticism (p 754)

The classic signs include depression, weakness, vomiting and diarrhea. However, GI signs do not occur in all cases, and the cause of the vomiting or diarrhea is unknown. Some cats will not develop concurrent mineralocorticoid deficiency with the glucocorticoid deficiency, and thus electrolyte disturbances will not be apparent.

NEOPLASTIC

- **Alimentary lymphosarcoma* (p 742)**

This is the most common neoplasm of the feline intestine, and because of the lymphocytic infiltrate and clinical presentation, is easily confused with IBD. Most cats with alimentary lymphoma are FeLV antigen negative. Aggressive chemotherapy is the only effective treatment, and may result in a 3–12-month survival time.

- Intestinal adenocarcinoma (p 750)

The intestinal tract is a much less common location for adenocarcinoma than the colon in cats. This tumor is the second most common intestinal tumor and tends to cause obstructive lesions of the ileum that frequently cause vomiting, but may also be associated with diarrhea. Siamese cats may be predisposed.

- Intestinal mast cell tumor (p 753)

Intestinal mast cell tumors are the third most common neoplasm affecting the feline small bowel, but are rare occurrences. This tumor is aggressive, poorly responsive to therapy and usually has metastasized by the time of diagnosis.

continued

continued

● Other small intestinal neoplasia (fibrosarcoma, carcinoids, plasmacytoma) (p 757)

Other malignant and benign neoplasms that may be associated with vomiting, diarrhea, weight loss or anorexia in cats include fibrosarcoma, plasmacytoma, hemangiosarcoma, leiomyosarcoma, etc. Clinical signs and prognosis are dependent on the location of the tumor, the type of tumor and its response to therapy. Tumors of the duodenum are rare and usually associated with extension of a local neoplasm.

● APUDomas (p 758)

Neoplasms of APUD cells are rare tumors in the cat. They include insulinomas, gastrinomas, pheochromocytomas and carcinoid tumors of the GI tract. Clinical signs will depend on the tumor type, but carcinoid tumors are most likely to cause diarrhea.

NUTRITIONAL

● Food intolerance*** (p 740)

Food intolerance is a non-immune-mediated condition associated with intermittent diarrhea or vomiting, with no pattern or association with eating, and it resolves when the food source is changed to omit the offending substance from diet. The clinical significance of food intolerance is unknown relative to other causes of diarrhea because of the difficulty in obtaining a definitive diagnosis.

IMMUNOLOGIC

● Food allergy (dietary hypersensitivity)*** (p 739)

Chronic vomiting appears to be more common than diarrhea in cats with food allergy, and cutaneous signs may also be present.

● Idiopathic inflammatory bowel disease (IBD)* (p 745)

IBD is a chronic inflammatory disease of the GI tract of unknown etiology. It affects cats of all ages, sexes and breeds, but is most commonly found in middle-aged, purebred adult cats. Lymphocytic plasmacytic enteritis is the most common histologic form of IBD, but eosinophilic and suppurative infiltrates occur as well.

INFLAMMATION (INFECTIOUS)

● Inflammatory hepatobiliary disease (cholangitis) (p 746)

The clinical presentation of cholangitis is non-specific and presenting signs include anorexia, lethargy, weight loss, vomiting, diarrhea, dehydration, hepatomegaly and icterus.

INFECTIOUS:

Viral:

● Feline coronavirus infections (feline enteric coronavirus/feline infectious peritonitis) (p 749)

Feline enteric coronavirus results in mild, self-limiting diarrhea or subclinical infection. In FIP, the GI tract is rarely affected singularly, and so, vomiting or diarrhea is often associated with the effects of the disease on other organs. Rarely, FIP causes intestinal granulomas that obstruct the GI tract and cause vomiting or diarrhea. Systemic signs of FIP may include lethargy, anorexia, pyrexia and CNS signs.

● Feline immunodeficiency virus (p 749)

Diarrhea is not a common presenting sign of cats with FIV, but diarrhea can occur secondary to the immunodeficiency disease or result from a purulent form of colitis that can occur in a small number of cats that are infected with FIV.

Bacterial:

- *Clostridium perfringens* enterocolitis/clostridial enterocolitis (p 748)

Diarrhea occurs due to sporulation of clostridial organisms and release of enterotoxin resulting in a secretory diarrhea that is usually small bowel in character, but may also have a large bowel component.

- Campylobacteriosis (p 750)

Campylobacter infection may cause mucoid, bloody diarrhea, weight loss, anorexia and fever in affected kittens or young cats. Most affected cats are from shelters or catteries that have crowded conditions and poor hygiene.

Protozoal:

- **Giardiasis* (p 744)**

Acute or chronic small bowel diarrhea is the most common clinical presentation. However, in some cats large bowel diarrhea also may occur.

Fungal:

- Histoplasmosis (p 755)

Diarrhea associated with intestinal histoplasmosis is uncommon in cats compared to dogs. The most common clinical signs in cats are associated with respiratory infection, or anorexia, fever and weight loss associated with systemic illness.

Parasitic:

- **Coccidiosis (isosporosis, cryptosporidiosis, toxoplasmosis)** (p 741)**

Infections that result in mild to moderate diarrhea are most common in neonates and immunosuppressed adults. Most adults have asymptomatic infestations. The species of coccidia most commonly associated with disease in cats are *Cystoisospora* spp., *Cryptosporidium parvum,* and occasionally *Toxoplasma gondii*. Toxoplasmosis has recently been observed in association with IBD.

Idiopathic:

- Idiopathic juvenile diarrhea (p 753)

This condition is associated with small bowel diarrhea and occurs in kittens or young cats less than a year of age. There is no known cause for the diarrhea and when the cat reaches adulthood, the diarrhea resolves.

- Protein-losing enteropathy (p 760)

This condition is much less common in cats than in dogs, but may result in chronic diarrhea, malabsorption, weight loss and hypoproteinemia. Primary lymphangiectasia is rare, but secondary causes of lymphatic obstruction, such as inflammation or neoplasia, are relatively more common and must be considered.

- Hypereosinophilic syndrome (p 758)

This rare disorder is associated with eosinophilic IBD and systemic eosinophilia (increased circulating eosinophils and eosinophilic infiltrate in the lymph nodes, etc). It is usually associated with chronic vomiting, diarrhea, and weight loss, and is poorly responsive to treatment.

INTRODUCTION

MECHANISM?

Chronic small intestinal diarrhea is distinct from acute diarrhea, in that the disease or disturbance causing the problem is **not self-limiting.**

Diarrhea is the **most consistent manifestation of intestinal disease.**

In cats with small bowel diarrhea for > 3 weeks duration, **an aggressive search for the cause** should be undertaken.

Characteristics of small bowel diarrhea include:
- **Large volume of watery or very soft feces.**
- **No mucus or hematochezia**, and if blood is present it occurs as **melena.**
- There is little or **no straining or tenesmus.**
- **Weight loss** and vomiting are commonly observed.
- The **frequency** of defecation is **normal to increased**.

Diarrhea occurs when there is an **increase in fecal water,** which can occur due to a variety of small or large intestinal disorders, but has been generally grouped into four categories: **osmotic, permeability, secretory and motility disturbances.**

Chronic diarrhea due to increased **osmotically active substances** present in the lumen is usually associated with **GI malabsorption syndromes** (EPI, liver failure, severe small intestinal disease, lymphangiectasia, etc.) **or dietary overload.**

Increased secretion of water and electrolytes is usually a cause of acute small bowel diarrhea, which occurs primarily as a result of activation of cellular second messenger pathways (cAMP, cGMP, etc.) by **enteric pathogens.** Conditions that cause diarrhea by increasing secretory mechanisms include bacterial infections with enterotoxigenic or endotoxin-producing species, the presence of unconjugated bile acids in the small bowel or increased secretion due to endocrine tumors.

The presence of **increased intestinal permeability** due to **inflammation, erosion/ulceration or necrosis** is also an important cause of both acute and chronic diarrhea. Inflammatory bowel disease, lymphatic obstruction (due to lymphangiectasia or mucosal inflammation), systemic diseases that alter GI blood flow or mucosal integrity, neoplasia, enteric pathogens and parasites, and toxins may all produce diarrhea by this mechanism.

Altered intestinal motility, either increased or decreased segmentation or propulsion movements will cause diarrhea. Unfortunately, evaluation of intestinal motility is a difficult process, and differentiating cause from effect in motility problems even more challenging. Diarrhea due to intestinal motility disturbances may be caused by stagnant loop syndrome, dysautonomia, ileus, loss of segmentation or peristalsis due to drugs, toxins, etc.

Chronic small bowel diarrhea is often a sign of a **serious small intestinal disease** (e.g. inflammatory bowel disease, neoplasia, lymphangiectasia, severe food intolerance, or a chronic infectious disease) which should be **thoroughly investigated.**

However, **systemic disorders** such as EPI, renal failure, liver disease and some endocrinopathies (e.g. hyperthyroidism, APUD tumors and hypoadrenocorticism) will also cause chronic diarrhea and should not be overlooked.

WHERE?

Small bowel diarrhea can be the result of **disease in the small intestine** (duodenum, jejunum, ileum) or occur secondary to **organ failure** (hepatic, renal or pancreatic disease) or **endocrinopathies** (hyperthyroidism, hypoadrenocorticism, or rarely APUD tumors).

A careful **history and physical examination** will determine whether the problem is likely related to the GI tract or a systemic problem.

Diagnostic tests that will aid localization of the problem include a **hemogram, chemistry profile, fecal analysis, intestinal function studies (fTLI, cob/folate) and abdominal imaging studies** (radiographs or ultrasound).

WHAT?

Cats with small bowel diarrhea of a chronic nature often have **severe intestinal disease** (neoplasia, inflammatory bowel disease), or **systemic illness/organ failure** (hepatitis, pancreatic disease such as EPI or hyperthyroidism).

Diagnosis is based upon history and physical examination findings, radiography, hematology and serum chemistry profiles, serology if indicated for FeLV/FIV, etc., serum TLI, fecal analysis, including cytology or alpha-1 protease inhibitor testing, and histopathology.

DISEASES CAUSING SIGNS OF CHRONIC SMALL BOWEL DIARRHEA (> 3 WEEKS DURATION)

FOOD ALLERGY (DIETARY HYPERSENSITIVITY)***

> **Classical signs**
>
> - Vomiting or diarrhea.
> - Anorexia and weight loss.
> - Pruritus or miliary dermatitis.
> - Alopecia.
> - Seborrhea.

See main reference on page 667, Food sensitivity, in "The Cat With Signs of Chronic Vomiting" for details.

Clinical signs

Food allergy is an adverse reaction to food that has a **proven immunologic component.**

Gastrointestinal signs are variable, but can include **vomiting, diarrhea, flatulence, weight loss or anorexia.** Diarrhea can be profuse and watery suggesting small bowel disease, or mucoid and hemorrhagic, consistent with colitis. The true incidence of GI signs associated with food sensitivity is unknown.

Signs tend to occur suddenly after the animal has been on a particular diet for **months or years.**

There may also be dermatologic signs, such as pruritus, alopecia, miliary dermatitis, seborrhea, pustules, etc., which affect the head, face, ears and inner thigh especially, and are non-seasonal in occurrence.

Dermatologic signs need not be present to attribute GI signs to food allergy.

Respiratory tract hypersensitivity is reported in humans but is poorly documented in cats. However, the propensity for cats to develop airway hypersensitivity may warrant further consideration of this possibility.

Most cats are **young adults when signs first develop,** but the signs can occur in **any age, breed or sex** of cat.

Diagnosis

The **definitive diagnosis** of food allergy is only obtained by **feeding an elimination diet**. The signs will resolve after **6–9 weeks** (there is usually a clinical response within **1–3 weeks**), with reintroduction of the offending diet resulting in the reappearance of signs within 4–10 days.

Other diagnostic tests, including intradermal skin testing, ELISA testing, RAST testing, and gastroscopic food testing have all been tried in an attempt to find easier methods of making the diagnosis. However, all of these tests are fraught with **false-negative and -positive results** that limit their usefulness. The only **reliable test currently available is the food elimination trial,** which is also used in humans.

In most cats, the **hemogram and chemistry profile will be completely normal** or have mild non-specific changes associated with inflammation (e.g. eosinophilia, proteinuria).

The **elimination diet** chosen to make the diagnosis will depend on the cat's preferences for food, the owner's willingness to make homemade foods, and the clinical situation. However, the **best elimination diet is a diet** containing a **single, novel protein source** (turkey, venison, duck, rabbit, ostrich, kangaroo, crocodile, whitefish, etc.) and a **single, novel carbohydrate source** (rice, potato, etc.), with no other additives except a pet vitamin. Use either a **commercial hypoallergenic diet or a homemade diet** (see page 741, Food intolerance, for details).

Intestinal biopsies will have **mild to severe infiltrates of inflammatory cells,** which may be lymphocytic, plasmacytic or eosinophilic or a combination of those cell types. There is currently **no way to differentiate the inflammatory infiltrates** present in cats with **food allergy** from those typically seen in cats with **IBD.**

Differential diagnosis

The presence of **dermatologic signs suggests that atopy and flea allergy as well as other dermatologic conditions** should be considered.

Some cats will have GI signs only, and thus other differentials such as food intolerance, parasites, and metabolic or neoplastic diseases should be considered. **Inflammatory bowel disease** is also a disease that **mimics food allergy** and is very difficult to differentiate from it.

Treatment

Once an **elimination diet** has been identified that successfully relieves the clinical signs, the cat should **remain on that diet indefinitely**. However, it is best to try to **identify a commercial diet that most closely resembles the elimination diet** so that the cat **receives a nutritionally complete and balanced diet.** Most homemade elimination diets are not nutritionally balanced and are not suitable for long-term maintenance.

Cats may develop a hypersensitivity to any diet, including the so-called hypoallergenic diet, and in that situation, another novel protein source will need to be selected.

Most cats with food allergy only respond partially or do not **respond at all to prednisolone therapy or antihistamines.**

The importance of **preventing access to any food other than the elimination diet** should be emphasized to the owners.

FOOD INTOLERANCE***

> **Classical signs**
> - Signs may range from intermittent vomiting or diarrhea to pruritus, dermatitis and other dermatologic signs.

See main reference on page 669, Food sensitivity in "The Cat With Signs of Chronic Vomiting" for details.

Clinical signs

Adverse reactions to foods may be **dermatologic or gastrointestinal** and the percentage of signs associated with either component is unknown.

Intermittent to persistent **vomiting (usually < 1 day) or diarrhea** are the most common GI signs. Flatulence and weight loss may occur.

Dermatologic signs may include pruritus, dermatitis or alopecia.

In contrast to food allergy, **food intolerance is a non-immunologic reaction, and can occur on the first exposure** to the offending food or additive. A wide variety of food ingredients may be responsible.

The relative occurrence of **GI versus dermatologic signs** and the importance of one or the other in the diagnosis of food intolerance is unknown. However, a combination of dermatologic and GI signs should raise the index of suspicion of a food-related problem.

Diagnosis

There is **no diagnostic test** for this problem other than to **observe a beneficial response to an appropriate dietary trial for 1 week.** Resolution of clinical signs is often apparent within 4 days.

The best elimination diet to obtain a diagnosis is made from **a single novel protein and novel carbohydrate source with no added colors or preservatives.** For the homemade diet, **boiled white rice or potato (1/3 cup) and a novel meat source** that the cat has not previously eaten (2/3 cups venison, rabbit, duck, ostrich, crocodile, kangaroo, tofu, turkey, whitefish, etc.) are good options. Use food intended for human consumption, not pet meat.

Alternatively, a **commercially available hypoallergenic diet** made from a single novel protein or protein hydrolysate is also a useful test diet. Once a diagnosis of food sensitivity (food intolerance or food allergy) has been made, a commercial hypoallergenic diet containing novel protein and carbohydrate sources should be used for long-term maintenance, as homemade diets are rarely balanced and complete.

Intestinal biopsies from cats with food intolerance may be normal, or may have **mild to moderate infiltrates of lymphocytes, plasma cells or eosinophils,** depending on the duration of intolerance and severity of clinical signs.

Differential diagnosis

Intermittent but unrelenting vomiting in an otherwise healthy cat suggests gastrointestinal motility disturbance, gastric parasites, early inflammatory bowel disease or antral pyloric hypertrophy.

In cats **where diarrhea is the presenting sign or occurs in addition to vomiting**, hyperthyroidism, chronic pancreatitis, early renal or liver disease, and other primary GI abnormalities such as neoplasia or intermittent intussusception, must be considered.

Treatment

Change to a diet that does not contain the offending substance. This may be as simple as changing from a grocery store brand to a premium brand food (or vice versa), but also may require changing to **a hypoallergenic food diet** (e.g. IVD's Limited Antigen diets, Hill's d/d or z/d, Eukanuba Response formula, Royal Canin Select Protein) or in some cases, formulating a **homemade diet** that is complete and nutritionally balanced.

Since the **abnormal gastrointestinal response is non-immunologic**, use of oral prednisolone is not likely to be beneficial.

COCCIDIOSIS (ISOSPOROSIS, CRYPTOSPORIDIOSIS, TOXOPLASMOSIS)**

Classical signs

- In young cats or kittens acute small bowel diarrhea occurs.

Classical signs—Cont'd

- Weight loss, anorexia and dehydration may occur if severely affected.
- Most adult cats will be asymptomatic or have subclinical infections.

See main reference on page 705 for details (The Cat With Signs of Acute Small Bowel Diarrhea).

Clinical signs

The principal clinical sign of coccidiosis is acute small bowel diarrhea, which may be bloody, mucoid or watery. It **usually occurs in young cats or kittens as acute diarrhea**, but may persist and present as chronic diarrhea. In severely affected kittens, weight loss, anorexia and dehydration may also occur.

Other signs that may be observed include **vomiting, weight loss, lethargy and dehydration**.

Adult cats that are infected with coccidian parasites (including cryptosporidia) are typically **asymptomatic**.

Young or immunocompromised cats with **cryptosporidiosis** will have **profuse, watery diarrhea and mesenteric lymphadenopathy** due to intestinal hypersecretion and malabsorption.

Toxoplasma infections are also **rarely associated with diarrhea**, but in cats with immunocompromise or other significant bowel conditions (e.g. IBD), quiescent toxoplasmosis may be re-activated and cause clinical signs.

Diagnosis

Diagnosis is made by identification of isosporoid oocysts in fresh feces.

The **oocysts of cryptosporidia are 1/10th the size of** *Isospora* (smaller than RBCs and 1/16th the size of a *Toxocara* cyst). *Toxoplasma* **oocysts are only slightly larger**.

Special flotation media (Sheather's sugar or zinc sulfate flotation) is required along with **special staining** (Kinyoun's carbolfuchsin negative) or **phase contrast microscopy**, to identify cryptosporidia.

Other methods of identification of fecal cryptosporidia include an **ELISA test**, but its effectiveness in identifying feline species of cryptosporidia is unknown. A **PCR test for *Cryptosporidium* DNA** in the feces, or **electron microscopy of intestinal biopsy** samples may also be used.

Fecal samples submitted to the laboratory **for identification of cryptosporidia** should be **preserved in formalin** to minimize the risk of human infection.

Toxoplasma titers (both IgG and IgM) can be submitted to determine the presence of **acute, chronic or previous infections**. See main reference on page 958.

ALIMENTARY LYMPHOSARCOMA*

Classical signs

- Chronic, progressive weight loss, anorexia, diarrhea and/or vomiting.
- More common in middle aged to older cats.

See main reference on page 317 for details.

Clinical signs

Chronic, progressive weight loss, anorexia, diarrhea and/or vomiting are the most common signs.

Lymphoma commonly causes diffuse **intestinal thickening due to infiltrative disease**, but sometimes there are focal areas of intestinal constriction due to mass lesions or luminal constriction.

Palpable thickening or **mesenteric lymphadenopathy** may be important clues to the problem.

Diagnosis

The **history and clinical signs** may be too **non-specific** to be of particular help.

Palpable intestinal thickening or mesenteric lymphadenopathy is suggestive of neoplasia, but does not rule out other possible causes, such as inflammatory bowel disease, alimentary histoplasmosis or other infectious intestinal diseases (FIP, FIV, severe giardiasis).

Hemogram and chemistry profile results may be normal or will reveal non-specific abnormalities such as chronic non-regenerative anemia, hyper- or hypoproteinemia, elevations in liver enzyme concentrations,

hypercalcemia or abnormal electrolytes due to vomiting or diarrhea.

Imaging studies, especially abdominal ultrasound, are important in identifying and localizing intestinal abnormalities. **Fine-needle aspirates** of lymph nodes or affected segments of bowel may point toward the diagnosis.

The **key to diagnosis is identification of neoplastic lymphocytes in the intestinal mucosa or wall**. This may be achieved by fine-needle aspirates, endoscopic brush cytology or histopathology. **Endoscopic biopsies** are an excellent method of obtaining tissue for diagnosis, but the biopsies must be of good quality to be useful. **Samples must include mucosa and muscularis layers, and extend to the submucosa** to be diagnostic.

In cats with early, or very **well-differentiated lymphosarcoma, it may be impossible to distinguish lymphoma from severe IBD**, even with full-thickness biopsy samples. In these cases, **immunohistochemistry** will be required to separate monoclonal neoplastic cells from the polyclonal cell of IBD. Unfortunately, this technique is currently available at only a few institutions.

Differential diagnosis

The primary differential for alimentary lymphoma, both clinically and diagnostically, is **lymphocytic plasmacytic inflammatory bowel disease.** However, other important differentials include food intolerance/allergy and severe giardiasis, and systemic diseases such as cholangitis and hyperthyroidism.

Treatment

The best approach is to use **multiple-agent chemotherapy**, using a **treatment regimen of stages**: (1) induction of remission, (2) intensification, (3) maintenance and (4) rescue.

Cats treated with **prednisolone alone may improve initially, but once the tumor escapes remission, it is very difficult to re-induce remission**.

There are several protocols available, but the **COAP protocol is commonly used to induce remission.** C = cyclophosphamide, O = vincristine (oncovin), A = cytosine arabinoside, P = prednisolone. The **induction protocol generally takes 6–8 weeks,** and **side effects** with this protocol are **minimal.** The dose-limiting toxicity is hematologic, and thus, **weekly hemograms are required**

before each treatment. Specific dosing protocols are described in detail under alimentary lymphoma in the chronic vomiting section.

Intensification is only used if the induction phase does not result in complete remission of the tumor.

The most common agents used for intensification in cats are **doxorubicin** or **mitoxantrone.**

The **COAP protocol is also used for maintenance in cats**, but the treatments are spread out to every other week or every third week for six treatments, with the goal to be able to maintain the cat with treatment once every 4 weeks. **Maintenance therapy is continued until the tumor relapses.**

Rescue, or re-induction of remission, **is necessary in almost all cats** and generally occurs **6–8 months after the start of induction. Rescue protocols are not as successful in cats** as they are in dogs. There have been a wide variety of protocols recommended, and the reader is referred to an oncology text for further details. In most cases, the rescue protocol will involve **mitoxantrone, doxorubicin and the other COAP drugs.** See the alimentary lymphoma section under chronic vomiting for specific protocol details.

Prognosis

Most (80%) cats with lymphoma treated with multiple-agent chemotherapy protocols are expected to **live 3–9 months. As many as 20% will live for longer than 1 year.**

Cats that are not treated will live for 4–8 weeks.

Feline leukemia-positive cats have a shorter survival time, not because they do not respond to chemotherapy, but due to development of other feline leukemia-associated disorders.

HYPERTHYROIDISM*

Classical signs

- Weight loss despite a good to ravenous appetite.
- Vomiting, diarrhea or voluminous feces.
- Polyuria/polydipsia.
- Poor coat condition.
- Hyperactivity.

See main reference on page 304 for details.

Clinical signs

Weight loss despite a good to **ravenous appetite** and **hyperactivity are the most common signs**.

Polyuria/polydipsia, poor coat condition, vomiting, **diarrhea or voluminous feces** individually occur in 30–50% of cats.

Gastrointestinal signs associated with hyperthyroidism are often **intermittent or relatively mild**, with the exception of weight loss and appetite changes. About **90% of cats have increased appetite**, but **a small number are depressed and have a reduced appetite** (apathetic hyperthyroidism).

Some cats will have **tachycardia, a gallop rhythm** or other signs associated with congestive heart failure (coughing, increased respiratory rate, weakness) secondary to **thyrotoxic heart disease**.

Diagnosis

The **definitive diagnosis** is an **elevated serum total thyroxine concentration** (total T_4). Other **non-specific abnormalities of the hemogram or chemistry profile** may include hemoconcentration, mild anemia, elevated serum alanine aminotransferase activity, or hyperglycemia.

A **thorough assessment of renal function** should be undertaken (BUN, creatinine, urinalysis) before initiating treatment of hyperthyroidism because the increased renal blood flow associated with hyperthyroidism may result in **acute renal decompensation when the thyroid disease is treated** (especially with surgical or radioactive iodine therapy).

Many cats will have a **palpable thyroid nodule**.

Cats with **signs of hyperthyroidism but serum T_4 concentrations in the upper ½ of the normal range** should be tested using **free (unbound) T_4 levels**, as false lowering of the T_4 level may occur due to non-thyroidal illness.

In cats with **suspected hyperthyroidism**, but **normal total or free T_4 levels,** radioactive thyroid scan can be performed to confirm the diagnosis. See page 305.

Cats with tachycardia or an abnormal rhythm should also have **thoracic radiographs and an echocardiogram** performed to determine the extent of thyrotoxic heart disease and evaluate the need for therapy.

Differential diagnosis

The major differentials for an older cat with weight loss, vomiting or diarrhea include neoplasia, hepatic or renal disease, inflammatory bowel disease and chronic pancreatitis. However, the presence of cardiovascular signs, a ravenous appetite or hyperactive behavior with the GI signs should point to hyperthyroidism first.

Treatment

Treatment for hyperthyroidism includes both control of the over-secretion of thyroid hormone as well as its effects on the remainder of the body (e.g. thyrotoxic heart disease).

There are **three commonly used therapeutic approaches** to treatment of the hyperthyroid condition in cats: (1) **medical management** with methimazole or carbimazole, (2) **surgical removal** of the adenomatous thyroid, and (3) **radioactive iodine treatment** of the cat to destroy thyroid follicular cells.

See pages 305 and 671 for details (in The Cat With Weight Loss and a good Appetite and The Cat with Signs of Chronic Vomiting).

GIARDIASIS*

Classical signs

- Liquid, to semiformed, diarrhea with increased frequency and urgency.
- Most cats are bright, alert and afebrile.
- Many cats are asymptomatic.

See main reference on page 707 for details (The Cat With Signs of Acute Small Bowel Diarrhea).

Clinical signs

Most adult cats infected with *Giardia* spp. remain **asymptomatic**.

The **most common signs observed are the presence of liquid to semi-formed diarrhea,** associated with **increased frequency and quantity of defecation,** in an otherwise healthy cat.

Most cats remain bright, alert and afebrile.

Vomiting, dehydration, lethargy and anorexia may be observed in severe cases, but are **uncommon.**

Occasionally, **chronic small bowel diarrhea** with weight loss and poor body condition are observed.

Cats are more likely to also have evidence of acute or chronic large bowel diarrhea (with hematochezia, increased mucus and tenesmus) than are other species affected.

Diagnosis

The **diagnosis** is made by appropriate **fecal examination techniques. Zinc sulfate flotation is considered to be the most accurate and practical test. Three consecutive zinc sulfate flotations will identify 95% of infected animals**.

Other methods include examination of **fresh fecal saline smears for trophozoites** (only 40% of infected animals will be identified), **duodenal aspiration of fluid** for examination for trophozoites (requires endoscopy or laparotomy, but is 88% effective), **or fecal ELISA testing** for *Giardia*-specific antigens (good sensitivity, but not specificity).

Fecal ELISA testing is highly sensitive (93% sensitivity) but has low specificity (60% specificity).

Differential diagnosis

Many other infectious, parasitic, dietary, toxic and idiopathic causes of small bowel diarrhea must be considered since many cats will have mild signs and be otherwise healthy.

Treatment

Metronidazole (25 mg/kg/q 12 h PO for 5 days) continues to be recommended for treatment of giardiasis in cats. However, resistant strains of the protozoan are increasingly being reported, and thus this therapy may not be effective in all cases.

Side effects associated with metronidazole therapy include **gastrointestinal upset and neurologic signs,** such as seizures, coma and behavioral changes. All of these are **less common in cats than in dogs** and are reversible with discontinuation of treatment.

Other drugs that have been recommended for treatment of giardiasis are **quinacrine and furazolidine**, but these drugs may not eliminate the infection, only improve the clinical signs.

Fenbendazole has been shown to be effective in treatment of giardiasis in cats and dogs. Another benzimadizole, **albendazole, is not approved** for use in cats in the United States and it may be **teratogenic, hepatotoxic or cause bone marrow toxicity. Fenbendazole (50 mg/kg/day × 5 days) has been recommended for treatment of giardiasis in cats, and especially those with other concurrent parasitic infections.**

Proper disposal of feces and good sanitation is essential to remove any environmental contamination.

IDIOPATHIC INFLAMMATORY BOWEL DISEASE (IBD)*

Classical signs

- Vomiting, anorexia and weight loss are the most common signs of upper GI IBD.
- Diarrhea can occur, but is more prevalent with colonic disease.
- Affected cats are usually middle-aged or older, with no particular sex or breed predisposition.

See main reference on page 768 for details.

Clinical signs

Vomiting, which may be intermittent or severe, **weight loss and anorexia** are the most common signs.

Diarrhea is also observed in some cats, but is more prevalent with **disease affecting the distal small intestine or colon**.

Most cats with IBD have intermittent, chronic signs of GI disease, and with time, the signs progress to become more persistent and severe.

The disease is **most prevalent in middle-aged to older cats**, but the range is from 6 months to 17 years.

There appears to be **no breed or sex predisposition to IBD** in most studies, but purebred cats and males appear to be over-represented in some studies.

Diagnosis

IBD is a diagnosis of exclusion, that requires two steps: (1) the **histopathologic confirmation** of an excessive inflammatory response in the intestinal mucosa, and (2) **the elimination of the multitude of potential causes for GI inflammation**.

The majority of cats with IBD will have a **normal hemogram and serum chemistry profile**. However, **abnormalities are not uncommon, but they are not specific for IBD**. These include leukocytosis, mild nonregenerative anemia, increases in liver enzyme concentrations, mild hypoalbuminemia and mild hyperglycemia.

Fecal examination (flotation, direct exam, cytology) is essential to rule out parasitism, especially giardiasis.

Ultrasound examination is very important, not only in evaluation of the abdomen for structural abnormalities, but especially for **assessing bowel wall thickness and lymph node enlargement**, which have recently been shown to correlate well with the severity of IBD. Ultrasound is also important, as it may allow **fine-needle aspiration** of abnormalities which facilitate diagnosis, but also will help determine the best approach to take when obtaining the biopsies (**full thickness vs. endoscopic**).

Radiography, including contrast studies, **has not been shown to be helpful** in differentiating cats with IBD and those with other diseases.

Ultimately, endoscopic examination or **a surgical exploratory** will be necessary to obtain biopsies of the GI tract. Endoscopy is less invasive and allows visualization of the mucosal surface, which may help obtain more diagnostic biopsy samples. **Multiple (6–8) biopsies should be taken from various sites** including the stomach, duodenum, ileum and colon, even if there is no visible evidence of disease.

Since there are no simple, easy tests for food intolerance or allergy, **dietary elimination trials** should be conducted in all cats with signs of IBD or that have inflammatory infiltrates of the GI tract.

Differential diagnosis

The list of diseases that may mimic, cause or complicate IBD (e.g. cause GI inflammation and similar clinical signs) is extensive:

- Systemic diseases (**hyperthyroidism, pancreatic disease, liver disease**, feline viral diseases, **toxoplasmosis**).
- Parasitic diseases (nematodes, *Giardia*, *Cryptosporidia*, other parasites such as coccidia, *Entamoeba*).
- **Bacterial infection** (*Helicobacter*, *Campylobacter*, *Salmonella*, *Clostridia*, etc.).
- Metabolic diseases (EPI, serum cobalamin or folate deficiency).
- Nutritional disorders (**food intolerance/allergy**).
- **Neoplasia** (**lymphoma**, adenocarcinoma, mast cell tumor).

Treatment

The first **key to successful treatment** of IBD is to have a **correct diagnosis**, and that is a real **challenge**.

Even if food allergy/intolerance has been ruled out, a **highly digestible, hypoallergenic or elimination diet is important in the treatment of IBD**. Cats with IBD have an abnormal gut immune system, thus the presence of additional dietary antigens may serve to exacerbate the inflammatory response. A "sacrificial" protein source may have to be used first, while the bowel is still subject to a strong inflammatory response, before moving onto a more permanent food choice.

The **mainstay of treatment** of IBD in cats is **immunosuppressive doses of prednisolone (2–4 mg/kg/day PO)**.

Metronidazole (10–15 mg/kg q 12 h PO) is also very effective, and in some cats, may be as effective as steroid therapy. Many clinicians start with metronidazole and dietary therapy, and then add prednisolone if the response to treatment is incomplete.

In cats with severe IBD that is not responsive to metronidazole, prednisolone and dietary therapy, **cytotoxic drugs may be considered**. However, **most cats with IBD do not require additional cytotoxic drug therapy** to manage their disease, so a careful re-evaluation of the patient is indicated to be sure you have the correct diagnosis. Drugs that may be considered include **chlorambucil** (2 mg/m^2), **azathioprine** (0.3 mg/kg EOD) and **cyclosporine** (5 mg/cat/day). **Hemograms should be monitored every 2–3 weeks** to detect myelosuppression, and if cyclosporine is used,

cyclosporine therapy must be monitored by checking trough and peak drug levels.

Cats with a **poor response to treatment** or recurrent disease should be **carefully re-evaluated**, including re-biopsy if indicated. **Lymphoplasmacytic enteritis can be mistaken for lymphoma in the early stage.** Cats with IBD have been reported to have concurrent reactivation of toxoplasmosis. Food allergy/intolerance is extremely difficult to differentiate from IBD and in some cats finding the appropriate diet is a true challenge.

INFLAMMATORY HEPATOBILIARY DISEASE (CHOLANGOHEPATITIS)

Classical signs

- With lymphoplasmacytic forms, chronic weight loss, anorexia, vomiting and icterus are common signs.
- In neutrophilic cholangitis, the disease is more acute in nature, and fever, depression and icterus are typical.

See main reference on page 427 for details (The Yellow Cat or Cat With Elevated Liver Enzymes).

Clinical signs

Weight loss (often dramatic), anorexia, intermittent vomiting, and icterus are the most common signs in cats with lymphocytic cholangitis. These cats often are **middle aged**, there is **no breed or sex predisposition**, and they have **hepatomegaly**. **Concurrent pancreatitis and/or IBD** is seen in some cats and their illness is more chronic and subacute. In some cats, there is a **waxing and waning course with periods of normalcy** and a good appetite following episodes of signs.

Ascites (high protein content) is more likely with the lymphoplasmacytic form, but it is rare.

Cats with **neutrophilic cholangitis** are more often **male, febrile, depressed, icteric and have an acute onset of illness** that is rapidly progressive.

The **diarrhea** may be mild, with soft to unformed feces in cats with lymphocytic cholangitis, to severe, liquid diarrhea in cats with neutrophilic cholangitis.

Diagnosis

The **presence of icterus** helps to narrow the differentials list to **hepatic, pre-hepatic and post-hepatic diseases**.

The **hemogram in cats with hepatic disease is often abnormal** (e.g. mild, non-regenerative anemia, with RBC morphology having schistocytes, leptocytes or target cells present), but the changes are **not specific for liver disease**. However, it does help **rule out pre-hepatic causes of icterus**.

Serum chemistry abnormalities may include **elevated liver enzyme activities** (sometimes dramatically), **hyperbilirubinemia, hypocholesterolemia, hypoalbuminemia**, decreased BUN, and electrolyte alterations consistent with vomiting or dehydration, e.g. hypokalemia, hypernatremia.

Bilirubinemia and bilirubinuria are both common.

Serum bile acid assay (pre- and 2 hours post-prandial) may show mild to moderate elevations.

Urine sulfated bile acids is a new test of hepatic function that may also become useful in the diagnosis of liver disease.

Coagulation function (platelet numbers and function, and coagulation factors) should be evaluated since liver disease often adversely affects these functions.

Ultrasonography is the most **useful imaging modality**, because it can also be used to obtain **fine-needle aspirates or biopsies**. However, **needle biopsies are only accurate for diagnosis of cholangitis < 40% of the time**. In cats with cholangitis, **the liver may be normal, decreased or increased in size**, but typically will have a **hyperechoic pattern** due to the presence of **inflammatory infiltrates**.

Liver biopsies taken via surgical exploratory or laparoscopy **are more accurate**, and will also allow **placement of a feeding tube** (gastrostomy or jejunostomy tube) during the procedure, which is **essential for any cat that has not eaten for 3–5 days**.

In addition to **liver histopathology**, samples of hepatic tissue should also be submitted for **aerobic and anaerobic culture**.

Differential diagnosis

Cats that have **vomiting, diarrhea, and weight loss in addition to icterus,** the list of differentials is narrowed to **pre-hepatic causes** (hemolysis), **hepatic causes** (hepatic lipidosis, hepatic necrosis, hepatic failure, etc.), and **post-hepatic causes** (pancreatitis, neoplasia of stomach, pancreas, duodenum or bile duct, and common bile duct obstruction).

In **cats that are not icteric,** the list of potential causes broadens extensively to include the spectrum of metabolic, neoplastic, toxic and infectious causes of both systemic and primary gastrointestinal origin.

Treatment

Therapy for cats with cholangitis is **largely supportive**, but the histopathologic findings are crucial in **determining severity, the type of inflammatory infiltrate** (which is essential to choosing appropriate therapy), and the overall **prognosis** for the disease.

Most cats with severe liver disease will require **fluid therapy** to replace deficits, provide maintenance fluid support during the recovery period, and induce diuresis to assist removal of hepatotoxins and prevent tubular sludging from bilirubinuria and casts.

The fluids should be **isotonic, balanced electrolyte solutions**, but preferably **not containing lactate** which is not converted to bicarbonate in cats with liver failure and thus serves as an **additional source of acid** (Ringers solution and Normosol-R are replacement electrolyte solutions without lactate).

Vomiting should be controlled with a combination of **anti-emetic therapy** (e.g. metoclopramide or dolasetron) and **acid-blocking therapy (H$_2$ antagonists** such as famotidine, ranitidine or cimetidine), since cats with liver disease are **prone to the development of hypergastrinemic gastritis**.

Diarrhea is rarely severe enough to require therapy and often resolves as the anorexia worsens.

Cholerectic agents (ursodeoxycholic acid) should be used to **reduce bile sludging and improve bile salt flow.**

Cats with **neutrophilic cholangitis** should be given **broad-spectrum parenteral antibiotics.** Penicillin or metronidazole, and fluorinated quinolones or aminoglycosides combined together provide a good spectrum of activity for enteric pathogens. Ideally, the antibiotic choice should be based upon culture results, but **if the culture is negative or the cat is systemically ill,** antimicrobial chemotherapy should be initiated and is **continued for 3–6 months.**

Lymphocytic cholangitis is believed to be an **immune-mediated** phenomenon and has recently been shown to occur in association with inflammatory bowel disease, inflammatory renal disease and pancreatitis. **Prednisolone therapy** (2–4 mg/kg/day) is indicated in cats with **lymphocytic plasmacytic hepatic infiltrates.** The decision of when to decrease the dose to 1 mg/kg/day or eventually every other day depends entirely on the cat, its clinical response to treatment and clinicopathologic evidence of improvement.

Metronidazole (10–15 mg/kg/day PO) for 2–4 weeks or indefinitely is also used, especially in cats with concurrent IBD.

Ursodeoxycholic acid supplementation is also recommended (10–15 mg/kg/day PO) indefinitely for its choleretic activity.

Nutritional support must be provided, and in the short term (1–3 days) **nasoesophageal feeding tubes** work well, but for longer periods, **esophageal feeding tubes** or a **percutaneous endoscopic gastrostomy (PEG) tube** should be placed to allow larger amounts of food per feeding, as well as feeding a blenderized cat food rather than liquid enteral diets.

Most anorectic or ill cats will benefit from **addition of B vitamins to the fluids.** However, fat-soluble vitamin deficiency may also develop in cats that are anorectic or have malabsorption. **Supplementation with vitamin K** (2.5–5 mg SC q 2 weeks) and in some cases, **vitamin E** should be considered in those cats.

In some cats with evidence of concurrent lipidosis, **supplemental taurine** (250–500 mg PO q 24 h) and **carnitine** (250 mg PO q 24 h) should be given.

Anti-oxidant therapy with S-adenosylmethionine (SAMe) 20 mg/kg/day PO should be instituted for hepato protection.

CLOSTRIDIUM PERFRINGENS ENTEROCOLITIS

> **Classical signs**
>
> - Typically, there is acute small bowel diarrhea with or without anorexia or lethargy.
> - Some cats develop chronic, intermittent diarrhea.

See main reference on page 721 for details (The Cat With Signs of Acute Small Bowel Diarrhea).

Clinical signs

The **most common clinical sign** is **severe, watery to mucohemorrhagic diarrhea.**

In most cats, the diarrhea only lasts a few days, but in some, it may persist and become chronic. Animals that have severe diarrhea will become dehydrated, lethargic and may be anorexic.

There is **no breed, sex or age predisposition,** but cats from **catteries or in stressed environments** are at increased risk.

Diagnosis

The **history and physical examination findings** help to focus the diagnostic approach toward infectious, parasitic and dietary causes of diarrhea.

The presence of the organism can be confirmed by **culture of fresh fecal specimens.** However, **because this bacterium is part of the normal flora, this is not definitive.**

Similar to the dog, the **presence of spores in large numbers** (> 5/hpf) on a stained fecal smear **does not correlate with the presence of enterotoxin.**

Reverse passive latex agglutination (RPLA) tests for clostridial enterotoxin are available and have been used in dogs and humans, but have **not been evaluated in cats.** In dogs, the test does not differentiate dogs with clostridial diarrhea from normal dogs. A **positive enterotoxin assay determined by ELISA** (Techlab, Inc., Blacksburg, VA) in the context of clinical signs consistent with clostridial infection is strongly supportive of clostridial-associated diarrhea in dogs. The **clinical utility of this assay in cats has not been evaluated.**

PCR tests are also utilized for testing feces for **enterotoxin,** but are not universally available.

FELINE CORONAVIRUS INFECTIONS (FELINE ENTERIC CORONAVIRUS/FELINE INFECTIOUS PERITONITIS)

Classical signs

- Variable and vague clinical signs including weight loss, fever and anorexia.
- Vomiting or diarrhea are less common.

See main references on page 372 for details.

Clinical signs

The clinical signs are quite **variable and depend a great deal upon the stage when the cat presents** for evaluation and whether they have **enteric coronavirus infection or FIP**.

Cats with **fulminant FIP** will likely be **severely depressed, pyretic, anorectic,** and have significant weight loss. Respiratory distress from **pleural effusion** is also common, as is the presence of ascites.

Cats with so-called **non-effusive,** or "dry" FIP, will have more **vague clinical signs**, including reduced appetite, fever, mild weight loss and general malaise. Some cats will have mild abdominal discomfort, respiratory signs and granulomatous retinal lesions.

In some cats, FIP **granulomas** will cause **more focal signs** associated with the body system that is affected.

Vomiting and/or diarrhea are usually secondary to the systemic effects of infection or due to granuloma formation in the GI tract.

Central nervous system signs range from ataxia to seizures, and behavior changes, are common in cats with the non-effusive form of FIP.

Most cats with enteric coronavirus have subclinical infections or only develop mild, self-limiting diarrhea.

Diagnosis

The **definitive diagnosis of FIP in cats is quite difficult,** especially in cases of focal or non-fulminant FIP.

Serologic tests are not useful, because most are **not specific for FIP rather than coronavirus infection.** The ELISA for the 7B protein of the FIP virus generates a relatively high number of false-negative and false-positive results. **Polymerase chain reaction (PCR) testing** is the best hope for a definitive test, but at present is **only definitive for confirmation that a cat does not have FIP**. The **PCR test still has false positives** that prevent it from being a good screening/diagnostic test.

Currently, **the definitive test for FIP remains histopathologic examination** and virus isolation.

FELINE IMMUNODEFICIENCY VIRUS

Classical signs

- Variable clinical signs which depend on the stage of the disease and its presentation (immunodeficiency disease, neoplasia, CNS disease, etc.).
- Chronic diarrhea sometimes occurs.

See main reference on page 339 for details.

Clinical signs

The **most common signs** in cats with FIV are **immunodeficiency diseases** such as **chronic or recurrent infections,** especially of the oral cavity (gingivitis/stomatitis), skin (dermatitis, neoplasia), ears (chronic otitis), urinary tract (cystitis) and GI tract.

Chronic enteritis or enterocolitis are associated with **chronic diarrhea, weight loss, anorexia and lethargy**.

In severe cases, the diarrhea is persistent and unresponsive to therapy.

Other clinical signs are associated with development of CNS disease, neoplasia or secondary infections that result in systemic illness.

FIV is **most prevalent in middle-aged, male cats that live outdoors** or are allowed to roam, and are prone to fighting.

Diagnosis

The **history and physical examination findings** are often suggestive of chronic immunodeficiency disease.

Hemogram and serum chemistry abnormalities are not specific, but **lymphopenia is a common finding.**

Diagnosis is made by determining the **presence of FIV antibody** on a commercially available ELISA test, as long as the cat has not been previously vaccinated with the FIV vaccine.

A western blot analysis or PCR test can be used to confirm the presence of the virus.

In cases where FIV is confirmed, a further search for **other infectious or parasitic causes** (*Cryptosporidia, Toxoplasma, Giardia, Campylobacter, Salmonella,* etc.) should be pursued because **concurrent infections with other agents are common with FIV.**

INTESTINAL ADENOCARCINOMA

Classical signs

- Weight loss, anorexia and vague signs of malaise.
- Vomiting is the more common than diarrhea.
- Most common in older, Siamese cats.

See main reference on page 677 for details.

Clinical signs

The **most common clinical signs are anorexia, weight loss and vague signs of malaise.**

Vomiting is more common than diarrhea because of the tendency of the tumor to produce an annular, obstructive lesion in the distal small intestine, however, diarrhea is not unusual. In general, the **GI signs occur late** in the course of the disease.

Abdominal pain may also occur, especially in cats with **metastatic disease**.

The disease is most common in **older, Siamese cats**.

Diagnosis

A history of persistent lethargy, weight loss or anorexia in an older cat, especially a Siamese, should raise suspicions of chronic GI disease and the need for further evaluation.

Abdominal palpation may reveal a thickened region of bowel or a firm mass.

A routine hemogram and chemistry profile is often **unremarkable** or has **non-specific abnormalities** associated with chronic disease, such as mild non-regenerative anemia, hypoproteinemia, or elevated liver enzyme concentrations.

Imaging studies such as **contrast radiography** or **ultrasound examinations** are useful in identifying and localizing the lesion. Ultrasound can also be used to obtain a **fine-needle aspirate of the mass or regional lymph nodes. A thoracic radiograph to check for metastasis** is also indicated.

Ultimately, the **definitive diagnosis is by histopathologic examination** of the tissue obtained either by **endoscopic or surgical biopsies**.

Surgical exploratory is often the best approach for both obtaining tissue for diagnosis, as well as allowing for surgical removal of the affected tissue. In addition, biopsies of regional lymph nodes can also be obtained.

CAMPYLOBACTERIOSIS

Classical signs

- Abdominal distention, colicky abdominal pain, and diarrhea are most common.
- Kittens are generally in poor body condition, or have other concurrent infections.

See main reference on page 726 for details.

Clinical signs

Campylobacter was isolated from **21% of cats with diarrhea and 4% of healthy cats** in one study. Other studies with and without diarrhea have reported isolation rates varying from 0–50%.

In cats, **clinical signs of campylobacteriosis are uncommon,** as most infections are asymptomatic in the absence of other pathogens. **Concurrent infections with other intestinal pathogens,** such as *Giardia* or *Salmonella* **may exacerbate signs.**

Affected cats are usually **less than 6 months** of age.

The primary clinical sign of infection is **diarrhea,** which may be watery, bloody, mucoid or a combination.

Some kittens will become systemically ill with lethargy, dehydration and anorexia observed.

Most kittens will have acute diarrhea, but in some cats, **chronic, recurrent bouts of diarrhea** are observed.

Diagnosis

History and physical examination findings are important to rule out other causes, but may be unremarkable.

Routine hematology, chemistry profiles and imaging studies are typically **within normal limits.**

Diagnosis can be confirmed by culturing freshly obtained fecal samples. Samples can be transported at room temperature without special handling, but **must be cultured in a microaerophilic atmosphere.**

A **specific request for culture of** *Campylobacter* should be submitted if it is suspected.

Dark-field or phase contrast microscopy can also be used to identify the motile, curved bacteria on fresh fecal samples. **Gram-stained samples** can also be used to identify the gull wing-shaped rods in the feces. However, these approaches are less sensitive and require more technical skill.

Differential diagnosis

Infectious (*Salmonella, Clostridium*), **parasitic** (*Giardia, Cryptosporidia,* etc.), and **dietary** (food intolerance or dietary indiscretion) agents should all be considered.

Treatment

Since most cats with *Campylobacter* infections are asymptomatic, or it is associated with other infections,

the effectiveness of antibiotics for treatment of this disease is unknown.

Several antibiotics appear to be effective in eliminating the organism, including erythromycin (10 mg/kg q 8 h PO), metronidazole (5–10 mg/kg q 12 h PO), cephalosporins (20 mg/kg q 12 h PO), and fluorinated quinolones (5 mg/kg q 12 h PO).

EXOCRINE PANCREATIC INSUFFICIENCY

Classical signs

- Weight loss despite a vigorous appetite, which may include pica and coprophagy.
- Fecal characteristics may be normal, soft and voluminous or watery diarrhea.
- Poor haircoat and greasy, flakey seborrhea are also common.
- Very rare in cats.

Pathogenesis

The **most common cause** of exocrine pancreatic insufficiency (EPI) in the cat is **chronic pancreatitis.**

A less common cause of EPI is infestation with the feline pancreatic fluke, *Eurytrema procyonis.*

Other, possible causes of EPI in cats include **pancreatic adenocarcinoma,** and congenital pancreatic acinar hypoplasia or aplasia.

Idiopathic pancreatic acinar atrophy, the most common cause of EPI in dogs, **has not been reported in cats.**

In humans with EPI caused by chronic pancreatitis, diabetes mellitus occurs concurrently. **It is unknown whether cats with chronic pancreatitis and EPI will also progress to develop diabetes mellitus** as well, however, diabetes mellitus has been reported in a cat with EPI.

EPI is believed to develop when **> 90% of the enzymes of the exocrine pancreas are destroyed.** These enzymes play an integral role in assimilating the major food components: proteins, lipids and carbohydrates.

Pancreatic enzymes increase the efficiency of breakdown of macromolecules in the digestive tract and enhance the transport mechanisms for sugars, amino acids and fatty acids. Thus, **without pancreatic enzymes, food substances are inefficiently broken down and cannot be readily transported across the intestinal lumen.**

Diarrhea occurs due to the **presence of large quantities of fats, protein and carbohydrates,** which are osmotically active.

Maldigestion of these important nutrients leads to **weight loss** and may also cause **deficiencies of vitamins, fatty acids or other essential nutrients.**

Clinical signs

This is a **rare disease in cats.**

The **most common clinical signs are polyphagia, diarrhea and weight loss**.

Vomiting and anorexia are also occasionally reported.

The feces are typically **pale, loose, voluminous**, and they may be quite **malodorous**.

Cats often have a **greasy, flaky haircoat due to the fat malabsorption**.

Deficiencies of fat-soluble vitamins can result in a bleeding disorder (vitamin K-responsive coagulopathy), which may present as excessive bleeding from venipuncture sites or spontaneous hemorrhage (nose bleeds, hematuria, melena, etc.).

Diagnosis

Results from **routine hematology and chemistry profiles will be normal** in most cats. Occasionally, elevations in hepatic enzymes or neutrophilia will be observed.

Routine **abdominal radiography and ultrasonography** is usually normal, and is **not diagnostic.**

Fecal proteolytic activity testing will reveal **undetectable levels of enzymes,** which is diagnostic for EPI, but the test is very labile, so **false-positive results may occur due to improper sample handling.**

A recently validated radioimmunoassay for **feline trypsin-like immunoreactivity (fTLI)** is available, much like the TLI test available for use in dogs.

Severely decreased fTLI concentrations (< 8 ug/L) are diagnostic for EPI in cats.

All cats with EPI should have a **serum cobalamin and folate assay,** since many cats with EPI are cobalamin deficient or have concurrent small bowel disease (folate levels will be low).

Differential diagnosis

The clinical signs are so non-specific that many other diseases that cause polyphagia, weight loss and diarrhea must be considered. **Hyperthyroidism**, diabetes mellitus, corticosteroid treatment or hyperadrenocorticism, **chronic renal failure**, heart failure, liver disease, dental disease, neoplasia, **and chronic intestinal diseases such as inflammatory bowel disease** are the main differentials.

Treatment

Most cats with EPI can be successfully treated by **dietary supplementation with pancreatic enzymes**. The powder products (1 tsp per meal) appear to be more clinically effective than tablets.

If the cat refuses to eat the food with pancreatic extract, raw pancreas can be offered, **but it is essential to use bovine pancreas to prevent transmission of Aujeszky's disease in porcine pancreas.**

A diet that contains **low amounts of insoluble fiber should be fed,** since insoluble fibers may interfere with pancreatic enzyme activity.

Some cats will not respond to enzyme supplementation alone, and this may be due to **concurrent cobalamin deficiency or small intestinal disease**. Cobalamin supplementation should be given **parenterally (100–250 µg SC once weekly** for 6–8 weeks, then monthly or bimonthly as needed).

In cats with **suspected vitamin K deficiency,** supplementation should also be initiated (vitamin K_1 1 mg/kg/day PO).

It is **unknown whether or not cats develop small intestinal bacterial overgrowth as a complication of EPI** (as is common in dogs). However, in cats that do not respond as anticipated to pancreatic enzyme supplementation, addition of metronidazole or tetracycline to the treatment regime is indicated.

Prognosis

Because EPI is associated with the **irreversible loss** of pancreatic acinar tissue, **complete recovery is not possible.**

However, with appropriate management, cats with EPI will gain weight, pass normal feces and can live a normal life.

Prevention

There is no known way to prevent the development of EPI, however, if cats with chronic pancreatitis can be recognized and appropriately managed, it may be possible to prevent the consequences of chronic pancreatitis and the development of EPI.

IDIOPATHIC JUVENILE DIARRHEA

Classical signs

- The only presenting sign is chronic diarrhea.

Pathogenesis

Unknown pathogenesis.

Clinical signs

Disorder occurs in **kittens and young cats under a year of age**.

The only clinical sign is presence of **chronic small bowel diarrhea**.

Kittens are **otherwise healthy, active and gain weight**.

Diagnosis

The diagnosis is one of exclusion. Thus, infectious, parasitic, dietary and mechanical disorders must all be ruled out.

Cats with this syndrome are **often purebred cats, and the diarrhea is self-limiting once they reach adult age.**

Differential diagnosis

Because this is a disease of kittens, bacterial, viral, parasitic, protozoal, dietary and toxic causes of diarrhea must all be carefully considered.

Treatment

There is **no known effective treatment for this condition,** but it appears to be self-limiting as the kitten reaches adult age. The reason for this is unknown, but may be due to development of an adult, fully competent immune system.

Prognosis

Good once the kitten reaches adult age.

INTESTINAL MAST CELL TUMOR

Classical signs

- Weight loss, decreased appetite or anorexia and chronic diarrhea.

See main reference on page 687 for details.

Clinical signs

Systemic mast cell tumors produce GI tract signs through **release of histamine and other vasoactive substances**, which result in **gastroduodenal ulceration**.

Intestinal mast cell tumors are typically poorly differentiated, highly malignant tumors that appear to consist of degranulated (e.g. non-functional) neoplastic mast cells. However, they produce GI tract signs through **local effects** (e.g. obstruction) or **surface ulceration** (bleeding) rather than through the release of vasoactive substances, as is the case with systemic mast cell tumors.

The most common clinical signs are **weight loss, anorexia or decreased appetite, and chronic diarrhea**. Other signs include lethargy, vomiting or acute abdominal pain.

Melena or chronic asymptomatic blood loss may result in anemia, and sometimes is severe enough to cause weakness or lethargy.

In some cats, **a palpable thickened intestinal segment or a mass** will be present.

Intestinal mast cell tumors are very small, difficult to palpate until late, and tend to be solitary. They occur as an infiltrating mass, but **metastasize early in the course of the disease**.

Intestinal mast cell tumors are not generally associated with development of massive splenomegaly or systemic mast cell infiltration like systemic mastocytosis.

Diagnosis

A **chronic history of weight loss or anorexia** in a middle-aged or older cat should raise the suspicion of intestinal neoplasia.

Routine hemogram and serum chemistry profiles will often be normal, but non-specific abnormalities such as mild non-regenerative anemia, hypoproteinemia or hypoalbuminemia, and electrolyte disturbances associated with chronic vomiting or diarrhea can be seen.

Other **tests of GI function** (e.g. fTLI, fecal alpha-1 protease inhibitor, cobalamin/folate assays, fecal analyses for parasites) should be considered or performed, but **will not be diagnostic.**

Imaging studies, especially ultrasound examination, will be the most helpful in localizing the lesion (which can be easily missed because they are often extremely small or focal). **Fine-needle aspirates** of focal masses can be obtained which will often help direct further diagnostic and treatment plans.

Endoscopy may be helpful, but in many cases, these tumors are present in the jejunum, and are unreachable by the endoscope.

If imaging studies are unavailable, or fine-needle aspirates are non-diagnostic, an **exploratory laparotomy is indicated**.

Differential diagnosis

The primary differentials for cats with chronic weight loss, anorexia and chronic diarrhea are IBD, neoplasia, lymphangiectasia, and systemic organ failure or dysfunction (renal disease, liver failure, etc.).

Treatment

Treatment is palliative and supportive for cats with intestinal mast cell tumors.

Surgical removal of the affected segment of bowel with **wide surgical margins** is the only therapy reported to be effective in prolonging survival. **Mesenteric, hepatic and splenic metastasis** are commonly observed by the time the tumor is diagnosed.

Chemotherapy has not been shown to increase survival time in cats with this disease, although **prednisolone** (2–4 mg/kg/day) and **histamine$_2$ blockers** (cimetidine, ranitidine, famotidine) are advocated to reduce secondary clinical signs associated with mast cell disease.

Nutritional support may be required in cats that refuse to eat, as they will develop hepatic lipidosis and protein calorie malnutrition.

The prognosis is poor, as the average survival time following diagnosis with this tumor is **4 months.**

HYPOADRENOCORTICISM

> ### Classical signs
>
> - Typically, lethargy, weakness and vomiting.
> - Regurgitation (megaesophagus), diarrhea and abdominal pain may occur.

See main reference on page 752 for details.

Clinical signs

Lethargy, weakness and vomiting are the classic presenting signs, but diarrhea and abdominal pain may also be observed.

Megaesophagus, with resultant regurgitation, may occur due to muscle weakness, but it is **very uncommon in cats.**

Hypoadrenal crisis is associated with an acute episode of collapse due to severe alterations in **sodium and potassium** that result in severe muscle weakness and cardiovascular collapse. This is a **rare occurrence in cats compared to dogs,** but requires rapid recognition and response to stabilize the patient.

Diagnosis

The **history and clinical signs** are often **too non-specific to be helpful,** but are still important in development of a diagnostic approach.

The **classic hemogram and biochemical changes** include eosinophilia, lymphopenia, azotemia, hypercalcemia, hyperkalemia, hyponatremia and low or isosthenuric urine specific gravity.

However, **some cats will not have mineralocorticoid deficiency,** thus, **no electrolyte changes** will be evident on the chemistry profile.

Cats with **severe hyperkalemia** (> 7 mEq/L) will have characteristic ECG abnormalities and bradycardia.

Definitive diagnosis is by performing an ACTH stimulation test. Cortisol levels will be low and will not respond to ACTH administration.

Differential diagnosis

Because the clinical signs and routine blood work are non-specific, **a wide variety of metabolic, neoplastic, infectious and idiopathic conditions must be considered.** In many cats, the ACTH stimulation test is performed based on clinical suspicion, not clear physical or biochemical findings that suggest hypoadrenocorticism.

Treatment

In cats that are clinically dehydrated, have pre-renal azotemia or in an acute adrenal crisis, **fluid therapy with isotonic saline** is the initial treatment of choice. If there are **cardiac arrhythmias** or ECG abnormalities associated with **severe hyperkalemia, regular insulin** (0.2–0.5 U/kg IV) **and dextrose therapy** (0.5–1.0 g/kg IV slowly), **intravenous bicarbonate** (body weight (kg) × 0.5 × base deficit, or 0.5–1.0 mEq/kg over 6 h), **or intravenous calcium gluconate therapy** (0.5–1.0 ml/kg, IV slowly) may be administered to rapidly lower extracellular potassium levels.

Parenteral corticosteroids (dexamethasone, methyl prednisolone, which have some mineralocorticoid effects as well) should be administered in physiologic doses (0.2–0.4 mg/kg) initially, and **continued daily** (oral or injectable) as replacement therapy until the cat is stable.

Once the cat is in stable condition, **replacement of mineralocorticoid hormones** can be achieved orally (fluorinef) or with repository forms of the hormone, such as desoxycorticosterone pivalate (DOCP).

Therapy for cats with this disease will be lifelong, and **frequent rechecks** to allow dose adjustments will be required. Most cats will have a good quality of life with proper management of this disease.

HISTOPLASMOSIS

Classical signs

- Signs may indicate respiratory, eye, CNS, bone marrow or GI tract involvement.
- Typically, respiratory signs such as wheezing, coughing or dyspnea predominate.
- GI signs are usually associated with protracted, watery diarrhea, that may contain blood or mucus.

Pathogenesis

Histoplasma capsulatum is a soil-borne fungus, which is found in many temperate and subtropical areas of the world, especially where it is moist and humid. The organism grows particularly well if there is bird or bat excrement in the soil.

In the States, it is most frequent in Southern and Central USA around the **Ohio, Missouri and Mississippi Rivers**.

The majority of infections are subclinical or cause only mild, transient clinical signs.

Cats are equally susceptible as dogs, and the **majority of symptomatic cats are young** (< 4 years of age).

Infection is contracted via inhalation, although the GIT may also be a route of infection. Signs occur approximately 12–16 days after exposure.

Initial infection is confined to the respiratory tract, **but dissemination often occurs** resulting in chronic disease over months or years with signs referable to spleen (splenomegaly), liver (hepatomegaly, icterus, ascites), GIT (chronic diarrhea and weight loss), peritoneum (omental or mesenteric masses); lymph nodes (peripheral or abdominal lymphadenopathy), bone marrow (anemia, thrombocytopenia, leukopenia), bones (lameness and proliferative or lytic boney lesions), eyes (conjunctivitis, exudative anterior uveitis, multifocal granulomatous chorioretinitis, optic neuritis), central nervous system (ataxia, seizures, circling, disorientation, anisocoria, paresis, decreased conscious proprioception), and occasionally skin (nodular or ulcerated lesions).

Clinical signs

The **most common clinical signs** of histoplasmosis in cats are **multisystemic**, including **depression, weight loss, anorexia, dyspnea or lameness**.

Other signs may include fever, pale mucous membranes, peripheral lymphadenopathy, icterus, hepatomegaly, skin nodules or splenomegaly.

The organism can be **most commonly found in the respiratory tract, bone, bone marrow, skin and GI tract**.

GI signs are not common in cats (as they are in dogs), but when they occur **chronic diarrhea, mesenteric lymphadenopathy and anorexia** are common.

Ocular changes may include conjunctivitis, anterior uveitis, retinal detachment or chorioretinitis.

Diagnosis

The clinical signs of disseminated histoplasmosis are consistent with **systemic illness** and are associated with a **wide variety of non-specific clinical and laboratory changes**.

Anemia of chronic disease is the **most common hematologic abnormality**.

Occasionally histoplasma organisms can be found in circulating mononuclear cells and eosinophils.

Thrombocytopenia is also a common abnormality.

Diagnosis of histoplasmosis by serology is unreliable as the sensitivity and specificity for the organism is poor.

The **best method of diagnosis** is to identify the organism in **cytologic or histopathologic examinations**. The **best tissues** for diagnosis of histoplasmosis in the cat are **bone marrow, lymph nodes, lung, liver or skin nodules if present**.

Differential diagnosis

There are a **wide variety of potential differentials** due to the different clinical presentation that may occur depending on the organ system affected.

Treatment

Itraconazole (10 mg/kg PO q 24 h) is the drug of choice for initial therapy. It is highly effective and has minimal toxicity, but is relatively expensive and treatment must be continued for 1 month (at least) beyond the resolution of clinical signs and evidence of disease (typically 6–9 months).

Other treatment options include fluconazole, ketoconazole and amphotericin B.

The **success rate with itraconazole therapy** is reported to be anywhere from 33% to >90%, but this depends in large measure on the severity of the infection at the time of diagnosis.

INTUSSUSCEPTION

> ## Classical signs
>
> - Abdominal pain, anorexia and vomiting.
> - Diarrhea, weight loss, and lethargy occur in long-standing cases.
> - Intussusceptions are usually seen in young cats or kittens.

See main reference on page 643 for details.

Clinical signs

With **high intussusceptions**, vomiting, abdominal discomfort, anorexia, lethargy, dehydration and hypovolemia leading to shock are the most common clinical signs.

Low intussusceptions (at the iliocolic junction) typically present with bloody, mucoid diarrhea, tenesmus, intermittent vomiting and weight loss. In many of these cases, the intussusception can be palpated.

Most intussusceptions are associated with acute disease, but **sliding intussusceptions** may result in chronic, intermittent signs.

A **palpable mass in the abdomen** may be evident, especially with low intussusceptions.

Diagnosis

Hemogram and serum biochemistry profiles will be variable depending on the severity and location of the intussusception, however, dehydration, electrolyte abnormalities, anemia and leukocyte changes have all been observed depending on the site, severity and precipitating cause of the intussusception.

Radiographs and/or ultrasound examination of the gastrointestinal tract are the best means of confirming the diagnosis. Radiographs may not be definitive, but in most cases, an obstructive pattern (dilated loops of bowel, different bowel loop sizes) will be apparent. However, an **ultrasound of the abdomen will often definitively identify the intussusception.** Contrast studies may be used but should not be done at the expense of delaying treatment in severely ill cases. In the case of sliding intussusceptions, the diagnostic procedures should be performed when the clinical signs are most prominent.

Endoscopic examination or colonoscopy can also be used to obtain a diagnosis, especially with low intussusceptions.

Exploratory laparotomy may be required to obtain a definitive diagnosis, and is essential for treatment, **so in cats with evidence of intestinal obstruction, or in cats with acute abdomen and shock, surgery should be performed early.**

Differential diagnosis

Many diseases that can precipitate an intussusception (e.g. viral enteritis, foreign bodies, gastroenteritis, intestinal parasitism, etc.) **also have clinical signs that mimic it.** Thus, a thorough physical examination, diagnostic evaluation, and close patient monitoring are essential. **Mesenteric volvulus** is a very difficult condition to differentiate from intussusception, both clinically and radiographically.

Treatment

Intussusception must be considered a **surgical emergency**. Cats with signs of shock or endotoxemia should be prepared for surgery by **correcting fluid and electrolyte imbalances,** administration of **broad-spectrum, parenteral antibiotics** (combinations such as ampicillin or cefazolin and enrofloxain, amikacin, cefoxitin or imipenam), and use of **histamine-2 blockers** (ranitidine or famotidine) or **protectants** if gastric erosions or ulceration is suspected.

Motility-enhancing drugs, such as metoclopramide, **are contraindicated** in patients with GI obstruction and should not be used.

After surgical correction, if gastric ulceration is not a complicating factor, oral alimentation should be instituted in the first 24 hours, to enhance the return of normal motility and reduce the possibility of postoperative ileus.

OTHER SMALL INTESTINAL NEOPLASIA (FIBROSARCOMA, CARCINOIDS, PLASMACYTOMA)

Classical signs

- Weight loss.
- Lethargy or depression.
- Anorexia.
- Vomiting and/or diarrhea.

Clinical signs

The **clinical signs observed will depend upon the tumor location** in the GI tract.

In cats, anorexia, weight loss and lethargy are the most common clinical signs of any gastrointestinal neoplastic disease.

Vomiting and/or diarrhea may be observed, but will be variable depending on whether the tumor is in the small intestine or colon, and whether it is diffuse or solitary in extent.

Diagnosis

Palpation of an intestinal mass is an important diagnostic tool, since many of these tumors are solitary and produce strictures or obstructions.

Hematology and serum biochemistry profiles may be within normal limits in cats with intestinal neoplasia.

Abnormalities associated with secondary effects of the tumor include dehydration, electrolyte imbalances, anemia of chronic disease, etc.

Radiographs of both the thorax and abdomen are an important, but sometimes non-diagnostic, tool.

Radiographs are best for assessment of pulmonary metastasis.

Ultrasound is an invaluable tool for **lesion localization**, determination of **lesion extent** and in some cases, obtaining a **fine-needle aspirate** or biopsy of the lesion.

Definitive diagnosis is by **histopathologic evaluation of a biopsy** or tissue obtained after surgical resection.

APUDOMAS

> ### Classical signs
>
> - Severe and in some cases intractable small bowel diarrhea.

Pathogenesis

Amine precursor uptake and decarboxylation (APUD) cells are a diffuse system of endocrine cells in the body (primarily associated with the GI tract and other endocrine organs) that are able to **secrete biogenic amines from amino acid precursors.**

APUD cells are responsible for the **potent secretory functions** that APUD tumors display (e.g. insulinomas, gastrinomas, pheochromocytomas and carcinoid tumors of the gut).

Clinical signs

The clinical signs are dependent on the tumor and effects, for example carcinoid tumors of the GI tract may produce **secretory diarrhea** in affected cats because of the vasoactive amines they produce.

These are **rare tumors,** and most tumors reported to date have been clinically silent.

Gastrinomas are also rare neoplasms that secrete gastrin, causing excessive secretion of hydrochloric acid by the stomach and resulting in **gastric and duodenal ulcer disease.**

Diagnosis

These are **rare neoplasms** that are extremely difficult to diagnose (because they are **very difficult to find**).

Some of these tumors (insulinoma, gastrinoma) can be **presumptively diagnosed by measuring the level of the hormone they produce,** but most APUDomas do not secrete hormones that are routinely measured.

Differential diagnosis

Because these tumors are so rare, **all other causes of chronic diarrhea should be considered** before pursuing the APUD tumors as the cause of diarrhea.

Treatment

The treatment of choice is to find and **surgically excise the tumor.** However, because **the tumors are often microscopic or extremely small,** they are often overlooked during an exploratory. In addition, by the time the tumor is large enough to find, it has often already metastasized.

Supportive care and symptomatic therapy are often the only avenue. For example, in cats with gastrinomas, histamine$_2$ blockers and proton pump inhibitors are used to help control the excessive secretion of acid.

Prognosis

Guarded to poor. These tumors are usually malignant, surgical excision is rarely curative and metastatic tumors are poorly responsive to chemotherapy.

HYPEREOSINOPHILIC SYNDROME

> ### Classical signs
>
> - Severe and in some cases intractable small bowel diarrhea.
> - Peripheral eosinophilia and infiltration of the bone marrow, spleen, liver, lymph nodes and other organs with eosinophils.

Pathogenesis

Hypereosinophilic syndrome is a **relatively common variant of eosinophilic enteritis** in the cat, but is **distinct from eosinophilic leukemia.**

The disease is characterized by **infiltration of eosinophils** in bowel, lymph nodes, spleen, liver and other organs, and **peripheral eosinophilia**, which separates this disease from eosinophilic IBD.

The **etiopathogenesis of this disorder is unknown**, but may be due to extensive antigenic dissemination or aberrant regulation of the normal eosinophilic response.

The disease is most common in middle-aged to older cats, and there is no breed or sex predisposition.

Clinical signs

The **clinical signs** are similar to those of cats with IBD except the **intestinal wall thickening** is more pronounced, **hepatosplenomegaly** is common, and **bloody diarrhea is common**.

Some cats will **cough**, have **skin lesions** (miliary dermatitis) and have **peripheral lymphadenopathy**, but these clinical signs are less common.

Diagnosis

The diagnosis is made by **histopathologic examination of liver, spleen, lymph node or intestinal biopsies** which will reveal infiltration of large numbers of normal eosinophils.

Differential diagnosis

The **primary differentials are eosinophilic IBD and eosinophilic leukemia**. Eosinophilic leukemia is differentiated from hypereosinophilic syndrome by its **localization of eosinophils to the peripheral circulation and bone marrow**. In **eosinophilic IBD**, eosinophils are found **only in the lamina propria of the intestine** and do not infiltrate other abdominal organs and lymph nodes.

Treatment

High-dose prednisolone therapy (3–6 mg/kg/day PO) is most commonly used, but **relapses are common,** even if the high doses of steroids are maintained.

An alternative therapy is with hydroxyurea (7.5 mg/kg q 12 h PO) for 3–14-day courses, as required to maintain the cat in remission.

Cats with hypereosinophilic syndrome often have **severe diarrhea,** and may require **nutritional or fluid support** until the disease is brought under control.

Prognosis

The prognosis is guarded to poor.

INTESTINAL DIVERTICULOSIS

> **Classical signs**
>
> - Moderate to severe, small or large bowel diarrhea, and weight loss, depending on the location and number of diverticuli.

Pathogenesis

Diverticuli may be congenital or occur secondary to intussusception or other intestinal obstructive processes.

Most clinical disease is associated with the diverticulitis and infection occurring at the site.

Clinical signs

Many intestinal diverticuli are **clinically silent** and are only found incidentally.

Diverticulitis may result in the development of **diarrhea, abdominal pain, lethargy or anorexia.**

Diagnosis

The **definitive diagnosis is made by imaging studies** (ultrasound, contrast rads) **or by visualization** (endoscopy or exploratory surgery).

Differential diagnosis

The **rarity of this problem** should suggest that all other possible causes of diarrhea and lethargy are ruled out before consideration of this condition.

Treatment

Surgical resection of the affected bowel segment in clinically affected patients. Cats with diverticuli but without signs of disease do not require surgery.

PROTEIN-LOSING ENTEROPATHY

Classical signs

- Weight loss, poor hair coat, inappetance, and chronic (may be intermittent) diarrhea.

Pathogenesis

Primary lymphangiectasia is rare as a cause of protein-losing enteropathy (PLE) in cats. Most cats have PLE secondary to **IBD or lymphosarcoma.**

PLE in cats may be associated with **other severe malabsorptive or infiltrative diseases** (e.g. histoplasmosis, exocrine pancreatic insufficiency), but these are **rare causes of protein loss in cats**.

Clinical signs

The clinical signs are **dependent on the primary cause** of the PLE. Cat may have anorexia and weight loss only, or have chronic unrelenting diarrhea, along with inappetance.

Most cats are **middle-aged to older,** typical of the age range for IBD or lymphoma. PLE is simply **another complication of the primary process** and is not a diagnostic entity in cats.

Diagnosis

Cats with PLE will have **decreased serum total protein and albumin levels**, in addition to other abnormalities consistent with their primary disease.

Urinary protein loss, third space loss, lack of adequate intake and severe hepatic disease must all be ruled out before considering a diagnosis of PLE. **Fecal alpha-1 protease inhibitor levels,** a test for abnormal GI protein loss available for dogs, **have not yet been validated for use in cats.**

As for many other GI conditions, the definitive diagnosis of the inciting cause of PLE is obtained by biopsy.

Differential diagnosis

Since **PLE is not a definitive diagnosis**, a search for the primary cause is **essential. Cats rarely develop** lymphangiectasia or idiopathic PLE as is reported in dogs.

Other causes for low albumin and serum protein levels must be considered when this abnormality is discovered, e.g. renal protein loss, severe hepatic disease, third space loss, and severe protein calorie malnutrition.

Treatment

Treatment of PLE is directed solely at **correction of the primary disease process.** Specific therapy for lymphoma or IBD will correct or at least control the cause of the protein loss.

Symptomatic therapy for severe intestinal protein loss includes a **highly digestible diet**. Alternative sources of protein for inclusion in the diet are **hydrolyzed protein diets** (Hill's z/d) and **elemental diets** (e.g. Vivonex).

Medium chain triglyceride (MCT) oil is not recommended for use in cats, as it is in dogs, because of the **increased risk of hepatic lipidosis.**

Prognosis

Guarded, as most cats with PLE have a disease that is difficult if not impossible to cure.

SHORT BOWEL SYNDROME

Classical signs

- Severe and in some cases intractable small bowel diarrhea.

Pathogenesis

Short bowel syndrome is classically due to **surgical resection of a large segment of the small intestine** that results in fluid overload to the colon and resultant diarrhea.

Other causes include ischemic intestinal diseases such as intussusception, bowel strangulation and intestinal volvulus.

Intestinal adaptation occurs in the large bowel, which ultimately results in a return to a soft or semi-formed fecal specimen, usually **within 2–6 weeks.**

If greater than 85% of the small intestine has been removed the chance for adaptation is poor.

Clinical signs

Diarrhea, **dehydration and weight loss** all occur as a result of short bowel syndrome.

Other signs are related to intestinal malabsorption, such as deficiencies of essential amino acids, vitamins or clotting factors.

Small intestinal bacterial overgrowth may also occur, resulting in vomiting or anorexia as well.

Diagnosis

The diagnosis is **presumptive if surgical resection is the cause**.

Cats are often **hypoproteinemic**, may be **hypocholesterolemic**, and have other **non-specific hemogram or chemistry abnormalities**.

Imaging studies can be used to confirm the diagnosis.

Differential diagnosis

Other diseases that may cause similar signs include **severe intestinal strangulation, intussusception and intestinal volvulus**, which is rare in cats.

Treatment

Tincture of **time** will allow the bowel to **adapt**.

Broad-spectrum antibiotics may be needed.

Low-fat, highly digestible diets are necessary to maximize absorption of nutrients.

Administration of vitamins and minerals is usually needed. Monitoring **prothrombin time and serum cobalamin levels** will help determine whether supplementation is needed. (Vitamin K_1 5 mg/kg once, then 2.5 mg/kg q 12–24 h, cobalamin or multi-B complex injection weekly).

Parenteral nutrition may be required in some cats in the early stages to support them until bowel function returns.

Prognosis

The prognosis is guarded in cats in which diarrhea persists for longer than 2 months after the resection, as by that time, the chances of a return to normal function are poor.

RECOMMENDED READING

August JR. Consultations in Feline Internal Medicine, 2001, WB Saunders, Philadelphia, PA.

Guilford W, Jones B, Markwell P, Arthur D, Collett M, Harte J. Food sensitivity in cats with chronic idiopathic gastrointestinal problems. J Vet Intern Med 2001; 15: 7–13.

Guilford WG, Center SA, Strombeck DR, Williams DA, (eds). Strombeck's Small Animal Gastroenterology, 1996,WB Saunders, Philadelphia, PA.

Marks SL, Kather EJ. Bacterial-associated diarrhea in the dog: a critical appraisal. Vet Clin North Am Small Anim Pract 2003; 33: 1029–1060.

Simpson KW. Vet Clin North Am 1999; 29(2).

34. The cat with signs of large bowel diarrhea (acute and chronic)

Debra L Zoran

> **KEY SIGNS**
>
> - Soft, mucoid, formed to semi-formed feces.
> - + Fresh blood or straining.

MECHANISM?

- Large bowel diarrhea is induced by **increased secretion of water and electrolytes** by colonic epithelial cells, **overload of substrate** (from small bowel) or by **altered motility** (e.g. decreased motility, loss of segmentation).
- **Increased fermentable substrate** (e.g. carbohydrates such as soluble fibers, lactulose, etc.) **may increase fecal water** and create a softer fecal mass.

Signs of large bowel diarrhea:

- Soft, mucoid, formed to semi-formed feces.
- Hematochezia.
- Straining to defecate.
- Increased urgency to defecate.
- Small volume of fecal material expelled.
- Vomiting or weight loss not typically observed.

WHERE?

- **Acute, large bowel diarrhea is uncommon in cats** and is less likely to be associated with parasites (e.g. whipworms) or clostridial enterocolitis compared to dogs.
- **Chronic or recurrent large bowel diarrhea** may be caused by **local** (e.g. large bowel) **or systemic disease,** and thus a **thorough evaluation** that includes a **minimum database, imaging studies** (radiographs, ultrasound, etc.), or **endoscopy with collection of biopsies** is required to determine the cause.
- **Irritant colitis** secondary to ingestion of hair, feathers or other foreign material is a **common cause of acute large bowel diarrhea.**
- **Cats usually do not lose weight or have vomiting episodes in association with large bowel diarrhea** unless a systemic disease is the cause of the problem.

WHAT?

- **The most common causes of large bowel diarrhea are inflammatory** (inflammatory bowel disease), **neoplasia, metabolic diseases** (hyperthyroidism) **and mechanical** (hair, feathers or bone-induced colitis).
- **Food intolerance** may be a common cause of colitis, but is **not well documented in cats.**
- **Clostridial enterocolitis** is the **most common infectious cause of colitis in adult cats,** but the **incidence in cats is low** compared to other causes of large bowel diarrhea.

QUICK REFERENCE SUMMARY
Diseases causing signs of large bowel diarrhea
ANOMALY

- Congenital malformations (e.g. diverticulum, short colon syndrome, vascular ectasia) (p 779)

All are rare conditions that are observed in young cats or kittens, with the severity depending on the anomaly (e.g. short colon syndrome causes severe signs, while vascular ectasia and diverticular formations may initially be clinically silent.

MECHANICAL

- **Irritant (foreign body) colitis** (p 765)

This is the acute development of colitis manifest by the presence of mucoid- to blood-streaked feces resulting from ingestion of hair, bones, string, feathers or other foreign material.

- Perineal hernia (p 776)

Perineal hernias cause perineal swelling associated with a mucoid- or blood-streaked fecal mass and straining to defecate. In long-standing cases, constipation may occur.

- Perianal tumors (p 777)

The tumor mass may cause straining to defecate and other signs of large bowel disease, or it may obstruct the passage of feces and cause constipation.

METABOLIC

- **Hyperthyroidism*** (p 771)

Hyperthyroidism may cause voluminous, soft and mucoid feces due to increased intake and reduced GI transit time, changes in metabolism (malassimilation of food) and motility disturbances.

- Pseudomembraneous colitis (antibiotic-induced colitis) (p 777)

Acute or chronic large bowel diarrhea may be caused by the use of anaerobic antibiotics resulting in overgrowth of pathogenic species that may be resistant to many or most antibiotics. Severe forms of this disease are rare in cats, but diarrhea due to antibiotic use is not uncommon.

NEOPLASTIC

- **Colonic adenocarcinoma*** (p 774)

This is the most common non-hematopoietic tumor of the GI tract and the most common colonic tumor in cats. It typically affects old cats (>10 years) and vomiting, weight loss and lethargy are more common signs than diarrhea.

- **Lymphosarcoma*** (p 773)

Lymphosarcoma tends to cause infiltrative disease that affects both the large and small intestine, but may be localized to the colon in some cases causing only signs of large bowel disease.

- Colorectal polyps (p 778)

These are benign growths that are clinically silent until they grow large enough to prevent normal fecal passage and cause large bowel diarrhea or constipation. Most cases reported in Siamese cats.

continued

continued

NUTRITIONAL

● **Food intolerance** (p 766)

Food intolerance is a non-immune-mediated condition associated with intermittent diarrhea or vomiting, with no pattern or association with eating, and it resolves when the food source is changed to omit the offending substance from the diet. The clinical significance of food intolerance is unknown relative to other causes of diarrhea because of the difficulty in obtaining a definitive diagnosis.

IMMUNOLOGIC

● **Food allergy (dietary hypersensitivity)*** (p 767)

Chronic vomiting appears to be more common than diarrhea in cats with food allergy, and cutaneous signs may also be present.

● **Idiopathic inflammatory bowel disease (IBD)*** (p 768)

This is a chronic inflammatory disease of the feline GI tract that has no known cause. Depending on the extent of the disease, the diarrhea may be entirely of large bowel character, small bowel character or may be a combination of both. Weight loss and vomiting are also frequently observed clinical signs.

INFECTIOUS

● *Infectious colitis (Clostridium spp., E. coli, Campylobacter spp.)** (p 770)

Clostridial spp. cause an enterocolitis characterized by acute onset of soft, mucoid- or blood-streaked feces that may become liquid, unformed small bowel diarrhea. Diarrhea is caused by overgrowth of clostridial spp. followed by subsequent sporulation and enterotoxin formation. *E. coli* is an uncommon cause of enterocolitis and large bowel diarrhea in cats.

● *Parasitic infections (Giardia, Tritrichomonas, Cryptosporidia, Isospora, Toxoplasma, Balantidium and Trichuris)* * (p 775)

Diarrhea is the primary clinical sign with *Tritrichomonas*, *Cryptosporidia* and *Cystoisosporidia* infections. Infections are inapparent except in young kittens and debilitated or immunocompromised adult cats. *Trichuris vulpis* is a rare cause of colitis or large bowel diarrhea in cats, but is occasionally found on fecal examination in cats from a contaminated environment.

Inflammatory:

● Chronic pancreatitis (p 776)

This disease is most often associated with vague, non-localizing signs, but hematochezia and diarrhea with a large bowel character are not unusual.

INTRODUCTION

MECHANISM

The signs of large bowel disease include:
- Increased mucus.
- Hematochezia.
- Straining or increased urgency to defecate.
- Soft to semi-formed feces.
- Normal or increased frequency of defecation but not increased volume.
- It is rarely associated with weight loss or vomiting.

The colon responds to inflammatory conditions by **producing increased amounts of mucus.**

Blood streaks or fresh blood is also a common presenting sign due to the proximity to the anus.

WHERE

Large bowel disease can result from disorders of **ileocecal region, colon or rectum**.

Historical and physical examination signs are important in localizing the problem to the large intestine.

Rectal examination is an especially important component of the physical examination when evaluating a cat for large bowel disease.

WHAT

Large bowel diarrhea can be caused by a variety of infectious, dietary, metabolic, mechanical, neoplastic or idiopathic disorders.
- **Acute large bowel diarrhea is often managed by empirical therapy** with anthelminitics, antibiotics or a diet change.
- The **most common causes of acute large bowel diarrhea are parasites, dietary or infectious agents**.

Chronic large bowel diarrhea is defined as the presence of signs for **more than 3 weeks**.
- Cats with chronic large bowel diarrhea should be **thoroughly evaluated to determine the diagnosis,** both for effective therapy to be initiated and for providing an accurate prognosis.
- The **minimum database** should include a **CBC, panel, urinalysis and complete fecal examination** (fecal flotation, direct, cytology).
- **Other diagnostic approaches** that may be required include radiography, ultrasonography, endoscopic examination (especially for biopsy).
- **Surgery** on the colon is difficult, but in some neoplastic conditions or obstructive diseases, it will be required.

DISEASES CAUSING SIGNS OF LARGE BOWEL DIARRHEA

IRRITANT (FOREIGN BODY) COLITIS**

> ### Classical signs
> - Mucus- or blood-streaked, soft (semi-formed) stools.
> - History of ingestion of feathers, hair, bones or other foreign objects (e.g. string, plants).

Pathogenesis

Colitis and large bowel diarrhea that is caused by the presence of **foreign objects** (e.g. hair, bones, feathers) is primarily due to the **irritation of the colonic epithelium.**

This results in **motility disturbances** and release of local **inflammatory mediators** that cause **secretory or motility changes** and ultimately, diarrhea.

Ingested hair, or a trichobezoar, is a **common cause of irritant colitis in cats**, especially in cats with long hair coats or with dermatologic disorders that result in excessive grooming.

Clinical signs

Irritant colitis causes large bowel diarrhea that is **intermittent and generally not severe** in nature. **Mucus- or blood-streaked, soft (semi-formed) stools** are the most common presenting signs.

The **history typically supports the presumptive diagnosis** (e.g. cat consumes prey, feces contains large amounts of hair or other foreign material).

Diagnosis

A **good history and visual examination of the feces** is especially helpful in making this diagnosis in cats with irritant colitis.

The **physical exam and minimum database** are usually **unremarkable** in these cats.

Survey radiographs may be helpful **if there is bony material** present in the colon, but **otherwise, imaging studies are not helpful.**

Fecal exams are not diagnostic, but may be helpful to **reveal the presence of large amounts of foreign material** in the fecal material.

Because the episodes are typically **intermittent, short lived** (few days at the most) and the **cat is normal in the intervening periods,** more **aggressive diagnostic evaluations are rarely indicated.**

Differential diagnosis

Other important differentials are infectious (clostridial enterocolitis), dietary indiscretion or food intolerance, and parasitic causes of large bowel diarrhea.

Treatment

Identification and removal of the offending substance is curative.

In cats in which the cause cannot be identified or removed:
- Addition of **bulk-forming laxatives** (e.g. psyllium, methylcellulose).
- **Lubricant laxatives** (petroleum-based laxatives found in hair ball remedies).
- **Foods that contain increased fiber** (canned pumpkin, coarse wheat bran) may be helpful.

Alternatively, feeding the cat a **diet that is high in insoluble dietary fiber** to **increase segmentation and propulsion movements in the colon,** may also be effective in decreasing occurrences of irritant colitis.

Prevention

Prevention is **most successful if the cause of the irritation is identified and removed**.

Removal of excess hair (grooming, brushing, clipping) from long-haired cats, **reduction of causes of excessive grooming** (management of pruritus, behavioral therapy), **prevention of prey consumption or ingestion of foreign objects** (e.g. string, rubber bands, etc.) are important measures in controlling foreign body colitis.

FOOD INTOLERANCE**

Classical signs

- Dietary indiscretion: Vomiting, small or large bowel diarrhea, inappetance.
- Food intolerance: Vomiting, small or large bowel diarrhea.

See main reference on page 669 (The Cat With Signs of Chronic Vomiting) for details.

Clinical signs

Dietary indiscretion is more commonly associated with vomiting, but colitis (**hematochezia, large bowel diarrhea, mucus-covered feces**) may occur if the substance ingested reaches the colon intact (hair, feathers, bones) or changes the colonic microflora due to bacterial overgrowth of *E. coli* or other pathogens.

The **signs are acute,** and often include **vomiting or inappetance** in addition to diarrhea.

Food intolerance is an adverse reaction to a food or food substance that is **not immunologic** in nature (e.g. reaction to protein, preservative, flavoring, etc.).

The **signs of food intolerance** may be acute, but **often are chronic and intermittent,** and can involve vomiting alone, diarrhea alone, or a combination.

Diagnosis

The diagnosis of food intolerance is based on cessation of clinical signs upon **elimination of the offending substance from the diet**, and recurrence of signs when the substance or diet is re-introduced to the cats.

A response should be seen with the non-offending diet, whether commercial or homemade, within 4 days if there is total compliance with the diet.

Dietary indiscretion is a presumptive diagnosis made based upon the history of eating lizards, beetles, plants, etc., lack of other physical examination or diagnostic (fecal examinations negative for parasites, normal fecal cytology, normal blood work and radiographs) findings.

Differential diagnosis

Food allergy is the major differential diagnosis for cats with food intolerance and it is very difficult to distinguish the two conditions clinically. Since the treatment for both food intolerance and food allergy is the same and the response to treatment should be identical, it is probably unnecessary in clinical practice to differentiate the two conditions.

Treatment

In most cats, **treatment of dietary indiscretion is symptomatic** (e.g. feeding a high-fiber diet for cats with large bowel signs, low-residue diet if both large and small bowel signs are present), with judicious use of antibiotics (for bacterial flora manipulation) and fluid support if needed. Prevent access to the offending material.

Treatment of food intolerance involves the removal of the offending substance from the diet, which is usually achieved by changing to a commercial diet containing different protein or carbohydrate sources, and no additives, flavorings, colorings, etc.

FOOD ALLERGY (DIETARY HYPERSENSITIVITY)*

Classical signs

- GI signs (vomiting, diarrhea, weight loss, inappetance) are most commonly associated with this condition.
- Dermatologic signs (pruritus, alopecia, papules) may accompany the GI signs in some cases.

See main reference on page 667 (The Cat With Signs of Chronic Vomiting) for details.

Clinical signs

Food allergy is an adverse reaction to food (usually protein, but may also be carbohydrate) that is **immunologic** (i.e. food allergy, hypersensitivity, delayed hypersensitivity).

The **signs are acute,** and often include **vomiting or inappetance** in addition to diarrhea.

The GI signs of food allergy **are usually chronic and may be intermittent.** They can involve vomiting alone, diarrhea alone, or a combination.

Clinical signs of food allergy may also involve the skin around the head and neck (pruritus, alopecia, dermatitis, otitis) as well as the GI tract, and vomiting or diarrhea is reported.

Those cats that develop GI signs usually have **vomiting or small bowel diarrhea,** however, some cats will develop **colitis** due to food allergy and have large bowel diarrhea, or episodes of mucoid feces.

Diagnosis

Diagnosis of food allergy is based on cessation of clinical signs upon **elimination of the offending substance from the diet**, and recurrence of signs when the substance or diet is re-introduced to the cats.

A response should be seen with the hypoallergenic diet, whether commercial or homemade, within 4 days if there is total compliance with the diet and the cat has not been previously sensitized to ingredients in the diet.

Intradermal skin testing and **measurement of food-specific IgE in the serum** have been advocated by some, but are fraught with both **false-negative and false-positive results** since most food allergies are not mediated by IgE. Also, IgE present in the skin does not correlate to IgE in the GI tract.

Gastroscopic food sensitivity testing has not been reported to be useful in cats.

Differential diagnosis

Colonic IBD is the major differential for cats with **severe or persistent signs,** and endoscopic biopsy will not distinguish between eosinophilia or inflammation due to food allergy and that due to other causes. Cats with food allergy usually have signs that resolve within 4 days on an appropriate hypoallergenic diet. Signs of IBD do not usually resolve solely with a change in diet, although they may improve.

Treatment

Food allergy is diagnosed and treated by feeding an elimination diet for the dietary trial period.

Homemade diets allow the use of a **single novel protein source** (turkey, duck, venison, etc.) and a novel, **highly digestible carbohydrate source** (rice, potato) without preservatives, flavorings, or other additives that may be cause of the problem. Alternatively, use a commercial hypoallergenic diet containing protein and carbohydrate the cat has been previously exposed to.

However, homemade diets are not recommended for **long-term management** of food allergy as they are **not balanced or nutritionally complete.**

There are a number of **commercial diets that have been formulated as "hypoallergenic" or limited antigen diets.** Many of these diets (Hill's, Innovative Veterinary Diets, Royal Canin, Iams, Nature's Recipe, Nutro, and Wysong to name just a few) will be quite effective and **should be used for long-term dietary management** of intolerance or allergy to prevent nutritional deficiencies or excesses.

IDIOPATHIC INFLAMMATORY BOWEL DISEASE (IBD)*

Classical signs

- Diarrhea ranges from soft, mucoid blood-streaked feces to liquid diarrhea (more characteristic of small bowel disease).
- Other signs may include vomiting, anorexia, weight loss and lethargy.

Pathogenesis

The **etiopathogenesis** of colitis or IBD is **unknown**.

A **diagnosis of colonic IBD is based on exclusion** of all other causes of colitis in conjunction with the **histologic presence of an increased number of inflammatory cells in the lamina of the crypts**.

The **histopathologic changes** associated with colonic IBD are **quite variable** and include infiltration of the lamina with **lymphocytes and plasma cells (most common)**, eosinophils, macrophages, neutrophils, or a combination of these cells.

An **immunologic mechanism is suspected** primarily because of the response to immunosuppressive therapy, but this has not been proven.

The **disease in cats is so heterogeneous** (compared to human IBD) that it likely represents a **combination of genetic** (purebred cats have a higher incidence), **environmental, infectious (bacterial), dietary and immunologic components**.

Clinical signs

Hematochezia is the most commonly observed clinical sign in colonic IBD.

When **large bowel diarrhea** occurs, it may be either **mild and intermittent** or **persistent and severe** in character.

Most cats with the colonic form of IBD do not have vomiting, weight loss or decreased appetite, but it can occur in cats with severe disease or disease affecting the small and large bowel together.

The presence or severity of diarrhea or hematochezia does not correlate with the histologic grade of disease.

Diagnosis

Hematologic abnormalities are uncommon, but are consistently associated with severe colonic IBD and usually represent a typical stress response.

The most common biochemical abnormalities (when they occur) are **elevated hepatic enzyme activities** and **hypokalemia**. Hyperglobinemia may also occur.

Fecal floatation should be performed to rule out intestinal parasitism, including giardiasis and coccidia.

Fecal cultures are rarely indicated in acute colitis, but in chronic or recurrent colitis they should be performed.

Imaging studies may reveal a **thickened colonic wall or abnormal gas patterns,** but these findings are **nonspecific.**

The **definitive diagnosis is achieved by histopathologic evaluation** of the colonic mucosa from biopsies obtained via endoscopy.

Endoscopic biopsies are less invasive, and are an accurate and rapid means of obtaining the diagnosis (if the biopsies are adequate), and they also allow examination of the mucosal surface.

Mild or moderate infiltrations of lymphocytes or plasma cells in the lamina of the colon are normal, or suggest inflammation that is due to normal response to a lumenal pathogen.

The amount of infiltration should be carefully graded and the presence of other **alterations in crypt architecture** should be found before concluding that the inflammatory cells present are pathologic or suggestive of IBD.

Differential diagnosis

A major differential for lymphoplasmacytic colitis is gastrointestinal lymphoma. Lymphocytic infiltration in the GI tract may be very difficult to distinguish from a well-differentiated neoplastic infiltration.

Differentiating lymphoma from IBD is an important step in the diagnostic process, both for appropriate treatment planning as well as for giving an accurate prognosis.

The **presence of inflammatory cells in the lamina propria is not diagnostic for IBD,** because almost all other causes of colitis can result in the influx of inflammatory cells.

Another differential for colonic IBD is food sensitivity (food intolerance and food allergy). Some cats will have an **eosinophilic infiltrate,** but this is not consistent. **Dietary trials** must be instituted to investigate the possibility of food intolerance or food allergy. In contrast to elimination diets used for dermatological trials,

the duration of the elimination diet in cats with GI disease need not exceed 7 days as signs in most cats resolve within 3–4 days. A single novel protein and carbohydrate source diet is the best choice.

Clostridial enterocolitis or overgrowth of other intestinal flora are important infectious causes of colitis. Testing for clostridial toxin or culture for specific pathogen is the best means of diagnosis.

Campylobacter spp. are more common in **young kittens or immunocompromised adult cats** and can be identified on **fecal cytology** (motile, "seagull"-shaped bacteria) or via culture (the definitive means of making the diagnosis).

Metabolic diseases should also be considered, as they may **mimic or complicate IBD.** The metabolic diseases that should be ruled out include hyperthyroidism and chronic pancreatitis.

Treatment

The best approach is to use a **combination of dietary (increased fiber, hypoallergenic or low-residue) and pharmacologic therapy.**

There is **no single diet that will be effective in all cases,** and sometimes dietary trials using different diet types is necessary.

Diets with **increased insoluble fiber** (Hill's r/d, Purina's OM formula, IVD's hifactor diet) increase normal segmentation, reduce fecal water and dilute luminal toxins, thus normalizing motility and reducing the stimulus for release of inflammatory mediators. In some cats signs are improved using high insoluble fiber and in others signs are worsened. High-fiber diets tend to be less palatable to cats and may cause constipation in some cats.

Diets that are **highly digestible, and hypoallergenic,** are also recommended for treatment of colonic IBD. By minimizing the opportunity to react to proteins in the diet, the response to therapy is often more predictable.

The **best hypoallergenic diet for ruling out food sensitivity is a homemade diet** (1/3 cup boiled rice or potato and 2/3 cup venison, rabbit, duck, ostrich, crocodile, kangaroo). For **long-term management of IBD,** commercial diets are recommended because they are nutritionally complete and balanced.

Low-residue diets are usually more appropriate for cats with small bowel IBD, but in some cases, providing a diet that will result in reduced colonic residue is more effective.

The key to choosing a diet is recognizing that not all cats respond the same and a willingness to try a different approach is necessary.
- Initial pharmacologic therapy includes prednisolone (2–4 mg/kg q 12 h) and metronidazole (10–15 mg/kg q 12 h).
- In cases that do not respond to these drugs, tylosin (5–100 mg/kg q 12 h), sulfasalazine (11–22 mg/kg q 12–24 h) or olsalazine (no dose established in cats, but 5–10 mg/kg may be reasonable), may be added.
- Chlorambucil and azathioprine have been used in refractory cases of small bowel IBD, but usually are not required in colonic IBD. Cats are particularly sensitive to the myelosuppressive side effects of azathioprine.

Most cats will respond to a combination of dietary and prednisolone or metronidazole therapy and eventually can be maintained with dietary management alone.

Prognosis

The prognosis for complete remission is only guarded to fair.

However, most cats with colonic IBD can be successfully managed with a combination of dietary and pharmacologic therapy, and thus, the prognosis for control is very good.

INFECTIOUS COLITIS* (*CLOSTRIDIUM SPP., E. COLI, CAMPYLOBACTER* SPP.)

Classical signs
- Diarrhea ranges from soft, mucoid blood-streaked feces to liquid diarrhea (more characteristic of small bowel disease).
- Other signs may include vomiting, anorexia and lethargy.

Pathogenesis

Disease is induced by changes in the diet, antibiotic therapy, ingestion of carrion or contaminated food, or stress that results in alteration of the normal colonic bacterial flora and changes in colonic motility.

These changes allow pathogens normally present (*Clostridia, Campylobacter, E. coli,* etc.) to overgrow or begin to secrete toxins that change permeability, increase secretions, or cause release of inflammatory mediators.

Campylobacter is much more common in young cats, while clostridial overgrowth is more commonly seen in adults.

Clinical signs

Hematochezia and large bowel diarrhea that is mucoid, soft and self-limiting is common.

Diarrhea may become more liquid with time and severity, and is more common with *E. coli* infections.

Vomiting may occur, but is uncommon.

Anorexia or lethargy are variably present, depending on the severity.

Fever and other signs of infectious disease rarely occur with infectious colonic diseases.

Weight loss is uncommon due to the acute nature of the condition.

Historical information is very important in establishing the presumptive diagnosis.

Diagnosis

A definitive diagnosis is difficult, because identification of these organisms in feces is not necessarily abnormal.
- *Clostridium perfringens* enterotoxicosis is best diagnosed by positively identifying the presence of enterotoxin in the feces (ELISA or RPLA assays are commercially available). Note: these assays have not been evaluated in cats, but the ELISA assay appears to be more specific in dogs. A positive enterotoxin test determined by ELISA

(regardless of spore numbers) in the context of clinical signs consistent with *C. perfringens* is strongly supportive of clostridial-associated diarrhea. In dogs, the RPLA test does not differentiate dogs with clostridial diarrhea from normal dogs and 25% of normal dogs have positive test results. In both cats and dogs, there appears to be poor correlation between the presence of fecal endospores and the presence of enterotoxin.

Campylobacter is also a **normal inhabitant** of the feline colon and thus, a **pure culture along with detection of the presence of enterotoxin is recommended for diagnosis**.

Pathogenic and nonpathogenic strains of *E. coli* can be cultured from feces and thus before a **diagnosis can be based upon the culture results and clinical presentation, the results should be confirmed by PCR testing for specific pathogenic strains**.

Once the diagnosis has been made, affected cats should be tested for FIV/FeLV, in case the condition is secondary to immunocompromise by viral disease.

Differential diagnosis

Dietary indiscretion.

Parasitic enterocolitis (e.g. protozoal agents such as *Giardia*, *Tritrichomonas*, etc.), and mechanical diseases of the large bowel (e.g. intussusception, cecal inversion, foreign bodies) should all be considered when formulating a differential diagnosis.

Treatment

Clostridial enterocolitis: ampicillin (22–33 mg/kg PO q 8 h), amoxicillin (10–22 mg/kg PO q 12 h), metronidazole (5–15 mg/kg PO q 12 h), tylosin 5–20 mg/kg PO q 12–24 h), clindamycin (5–10 mg/kg q 12 h).

Campylobacteriosis: tetracycline (20 mg/kg q 8 h PO) tylosin (20 mg/kg PO q 12 h) or fluorinated quinolones (e.g. enrofloxacin).

E. colibacillosis: trimethoprim-sulfonamide (15 mg/kg PO q 12 h), cephalosporins (10–30 mg/kg PO q 12 h), doxycycline (5–10 mg/kg PO q 12–24 h), or fluorinated quinolones (e.g. enrofloxacin, orbifloxacin, ciprofloxacin, etc.).

Dietary management should include feeding a **high-fiber diet, unless the signs also involve the small intestine.** In those cases, a low-residue diet is recommended.

Most cases in adults are self-limiting, but respond rapidly to antibiotics and dietary intervention. **In neonates or debilitated cats, additional supportive care** (e.g. fluid therapy) **may be required in severe cases.**

Prognosis

Good to excellent, especially with appropriate antibiotic therapy.

Prevention

In kittens or colonies of cats that have recurrent problems with infectious colitis, **minimizing stress, improving sanitation, and maximizing nutrition** will all help to reduce the occurrence of these stress-related diseases.

All cats should be tested to be sure that they are FeLV/FIV negative.

HYPERTHYROIDISM*

Classical signs

- Weight loss despite a good appetite.
- GI signs (vomiting or diarrhea).
- Unkempt hair coat and increased dander are common.
- Tachycardia secondary to thyrotoxic heart disease.
- Hyperactivity or restlessness.

See main reference on page 304 for details.

Clinical signs

This disease is most commonly observed in **middle-aged to old cats** (> 8 years).

Weight loss is a very common feature of the disease.

Polyphagia, normal or decreased appetite, are all observed, but **ravenous appetite is the classic presentation**.

Hyperthyroidism may cause **hyperactive or restless behavior** and some cats are also irritable.

Decreased grooming habits, unkempt hair coat and increased dander are often reported.

Vomiting or diarrhea may be observed. Feces are usually voluminous due to increased intake and decreased gut transit time.

Tachycardia, and sometimes a **gallop rhythm** are present secondary to thyrotoxic effects on the myocardium that leads to **thyrotoxic heart disease** and heart failure.

Diagnosis

This is confirmed by presence of **elevated serum total thyroxine (T4) levels**.

Other diagnostic methods that may be used if the serum total T4 is in the upper half of the normal range, but the cat has clinical signs of hyperthyroidism include **radionuclide scanning, serum free T4 test, or a T3 suppression test**.

Abnormalities may be observed in routine blood screening tests (e.g. erthyrocytosis, elevated liver enzyme activities) but these are not specific for thyroid disease.

If the cat has an **elevated heart rate or gallop rhythm** consistent with heart disease, **thoracic radiographs and echocardiography are indicated to assess the severity**.

Differential diagnosis

Other **metabolic diseases** and **extra-intestinal causes of GI signs, weight loss or tachycardia** that affect older cats should be considered carefully.

Differentials for chronic large bowel diarrhea include IBD, neoplasia and food intolerance or food allergy.

Major differentials associated with the systemic signs of hyperthyroidism are diabetes mellitus, chronic renal failure, neoplasia, IBD and hypertrophic or restrictive cardiomyopathy.

Treatment

Anti-thyroid drug therapy includes **methimazole (2.5–5 mg/cat q 12–24 h)**, with a maximum dose of 15 mg/day. Occasionally, side effects such as anorexia, vomiting, lethargy, pruritus, hepatotoxicity and hematologic changes may be observed, but will resolve if the drug is stopped. Carbimazole (5 mg PO q 8–12 h) is metabolized to methimazole.

Radioactive iodine therapy: if available is the treatment of choice. Iodine-131 is concentrated in adenomatous thyroid but spares normal tissue. Note: Use with extreme caution if the cat has concurrent renal disease as reduced renal perfusion post-treatment may worsen the condition, or unmask subclinical renal failure.

Cats treated with I-131 must be **isolated for a variable period (up to 3 weeks)** of time (depending on local laws) following treatment.

Surgical removal of a hyperplastic or neoplastic thyroid nodule is only **indicated if the disease is unilateral** (70% of cats have bilateral disease).

The **risk of anesthesia is reduced by prior treatment with methimazole** to make the cat euthyroid and also by **careful selection of anesthetic agents.** Xylazine, ketamine or other arrhythmogenic agents should not be used.

Bilateral thyroidectomy should be staged to minimize risk of hypoparathyroidism.

Management of thyrotoxic heart disease with beta-adrenergic antagonists (atenolol, 6.25–12.5 mg PO q 12–24 h) may be necessary in some cases, although cardiac complications usually resolve when the hyperthyroidism is treated. Other agents that may be considered include calcium channel blockers e.g. diltiazem (1.5–2.5 mg/kg q 8–12 h).

LYMPHOSARCOMA*

Classical signs

- Vomiting, small bowel diarrhea, weight loss and anorexia are the most common presenting signs.
- Large bowel diarrhea alone is rarely observed because the tumor is typically infiltrative throughout the GI tract.

See main reference on page 317 for details.

Clinical signs

Vomiting, small bowel diarrhea, weight loss and anorexia are the most common presenting signs.

Large bowel diarrhea alone is rarely observed because the tumor is typically **infiltrative throughout the GI tract.**

Palpation may reveal **thickened loops of bowel**.

Most cats with alimentary lymphoma are **FeLV negative** so associated clinical disease is uncommon.

Occasionally, lymphoma will present as a **solitary mass in the small intestine or colon, which obstructs the GI tract** and must be differentiated from adenocarcinoma and other neoplastic or granulomatous diseases.

Diagnosis

Routine hematology and chemistry profiles are often **within normal limits**.

Survey radiographs of the abdomen may reveal **thickened bowel loops or abnormal gas patterns**, but they also may be interpreted as normal.

Ultrasound examination of the abdomen is especially helpful in identifying **enlarged lymph nodes, liver or splenic changes** in echogenicity, and **measurement of intestinal wall thickness**.
- **Fine-needle aspirates** may be obtained via ultrasound guidance that will **facilitate a definitive diagnosis and staging**.

Endoscopy is also an important diagnostic tool in making a definitive diagnosis, because **multiple samples can be obtained for histopathologic examination.**

Differential diagnosis

The **primary differential** for lymphoma in cats is **severe lymphocytic plasmacytic IBD**, and it is suspected that this may be a precursor lesion to lymphoma in some cats.

Other **extra-intestinal causes of weight loss and vomiting** must also be considered, including pancreatitis, renal or liver disease, hyperthyroidism, diabetes mellitus, etc.

Other less-common neoplastic diseases to consider in cats are mast cell tumors, leiomyosarcomas and carcinoids.

Treatment

Combination chemotherapy with cyclophosphamide, vincristine and prednisolone (**COP protocol**) is the most commonly recommended regimen. Most cats treated with this protocol are expected to live 6–9 months, with 20% living longer than 1 year. Asparaginase or doxyrubicin can be added to increase the remission times or serve as the rescue.
- Cyclophosphamide (300 mg/m^2 PO q 3 weeks).
- Vincristine (0.75 mg/m^2 IV weekly for 4 weeks).
- Prednisone (2 mg/kg/day).
- Doxyrubicin (25 mg/m^2 IV q 3 wk).
- L-Asparaginase (10 000 IU/m^2 IM).

Other protocols exist for induction, maintenance and rescue, but the reader is referred to oncology texts for additional information.

Supportive care in the form of nutrition is essential for cats with alimentary lymphoma because they tend not to eat and often vomiting precludes oral alimentation.

Placement of **jejunostomy tubes** may be required in these cats.

Prognosis

Guarded to poor. Survival times are shorter for cats with alimentary lymphoma than other forms of lymphoma (e.g. multicentric or mediastinal), primarily because **response to chemotherapy is more variable** with these tumors.

In one recent report, mean survival was 230 days, but median survival was only 50 days.

COLONIC ADENOCARCINOMA*

Classical signs

- Vomiting, weight loss and anorexia are classical signs.
- Hematochezia, tenesmus or large bowel diarrhea occur with a distal location.

Pathogenesis

Adenocarcinoma is the most common tumor of the feline colon and most common non-hematopoietic tumor of the GI tract.

It usually occurs in **old cats (>10 years)** and has **a higher incidence in Siamese cats**.

It most commonly occurs as a solitary lesion causing signs of bowel obstruction due to a large mass or annular growth around the circumference of the bowel.

Malignant behavior with metastasis to regional lymph nodes, mesentery, liver and other abdominal organs is typical of this neoplasm.

However, it **rarely metastasizes to the lungs**.

Clinical signs

Vomiting, weight loss and anorexia are the classical signs.

Hematochezia, tenesmus or large bowel diarrhea are observed the more distal the tumor location.

Some cats may only have **lethargy, decreased appetite or weight loss without GI signs, so history and signalment** (old, Siamese cat) **are important clues**.

Physical examination may reveal an **abdominal mass or abdominal discomfort** upon palpation.

Diagnosis

Careful **abdominal palpation** may reveal a **mass or thickened bowel loop**.

Routine hematology and serum chemistry profile are **often within normal limits in the early stages of disease**.

Late changes may include **hypoproteinemia, hypoalbuminemia, electrolyte disturbances** due to vomiting or elevations in **liver enzyme** activities due to metastasis.

Imaging studies (radiography, **ultrasound**) are useful in identifying the abdominal mass and a preliminary diagnosis can be made via ultrasound-guided **fine-needle aspiration** of the mass in many cases.

Ultrasonography is also especially useful in **assessing regional lymph nodes and liver** for evidence of **metastatic disease**.

The **definitive diagnosis is obtained by histopathology**.

Endoscopy may be used to obtain biopsies, but **exploratory surgery with resection of the affected area and biopsy of regional lymph nodes or liver is diagnostic, prognostic and therapeutic**.

Differential diagnosis

Other intestinal diseases such as IBD, lymphoma, other tumors, or intussusception may have a similar clinical presentation.

Extra-intestinal diseases should also be considered when the clinical signs are vague. These include pancreatitis, hyperthyroidism, chronic renal failure, hepatic disease and neoplasia in other locations.

Treatment

The **treatment of choice** for colonic adenocarcinoma is **wide surgical excision**, even if the tumor has metastasized, which it usually has at the time of surgery.

Chemotherapy for metastatic disease has not been reported, but would **not be expected to be successful**.

Mean survival time following surgical resection is generally less than one year but this is not correlated with the presence of metastatic disease. Survival time is shorter without treatment.

Extensive surgical removal of the colon will require that the cat be fed a **highly digestible, low-residue diet** to minimize clinical signs of short bowel syndrome.

Prognosis

Long-term prognosis is poor. However, many cats will have lengthy (up to 15 months) periods of good-quality life following surgical resection.

PARASITIC INFECTIONS (*GIARDIA, TRITRICHOMONAS, CRYPTOSPORIDIA, ISOSPORA, TOXOPLASMA, BALANTIDIUM AND TRICHURIS*)*

Classical signs

- Mucus- or blood-streaked, soft (semi-formed) feces.
- Rarely, overt large bowel diarrhea in immunocompromised or very young cats.

Pathogenesis

There are **no major parasitic causes of large bowel diarrhea in the cat**.

However, **occasional infections with *Giardia, Tritrichomonas, Cryptosporidia, Isospora, Toxoplasma*, and *Balantidium*** may be observed.

Each of these parasites has a different life cycle and degree of pathogenicity in the host, but **none of these is a strictly large bowel parasite** and **most cause disease only in the very young, the very old, or sick, debilitated cats** (especially FIV- or FeLV-positive cats).

Whipworm eggs (*Trichuris serrate* and *T. campanula*) are **occasionally observed in cats**, but **do not cause clinical disease** and are believed to be either **mis-diagnosed** (e.g. *Capillaria* spp.) or are present because the **cat ingested rodent or canine whipworm eggs in the environment**.

Most of these **protozoan parasites** (e.g. *Giardia, Toxoplasma, Cryptosporidia*) are **pathogenic** (**zoonotic**) to humans.

Clinical signs

Most infections of these parasites in cats are **asymptomatic** and are accidentally found on a routine fecal examination.

Tritrichomonas is the exception, as kittens or young cats with *Tritrichomonas* infection will have persistent foul-smelling diarrhea.

Hematochezia, mucoid stools, large bowel diarrhea and flatulence have all been infrequently reported in cats with these parasites, but are **secondary to the primary disease (often FIV)**.

Diagnosis

Fecal floatation, direct smears of feces, and fecal cytology have all been used to identify these parasites.

Multiple (at least three) zinc sulfate solutions on consecutive days are best to float *Giardia* and *Cryptospordia* oocyts.

Cryptosporidia **are so small** that identification is difficult without **special stains or advanced microscopy techniques**.

Cryptosporidia can also be identified by use of a **fecal ELISA test** (human test but effective in cat feces).

Toxoplasma will float in salt solution but are **very small (< 5 micron)** and may be missed without careful examination of the slide.

Diagnosis of *Tritrichomonas* is best confirmed by PCR testing or culture of the organism in feces using a special technique.

Differential diagnosis

Because these are **rare causes of large bowel disease in cats,** all other, more common, causes of colitis should be ruled out first.

If these parasites are found in the feces of an adult cat that is symptomatic, an immediate search for an **immunosuppressive disease** should be initiated (**ie. rule out FeLV, FIV, FIP, etc.**).

Treatment

Tritrichomonas: **Ronidazole** (30–50 mg/kg PO q 12h)

Giardia: **Metronidazole** (10–25 mg/kg PO q 12 h for 5–10 days) or **fenbendazole** (25–50 mg/kg PO q 24 h for 5–7 days)

Isospora: **Sulfadimethoxine** (25 mg/kg PO q 24 h for 10–14 days)

Cryptosporidia: **Azithromycin** (5 mg/kg q 24 h PO for 5 days then q 48 h)

Toxoplasmosis: Clindamycin (10–25 mg/kg PO q 12 h) (high dose recommended but often causes GI side effects), or **azithromycin** 5 mg/kg q 24 h for 5 days then q 48 h.

CHRONIC PANCREATITIS

Classical signs

- Clinical signs are vague and non-localizing in cats (e.g. lethargy, anorexia).
- Vomiting or diarrhea are less common.
- Hematochezia or large bowel diarrhea occur more often with chronic pancreatitis.

See main reference on page 318 for details.

Clinical signs

Anorexia and lethargy are the most common signs associated with feline pancreatitis.

Vomiting is less common (< 50% of cats vomit) and thus, dehydration is less common.

Chronic pancreatitis is also associated with vague clinical signs, but **hematochezia or large bowel diarrhea** may be observed.

Diagnosis

There is **no single, definitive test for pancreatitis** in cats.

Non-specific abnormalities on the hemogram may include neutrophilia or mild, non-regenerative anemia.

Serum chemistry abnormalities may include elevated liver enzyme activities and/or hyperbilirubinemia.

Serum amylase and lipase are of no use in the cat for diagnosis of pancreatitis due to false-negative and -positive results.

Loss of visceral detail or increased duodenal gas are sometimes observed on **survey radiographs**, but this is **not consistent**.

Ultrasonographic examination of the pancreas is a good method of detecting pancreatic abnormalities. However, this is still **not a specific or sensitive test for pancreatitis**.

Elevations in serum trypsin-like immunoreactivity (TLI) have been used as a screening test, but caution is advised because the assay often has **false-negative and -positive results**.

Feline pancreatic lipase immunoreactivity (fPLI) is the most specific and sensitive serum test for pancreatitis currently available. fPLI is 100% specific for pancreatitis.

fPLI and ultrasound examination, when used together, have a sensitivity of >90%.

PERINEAL HERNIA

Classical signs

- Straining to defecate.
- Large bowel diarrhea.
- Irritation or perineal swelling.

Pathogenesis

Perineal hernia occurs when there is failure of the pelvic diaphragm musculature to support the rectal wall. A peritoneum-lined sac protrudes through the defect and may contain pelvic and abdominal contents. The rectal wall stretches and deviates into the sac.

Feces are retained in the divided section of the rectal wall resulting in straining and difficulty defecating.

Weakness of the pelvic diaphragm musculature and herniation is often idiopathic but may be associated with previous perineal urethrostomy, megacolon, perineal mass or chronic colitis.

Clinical signs

Straining to defecate, constipation or less commonly, large bowel diarrhea, irritation or perineal swelling are all typical signs of perineal hernia.

Usually older cats are affected.

On rectal examination there are impacted feces in a rectal dilation or sacculation, and evidence of a defect in the pelvic diaphragm musculature.

Diagnosis

The diagnosis may be suggested by the **history or appearance of the perineal area and a rectal examination will confirm the problem** in many cases.

In cases where the diagnosis is in doubt, a **barium enema will outline the herniated rectal tissue**.

These hernias are rare in cats compared to dogs.

Treatment

Medical management using low-residue food and fecal softeners (e.g. lactulose) or enemas may help in cats with small hernias.

Surgery is considered the preferred treatment and several herniorrhaphy techniques have been described, although recurrence rates can be high (10–50%). In cats with megacolon, subtotal colectomy may resolve the constipation and tenesmus. Herniorraphy can be performed in cats that do not improve with medical therapy.

PERIANAL TUMORS

Classical signs

- Straining to defecate.
- Large bowel diarrhea or constipation.
- Perineal swelling.
- Licking excessively at the perineum.

Pathogenesis

These tumors occur more commonly in **older cats.**

Tumors of the perianal region in cats, unlike those in dogs, are usually **adenocarcinomas**. Perianal tumors are very rare in cats compared to dogs.

Clinical signs

Straining to defecate, large bowel diarrhea, perineal swelling, or constipation may all occur due to large perianal mass(es).

Cats often will lick at the area frequently which may draw attention to the region.

Diagnosis

In the majority of cases, the **presence of a perianal mass** will be the obvious cause of the intestinal disturbance.

Perianal tumors may **metastasize locally** (to regional lymph nodes or bones) **or to distant sites** (liver, lung or abdominal sites) and so, a **routine database, radiographs and ultrasound, and fine-needle aspirates** of **regional or enlarged lymph nodes should be performed.**

Fine-needle aspirates of the tumor can be used to identify the tumor type prior to surgical biopsy.

Differential diagnosis

The **primary differential** for this problem is **anal sacculitis or abscess**, which are more common problems, but **generally are less likely to cause problems with fecal passage**.

Treatment

Surgical resection of tumor with **wide margins to prevent recurrence**.

Histopathologic examination of the tumor as well as **biopsies of regional lymph nodes** is recommended for **confirmation of the diagnosis** and determination of the **prognosis**.

Fecal softeners (e.g. lactulose or docusate sodium) may be helpful if fecal material is difficult or painful to pass.

PSEUDOMEMBRANEOUS COLITIS (ANTIBIOTIC-INDUCED COLITIS)

Classical signs

- Mucus- or blood-streaked, soft (semi-formed) feces.
- Progression to severe large bowel diarrhea.

Pathogenesis

This disease is **caused by the use of antibiotics (especially clindamycin or cephalosporins)** that disturb the normal bacterial flora of the colon resulting in **overgrowth of antibiotic-resistant, pathogenic species**.

Diarrhea due to clostridial spp. is not uncommon, but it is **usually due to** *Clostridium perfringens*. *Clostridium difficile* **are not common inhabitants of the feline colon**, but may populate and overgrow in the right circumstances (primarily chronic antibiotic use).

This is a very **uncommon problem** in cats.

Clinical signs

Mucus- or blood-streaked feces which may progress to **severe large bowel diarrhea**.

In **some cases**, the diarrhea is **poorly responsive to treatment**.

Diagnosis

Historical correlation between the **development of mucoid diarrhea and the use of antibiotics that have an anaerobic spectrum**.

Confirmation of the diagnosis requires **fecal culture** (requiring special handling) **or colonic biopsies** that confirm the presence of **pseudomembrane formation**.

Fecal analysis for Clostridial toxins A and B is very important for confirmation.

Differential diagnosis

Clostridial enterocolitis due to *Clostridium perfringens* is the primary differential, but **simple diarrhea** due to antibiotic therapy, diet changes or infectious or parasitic agents should be considered carefully.

Treatment

The **choice of antibiotic should be based upon culture results** due to resistance. **Metronidazole** has been used successfully in some cases.

Non-specific therapy for this disorder includes use of a **high-fiber diet** (or addition of insoluble fiber to the diet) **to normalize colonic function** (secretion and motility).

In **severe cases, long-term (weeks) antibiotic therapy** will be required to achieve control.

Prevention

Cautious use of antibiotics that have an anaerobic spectrum over a long period (weeks).

COLORECTAL POLYPS

> **Classical signs**
>
> • Mucus- or blood-streaked, soft (semi-formed) feces.

Pathogenesis

Benign growths of the **colonic epithelium**.

Rare in cats, but reported occasionally.

Most are found in the upper duodenum, near the pylorus or in the **ileum or proximal colon**, and **Siamese cats** are over-represented.

Clinical signs

May be clinically silent.

May cause **intermittent large bowel signs**: increased **tenesmus, mucus- or blood-streaked feces, or difficulty in passing feces** (constipation is possible).

Diagnosis

No changes in hematology or serum chemistries will occur.

Contrast radiography or ultrasound examination will delineate them, but **colonoscopy is the best diagnostic method**, and will allow visualization, biopsy and in some cases assist removal (if distal enough).

Differential diagnosis

Other neoplastic diseases of the large bowel: i.e. adenocarcinoma, focal lymphoma, mast cell tumors, carcinoids, etc.

Sliding or intermittent intussusception.

Granuloma due to **fungal or infectious disease (e.g. FIP).**

Treatment

Surgical removal is curative.

Recurrence is unusual.

Prognosis

Excellent.

CONGENITAL MALFORMATIONS (SHORT COLON SYNDROME, VASCULAR ECTASIA, DIVERTICULUM)

> ### Classical signs
>
> - Signs depend on the location of the anomaly.
> - Large bowel diarrhea, constipation or abdominal pain (typhilitis).
> - Young cats or kittens, and do not worsen with age, except with short colon syndrome.

Pathogenesis

The **etiopathogenesis** of the congenital malformations affecting the large bowel is **unknown.**

The **most frequently reported malformations** affecting the large bowel are **vascular ectasia, short colon syndrome and enterocyst formation**.

Vascular ectasia is a syndrome of **abnormal blood vessel formations** that results in abnormal bowel function (especially motility) due to the lack of a normal blood supply.

Short colon syndrome can be **congenital or iatrogenic** (secondary to surgical removal of the colon due to neoplasia or other disease). Cats with short colon syndrome are **unable to reabsorb water and electrolytes** and thus, are not able to form normal feces without providing very highly digestible diets that reduce the amount of ingesta that reaches the colon.

Diverticular formations are also found, however, they can be **congenital or secondary to chronic disease.**

Many diverticular formations are **incidental findings** and are not associated with abnormal colon function unless they are large or become diseased.

Clinical signs

Large bowel diarrhea and flatulence.

Constipation.

Abdominal pain (due to typhilitis or gas distention).

Diagnosis

These are **rare congenital diseases**.

Kittens are usually presented at just **weeks of age**.

Blood work (CBC, profile) will usually be completely **normal**.

Survey radiographs will **generally not be helpful, except in cases of short colon syndrome**, where the colon may be visibly abnormal.

Contrast radiographs may be very helpful in identifying **short colon syndrome**.

Ultrasonography is very useful in identifying an **abnormal enterocyst**, but **colonoscopy or surgical exploration** may be required to make the **definitive diagnosis**.

Differential diagnosis

The differentials are usually limited to **those things causing colonic disease in kittens**, e.g. parasites, infectious, mechanical (foreign objects) and dietary indiscretion or food intolerance.

Treatment

Treatment of **vascular ectasia and enterocysts** is via **surgical resection of the affected area(s)**.

Short colon syndrome must be managed medically by providing a **low-residue diet** (e.g. Hill's i/d diet, Iam's low residue diet or IVD neutral formula), **use of motility-modifying drugs as needed** (e.g. lomotil, loperamide), and **antibiotics when they are indicated**.

Prognosis

The prognosis is **guarded to good, depending on the anomaly** that is present.

Cats with **vascular ectasia or enterocysts that can be corrected surgically** have a **very good prognosis**.

Cats with **short bowel syndrome** have a very **guarded prognosis** and will require **life-long therapy**.

RECOMMENDED READING

Guilford WG. The gastrointestinal tract and adverse reactions to food. Consult Feline Intern Med 2001; 4.

Guilford W, Jones B, Markwell P, Arthur D, Collett M, Harte J. Food sensitivity in cats with chronic idiopathic gastrointestinal problems. J Vet Intern Med 2001; 15: 7–13.

Guilford WG, Center SA, Strombeck DR, Williams DA, (eds) Strombeck's Small Animal Gastroenterology, 3rd edn 2000, WB Saunders, Philadelphia, PA.

Jergens AE. Feline idiopathic inflammatory bowel disease. Comp Cont Ed 1992; 14(4): 509–520.

Simpson, KW. Vet Clin North Am Small Anim Pract 1999; 29(2): 441–470, 501–522, 577–588.

Steiner J. Diagnosis of pancreatitis. Vet Clin North Am Small Anim Pract 2003; 33: 1181–1195.

35. The constipated or straining cat

Albert E Jergens and Annette Litster

KEY SIGNS

- Reduced frequency of defecation.
- Tenesmus or painful defecation.
- Hard, dry, low-volume feces, sometimes with mucus.

MECHANISM?

- Constipation denotes infrequent or difficult defecation and is a common problem in cats. Straining (tenesmus) occurs when there is ineffectual defecation or urination, or irritation of the bowel or bladder wall.
- Straining may also be associated with conditions affecting the lower urinary tract. Refer to p. @ (The Cat Straining to Urinate).

WHERE?

- Disorders of the large intestine are the most common causes of constipation.

WHAT?

- Constipated cats may have underlying orthopedic or neurologic diseases which cause fecal impaction and clinical signs.

QUICK REFERENCE SUMMARY

Diseases causing a constipated or straining cat

DEGENERATIVE

● **Constipation (including idiopathic megacolon)***(p 783)**

The hallmarks are reduced, painful, or absent defecation +/– tenesmus. Idiopathic megacolon denotes diffuse colonic dilatation with colonic hypomotility.

● Dysautonomia (p 792)

This is a rare cause of constipation, and associated clinical signs include sudden onset of depression and anorexia coupled with a variety of signs including regurgitation, mydriasis, constipation, brady-cardia and dysuria. Dysautonomia was of regional importance in the UK in the early 1980s and more recently in the USA.

MECHANICAL

● Hair matting* (p 789)

Matting of the hair around the anus with feces is associated with poor grooming, and may cause perianal dermatitis and discomfort with defecation. It may also obstruct fecal passage through the anus. It occurs more often in obese cats, and long-haired cats.

METABOLIC

● Dehydration and hypokalemia* (p 787)

Metabolic conditions such as dehydration or hypokalemia can predispose to constipation by reducing fecal moisture and colonic muscle activity. Signs of dehydration, inability to jump, or ventroflexion of the neck may be evident.

NEOPLASIA

● Neoplasia (p 791)

Intraluminal or extraluminal tumors may cause mechanical obstruction to the passage of feces. Signs may include straining to defecate and evidence of fresh blood on the feces.

PSYCHOLOGICAL

● Litter box dissatisfaction* (p 789)

Litterbox dissatisfaction, caused by poor litterbox hygiene or inadequate litterbox access, may discourage regular defecation and result in constipation.

INFLAMMATION

● Acute non-specific colitis** (p 786)

This condition presents with an abrupt onset of large bowel diarrhea which is usually self-limiting. Signs include tenesmus, mucoid feces and hematochezia. Vomiting may occur.

● Chronic colitis** (p 787)

Chronic colitis causes hematochezia, large bowel diarrhea, and tenesmus, which are attributable to infectious, inflammatory, neoplastic and benign infiltrative mucosal diseases.

● Perineal inflammation/infection (p 792)

Conditions such as perineal abscesses, perianal fistulae and anorectal foreign bodies may cause pain, discouraging regular defecation and lead to constipation and/or tenesmus.

● Lower urinary tract disease* (p 790)

Hematuria, strangiuria and pollakiuria caused by lower urinary tract disorders must be differentiated from constipation by history and physical examination.

IATROGENIC

● Drugs (p 791)

Drugs such as opioid agonists, cholinergic antagonists, diuretics, phenothiazines and barium sulfate can cause constipation.

TRAUMA

● Pelvic fractures* (p 788)

Pelvic fractures may reduce the size of the pelvic canal, causing obstruction. In the acute phase following trauma, painful defecation may lead to constipation.

INTRODUCTION

MECHANISM?

Constipation may be suspected when a cat has chronic difficulty or pain while defecating; defecation is reduced in frequency; or reduced amounts of hard dry feces are passed. The **proximal colon in cats is particularly efficient at water reabsorption**, so prolonged transit times predispose to constipation. **Common signs** of constipation include:
- **Reduced or absent defecation**.
- **Marked tenesmus**.
- **Painful defecation may be evidenced by crying out on defecation, numerous aborted attempts to defecate, or prolonged attempts to defecate**.
- **Reduced amounts of hard, dry feces which may have a mucus covering**.
- **Anorexia, lethargy, vomiting and weight loss are systemic manifestations** observed in cats with severe constipation.

Obstipation is the presence of **chronic intractable constipation with massive fecal impaction and inability to defecate**.

Idiopathic megacolon denotes **severe generalized colonic dilatation which is irreversible** and poorly responsive to aggressive medical therapy.

Tenesmus (straining) may also be associated with other colonic disorders that cause inflammation and diarrhea.

Cats with tenesmus may be straining to urinate, and if signs or physical examination findings suggest a urinary tract problem, the reader is referred to page 173 (The Cat Straining to Urinate).

WHERE?

Signs of constipation and straining result from problems involving the following sites:
- **Colonic lumen and mucosa**.
- **Urinary bladder and/or urethra**.

Physical examination (especially abdominal palpation) and history help localize the cause. **Posture** while straining often differentiates a problem with defecation from a urinary tract problem. **Defecation posture is a high squat with an arched tail**, while **urination posture is a low squat with a straight tail**.
- Other signs suggesting a urinary tract problem include a small or large firm bladder, normal amounts of fecal material on abdominal palpation, and a history of small amounts of urine being produced associated with tenesmus. The urine may be discolored; typically there is hematuria.

Abdominal radiography and routine urinalysis most readily differentiate constipation from lower urinary tract disorders.

WHAT?

Causes for constipation are diverse and may include **orthopedic, neoplastic, pharmacologic, metabolic and neurologic etiologies** or they may be **idiopathic** in origin.

Abnormal evacuation of feces leads to constipation, colonic impaction and clinical signs.

The most common causes of straining to urinate include lower urinary tract disease or idiopathic cystitis, bacterial cystitis in older cats, neoplasia and uroliths.

Diagnosis of the constipated/straining cat is based on **history, physical examination findings, radiography, urinalysis and histopathology of colonic biopsy specimens**.

DISEASES CAUSING CONSTIPATION OR STRAINING

CONSTIPATION*** (INCLUDING IDIOPATHIC MEGACOLON)

Classical signs
- Most common in middle-aged male cats, but may occur in any age, or gender.
- Reduced, painful, or absent defecation +/– tenesmus.
- Feces are hard, dry and low-volume, with or without mucus.
- +/– Anorexia, lethargy, weight loss, and vomiting with chronicity.

Pathogenesis

Etiologies for constipation are diverse. While the majority of cases are idiopathic, pelvic canal stenosis, nerve injury and Manx sacral spinal cord deformity are also regularly diagnosed.

- **Idiopathic megacolon** is likely a **generalized dysfunction of colonic smooth muscle**. The disorder involves a **disturbance in the intracellular activation of smooth muscle myofilaments**, and affects both longitudinal and circular smooth muscle from both the proximal and distal colon. **Histologic evaluation is unhelpful** in the diagnosis of this condition. **Burmese are over-represented** with idiopathic megacolon.
- **Orthopedic causes** for constipation include pelvic fractures and pelvic canal stenosis.
- **Mechanical (extraluminal) obstruction** may be caused by **intra-abdominal tumors**.
- **Anal inflammation** may discourage defecation because of pain.
- **Perineal hair–fecal mats** may impede fecal passage, especially in obese cats that are unable to groom effectively. Long-standing mats are associated with perianal dermatitis which may contribute to the discomfort of defecating.
- **Nerve injury** may manifest as spinal cord injury or sacral spinal cord deformities (e.g. Manx cats). Affected cats usually present with accompanying clinical signs of nerve injury, such as urinary incontinence, poor anal sphincter tone, reduced perineal sensation or poor tail sensation, with reduced motor function of the tail in more severe cases.
- Constipation may be one manifestation of feline **dysautonomia**.

Abnormal evacuation of feces leads to constipation, colonic impaction and associated clinical signs.

Idiopathic megacolon in some cats has been reported in association with either intestinal pyogranuloma due to feline infectious peritonitis virus infection, or intestinal lymphosarcoma. Refer to the main references for these conditions.

Clinical signs

Constipation is most common in **middle-aged male cats,** but may be observed in cats of any age, gender or breed. Burmese cats are over-represented with idiopathic megacolon.

Reduced, absent or painful defecation occurs over days to weeks.

Tenesmus is frequently noted.

Feces are **hard, dry and low-volume**, with or without **mucus**.

Systemic signs including lethargy, dehydration, anorexia, weight loss, vomiting, and mild to moderate mesenteric lymphadenopathy, are often seen in chronic cases.

Occasionally, small amounts of **brown mucoid liquid** are passed and can be **mistaken for diarrhea.**

Diagnosis

Cats with **megacolon** often have a **previous history of episodes of constipation**.

Careful history taking is necessary to identify any underlying causes. Check the frequency of litterbox cleaning, litterbox accessibility, drug administration, diet, and history of previous injuries. **Details of posture while straining are often helpful** in differentiating problems of defecation and urination.

Abdominal palpation reveals firm fecal masses in constipation, or severe, generalized colonic distention with impacted feces if megacolon is present. The perineal area should be checked for inflammation or hair matting.

Abdominal radiography serves to delineate the severity of fecal impaction.

Abdominal ultrasound examination may identify intra-abdominal tumors.

Digital rectal examination should be performed to detect/rule out intraluminal and pelvic causes for constipation.

Neurologic examination is completed to assess caudal spinal cord integrity and function.

- A diminished or absent perineal reflex with reduced anal sphincter tone is found with lower motor neuron lesions involving S_1–S_3 spinal cord segments, or pudendal nerve and/or pelvic nerve disorders.

Serum biochemistry analysis may detect electrolyte disturbances (e.g. hypokalemia) contributing to reduced evacuation of feces.

Differential diagnosis

Constipation can usually be easily differentiated from other causes of straining, such as lower urinary tract disorders, by physical examination.

Treatment

Therapy is dependent on the severity of constipation and the underlying cause. Any underlying causes such as litterbox problems, intraluminal or extraluminal obstructions, orthopedic disorders, anal inflammation or perineal hair matting should be corrected.

Animals with **mild to moderate constipation** may be treated as **outpatients**.

- **Tepid water enemas** (5–10 ml/kg q 8–24 h) or **commercially available pediatric enemas** (Microlax, 1–2 tubes/cat) should be administered as needed to facilitate fecal breakdown and passage.
- **Dietary fiber** serves to enhance fecal bulk, and has laxative effects. These effects are due to increased fecal water content, decreased intestinal transit time and increased frequency of defecation. A number of fiber supplements are available, including **psillium** (Metamucil, 1–4 tsp mixed with food at each meal), or **wheat bran** (1–2 tsp mixed with food at each meal). Some cats find the sweetness of **canned pumpkin or canned creamed corn** (1–4 tbsp mixed with food at each meal) makes a more palatable fiber supplement.
- **Lactulose** (0.5 ml/kg PO q 8–12 h) is a hyperosmotic laxative which softens feces by reducing water absorption in the colon. **Milk** may be a more palatable alternative, as the lactose in milk is indigestible in most cats, causing it to act as a hyperosmotic agent.
- **Cisapride** (2.5 mg PO q 12 h) is a gastrointestinal prokinetic agent, which stimulates colonic motility from the gastroesophageal sphincter to the descending colon. It is believed to **enhance cholinergic neurotransmission in the gastrointestinal tract via stimulation of enteric neuronal serotonin receptors**. Cisapride may be used alone for the treatment of mild to moderate constipation, or with

lactulose on a daily basis for the prevention of constipation.

- **Emollient laxatives** act as anionic detergents to **increase the miscibility of water and lipid in the bowel contents**, enhancing lipid absorption but impairing water absorption. Dioctyl sodium sulfosuccinate (Colace, 50 mg PO q 24 h) and dioctyl calcium sulfosuccinate (Surfax, 50 mg PO q 12–24 h) are two examples of this class of drugs. **Care should be taken that the cat is well hydrated prior to the administration of these agents,** as they retard the absorption of water from the intestine.
- **Lubricant laxatives** act by easing fecal passage and decreasing water absorption from the colon by creating a coating layer on the mucosa. These agents (e.g. mineral oil or petrolatum products such as Laxatone or Kat-A-Lax) are **suitable only for mild constipation**, or for regular use to prevent constipation in mildly affected cats.

If there is **obstipation, manual extraction of feces** under general anesthesia is usually required to treat obstipation, as the condition is too severe to respond to enemas alone.

- **Balanced fluids** (e.g. Lactated Ringer's Solution, Plasma-Lyte A or Normisol-R) should be administered to rehydrate and correct fluid deficits. This is particularly important in older cats or if general anesthesia is required for treatment. An **endotracheal tube** should be placed to prevent inhalation pneumonia as manipulation of the colon may induce vomiting.
- After the distal colon has been lubricated by a warm water or saline infusion, forceps are inserted and used to carefully grasp or break down fecal material. A **constantly twisting motion**, clockwise and counterclockwise, should be used **to prevent the forceps accidentally grasping the colonic mucosa**. Alternatively, a spoon-shaped instrument, specifically designed for the purpose, may be used to gradually break down the fecal mass, while connected to a faucet to provide a steady trickle of warm water into the colon.
- **If any bleeding is noted on manual fecal extraction, the procedure should be aborted** to minimize the risk of intestinal perforation or devitalization of the colonic mucosa. It **may be preferable to perform manual extraction over**

short periods on consecutive days, rather than risk prolonged anesthesia and intestinal mucosal damage.

Severe constipation or megacolon is usually **nonresponsive to aggressive medical management. Colotomy** may be required if manual fecal extraction is unsuccessful. Recurrent severe obstipation, refractory to dietary therapy, enemas or manual extraction, may be treated by subtotal colectomy.

Assessment of **serum electrolyte status** and administration of intravenous fluid therapy are particularly important in severely affected cats and in older cats. **Subtotal colectomy** is the preferred therapy in severe chronic constipation or megacolon.

While subtotal colectomy is a major surgical procedure, it provides a **permanent cure for idiopathic megacolon**. Postoperative diarrhea should be expected and usually lasts for about 2 weeks, although it may persist for 4–6 weeks in some cases. Post-operative diarrhea is less likely to occur if the ileocolic junction is not removed during the surgical procedure (i.e. subtotal colectomy rather than total colectomy).

Prognosis

Generally **good to excellent in cats with mild to moderate constipation**.

Cats with **severe constipation or megacolon** have a **favorable long-term prognosis following total or subtotal colectomy**.

ACUTE NON-SPECIFIC COLITIS**

Classical signs

- Acute onset of large bowel diarrhea (tenesmus, mucoid feces, hematochezia) predominates.
- +/− Vomiting with diarrheic episodes.
- Signs are usually mild and often self-limiting.

See main reference on page 762 (The Cat With Signs of Large Bowel Diarrhea) for details.

Pathogenesis

Acute colitis may be caused by **hair ingestion, infectious agents, dietary factors (indiscretion, additives) and/or parasites**.

The **cause is rarely identified** as **most animals spontaneously resolve or respond to symptomatic therapy**.

Clinical signs

There is an **acute onset of large bowel diarrhea** characterized by small-volume, high-frequency feces, sometimes accompanied by mucus or blood.

Straining to defecate is a common clinical sign.

Vomiting may accompany diarrheic episodes.

Signs are usually **mild and often self-limiting.**

Diagnosis

An **underlying cause** for gastrointestinal signs is **rarely identified.**

Signs tend to be **self-limiting** or they **respond to symptomatic therapy in 3–5 days.**

Perform **fecal flotation and direct fecal examinations** for intestinal parasites.

Fecal cytology is useful in identification of infectious agents (bacteria) and leukocytes may be seen with acute mucosal inflammation.

Culture feces if infectious (bacterial) colitis is suspected.

Differential diagnosis

The history and clinical features of acute non-specific colitis make most other diseases unlikely.

Treatment

Provide intravenous or **subcutaneous fluids** lactated ringers solution if dehydration is evident.

Feed **small but frequent meals** of an easily digested food.

Administer an appropriate **broad-spectrum anthelmintic** to eliminate parasitic infestations.

Antibiotics are **only used in culture-proven cases** of infectious colitis.

If the cat is long-haired or over-grooms, consider clipping the coat if other causes of colitis cannot be identified.

Prognosis

The prognosis for full recovery is **excellent** in most instances.

CHRONIC COLITIS** (INFECTIOUS, NEOPLASTIC, AND BENIGN INFILTRATIVE MUCOSAL DISEASE)

Classical signs

- Chronic large bowel diarrhea (tenesmus, small-volume mucoid feces, hematochezia).
- +/- Systemic signs (lymphadenopathy, anorexia, weight loss, +/- fever) if infectious cause.

See main reference on page 762 (The Cat With Signs of Large Bowel Diarrhea) for details.

Clinical signs

Hematochezia, small-volume, high-frequency feces, and straining are observed.

Systemic signs (lymphadenopathy, anorexia, weight loss, +/- fever) may be seen with infectious viral diseases (FeLV and FIV) and systemic mycoses.

Cats with **benign infiltrative mucosal disease** (e.g. lymphocytic-plasmacytic colitis) rarely have systemic signs except with concurrent small intestinal involvement.

Diagnosis

Laboratory testing detects evidence of infectious viral diseases.

Screen susceptible cats for **FeLV antigenemia and serum antibodies to FIV.**

Mucosal biopsies are required for definitive diagnosis of neoplastic, mycotic and benign infiltrative mucosal diseases causing chronic colitis.

Differential diagnosis

Chronic colitis should be **differentiated from more acute causes of tenesmus**, such as acute non-specific colitis, **and conditions causing small intestinal diarrhea**, because some causes of chronic colitis also involve the small intestine, resulting in signs of both large and small bowel involvement.

Treatment

Treatment for this condition is **based on treating the primary cause.** Lymphocytic-plasmacytic colitis may require a **food trial** to investigate a dietary etiology, combined with **oral prednisolone therapy at immunosuppressive dose rates** (2–4 mg/kg/day).

DEHYDRATION AND HYPOKALEMIA*

Classical signs

- Skin tenting, tacky mucus membranes, increased plasma protein and PCV.
- ± Muscular weakness, reluctance to jump, ventroflexion of the neck associated with hypokalemia.
- Reduced, painful or absent defecation +/- tenesmus.
- Feces are hard, dry with or without mucus.
- +/– Anorexia, lethargy, weight loss and vomiting depending on the cause.

See main reference on page 557 (The Polycythemic Cat (for dehydration)) and page 945 (The Cat With Generalized Weakness) and page 893 (The Cat With Neck Ventroflexion) for hypokalemia)) for details.

Pathogenesis

Both dehydration and hypokalemia may be caused by either **reduced intake** in anorexia, or by **increased losses, or by a combination of both**. This most commonly occurs in **chronic renal failure** in older cats. Other causes of **vomiting and/or diarrhea** may also result in dehydration and/or hypokalemia and constipation.

Dehydration exacerbates the already efficient reabsorption of water from the feline colon, and hypokalemia results in weakness of the colonic smooth muscle, slowing the passage of fecal material to the rectum. The **increased fecal volume** that occurs over the extended time in the colon, and **fecal dryness**, worsen the condition.

The differential diagnosis of dehydration depends on the **primary cause**. Hypokalemia may be caused by any condition which causes **reduced intake from anorexia**, or **increased losses via the urinary or gastrointestinal tract.** Conditions commonly associated with increased loss of potassium include **chronic renal failure**, and any causes of **vomiting and/or diarrhea.**

Clinical signs

Depending on the severity of dehydration, signs progress from **subtle loss of skin tenting** to **dry mucous membranes** and **sunken eyeballs**. There are **signs of shock** in advanced cases.

Hypokalemic cats are **weak**, and may show a **reluctance to jump** or climb stairs, **ventroflexion of the head** and **poor limb tone.**

Reduced, absent or painful defecation may be present, and **tenesmus** is frequently noted.

Feces are **hard, dry** and may or may not be covered in mucus.

Systemic signs including lethargy, anorexia, weight loss and vomiting may be present, depending on the underlying cause.

Diagnosis

Clinical signs of **loss of skin elasticity and tacky mucous membranes**, accompanied by **elevations in PCV and total protein** are indicative of dehydration, together with evidence of **constipation** (**hard, dry feces and tenesmus**).

Serum potassium concentration is low, determined by in-house or laboratory analysis.

Differential diagnosis

Severe constipation or megacolon can result in depression, anorexia and dehydration. Constipation resulting from dehydration and hypokalemia is more likely when an underlying disease with the potential to cause dehydration and hypokalemia is detected, and the constipation or megacolon is not severe.

Treatment

Treatment of dehydration is by **administration of fluid therapy** to correct hydration, electrolyte and acid–base status.

Potassium deficits can be corrected by **oral and/or IV supplementation**, depending on the severity of the problem. Fluid therapy may initially worsen hypokalemia because of expansion of blood volume and diuresis, so it may be beneficial to supply oral K^+ concurrently. **Oral potassium should ideally be supplied as gluconate or citrate**, as KCl may worsen concurrent metabolic acidosis. Please refer to the main reference for correction of K^+ deficits in dehydration on page 557.

Maintainence fluid rates are 70 ml/kg/day. **Fluid deficits and ongoing losses** should be estimated and added to maintenance rates so that the deficit can be corrected over the first 12–24 hours. Please refer to the main reference for treatment of dehydration on page 558.

Prognosis

The prognosis for constipation from dehydration and hypokalemia depends on the **primary cause** of the problem.

PELVIC FRACTURES*

> ### Classical signs
>
> - Inability to walk and severe pain on palpation of the pelvic area in a cat with a recent history of trauma.
> - Dry hard feces and straining to defecate in a cat with evidence of healed pelvic fractures.

Clinical signs

Cats with recent pelvic fractures may be able to sit up, but are **rarely able to walk normally.** Attempts at abdominal and especially pelvic palpation elicit a **pain response**. When the tuber ischii are palpated from behind, there may be asymmetric movement in an anteroposterior direction. Attempts to defecate may be absent.

Cats with **old healed pelvic fractures** may have asymmetry on pelvic palpation, and differences in length of pelvic limbs when they are compared with each other in full extension.

Constipation may result either from **pain associated with defecation, or obstruction from a narrowed pelvic cavity.**

Diagnosis

The pelvis should be **radiographed in two views** (lateral and DV or VD) to detect fractures and gauge pelvic narrowing.

Differential diagnosis

Any conditions that cause pain in the hindquarters and lumbosacral region, such as **severe bruising,** should be considered.

Conditions causing hindlimb paresis or paralysis may present as a refusal to move, as do pelvic fractures. A physical and **neurological examination** should be performed to differentiate these conditions.

Treatment

Pelvic fractures **often require surgical repair,** but depending on the position and degree of distraction of the bone fragments, **some may heal with extended cage rest** (4–6 weeks).

Laxatives and/or dietary fiber supplements should be provided to produce a soft stool that is easy to pass. See page 785 (Constipation) for details.

HAIR MATTING*

Classical signs

- Hair is matted with feces over the perineal region, usually in a long-haired or obese cat.
- Constipation or obstipation.

Clinical signs

Long-haired cats in unkempt condition may be presented with hair matted with feces over the perineal region. An **underlying cause** should be established for this lack of grooming, such as **inability to reach the perineal region** because of severe obesity, or an underlying condition causing **diarrhea or lethargy,** because

cats should normally be able to groom well enough to prevent this happening.

Morbidly obese cats frequently are unable to groom effectively around the anal region and may develop mats of feces adhered to hair. These result in perianal dermatitis if they are not removed. The discomfort and obstruction to defecation promote constipation.

Concurrent signs of constipation or obstipation are present including tenesmus and infrequent passage of hard dry feces.

Diagnosis

The diagnosis is made by an **inspection of the perineal region**. More information should be obtained to investigate an underlying cause by performing a **general physical examination and neurological examination**, and if indicated, **more specific blood and/or fecal tests**. The perineum should also be clipped and inspected.

Differential diagnosis

This condition is **self-evident on perineal examination,** but should be differentiated from **other conditions that cause inability to groom and reluctance to defecate,** such as pelvic fractures and perineal abscesses.

Treatment

The **perineum should be clipped and cleaned. Corticosteroid/antibiotic cream** may be applied morning and night if there are signs of perineal inflammation. Purulent skin infections should be treated with **oral antibiotics** such as doxycycline (5 mg/kg PO q 12 h 8 days).

Any **underlying cause** should be **treated appropriately.**

LITTERBOX DISSATISFACTION*

Classical signs

- Cats may urinate and defecate in inappropriate places.
- History of poorly cleaned litter box or insufficient litter boxes for the number of cats.
- Straining, hard dry feces.

Clinical signs

Litterbox dissatisfaction often results in **both defecation and urination in inappropriate places**.

Because of reluctance to use the litter tray, the cat may defecate infrequently, predisposing it to **chronic constipation**.

On close questioning of the owner, **litterbox hygiene may be unacceptable**. Alternatively, the **position of the litterbox may be unacceptable to the cat** because of noise or accessibility by other animals.

Diagnosis

The **owner must be questioned closely but tactfully** about the **frequency and method of litterbox cleaning**, and the **position of the litter tray**, especially in relation to noise levels and accessibility by other animals. **Type of litter material** and the cat's previous history in this regard should also be determined, as some cats do not accept a change in litter material readily. A **house call** may be required to fully assess the situation.

Differential diagnosis

Litterbox dissatisfaction must be differentiated from **other conditions causing reluctance to defecate**, such as painful pelvic or perineal conditions.

Treatment

The litterbox must be placed in a **quiet, secluded area easily accessed by the cat**, but not by other animals such as dogs. There should be **at least one litter tray provided per cat in the household**. The **litter should be completely changed and the tray scrubbed every day**. Just a **small amount** of the type of litter acceptable to the cat should be placed in the tray, **to facilitate frequent cleaning during the day**. Automatic litter trays may also be helpful.

LOWER URINARY TRACT DISEASE*

> ### Classical signs
>
> - Pollakiuria, dysuria and hematuria if non-obstructed.

> ### Classical signs—Cont'd
>
> - Affected cats may urinate in inappropriate places.
> - Anorexia, weakness and anuria with urinary obstruction.

See main reference on page 176 (The Cat Straining to Urinate) for details.

Clinical signs

Pollakiuria, hematuria, stranguria and inappropriate urination are the most common signs. The bladder is typically small on palpation.

Anorexia, depression, vomiting and anuria occur with **urinary obstruction. Typically the bladder is distended and firm on palpation.**

Diagnosis

The diagnosis of non-obstructive LUTD is often based on **relevant history and a normal physical examination.** The majority (55–69%) of cats with signs of lower urinary tract disease have **idiopathic cystitis;** some have **struvite or calcium oxalate uroliths** (20%); and the remainder have a variety of conditions including anatomical defects, urethral obstruction, tumors and bacterial infection.

Urinalysis reveals hematuria, and is usually sterile. Depending on the cause, struvite crystalluria, bacteria or neoplastic cells may be evident.

A diagnosis of **obstructive LUTD** is based on history and palpation of a **turgid, distended bladder,** which is difficult or impossible to express. Radiography, including contrast radiographs, and ultrasonography will help to identify uroliths, neoplasia, anatomical defects and urethral obstruction.

Differential diagnosis

Distinguish LUTD from **other causes of straining associated with the gastrointestinal tract**.

Treatment

Non-obstructive LUTD generally resolves spontaneously or with symptomatic therapy in **5–7 days**.

- Modify the **diet** to minimize urine concentration by using canned food or add water to dry food. If urine pH is > 6.5 and there is struvite crystalluria, maximize urine acidity, and minimize magnesium intake using a diet designed to reduce struvite formation.
- Amitriptyline (2.5–12.5 mg/cat PO q 24 h) may be effective in reducing clinical signs in cats with idiopathic cystitis.
- Empirical use of antibiotics, anti-inflammatory agents and antispasmodics is **controversial**.

Obstructive LUTD is a **medical emergency**.

- Therapeutic strategies are directed at **relief of the obstruction and supportive therapy as needed. For prevention, use specific diets for struvite and calcium oxalate uroliths, and maximize dietary water intake**.

See a detailed discussion on obstructive LUTD see page 179 (The Cat Straining to Urinate).

NEOPLASIA

Classical signs

- ± Palpable abdominal mass.
- Straining, hard, dry feces.

Clinical signs

Abdominal neoplasms may obstruct the passage of feces along the large intestine.

Signs of neoplasia, such as **weight loss and a palpable abdominal mass**, may accompany the clinical signs of constipation and straining.

An abdominal mass may be palpable.

The abdominal neoplasms that have the potential to cause constipation because of their anatomical position and prevalence in cats are **lymphosarcoma** of the intestine or abdominal lymph nodes, **intestinal adenosarcoma** and intestinal mast cell tumor.

Diagnosis

Abdominal neoplasms are most readily diagnosed by **abdominal ultrasound** followed by **fine-needle aspirate biopsy or surgical biopsy and histopathology.**

Abdominal radiographs may also be useful in visualizing the mass. The obstruction may be caused by **intraluminal or extraluminal masses**.

Differential diagnosis

Abdominal neoplasia must be differentiated from **other causes of abdominal masses** such as an **obstructed bladder or trichobezoars** (hairballs). This can be done by **abdominal ultrasonography or radiographs,** and clinical signs.

Treatment

Treatment of abdominal neoplasia **depends on the type of tumor identified on histopathology. Surgical excision** should be performed, sometimes followed by a **chemotherapeutic protocol**, depending on the histopathological diagnosis.

DRUGS

Classical signs

- History of drug use, such as opiates or kaolin/pectin.
- Signs of constipation.

Clinical signs

There are signs of constipation, such as **reduced frequency of defecation, and straining**, with an **appropriate drug history**, such as the administration of **opiates or kaolin/pectin**.

Overzealous use of **furosemide** promotes dehydration which predisposes to constipation.

Diagnosis

The diagnosis is made by a **thorough drug history** and **evidence of constipation** on abdominal palpation or radiographs.

Differential diagnosis

Drug-related causes of constipation should be differentiated from **other causes of constipation that do** not have overt accompanying clinical signs on physical examination, such as idiopathic megacolon, acute or chronic colitis, and litterbox dissatisfaction. This is done by taking a thorough drug and litterbox history.

Treatment

The condition resolves once the causative drug is withdrawn.

PERINEAL INFLAMMATION/INFECTION

Classical signs

- History of pain or sensitivity in the perianal region or evidence of perianal wound or abscess.
- Signs of constipation.

Clinical signs

Cats are presented with a history of pain or sensitivity in the hindquarters, and sometimes a reluctance to sit or an unusual sitting posture. On inspection of the perineum, there may be hair loss and/or matting, and wounds or abscessation. Sometimes, an abscess is associated with one of the anal sacs.

Signs or history of constipation are present because pain associated with defecation promotes fecal retention.

Diagnosis

The condition is self-evident, but in some cats, heavy sedation or general anesthesia may be required to thoroughly inspect the area.

Differential diagnosis

Perineal inflammation or infection should be differentiated from other conditions causing matting of the perineal hair, such as chronic diarrhea or conditions causing poor grooming. This is done by performing a thorough physical examination including the perineal region.

Treatment

The perineal area should be clipped and cleaned. Wounds and/or abscesses should be debrided and flushed with saline or an aqueous iodine solution. Feces should be kept soft by the use of laxatives and/or dietary fiber supplements until healing has occurred. See page 785 (Constipation (including idiopathic megacolon)).

Oral antibiotics, such as doxycycline (5 mg/kg q 12 h 8 days) should be prescribed.

DYSAUTONOMIA

Classical signs

- Mostly young adult cats (< 3 years of age).
- Acute onset of depression and anorexia over 48 h.
- Constellation of signs including regurgitation, constipation, mydriasis and dry eyes.
- ± Protrusion of the third eyelids, bradycardia and dysuria.

Pathogenesis

Dysautonomia is an idiopathic condition characterized by widespread degeneration of the autonomic ganglia.

The condition was originally reported in the UK and Europe, but is rarely recognized at this time. There are rare reports of affected cats in the USA. While some of these cats were imported from the UK, a small number were bred in USA.

Recent evidence suggests that *Clostridium botulinum* type C neurotoxin may be involved. The toxin was detected in the feces or ileum contents in affected cats, and also in their dry food, but not in healthy control cats. Fourteen weeks after the outbreak, IgA antibodies to the toxin and organism were significantly higher in the feces of affected cats compared to unaffected cats.

Both sympathetic and parasympathetic nervous systems are affected.

The predominance of gastrointestinal signs relates to failure of parasympathetic stimulation of esophageal, gastric and colonic motility.

Loss of autonomic control to the eye and heart result in dilated fixed pupils and a fixed heart rate.

Tenesmus is attributable to **constipation and/or dysuria**.

Clinical signs

Dysautonomia is primarily seen in **young cats (< 3 years old).**

Outbreaks in multicat households and single isolated cases have been reported.

Signs often develop **acutely** over 48 h, with nearly all cats **showing depression** and **anorexia.** In some cats, signs develop over several weeks, and weight loss may be evident.

Regurgitation associated with megaesophagus, vomiting, constipation, weakness and **dry mucous membranes** of the mouth, nose and eye, are the most commonly reported clinical signs.

Pupils are dilated and fixed, but the cat is visual. There is **protrusion of the third eyelids** in more than 90% of affected cats, and the eyes appear dry.

Braycardia of 90–120 beats per minute occurs in about 60% of cats.

Loss of anal tone and fecal incontinence may be evident.

Dysuria and a distended bladder are less common signs. Urinary incontinence may also occur.

Occasionally **constipation or obstipation is the major presenting sign,** and the other signs are less obvious.

Diagnosis

A presumptive diagnosis is usually made based on the **characteristic clinical presentation**.

Survey and/or contrast radiography demonstrate **megaesophagus, delayed gastrointestinal transit and/or bladder distention.**

Confirmation of **abnormal autonomic function tests** may be pursued if indicated. **Ocular (pupillary) response tests** to 0.1% pilocarpine and 0.25% physostigmine may be performed.
- **Pilocarpine** is a direct-acting parasympathomimetic agent, which when applied topically will result in **miosis and retraction of the third eyelid to a normal position in a cat with dysautonomia, but will have no effect on a normal cat**.
  - This results from the phenomenon of **denervation hypersensitivity** in the dysautonomic cat, causing an **enhanced response to direct-acting agents.**
- By contrast, **topical physostigmine** is an indirect-acting parasympathomimetic agent, which acts by inhibiting cholinesterase to prevent local degradation of acetylcholine, causing **rapid miosis in a normal cat, but no response in a cat with dysautonomia.**

Determination of **plasma and urinary catecholamine concentrations** may also be useful. Plasma epinephrine and norepinephrine concentrations and urinary catecholamine levels are **reduced in cats with dysautonomia compared to normal cats**.

Differential diagnosis

The clinical features of classical feline dysautonomia make **most other diseases unlikely**.

Atypical cats may present with constipation or obstipation as the major sign. Careful physical examination, and an index of suspicion for dysautonomia are required to make a diagnosis in these cats.

Treatment

Treatment is **supportive but palliative** in most instances. Approximately 20–40% recover with supportive therapy. Recovery is over 2–12 months, and may not be complete.

Correct dehydration if present.

Prolonged nutritional support should be provided via parenteral or enteral means if there is persistent vomiting or regurgitation.

Parasympathomimetic drugs may be administered to improve oronasal secretion, and treat the ocular manifestations of the condition, especially decreased lacrimation.
- **Pilocarpine drops** (**0.25–1%** solution 1 drop q 6–8 h).
- **Physostigmine drops** (0.5% 1 drop q 12 h).

Metoclopramide (Reglan, 0.2–0.4 mg/kg PO or SC q 8 h) enhances gastrointestinal motility. The aim is to decrease esophageal dilation and increase gastric emptying, and hence reduce vomiting and regurgitation.

- **Cisapride** (Propulsid, 2.5–5 mg/cat q 8–12 h) is thought to be more effective than metoclopramide, and can be combined with metoclopramide to improve gastric emptying and small intestinal motility. Cisapride is indicated in cats with esophagitis from vomiting. Cisapride is currently unavailable in the USA. Nizatadine (2.5–5 mg/kg PO once daily) or ranitidine (1–2 mg/kg PO q 8–12 h) may be used instead as colonic prokinetic agents.

Dysuria, urinary bladder emptying, and gastrointestinal motility may be improved with **bethanecol** (2.5–5.0 mg PO q 8–12 h, or 0.0375 mg/kg SC q 8–12 h). Start with the lower dose and increase if necessary, but beware of adverse effects such as bradycardia and arrhythmias).

Relieve constipation using **laxatives and enemas.** See page 785 (Constipation (including idiopathic mega-oesphagus)).

Manual emptying of the bladder and colon may be required if drug therapy is ineffective. Urine should be monitored for bacterial infection, and infection treated promptly.

Prognosis

Initial severity of clinical signs is not necessarily correlated with survival, and **response to treatment is a better indication of prognosis**.

The prognosis is **guarded to poor**, especially in cats with megaesophagus. If cats continue to regurgitate fluids after 1–2 weeks of treatment, consider euthanasia.

The mortality rate is approximately 60%, and surviving cats may have residual signs.

RECOMMENDED READING

Firth M, Fondacaro JV, Greco DS. Challenging cases in internal medicine: What's your diagnosis? Vet Med 2000; 95(8): 606–614.

Grauer GF. Feline lower urinary tract inflammation. In: Nelson RW, Couto CG (eds) Small Animal Internal Medicine, 3rd edn. Missouri, Mosby, 2003, pp. 642–649.

Washabau RJ, Hasler AH. Constipation, obstipation and megacolon. In: August JR (ed) Consultations in Feline Internal Medicine, 3rd edn. Philadelphia, PA, W.B. Saunders, 1997, pp. 104–112.

White RN. Surgical management of constipation. J Feline Med Surg 2002; 4(3): 129–138.

PART 10

Cat with signs of neurological disease

36. The cat with seizures, circling and/or changed behavior

Andrée D Quesnel[†] and Joane M Parent

MECHANISM?

- **Seizures** occur when a forebrain lesion irritates the surrounding neurons or when there is diffuse neuronal hyperexcitability as a result of a genetic predisposition (primary epilepsy), metabolic disturbance (e.g. hypoglycemia) or intoxication.
- **Circling** may occur with forebrain disease and is compulsive and obsessive in nature.
- **Changed behavior** arises from intellectual dysfunction, psychic perturbations, learning disabilities and memory losses.

continued

continued

WHERE?

- Most cats with seizures, compulsive circling or changed behavior from neurological disease have a **forebrain (thalamocortex) lesion.**

WHAT?

- Seizures are most often associated with tumors, encephalitides and inactive lesions (e.g. glial scar), while extracranial causes (metabolic and toxic) and idiopathic epilepsy are rare.
- Compulsive circling is caused by any kind of lesion located in the frontal lobe or rostral thalamus, although trauma, tumors and ischemic encephalopathy are the most common causes. Circling is usually toward the side of the lesion.
- Changed or abnormal behavior usually consists of subtle personality changes, and is most often associated with tumors, head trauma, ischemic encephalopathy, congenital and inherited forebrain anomalies, hepatic encephalopathy, feline infectious peritonitis, and feline immunodeficiency encephalopathy.

QUICK REFERENCE SUMMARY

Diseases causing seizures, circling and/or changed behavior

DEGENERATIVE

- **Likely symptomatic epilepsy*** (p 800)**

Recurrent seizures typically beginning as single seizures at intervals of several weeks to months. Frequency may remain low or progressively increase over time. Seizures are partial in onset (± aura, unilateral or localized motor activity, ± localized post-ictal motor deficits) with or without secondary generalization (to violent tonic-clonic motor activity involving the whole body) which may obscure the partial signs.

- **Feline ischemic encephalopathy*** (p 804)**

Peracute onset of unilateral forebrain signs (mental depression and confusion, compulsive circling, hemiparesis) and rarely, severe cluster seizures or status epilepticus. Personality changes and/or post-ischemic epilepsy may be the only manifestation of the milder atypical form.

- **Cerebrovascular accidents** (p 808)**

Peracute onset of focal cerebral signs attributable to the forebrain (confusion, circling, pacing) or brainstem (depression, head tilt, loss of balance, nystagmus, facial paresis) or cerebellum (hypermetria, intentional tremors). Occasionally, seizures occur either as immediate cluster seizures or status epilepticus, or later as secondary epilepsy.

ANOMALY

- **Congenital and inherited forebrain anomalies*** (p 805)**

Developmental abnormalities, such as mental retardation, learning disability or loss of training are often evident historically in kittens and young adult cats (< 2 years old) presenting with abnormal mentation and behavior, central visual deficits and occasionally, secondary epilepsy.

METABOLIC

● Hepatic encephalopathy*** (p 806)

Episodes of mental alteration including depression, confusion, agitation, dementia or stupor occur together with bizarre behavior, hypersalivation and rarely, seizures. Mostly in young animals (< 1–2 years of age) with congenital portosystemic shunt.

● Hypoglycemia** (p 809)

Mental confusion, muscles tremors, weakness, ataxia and occasionally, seizures or coma. Typically, there is history of a diabetic cat receiving insulin therapy or hypoglycemic drugs.

● Hypocalcemia* (p 817)

Progressive neuromuscular hyperexcitability evidenced as muscle fasciculation, tremors or generalized tetany. Rarely culminates in terminal convulsive status epilepticus.

● Uremia (p 819)

CNS depression; occasionally, seizures. Typically, there are other signs of severe acute or chronic renal failure, for example anorexia, vomiting, dehydration, polydipsia, polyuria or anuria.

NEOPLASTIC

● Forebrain tumors** (p 810)

Typically middle-aged and older cats with progressive focal forebrain signs such as personality changes, mental depression, confusion, pacing, compulsive circling and subtle hemiparesis. Seizures may also occur.

NUTRITIONAL

● Thiamine deficiency*** (p 808)

Central vestibular signs (head tilt, loss of balance), mydriasis, spasmodic ventroflexion of the neck with whole-body contorsions, which may be misinterpreted as seizures. Terminally, opisthotonos, coma and death.

INFLAMMATORY

● Feline non-suppurative meningoencephalitis*** (p 803)

Focal or multifocal neurological signs attributable to any portion of the CNS (hindlimb paresis and ataxia, head tilt and loss of balance, seizures) ± systemic (fever, inappetence, lymphadenopathy) and/or ocular (chorioretinitis) signs.

INFECTIOUS:
VIRAL

● Feline infectious peritonitis** (p 811)

CNS signs (typically head tilt, balance losses, intentional tremors) accompanied by systemic (fever, lethargy, inappetence, weight loss) ± ocular signs (anterior uveitis, chorioretinitis) in cats usually younger than 3 years of age.

● Rabies (p 819)

Variable prodromal signs progressing often to a furious phase characterized by vicious and aggressive behavior +/– dysphagia, paralysis, convulsions, coma and death.

continued

continued

● Feline immunodeficiency virus encephalopathy (p 819)

Usually asymptomatic, but may cause subtle and non-specific behavioral changes such as depression, social withdrawal and roaming.

PROTOZOAL

● **Toxoplasmosis** (p 815)

Focal or multifocal CNS signs are rare signs accompanying the more common systemic signs such as fever, or dyspnea or ocular manifestations (anterior uveitis, chorioretinitis) of the disease.

FUNGAL

● **Cryptococcosis** (p 812)

Cerebral signs such as depression, circling and ataxia are often accompanied by chronic nasal discharge, cutaneous nodules or ulcers, or ocular signs including chorioretinitis, retinal detachment and panophthalmitis.

IDIOPATHIC

● **Idiopathic epilepsy*** (p 816)

Rare in cats and occurs as recurrent generalized motor seizures starting with single seizures at several week intervals in a young adult animal that has no other neurological signs or deficits.

TRAUMA

● Head trauma (p 806)

Peracute onset of cerebral signs such as confusion to dementia, pacing, circling or hemiparesis. Immediate onset of seizures and/or post-traumatic epilepsy may occur.

TOXIC

● **Intoxications** (p 812)

Typically present with signs of depression or stimulation of the CNS (depression, agitation), together with autonomic system signs (miosis, hypersalivation) and neuromuscular signs (weakness, muscle tremors). Occasionally, convulsive status epilepticus.

INTRODUCTION

MECHANISM?

Seizures are generated by paroxysmal excessive discharge of thalamocortical neurons which are rendered focally or diffusely hyperexcitable by several mechanisms:

● **Structural brain lesions**, either active (e.g. encephalitis, tumor) or inactive (e.g. glial scar), irritate the surrounding neurons and transform them into transient or permanent epileptic foci; some areas of the brain are more likely to generate seizures (e.g. frontal and temporal lobes) than others (e.g. occipital lobe).

● In **idiopathic epilepsy**, no causes other than a genetic predisposition underlie the intrinsic neuronal disturbances.

● **Extracranial causes** of seizures (metabolic and toxic) diffusely affect the brain.

The clinical appearance of seizures varies a great deal, depending on the origin and extent of spreading of the seizure discharge within the brain.

Primary generalized seizures have a diffuse onset within both cerebral hemispheres.

● They manifest with a complete loss of consciousness and generalized, symmetrical and usually violent tonic and/or clonic motor activity that results in complete recumbency often with thrashing and limb paddling. This is often accompanied by jaw champing, facial twitching and autonomic signs (e.g. mydriasis, hypersalivation, piloerection, micturition).

- In partial (focal) seizures with secondary generalization, the seizure is preceded by behavioral change (aura) or localized or lateralized motor signs or followed by motor deficits.

Partial (focal) seizures have a focal onset in one cerebral hemisphere and a limited propagation within one or both hemispheres.

- They manifest with variable degrees of alteration of consciousness ranging from normal to totally absent awareness and responsiveness.
- **Partial (focal) seizures have motor signs that may be either lateralized** to one side of the body, **localized** to one part of the body, or may even be **generalized** but not violent enough to cause complete recumbency (e.g. mild tremors of the whole body).
  - **Lateralized signs** include unilateral facial twitching, tonic or clonic movements of one or both limbs on one side, and spasmodic turning of the head to one side.
  - **Signs localized to one part of the body** include hindlimb weakness causing difficulty or inability walking, and bilateral facial twitching with or without spasmodic head bobbing.
- **Partial (focal) seizures of cats are often subtle and/or bizarre** and may be difficult to recognize as being seizure activity.
- Some partial (focal) seizures previously called psychomotor seizures mainly manifest with bizarre stereotypical and behavioral activities (e.g. hallucinatory prey or predator behavior with running fits).
- **Seizures preceded by an aura** (behavioral changes within a few seconds or minutes of the ictus onset) or followed by **localized post-ictal motor deficits** (e.g. hemiparesis) **are partial in onset**, even if they appear to be generalized from the beginning of the ictus.
- **Partial (focal) seizures may secondarily generalize** to tonic-clonic generalized seizures and this may occur so quickly that their initial partial phase may not be observed clinically; most generalized seizures of cats are probably within that category.
- The occurrence of partial seizures usually indicates that there is a **focal forebrain lesion** which excludes the possibility of idiopathic (genetic) epilepsy and extracranial (metabolic and toxic) causes of seizures.

Seizures must be differentiated from seizure-like events such as syncopes, sleep disorders (e.g. excessive dream-like movements), movement disorders (e.g. myoclonia, tremors-tetany), narcolepsy-cataplexy, episodic behavioral disorders (e.g. fly catching, feline hyperesthesia), dysphoric and agitated anesthetic recovery, and paddling associated with decerebration.

Compulsive circling is usually accompanied by mental confusion with either depression or agitation. It is often associated with wandering, pacing and sometimes with an abnormal posture (head and eye deviation or turning, leaning).

- **Compulsive circling must be differentiated from vestibular circling** which is due to marked loss of balance.
  - The cat with compulsive circling does not have a head tilt (its head may however be turned), loss of balance, nystagmus and other vestibular signs. It usually has a normal gait (no detectable ataxia nor paresis) and often can walk in a straight line when it is motivated to do so (e.g. reach a specific goal such as a food plate).

Personality and behavioral changes due to forebrain diseases must be differentiated from pure behavioral disorders.

WHERE?

Forebrain (thalamocortex) diseases can cause any of the following signs:

- **Mentation abnormalities** ranging from depression to semi-stupor, or confusion.
- Subtle **personality changes** (e.g. loss of good or bad habits) to obvious **behavioral abnormalities** (e.g. dementia, aggression).
- Abnormal activities such as **wandering**, propulsive **pacing**, **head pressing** and compulsive **circling**.
- **Seizures**.
- Mild contralateral **hemiparesis** and **proprioceptive loss** causes either subtle gait abnormalities (e.g. knuckling) or is only detected as **postural reaction deficits** (e.g. proprioceptive positioning, hopping, lateral tactile limb placing).
- Central **visual loss** either causes the cat to bump into things, or is only detected by a **deficit in the menace response** together with normal pupillary light reflexes in the contralateral eye when the affected eye is tested.

- Impaired **facial sensation** is detected by decreased head withdrawal when the contralateral nasal septum, upper lip or whiskers are touched.

Large or diffuse forebrain lesions (e.g. tumors, edema) may cause signs of **increased intracranial pressure** (e.g. marked depression, bilateral miosis); this may evolve to **tentorial herniation** with signs of brainstem compression (e.g. coma, unresponsive mydriasis, abnormal respiratory patterns and death by respiratory arrest).

WHAT?

Most cats with **seizures** have a **structural forebrain lesion** that may be active (e.g. encephalitis, tumor, ischemic encephalopathy) or inactive (e.g. post-ischemic glial scar). Extracranial causes of seizures (e.g. metabolic, toxic) and idiopathic epilepsy are rare.

Compulsive circling may be caused by lesions affecting the **rostral thalamus or frontal lobe** and is usually toward the side of the lesion. Most common causes are neoplasia, trauma and ischemic encephalopathy.

Personality and behavioral changes result from lesions affecting the **limbic system** and associated areas of frontal and temporal lobes. Most common causes are neoplasia, trauma, ischemic encephalopathy, feline infectious peritonitis and hepatic encephalopathy.

Diagnosis is based on history, clinical examinations, CSF analysis (reference values in cats are a protein concentration ≤ 0.36 g/L (0.036 mg/dl) and a leukocyte count ≤ 0.002 cells/10^9(2/μl) with the majority of cells being mononuclear cells), brain imaging and other ancillary tests.

DISEASES CAUSING SEIZURES, CIRCLING AND/OR CHANGED BEHAVIOR

LIKELY SYMPTOMATIC EPILEPSY***

Classical signs

- Recurrent seizures are the only problem.
- The initial seizure frequency is low but may increase over time.
- Seizures are partial in onset with or without secondary generalization.

Pathogenesis

Likely symptomatic epilepsy is **common** in cats.

It is most often caused by an **acquired** focal thalamo-cortical lesion that is no longer active but has transformed into an **epileptic focus** by irritating the surrounding neurons.

- Following an insult to the brain such as trauma, encephalitis or ischemia, the glial reaction may result in a persistent glial focus, which irritates the surrounding neurons.
- Seizure onset is usually delayed by a few to several months from an **initial brain insult.** The insult may have occurred in utero (e.g. porencephalic [cystic] lesions due to fetal encephalitis), at birth (e.g. dystocia-related cerebrovascular accidents) or later in life at any age. Post-natal diseases may have been symptomatic (e.g. encephalitis, ischemic encephalopathy, head trauma) or asymptomatic (e.g. atypical form of ischemic encephalopathy, non-suppurative meningoencephalitis).
- Symptomatic seizures occurring during the active phase of a cerebral disease may or may not lead to likely symptomatic epilepsy, depending on the extent of secondary gliosis.

Other rare **congenital or inherited** focal cerebral anomalies may also act as epileptic foci. These include lesions associated with surrounding gliosis (e.g. vascular malformations such as angiomas and arteriovenous malformations) or with intrinsic neuronal hyperexcitability (e.g. disorders of neuronal migration such as cortical dysplasia and heterotopias).

- Seizures usually start during adolescence or young adulthood.

Clinical signs

The initial **seizure frequency** usually is low with single seizures occurring at intervals of several weeks to months. The subsequent seizure frequency often remains low but may progressively increase over months or years due to a self-perpetuating electrical kindling-like phenomenon. This sometimes leads to intractable seizures with frequent and severe cluster seizures and status epilepticus.

Seizures are partial (focal) with or without secondary generalization. Secondary generalization may sometimes occur so quickly that no features of partial seizures may be detected clinically.

Seizures preceded by an **aura** (behavioral changes a few seconds or minutes before the onset of ictus) or followed by **localized post-ictal motor deficits** (e.g. hemiparesis) are partial, even if they appear to be generalized from their onset.

Other static **neurological signs** (e.g. personality changes) and/or **thalamocortical deficits** (e.g. menace, facial sensation, postural reactions) may or may not be present, depending on the size and location of the lesion.

Diagnosis

There may be a **history** of neurological signs a few to several months before the seizure onset (initial cerebral insult). These signs should have improved or resolved; if not, an active brain disease is likely.

Neurological examination may be normal or reveal thalamocortical deficits that are often subtle; the responses obtained from both sides of the body must be carefully compared.

CSF analysis is usually normal. Mild non-specific degenerative changes such as an increased proportion of macrophages despite a normal leukocyte count may sometimes persist for months after the initial cerebral insult (e.g. trauma, ischemic encephalopathy).

Brain imaging may identify an inactive lesion; magnetic resonance imaging (MRI) is more sensitive than computed tomography.

In many cases with clinical evidence of likely symptomatic epilepsy (e.g. partial seizures, non-progressive focal thalamocortical deficits), the underlying cause remains unknown because the CSF analysis and brain MRI are normal. Such epilepsy previously classified as cryptogenic (hidden cause) is now called "likely symptomatic" epilepsy.

Differential diagnosis

Exclusion of other causes of seizures is often possible based on the **history** and **clinical examination**, even before any ancillary tests are performed.

- **Active brain diseases** often cause a higher initial seizure frequency, including cluster seizures and status epilepticus, and a rapid progression toward high-frequency seizures within the first few weeks

or months. A regressive course may occur with self-limiting conditions. Other progressive (or regressive) neurological signs and deficits, and abnormal CSF and/or brain imaging findings reflecting an active disease process are also likely to be present.

- **Idiopathic (genetic) epilepsy** causes primary generalized seizures that begin in young adult cats that have no other neurological signs and deficits (see page 816).
- **Intoxications** typically cause an acute onset of severe convulsive status epilepticus or cluster seizures that is usually preceded by signs of other body systems (e.g. vomiting) as well as diffuse neurological signs (e.g. mental depression, hyperexcitability, tremors). There are no periods of normalcy in between the seizures, which continue until appropriate treatment is provided or until death occurs (see page 812).
- **Metabolic causes** produce a high initial seizure frequency. Metabolic causes may be excluded when there are no other signs of metabolic disorders preceding and following the seizures (e.g. severe and classical signs of hepatoencephalopathy, hypocalcemic tremors – tetany, hypoglycemic weakness and confusion). They can also be excluded when there are partial seizures or focal (unilateral, asymmetrical) neurological signs or deficits. Metabolic diseases, like intoxications, produce generalized seizures and bilateral and symmetrical neurological dysfunction.

Treatment

Aggressive but rational **anti-epileptic drug therapy** is mandatory **if there is more than one single seizure every 6–8 weeks**.

- **Start phenobarbital** 1.5–2.5 mg/kg PO q 12 h.
  - Measure serum phenobarbital concentration **14 days after treatment initiation** and after any dosage modification. Measure trough level, that is, just prior to next treatment. Adjust the dosage to obtain an optimal phenobarbital concentration of 100–130 µmol/ml (23–32 µg/ml) using the formula: optimal dosage = optimal phenobarbital concentration ÷ actual phenobarbital concentration × actual dosage.
- **Add diazepam** (0.5–1.0 mg/kg q 12 h) if seizures are not well controlled (if > 1 seizure/6–8 weeks) despite an optimal phenobarbital concentrations 14 days after treatment initiation or change in drug dose.

- Measure serum benzodiazepine concentration at steady state (reached within 4–5 days) and adjust the dosage to obtain at least 500–700 nmol/L (ng/L); use the same formula as for phenobarbital.
  - Also measure liver enzymes to detect rare idiosyncratic acute hepatic necrosis induced by diazepam in cats.
- **Add gabapentin 10–40 mg/cat q 8 h** if seizures are still not well controlled despite optimal phenobarbital concentrations and benzodiazepine concentrations.
  - **Potassium bromide (KBr) is contraindicated in cats;** in a study of 26 cats treated with KBr, 42% developed respiratory signs from 7 weeks to 14 months after onset of therapy. Two cats died of their airway disease. **The safety of potassium bromide use in the cat remains a serious issue.** If there are no other options, monitoring monthly by way of thoracic radiographs should be done. The clinical signs resolve with the arrest of treatment (up to 17 months are required for full recovery).

Anti-epileptic drug therapy is likely to be required for life. Only if the cat remains seizure-free for longer than 6–12 months should **slow weaning** from drugs be attempted. Weaning should occur over a few months with one drug at a time. If more than one seizure/8 weeks recurs during or after drug withdrawal, resume treatment.

- **Status epilepticus and cluster seizures require emergency treatment**.
  - **First give a diazepam bolus of 0.5 mg/kg IV.** Repeat if the seizure has not stopped within 1–2 minutes or if another one begins.
  - **Immediately start a diazepam constant rate IV infusion** of 0.5 mg/kg/h to prevent seizure recurrence.
  - Mix the diazepam in an in-line burette with maintenance fluids. Prepare only 1–2 hour supply at a time as diazepam is rapidly adsorbed into the plastic tubing and is inactivated by exposure to light.
  - When no seizures have occurred after 4–6 hours, slowly decrease the infusion rate (25% steps every 4–6 hours).
  - **If > 2 seizures occur during the diazepam infusion, either give another diazepam bolus (0.5 mg/kg) and increase the diazepam infu-** sion (to 0.75–1.0 mg/kg/h), **or give a phenobarbital IV bolus** (2–5 mg/kg) and add phenobarbital to the diazepam infusion (0.5–1 mg/kg/h) for at least 4–6 hours before attempting to decrease it. Because it takes at least 20 minutes for a phenobarbital IV bolus to exert its anticonvulsant effect, sustained seizure activity must be controlled with diazepam in the mean time.
  - **If phenobarbital is to be started as a maintenance anti-epileptic drug, a loading dose of 15–20 mg/kg (slow IV bolus) may be given to immediately** achieve a therapeutic serum concentration of 60–110 µmol/L (15–25 µg/ml). Maintenance dosing should be continued afterwards (2.5 mg/kg q 12 h PO or IM if the cat is sedated to the point it is unable to safely swallow). Phenobarbital is potentiated by diazepam. Close monitoring of the patient must be done when adding phenobarbital to diazepam.
  - If the cat is already treated with chronic oral phenobarbital therapy and its phenobarbital concentration is known to be sub-therapeutic, it can be immediately increased by administering an IV bolus; each 1 mg/kg IV bolus will increase the phenobarbital concentrations by 5 µmol/L (1 µg/ml).
- **If seizures are not adequately controlled, propofol at sub-anesthetic dosage can be administered.** Use an IV bolus of 1.0–3.5 mg/kg plus a continuous IV infusion of 0.01–0.25 mg/kg/min, to effect, for several hours (up to 12–48 hours, if necessary) before attempting weaning.
- **If high-frequency or sustained convulsive seizures persist** despite the above treatment, proceed to **general anesthesia with pentobarbital** (5–15 mg/kg slow IV over several minutes, to effect; wait 10 minutes to see maximal effect before giving more).
  - Add an IV continuous rate infusion of 5 mg/kg/h for at least 6 hours if other seizures occur afterwards.
  - **Intubation and ventilation are recommended** as well as close anesthetic monitoring (temperature, blood pressure, etc.).
  - **Isoflurane anesthesia is the last resort** for refractory seizures. It should be done for at least a few hours.

Prognosis

Good seizure control is often obtained with appropriate anti-epileptic drug therapy. Progression toward intractability may however occur despite adequate treatment and indicates a poor prognosis.

FELINE NON-SUPPURATIVE MENINGOENCEPHALITIS***

> **Classical signs**
>
> - Focal or multifocal CNS signs.
> - Seizures.
> - Occasionally, generalized tremors ("shaker cat syndrome").

Pathogenesis

A viral infection is suspected even though the condition does not appear to be contagious. Signs are usually confined to a single cat in a household.

- Several feline **(e.g. herpesvirus type I)** and non-feline **(e.g. arboviruses)** viruses may infect the CNS of cats and produce a subclinical or clinical meningoencephalitis.

An **immune-mediated** process is also possible. This can be primary (idiopathic autoimmune) or secondary to various antigenic stimulation such as vaccination, CNS infection with a non-pathogenic virus or infection in another system.

Cats of **any age** and with or without outdoor access may be affected.

Clinical signs

The clinical course is variable with an acute or insidious onset and a static, progressive or regressive course.

The disease can produce **focal or multifocal signs** of variable severity attributable to **any portion of the CNS**; **central vestibular** (head tilt, balance losses, mental depression, postural reaction deficits), **spinal cord** (hindlimb proprioceptive ataxia and paresis), cerebellar and cranial nerve signs are most common and may occur alone or in any combination.

- **Seizures may occur** alone or with other signs during the active phase of the disease. They may present with the full spectrum of severity.
- **Delayed onset post-encephalitic secondary epilepsy** may also occur after a symptomatic or an asymptomatic course of the disease.

A steroid-responsive **"shaker cat syndrome"** similar to the "little white dog shaker syndrome" has been observed as the only clinical manifestation of the disease in a few cats.

Systemic signs including fever, inappetence, lymphadenopathy and mild hematological abnormalities (e.g. leukopenia, lymphocytosis, anemia) may sometimes precede or accompany the neurological signs. **Ocular signs** (e.g. chorioretinitis) may also be seen.

Diagnosis

CSF analysis may be normal or reveal a mild increase of the protein concentration (< 0.70 g/L) and/or a mononuclear pleocytosis (< 50 cells/µl) with numerous small lymphocytes and/or large foamy mononuclear cells.

Brain imaging (MRI) **may be normal or show inflammatory lesions** with contrast uptake. Obstructive or compensatory hydrocephalus and porencephalic (cystic) lesions may sometimes be seen.

Differential diagnosis

Other infectious encephalitis (e.g. FIP, toxoplasmosis, cryptococcosis) when there are other systemic signs, ocular involvement or a progressive course.

- **CSF analysis** is the best test to differentiate the disease from FIP. **Cats with FIP** usually have a higher CSF protein concentration and cell count with a predominance of neutrophils (see page 844). **Toxoplasmosis** can however produce similar CSF changes. Rarely, **cryptococcosis** may produce only mild CSF inflammation but culture and titers help with diagnosis when the organism is not visible in the CSF. Usually signs are rapidly progressive with cryptococcosis.

Other causes of seizures in cats should be considered when seizures are the only sign of the disease (e.g. **idiopathic and likely symptomatic epilepsies**).

Treatment

Treatment is generally **supportive to ensure fluid, electrolyte and nutritional requirements are met**.

Symptomatic anti-epileptic drug therapy should be instituted in cats with seizures (see Likely symptomatic epilepsy, page 802).

Glucocorticosteroids such as dexamethasone (0.25 mg/kg q 24 h to be decreased over a few weeks to months) may be beneficial in immune-mediated cases, but could be deleterious if a pathogenic virus is involved.

Prognosis

The prognosis is often excellent as signs resolve spontaneously over weeks or months. Sometimes it is poor because of progressive deterioration leading to death or euthanasia.

FELINE ISCHEMIC ENCEPHALOPATHY***

> ### Classical signs
>
> - Peracute onset unilateral forebrain signs (mental depression/confusion, compulsive circling, hemiparesis) ± seizures.
> - Personality changes and/or post-ischemic epilepsy several months later.

Pathogenesis

An **ischemic cerebral infarction** typically occurs in the parietal-temporal field of one cerebral hemisphere which controls contralateral sensorial (proprioceptive, nociceptive) and motor function as well as behavior. Secondary edema and necrosis lead to atrophy and gliosis.

- The lesion is usually unilateral, although it can be bilateral but markedly asymmetrical.
- A vasospasm phenomenon of the middle cerebral artery is suspected but its pathogenesis remains unknown. Cuterebra larval migration has been incriminated as a cause.

Young adults to middle-aged cats are usually affected.

Clinical signs

The **classical form** of the disease is seen with large ischemic lesions that may involve up to two thirds of an hemisphere.

Typically, there is **peracute onset of severe and uni-lateral forebrain signs** usually including mental depression, pacing, circling, hemiparesis, and deficits in the menace response, facial sensation and postural reactions.

- Rarely, seizures occur and may initially be difficult to control (e.g. cluster seizures or status epilepticus).
- **Rapid neurological improvement** occurs in the first 24–72 hours. Good recovery and **minimal residual signs and deficits** occur within a few weeks in most cases.
  - Rare complications that lead to neurological deterioration in the first 24 hours and sometimes to death or euthanasia include hemorrhage, increased intracranial pressure, tentorial herniation and intractable seizures.
  - **Personality changes, especially a more or less affectionate behavior** and tolerant attitude towards other animals, or for grooming, nail cliping, etc., may become apparent as the initial signs resolve.
  - Persistent seizures or delayed onset of post-ischemic secondary epilepsy may occur, but appear to be unusual.

The atypical form of the disease is caused by small and superficial ischemic lesions that often do not cause any clinical signs at the time of the infarction.

- A few **seizures** and/or **personality changes** may however occur.
- **Delayed onset post-ischemic secondary epilepsy** may be the only clinical manifestation. This may be a common cause of seizure disorders in cats.
  - The seizures are usually of low to moderate frequency initially and subsequently.
- No or only subtle unilateral or occasionally asymmetric bilateral **thalamocortical deficits** may be detected in these cats.

Diagnosis

CSF analysis may be normal or reveal mild non-specific degenerative changes (**increased proportion**

of large foamy mononuclear cells) that may persist for several months after the infarction.

Brain imaging (MRI is optimal) is the only means of antemortem diagnosis. It typically reveals the lesion in the parietal-temporal field of one cerebral hemisphere. A similar but much milder lesion may be seen in the other hemisphere.

Differential diagnosis

The typical form of the disease must be differentiated from the following:

- **Cerebrovascular accidents** are rare in cats and older animals are at greater risk. They may be associated with hypertension due to renal insufficiency, hyperthyroidism or blood hyperviscosity due to polycythemia vera.
- **Head trauma** is differentiated by the history and external signs of trauma to the head and face area.
- **Sudden decompensation or hemorrhage associated with a cerebral tumor** is usually seen in older cats with other preceding neurological signs, especially mentation and behavioral changes. A progressive rather than a regressive course would be expected afterwards.
- **Acute and severe encephalitides** (infectious and non-infectious) are more likely to produce initially progressive multifocal or diffuse signs.

In cats with the atypical form of ischemic encephalopathy with personality changes or seizures as the only sign, **behavioral disorders** and other **intracranial causes of seizures** such as idiopathic epilepsy, active brain diseases must be investigated.

Treatment

Treatment is symptomatic.

- To reduce cerebral edema and intracranial pressure in the typical form of ischemic encephalopathy, give:
  - **Glucocorticosteroids** (methylprednisolone sodium succinate [SoluMedrol®] 30 mg/kg IV or dexamethasone phosphate 0.25 mg/kg IV).
  - **Furosemide** (0.5–2.0 mg/kg IV) may be preferred to or combined with glucocorticosteroids when neurological signs are mild (mental depression/confusion, miotic pupils).

  - **Mannitol** 25% (0.5–2.0 g/kg slow IV over 20–30 minutes) may be **indicated in severe cases** (semi-stupor, pinpoint pupils).
- To control seizures, give anti-epileptic drugs (see Likely symptomatic epilepsy, page 802).

Prognosis

The prognosis is **excellent** in most cases.

- **Persistent personality changes** are usually mild, but rarely they may make the animal unsuitable as a pet, for example severe aggression.
- **Post-ischemic epilepsy** is usually well controlled with adequate anti-epileptic drug therapy.

Recurrences of infarction are not reported to occur.

CONGENITAL AND INHERITED FOREBRAIN ANOMALIES***

Classical signs

- Focal or diffuse forebrain signs (mentation depression and confusion, central visual deficits with normal pupillary light reflexes, proprioceptive positioning and hopping deficits).
- Abnormal development and behavior.
- Occasionally, seizures.

Pathogenesis

Congenital hydrocephalus is uncommon and rarely symptomatic in cats. It may be primary (e.g. inherited) or secondary, for example obstructive and/or compensatory following fetal encephalitis. Signs are diffuse and mainly due to a lack of formation or loss of cerebral tissue, although intracranial pressure elevation may sometimes contribute to the signs.

Lysosomal storage diseases are inherited, progressive and lethal multisystemic degenerative disorders that often involve the CNS of young to adolescent kittens under 1 year of age. Initial signs are often attributable to cerebellar dysfunction.

Lissencephaly-pachygyria is due to an abnormal migration of cerebrocortical neurons. It usually causes learning disabilities, sometimes with behavioral abnormalities and seizures.

Dermoid cysts and other tumors of embryonic origin, for example teratomas and germ cell tumors, produce progressive focal forebrain signs that often become complicated by an increased intracranial pressure and/or secondary obstructive hydrocephalus.

Likely symptomatic **epilepsy** may be the only neurological sign in cats with small focal and inactive brain lesions (e.g. cysts, cortical dysplasia) (see Likely symptomatic epilepsy, page 801).

Clinical signs

Forebrain signs including mentation abnormalities, compulsive pacing or circling, central visual deficits with normal pupillary light reflexes and hemiparesis are present since birth, young kittenhood or early adult life. Neurological deficits and signs can be focal or diffuse, and static or progressive, depending on the underlying pathological process.

- Extensive or diffuse forebrain anomalies such as hydrocephalus or lissencephaly-pachygyria may manifest with **retarded development, learning disability**, loss of training, mental depression, abnormal behavior and visual deficits.
  - Severe hydrocephalus may also cause gait abnormalities as a result of cerebellar and brainstem distortion, as well as pacing and head pressing, especially when the intracranial pressure is elevated.

Symptomatic seizures may occasionally occur but usually are preceded by other signs of the anomaly (e.g. of hydrocephalus, tumors of embryonic origin, lysosomal storage diseases, lissencephaly-pachygyria).

Likely symptomatic **epilepsy** may occur. Seizures typically are initially of low frequency and are partial in origin, but can secondarily generalize to tonic-clonic seizures (see Secondary epilepsy, page 800).

Diagnosis

Facial and head deformities may be apparent with hydrocephalus, for example a domed calvaria with open suture lines and fontanelles.

CSF analysis is likely to be normal or only reveal mild non-specific degenerative changes.

Brain MRI will often show the underlying anomaly, for example porencephalic lesions.

Other specific tests, for example, ultrasonography through open fontanelles for hydrocephalus, enzymatic assays and biopsies of peripheral nerves or other organs for some lysosomal storage diseases, are useful for obtaining a definitive diagnosis.

Differential diagnosis

Acquired forebrain diseases affecting young cats such as FIP and non-suppurative meningoencephalitis usually have a subacute onset and a rapidly progressive (or regressive) clinical course.

Hepatoencephalopathy due to portosystemic shunting would be distinguished by its episodic nature.

Treatment

Anti-epileptic drug therapy should be instituted for likely symptomatic epilepsy (see Likely symptomatic epilepsy, page 802).

Symptomatic medical treatment including glucocorticosteroids and surgical shunting for hydrocephalus is poorly documented in cats.

Lysosomal storage diseases are currently untreatable.

Prognosis

Prognosis is usually guarded to poor, with the exception of secondary epilepsy, which may be successfully controlled with anti-epileptic drugs.

HEPATIC ENCEPHALOPATHY***

> **Classical signs**
>
> - Episodes of hypersalivation, abnormal mentation and bizarre behavior.

Pathogenesis

Hepatic encephalopathy results when endogenous toxins produced by the action of the gut microflora on alimentary proteins are not removed from the systemic circulation by the liver. When a critical toxin level is reached, diffuse cerebral dysfunction ensues.

Hepatic encephalopathy is **most often due to a congenital portosystemic vascular shunt** and signs are usually noticed during the first year of life.

Severe acquired liver diseases also very occasionally cause hepatic encephalopathy in cats of any age. Other signs of liver disease will usually predominate including anorexia, weight loss and sometimes jaundice.

Clinical signs

Neurological signs are episodic. They develop then regress progressively over periods of a few to several hours.

- **Episodes may be precipitated by feeding**, especially when a high-protein diet is ingested in large amounts. Several (up to 8–10) hours may however elapse between meal times and onset of signs. Signs do not follow each meal, especially early in the course of the disease. Several days and sometimes a few weeks may elapse between episodes.

Neurological signs are of diffuse thalamocortical dysfunction:

- **Mentation abnormalities** include depression, confusion, staring into space.
- **Bizarre behavioral activities** may occur, for example pacing, head pressing, dementia with running fits, frantic vocalization and aggression.
- **Profuse salivation** is common. This may last for several minutes to hours and may be the first and only sign early in the course of the disease.
- Fine generalized muscle tremors (shivering).
- **Central blindness** and ultimately stupor and coma may develop in the advanced stage of hepatic encephalopathy.
- Episodes of dementia with frantic behavioral activities such as running fits, attacking inanimate objects and profuse salivation sometimes are misinterpreted as being seizure activity. **True seizures are rare** and usually occur as clustered seizures after the other classical and severe signs of hepatic encephalopathy have developed.

Systemic signs may include polyuria, polydipsia, vomiting, diarrhea, dysuria with hematuria (due to urate calculi) and delayed anesthetic recovery.

- Cats with congenital portosystemic shunts may be thin and small for their age.

Other physical and laboratory signs of liver failure will be obvious in cats with severe liver pathology.

Diagnosis

Pre- and post-prandial bile acids are usually markedly increased.

Laboratory abnormalities may include microcytic non-regenerative anemia, low albumin, urea and cholesterol concentrations, and urinary ammonium biurate crystals.

Fasting blood ammonia is markedly elevated in most (90%) cats with a portosystemic vascular shunt, especially during episodes of hepatoencephalopathy. This test is however inconvenient in most practices because blood samples must be drawn in cold heparinized tubes and immediately transported to an appropriate laboratory on ice for refrigerated centrifugation and assay, preferably within an hour of collection. False blood ammonia values may occur with hemolysis, prolonged venous occlusion and struggling at the time of venipuncture.

- An **ammonia tolerance test** identifies virtually all cats with a portosystemic vascular shunt but may precipitate severe signs of hepatoencephalopathy. Cats with a shunt have a blood ammonia concentration 30 minutes post-challenge that is > three times higher than the fasting values.

Abdominal radiographs may show a small liver in cats with congenital portosystemic shunt.

Abdominal echography may allow visualization of a congenital portosystemic shunt or may detect diffuse liver disease.

Differential diagnosis

Cats presented for bouts of hypersalivation are often erroneously diagnosed with a **stomatitis,** even though they may have no oral lesions. **Ingestion of irritant substances or plants** is another common misdiagnosis.

Some intoxications may produce signs similar to those of hepatic encephalopathy including depression or agitation, but are not recurrent unless re-exposure to the toxin occurs.

Treatment

Medical treatment is aimed at reducing the production and absorption of endogenous colonic toxins. Maintenance therapy includes a low-protein diet (e.g.

Prescription Diet feline k/d, Hill's Pet Nutrition), with added carnitine, taurine and arginine, antibiotics (e.g. metronidazole 7.5 mg/kg PO q 12 h, or neomycin 22 mg/kg PO q 8–12 h, or amoxicillin 22 mg/kg PO q 12 h) and lactulose (0.25–0.5 ml/kg PO q 8–12 h). See page 821, The Cat With Stupor or Coma, for further details.

Surgical treatment including ligation or use of an occlusive device offers the best chance for long-term control of clinical signs. This must be performed by an experienced surgeon to decrease the risk of excessive ligation which may cause rapid post-operative death due to portal hypertension and bowel ischemia. Like in dogs, severe seizures may develop in the first few post-operative days, and some cats have remained epileptic for months and years afterwards.

Prognosis

Prognosis is good if surgical treatment is feasible, for example with a single extrahepatic shunt, and is not complicated by portal hypertension. Recurrence of signs appears to be more common in cats than in dogs and occurs in more than 40–50% after a few years. It may be due to the persistence of shunting through a partially ligated vessel or the development of multiple secondary shunts because of chronic portal hypertension.

Prognosis is guarded with medical treatment as the condition often worsens over time.

THIAMINE DEFICIENCY***

Classical signs

- Inappetence, depression, intermittent vomiting.
- Central vestibular signs (reluctance to walk, nystagmus, loss of balance).
- Mydriasis with poor pupillary light reflexes.
- Spasmodic ventroflexion of the neck or opisthotonos.

See main references on page 848 (The Cat With Head Tilt, Vestibular Ataxia or Nystagmus) and page 899 (The Cat With Neck Ventroflexion).

Clinical signs

History of feeding all-fish diets (containing thiaminase), diets consisting of **entirely cooked meat** (thiamine destruction by heating), poor-quality, thiamine-deficient commercial diets, commercial food stored for long periods of time or in excessively hot conditions or, **pet meat preserved with sulfur dioxide** which destroys thiamine.

Depression and inappetence are initial signs. Later **mydriasis** with poor pupillary light response, but usually without blindness and **central vestibular dysfunction** occur with head tilt, loss of balance, spastic gait and tremors. Terminally, semicoma, crying, opisthotonos with limb spasticity and death result.

True seizures are uncommon and must be differentiated from periods of opisthotonic posturing with paddling, and from the spasmodic ventroflexion of the neck and body contorsions that may be induced when the cat is picked from the ground. These are likely due to marked spatial disorientation because of the bilateral vestibular dysfunction.

Diagnosis

Diagnosis is based on a **history of dietary deficiency and response to thiamine supplementation** (10–20 mg thiamine IM q 8– 12 h, then orally).

CEREBROVASCULAR ACCIDENTS**

Classical signs

- Peracute and rapidly resolving cerebral signs.

Pathogenesis

Cerebrovascular accidents are rare in cats.

Vascular events result in acute ischemic lesions. Vascular events include spontaneous hemorrhage from coagulopathies, thrombocytopenia and hypertension associated with chronic renal failure and hyperthyroidism. They also include thrombosis (e.g. polycythemia hyperviscosity syndrome) and embolization including septic and metastatic from rapidly growing cell type tumors.

Clinical signs

Peracute onset of non-progressive and rapidly regressive focal cerebral signs, including seizures alone or with other signs.

- Slight deterioration may occur over the first 24 hours as a result of edema or increased intracranial pressure before the condition improves. A rapidly progressive course is expected with septic and metastatic embolization.

Diagnosis

Diagnosis is based on a clinical course suggestive of a vascular event, that is, a peracute, onset of signs that improve rapidly.

Neurological signs and deficits are attributable to a focal CNS lesion. Multifocal lesions are however possible, for example, hemorrhage due to coagulation disorders or thrombocytopenia, or multiple metastasis.

Evidence of historical, clinical, laboratory and imaging findings related to the underlying cause such as polycythemia, hypertensive retinal changes, hyperthyroidism, abdominal tumor increase the index of suspicion when neurological findings are consistent with a vascular accident.

Differential diagnosis

The classical form of the feline ischemic encephalopathy is a cerebrovascular accident that occurs in young adult to middle-aged healthy cats.

Acutely decompensated brain tumor as occurs following spontaneous hemorrhage, or tentorial herniation may appear clinically similar.

Treatment

Treatment is specific if the cause is known and treatable.

Supportive and symptomatic therapy is indicated to control secondary brain edema and increased intracranial pressure (see Feline ischemic encephalopathy, page 805 and Head trauma, page 818).

Prognosis

The prognosis **depends on the severity** of the neurological signs and the underlying cause and whether it is treatable or not.

Recurrences may occur if the underlying cause persists (e.g. hypertension). The lesion localization is however likely to be different from one event to another.

Post-ischemic gliosis may result in **epilepsy**.

HYPOGLYCEMIA**

> ### Classical signs
>
> - Mental alteration, weakness, ataxia, visual loss.
> - Seizures.

PATHOGENESIS

Because blood glucose is the primary energy source for the CNS, hypoglycemia causes **diffuse CNS dysfunction**. The nature and severity of the neurological signs depend on the rate of blood glucose decrease, level of glucose attained and duration of hypoglycemia.

Severe and symptomatic hypoglycemia is rare in cats except as a result of insulin over-dosage in diabetic cats. Rarely reported causes include insulin-secreting tumors, other tumors secreting insulin-like growth factor (IGF), sepsis and terminal hepatic disease.

Clinical signs

Signs may be episodic or persistent and include mentation abnormalities (e.g. depression, confusion, stupor), weakness, ataxia, central visual impairment and generalized seizures. Nervousness, muscle fasciculations and tremors may also occur.

- Seizures more often occur when there is a sudden and marked decrease in the glucose concentration, and are usually preceded by other more subtle signs of hypoglycemia such as confusion and weakness.

Severe and sustained hypoglycemia may cause diffuse cerebral anoxic injuries resulting in stupor-coma, decerebrate rigidity and miotic pupils. This may progress to irreversible damage (cortical necrosis) and permanent neurological sequela including blindness and secondary epilepsy.

Diagnosis

Serum glucose concentration is usually < 2.2 mmol/L (40 mg/dl).

Other historical, clinical and laboratory abnormalities may be evident, depending on the underlying cause.

More commonly, there is a history of diabetes mellitus treated with insulin or hypoglycemic drugs.

Differential diagnosis

Other episodic or peracute conditions such as metabolic disturbances, intoxications and encephalomyelitis should be considered depending on the clinical presentation.

Treatment

Treatment involves glucose administration (food, sugar water, corn syrup or dextrose 50% IV [1/2–4 ml/kg], according to the severity of hypoglycemic signs) and specific treatment of the underlying cause. See page 956 (The Cat With Generalized Weakness) and page 832 (The Cat With Stupor or Coma).

Diabetic cats need re-evaluation of their treatment regime. Some cats presenting with hypoglycemia are in diabetic remission and do not require further insulin or oral treatment.

Prognosis

Prognosis is good unless the underlying cause is associated with a poor prognosis (e.g. neoplasia) or significant structural cerebral damage has occurred.

FOREBRAIN TUMORS**

> **Classical signs**
>
> - Progressive forebrain signs (personality changes, circling, pacing) in middle-aged and older cats.
> - Seizures.

PATHOGENESIS

Forebrain neoplasms cause **progressive focal neurological signs**, the nature and severity of which depend on the tumor location and growth rate.

- **Meningiomas are the most common.** Other brain tumors of cats include gliomas, pituitary tumors, extension of nasal cavity and paranasal sinus neoplasms and metastatic brain tumors.

Clinical signs

Initial signs often include subtle personality and behavioral changes, mental depression, pacing and circling.

Seizures may manifest as the first and only sign, occur concurrently with other signs or develop later. The initial seizure frequency is variable but is inevitably progressive.

Focal signs such as contralateral hemiparesis with postural reaction deficits, **visual loss** and **decreased facial sensation** are often detected upon examination.

Tumors complicated with obstructive hydrocephalus and **increased intracranial pressure** cause more diffuse signs (e.g. **profound depression, bilateral miosis**). This may also lead to tentorial herniation which **often develops slowly and remains asymptomatic until an acute decompensation** is triggered by further tumor growth, spontaneous hemorrhage in or around the tumor, concomitant disease or stress, anesthesia and CSF collection.

- **Tentorial herniation** resulting in brainstem compression produces **coma, unresponsive mydriasis, abnormal respiratory patterns** and death from respiratory arrest.

Diagnosis

Skull radiographs are likely to be unrewarding except for some **meningiomas** which may result in thinning or thickening of the adjacent calvaria and increased density of adjacent soft tissue, and **neoplasms of the nasal cavity and paranasal sinus** which produce soft tissue density, osteolysis and bone proliferation.

CSF analysis may reveal mild to moderate increase of the protein concentration and/or pleocytosis (elevated leukocyte count); **CSF may be normal** with small and deeply seated tumors.

- **CSF collection is contraindicated in cats with signs of increased intracranial pressure** (marked mental depression, inappropriate miosis) because it may cause or exacerbate a tentorial herniation leading to death.

Brain imaging is essential to confirm the diagnosis and to localize the tumor when surgical or radiation therapy is considered.

Differential diagnosis

Other focal and slowly progressive brain diseases are uncommon in cats (e.g. **toxoplasma granuloma, cerebral abscess**).

Multiples tumors (e.g. meningiomas, metastases) may cause multifocal signs and must be differentiated from **encephalitides**.

Treatment

Surgical excision may be possible if the tumor is surgically accessible. Meningiomas on the dorsal surface of the cerebral hemispheres can be successfully removed.

Radiation therapy is a useful adjunct to surgical debulking, or can be used alone when surgical excision is not possible.

Chemotherapy is poorly documented for brain tumors of cats. Lomustine (a nitrosourea) has been safely used in the cat.

Palliative medical treatment using dexamethasone (0.12–0.25 mg/kg q 24–48 h) to decrease peritumoral edema.

Symptomatic anti-epileptic drug therapy should be instituted in cats with seizures (see Secondary epilepsy, page 801).

Prognosis

Long-term prognosis is poor except for convexity meningiomas (located on the dorsal surface of the cerebral hemispheres), which can often be completely excised with good survival, rapid recovery and low incidence of recurrence.

FELINE INFECTIOUS PERITONITIS**

> ### Classical signs
>
> - Multifocal CNS signs (head tilt, nystagmus, intentional tremors, ataxia, paresis).
> - Systemic signs (fever, lethargy, inappetence, weight loss) +/− ocular signs.

See main references on page 844 (The Cat With Head Tilt, Vestibular Ataxia or Nystagmus) and page 352 (The Thin, Inappetent Cat).

Clinical signs

FIP causes multifocal or focal neurological signs attributable to any portion of the CNS. **Central vestibular signs** (head tilt, balance losses, nystagmus, mental depression, postural reaction deficits) are the most common and are often accompanied by **cerebellar signs** (intentional tremors, hypermetria).
- Seizures are unusual and do not occur as the only sign.

Affected cats usually have **other clinical and laboratory evidence of systemic involvement** (e.g. lethargy, inappetence, weight loss, fever, anemia, renal and hepatic signs).

Ocular signs are also common (e.g. chorioretinitis, anterior uveitis).

Typically, there is an insidious onset and a slowly progressive course over weeks.

Usually, **cats are less than 3 years old** and were obtained from a **large multiple-cat household, breeder** or **pet store**.

Diagnosis

CSF analysis is the most useful test when there are CNS signs; typically, there is a marked increase of the protein concentration (> 1 g/L; 100 mg/dl and often > 2 g/L; 200 mg/dl) and leukocyte count (> 100 cells/µl) with a large proportion of non-lytic neutrophils.

Serological testing has been of little diagnostic value except that a negative test suggests the disease is unlikely to be FIP. However, negative test results do occur rarely in cats with FIP, especially in the terminal stages.

The ELISA that detects antibody to the 7B protein, which is specific to the coronavirus strains causing FIP has not been shown to improve accuracy of diagnosis in clinical practice. Newer PCR methods may be useful.

Differential diagnosis

Other infectious and non-infectious encephalitides, for example non-suppurative meningoencephalitis and toxoplasmosis need to be differentiated from FIP. CSF analysis may help to differentiate theses diseases.

Treatment

No treatment is effective once neurological signs are present. Glucocorticosteroid may temporarily improve the neurological signs.

CRYPTOCOCCOSIS**

Classical signs

- Chronic nasal discharge, often with nasal distortion.
- Cutaneous lesions – nodules or ulcers.
- Occasionally, ocular and CNS signs.

See main reference on page 19 for details (The Cat With Signs of Chronic Nasal Disease).

Pathogenesis

Infection is by inhalation of the organism contained in high concentration in soil contaminated by **pigeon droppings** or **eucalyptus tree debris**.

CNS infection occurs by direct extension through the cribriform plate or by hematogenous spread. A diffuse or focal granulomatous meningoencephalitis results.

Clinical signs

CNS signs can occur alone or with other signs (e.g. rhinitis, cutaneous lesions) and are usually rapidly progressive.

- Most commonly, cats exhibit **cerebral signs such as mental depression, behavioral changes**, circling, head pressing and ataxia; **seizures** may occur with forebrain involvement but are unlikely to be the only sign.
- Blindness with dilated and unresponsive pupils may occur due to optic neuritis.

Ocular signs including chorioretinitis, panophthalmitis, and retinal detachment are often associated with CNS involvement.

Diagnosis

CSF analysis may reveal mild to marked inflammatory changes, often with numerous cryptococcal organisms.

Serology from blood, CSF, aqueous humor and urine is highly specific and sensitive.

Identification of the organism may be made by cytology, histology or culture of various body fluids and tissues including CSF, nasal discharge and polyp-like masses, skin lesions, enlarged lymph nodes.

Differential diagnosis

Other infectious encephalitides such as FIP and toxoplasmosis need to be differentiated from cryptococcosis. With cryptococcosis the organism is usually evident in CSF, although occasionally culture may be required to demonstrate it.

Treatment

Fluconazole (2.5–10 mg/kg PO q 12 h) is best for CNS infections, or itraconazole (5 mg/kg PO q 12 h). See main reference on page 26 for treatment details.

Prognosis

The prognosis is guarded once CNS involvement occurs.

INTOXICATIONS**

Classical signs

- Signs of CNS, autonomic or neuromuscular stimulation or depression.
- Rarely and terminally, convulsive status epilepticus.

Pathogenesis

Signs of intoxications usually occur shortly after acute and accidental ingestion or topical contact. Cats' selective eating behavior is protective but their grooming habits may increase exposure.

Most intoxicants cause functional disturbances for example conduction failure or neurotransmitter imbalance in various portions of the nervous system, although others cause structural damage.

Intoxicants that may cause seizures include the following:

- **Pyrethrins and pyrethroids** (e.g. fenvalerate, allethrin, tetramethrin, deltamethrin). Signs of intoxication usually occur a few minutes to hours after excessive topical application of anti-flea and tick sprays, powders, foam, dips and shampoos.
- **Organochlorines** are used for pest control (e.g. lindane, methoxychlor, endosulfan, DDT, aldrin, chlordane, dieldrin, heptachlor, dicofol, endrin, perthane, toxaphen) and may contaminate water or food, or be absorbed through the skin and the mucous membranes.
- **Organophosphates** (e.g. dichlorvos, malathion, chlorpyrifos, fenthion, parathion, phoxime, cythioate, diazinon, safrotin, phosmet, tetrachlorvinphos, diazinon) **and carbamates** (e.g. propoxur, carbaryl, bendiocarb, chlorprophane, buphame methomyl) are insecticides used in various formulations to control fleas, ticks and mites on pets, in the house and yard, on crops, stored grains, soils, and have also been used as fly, ant and roach baits. Intoxication occurs by ingestion, dermal exposure and after inhalation.
- **Bromethalin** is a non-anticoagulant rodenticide available in bait form. Secondary intoxication due to the ingestion of bromethalin-poisoned rodents may occur.
- **Strychnine** is a rodenticide marketed as pellets or treated seeds.
- **Methaldehyde** is a molluscicide often mixed with bran flakes or pellets.
- **Lead** is ingested in old paint flakes or paint dust from sanding, linoleums, roofing materials, plaster board, putty, artist paint, lead objects (drapery and fishing weights, sinkers, bullets), used motor oils from leaded gasoline-burning engines, greases leaded gazoline, eating or drinking from improperly glazed bowls.
- **Other intoxicants potentially dangerous for cats** include penitrem mycotoxins (produced in spoiled dairy products such as cottage cheese), nicotine (gum and skin patches), caffeine, chocolate (theobromine) and illicit drugs (e.g. cocaine).

Clinical signs

Most intoxications are **acute** and produce **diffuse and rapidly progressive neurological signs**. These may be accompanied by signs of stimulation of other body systems, for example gastrointestinal with vomiting and/or diarrhea.

- **Neurological signs vary according to the intoxicant** and include various combinations of **CNS signs** (e.g. mental depression to coma, hyperexcitability, tremors, ataxia, paresis), **autonomic signs** (e.g. hypersalivation, miosis, diarrhea) and **neuromuscular signs** (e.g. muscle fasciculations-tremors, LMN signs).
- **True seizures are less common** than generally believed and must be differentiated from other seizure-like features of poisoning such as tremors, tetany or hysterical behavior. Seizures usually manifest as convulsive status epilepticus that continues until treatment is provided or until death ensues.
  - **Pyrethrins and pyrethroids** intoxications are usually mild and resolve in most cases within 24–72 hours. **Signs include depression, salivation**, anorexia, vomiting, muscle tremors (ear flicking, contractions of the cutaneous muscles, paw shaking), hyperexcitability or hyperactivity, disorientation, weakness, ataxia, dyspnea and rarely, seizures and death.
  - **Organochlorines** produce progressive or explosive onset of hyperesthesia, nervousness, agitation, hyperexcitability, salivation, vomiting, tremors, ataxia, nystagmus, blindness, opisthotonos, convulsive seizures, depression, coma and death.
  - **Organophosphates and carbamates** inactivate acetylcholinesterase resulting in excessive activity and fatigue of cholinergic end-organs and muscles. This includes **muscarinic signs** (miosis, bradycardia, vomiting, diarrhea, hypersalivation, lacrimation, dyspnea due to excessive bronchosecretions and bronchoconstriction, anorexia), **nicotinic signs** (muscle tremors, weakness), as well as **CNS signs** depression, behavioral changes, ataxia, hyperactivity, seizures).
  - **Strychnine** toxicity results in anxiousness and nervousness, extreme sensitivity to external stimuli (e.g. noise, bright light), muscle tremors, intermittent then sustained extensor rigidity with opisthotonos and tetany (pseudo-convulsions), hyperthermia and death by respiratory apnea and hypoxia.
  - **Methaldehyde** causes anxiety, restlessness, ataxia, tremors, salivation, vomiting, diarrhea, mydriasis, nystagmus, opisthotonos, tetanic convulsions, hyperthermia and death from respiratory muscle spastic paralysis.

- **Lead** poisoning induces gastrointestinal (anorexia, vomiting, diarrhea, constipation), renal (polyuria, polydipsia) and neurological (depression, central blindness, hyperexcitability, running fits, seizures, vocalization, ataxia, head pressing, opisthotonos, paraparesis) signs. Megaesophagus with regurgitation and pharyngeal/laryngeal paresis has been observed with chronic lead poisoning in cats.
- **Bromethalin** acute toxicity causes tremors, hyperexcitability, hyperesthesia, depression, fever, anisocoria, positional nystagmus, extensor rigidity, opisthotonos and seizures (running fits and generalized). Death may sometimes be delayed up to 2–3 weeks in cats. Chronic intoxication with lower dosages causes occasional vomiting, ascending paresis and ataxia with proprioceptive deficits, depressed spinal reflexes (patellar and withdrawal), tremors, depression and lateral recumbency. Recovery is possible after exposure is discontinued.
- Penitrem mycotoxins.

Diagnosis

Diagnosis is based on a **history of exposure** to a toxin capable of producing the observed signs within the documented time for exposure.

Toxicologic analysis may be diagnostic when performed on the following:
- **Tissues** (e.g. liver, kidney, fat, brain) for organochlorines, organophosphates, strychnine, lead, etc.
- **Vomitus and stomach content** (for bromethalin, strychnine, methaldehyde).
- **Urine** (for strychnine).
- **Blood** for lead concentration and acethylcholinesterase activity (organophosphate poisoning).

Toxicity as a cause of seizures can be excluded when (a) there are no other diffuse neurological signs preceding the seizure onset (e.g. tremors, hyperexcitability), (b) when partial seizures occur, (c) when isolated seizures are interspersed with periods of normalcy, or (d) when focal neurological signs or deficits are present.

Differential diagnosis

Metabolic disturbances that are severe enough to cause obvious neurological signs including seizures in cats are rare. Hypoglycemia is typically associated with insulin overdose in a diabetic patient, hypocalcemia is mainly seen after bilateral thyroidectomy, and hepatoencephalopathy causes episodic signs, which rarely occur in intoxications.

Inflammatory conditions (e.g. encephalitides, polyneuropathies) need to be ruled out. Usually history and physical examination findings differentiate these from intoxications.

Treatment

With dermal exposure it is important to bath the cat with soap or detergent to remove the toxin from the hair and skin. Intoxication with anti-flea and -tick sprays, dips, and aerosols containing insecticides such as pyrethrins, carbamates, organophosphates often occurs via dermal exposure.

When ingestion has occurred within the previous 2 hours, emesis may be indicated or contraindicated, according to the specific toxin and formulation that was ingested. Emesis may be induced with hydrogen peroxide 3% (2 ml/kg PO) or apomorphine (0.03–0.04 mg IV or 0.04–0.08 mg/kg IM). **Gastric lavage** performed under general anesthesia may be beneficial if emesis is not effective. Enemas also may be useful. **Activated charcoal** (0.1–1.0 mg/kg q 8–12 h) preferably administered with a cathartic such as magnesium sulfate (250 mg/kg) or 70% sorbitol (3 ml/kg) is also indicated to reduce gastrointestinal absorption.

Atropine sulfate (0.02–0.04 mg/kg IM or SC) will decrease salivation and muscarinic signs associated with organophosphate and other poisoning, but because of the risk of fatal bronchospasm it is only recommended if marked bradycardia is present.

Pralidoxime chloride (2-PAM, Protopam chloride) is useful to reactivate cholinesterase (10–15 mg/kg IM or SC q 8–12 h) and control nicotinic signs of organophosphate poisoning. It is most effective if exposure was within the previous 24–48 hours, if exposure was by the dermal route and if a slowly eliminated compound was involved (e.g. fenthion, chlorpyrifos).

Diphenhydramine also has antinicotinic activity.

Chelation therapy (e.g. calcium EDTA and/or penicillamine) is indicated for lead poisoning.

Treat cerebral edema (e.g. bromethalin, lead) with mannitol and/or glucorticosteroids, and control seizures or pseudo-seizures with diazepam, phenobarbital, propofol and pentobarbital. See page 801 (Likely symptomatic epilepsy) for treatment details.

Provide supportive care including fluids, which also promote excretion of the toxin.

Prognosis

Prognosis is variable and depends on the severity of the signs and time between intoxication and treatment.

TOXOPLASMOSIS**

Classical signs

- Pneumonia, hepatitis, pancreatitis, myositis.
- Often, uveitis or chorioretinitis.
- Occasionally, focal or multifocal neurological signs.

See main reference on page 705 for details (The Cat With Signs of Acute Small Bowel Diarrhea).

Pathogenesis

Toxoplasma gondii is an opportunistic pathogen. Although subclinical infection is common in cats, **clinical disease rarely develops**.

- Clinical toxoplasmosis causing neurological signs in adult cats is believed to be mainly associated with concurrent stress, illness or immunosuppression that **reactivate a latent infection acquired at a young age by carnivorism associated with hunting.**

Toxoplasma gondii **causes a non-suppurative encephalomyelitis** that may be widely scattered throughout the CNS or localized in one area as a granuloma.

Clinical signs

Systemic signs including lethargy, anorexia, fever are most often related to pneumonia, dyspnea, tachypnea. Hepatitis, pancreatitis, myositis and myocarditis may also occur.

The enteroepithelial cycle with oocyst shedding almost exclusively occurs in young weanling kittens and rarely results in gastrointestinal signs.

Sudden death associated with acute *Toxoplasma* encephalitis may occur in approximately 30% of kittens infected at 6–12 weeks of age.

Ocular signs such as anterior uveitis and chorioretinitis are also common.

Neurological signs manifest rarely even though the organism is frequently found in the CNS.

- Acute to subacute multifocal or focal cerebral signs are more common. Seizures are unlikely to occur as the only sign.

Diagnosis

The antemortem diagnosis of clinical toxoplasmosis is difficult; it relies on serological demonstration of previous exposure and perhaps of recent or active infection, exclusion of other causes, and positive response to treatment.

CSF analysis may reveal a **mild to moderate increase of the protein concentration** (< 1.0 g/L) with normal or only slightly elevated leukocyte count (<50/μl). Organisms are only rarely seen on cytologic examination of CSF and other body fluids.

Demonstration of the organism in tissue biopsy sections will confirm the diagnosis only if inflammation is present.

Fecal examination is likely to be unrewarding because of the short period of oocyst shedding that occurs for only a few weeks after infection.

Serologic testing often cannot distinguish latent asymptomatic from active clinical infection. A positive IgM titer or a 4-fold increase in IgA or IgG titer suggests recent infection. However, in some cats, IgM titers remain positive for months to years after infection, and 20% of cats may not develop IgM titers. IgG titers may take 4–6 weeks to develop and high IgG titers (> 30 000) are commonly detected 6 years after infection. Positive titers occur in 30–60% of cats. Many adult cats with neurological signs are believed to have reactivation of a latent infection, rather than a newly acquired infection, which is typically detected by a positive 1 IgM titer or rising IgG titer.

Differential diagnosis

Other infectious and non-infectious causes of encephalomyelitis including FIP and non-suppurative meningoencephalitis should be considered.

Treatment

Clindamycin 12.5 mg/kg PO q 12 h doses for a minimum of 4 weeks.

Clarithromycin (7.5 mg/kg PO q 12 h) and **azithromycin** (7–15 mg/kg q 12 h) are newer macrolides which may be useful.

Prognosis

Prognosis is guarded with CNS involvement. Clinical signs of systemic illness usually begin to resolve within 24–48 h of beginning therapy but neurological signs may take weeks to improve and major neurological abnormalities may remain. Response may be poor, slow, incomplete, and recurrence may occur.

IDIOPATHIC EPILEPSY*

Classical signs

- Recurrent primary generalized tonic-clonic seizures.
- The initial seizure frequency is low (< 1 single seizure every 6–8 weeks) but may later increase.
- Seizures begin in young adult cats (6 months to 5 years of age) that have no other neurological signs and deficits.

Pathogenesis

This is believed to result from a **diffuse imbalance between neuronal excitatory and inhibitory mechanisms** that has no underlying cause other than a **genetic predisposition**.

Idiopathic epilepsy is rare and poorly documented in cats.

Clinical signs

Recurrent primary generalized tonic-clonic seizures should be the only sign.

- **There is no aura, no localized or unilateral signs** during the ictus and in the post-ictal phase.

The **initial seizure frequency** should be low with isolated single seizures at more than 6–8 week intervals.

- The **subsequent seizure frequency** could remain low or progressively increase, perhaps to the point of intractability, but this should not occur before several months to a few years from the seizure onset.

Onset of seizures should be during adolescence or young adulthood (probably between 6 months and 5 years).

Diagnosis

Diagnosis is by exclusion of other causes.

Physical and ophthalmological examinations should be normal. Abnormal findings would indicate the presence of another pathological process possibly related to the seizure disorder (e.g. fever, chorioretinitis).

Neurological examination should be normal. Other neurological signs or deficits would indicate that an active or inactive structural brain lesion is present.

CSF analysis should be normal. Abnormalities would reveal the presence of an active or a resolving brain disease.

Brain imaging (MRI) should be normal. Any abnormality could be related to the seizure disorder (e.g. active or inactive lesions).

Idiopathic epilepsy should be excluded when there are **partial seizures** (including seizures that appear to be generalized from their onset but that are preceded by an aura or followed by localized post-ictal signs), **a seizure onset before 6 months or after 5 years of age, an initially high seizure frequency, a rapid increase of the seizure frequency** within the first few weeks or months, other neurological signs or deficits, CSF changes or MRI abnormalities.

Differential diagnosis

Extracranial causes of seizures such as metabolic, toxic and hypoxic causes usually produce a sudden onset of high-frequency seizures, often cluster seizures or status epilepticus, and other diffuse neurological and/or systemic signs before and in between the seizures.

Active brain diseases often cause a higher seizure frequency, interictal neurological signs and deficits, and abnormal findings upon CSF analysis or brain imaging.

Likely symptomatic **epilepsy** may sometimes be distinguished from idiopathic epilepsy only by the occurrence of partial seizures and/or the presence of focal neurological deficits because CSF analysis and MRI may also be normal.

Treatment

Symptomatic anti-epileptic drug therapy for life (see Likely symptomatic epilepsy, page 801).

Prognosis

Good seizure control should be obtained in most cases, although some cats can progress toward refractoriness, despite adequate anti-epileptic drug treatment.

HYPOCALCEMIA*

Classical signs

- Muscle fasciculation, especially involving the head and ears.
- Generalized weakness.
- Stiffness, tremors, tetany.
- Rarely, convulsive status epilepticus.
- Vomiting.

See main reference on page 962 for details (The Cat With Generalized Weakness).

Clinical signs

Symptomatic hypocalcemia is rare in cats. It is usually iatrogenic following bilateral thyroidectomy.

Signs are episodic or persistent and include multifocal muscle fasciculations, which often involves the face and ears. This may progress to generalized weakness with stiffness, panting, tremors and tetany. Terminally, convulsive status epilepticus may occur.

Diagnosis

Diagnosis is based on finding a **total serum calcium concentration < 1.6 mmol/L** (6.5 mg/dl) and ionized calcium level < 0.6 mmol/L (2.5 mg/dl).

Other historical, clinical and laboratory abnormalities may reflect the underlying cause, including idiopathic or post-thyroidectomy hypoparathyroidism, puerperal tetany, renal failure and phosphate enema.

Differential diagnosis

Other causes of neuromuscular hyperexcitability such as intoxications should be considered. With organophosphate toxicity, muscarinic signs are usually present (miosis, salivation, vomiting, bradycardia). Fenthion has few muscarinic signs and mainly produces muscle weakness.

Tetany must be differentiated from convulsive status epilepticus of hypocalcemia. The cat with tetany is conscious although it is very anxious.

Treatment

Calcium supplementation and specific treatment of the underlying cause is required.
- Use 0.5–1.5 ml/kg IV of 10% calcium gluconate. Infuse slowly over 10 minutes while monitoring heart rate. Stop if bradycardia develops. See Hypocalcemia, page 962 in "The Cat With Generalized Weakness" for treatment.

HEAD TRAUMA

Classical signs

- Peracute onset of cerebral signs ± seizures.
- Signs of head trauma, including hemorrhage in eyes, ears, nose.
- Delayed onset epilepsy.

Clinical signs

Concussion manifests with immediate and brief (a few seconds to minutes) mental confusion or loss of consciousness. Recovery is rapid and complete with no residual neurological signs as there are no parenchymal lesions.

Contusions and lacerations produce parenchymal lesions and signs that may worsen over the initial 24 hours because of edema and increased intracranial pressure, but improve afterwards.

- **Forebrain signs include mentation abnormalities** such as depression to semi-stupor and confusion, **behavioral manifestations** such as agitation and dementia, **compulsive activities** including restlessness with propulsive pacing and circling. Hemiparesis and central blindness may also occur.

Seizure onset is often with cluster seizures or status epilepticus occurring immediately or within the first 12–24 hours after trauma. These may initially be difficult to control.

Delayed onset post-traumatic epilepsy (see Likely symptomatic epilepsy, page 800) may occur a few to several months later.

Diagnosis

History and external signs of severe head trauma as a result of a road accident, fall from several stories or mistreatment by humans.

Post-traumatic epilepsy should be excluded if there were no serious forebrain signs and deficits at the time of a reported trauma, as well as when the seizure onset occurs more than 2 or 3 years after trauma.

- **Brain imaging** may demonstrate a parenchymal lesion. A skull fracture may or may not be present.

Differential diagnosis

Cerebrovascular accident may also manifest with an acute onset of severe focal cerebral signs but there are no history or external signs of trauma.

Onset of seizures with low to moderate frequency a few to several months after major head trauma has occurred is highly suggestive of post-traumatic epilepsy but other causes of seizures must be ruled-out.

Treatment

Re-establish or maintain adequate cerebral perfusion.

- **First treat hypotension and systemic shock**, if present, by giving **volume replacement fluids**:

  - **Hetastarch** 6%, 10–20 ml/kg to effect, to be given in 5 ml/kg increments over 5–10 minutes to avoid nausea and vomiting,

  OR

  - **Hypertonic saline** (NaCl 7%), 4–5 ml/kg slow IV over 3–5 minutes.

- If volume replacement fluids are not available, give isotonic **crystalloid fluids** (e.g. NaCl 0.9%, LRS) 40–60 ml/kg/h IV, to effect administering just enough to re-establish euvolemia and mean arterial blood pressure.

- **Whole blood transfusion or plasma administration** may be indicated when significant blood loss has occurred.

- **Administer supplemental oxygen** via a nasal or transtracheal catheter. If the cat is unconscious, intubate and ventilate at 10–20 breaths/minute to keep $PaCO_2$ around 30–35 mmHg.

Control secondary brain edema to prevent or reduce intracranial hypertension.

- If shock treatment has not sufficiently improved the cat's neurological status, if the cat is mentally very depressed or stuporous, or if its neurological status deteriorates (mental status, pinpoint pupils or progression to mydriatic and non-responsive pupils):

  - **Give furosemide** 0.5–2 mg/kg IV.

  - A few minutes later, **give mannitol** 0.5–1.0 g/kg IV slowly over 10–20 minutes. A dramatic decrease of the intracranial pressure and neurological improvement usually occurs within 15 minutes and lasts for 2–5 hours. If neurological deterioration occurs afterwards, mannitol can be repeated for a maximum of three doses over a 24-hour period. Careful monitoring of serum osmolality and electrolytes is mandatory.

- **Keep the head elevated at 15–30 degrees**, avoid pressure on the jugular veins from IV lines, bandage and bedding, and monitor mental status and pupil size continuously.

Glucocorticosteroid administration in the head trauma patient is controversial because of few documented beneficial effects and potential deleterious effects, etc. If the patient does not respond adequately to appropriate fluid, oxygen and mannitol administration, methylprednisolone (Solu-Medrol) may be given if hyperglycemia is not already present (30 mg/kg at time 0, and 15 mg/kg at 2 and 6 hours, followed or not with a continuous intravenous infusion of 2.5 mg/kg/h for 24 hours).

Control cluster seizures and status epilepticus with anti-epileptic drugs (see Likely symptomatic epilepsy, page 801).

Emergency craniectomy may be indicated when aggressive medical treatment has not succeeded in stabilizing a patient with a depressed skull fracture, calvarial penetration with contaminated bone fragments or foreign material, and focal hemorrhage as documented by brain imaging (CT scan or MRI). Craniectomy with durotomy solely as a decompressive procedure may also be attempted.

RABIES

Classical signs

- Progression from mild behavioral changes, to aggression and vicious behavior, to paralysis and death.

Clinical signs

The development of the disease often follows three stages; an early short prodromal phase (1–2 days) characterized by a non-specific change in mental status; the cat may become shy and withdrawn or affectionate and unpredictable. This progresses into an aggressive and furious form (2–4 days) where the cat may viciously attack anything in sight. This may be accompanied by excessive drooling secondary to dysphagia. Convulsions may also occur. In the later stage (1–4 days) of the illness, the animal develops paralysis, coma and death.

Diagnosis

Any cat presented with an acute onset of aggression or with unusually fractious behavior, should be considered as a rabies suspect and handled with caution.

The diagnosis is made on post-mortem tissue using immunofluorescence antibody (IFA), ELISA and more recently polymerase chain reaction (PCR) testing.

The strain of rabies can be further diagnosed using monoclonal antibody testing.

Routine laboratory tests are unrewarding.

UREMIA

Classical signs

- Mental alterations, abnormal motor function and occasionally, seizures.
- Depression, anorexia.
- Polyuria, polydipsia, weight loss.

See main reference on page 334 (The Thin, Inappetent Cat) and page 231 (The Cat With Polyuria and Polydipsia).

Clinical signs

Neurological signs occur mainly in severely ill patients with advanced stage of acute or chronic renal failure.

Signs are often vague and include mental disturbances such as depression, confusion, restlessness, hyper-reactivity to various stimuli, delirium. Weakness may be evident sometimes with muscle spasms, myoclonia or tremors. Ataxia, head-bobbing and muscle fasciculations may also occur. The signs are likely caused by the debilitating effects of renal failure, uremic encephalopathy and associated metabolic disturbances including hypocalcemia, hypoglycemia, acid–base disturbances, anemia.

- **Seizures occur in severely ill cats** and more often with acute than chronic renal failure.

Diagnosis

Other historical, clinical and laboratory abnormalities consistent with severe renal failure and perhaps related to the underlying cause (e.g. ethylene glycol intoxication) are present. **There is no correlation between the degree of azotemia and the severity of the neurological signs.**

FELINE IMMUNODEFICIENCY VIRUS ENCEPHALOPATHY

Classical signs

- Usually asymptomatic.
- Rarely, behavioral abnormalities.

Clinical signs

Subtle and non-specific changes in behavior including depression, social withdrawal, compulsive roaming and psychotic behavior have been attributed to FIV encephalopathy. Signs have mainly been observed in the advanced stage of infection.

Diagnosis

Other systemic signs of FIV infection for example, weight loss, fewer immunodeficiency-related infections of the skin, respiratory or gastrointestinal tracts should have manifested by the time neurological signs develop.

CSF analysis may reveal a mild non-specific mononuclear pleocytosis (5–10/µl) with normal protein concentration. **A positive antibody test** on a **CSF sample not contaminated with blood** indicates CNS infection.

Unrelated CNS pathologies and secondary opportunistic infections (e.g. FIP, toxoplasmosis) would likely be responsible for neurological signs other than behavioral changes in FIV-positive cats.

Treatment

No effective treatment is known.

RECOMMENDED READING

Parent JM, Quesnel AD. Seizures in cats. Vet Clin North Am 1996; 26: 811–825.

Quesnel AD. Seizures. In: Ettinger JE, Feldman EC (eds) Textbook of Veterinary Internal Medicine – Diseases of the Dog and Cat, 5th edn. Philadelphia, WB Saunders Co., 2000, pp. 148–152.

Quesnel AD, Parent JM. Diagnostic approach and medical treatment of seizure disorders. In: August T (ed) Consultations in feline internal medicine 3. Philadelphia, WB Saunders Co., 1997, pp. 389–402.

Quesnel AD, Parent JM, McDonell W, Percy D, Lumsden JH. Diagnostic evaluation of cats with seizure disorders: 30 cases (1990–1993). J Am Vet Med Assoc 1997; 210: 65–71.

Quesnel AD, Parent JM, McDonell W. Clinical management and outcome of cats with seizure disorders: 30 cases (1991–1993). J Am Vet Med Assoc 1997; 210: 72–77.

37. The cat with stupor or coma

Rodney S Bagley

KEY SIGNS

- Moderate to marked decrease in consciousness and wakefulness.
- Reduced or absent response to external stimuli.

MECHANISM?

- Stupor and coma result from diseases that alter consciousness and wakefulness.

WHERE?

- Disease of the intracranial nervous system including the supratentorial structures (cerebral cortex, thalamus) and the brain stem (midbrain, pons or medulla oblongata) may result in stupor or coma.
- Systemic (metabolic) disease may affect these areas secondarily and result in stupor or coma.

WHAT?

- Diseases of the intracranial nervous system resulting in coma include head trauma, brain tumor, encephalitis, vascular-based diseases and severe hypoglycemia.
- Many of these diseases result in increased intracranial pressure that perpetuates the clinical signs.
- These diseases are often severe.

QUICK REFERENCE SUMMARY

Diseases causing stupor or coma

ANOMALY

- **Hydrocephalus** (p 826)**
If hydrocephalus is congenital, cats may have an enlarged, "dome-shaped" skull. A fontanelle that persists during maturation may be palpable. Acquired hydrocephalus in adults will show no outward anatomical signs. Clinical signs include seizures, poor learning ability, behavior changes, paresis, cranial nerve deficits and changes in consciousness.

continued

continued

METABOLIC

● Metabolic encephalopathy* (p 830)

Metabolic encephalopathies secondary to hypoglycemia, hepatic or renal disease may be associated with signs of cerebrocortical dysfunction including seizures, behavior abnormalities and limb dysfunction. Neurological signs tend to be symmetrical. Other signs of a polysystemic disease such as vomiting and diarrhea may be present. Hypoglycemia results in a dazed cat with a drunken, wobbly gait and muscle trembling, which may progress to seizures and coma if severe and untreated.

● Feline ischemic encephalopathy* (p 828)

Clinical signs begin acutely and rapidly evolve. Clinical signs usually include circling, blindness and seizures.

NEOPLASTIC

● Brain tumor*** (p 824)

Tumors occur most often in older cats. Clinical signs may be acute in onset or slowly progressive. Seizures, circling, paresis, head tilts and nystagmus are most common.

NUTRITIONAL

● Thiamine deficiency* (p 832)

Decreased thiamine can result in brain stem disease in cats. Clinical signs initially begin with lethargy, inappetence and reluctance to walk. Later there is vestibular ataxia and episodes of spastic ventroflexion of the neck or opisthotonus, dilated pupils, stupor and coma.

INFLAMMATORY (INFECTIOUS)

● Encephalitis* (p 829)

Clinical signs are often diffuse and may not localize to a single area within the nervous system. Fever and leukocytosis are inconsistent findings. Systemic signs of disease such as fever, coughing, vomiting and diarrhea may accompany the neurologic signs. Feline infectious peritonitis, toxoplasmosis and *Cryptococcus* are more common causes of encephalitis. The systemic signs are consistent with the disease process.

TRAUMA

● Head trauma*** (p 823)

Usually associated with an acute onset of clinical signs reflective of an intracranial problem. Signs present often include alterations in consciousness, paresis and cranial nerve abnormalities. Fresh blood from lacerations on or around the head, skull fractures, blood in the ear canals, and scleral hemorrhage may be clues to a previous traumatic incident.

TOXICITY

● Lead toxicity* (p 833)

Rare in cats because of eating behavior, but they may be exposed through aerosolized paint dust during house renovations. Inappetence and weight loss are early signs. In addition to central nervous system signs of behavioral abnormalities and alterations in mentation, blindness, vomiting, diarrhea and hematologic abnormalities may be found.

INTRODUCTION

MECHANISM?

Stupor and coma result from diseases that primarily or secondarily affect the cerebral cortex and thalamus and/or the reticular activating system of the brain stem responsible for consciousness and wakefulness.

Systemic (metabolic) disease may affect these areas indirectly and result in stupor or coma.

WHERE?

Disease of the intracranial nervous system including the supratentorial structures (cerebral cortex, thalamus) and the brain stem (midbrain, pons or medulla oblongata) may result in stupor or coma.

WHAT?

Diseases of the intracranial nervous system resulting in coma include head trauma, brain tumor, encephalitis and vascular-based diseases.

Many of these diseases result in increased intracranial pressure that perpetuates the clinical signs.

These diseases are often severe.

The most common metabolic diseases producing stupor or coma are hypoglycemia secondary to insulin overdose in a diabetic cat and hepatic encephalopathy secondary to a congenital portosystematic shunt.

DISEASES CAUSING STUPOR OR COMA

HEAD TRAUMA***

Classical signs

- Acute onset of signs including stupor, coma, paresis, gait abnormalities and cranial nerve deficits, especially those involving pupillary responses.

Classical signs—Cont'd

- Evidence of external trauma to the head and face such as facial lacerations, bleeding from the nose and mouth, bruising, retinal hemorrhage or hemorrhage in the external ear canals.

Pathogenesis

Traumatic injury to the brain occurs most commonly from automobile trauma, although gunshot wounds and falls may also occur.

All of these disease processes result in mechanical disruption of intracranial tissues (primary injury) such as axonal shearing.

Primary injuries to the brain may initiate a number of secondary pathophysiological sequelae such as metabolic alterations in neuronal or glial cells, impairment of vascular supply to normal tissue (ischemia), impairment of cerebrovascular autoregulation, hemorrhage (intraparenchymal, intraventricular, extradural or subdural), irritation (seizure generation), obstruction of the ventricular system; edema formation, production of physiologically active products, and finally, increased intracranial pressure (ICP).

Hemorrhage, either within or around the brain, may result in rapid cerebral dysfunction.

In an experimental study of blunt craniocerebral trauma in cats, all had some degree of subarachnoid hemorrhage, and many had subdural hemorrhage. Fifteen percent of cats had subdural hematomas that displaced the corresponding cerebral hemisphere.

- Many also had cortical contusion. Intraparenchymal hemorrhage and petechiation were common, most often in the hemisphere directly receiving the blunt force.
- One-fifth of the cats had tentorial herniation.

Clinical signs

Signs usually begin acutely after trauma.

Intracranial signs most commonly seen include stupor and coma, paresis and gait abnormalities, and cranial nerve deficits, especially those involving pupillary responses.

Evidence of external trauma to the head and face such as facial lacerations, bleeding from the nose and mouth, bruising, or hemorrhage in the external ear canals may be clues to the traumatic etiology.

Diagnosis

The diagnosis of trauma is usually straightforward when the trauma is witnessed.

In some instances, when animals are presented with an acute onset of neurological signs and an unknown history, examining for external signs of trauma such as lacerations or skull fractures is important.

Evaluating the retinas and external ear canals for acute hemorrhage may also provide clues to the diagnosis.

Advanced imaging studies such as CT or MR imaging are useful, primarily for determining structural damage to the brain.

Differential diagnosis

External evidence of a traumatic incident is helpful to separate traumatic causes of stupor and coma from other intracranial diseases.

Sometimes cats with intracranial disease are unbalanced, weak or have seizures and fall. This may result in external injuries being misconstrued as the actual cause of the intracranial signs.

Treatment

Basic life support measures may be necessary including **blood or isotonic fluid administration**.

Corticosteroid administration for treatment of head trauma is commonly used but efficacy is often based upon anecdotal evidence. Beneficial effects of **methylprednisolone sodium succinate (30 mg/kg IV slowly)** in nervous system injury include inhibition of lipid peroxidation and its associated detrimental effects. The role of corticosteroids in the treatment of head trauma, however, is unclear and are currently not recommended in humans suffering from head trauma.

Hyperventilation keeping **$PaCO_2$** concentrations **between 28 and 32** mmHg can **decrease ICP** due to the established effects of $PaCO_2$ concentrations on cerebral blood flow.

Mannitol is used to decrease cerebral edema and ICP. Mannitol has been thought to decrease cerebral edema primarily through its associated **osmotic effects**, although other effects such as concurrent **decreases in blood viscosity** and **free-radical scavenging** may, in fact, be more beneficial. By decreasing blood viscosity, cerebral perfusion will be increased at the same level of systemic blood pressure. Vasoconstriction will result, lowering cerebral blood volume and concurrently lowering ICP. Mannitol is administered at 1 g/kg IV over 5–10 minutes. **Maximal lowering of ICP** most often **occurs in 10–20 minutes**.

Furosemide (0.7 mg/kg IV) is a loop diuretic that may help to lower ICP primarily or may **potentiate the effects of mannitol**. Furosemide given 15 minutes after mannitol administration potentiates the intracranial pressure-lowering effects of the latter.

The **antioxidant drug, desferoxamine mesylate** has been shown to reduce cold-induced brain edema in cats.

Surgical treatment centers on evacuation of subdural hematomas, removal of depressed skull fractures, or debridement of damaged tissue and foreign material.
- Craniectomy and durotomy has been shown to lower ICP acutely by 15–65%, respectively, in cats, however, long-term benefits are uncertain.

Prognosis

Prognosis for life is good if signs are not severe.

Cerebrocortical and cerebellar injuries are more readily recoverable from than brain stem injuries.

Prevention

Keep cats in a controlled environment and prevent free-roaming.

BRAIN TUMOR***

Classical signs
- Middle-aged to older cats.
- Signs include seizures, circling, blindness, behavior changes, and may progress to stupor and coma.

Pathogenesis

Neoplasia can arise from structures within or surrounding the brain (primary brain tumors).

Neoplasia secondarily involves the brain via **metastasis** or via direct **extension from extraneural sites**. Primary tumors within the **skull**, **nasal cavity** or **frontal sinuses** can extend directly into the brain.

Meningioma is the **most common brain tumor** in cats. Meningiomas arise from the arachnoid layer of the meninges. Meningiomas are usually histologically benign, but occasionally are malignant.

Some younger cats with mucopolysaccharidosis have a high incidence of meningiomas.

Gliomas arise from cells of the brain parenchyma. These include **astrocytes and oligdendrogliocytes**.

Choroid plexus tumors arise from areas where the choroid plexus is concentrated (the lateral, third and fourth ventricles).

Signs reflect either primary nervous parenchymal damage from the tumor, or secondary pathophysiological sequelae such as **hemorrhage and edema**. Frequently, these secondary sequelae are more devastating to intracranial function than the primary disease itself.

Clinical signs

Middle-aged to older cats are most commonly affected. Cats are usually older than 5 years of age with a median age of onset of clinical signs at 9 years of age.

Clinical signs are often slowly progressive, however, they can also occasionally begin acutely and be rapidly progressive.

Signs reflect the intracranial location of the lesion.
- Signs include seizures, circling, blindness, behavior changes, cranial nerve abnormalities, and may progress to **stupor and coma.**
- If the brain stem is involved, head tilt, nystagmus and paresis are most common.

Diagnosis

Routine laboratory evaluations (CBC, biochemistry profile) are not affected by intracranial neoplasia.

Hyperostosis of the skull is occasionally present on survey radiographs of the skull, especially with meningiomas. A "sky-line" view may be necessary to image this abnormality.

Diagnosis of a structural intracranial abnormality in the brain is most readily accomplished with **magnetic resonance (MR) imaging** or **computed tomography (CT) of the brain**.
- A broad-based, extra-axial (arising outside and pushing into the parenchyma) **contrast-enhancing mass** on CT or MR imaging is found in most instances of **meningioma**.
- The CT and MR appearance of gliomas is varied and enhancement after contrast administration may not be present. As these tumors arise from brain parenchymal cells, they are found within the neuroaxis (intra-axial).
- **Choroid plexus tumors**, because of the increased concentration of blood vessels within the tumor, **often enhance markedly** after contrast administration. Because of their association with the ventricular system, associated **hydrocephalus is common**.

Cerebrospinal fluid often contains **elevations in protein** content but this finding is not pathognomonic for brain tumors.
- Cerebrospinal fluid can contain **evidence of inflammation** (contains elevations in nucleated cells and protein content). If CSF is the only assessment made, an erroneous diagnosis of encephalitis may be made.
- **Cerebrospinal fluid** collection may be associated with an **increased mortality** in cats with space-occupying mass lesions within the intracranial space, because of the sudden decrease in pressure at the cisterna magna.

Differential diagnosis

Cats with intracranial tumors may present with signs similar to other intracranial diseases.

There are no pathognomonic clinical signs for intracranial tumor.

Congenital hydrocephalus may be associated with changes in the skull ("Dome-shaped" skull, persistent fontanelle), but these will not be present with acquired hydrocephalus.

Feline ischemic encephalopathy is usually associated with an acute onset of clinical signs localizing to the cerebral cortex.

Encephalitis may be associated with systemic diseases causing chorioretinitis, fever and leukocytosis.

Treatment

Corticosteroids (prednisolone 1–2 mg/kg q 12 h) may **reduce peritumoral edema** and improve clinical signs.

Surgical removal of primary brain tumors may be accomplished, especially with **meningioma.**

A well-encapsulated, firm whitish mass is most often encountered at surgery in cats. Cortical parenchyma is usually not infiltrated but rather compressed in cats, leaving indentations in the nervous tissue parenchyma after resection.

Radiation therapy at a total dose of 45–48 GY may control tumor growth.

Prognosis

Prognosis for life is good (22–27 months median survival) after surgical removal of meningiomas in cats.

Uncontrolled or untreated brain tumors usually result in **death of the cat in less than 6 months**, however, the natural course of affected cats has not been accurately determined.

Prevention

There is no known way to prevent these diseases.

HYDROCEPHALUS**

Classical signs

- Young cats may have a dome-shaped or bossed appearance to the head or persistent fontanelles.
- Other signs of hydrocephalus include seizures, poor learning ability, behavior changes, paresis, cranial nerve deficits and changes in consciousness.

Pathogenesis

Hydrocephalus is the term commonly used to describe a condition of **abnormal dilation** of the **ventricular system** within the brain.

Hydrocephalus can result from obstruction of the ventricular system, irritation of the ventricular lining (from inflammation or hemorrhage), loss of brain parenchyma (hydrocephalus ex vacuo), be present without an obvious cause (congenital), or rarely, be the result of overproduction of CSF associated with a choroid plexus tumor.

If the ventricular system is obstructed, CSF will be trapped behind the level of obstruction.

Anatomically **smaller areas of the ventricular system are common sites of obstruction**. These include the **interventricular foramen** and the **mesencephalic aqueduct**.

Obstruction can result from **tumor, granuloma, hemorrhage or inflammation**.

- With infectious diseases that affect the ventricular system, the ependymal layer may be damaged predisposing the underlying parenchyma to be penetrated by the agent or associated products.
- An inflammatory reaction ensues, further damaging local tissues.
- The ependymal cells may be lost and replaced by subependymal microgliacytes or astrocytes. The end stage is a **granular ependymitis**.
- **Feline infectious peritonitis virus** infection is a common cause.

In **Siamese cats hereditary hydrocephalus** in transmitted as an **autosomal recessive trait**.

The cause of congenital hydrocephalus, however, is not always apparent. Speculation suggests that this abnormality may be due to an **obstruction of the ventricular system** during a **critical stage in development** and subsequent damage to the vulnerable maturing nervous parenchyma.

Feline cerebellar hypoplasia is caused by in utero infection with the panleukopenia virus (parvovirus), which affects the external germinal layer of the cerebellum and prevents the formation of the granular layer. Some affected cats have a concurrent hydrocephalus and hydranencephaly.

Hydrocephalus can result in **clinical signs due to loss of neurons** or neuronal function, **alterations in intracranial pressure**, or the associated pathophysiological effects of intracranial disease.

Clinical signs

In young cats prior to ossification of the cranial sutures, hydrocephalus may contribute to abnormalities of skull development such as a thinning of the bone structure, a **dome-shaped or bossed appearance** to the head or persistent fontanelles.

Clinical signs of hydrocephalus reflect the anatomical level of disease involvement.

Supratentorial, vestibular and cerebellar signs are most common.

As the supratentorial structures are often involved with hydrocephalus, **alterations in awareness and cognition are common.**

Many animals affected congenitally may appear to be **less intelligent** than normal.

Circling, paresis and seizure may also be seen.

Severity of clinical signs is not dependent upon the degree of ventricular dilation, but rather on a host of concurrent abnormalities including the underlying disease process, associated intracranial pressure changes, intraventricular hemorrhage, and the acuity of ventricular obstruction.

Diagnosis

Routine laboratory evaluations are normal.

Historical, invasive techniques for diagnosis of hydrocephalus such as pneumo- or contrast ventriculography have been replaced by non-invasive diagnostic modalities.

Survey radiographs may suggest the presence of hydrocephalus, however, are usually not helpful for definitive diagnosis. Findings associated with **congenital hydrocephalus** include loss of gyral striations, separation of cranial sutures (diastasis), and **persistent fontanelles**. If hydrocephalus is acquired **after the skull has formed, abnormalities are rarely encountered**.

Electroencephalography has been used to diagnosis hydrocephalus, primarily prior to advanced imaging.

Classically, **slow-frequency, high-voltage** (amplitude) activity is noted. This pattern, however, can be seen with **other encephalopathies** that destroy cortical parenchyma. Because of this, EEG is rarely used as the sole means of diagnosing hydrocephalus.

Ultrasound can be used to diagnosis hydrocephalus.
- This is most readily accomplished **when a fontanelle is present** providing an "acoustic window" as ultrasound waves do not usually penetrate the skull well enough.
- If the bone is intact, a craniotomy defect can be created.
- For imaging of the lateral and third ventricles, the bregmatic fontanelle may be used.
- Often, ultrasound can be performed in awake cats as a screening test to determine ventriculomegaly.
- Depending upon the size of the fontanelle, the **lateral and third ventricles** as well as the **mesencephalic aqueduct** are usually easily identified.

Computed tomography (CT), as a non-invasive intracranial imaging modality, is often useful in defining ventricular size.

Magnetic resonance (MR) imaging also affords evaluation of the ventricular system. This modality provides better parenchyma resolution than CT, and is especially useful for evaluation of the infratentorial structures.

Diffuse ventricular enlargement suggests congenital ventricular dilation or obstruction at the level of the lateral apertures or foramen magnum. **Focal ventricular enlargement** suggests **focal obstruction** or **parenchymal cell loss.**

Animals with an **asymmetric appearance** of the ventricles should be critically evaluated for **focal obstruction** of or impingement on the ventricular system due to **mass effect**.

Differential diagnosis

Congenital hydrocephalus may be associated with changes in the skull ("dome-shaped" skull, persistent fontenelle), but these will not be present with acquired hydrocephalus.

Cats with hydrocephlaus may present with signs similar to other intracranial diseases. Rule out other **inflammatory, neoplastic and traumatic causes of intracranial disease.**

There are no pathognomonic clinical signs for acquired hydrocephalus in adult animals.

Correlation of degree of ventricular enlargement and clinical signs is poor.

Treatment

Medical treatment may include general supportive care, and medications to limit CSF production and reduce intracranial pressure.

Glucocorticoids are used to decrease CSF production, thereby, limiting intracranial pressure and further neurologic injury. Prednisone at 0.25–0.5 mg/kg is given orally twice daily. The dose is gradually reduced at weekly intervals to 0.1 mg/kg every other day. This dose is continued for at least one month. Then the medication is discontinued if possible.

Alternatively, **dexamethasone** may be given orally at 0.25 mg/kg every 6–8 hours. The dose can be gradually reduced over 2–4 weeks.

Some animals can be adequately managed with long-term glucocorticoid administration at low doses.

If no clinical benefits are observed within 2 weeks, or if side effects develop, other forms of therapy should be tried.

Surgical procedures where a shunt is placed in the ventricle are designed to provide controlled CSF flow from the ventricles of the brain to the peritoneal cavity. Commercial pediatric ventriculoperitoneal shunts are available for thus purpose.

Prognosis

Generally poor unless definitive surgical correction is successful. In some cats, clinical signs can be managed on a long-term basis with medication therapy alone.

FELINE ISCHEMIC ENCEPHALOPATHY*

Classical signs

- Signs occur acutely and reflect a unilateral cerebrocortical abnormality.
- Signs include seizures, circling, blindness, behavior changes and may progress rapidly to stupor and coma.

Pathogenesis

Feline ischemic encephalopathy is an **ischemic necrosis** of the **cerebral hemisphere** of cats.

The distribution of the vascular change is usually in the area supplied by the **middle cerebral artery.**

Vascular lesions, however, are infrequently found at necropsy.

Some authors have speculated that this disease is the result of a Cuterebra migration.

One 7-year-old Siamese cat has been reported with an intravascular malignant T-cell lymphoma occluding the middle cerebral artery.

Clinical signs

Clinical signs **begin acutely.**

Signs often reflect a **unilateral cerebrocortical abnormality.**

Signs include **seizures, circling, blindness, behavior changes** and may progress to stupor and coma.

Diagnosis

Routine laboratory evaluations are normal.

Cerebrospinal fluid often contains **elevations in protein content** but this finding is not pathognomonic for this disease.

CSF may contain mild increases in nucleated cells (usually < 10 cells/μl). Neurophils, macrophages and mononuclear cells are possible.

Diagnosis of a structural intracranial abnormality in the cerebral hemisphere is most readily accomplished with **magnetic resonance imaging** of the brain. Minimal changes, however, may be seen on MR studies with this disease.

Cerebral angiography would theoretically aid in the diagnosis of this disease, but is rarely performed.

Differential diagnosis

Rule out brain tumor, encephalitis, head trauma and hydrocephalus.

Treatment

No treatment has been shown to be effective.

Prognosis

Prognosis for life is good after the first 48 hours as this is a non-progressive disorder.

Residual neurologic deficits, most notably seizures, may persist throughout life. Behavioral changes, such as aggression or irritability may persist and make the cat less acceptable as a pet.

Prevention

None.

ENCEPHALITIS*

Classical signs

- Neurological signs are often diffuse or multifocal.
- Cervical pain can be present.
- Fever is an inconsistent finding.
- Chorioretinitis is often present on fundic examination.
- Other signs of polysystemic disease such as coughing, vomiting and diarrhea may be associated.

See main reference on page 859 for details (The Cat With Tremor or Twitching).

Clinical signs

Numerous infectious agents have been incriminated, with the incidence of infectious agents causing meningitis varying with geographic location. Systemic signs reflect the specific agent.

- Infectious agents causing brain disease include viral (**feline infectious peritonitis**), fungal (**cryptococcosis**, blastomycosis, histoplasmosis, coccidioidomycosis, aspergillosis), protozoal (**toxoplasmosis**, neosporosis), bacterial, rickettsial, and unclassified organisms (protothecosis).
- Involvement of the intracranial nervous system can occur with parasites such as **Cuterebra larvae, toxocara**, and aberrant **heartworm** migration.

Clinical signs are often diffuse or multifocal and may not localize to a single area within the nervous system. Clinical signs often reflect multiple levels of neurological involvement

Cervical pain can be present.

Fever is an inconsistent finding.

Fundic examination is important to look for clues of systemic inflammatory disease, as **chorioretinitis** is often present.

Other signs of a **polysystemic disease** process such as inappetence, weight loss, **nasal discharge, coughing, vomiting, and diarrhea** may be associated.

Diagnosis

Complete blood cell count may show evidence of systemic inflammation (e.g. leukocytosis).

Serum biochemical analysis may show evidence of systemic abnormalities if the disease diffusely affects the body (e.g. vasculitis) such as elevated globulin, CK, liver enzymes or creatinine.

Evaluation of titers for the infectious diseases often helps to rule in or out the diseases.

Cerebrospinal fluid analysis (CSF) will usually show evidence of **increased nucleated cells** and/or **elevated protein content**. Occasionally, CSF will be normal.

- Evidence of inflammation on CSF evaluation alone, however, is not specific for primary encephalitis as other CNS disease (e.g. **neoplasia**) **may result in a CSF pleocytosis** and protein increases.
- With feline infectious peritonitis (FIP), cerebrospinal fluid analysis may show a pleocytosis, with either **mononuclear** or non-lytic **neutrophils** as the predominant cell type and **elevated protein** concentration, often > 1 g/L (0.1 g/dl).
- With **toxoplasmosis**, cerebrospinal fluid frequently contains a pleocytosis, usually with mononuclear cells, and occasionally, eosinophils. Increasing IgG or a single positive IgM serum antibody titer is suggestive of active infection. Animals with **neurologic signs and positive IgM titers warrant treatment** for the disease.

With **cryptococcosis**, identification of the organism from cytological evaluation of samples such as CSF, nasal discharge, and skin lesions supports the diagnosis.

A neurophilic pleocytosis, and occasionally an eosinophilic pleocytosis may be found on CSF analysis. If positive, detection of the cryptococcal capsular antigen in serum is usually diagnostic. Tissue biopsy and fungal culture or fungal culture of CSF may be more definitive in the diagnosis as occasionally the serum titer is negative.

With parasites such as Cuterebra larvae, toxocara and aberrant heartworm migration, CSF may show inflammation with eosinophils is some instances.

Imaging studies (CT and MR) are helpful for defining structural lesions. **Multifocal, contrast-enhancing lesions** are usually seen. Occasionally, non-contrast-enhancing lesions are present, especially with toxoplasmosis.

Differential diagnosis

Multifocal signs are more suggestive of **encephalitis**.

Cats with encephalitis may present with signs similar to other intracranial diseases such as brain tumor, trauma, hydrocephalus and cerebrovascular disease.

Treatment

Treatment is directed at a specific infectious cause if found.

Without a definable cause of the encephalitis, the author uses **trimethoprim-sulfadiazine** (30 mg/kg PO q 12 h), **clindamycin** (25 mg/kg q 12 h), and **corticosteroids** (prednisone 1–2 mg/kg PO q 12 h) in combination.

While corticosteroids are contraindicated with infectious diseases, they are often beneficial in the acute treatment of brain inflammation and edema. These associated pathophysiological events often lead to more neurologic deterioration than the organism itself.

If rickettsial diseases are endemic, **chloramphenicol** or **doxocycline** can be substituted or added to the regime.

If the animal is receiving phenobarbital, do not use chloramphenicol as this drug will decrease the metabolism of the barbiturate and the animal will become comatose and possible die. Also, chloramphenicol may result in bone-marrow suppression in cats.

With feline infectious peritonitis (FIP), no specific treatment is effective. Immunosuppressive therapy may result in short-term improvement of clinical signs.

With **toxoplasmosis**, treatment includes **clindamycin and trimethoprim** sulfa antibiotics.

For **cryptococcosis**, treatments that have had some success for cryptococcosis in cats include amphotericin B, fluconazole, itraconazole, and flucytosine. See page 26 (The Cat With Signs of Chronic Nasal Disease for treatment details).

With CNS parasites, treatment has not been attempted uniformly and treatment recommendations are anecdotal.

Prognosis

Many of the encephalities are poorly responsive to treatment, and therefore morbidity and mortality is > 50%.

Some infectious encephalities (e.g. toxoplasmosis) may be cured with appropriate treatment.

METABOLIC ENCEPHALOPATHY*

Classical signs

- Hepatic encephalopathy usually occurs in younger cats. Clinical signs include seizures, ptyalism and mentation changes.
- Cats with diabetic ketoacidosis may have cerebral signs (depression).
- Cats with hypoglycemia may show depression, seizures and tremors.

Pathogenesis

Various metabolic imbalances within the body may produce physiologic alterations, toxins or by-products that effect nervous system functions.

Hepatic encephalopathy (HE) results when numerous putative neurotoxins reach the brain unmetabolized as they pass through an abnormally functioning liver or bypass hepatic detoxification.

Younger animals with HE usually have congenital portosystemic shunts, however, some animals do not have clinical signs of this disease until later into adulthood.

Hepatic encephalopathy in older animals can be associated with liver failure such as with cirrhosis.

Hypoglycemia can occur secondary to some endocrine disorders such as hypoadrenocorticism and insulinoma or from lack of production by the liver in young kittens or in cats with liver failure, and some tumors. However, it is **most common following overdose of insulin in diabetic cats**.

Because the central nervous system (CNS) requires a constant supply of glucose, clinical signs of hypoglycemia relate to CNS dysfunction and activation of the sympathetic nervous system and include depression, seizures and tremors.

Cats with **diabetic ketoacidosis** may have cerebral signs (depression), but whether these changes relate to the hyperglycemia or other physiologic derangements such as hyperosmolality is unknown.

Hypernatremia can result in abnormal mentation progressing to stupor and coma.
- Hypernatremia usually results from inadequate drinking. This may occur due to alterations in awareness of thirst or inability to physically move to water.
- Idiopathic adipsia can occur, usually in younger cats.

Hypernatremia and adipsia in an older animal should warrant an evaluation for structural intracranial disease such as hydrocephalus and brain tumor.

Renal failure and pancreatitis may affect cerebral function if severe, producing depression, stupor, tetany or seizures.

Clinical signs

Neurologic signs often include seizure, alterations in mentation, behavior abnormalities and paresis.

Neurologic signs are **often symmetrical** and **may be episodic.**

Clinical signs of **hepatic encephalopathy** include **seizures, ptyalism and mentation changes**.

In hypoglycemia, clinical signs occur due to decreased CNS glucose supply (neuroglycopenic signs) or because of sympathetic nervous system activity.

- Weakness and seizures are most common. Affected animals may be depressed, and have intermittent twitches or tremors.

Clinical signs of hypernatremia include adipsia, depression, seizures progressing to stupor and coma.

Uremic encephalopathy may result in depression, stupor, myoclonic movements, generalized weakness and partial or generalized seizures.

Diagnosis

Diagnosis of metabolic encehalopathy is suggested by metabolic abnormalities on routine physical examination or laboratory evaluations (CBC, serum biochemical analysis, urinalysis).

Diagnosis of hepatic encephalopathy is supported by **abnormal liver function studies** such as elevated pre- or post-prandial **bile acids** or elevated fasting **ammonia**. Ammonia chloride challenge is rarely required in cats to make a diagnosis.
- Abdominal ultrasound may show abnormal liver vasculature.
- Portal vein angiography or direct visualization at surgery may be needed for accurate diagnosis.

Diagnosis of hypoglycemia is based upon finding **hypoglycemia** (blood glucose < 3.3 mmol/l: 60 mg/dl) in the face of clinical signs.
- Concurrent measurement of **serum insulin concentration** will help identify an insulin-secreting tumor, by demonstrating inappropriately high insulin concentration in the presence of hypoglycemia. Non-beta cell tumors producing hypoglycemia have low to undetectable insulin concentration during hypoglycemia.
- Insulin-treated diabetic cats with clinical hypoglycemia need re-evaluation. Some cats will be in **diabetic remission** and do not need **insulin**. Other cats have accidentally received a higher than normal dose. This may occur when insulin syringes are changed from U100 to U40 or from 0.5 ml to 1 ml syringes. Accidental overdose may also occur when someone other than the owner gives the insulin. Careful history taking will identify these problems.

Diagnosis of hypernatremia is based upon finding elevated serum sodium (> 165 mmol/l: 165 mEq/l) in the face of clinical signs.

- Diagnosis of a structural intracranial abnormality in the hypothalamus or pituitary region is most readily accomplished with computed tomography or magnetic resonance imaging of the brain.

Differential diagnosis

Rule out other inflammatory, neoplastic and traumatic causes of intracranial disease.

Treatment

Treatments should be directed at the underlying metabolic abnormality.

Medical treatment of hepatic encephalopathy centers on frequent small meals of a **low-protein diet**, **antibiotics** (metronidazole 7.5 mg/kg PO q 12 h and neomycin sulfate 20 mg/kg PO q 8–12 h), **l-carnitine** (250–500 mg/cat/day PO as aqueous solution), **taurine** (250–500 mg/cat/day in food), arginine (250 mg q 12 h in food), vitamins B, K₁ and E and **lactulose** (1–3 ml/cat PO q 8–12 h to produce a soft stool, beginning at the lowest dose and increasing as necessary). If the cat is severely depressed, lactulose should be given as a retention enema for the first 1–2 days. A solution of three parts lactulose to seven parts water is dosed at 18 ml/kg q 4–6 h. The solution is instilled via a Foley catheter as cranially in the colon as possible. The solution must be aspirated after 15–20 minutes. Fluid and electrolyte status should be monitored carefully to avoid dehydration and hypernatremia. Benzodiazepine receptor antagonists (e.g. flumazenil) may be useful in cats with severe encephalopathy, but are unproven.

If the clinical signs of hepatic encephalopathy are severe, or do not improve within 4–6 hours after institution of medical treatment, and if the animal is not dehydrated, mannitol (1–2 g/kg IV) followed by furosemide (0.7 mg/kg IV) can be administered as a treatment for possible secondary cerebral edema.

Surgical correction of a congenital portosystemic shunt may result in a permanent cure.

Diabetic cats with marked signs of hypoglycemia should be treated initially at home with **honey or a sugar-solution designed for human diabetics** poured on the owner's finger and rubbed on the cat's buccal mucosa. In hospital, treatment is with dextrose

(1/2–2 ml IV, 20–50% dextrose) to effect. The insulin dose should be decreased by 50% or stopped if the cat is in remission. Accidental causes of overdose should be resolved.

Cats with hypoglycemia associated with neoplasia, including insulinoma should be managed with frequent feeding and corticosteroids (0.5–6 mg/kg/day in divided doses) to antagonize insulin action. See page 962 (The Cat With Generalized Weakness) for further treatment details. Surgical removal of a pancreatic insulin-secreting tumor may normalize serum glucose concentrations.

Treatment for hypernatremia centers on **slowly decreasing serum sodium through fluid administration**. This is most safely accomplished with **oral administration of water**. If the hypernatremia has evolved slowly, extreme caution should be exercised when attempting to decrease serum sodium with fluid therapy. As a rule, slowly **decreasing serum sodium concentrations (over 2–3 days)** is safe, however, serum sodium should be measured frequently to avoid rapid decreases in sodium which can result in life-threatening cerebral edema. Do not decrease serum sodium by more than 0.5 mmol (mEq)/L/h (12 mmol/L/day) if the hypernatremia is chronic.

If metabolic encephalopathy results in cerebral edema, mannitol (1 g/kg IV bolus) and furosemide (0.7 mg/kg IV) can be given provided the cat is not dehydrated. Indications for therapy are severe signs or lack of improvement after 4–6 hours of appropriate medical treatment.

Prognosis

Prognosis depends upon the ability to treat the underlying disease process.

THIAMINE DEFICIENCY*

Classical signs

- Initially, lethargy, inappetence and ataxia.
- Later signs include weakness, ventral flexion of the neck, dilated pupils, stupor, and coma.

See main reference on page 848 for details (The Cat With a Head Tilt, Vestibular Ataxia or Nystagmus).

Pathogenesis

Occurs in **anorexic cats** or cats that are **fed all-fish diets** containing thiaminase.

This deficiency results in polioencephalomalacia of the oculomotor and vestibular nuclei, the caudal colliculus and the lateral geniculate body.

Clinical signs

Early non-specific signs are **typically lethargy and inappetence**.

The earliest localizing sign is **bilateral vestibular ataxia**, which appears as **an abnormal broad-based stance**, loss of balance and vertigo.

There is weakness and an **inability or reluctance to walk**. The cat sits **crouched with ventral flexion of the neck**.

Pupils are dilated and non-responsive or poorly responsive to light reflexes.

If untreated, signs **progress to semi-coma**, persistent vocalization, opisthotonus and death.

Episodes of spastic opisthotonus or ventroflexion of the neck and generalized muscle spasm may occur especially when the cat is lifted or stressed. They may be interpreted as seizures, but true seizure activity rarely occurs.

Diagnosis

No antemortem diagnostic test is available.

Diagnosis is based on **clinical signs** and **rapid response to thiamine**.

Differential diagnosis

Other **encephalopathies** and **encephalitis** are differentiated on history, CSF findings and lack of response to thiamine.

Head trauma may appear similar to late signs of thiamine deficiency, but can usually be differentiated on history and evidence of trauma. Thiamine-deficient cats are lethargic and inappetent days and weeks before signs are severe.

Hydrocephalus can present with central blindness and ataxia, but there is no response to thiamine.

Dysautonomia is a consideration in countries where it occurs. The bilateral non-responsive pupils and ventroflexion of the neck may appear similar to thiamine deficiency, but there is no response to thiamine.

Hypokalemic myopathy, **myasthenia gravis**, **polymyositis** and **organophosphate** toxicity can all cause ventral flexion of the neck. However, **ventral neck flexion in thiamine deficiency is the result of active muscle contraction** associated with increased muscle tone rather than passive ventroflexion from weakness. Thiamine deficiency responds to thiamine supplementation unless in terminal stages.

Treatment

Treatment is **administration of thiamine** dosed typically at 5–30 mg/cat/day per os. Maximum dose up to 50 mg/cat/day.

Severely affected cats should receive at least **1 mg parenterally**.

Change the diet to one with adequate thiamine and **supplement with thiamine for at least a week**.

Prognosis

Mildly affected cats usually recover rapidly following administration of thiamine.

Cats that have progressed to a comatose state have a poor prognosis.

LEAD TOXICITY*

Classical signs

- Rare in cats compared to dogs.
- Nervous system signs include mentation changes, seizures, ataxia, blindness.
- Gastrointestinal signs and hematologic abnormalities may accompany the CNS signs.

Pathogenesis

Lead toxicity usually results from ingestion of lead-containing products.

Removal of **lead-containing paint via sanding** may allow for lead-laden dust to be produced. If this dust contaminates the cat's fur or adheres to the feet, enough lead may be ingested during normal grooming to cause toxicity.

Clinical signs

Early signs are lethargy, inappetence and weight loss.

Gastrointestinal signs (vomiting, diarrhea) and **hematologic** abnormalities (obvious basophilic stippling or nucleated red cells occur in less than 50% of cats with lead poisoning) may accompany the CNS signs.

Nervous system signs include **depression**, behavioral changes, tremors, seizures, ataxia, **blindness** and weight loss.

Diagnosis

Increased **lead levels** in the cat's **blood** best supports a diagnosis.

Differential diagnosis

Rule out other encephalopathies, encephalitis, head trauma, hydrocephalus and tumor.

Treatment

Chelation therapy with **calcium EDTA** (25 mg/kg SC, IM or IV q 6 h for 2–5 days) or **penicillamine** (10–15 mg/kg PO q 12 h) may be necessary to improve clinical signs.

Prognosis

Variable depending upon the degree of toxicity.

Prevention

Prevent exposure to the toxin.

RECOMMENDED READING

Braund KG. Clinical Syndromes in Veterinary Neurology, 2nd edn. St. Louis, Mosby, 1994.

Bunch SE. Acute hepatic disorders and systematic disorders that involve the liver. In: Textbook of Veterinary Internal Medicine, 5th edn. WB Saunders, Philadelphia, 2000, pp. 1326–1340.

Chrisman CL. Problems in Small Animal Neurology, 2nd edn. Philadelphia, Lea & Fabiger. 1991.

deLahunta A. Vetcrinary Neuroanatomy and Clinical Neurology, 2nd edn. Philadelphia, WB Saunders, 1983.

Greene CE (ed) Infectious Diseases of the Dog and Cat, 2nd edn. Philadelphia, WB Saunders, 1998.

Oliver JE, Hoerlein BF, Mayhew IG. Veterinary Neurology. Philadelphia, WB Saunders, 1987.

Oliver JE Jr, Lorenz MD. Handbook of Veterinary Neurologic Diagnosis. Philadelphia, WB Saunders, 1993.

Wheeler SJ. Manual of Small Animal Neurology. West Sussex, British Small Animal Veterinary Association, 1989.

38. The cat with a head tilt, vestibular ataxia or nystagmus

Joane M Parent

> **KEY SIGNS**
>
> - Cat leans, drifts, falls or rolls to the side of the head tilt.
> - Rapid eyeball movement, either horizontally, vertically or rotatory.
> - Reluctance to walk, crouched stance, exaggerated swaying of head, poor to absent normal nystagmus.

MECHANISM?

- Any disease affecting the vestibular system, peripherally or centrally, results in a head tilt that may or may not be associated with vestibular ataxia and nystagmus.
- Pendular (described as oscillatory) nystagmus is not vestibular in origin. It is the result of a defect in the visual pathways. It is always congenital.

WHERE?

- The vestibular system is affected either peripherally, in the inner ear within the petrosal bone, or centrally, within the cranial vault, in the brainstem, at the level of the rostral medulla.

WHAT?

- The diseases of the peripheral vestibular apparatus are the most common. They include idiopathic vestibular disease and otitis media-interna.
- Involvement of the central vestibular system occurs less frequently. The meningoencephalomyelitides, including principally feline infectious peritonitis and fungal conditions, are the most common causes.

QUICK REFERENCE SUMMARY

Diseases causing head tilt, vestibular ataxia or nystagmus

ANOMALY

- Congenital vestibular disease (p 848)

Varying degrees of head tilt, falling and rolling are present from birth. Reported in Siamese and Burmese kittens.

continued

continued

• Congenital pendular nystagmus (p 848)

Nystagmus is due to a congenital defect in the visual pathways observed mainly in Siamese and Himalayan cats. Nystagmus persists for life and is oscillatory in character.

NEOPLASTIC

• Neoplasia (p 845)

Chronic and progressive onset of a head tilt. The head tilt may be associated with facial nerve paralysis, decreased lacrimation and/or Horner's syndrome if the tumor is invading the tympanic bulla (squamous cell carcinoma is the most common tumor of the middle ear), or with somnolence, +/– ipsilateral proprioceptive deficits, +/– trigeminal and facial nerve deficits may occur if the tumor is intracranial at the level of the brainstem.

NUTRITIONAL

• Thiamine deficiency (p 848)

Acute onset of bilateral central vestibular signs (lethargy, pupillary dilatation, poor to absent physiological nystagmus, reluctance to move, and side-to-side exaggerated head movements), in cats fed a fish-based diet containing thiaminase or pet mince containing the preservative sulfur dioxide. Signs may also occur following a period of anorexia. A characteristic posture with ventro-flexion of the neck is present.

INFLAMMATORY (INFECTIOUS)

• Otitis media–interna (p 840)

Ipsilateral head tilt, with or without nystagmus, and with varying degrees of ataxia. Unilateral deafness may result. Neurological structures in the middle ear may also be affected leading to an ipsilateral facial paresis/paralysis, decreased lacrimation and/or a Horner's syndrome. Signs may appear 48–72 hours after an ear flush. Very rarely extension of the infection to the central nervous system occurs.

• Feline infectious peritonitis (FIP) (p 844)

History of chronic illness (fever, inappetence, weight loss, lethargy) that has been unresponsive to antibiotics. Ocular lesions may be present. The neurological disease is variable and depends on the location and extent of the central nervous system lesion. Seizures, changed behavior and head tremor are common. If head tilt is present it is always associated with somnolence, with or without cerebellar signs.

• Cryptococcosis (p 847)

Head tilt and altered mental status are associated with systemic manifestations such as anorexia, upper respiratory tract disease or skin disease. Chorioretinitis and optic neuritis often observed. The neurological disease is variable and depends on the location and extent of the central nervous system lesion.

INFLAMMATORY (NON-INFECTIOUS)

• Middle ear polyps (p 842)

Chronic, progressive onset of a head tilt, facial paresis/paralysis, decreased lacrimation, Horner's syndrome and unilateral deafness. Polyps can occur bilaterally. Upper respiratory signs may be present. A mass may be visualized in the external ear canal or the oropharynx.

IDIOPATHIC

- Idiopathic vestibular syndrome (p 839)

Acute to peracute non-progressive onset of a head tilt with ipsilateral falling or rolling in an otherwise healthy cat. The disorientation may be severe. If the disease is bilateral, the head tilt is not evident, the physiological nystagmus is poor to absent, and the cat moves in a crouched posture, low to the ground. The head swings from side to side in exaggerated motions.

IATROGENIC

- Aminoglycosides (p 849)

Acute onset of peripheral vestibular signs uni- or bilaterally following systemic or topical therapy with aminoglycosides. Deafness may accompany the vestibular signs.

- Ear flush (p 846)

Peripheral vestibular signs that appear immediately or in the 72 hours following an ear flush.

TOXIC

- Blue-tailed lizard ingestion (p 848)

In southeastern United States, ingestion of a blue-tailed lizard is thought to be the cause of an acute unilateral peripheral vestibular syndrome.

TRAUMA

- Fracture of the petrous temporal bone or tympanic bulla, and ethmoid fracture (base of the skull) (p 848)

Peripheral and central vestibular signs following a road accident.

INTRODUCTION

MECHANISM?

The presence of a **head tilt**, ipsilateral to the lesion, is the salient **feature of vestibular disease**. **Nystagmus and/or vestibular ataxia may accompany the head tilt**. The more acute the disease process, the more likely that nystagmus and ataxia are present. In vestibular ataxia, the animal leans, drifts, falls or rolls toward the side of the lesion. The **nystagmus can be resting or positional** (induced by holding the head in full extension), and, vertical, horizontal or rotatory in direction. The direction may change in time. **Pendular nystagmus** (oscillatory with rapid, short excursions) is **not a sign of vestibular disease**.

Occasionally, there is **bilateral vestibular disease**. The animal may be reluctant to move because of severe disorientation. If able to walk, there are **characteristic**

exaggerated motions of the head and neck and the cat moves in a crouched posture close to the ground. Physiological nystagmus is poor to absent. In these instances, a head tilt may not be present, or if present, is subtle on the most affected side.

Circling is not a feature of vestibular disease but is frequent with thalamic and cerebral diseases.

The most important diagnostic step is to differentiate if the disease involves the peripheral OR the central portion of the vestibular system.

Peripheral vestibular disease:
- The head tilt is toward the side of the lesion. The nystagmus is horizontal or rotatory but never vertical, and never changes in direction. The ataxia, if present, is on the side of the head tilt.
- By close proximity, the neurological structures associated with the middle ear may be affected leading to facial nerve paresis/paralysis, dry eye from decreased to absent lacrimation, and/or

Horner's syndrome, partial or complete. The cochlear part of the vestibulo-cochlear nerve may be affected leading to ipsilateral deafness.
- If the disease is **bilateral**, there is no head tilt or only a mild one on the side that is the most severely affected. The more acute the disease, the more severe the disorientation. The cat is reluctant to walk and has a crouched posture, low to the ground. The head characteristically moves from side to side in exaggerated motions and there is often ventroflexion of the head and neck. The physiological nystagmus (normal involuntary rhythmic typewriter-like movements of the eyes initiated by side-to-side movements of the head) is poor to absent.

Central vestibular disease:
- **The most consistent feature indicating central vestibular disease is the concomitant presence of somnolence, or quietness of the animal**. This may or may not be obvious at time of examination, **but will be evident with good history taking**.
- The head tilt is toward the side of the lesion. The **nystagmus is horizontal, rotatory or vertical and may change in direction**.
- Due to their close proximity, **other central nervous system structures may be involved ipsilaterally**. These include the ascending reticular activating system or ARAS (**somnolence**) and the ipsilateral trigeminal nerve (**loss of facial sensation and/or masticatory muscle atrophy**), abducent nerve (**strabismus**), facial nerve (**facial paresis/paralysis**), cerebellum (**tremors, hypermetria**), ascending sensory pathways (**proprioceptive deficits**) and descending motor pathways (**upper motor neuron weakness**).
- Bilateral involvement of the central vestibular system appears clinically similar to bilateral peripheral vestibular disorders in the early phase, except that the animal is more quiet or somnolent. If the cause is not corrected, involvement of other structures of the brainstem and/or cerebellum ensues.

Paradoxical vestibular syndrome.
- In this rare syndrome of central vestibular disease, the head tilt is contralateral to the lesion. The diagnosis is made on the presence of cerebellar signs or

postural reaction deficits ipsilateral to the lesion but contralateral to the head tilt.

WHERE?

Peripheral vestibular disease results from a problem in the petrosal bone or tympanic bulla.
- The peripheral part of the **vestibular apparatus** (receptors and nerve) is **situated in the inner ear**, in close proximity to the middle ear. The inner and middle ear are located within the petrosal bone or tympanic bulla. The **facial nerve, the parasympathetic innervation of the lacrimal glands** and the **sympathetic nerve for pupillary dilatation** are the neurological structures associated with the **middle ear**.
- Diseases of the inner ear can by extension reach the middle ear and vice versa.
- The neurologic structures of the middle ear are more resilient to insult than the receptors in the inner ear (receptors vs axons). As a result, middle ear disease may be present without neurological deficits. With time, facial paresis/paralysis and/or Horner's syndrome may appear.
- The **auditory receptors** are situated in the **inner ear** as well. Unilateral deafness goes unnoticed clinically but is diagnosed with electrodiagnostic testing (brain auditory-evoked potentials).

Central vestibular disease results from an intracranial problem in the brainstem, at the level of the rostral medulla. This area is in close proximity to the cerebellum and pons. This anatomical location is called the cerebello-ponto-medullary angle.

WHAT?

The most common causes of vestibular disease are peripheral and include:
- Idiopathic vestibular disease.
- Otitis media-interna.
- Less common causes are the middle ear polyps and tumors.

Central vestibular diseases are not as frequent as peripheral diseases.
- Inflammatory diseases are the most common, with the clinical signs directly related to the location and

severity of the inflammation. Although inflammatory diseases are multifocal or diffuse pathologically, this is often not the case clinically, where the neurological deficits in most cases can be assigned to one location.

Diagnosis is based on careful history taking (to disclose if there is somnolence or quietness of the animal), physical, neurological, otoscopic and ophthalmoscopic (including Schirmer tear test) examinations, serum protein concentration, cerebrospinal fluid analysis (CSF), CSF anti-coronavirus IgG titer, electrodiagnostic testing (brain auditory-evoked responses), bullae radiography, computed tomography (CT) and magnetic resonance imaging (MRI) scan.

Reference ranges for feline CSF.
- **RBC** < 0.030×10^9/L (30/µl)
- **WBC** ≤ 0.002×10^9/L (2/µl)
- **Cytology (%)**
  - Monocytoid cells 69–100%
  - Lymphocytes 0–27%
  - Neutrophils 0–9%
  - Eosinophils 0
  - Macrophages (large foamy mononuclear cells) 0–3%
- **Protein** 0.036 g/L (36 mg/dl)

It is good practice to request electrodiagnostic testing (BAER) to evaluate for deafness. If deafness is concomitantly present, it is an indication of a more aggressive disorder and a thorough diagnostic work up should be pursued.

When a head tilt is present, or when there is facial paresis/paralysis or a Horner's syndrome, **bulla radiography is recommended** to evaluate the middle ear cavities. An open mouth view is best to compare the density between the bullae. Bulla radiography is not a sensitive tool. It may be normal despite the presence of disease. Computed tomography (CT) scan of the bullae is superior and should be done when available.

Regardless of the cause of the vestibular signs, nystagmus and vestibular ataxia usually resolve, but the **head tilt usually persists for the life of the animal**. It may be barely noticeable but may be **exacerbated after a general anesthetic or when the cat is ill**.

DISEASES CAUSING A HEAD TILT, VESTIBULAR ATAXIA OR NYSTAGMUS

IDIOPATHIC VESTIBULAR SYNDROME***

Classical signs

- Acute to subacute onset of a head tilt, falling, rolling and nystagmus.
- Disorientation can be severe with the cat unwilling to move and crying out with anxiety.
- Otherwise healthy cat.

Pathogenesis

Unknown.

Clinical signs

Possibly higher incidence in July and August in northeast United States.

Cats of **any age** or sex, median age is 4 years old.

Acute, non-progressive, unilateral and occasionally bilateral, **peripheral vestibular disturbance**.

The head tilt, ataxia and nystagmus (most often horizontal) can be severe with the animal crying out with anxiety, reluctant to walk, remaining in a crouched posture or with wide abduction of the limbs.

Rarely, can be bilateral.

Vomiting occasionally occurs, usually soon after onset of signs.

Affected cats are otherwise healthy.

Diagnosis

History of an acute to subacute onset, in a previously healthy cat, of severe disorientation, falling and rolling, that **improves rapidly (a few days to 2 weeks)** and without treatment.

The cat is otherwise healthy and has no other neurological signs.

The otoscopic examination is unremarkable.

Diagnosis is usually by exclusion of other diseases causing similar acute signs.

With currently available diagnostic techniques it may not be possible initially to differentiate this syndrome from otitis media-interna, but the **vestibular signs in otitis media-interna do not usually occur so acutely and severely**.

It is advisable to **perform BAERs**. If there is concomitant deafness, the idiopathic syndrome is ruled out as **only the vestibular system should be affected**.

Differential diagnosis

Otitis media-interna usually has a more progressive history. On otoscopic examination there may be otitis externa, mite infestation and/or a ruptured tympanic membrane. Signs of middle ear disease such as facial paresis/paralysis, decreased lacrimation and/or Horner's syndrome are often present. Radiographic changes in the tympanic bulla are rarely observed. Computed tomography and MRI scans are more sensitive for detecting changes.

Middle ear polyps can cause peripheral vestibular disturbance uni- or bilaterally but since the polyps originate from the middle ear, facial and/or sympathetic nerve deficits are present. The onset is mild and progressive. **Blue-tailed lizard** ingestion is believed to cause similar signs in the southeastern United States. Vomiting, salivation, irritability and trembling are also observed. Signs may be indistinguishable from idiopathic vestibular syndrome.

Aminoglycoside toxicity, especially topical streptomycin, can cause uni- or bilateral peripheral vestibular disturbance but the history reveals use of the drug.

Treatment

Supportive. In a few cats, fluid therapy, intravenously or subcutaneously, may be necessary initially.

Sedation (acepromazine 0.05–0.10 mg/kg IM, SC, IV to a maximum of 1 mg) may occasionally be required if the rolling is severe.

Antibiotics such as amoxicillin or cephalosporine for 10 days are indicated if otitis media-interna cannot be ruled out.

Glucocorticoids are not indicated.

Prognosis

Excellent.

Rapid improvement of the clinical signs within the first 2 weeks in all cats.

Most cats recover entirely but frequently have a mild residual head tilt.

OTITIS MEDIA-INTERNA***

Classical signs

- Acute to chronic history.
- Variable degree of peripheral vestibular disturbance.
- Signs of otitis externa often present.
- Facial paresis/paralysis, decreased lacrimation and/or Horner's syndrome often present.

Pathogenesis

The **infection** extends **from an otitis externa** or **from the oro- and nasopharynx** by way of the eustachian tubes, **or hematogenously**.

Most infections are caused by *Staphylococcus* spp., *Streptococcus* spp., *Proteus* spp., *Pseudomonas* spp. or *Escherichia coli*.

Frequently, mites are the instigating factor for the otitis externa, which leads to secondary microbial infection with spread to the middle ear.

Clinical signs

The diagnosis of otitis media-interna is difficult as, except for surgical exploration of the tympanic bulla, the tests performed have a low diagnostic yield.

The cat may have a history of chronic otitis externa. The ear may be sore to touch. There may be head shaking or scratching and frequent pawing at the ear.

There may be **difficulty in prehension** or chewing food due to pressure on the petrosal bone region upon jaw opening as the temporo-mandibular joint is in the vicinity of the petrosal bone.

The corner of the mouth may be wet with saliva.

On otoscopic examination, the external ear canal may be red and inflamed with a brownish discharge. Mites may be present. The **tympanic membrane may be red and bulging or perforated**.

The onset and the neurological deficits depend on the extension and severity of the infection. The onset of the vestibular signs may be acute with a marked head tilt, disorientation and nystagmus, or, chronic with nothing else other than a mild head tilt.

The **concomitant** presence of **facial nerve paresis/ paralysis, decreased lacrimation and/or Horner's syndrome confirms involvement of the middle ear**. The facial weakness may be subtle. Look for a complete closure of the lids following a single stroke of the finger on both lids at once. Look for saliva-stained hair at the commissure of the lips or for a droop of the lips on the side affected. The symmetry of the pupils is best assessed in a dark room to evaluate for the presence of a partial Horner's syndrome.

Facial nerve paralysis may be accompanied by **kerato- conjunctivitis sicca** because innervation of the lacrimal glands is carried by the facial nerve. A Schirmer tear test should be routinely done in these cases to avoid the formation of corneal ulcer.

Unilateral deafness is often present, but can be substantiated only with electrodiagnostic testing (BAER).

Diagnosis

Otoscopic examination may disclose an otitis externa, mite infestation or tympanic membrane bulging/perforation.

If there is an otitis externa, cytology and culture with sensitivity testing should be done. The same organism may be causing the middle-inner ear infection.

The presence of facial paresis/paralysis, decreased to absence of lacrimation or Horner's syndrome is a strong indicator of concomitant middle ear disease, but is not specific for infection.

On physical examination, there may be pain on opening the mouth or pain upon manipulation of the head.

Hearing should be evaluated with BAERs:
- Concomitant deafness indicates a more significant disease process such as in middle-inner ear infection, but is not specific for the disease. It is an indi-

cation that a more thorough diagnostic work up should be performed.
- Normal hearing does not rule out middle-inner ear infection because the auditory receptors are in the inner ear.

Bullae radiographs have a low sensitivity:
- It is important to obtain an open mouth view to visualize both bullae simultaneously for comparison.
- A normal study does not rule out middle-inner ear disease.
- The tympanic bulla may appear denser if there is an effusion.
- Thickening of the bulla or bone lysis may be observed in more severe and chronic infections.

Cytological examination and culture with sensitivity testing of the middle ear fluid is indicated when an effusion is suspected:
- The myringotomy is done using an otoscope to guide a 2½" spinal needle through the tympanic membrane.

CT or MRI scans are superior to radiographs to confirm tympanic bulla disease, but the changes detected are not specific for infection.

Surgical exploration of the middle ear with cytological examination and culture with sensitivity testing is the only definitive diagnostic tool in middle-inner ear disease.

Differential diagnosis

Idiopathic vestibular disease has an acute to per-acute onset in a cat that is otherwise healthy. There is no facial paresis/paralysis, decreased lacrimation, deafness or Horner's syndrome because the disease is limited to the vestibular part of the inner ear. Signs resolve over 1–2 weeks without treatment.

Neoplasia and middle ear polyps can be difficult to differentiate from middle-inner ear infection without an exploratory bulla osteotomy. If a polyp is visible in the external ear canal or in the oro-nasopharynx, a diagnosis of middle ear polyp is likely.

Treatment

If a bacterial middle-inner infection is suspected, early and aggressive treatment with antibiotics is best. If culture and sensitivity are not available, a broad-spectrum antibiotic is chosen such as trimethoprim-sulfa, cephalosporin or a penicillinase-resistant penicillin (enrofloxacin).

Antibiotic treatment should be continued for **6–8 weeks**.

If otitis externa is present, the antibiotic is chosen based on the culture and sensitivity of the external ear canal. The otitis externa should be treated as well. **Systemic treatment is preferable if the tympanic membrane is perforated or cannot be visualized**. Avoid topical drugs that are toxic for the vestibular and/or auditory system (gentamycin, neomycin). Selamectin (Revolution®) or systemic ivermectin (200–300 μg/kg IM, SC, PO) is preferable as a miticide rather than topical treatment.

Cats with radiographic changes in the bullae are treated with **surgical curettage of the tympanic bulla to allow drainage**, followed by long-term antibiotherapy based on the culture and sensitivity obtained from the sample collected at time of surgery. If the culture is negative, a broad-spectrum antibiotic as listed above is administered for 2–4 weeks.

If there is chronic or recurrent otitis externa, ablation of the external ear canal is indicated.

In the presence of paralysis of the eyelids, artificial tears arc unnecessary if tear secretion is normal as the spread of the tear film is taken over by the third eyelid. **Artificial tears** should be administered 2–6 times daily in the affected eye, **if the Schirmer tear test is abnormal** (< 10 mm/minute), to avoid development of a corneal ulcer.

Prognosis

Facial paralysis and partial Horner's syndrome often remain, although the severity is much improved. An ipsilateral mild deviation of the face occurs over time.

The vestibular signs resolve in most cases, except for the head tilt, which frequently remains for the life of the animal.

The cases managed medically may recur and require surgical curettage at later date.

Prevention

Treat otitis externa effectively when it occurs.

Treat ear mites.

MIDDLE EAR POLYPS**

Classical signs

- Mild and slowly progressive head tilt.
- +/− respiratory signs.
- +/− signs of otitis externa.
- +/− facial paresis/paralysis, +/− Horner's syndrome +/− keratoconjunctivitis sicca, +/− deafness.

Pathogenesis

The pathogenesis is incompletely understood.

The polyp **originates from the middle ear cavity** and is **composed of inflammatory granulation tissue** covered by respiratory epithelium.

The instigating cause is not exactly known. Some believe that it is congenital, to explain its frequency in very young cats. Others postulate that it results from chronic inflammatory middle ear disease, secondary to upper respiratory infections. The respiratory infection would create abnormalities in the eustachian tube epithelium, resulting in poor middle ear ventilation and secondary inflammation.

Most cats with middle ear polyps have a **bacterial infection**. The most common bacterial isolates are *Pasteurella multocida*, *Streptococcus*, *Staphylococcus*, *Bacteroides* and *Pseudomonas*.

The polypoid growth has a tendency to exit the middle ear cavity. It can do so by rupturing the tympanic membrane and **emerging into the external ear canal**, causing characteristic signs of otitis externa, or it **enters the eustachian tube to exit into the nasopharynx** with subsequent upper respiratory signs. The frequency of each end location versus the other is unknown.

The polypoid growth within the middle ear cavity may **encroach on the inner ear leading to vestibular signs**.

Clinical signs

Typically occurs in **young cats**, but any age can be affected (**mean age 1–5 years**; range 6 months to 15 years).

The most common signs associated with a middle ear polyp, which extends into the nasopharynx, are upper respiratory signs including **noisy breathing**, **dyspnea with or without nasal discharge**, **sneezing or coughing** and gagging.

Less often are signs characteristic of otitis externa.

Rarely a head tilt may be present. The head tilt may occur without other signs, or with upper respiratory signs, or with a visible external ear canal polyp.

Since the polyp originates within the middle ear cavity, the neurological structures of the middle ear may be affected causing facial paresis/paralysis, keratoconjunctivitis sicca and/or partial or complete Horner's syndrome. These can also occur without other signs.

Diagnosis

A mild and transient head tilt may be the only abnormality on neurological examination.

The concomitant presence of a **fibrous mass in the external ear canal**, or **upper respiratory signs**, is pathognomonic for middle ear polyp.

The concomitant presence of facial paresis/paralysis, decreased lacrimation and Horner's syndrome with a head tilt is indicative of middle and inner ear disease but is not diagnostic for the type of disease.

If there are upper respiratory signs, **visualization of the polyp in the nasopharynx** under anesthesia is the most efficient way of reaching a diagnosis.
- A glistening, red or pinkish mass filling the nasopharynx, or originating from the eustachian tube may be found.

Otoscopic examination, which may necessitate sedation/anesthesia to evaluate both ear canals and tympanic membranes should be performed.
- Aural inflammation may be present.
- A pedunculated red, pink or grayish mass may be observed in the ear canal.

The polyp may also affect hearing. Presence of deafness is evaluated by doing BAERs.

When a head tilt is present and there is facial paresis/paralysis, decreased lacrimation or a Horner's syndrome, bulla radiography is recommended to evaluate the middle ear cavities. An open mouth view is best to compare the density between the bullae. Bulla radiography is not a sensitive tool. It may be normal despite the presence of uni- or bilateral polyps. CT and MRI scans are superior in the diagnosis of middle ear cavities, and one of these scans should be performed if available.

CT and MRI scans are the most sensitive imaging techniques to reach a diagnosis of middle ear disease, but are not specific for the type of disease.

The final diagnosis is obtained at the time of surgery. **Surgical exploration of the middle ear is the only reliable test to reach a diagnosis. Cytology and culture** and sensitivity of the curetted tissue should always be done.

Differential diagnosis

If the disease process involves the middle ear, otitis media-interna, middle ear polyp and neoplasia of the middle ear cavity cannot be differentiated without biopsies taken at the time of surgical bulla exploration.

Treatment

Removal of the polyp from its origin through a ventral bulla osteotomy is the best therapeutic approach to avoid recurrence. Removal by grasping the polyp and cutting it at the base from the nasopharyngeal or aural location leads to a high recurrence rate.

Horner's syndrome is a frequent complication of bulla osteotomy. It resolves in most cases in 1–3 weeks, but even if it remains, it does not alter the patient's quality of life.

The head tilt, if present at onset, usually remains for the life of the patient. Occasional transient vestibular ataxia is rarely reported as a surgical sequella of polyp removal.

The cat should be treated for 6–8 weeks with an **antibiotherapy** based on the culture and sensitivity done at the time of surgery.

Prognosis

Removal of the polyp by a ventral bulla osteotomy minimizes the risk of recurrence. Recurrence is frequent using oral or aural access to the polyp.

The head tilt usually remains but the other vestibular signs (ataxia and nystagmus) usually resolve.

If facial paralysis is present, ipsilateral deviation of the face ensues.

If a Horner's syndrome is present, it usually improves and the residual deficit (aniscoria) is of no clinical significance.

FELINE INFECTIOUS PERITONITIS**

Classical signs

- Head tilt in a cat systemically ill for a few weeks.
- Non-specific systemic signs such as fever, weight loss and lethargy.
- Chronic progressive disease.
- There may be neurological deficits other than a head tilt.

See main references on page 372 for details (The Pyrexic Cat).

Pathogenesis

The causative virus is a macrophage-tropic mutant of the ubiquitous feline enteric coronavirus.

The clinical disease **results from an immune-mediated response of the host** to macrophage-infected feline infectious peritonitis virus (FIPV). The severity of the disease is based on host susceptibility and strain virulence.

Clinical signs

Affected cats are **usually less than 3 years of age** and **from large multiple-cat households** or breeders.

The most common non-specific systemic signs are **fever, weight loss and lethargy**.

Thirty-five percent of the cats with FIP have neurological signs. These vary with the lesion location. Behavioral changes, head tremor, seizures, depression, compulsive walking and decreased menace are some of the signs that may be observed.

Clinically, the disease frequently appears to be focal, although this is not the case at postmortem.

The head tilt is always associated with somnolence, with or without cerebellar signs, because the cerebellum is closely situated.

Chorioretinitis may be present (see The Blind Cat or Cat with Retinal Lesions).

Diagnosis

The history of **a young cat originating from a multi-cat household** or breeder, with a **protracted disease, vague systemic signs and neurological abnormalities** raises the index of suspicion for FIP.

The cerebrospinal fluid analysis on its own is not sensitive for a diagnosis of FIP.
- Cell counts and protein concentration can be within reference range especially if the disease is focal. Typically, there is a moderate to severe pleocytosis, with mononuclear cells or neutrophils as the predominating cell type, and a marked increase in protein concentration.
- **Protein concentration > 2 g/L increases the likelihood of FIP**.

MRI scan of the brain is helpful, as frequently there is **periventricular enhancement** suggestive of ependymitis, and hydrocephalus with ventricular dilatation. The MRI findings are more representative of the neuropathological extent of the disease than is the clinical presentation, which is often focal in nature.

Hematology and chemistry abnormalities are non-specific except for a high serum total protein concentration, which is frequent.

The **anti-coronavirus IgG titer in CSF is consistently positive**.

The polymerase chain reaction (PCR) test detects the presence of feline coronaviruses but is not specific to FIP coronavirus.

Immunohistochemistry and immunocytochemistry are techniques which appear promising for diagnosis of FIP. They use monoclonal antibody targeted against feline coronavirus to demonstrate coronavirus within macrophages in tissue or effusions. The concentration of infected monocytes in CSF fluid may make the test less sensitive for diagnosis of FIP than if used for tissue sections.

At this point in time, no single test is diagnostic for the neurological form of FIP, but when the history, signalment, serum protein concentration, CSF results, CSF serology and MRI findings are combined, an antemortem diagnosis can be reached.

Differential diagnosis

Other inflammatory infectious diseases of the central nervous system may produce similar neurological abnormalities. However, no other central nervous system infections are typically presented with the gamut of abnormalities mentioned above.

Treatment

There is **no effective treatment for FIP**. Patients almost invariably die. Therapy is based on supportive care. Immunomodulating and antiviral agents seem promising in vitro but have not shown good results in cats.

Prognosis

Poor. Most cats **die of their disease from 6 weeks to 6 months** after the onset of the neurological signs.

Prevention

Since most cats with FIP are from a multiple-cat household or breeder, adequate cleanliness is essential to prevent fecal–oral spread of virus.

Vaccination may be preventive.

NEOPLASIA*

> ### Classical signs
>
> - Otitis externa initially.
> - Subsequent development of peripheral vestibular signs.
> - Swollen face.
> - Facial nerve paresis/paralysis and Horner's syndrome are frequent.

Pathogenesis

The most **common tumor** affecting the middle-inner ear is the **squamous cell carcinoma**. The tumor arises from the epithelial lining of the ear canal and is usually aggressive, invading the adjacent tissue (middle and inner ears) then the skull. Squamous cell carcinomas of the ear canal are most commonly presented with neurological signs.

Ceruminous gland adenocarcinomas are also reported with some frequency in the middle-inner ear.

Clinical signs

Middle-aged to older cats.

Initially, the **signs relate to otitis externa**. There is a more or less rapid progression depending on the tumor type, to cause peripheral vestibular signs, i.e., a **head tilt, with or without nystagmus or vestibular ataxia**.

Due to the invading nature of the squamous cell carcinoma and the ceruminous gland adenocarcinoma, the facial nerve and the sympathetic chain in the middle ear are involved leading to **facial paralysis, decreased lacrimation and Horner's syndrome**.

There is **pain when the mouth is open**, which may result from involvement of the temporo-mandibular joint, soft tissue pain, microfractures (pathological), bone pain from lysis or involvement of the bulla structures.

The face may be swollen and firm on palpation.

Diagnosis

The history of an older cat presented with a **rapid onset of neurological signs** relating to the inner (vestibular signs and deafness) and **middle ear** (facial paralysis, decreased lacrimation and Horner's syndrome) with pain upon jaw opening and a swollen face increases the index of suspicion.

In most cases, **bulla radiography is diagnostic** for the presence of a destructive process. There is opacity in the tympanic bulla with sclerosis and lysis of the bone. Depending on the tumor and how invasive it is, adjacent bony tissue such as the temporo-mandibular joint and the zygomatic arch may also be affected.

Differential diagnosis

As in most cases of middle-inner ear disease, if there is no swelling of the face, surgical exploration of the bulla is the only reliable approach to reach a definitive diagnosis.

Middle ear polyp is usually in young cats, but can be in older cats. Typically, **the progression is slower**. The polyp may be visible in the ear canal or oro-nasopharynx. There is no pain, and no swelling of the face.

Treatment

Aggressive excision including ear canal ablation and lateral bulla osteotomy is the treatment of choice for malignant ear canal tumors. If excision is incomplete, radiation therapy can be a useful adjunct to surgery.

Prognosis

Prognosis is guarded because of the invasive nature of the tumor and advanced stage of the disease by the time neurologic signs are present.

Cats with ceruminous adenocarcinoma have a 75% 1-year survival rate following aggressive ear ablation and bulla osteotomy compared to a 33% 1-year survival after conservative surgical resection. The prognosis is more guarded for squamous cell carcinoma.

EAR FLUSH*

> **Classical signs**
>
> - Acute onset of peripheral vestibular signs that develop immediately or in the 72 hours following an ear flush.

Pathogenesis

The exact pathogenesis is unknown, but several mechanisms have been postulated to be involved. An ear flush that leads to such consequences is usually done under anesthesia or heavy sedation. If the signs develop immediately after the flush, it is possibly due to: (1) a **change in the temperature of the endolymph**; (2) **flooding of the inner ear** through a perforated tympanic membrane; or (3) **a toxic effect on the vestibu-**

lar receptors by the product used to flush the ear (e.g. chlorhexidine, quaternary ammonium compounds).

If the peripheral vestibular signs develop 48–72 hours following an ear flush, **an inner ear infection** is suspected. Bacteria may have been introduced through a perforated tympanic membrane at the time of the flush. The ear flush may not be vigorous for this to occur because the tympanic membrane may have already been ruptured secondary to an otitis externa. Alternatively, topical (e.g. gentamycin-containing ear drops) or systemic treatment administered after the ear flush may be toxic to the vestibular receptors.

Clinical signs

Acute onset of peripheral vestibular signs in the 72 hours **following an ear flush**. The flush may have been an elective procedure or therapeutic for a severe otitis externa.

Diagnosis

Diagnosis is based on the history of acute vestibular signs following a recent ear flush.

Differential diagnosis

Idiopathic vestibular syndrome cannot be differentiated from the iatrogenic cause if the signs appear 2–3 days following the flush.

Treatment

Whenever acute vestibular signs appear to be associated with an ear flush, a **broad-spectrum antibiotic** such as trimethoprim-sulfa, a cephalosporine or amoxicillin should be administered for 2–6 weeks.

Prognosis

If the onset was immediate and due to a change in the temperature or flooding of the inner ear, then the **signs may disappear within a few hours**.

If the signs are the result of toxicity, **the head tilt may remain**.

If the signs appeared 2–3 days later, most vestibular signs resolve except for the head tilt, which usually persists for the life of the animal.

Prevention

If an elective ear flush is to be performed under anesthesia or with heavy sedation, **ensure the tympanic membrane is intact prior to the procedure**.

If the tympanic membrane cannot be visualized, **use only sterile normal saline**, as most ear-cleaning solutions contain components that are potentially ototoxic, such as propylene glycol, salicylic acid, malic acid, lactic acid detergents and dioctols.

Perform ear flush with extreme care. Cleansing the ear with rubber bulb syringes, plastic syringes or water-jet appliances may rupture the tympanic membrane.

If the ear needs cleaning in the consultation room, avoid using solutions that are acidic or potentially ototoxic. Instead of removing the debris manually, let the animal shake its head and dislodge the debris itself after the medication had been put and massaged into the external ear canal.

CRYPTOCOCCOSIS*

Classical signs

- Lethargic cat with a head tilt, +/- ataxia, +/- nystagmus.
- Concomitant upper respiratory tract signs.
- Anorexia, weight loss.

See main reference on page 26 for details (The Cat With Signs of Chronic Nasal Disease).

Clinical signs

Typically, the cat has usually **been ill for a few weeks prior to the development of the neurological signs**.

The systemic signs may have been vague such as **decreased appetite, weight loss, lethargy**, or signs may relate to a specific system such as the upper respiratory tract, the skin or a combination of both.

Chorioretinitis may be present (see The Blind Cat or Cat With Retinal Lesions).

Diagnosis

The development of central nervous system signs in a cat **systemically ill for a few weeks** or having upper respiratory tract signs and/or draining skin lesions should raise the index of suspicion for this infection.

A latex agglutination test measuring the cryptococcal polysaccharide capsular antigen can be performed on the serum, cerebrospinal fluid or urine. However, negative results do not exclude the possibility of disease.

The CSF analysis is often diagnostic because the characteristic budding yeast forms are visible. This is best seen using India ink, but new methylene blue, Diff Quick, and Gram's stain preparation are adequate. Sometimes organisms are not evident, but grow when the CSF is cultured.

- The CSF inflammatory response associated with *Cryptococcus neoformans* **varies greatly**. The CSF may be normal to grossly abnormal with WBC counts ranging from 0 to > 500 cells × 10^6/L (0–0.5 × 10^9/L).
- In mild inflammation, lymphocytes and monocytes predominate. In severe inflammatory responses, neutrophils and occasionally eosinophils are present.
- The protein concentration varies from mildly to markedly increased (> 2 g/L).

If the disease is suspected, but the organism is not visible in the CSF, **CSF culture and/or serology** may provide a definitive diagnosis.

Cats may be simultaneously positive for feline leukemia virus (FeLV) and/or feline immunodeficiency virus (FIV), increasing their susceptibility to infection.

Differential diagnosis

Cryptococcosis cannot be differentiated from **feline infectious peritonitis** in cats presented with a protracted illness and vague systemic signs on history, physical and neurological examination alone. If *Cryptococcus* organisms are not visible, culture or serology may be necessary to establish the diagnosis.

Treatment

Fluconazole is the drug of choice because of its broad antifungal spectrum, its meningeal penetration even in the absence of inflammation, and the fact that serious side effects are uncommon. The recommended dose is 10 mg/kg/day divided twice daily for a period that extends beyond the resolution of all signs by 2–3 months. The drug should be given with food.

Ketoconazole should not be used. It does not penetrate the blood–brain barrier effectively and is hepatotoxic.

See page 26 (The Cat With Signs of Chronic Nasal Disease) for further details on treatment of cryptococcosis.

THIAMINE DEFICIENCY*

Classical signs

- Bilateral vestibular signs, i.e., a characteristic ventro-flexion of the neck associated with a crouched body posture and reluctance to move.
- Bilateral pupillary dilatation with poor light reflexes.

Pathogenesis

Thiamine is a co-enzyme in the oxidative metabolism for energy production in the central nervous system. Thiamine deficiency typically **produces lesions (polioencephalomalacia) in the brainstem gray matter** and more specifically in the vestibular, oculomotor and lateral geniculate nuclei. Focal, bilaterally symmetric hemorrhages are present in affected areas.

The deficiency occurs in cats that are fed an **uncooked all-fish diet** (due to the thiaminase content of the viscera), **diets entirely made of cooked meat** (where the thiamine is destroyed by heating), poor-quality thiamine-deficient commercial diets, or commercial food stored for long periods of time or in excessively hot conditions. In addition, the **meat preserver sodium metabisulfite** releases sulfur dioxide, which **destroys thiamine**. Pet mince meat containing this preserver is thiamine-deficient, and even when mixed with other food may have sufficient preserver to destroy all dietary thiamine.

Anorexia in a sick cat especially associated with polydipsia and polyuria or fluid diuresis **may precipitate thiamine deficiency** and complicate the primary illness.

Clinical signs

Lethargy and decreased appetite, sometimes with increased salivation, occur after 2–4 weeks on a deficient diet.

The cat has an **inability or a reluctance to walk** and therefore may appear weak. This is associated with a characteristic **rigid ventro-flexion of the neck**, a **crouched body posture** and loss of righting responses.

There is **bilateral mydriasis with poor light reflexes** from the involvement of the oculomotor and geniculate lateral nuclei.

Physiologic nystagmus is poor to absent.

Brief **episodes of opisthotonus or neck ventroflexing and muscle rigidity** may appear like seizures.

Bradycardia, and marked sinus arrhythmia may also occur.

If untreated, the cat becomes **comatose and dies**. The time of death varies from 1 week to a few weeks to months depending on the health status of the animal and the amount of thiamine in the diet.

Diagnosis

Diagnosis is based on a combination of a history that the cat has been quiet and anorexic, signs of a characteristic posture with poor to absent physiologic nystagmus indicative of bilateral vestibular disease and **documentation of a thiamine-deficient diet** (usually large quantities of uncooked fish).

Rapid response (within 24 hours) to treatment confirms the diagnosis.

Differential diagnosis

In bilateral idiopathic vestibular syndrome, the cat is healthy just prior to the development of the clinical signs. Thiamine-deficient cats are typically lethargic and anorexic.

Treatment

Injectable thiamine at 10–20 mg intramuscularly. For supplementation, give 5–30 mg/cat/day PO to a maximum of 50 mg/cat/day.

Change diet.

Prognosis

Prognosis is good if treatment is given early when the only clinical signs are bilateral vestibular signs.

Prognosis is poor in the late stage of the disease when the animal's consciousness is significantly altered.

CONGENITAL PENDULAR NYSTAGMUS*

Classical signs

- Siamese, Himalayan and white tiger cats.
- Pendular nystagmus, i.e., the phase of the nystagmus is equal on both sides.
- Present from birth.

Clinical signs

Typically, the **nystagmus has a rapid, short and oscillatory motion that is equal bilaterally**. It is observed especially when the cat is fixing its gaze.

The **defect is within the visual pathways** and **not the vestibular pathways**. No obvious visual impairment is present.

The nystagmus is **always congenital** and is **evident in the first few weeks of life**.

It occurs primarily in **Siamese**, **Himalayan** and white tiger cats.

Medial strabismus is usually simultaneously present.

Diagnosis

Diagnosis is based on the characteristic oscillatory nystagmus.

FRACTURES OF THE PETROUS TEMPORAL BONE OR TYMPANIC BULLA, AND ETHMOID FRACTURE (BASE OF THE SKULL)

Classical signs

- Altered consciousness and head tilt after a recent accident.
- +/– Facial nerve paresis/paralysis and Horner's syndrome.
- +/– Signs of brainstem involvement such as proprioceptive deficits.

Clinical signs

Sudden onset of head tilt associated with **somnolence or stupor** following a road accident or other trauma that caused a fracture at the base of the skull affecting the petrosal and ethmoid bones.

Facial paresis/paralysis and/or Horner's syndrome may be present if there is hemorrhage in the middle ear.

If the injury is primarily intracranial, facial paresis/paralysis and/or ipsilateral proprioceptive deficits may be present.

On otoscopic examination, **blood may be observed in the ear canal**.

Diagnosis

History of a road accident.

Brain auditory-evoked responses (BAER) may be helpful in localizing the lesion to mainly a peripheral or central location.

Survey radiographs of the skull are difficult to interpret because of the juxtaposition of multiple structures.

DRUG-INDUCED

Classical signs

- Unilateral or bilateral peripheral vestibular signs, following the use of drugs that are toxic for the vestibular receptors.
- Concomitant deafness is frequent.

Pathogenesis

Multiple drugs cause damage to the vestibular and/or auditory receptors separately or simultaneously.

Aminoglycosides especially streptomycin, **chloramphenicol, chlorhexidine, cisplatin, furosemide, salicylates and ceruminolytic agents** are a few of a long list of agents that may cause damage to these receptors.

Clinical signs

Toxicity occurs following **systemic or topical administration**.

The vestibular signs are peripheral and can be **unilateral, or bilateral**.

The signs may develop acutely following exposure to a high dose or after prolonged administration (> 14 days). Cats with renal dysfunction are at risk because decreased renal excretion of many drugs results in higher plasma concentrations.

The **vestibular signs may disappear** following discontinuation of the drug.

Diagnosis

The history of use of a drug potentially toxic for the vestibular receptors, topically or systemically.

The vestibular signs may appear immediately following an ear flush, or following topical treatment with a toxic medication, in a cat that has a perforated tympanic membrane.

Prevention

Avoid using any medication in the external ear canal if the tympanic membrane is perforated or cannot be visualized. This includes ceruminolytic agents and detergents.

CONGENITAL VESTIBULAR DISEASE

Classical signs

- Unilateral or bilateral vestibular signs present at birth or developing in the first 12 weeks of life.
- Siamese, Burmese and Tonkinese cats.
- Head tilt and tipping or rolling.

Clinical signs

Reported in **Siamese, Burmese and Tonkinese** cats.

Usually **unilateral vestibular signs**, but **can be bilateral**.

Head tilt with tipping, rolling or falling developing at birth or in the first 12 weeks of life. The head tilt can be marked and may vary with time.

The clinical **signs are non-progressive** and decrease in severity with time, but usually persist for life.

Diagnosis

Diagnosis is based on characteristic signs in a kitten from a susceptible breed.

BLUE-TAILED LIZARD INGESTION

Classical signs

- Southeastern United States.
- Unilateral peripheral vestibular signs following the ingestion of a blue-tailed lizard.
- The cat also salivates, vomits, trembles and is irritable.

Clinical signs

Acute onset of unilateral peripheral vestibular disturbance following ingestion of the blue-tailed lizard. The syndrome has not been well substantiated.

Varying degrees of vestibular signs associated with salivation, vomiting, trembling and irritability.

Spontaneous recovery occurs in most cats.

Death may occur.

Diagnosis

Acute onset of unilateral peripheral vestibular signs in a cat living in southeastern United States with access to lizards. Signs are indistinguishable from the idiopathic vestibular syndrome although salivation, vomiting and trembling are less common with the idiopathic disease.

RECOMMENDED READING

Burke EE, Moise NS, de Lahunta A, Erb HM. Review of idiopathic feline vestibular syndrome in 75 cats. J Am Vet Med Assoc 1985; 187: 941–943.

Faulkner JE, Budsberg SC. Results of ventral bulla osteotomy for treatment of middle ear polyps in cats. J Am Anim Hosp Assoc 1990; 26: 496–499.

Foley JE, Lapointe J, Koblik P, Poland A, Pedersen C. Diagnostic features of clinical neurologic feline infectious peritonitis. J Vet Intern Med 1998; 12: 415–423.

Hammond GJC, Sullivan M, Weinrauch S, King AM. A comparison of the rostrocaudal open mouth and rostro 10° ventro-caudodorsal oblique radiographic views for imaging fluid in the feline tympanic bulla. Vet Radiol Ultrasound 2005; 46: 205–209.

Little CJL. Nasopharyngeal polyps. In: August JR (ed) Consultations in Feline Medicine, 3rd edn. W.B. Saunders, Philadelphia, 1997, pp. 310–316.

London CA, Dubilzeig RR, Vail DM, et al. Evaluation of dogs and cats with tumors of the ear canal: 145 cases (1978–1992). J Am Vet Med Assoc 1996; 208: 1413–1418.

Rand JS, Parent J, Jacobs R, Percy D. Reference intervals for feline cerebrospinal fluid: Cell counts and cytologic features. Am J Vet Res 1990; 51: 1044–1048.

Rand JS, Parent J, Jacobs R, Johnson R. Reference intervals for feline cerebrospinal fluid: Biochemical and serologic variables, IgG concentration, and electrophoretic fractionation. Am J Vet Res 1990; 51: 1049–1054.

Remedios AM, Fowler JD, Pharr JW. A comparison of radiographic versus surgical diagnosis of otitis media. J Am Anim Hosp Assoc 1991; 27: 183–191.

39. The cat with tremor or twitching

Rodney S Bagley

KEY SIGNS

- Head and/or body tremor.
- Twitching.

MECHANISM?

- Tremor is an involuntary, rhythmic, oscillatory movement of all or part of the body. It results from the alternate or synchronous contraction of reciprocally innervated, antagonistic muscles.

WHERE?

- Disease of the nervous system (central and peripheral) and muscle may result in tremor, shaking or twitching.
- Usually tremors with increased amplitudes and slower frequencies (coarse tremor) are associated with cerebellar disorders. Those tremors with decreased amplitudes and faster frequencies (fine tremor) are associated with diffuse central nervous system disease or muscle weakness.
- Tremor can have differing amplitudes (the distance traveled during the movement) and frequencies (how fast the tremor is).

WHAT?

- Disease of the nervous system that results in persistent, generalized (whole body) tremor is usually diffuse (encephalitis).

QUICK REFERENCE SUMMARY

Diseases causing tremor or twitching

COARSE TREMOR AND TWITCHING (INTENTIONAL)

DEGENERATIVE

- Degenerative cerebellar diseases (p 857)

Using storage diseases as an example, these diseases tend to be breed-associated. Clinical signs usually begin in cats less than 1 year of age. Slowly progressive signs are typical and there is no hyperesthesia. When the disease involves the cerebellum, ataxia and hypermetria are most common.

NEOPLASIA

- Neoplasia (p 858)

Tumors involving the cerebellum usually occur in middle-aged to older cats. Clinical signs of cerebella dysfunction may occur acutely or be more chronically progressive.

INFECTIOUS/INFLAMMATORY

- **Cerebellar hypoplasia** (p 855)**

Cats are born with or develop this disease immediately after birth. Clinical signs become apparent when the cat begins moving and are most obvious when the animal begins walking (somewhere between 4–8 weeks of age). Intention tremor, ataxia and hypermetria are often found.

- Encephalitis (p 859)

Viral, fungal, protozoan, bacterial, rickettsial and parasitic agents are potential causes. Multifocal central nervous system signs are most common. Fever and leukocytosis are inconsistent findings. Other signs of a polysystemic disease such as coughing, vomiting or diarrhea may be associated.

TRAUMA

- **Head trauma* (p 856)**

Usually associated with an acute onset of clinical signs reflective of an intracranial problem. Signs present often include alterations in consciousness, paresis and cranial nerve abnormalities. Fresh blood from lacerations on or around the head, skull fractures, blood in the ear canals and scleral hemorrhage may be clues to a previous traumatic incident.

FINE TREMOR AND TWITCHING (UNINTENTIONAL)

DEGENERATIVE

- Degenerative diseases of the nervous system (p 867)

Some of these diseases are inherited with clinical signs beginning in cats less than 1 year of age. Examples include hypomyelination or dysmyelination and motor neuronopathies. Affected animals tend to have a "bouncy" movement. With other degenerative diseases, such as encephalomyelopathy of young cats and spongiform encephalopathy, tremoring may be acquired in young to middle-aged cats.

ANOMALY

- Myotonia (p 866)

Clinical signs are most often recognized in cats between 1–12 months of age. Classically affected cats have a stiff-stilted gait with increased size of the muscles. Tremor, if present, is usually of short duration and episodic.

METABOLIC

- **Hypocalcemia* (p 862)**

Most often occurs after thyroidectomy. Muscle weakness, tetany and tremors are typical. Preparturient hypocalcemia presents as anorexia, lethargy, trembling, muscle twitching and weakness. Primary hypoparathyroidism occurs in young to middle-aged cats and can result in similar clinical signs.

continued

continued

● Hypokalemia (p 865)

Typically older cats or Burmese < 1 year of age. Signs include weakness, inability or reluctance to walk or jump, stiff, stilted gait, neck ventroflexion and sensitivity to palpation of larger muscle groups. A short duration tremor may be present episodically and usually when the cat attempts purposeful movement.

NEOPLASTIC

● Neoplasia (p 869)

A 2-year-old cat has been reported with diffuse tremor resulting from multiple meningiomas. Clinical signs progressed to paresis and ataxia.

INFLAMMATORY

● Encephalomyelitis (p 864)

Clinical signs are often diffuse and may not localize to a single area within the nervous system. Fever and leukocytosis may be present but are inconsistent findings. The associated tremor tends to involve the entire body and is rapid and of low amplitude (fine).

● Myasthenia gravis (p 866)

Typically adult cats or Siamese < 1 year of age. Tremor usually is episodic and occurs during movement. Generalized weakness, a stiff, stilted gait prior to collapse, ventral neck flexion and decreased palpebral reflexes may also be seen. The gait improves with rest.

● Polioencephalomyelitis (p 868)

This is a diffuse nervous system disease that primarily affects the spinal cord. A viral cause is suspected. Signs have a slow onset and are chronically progressive. They include pelvic limb ataxia, paresis, hypermetria, intention tremors, decreased pupillary light reflexes, seizures and hyperesthesia over the thoracolumbar area.

IDIOPATHIC

● **Feline hyperesthesia syndrome* (p 862)**

A syndrome in which cats become suddenly startled, agitated and often run madly, usually when stimulated over the thoracolumbar area of the spine. Skin rippling and spasms occur usually over the lumbar region and the cat may lick or bite this area.

TOXICITY

● **Toxins* (p 861)**

Toxins such as organophosphate, hexachlorophene and ivermectin can affect nervous system transmission and result in tremor. Other signs such as miosis, salivation, urination, defecation and weakness may be present with OP toxicity. Ivermectin resulted in ataxia, tremor and weakness in a kitten.

INTRODUCTION

MECHANISM?

Tremor is an involuntary, rhythmic, oscillatory movement of all or part of the body. It results from the alternate or synchronous contraction of reciprocally innervated, antagonistic muscles.

True tremor ceases with sleep.

Tremor can be **localized to one body** area or be **generalized** and involve the whole body.

Tremors usually have a characteristic distance of travel (amplitude) and speed of travel (frequency). Tremors can be categorized generally into those that have an increased amplitude with a slower frequency (**coarse tremor**) or a decreased amplitude with a faster frequency (**fine tremor**).

WHERE?

Disease of the **nervous system (central and peripheral)** and **muscle** may result in involuntary tremor, shaking or twitching.

Cerebellar disease usually results in a **coarser tremor** that worsens (increases in frequency or amplitude) **when the animal moves** in a goal-oriented fashion (intention tremor).

Other signs of cerebellar disease that accompany cerebellar tremor include **ataxia** (incoordination; swaying from side to side), **dysmetria** ("goose-stepping"; overflexing of the limbs when walking), **menace deficits** (with normal vision, palpebral, and pupillary light reflexes), **head tilt** and **nystagmus.**

Fine tremor (decreased amplitude and increased frequency) is more often associated with **diffuse neuronal disease** or **muscle weakness** that result in involuntary muscle contraction.

WHAT?

Diseases of the intracranial nervous system (primarily the **cerebellum**) resulting in tremor include **storage diseases, brain tumor, encephalitis** and **vascular-based diseases.**

Systemic metabolic diseases altering neuronal or muscle membrane potentials (such as hypoglycemia, hypocalcemia, hypokalemia) can result in tremor.

Diseases that **decrease neuronal impulse conduction via abnormalities of myelin** (hypomyelination) often result in tremor.

Diseases of the nervous system that result in **persistent, fine tremor** are usually **diffuse (encephalitis).**

DISEASES CAUSING COURSE TREMOR

CEREBELLAR HYPOPLASIA**

Classical signs

- Signs are present from the early prenatal period.
- Clinical signs usually remain unchanged or may improve during life.
- Coarse tremor that worsens when the cat moves in a goal-oriented fashion (intention tremor).
- Other signs include ataxia, hypermetria, menace deficits, head tilt and nystagmus.

Pathogenesis

Cerebellar hypoplasia results from **in utero or immediately postnatal infection with the panleukopenia** virus (parvovirus).

Infection of the fetus may occur when a pregnant queen is **vaccinated with a modified-live** panleukopenia virus **vaccination**.

This virus **destroys the external germinal layer of the cerebellum** and prevents the formation of the granular layer.

Some affected cats have a concurrent hydrocephalus and hydranencephaly.

Clinical signs

Clinical signs are most apparent when the animal begins purposeful movement and attempts to walk.

Tremor accompanying the disease usually has a **slower frequency** (2–6 times/second) and **larger amplitude**. The tremor **worsens** (increases in frequency or amplitude), **when the cat moves** in a goal-oriented way (e.g. bends down to eat), which is termed an intention tremor.

Other signs include **ataxia** (incoordination; swaying from side to side), **hypermetria** ("goose-stepping"; overflexing of the limbs when walking), **menace deficits** (with normal vision and pupillary light reflexes), **head tilt**, and **nystagmus** (combination quick followed by slow movement of the eyes).

Clinical **signs** usually **remain static** or **improve with growth** as the cat compensates, causing the tremor to become less apparent.

Diagnosis

Antemortem testing for this disease often results in negative or normal findings.

Routine laboratory investigations are normal.

Definitive diagnosis is usually rendered only at **necropsy** and histopathological examination of the nervous tissue.

In some instances of cerebellar atrophy, a **smaller than normal cerebellum** may be seen on **magnetic resonance imaging** of the intracranial nervous system. This is most readily seen on the sagittal view.

Occasionally, inflammatory cells may be present in cerebrospinal fluid examination in cats with active panleukopenia viral infection. Cerebrospinal fluid with the other degenerative cerebellar conditions and with previous panleukopenia infection is usually normal.

Differential diagnosis

In this age of cat, other inflammatory central nervous system abnormalities such as **toxoplasmosis** infection is possible.

Congenital anatomical defects of the cerebellar may be present.

Trauma occurring at a young age may permanently damage the cerebellum.

Treatment

No treatment is currently helpful for cats affected with this disease.

Prognosis

Clinical signs associated with previous panleukopenia virus infection of the developing cerebellum usually remain static or improve with growth, causing the tremor to become less apparent.

Prevention

Do not vaccinate queens with modified live panleukopenia virus vaccine.

HEAD TRAUMA*

Classical signs

- Acute onset of signs following a traumatic event.
- Evidence of external trauma to the head and face such as facial lacerations, bleeding from the nose and mouth, bruising, retinal hemorrhage, or hemorrhage in the external ear canals.
- Cerebellar involvement may result in intention tremor, decerebellate rigidity, ataxia, hypermetria, head tilt and nystagmus.

See main reference on page 823 for details (The Cat With Stupor or Coma).

Clinical signs

Exogenous injury to the brain occurs most commonly from automobile trauma, although gunshot wounds and falls may also occur.

Cerebellar involvement may result in **intention tremor**, **decerebellate rigidity** (extension of all four limbs and the trunk), ataxia, hypermetria, head tilt and nystamus.

Signs usually begin acutely after trauma.

Intracranial signs most commonly seen include **stupor and coma**, **paresis and gait abnormalities**, and cranial nerve deficits.

Evidence of **external trauma to the head and face such as facial lacerations**, bleeding from the nose and mouth, bruising or **hemorrhage in the external ear** canals may be clues to the traumatic etiology, however, some animals that are uncoordinated may fall and injure themselves secondarily.

Diagnosis

The diagnosis of trauma is usually straightforward when the trauma is witnessed.

In some instances, animals are presented with an acute onset of neurological signs and an unknown history, examining for external signs of trauma such as lacerations or skull fractures is important.

Evaluating the retinas and external ear canals for acute hemorrhage may also provide clues to the diagnosis.

Advanced imaging studies such as CT or MR imaging are useful, primarily for determining structural damage to the brain.

DEGENERATIVE CEREBELLAR DISEASES

Classical signs

- Signs usually begin or are present in cats less than 1 year of age.
- Signs usually are slowly progressive or remain unchanged.
- Signs include coarse tremor, hypermetria, ataxia, intention tremor and menace deficits.

See main reference on pages 934 and 935 for details (The Cat With Ataxia Without Weakness).

Pathogenesis

Cerebellar degeneration is usually an inherited disease.

A hereditary cerebellar degeneration has been described in Japan in cats. An autosomal recessive mode of inheritance was presumed.

Cerebellar degeneration with neuroaxonal dystrophy has been reported in domestic tricolored cats. This is inherited as an autosomal-recessive trait.

Storage diseases result from inherited (or less commonly, acquired) intracellular metabolic derangements that result in abnormal metabolism of cellular products. Cellular products accumulate and afferent neuronal cells physiologically or mechanically, resulting in cellular dysfunction, and hence, clinical signs. Examples include gangliosidosis, sphingomyelinosis, globoid cell leukodystrophy and mannosidosis.

Clinical signs

Clinical signs usually begin between 3–12 months of age.

Cerebellar disease usually results in a coarse tremor that worsens (increases in frequency or amplitude) when the animal moves in a goal-oriented fashion (intention tremor).

Other signs of cerebellar disease that accompany cerebellar tremor include ataxia (incoordination; swaying from side to side), dysmetria ("goose-stepping"; overflexing of the limbs when walking), menace deficits (with normal vision and pupillary light reflexes), head tilt, and nystagmus (combination quickly followed by slow movement of the eyes).

Clinical signs of the hereditary cerebellar degeneration described in Japan in cats begin around 7–8 weeks of age and include head tremor along with ataxia, dysmetria, and intention tremor.

Cerebellar degeneration with neuroaxonal dystrophy in domestic tricolored cats results in head tremors and shaking. Clinical signs begin at 5–6 weeks of age and progress to ataxia and hypermetria. Affected kittens have a lilac color that darkens with age.

In cats with sphingomyelinosis (Niemann–Pick type C disease) clinical signs begin early in life (< 6 months) and progress to ataxia and hypermetria, absent menace responses, and occasionally positional nystagmus. Death usually occurs by 8–10 months of age.

Niemann-Pick type A disease occurs in Siamese and Balinese cats. Head tremor, head bobbing and dysmetria begin at 3–4 months of age. Clinical signs progress to ataxia and paresis, worse in the pelvic limbs.

Diagnosis

Antemortem testing for these diseases often results in negative or normal findings.

Routine laboratory investigations are normal.

Definitive diagnosis is often rendered only at **necropsy** and histopathological examination of the nervous tissue.

In some instances of cerebellar atrophy, a **smaller than normal cerebellum** may be seen on **magnetic resonance imaging** of the intracranial nervous system. This is most readily seen on the sagittal view.

Cerebrospinal fluid with these degenerative cerebellar conditions is **normal.**

With hereditary cerebellar degeneration described in Japan in cats there is marked loss of Purkinje cells upon histologic evaluation of the cerebellum.

In cats with sphingomyelinosis (Niemann–Pick type C disease) cerebellar atrophy, **Purkinje cell loss,** and **neuroaxonal dystrophy** are the **predominant pathological changes.**

Differential diagnosis

In this age of cat, other inflammatory central nervous system abnormalities such as **toxoplasmosis** infection is possible.

Congenital anatomical defects of the cerebellar may be present.

Trauma occurring at a young age may permanently damage the cerebellum.

Treatment

No treatment is currently helpful for affected cats.

Prognosis

Clinical signs associated with **degenerative cerebellar diseases progressively worsen**.

Animals are commonly euthanized due to the progressive incapacitation.

Prevention

Do not breed cats affected that have produced kittens with a presumed genetic or congenital cerebellar disease.

NEOPLASIA

Classical signs

- Signs usually begin in cats 5 years of age or older.
- Signs usually are progressive over weeks to months.
- Occasionally, clinical signs begin acutely.
- Intention tremor is often associated with other signs of cerebellar disease including ataxia, dysmetria, menace deficits, head tilt and nystagmus.

See main reference on page 824 for details (The Cat With Stupor or Coma).

Clinical signs

Signs reflect either **primary nervous parenchymal damage** from the tumor or **secondary** pathophysiological **sequelae** such as **hemorrhage and edema**.

Meningiomas are the **most common brain tumor** in cats and are usually histologically benign.

Less frequent tumors arise from astrocytes, oligdendrogliocytes, ependymal cells and choroid plexus cells.

Neoplasia may secondarily involve the brain via **metastasis** or via **direct extension** from extraneural sites.

Clinical signs usually begin in **cats 5 years of age or older.**

Clinical signs usually are **progressive over weeks to months.**

Occasionally, clinical signs begin acutely.

Intention tremor is often associated with other **signs of cerebellar disease** including ataxia (incoordination; swaying from side to side), dysmetria ("goose-stepping"; overflexing of the limbs when walking), **menace deficits** (with normal vision and pupillary light reflexes), **head tilt**, and **nystagmus** (combination quick followed by slow movement of the eyes).

Diagnosis

Routine laboratory investigations are normal.

Diagnosis of a structural intracranial abnormality in the brain is most readily accomplished with **magnetic resonance (MR) imaging** or **computed tomography (CT)** of the brain.

A **broad-based**, **extra-axial** (arising outside and pushing into the parenchyma) **contrast-enhancing mass** on CT or MR imaging is found in most **instances of meningioma**.

The CT and MR appearance of gliomas is varied and enhancement after contrast administration may not be present. As these tumors arise from brain parenchymal cells, they are **found within the neuroaxis (intra-axial)**.

Choroid plexus tumors, because of the increased concentration of blood vessels within the tumor, often **enhance markedly** after contrast administration. Because of their association with the ventricular system, associated **hydrocephalus is common.**

Cerebrospinal fluid often has **increased protein concentration** but this finding is not pathognomonic for neoplasia.

Cerebrospinal fluid can contain **evidence of inflammation** (contains elevations in nucleated cells and protein content). If CSF is the only assessment made, an erroneous diagnosis of encephalitis may be rendered.

Differential diagnosis

Congenital and inherited cerebellar diseases occur in younger animals.

Cerebrovascular, traumatic and inflammatory conditions can mimic the signs of a brain tumor.

Treatment

Corticosteroids (prednisolone 1–2 mg/kg q 12 h) may reduce peritumoral edema and improve clinical signs.

Surgical removal of primary brain tumors may be accomplished, especially with meningioma.

A well-encapsulated, firm whitish mass is most often encountered at surgery in cats. Cortical parenchyma is usually not infiltrated but rather compressed in cats, leaving indentations in the nervous tissue parenchyma after resection.

Radiation therapy (45–48 Gy) may control tumor growth of some brain tumors.

ENCEPHALITIS

Classical signs

- Diffuse or multifocal neurological signs.
- Cerebellar signs such as intention tremor, ataxia, hypermetria, head tilt and nystagmus.
- Cervical pain can be present.
- Fever is an inconsistent finding.
- Clues of systemic inflammatory disease such as chorioretinitis are often present.
- Other signs of polysystemic disease such as coughing, vomiting or diarrhea may be present.

Pathogenesis

The source of the inflammatory reaction includes both infectious and non-infectious etiologies.

Numerous infectious agents have been incriminated, with the incidence of infectious agents causing meningitis **varying with geographic location**.

Infectious agents causing brain disease include **viral (feline infectious peritonitis), fungal (cryptococcosis,** blastomycosis, histoplasmosis, coccidioidomycosis, aspergillosis), **protozoal (toxoplasmosis), bacterial, rickettsial** and unclassified organisms (**prototothecosis**).

Feline infectious peritonitis (FIP) is caused by a coronavirus infection in cats. This virus can involve various areas of the nervous system including the intracranial structures and spinal cord. Very young and, conversely, very old cats seem predisposed. Of the two forms of FIP that exist in cats, the "dry" form commonly affects the nervous system. This viral infection results in an immune complex vasculitis, which is responsible for most of the pathological effects.

Toxoplasmosis (*Toxoplasma gondii*) can affect the nervous system at any level including the brain and spinal cord.

Neosporosis results in **necrotizing encephalitis** in cats experimentally inoculated with *Neospora caninum*. Only those cats that were concurrently immunosuppressed by administration of methylprednisolone had severe histological brain lesions.

Of the fungal diseases of the brain in cats, cryptococcosis caused by *Cryptococcus neoformans* is the most common. The central nervous system is often affected through **direct extension of the infection from the nasal passages** or from disseminated infection from other organs.

Involvement of the intracranial nervous can occur with parasites such as Cuterebra larvae, toxocara, and aberrant heartworm migration.

Clinical signs

Depression, inappetence or anorexia and weight loss are common.

Clinical signs often reflect multiple levels of neurological involvement. Neurological signs may indicate diffuse or multifocal disease and often do not localize to a single area within the nervous system.

Paresis, gait abnormalities, proprioceptive deficits, cranial nerve defects, and occasionally stupor or coma may occur.

Cerebellar signs such as intention tremor, ataxia, hypermetria, head tilt and nystagmus may occur with involvement of the cerebellum.

Cervical pain can be present.

Fever is an inconsistent finding.

Fundic examination is important to look for clues of systemic inflammatory disease as chorioretinitis, which is often present with diseases causing systematic infection.

Other systemic signs such as vomiting, coughing, and diarrhea may be seen concurrently.

Diagnosis

Complete blood cell count may show evidence of systemic inflammation (e.g. leukocytosis).

Serum biochemical analysis may show evidence of systemic abnormalities if the disease diffusely affects the body (e.g. vasculitis) such as elevated globulin, CK, liver enzymes or creatinine.

Evaluation of titers for the infectious diseases often helps to rule in or out the diseases.

Cerebrospinal fluid analysis (CSF) will usually show evidence of **increased nucleated cells** and/or **elevated protein content**. Occasionally, CSF will be normal.

- Evidence of inflammation on CSF evaluation alone, however, is not specific for primary encephalitis as other CNS disease (e.g. **neoplasia**) **may result in a CSF pleocytosis** and protein increases.
- With feline infectious peritonitis (FIP), cerebrospinal fluid analysis may show a pleocytosis, with either **mononuclear** or non-lytic **neutrophils** as the predominant cell type and **elevated protein** concentration, often > 1 g /L (0.1 g/dl).
- With **toxoplasmosis**, cerebrospinal fluid frequently contains a pleocytosis, usually with mononuclear cells, and occasionally, eosinophils. Increasing IgG or a single positive IgM serum antibody titer is suggestive of active infection. Animals with **neurologic signs and positive IgM titers warrant treatment** for the disease.

With **cryptococcosis**, identification of the organism from cytological evaluation of samples such as CSF, nasal discharge and skin lesions supports the diagnosis. A neutrophilic pleocytosis, and occasionally an eosinophilic pleocytosis may be found on CSF analysis. If positive, detection of the cryptococcal capsular antigen in serum is usually diagnostic. Tissue biopsy and fungal culture of CSF may be more definitive in the diagnosis as occasionally the serum titer is negative.

With parasites such as Cuterebra larvae, toxocara, and aberrant heartworm migration, CSF may show inflammation with eosinophils is some instances.

Imaging studies (CT and MR) are helpful for defining structural lesions. **Multifocal, contrast-enhancing lesions** are usually seen. Occasionally, non-contrast-enhancing lesions are present, especially with toxoplasmosis.

Differential diagnosis

Multifocal signs are more suggestive of **encephalitis**.

Cats with encephalitis may present with signs similar to other intracranial diseases such as brain tumor, trauma, hydrocephalus and cerebrovascular disease.

Treatment

Treatment is directed at a specific infectious cause if found.

Without a definable cause of the encephalitis, the author uses **trimethoprim-sulfadiazine** (30 mg/kg PO q 12 h), **clindamycin** (25 mg/kg q 12 h), and **corticosteroids** (prednisone 1–2 mg/kg PO q 12 h) in combination.

While corticosteroids are contraindicated with infectious diseases, they are often beneficial in the acute treatment of brain inflammation and edema. These associated pathophysiological events often lead to more neurologic deterioration than the organism itself.

If **rickettsial diseases** are endemic, **chloramphenicol** or **doxocycline** can be substituted or added to the regime.

If the animal is receiving phenobarbital, do not use chloramphenicol as this drug will decrease the metabolism of the barbiturate and the animal will become comatose and possible die. Also, chloramphenicol may result in bone-marrow suppression in cats.

With feline infectious peritonitis (FIP), no specific treatment is effective. Immunosuppressive therapy may result in short-term improvement of clinical signs.

With **toxoplasmosis**, treatment includes **clindamycin and trimethoprim sulfa** antibiotics.

For **cryptococcosis** treatments that have had some success for cyrptococcosis in cats include amphotericin B, fluconazole, itraconazole and flucytosine. See page 26 (The Cat With Signs of Chronic Nasal Disease) for treatment details.

With CNS parasites, treatment has not been attempted uniformly and treatment recommendations are anecdotal.

Prognosis

Many of the encephalities are poorly responsive to treatment, and therefore morbidity and mortality is > 50%.

Some infectious encephalities (e.g. toxoplasmosis) may be cured with appropriate treatment.

DISEASES CAUSING FINE TREMOR

TOXINS*

Classical signs

- Tremors may be persistent or intermittent.
- A history of exposure to a toxin is most helpful in diagnosis.
- Diffuse CNS is often present in association with other systemic signs such as vomiting and diarrhea.

Pathogenesis

Toxins may **lower the threshold** for stimulation or **directly stimulate muscles and nerves** to result in tremor.

Organophosphate intoxication potentiates the effect of acetylcholine at the neuromuscular junction and other synapses, by binding with and inactivating acetylcholinesterase. This leads to increased acetylcholine concentrations at the neuromuscular junction, increased receptor stimulation and fatigue.

Hexachlorophene causes vacuolation of white matter that leads to abnormal impulse generation.

Ivermectin increases **GABA** (**inhibitory neurotransmitter**) concentrations and effects in the CNS.

Clinical signs

Cats with **acute organophosphate intoxication** may have signs including **miosis, salivation, urination, defecation**, as well as **muscle weakness**.

A more persistent weakness without associated autonomic signs can occur with **chronic organophosphate toxicity**. Cats may attempt to **walk a few steps**, then **collapse in sternal recumbency** mimicking catoplexy/narcolepsy.

Hexachlorophene toxicity results in **tremors** as the primary clinical sign.

Ivermectin toxicosis has resulted in generalized ataxia, tremor, weakness, incoordination and miosis in a kitten.

Diagnosis

History of exposure to a toxic product is most helpful in establishing a diagnosis.

For organophosphate toxicity, decreased concentration of **serum cholinesterase activity** may lend support to the diagnosis. Depending upon the laboratory, values less than 500 IU/L (normal 900–1200 IU/L) are considered consistent with organophosphate toxicity. Cats with polyneuropathy from chronic OP toxicity may have normal serum cholinesterase activity.

Differential diagnosis

Rule out other diffuse causes of tremor such as metabolic disease.

Physiological functions such as shivering from cold or apprehension should be considered.

Treatment

For organophosphate toxicity, treatment includes protopam chloride **2-PAM** (20 mg/kg q 12 h IV) which reactivates cholinesterase and **diphenhydramine** (1–2 mg/kg PO q 8–12 h) which reduces muscle fasciculations.

- Atropine (0.2–0.4 mg/kg) can be given with acute toxicity to decrease autonomic signs. Current recommendations are that it **only be used if marked bradycardia** is present, because it may **precipitate respiratory arrest**. Salivation and defecation are not life threatening and generally do not require atropine.
- **Diazepam should be avoided** in these cats as it may result in generalized muscle tremor, hypersalivation, miotic pupils, and vomiting similar to acute muscarinic signs of organophosphate toxicosis.

No specific antidote exists for the other toxicities described here.

FELINE HYPERESTHESIA SYNDROME*

Pathogenesis

The cause is unknown.

One theory is that this activity is a manifestation of a focal seizure.

Another theory suggests that it is similar to the obsessive-compulsive behavior associated with Tourette's syndrome in humans, which is the result of dopaminergic hyperinnervation.

Similar clinical signs have been associated with a vacuolar myopathy in cats and toxoplasmosis.

Others have suggested that this may be behavioral disorder.

Some believe that it begins with an inflammatory stimulus such as flea or food allergy dermatitis.

Clinical signs

Cats may become agitated and aggressive and show **skin rippling and muscle spasms**, **usually over the lumbar** area with stimulation such as stroking over the thoracolumbar region.

Cats may appear as though they were **startled**, then exhibit frenzied behavior such as **licking or biting** at the flanks, back and tail or running.

Cats may appear as though they are **hallucinating** and have dilated pupils.

Sudden startling, **running, frantic meowing**, growling, hissing, **swishing of the tail** may also occur.

Episodes may occur multiple times in a day and last 1/2 min to 5 minutes.

Diagnosis

Diagnosis is usually made solely on clinical signs.

A complete neurological examination should be performed to identify pain or deficits suggesting an underlying spinal lesion.

Spinal radiographs should be performed to rule out lumbar and lumbosacral lesions.

Biopsy of the paraspinal muscles should be used to rule out vacuolar myopathy.

IgM and paired IgG titers 3–4 weeks apart can be used to help rule out active toxoplasmosis.

Differential diagnosis

Rule out **dermatitis, lumbosacral spinal or nerve root compression and intracranial disease.**

Determine if the cat is exhibiting normal behavior during **estrus**.

Treatment

Initial treatment should be with anti-inflammatory drugs. Corticosteroid therapy (prednisolone) may help if a flea allergy or other inflammatory stimulus is suspected. NSAIDs like piroxicam or meloxicam or megestrol can also be tried.

Strict flea control may improve clinical signs.

Behavior-modifying drugs such as the tricyclic antidepressants amitryptyline (2 mg/kg or 5–10 mg/cat PO q 24 h), clomipramine (1–5 mg/cat PO q 12–24 h) or the selective seritonin uptake inhibitors fluoxetine (Prozac 0.5–4 mg/cat PO q 24 h) or paroxetine (Paxil, 0.5 mg/kg PO q 24 h) may be helpful in some cats.

Anticonvulsants (phenobarbital beginning at 3 mg/kg PO q 12 h with dose adjustments to maintain trough serum levels at 20–35 µg/ml) may help if anti-inflammatory and behavior-modifying drugs are unsuccessful.

Feeding food without preservatives has been suggested as helpful.

Carnitine/coenzyme Q12 may help cats with vacuolar myopathy. Also antioxidants and omega-3 fatty acids may be useful.

Decrease environmental stress.

Prognosis

Consistent results with any treatment have not been obtained.

Prevention

Flea prevention.

Decrease stress in the environment.

HYPOCALCEMIA*

Classical signs

- Tremor associated with this disorder is usually of short duration and episodic.
- Stiffness and muscle spasm may also occur.
- Twitching of the ears or facial muscles may be present.
- Weakness, lethargy and anorexia are typical.

Pathogenesis

Decreases in calcium **decrease the threshold for neuronal and muscle depolarization**.

Hypocalcemia most often results from **iatrogenic injury to the parathyroid gland** during surgical removal of thyroid tumors.

Primary hypoparathyroidism is reported but is rare.

Hypocalcemia associated with **queening (eclampsia)** is rarely reported but occurs.

Clinical signs

Clinical signs include **weakness, tetany and tremors**.

Spontaneous muscle depolarization can manifest as muscle fasciculation, cramping, rigidity and twitching.

Queens with **preparturient hypocalcemia** present with **anorexia, lethargy, trembing, muscle twitching and weakness**. They resemble the clinical picture of hypocalcemia in cows (**predominantly weakness**), rather than the violent muscle tremor of eclampsia in dogs.

Cats with primary hypoparathyroidism are more often male and typically range from 6 months to 7 years of age. Signs include lethargy and anorexia and a sudden or gradual onset of neuromuscular signs including focal (e.g. ears or facial muscles) or generalized muscle tremors, seizures, weakness or ataxia.

Diagnosis

Diagnosis is confirmed by finding decreased (usually less than < 1.5 mmol/l (6 mg/dl) serum calcium on serum biochemical analysis.

Differential diagnosis

Rule out other **inflammatory causes of muscle disease** and **acute organophosphate toxicity** (history of exposure, signs and low cholinesterase activity).

Physiological functions such as shivering from cold or apprehension should be considered.

Treatment

Treatment involves calcium supplementation and vitamin D therapy.

If clinical signs are present, rapid institution of treatment is indicated with 0.5–1.5 ml/kg IV of 10% **calcium gluconate. Infuse calcium slowly over 10 minutes while monitoring heart rate. Stop infusion if bradycardia occurs.**

Short-term maintenance involves either **SC calcium** (1–2 ml of 10% calcium gluconate diluted 1:1 in 0.9% saline q 8 hours) or **IV calcium** (10–20 ml of 10% calcium gluconate in 500 ml of 0.9% saline) with rate adjusted to maintain normocalcemia. Monitor calcium 2–3 times daily initially.

Longer-term maintenance includes **oral calcium** (25 mg/kg q 8–12 hours) and **vitamin D.** The active form of endogenous vitamin D_3 (called calcitriol or 1,25 dihydroxycholecalciferol) is used at 2.5–10 ng/kg q 24 hours or synthetic vitamin D_3 (dihydrotachysterol) at 0.02–0.03 mg/kg q 24 hours for 3 days, then 0.01–0.02 mg/kg q 6–24 hours.

Calcium should be monitored carefully, as hypercalemia is nephrotoxic.

Adjustments to doses should be made every 1–3 days based on calcium concentrations.

If hypocalcemia is the result of thyroidectomy, calcium and vitamin D therapy can be reduced gradually over 2–3 weeks, and stopped if calcium remains in the normal range.

Prognosis

Acute hypocalcemia following bilateral thyroidectomy can be fatal if not recognized early and appropriate therapy instituted.

Prevention

When performing bilateral thyroidectomy, allow 3–4 weeks between removal of each lobe.

ENCEPHALOMYELITIS

> ### Classical signs
>
> - Any aged cat may be affected.
> - A diffuse, whole-body, low-amplitude, higher-frequency tremor is present
> - Animals may twitch periodically.
> - Neurological signs are often diffuse.

Pathogenesis

This syndrome is associated with histological evidence of inflammation of the CNS. However, a consistent infectious etiology has not been identified.

Encephalomyelitis is a much rarer cause of tremor in cats compared to dogs.

Clinical signs

Any age of cat may be affected.

A diffuse, whole-body, low-amplitude (fine), higher-frequency tremor is present.

Animals may also twitch periodically.

Other neurological signs that may be present in cats with encephalomyelitis include seizures, blindness, conscious proprioceptive deficits and cranial nerve deficits.

Neurological signs may not localize to a single area within the nervous system.

Fever and leukocytes may be present but are inconsistent findings.

Evidence of chorioretinitis may be present on fundic examination.

Diagnosis

Cerebrospinal fluid may contain **increased numbers of nucleated cells** and/or **elevated protein** concentrations.

Nucleated cell counts can vary from mildly inflammatory (0.005–0.020×10^9 cells/L [5–20 cells/µl]; normal < 0.002–0.005×10^9 cells/L [2–5 cells/µl]) to greatly inflammatory ($> 0.05 \times 10^9$ cells/L [50 cells/µl]).

The nucleated cell type is variable, but most often is a mononuclear cell population. Neutrophils may also be seen.

In cats with FIP, CSF protein concentrations are usually elevated at greater than 2 g/L (200 mg/dl), and nucleated cell counts are greater than 0.1×10^9 cells/L (100 cells/µl).

In cats with FIP the predominant nucleated cell type present in the CSF is neutrophils

In cats with encephalitis from other suspected viral etiologies, CSF protein concentrations are usually less than 1 g/L (100 mg/dl), and nucleated cell counts are less than 0.05×10^9 cells/L (50 cells/µl).

Advanced **imaging** studies (CT or MR) may show **multifocal lesions**. Often these **lesions are enhanced** by intravenous contrast administration.

Differential diagnosis

Rule out other inflammatory, metabolic, and degenerative causes of tremor.

Physiological functions such as shivering from cold or apprehension should be considered.

Treatment

Treatment with **corticosteroids** (prednisolone 2 mg/kg q 12 h initially) may improve clinical signs.

If clinical signs improve, the corticosteroid therapy should be slowly tapered (over months) to prevent recurrence.

Prognosis

Clinical response to corticosteroid is variable.

HYPOKALEMIA

Classical signs

- A short duration tremor may be present episodically and usually when the cat attempts purposeful movement.
- Aged cats or Burmese < 1 year.
- Ventral neck flexion.
- Stiff, stilted gait.
- Reluctance to walk or jump, and physical inactivity.
- +/− Sensitivity to palpation of larger muscle groups.

See main reference on page 893 for details (The Cat With Neck Ventroflexion) and on page 945 (The Cat With Generalized Weakness).

Clinical signs

Signalment is typically **aged cats > 8 years** or **young Burmese** < 1 year (usually 2–6 months).

Typically there is a history of **acute onset of weakness**. However, **decreased activity and inappetence** are often present for **weeks to months** prior to presentation.

A **short-duration tremor** may be present **episodically** and **usually when the cat attempts purposeful movement**

Clinical signs include **ventral neck flexion**, **stiff, stilted gait**, and **a reluctance to walk or jump**. Typically, weak cats do not walk far, but soon sit or lie, flopping down, instead of carefully sitting as normal cats do. Sensitivity to palpation of larger muscle groups may be noticed.

Dyspnea occurs when the potassium is very low (2.0–2.5 mmol/L), because of weakness of the respiratory muscles. It may occur after fluid administration because volume dilution and increased urinary potassium loss induced by diuresis may lead to further worsening of the hypokalemia.

Young Burmese cats are susceptible to this disease, and potassium depletion may have played a role in the previously described myopathy of Burmese cats.

Transient episodes of weakness may occur beginning between 2–12 months of age.

Diagnosis

Diagnosis is made by finding **decreased serum potassium concentrations** (usually < 3.5 mmol/L) in association with clinical signs. The severity of signs varies between cats when potassium is 2.5–3.5 mmol/L. Below 2.5 mmol/L and especially below **2.0 mmol/L, signs are life threatening**, with death occurring from respiratory muscle failure.

Serum creatine kinase (CK) may be elevated reflecting the mypoathy associated with hypokalemia.

Electrodiagnostic evaluation is rarely performed. Abnormalities that may be found include increased insertional activity, fibrillation potentials and positive sharp waves, and some bizarre high-frequency discharges.

Muscle biopsies often have minimal change present. Mild myonecrosis is possible.

MYOTONIA

> ### Classical signs
>
> - Usually present in young cats as a congenital problem.
> - Stiffness and muscle spasm found at gait.
> - Steps are short and the limbs are stilted.
> - There is an increase in muscle size.

Pathogenesis

Cats with myotonia have **sustained muscle contraction**, which is initiated voluntarily or with stimulation, and sustained involuntarily.

Myotonia most often occurs as a **congenital problem**.

Excessive muscle contraction is thought to be due to an **abnormal muscle cell membrane** that **supports persistent depolarization.**

Clinical signs

Signs are first evident in young cats < 1–2 years of age.

Affected cats often have a **stiff, stilted gait** and have **large, bulky muscles on palpation.**

Muscle dimpling may occur with **direct muscle percussion**.

Tremor, if present, is usually of short duration and episodic.

Diagnosis

Electromyography demonstrates the characteristic **myotonic potentials** (sounds like a motorcycle revving its engines), and **muscle biopsies** may be supportive of the diagnosis.

Differential diagnosis

Rule out other myopathies such as **X-linked muscular dystrophy** (increased serum creatine kinase, typical muscle biopsy findings). Myotonia has characteristic EMG findings.

Treatment

No treatment has been described in cats.

MYASTHENIA GRAVIS

> ### Classical signs
>
> - Adult cats or Siamese < 1 year of age.
> - Tremor with this disease is usually episodic and occurs during attempts at movement, muscle weakness induced by movement.
> - Ventral neck flexion may also be seen.
> - Decreased palpebral reflex is a helpful clinical sign.

See main reference on page 955 for details (The Cat With Generalized Weakness) and page 896 (The Cat With Neck Ventroflexion).

Clinical signs

Muscle tremors are usually episodic and occur in muscles that are being used.

This is a rare disease in cats. Generally a disease of **adult cats**, except for the **congenital form in Siamese** which presents at < 6 months of age.

Exercise intolerance and **episodic weakness induced by walking** or playing are typical signs. The cat may walk a few steps and flop down. Recovery occurs with rest.

A **stiff, stilted gait** is often noted prior to collapse.

Weakness of facial muscle may also be seen, and this is most evident as a **decrease in the palpebral reflex** and narrowing of the palpebral fissure. This appears to be a more consistent finding in cats versus dogs.

Megaesophagus is uncommon and may lead to aspiration pneumonia.

One cat has been reported with a **jaw-drop and dysphagia** as the only clinical signs.

Diagnosis

Diagnosis is based upon clinical signs of **exercise-induced weakness** that is **resolved with edrophonium**.

An edrophonium response test may suggest the disease if strongly positive. Edrophonium is an anticholinesterase that potentiates acetylcholine (ACH) at the neuromuscular junction. When given IV (0.1 mg/kg), this drug can reverse the clinical weakness seen with myasthenia gravis for a short period of time.

Electromyography and nerve conduction studies will be normal. A decremental response may be seen during repeated stimulation of a peripheral nerve in some, but not all cats.

Single-fiber EMG is a relatively new technique that may aid diagnosis of this disease in the future.

Documentation of **antibodies to the acetylcholine receptor** in serum appears to be the most definitive diagnostic test. In congenital disease, however, these antibodies will not be present.

DEGENERATIVE DISEASES OF THE NERVOUS SYSTEM

Classical signs

- Some degenerative diseases occur in younger animals and some in older animals.

Classical signs—Cont'd

- With the encephalomyelopathy of young cats reported in the United Kingdom, cats 3–12 months were affected, however, the disease was seen in cats up to three years of age. Clinical signs usually are progressive over weeks to months.
- With spongiform encephalopathy of older cats, muscle tremors may be seen in association with ataxia and pupillary dilation.
- Clinical signs of hypomyelination or dysmyelination consist of diffuse tremor accompanied by frenzied behavior and indiscriminate biting. Clinical signs are worsened with activity.
- Motor neuronopathies were in adult cats. Clinical signs included tremor, progressive weakness, cervical ventroflexion, dysphagia and muscle atrophy.

Pathogenesis

A number of degenerative nervous system diseases have been reported in various locations around the world. These include encephalomyelopathy, spongiform encephalopathy, hypo or dysmyelination and motor neuronopathies.

Some degenerative diseases occur in younger animals and some in older animals. Some of the degenerative diseases are inherited and signs begin in cats less than a year of age.

An **encephalomyelopathy of young cats** has been reported in the United Kingdom. Wallerian degeneration was noted primarily involving the spinocerebellar pathways and the ventral funiculus of the spinal cord. A viral etiology was suggested but not proven.

A **spongiform encephalopathy** occurs in **older cats** in the United Kingdom and a prion may be the cause.

Hypomyelination or dysmyelination of the CNS has been reported in two **Siamese cats**. Pathologically there was a deficiency of myelin primarily in the ventral and lateral aspects of the spinal cord. Abnormal oligodendrocyte numbers or function is the suggested pathogenic mechanism.

Motor neuronopathies are diseases that affect the **cell bodies** of the **lower motor neuron** leading to degeneration of the cell in the ventral horn of the spinal cord and occasionally the cranial nerve nuclei. Histologic lesions are most severe in the ventral spinal gray matter and consist of neuronal cell loss and gliosis.

Clinical signs

With the **encephalomyelopathy of young cats** reported in the United Kingdom, cats **3–12 months** were affected, however, the disease was seen in cats **up to 3 years** of age. Clinical **signs usually are progressive** over weeks to months.

Signs include **ataxia, paresis, and "head shaking"**. **Ataxia of the pelvic limbs** was the **initial clinical sign** noted.

Spongiform encephalopathy occurs in older cats, and clinical signs include **muscle tremors, ataxia, dilated unresponsive pupils**, jaw champing, salivation, and behavior abnormalities. In one additional cat the tremor was most obvious in the pelvic limbs. Signs progressed to **severe ataxia and hypermetria.**

Clinical signs of **hypomyelination or dysmyelination** consist of **diffuse tremor** accompanied by **frenzied behavior** and **indiscriminate biting**. Clinical signs are worsened with activity. Reported cats were young Siamese < 1 year of age.

Motor neuronopathies were reported in **adult cats** and signs included **tremor, progressive weakness, cervical ventroflexion**, dysphagia, and **muscle atrophy**.

Diagnosis

Antemortem testing for many of these diseases often results in negative or normal findings.

Definitive diagnosis is often rendered only **at necropsy** and histopathological examination of the nervous tissue.

In some instances of motor neuronopathies, mild to moderate fibrillation potentials were found in the appendicular and paraspinal muscles with electromyography.

Cerebrospinal fluid with these degenerative conditions is normal.

Differential diagnosis

Rule out other metabolic, inflammatory, and toxic causes of tremor.

Physiological functions such as shivering from cold or apprehension should be considered.

Treatment

No treatment is currently helpful or has been attempted for affected cats.

Prognosis

Clinical signs associated with **degenerative diseases progressively worsen**.

Animals are commonly euthanized due to the progressive incapacitation.

Prevention

Do not breed cats affected that have produced kittens with a presumed inherited disease.

POLIOENCEPHALOMYELITIS

Classical signs

- Young to middle-aged cats have been affected.
- Clinical signs have a slow onset and are chronically progressive.
- Signs are variable but include pelvic limb ataxia, seizures, paresis, hypermetria, intention tremors, decreased pupillary light reflexes, and hyperesthesia over the thoracolumbar area.

Pathogenesis

Lesions primarily occur in the **spinal cord** and include **severe degeneration and loss of neurons**, perivascular mononuclear cuffing, lymphocytic meningitis, neuronphagia and glial nodules.

A viral etiology was suggested but not proved.

Clinical signs

Young to middle-aged cats have been affected.

Clinical **signs have a slow onset** and are **chronically progressive**.

Signs are variable but include **pelvic limb ataxia, seizures**, paresis, **hypermetria, intention tremors**, decreased pupillary light reflexes, and **hyperesthesia** over the thoracolumbar area.

Seizures were noted during sleep and were characterized by staring, clawing, biting and hissing.

Diagnosis

Two affected cats were leukopenic, with one having bone marrow hypoplasia.

Cerebrospinal fluid from one cat contained an elevated protein content.

One cat had diffuse, hyper-reflective tapetal areas and subretinal infiltrative lesions upon fundic evaluation.

Definitive diagnosis is often only made at **necropsy.**

Histological lesions are most severe in the spinal cord and included severe degeneration and loss of neurons, perivascular mononuclear cuffing, lymphocytic meningitis, neuronphagia and glial nodules.

Differential diagnosis

Rule out other inflammatory, metabolic and degenerative causes of tremor.

Treatment

No treatment has been attempted.

Prognosis

Clinical signs where progressive up until euthanasia.

NEOPLASIA

> **Classical signs**
> - A cat with multiple meningiomas presented with generalized tremors.

Pathogenesis

A 2-year-old cat with multiple meningiomas presented with generalized tremors. This cat was receiving chemotherapy for a previously diagnosed lymphoma.

Diffuse neoplastic involvement was present pathologically.

Clinical signs

Tremor was the **initial clinical sign** seen.

Clinical signs **progressed rapidly to ataxia and paresis**.

Diagnosis

Multiple tumors were found at necropsy extending from the parietal lobes of the brain to the lumbar spinal cord.

Differential diagnosis

Rule out other inflammatory, metabolic and degenerative causes of tremor.

Treatment

No definitive treatment was attempted.

RECOMMENDED READING

Braund KG. Degenerative and developmental diseases. In: Oliver JE Jr, Hoerlein BF, Mayhew IB (eds) Veterinary Neurology. Philadelphia, WB Saunders, 1987, p. 186.

deLahunta A. Comparative cerebellar disease in domestic animals. Compend Continu Edu 1980; 2: 8.

Forbes S, Nelson RW, Guptill L. Primary hypoparathyroidism in a cat. J Am Vet Med Assoc 1990; 196: 1285–1287.

Inada S, Mochizuki M, Izumo S, et al. Study of hereditary cerebellar degeneration in cats. AJVR 1996; 57: 296–301.

March PA. Degenerative brain disease. Vet Clinic North Am 1996; 26: 945–971.

Palmer AC, Cavanagh JB. Encephalomyelopathy in young cats. J Small Anim Pract 1995; 36: 57–64.

Peterson ME, James KM, Wallace M, et al. Idiopathic hypoparathyroidism in five cats. J Vet Int Med 1991; 5: 47–51.

Shelton GD, Hopkins AL, Ginn PL, et al. Adult-onset motor neuron disease in three cats. J Am Vet Med Assoc 1998; 212: 1271–1275.

40. The cat with anisocoria or abnormally dilated or constricted pupils

Rodney S Bagley

KEY SIGNS

- Inequality of pupil size.
- Inappropriately dilated or constricted pupils.

MECHANISM?

- **Anisocoria** is a resting inequality in pupil size.
- **An abnormally constricted pupil is referred to as a miotic pupil** and results from either excessive parasympathetic tone or decreased sympathetic tone.
- **An abnormally dilated pupil is referred to as a mydriatic pupil** and results from either decreased parasympathetic tone or excessive sympathetic tone.
- Mechanical abnormalities of the iris may also result in abnormal pupil size.

WHERE?

- Disease of the eye, the visual pathways, or the pathways innervating the pupil may result in anisocoria.

WHAT?

- Cats with anisocoria usually have primary ocular disease or abnormalities of iris innervation. Disease of the iris may also be present such as iris atrophy. Systemic disease that alters autonomic nervous system tone may also cause anisocoria.

QUICK REFERENCE SUMMARY

Diseases causing anisocoria or abnormally dilated or constricted pupils

MIOTIC (CONSTRICTED) PUPIL(S)

NEOPLASIA

- **Neoplasia* (p 881)**

Tumors involving the sympathetic nerves may result in miosis. Other signs consistent with Horner's syndrome are usually present. Signs of systemic disease (for example vomiting, diarrhea, enlarged lymph node size) may be found with diffuse diseases such as lymphoma and leukemia. Tumors of the middle/inner ear, which affect the sympathetic nerves, may result in pain, swelling and abnormal discharge from the affected ear.

INFECTIOUS/INFLAMMATORY

● Anterior uveitis** (p 879)

Infection or inflammation of the anterior chamber of the eye may result in miosis as a reflex response to pain or due to vascular congestion of the iris. Conjunctivitis, corneal edema and hypopyon often occur concurrently.

● Spastic pupil syndrome** (p 878)

Cats may have miotic or unresponsive pupils in association with feline leukemia virus (FeLV) infection. Usually the affected pupils do not dilate with dark adaptation and constrict poorly to light stimulation. Other signs of FeLV infection may be evident such as anemia, recurrent infections or neoplasia.

● Middle/inner ear infection** (p 877)

Otitis media/interna infection may affect the sympathetic innervation to the pupil and cause miosis. Other signs of Horner's syndrome such as prolapse of the third eyelid and enophthalmos are usually also present. Discharge from the ear or an abnormally appearing tympanic membrane are usually present.

IDIOPATHIC

● Horner's syndrome*** (p 875)

Horner's includes signs of miosis, enophthalmos, prolapse of the third eye, ptosis and vasodilation. Miosis and prolapse of the third eyelid are most consistent.

TRAUMA

● Brachial plexus avulsion* (p 880)

Characterized by decreased to absent movement, spinal reflexes, and muscle tone in a thoracic limb following being struck by a car or a fall. Miosis as well as other signs of Horner's syndrome can occur in the ipsilateral eye with damage to this area.

● Head trauma** (p 879)

Usually associated with an acute onset of clinical signs reflective of an intracranial problem. Signs present often include alterations in consciousness, paresis and cranial nerve abnormalities. Fresh blood from lacerations on or around the head, skull fractures, blood in the ear canals, and scleral hemorrhage may be clues to a previous traumatic incident.

TOXICITY

● Toxins (organophosphate)** (p 880)

Toxins such as organophosphates that interrupt or override sympathetic impulse transmission or stimulate parasympathetic nerve transmission can result in miosis. Often there are diffuse clinical signs present including salivation, urination, defecation, vomiting or diarrhea. Historical exposure to these toxins is important to ascertain.

● Parasympathomimetic drugs (p 882)

Miotic pupils can occur when drugs that stimulate the parasympathetic system centrally or peripherally are administered. If the drugs result in systemic parasympathomimetic signs, salivation, urination, defecation, vomiting, diarrhea or weakness may be present.

continued

continued

MYDRIATIC (DILATED) PUPIL(S)

DEGENERATIVE

● **Iris atrophy*** (p 883)**

Degeneration of the iris with age may result in a dilated pupil. Irregular pupil margins, tears in the iris and dyscoria are clues. Animals older than 5 years of age are most often affected.

● Spongiform encephalopathy (p @)

Rare in cats. Other clinical signs in addition to dilated pupils include muscle tremors, ataxia, jaw clamping, salivation and behavior abnormalities.

INFECTIOUS/INFLAMMATORY

● **Encephalitis* (p 888)**

Signs of diffuse intracranial nervous system dysfunction are often present including alteration in consciousness, gait abnormalities, paresis and cranial nerve abnormalities. Spinal hyperesthesia may also be found. If the disease affects diffuse body systems, anterior uveitis or chorioretinitis is often concurrently present. Fever and leukocytosis are inconsistently found.

NEOPLASIA

● **Neoplasia* (p 885)**

Tumors within or compressing cranial nerve III may result in ipsilateral mydriasis. If a space-occupying brain lesion is present, other signs seen may include circling, seizures, paresis and abnormalities of vision.

NUTRITIONAL

● **Thiamine deficiency** (p 884)**

Thiamine deficiency may result in dilated pupils. Anorexia and depression are early signs, ventral neck flexion and a crouched body position with reluctance to move are typical. Episodes of seizures – like muscle spasms with neck ventroflexion or opisthotonos may occur. Anorexic cats or cats on all-fish diets are at the highest risk for development.

IDIOPATHIC

● **Dysautonomia** (p 885)**

Reported most commonly in Europe, although the frequency has decreased. Sudden onset of depression and anorexia occur together with signs consistent with a lack of autonomic innervation. In addition to mydriasis, weakness, dry eye, xerostomia, prolapsed third eyelids, bradycardia, loss of anal reflex, incontinence and constipation may be seen.

TRAUMA

● **Head trauma** (p 883)**

Usually associated with an acute onset of clinical signs reflective of an intracranial problem. Signs present often include alterations in consciousness, paresis and cranial nerve abnormalities. Fresh blood from lacerations on or around the head, skull fractures, blood in the ear canals, and scleral hemorrhage may be clues to a previous traumatic incident. Unilateral caudal transtentorial brain herniation results in similar signs.

TOXICITY

- **Toxins* (p 887)**

  Toxins that interrupt parasympathetic nerve transmission or stimulate sympathetic nervous impulses can result in mydriasis. Bites from Elapid (cobra type) snakes often result in mydriasis. Often there are diffuse clinical signs present including weakness, ataxia and prolonged bleeding from venipuncture sites. Fluoroquirolone toxicity may result in a sudden onset of bilaterally dilated, non-responsive pupils. Historical information regarding exposure to these toxins is important to elucidate.

- **Parasympatholytic drugs (p 888)**

  Dilated pupils are most commonly seen following either systemic or topical administration of atropine. With systemic administration tachycardia is often also present. Historical administration of or exposure to these drugs is an important clue.

INTRODUCTION

MECHANISM?

Diseases that affect the iris muscle, other ocular structures, the visual pathways, the nervous system innervation to the iris, or systemic autonomic nervous system functions may result in pupillary abnormalities.

Mechanical abnormalities of the iris such as synechia and iris atrophy are commonly associated with anisocoria.

Abnormalities in the parasympathetic or sympathetic input to the eye often are associated with abnormal pupil size.

Intraocular causes of aniscoria are covered in The Cat With Abnormal Pupil Size, Shape or Response (page 1287) and The Cat With Abnormal Iris Appearance (page 1292).

WHERE?

Disease of the eye, the visual pathways, or the pathways innervating the pupil may result in anisocoria.

The visual pathway includes the retina, optic nerve, optic chiasm, optic tract, lateral geniculate body, optic radiations and the occipital cortex.

Sympathetic innervation to the pupil is responsible for pupillary dilation and innervation to the vessels of the iris (Figure 40.1).
- Sympathetic control is initiated in the hypothalamus of the diencephalon.

- The impulse then descends through the brain stem and cervical spinal cord in the lateral tectotegmental spinal pathway.
- **This upper motor neuron (UMN) pathway synapses** on the cell bodies of the preganglionic sympathetic nerves located in the intermediolateral horns **in the T_{1-3} spinal cord segments.**
- The preganglionic sympathetic nerves exit the spinal cord and run cranially in the cervical sympathetic trunk in the cranial thorax.
- **This pathway continues through the cervical area** with the vagus nerve forming the vagosympathetic trunk.
- The preganglionic nerves synapse in the **cranial cervical ganglion located just caudal to the ear. The postganglionic nerves run through the middle ear**, course with cranial nerve (CN) IX (glossopharyngeal nerve) and then with the carotid artery to enter the skull.
- These nerves then course in the cavernous sinus with the carotid artery, and **exit the skull through the orbital fissure.**
- The postganglionic sympathetic fibers travel with the ophthalmic branch of CN V (trigeminal nerve) to the eye and via the short ciliary nerve synapse on the dilator muscle of the pupil.
- Some postganglionic fibers innervate the smooth muscle fibers in the orbital sheath (musculus orbitalis).
- **Sympathetic innervation to eye includes** the muscle of the periorbita, eyelids (Muller's muscle), the third eyelid, the dilator muscle of the iris, and the

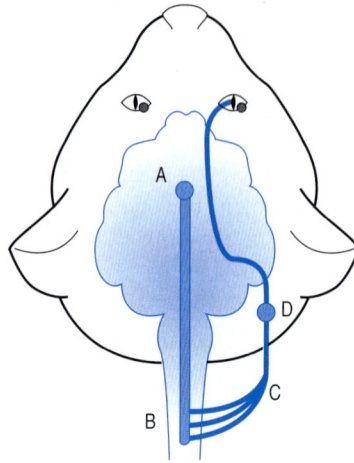

Figure 40.1. Schematic of the sympathetic innervation to the pupil. The information is initiated in the hypothalamus (A), travels caudally bilaterally in the spinal cord to the T1–T3 spinal segments (B), where the preganglionic fibers exit and travel cranially in the vagosympathetic trunk (C). The postganglionic fibers originate in the cranial cervical ganglion (D) and travel to the pupil.

vasomotor fibers to the blood vessels and chromatophores of the uveal tract.

Parasympathetic innervation to the eye occurs through cranial nerve (CN) III (oculomotor nerve) for pupillary constriction (Figure 40.2).

- The afferent pathway for pupillary constriction during light stimulation is the same as for vision from the globe to the lateral geniculate body.
- Prior to synapse in this region, the fibers responsible for the pupillary light reflex (PLR) leave the visual pathway and travel to the pretectal nucleus in the midbrain.
- These fibers project to the ipsilateral and contralateral parasympathetic nucleus of CN III (PSN CN III).
- Contralateral projection is functionally greater than the ipsilateral projection for this reflex, making **the direct pupillary light reflex stronger than the indirect**.
- **The parasympathetic nucleus of CN III is excited bilaterally** with impulses traveling from one eye. Cranial nerve III exits the skull through the orbital fissure and projects to the globe.
- The preganglionic portion of CN III synapses on the short ciliary nerves, which are the ultimate effector of pupil constriction.

- In cats, there are only two short ciliary nerves, a nasal (medial) and malar (lateral), compared to 5–8 in dogs.

WHAT?

Primary disease of the eye such as synechia, iris atrophy or glaucoma can result in an abnormal pupil.

Primary ocular disease of the eye such as uveitis can result in a constricted pupil.

Miotic pupils can result from parasympathetic overstimulation or lack of sympathetic influence.

Miotic pupils can result from an abnormality of sympathetic innervation to the eye. This can cause a miotic pupil alone (Horner's pupil) or in signs of complete sympathetic denervation of the orbit (Horner's syndrome: miotic pupil, prolapsed third eyelid, ptosis, enophthalmos, peripheral vasodilation, decreased sweating).

A large, poorly responsive or unresponsive pupil(s) is indicative of **parasympathetic denervation** of the iris. This can result from disease of cranial nerve III or its nucleus.

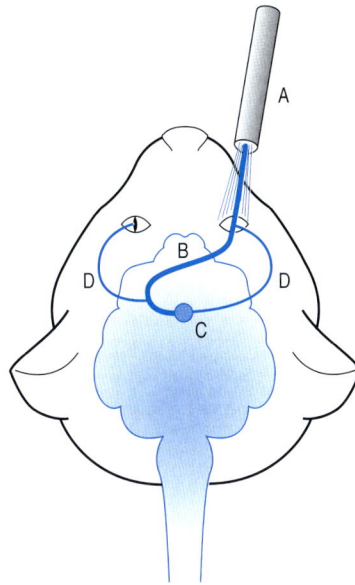

Figure 40.2. Schematic of the parasympathetic innervation to the pupil. The information is initiated by a light stimulus (A), travels caudally in the optic nerve, chiasm and optic tract (B), to the parasympathetic nucleus of cranial nerve III (C). The preganglionic and postganglionic fibers travel to the pupil with cranial nerve III (D).

A larger pupil can be seen ipsilateral to a prechiasmic lesion causing decreased vision. Examples include retinal disease and optic nerve disease (optic neuritis).

A larger pupil can be seen contralateral to an optic tract lesion.

Cerebellar disease may occasionally be associated with anisocoria.
- With unilateral lesions of the fastigial or interposital nuclei, pupillary dilation which is slowly responsive to light may be seen.
- Occasionally, the third eyelid may protrude and the palpebral fissure may be enlarged.
- The pupillary dilation occurs in the eye ipsilateral to an interposital nuclear lesion and contralateral to a fastigial nuclear lesion.

Dyscoria is an abnormality of the form or shape of the pupil or an abnormal reaction of the two pupils to light.

Enophthamos is a backward displacement of the eyeball in the orbit.

Ptosis is drooping of the upper eyelid from paralysis of CNIII or sympathetic innervation.

DISEASES CAUSING MIOSIS

HORNER'S SYNDROME***

Classical signs
- Miosis occurs in association with prolapsed third eyelid, enophthalmos and ptosis.
- Any aged cat may be affected.

Pathogenesis

Horner's syndrome occurs because of an abnormality of, or injury to, the sympathetic innervation to the eye and surrounding structures.

Normal sympathetic innervation is responsible for pupillary dilation.

Any disease that interrupts sympathetic transmission to the eye can result in Horner's syndrome.
- **Infiltration** of these nerves by lymphoma or leukemia cells is possible.
- **Traumatic damage** to the sympathetic system can occur.

Many instances of Horner's syndrome in cats do not have a definable cause.

Clinical signs

Unilateral or bilateral miosis is the most consistent clinical sign of sympathetic denervation.

The affected pupil will not dilate normally in a dark environment.

Other clinical signs constituting a diagnosis of Horner's syndrome include prolapsed third eyelid, enophthalmus, ptosis, and rarely, vasodilation of uveal tract vessels.

If middle or inner ear disease is present, pain and swelling around or ventral to the bulla may be present. There may also be pain upon opening the mouth, swelling in or around the ear, and abnormal discharge in the ear canal may be present.

Diagnosis

The clinical diagnosis is based upon the presence of this constellation of characteristic clinical signs however, these clinical signs are not pathognomonic for any particular disease.

Pharmacologic testing of the eye to determine the location (pre- or postganglionic) of the disease is rarely helpful.

An otoscopic examination should be performed to examine for signs of middle ear disease.

Palpation in the cervical area around the vagosympathetic trunk should be performed to check for masses or other abnormalities.

Radiographs of the bulla may show increased opacity or bony abnormalities if middle ear disease is present.

Advanced imaging studies (computed tomography (CT) or magnetic resonance (MR) imaging) are used to look for intracranial, middle ear or spinal disease.

Cerebrospinal fluid should be collected and evaluated for protein content and cellularity.

If a cervical spinal cord problem is suspected, spinal radiographs, myelography, or advanced imaging (CT, MR) may be needed.

Differential diagnosis

Primary disease of the eye such as anterior uveitis **should be ruled out** by performing a thorough ocular examination.

A neurologic examination should be performed to rule out associated intracranial or spinal disease.

Treatment

As **Horner's syndrome is a clinical diagnosis** and not an etiological diagnosis, any disease of the sympathetic system should be treated specifically.

No treatment is available for idiopathic Horner's syndrome.

Prognosis

The ultimate prognosis will depend upon the underlying cause.

The prognosis for otitis media is good with appropriate surgical or antimicrobial treatment.

The prognosis for brain and spinal cord disease depends upon the nature of these diseases.

Cats with idiopathic Horner's syndrome may improve with time.

Idiopathic Horner's syndrome is not life threatening.

While being a cosmetic abnormality, Horner's syndrome is infrequently irritating to the cat.

MIDDLE/INNER EAR INFECTION**

Classical signs

- Miotic pupil and other signs of Horner's syndrome on affected side.
- Pain on palpation or swelling around or ventral to the bulla may be present.
- Otits externa may be noted but is not constantly present.
- Pain upon opening the mouth and abnormal discharge in the ear canal may be present.
- Head tilt, facial nerve paralysis and nystagmus can result from middle ear disease.
- Abnormal odors may emanate from the ear canal.

Pathogenesis

Inflammation of the middle ear may result in damage to the sympathetic nerve for pupillary dilation, as well as damage to the VIIth (facial) cranial nerve. Extension to the inner ear may damage the VIIIth (vestibular) cranial nerve and receptors resulting in a head tilt, vestibular ataxia and nystagmus. See page 838 (The Cat With a Head Tilt, Vestibular Ataxia or Nystagmus).

Infection or inflammation of the middle ear can result via extension of these processes from the external ear or eustachian tube.

Infection can also occur secondary to systemic infections.

Allergic skin conditions, neoplasia, foreign bodies and trauma to the ear may be associated with middle ear infections.

Organisms present mainly are bacteria and fungi.

Grass awn migration into the middle ear is common in some geographic locations.

Clinical signs

On the affected side there is evidence of Horner's syndrome with a constricted pupil that does not dilate normally in a dark environment.

Pain on palpation or swelling around or ventral to the bulla may be present.

Otits externa may be noted but is not consistently present.

Pain upon opening the mouth and abnormal discharge in the ear canal may be found.

Head tilt, vestibular ataxia with leaning, rolling, rolling to the side of the lesion and nystagmus result from inner ear disease. **Facial nerve paralysis** may result from middle ear disease, and is evidenced by an inability to close the eyelids and loss of sensory innervation to the inner surface if the pinna.

Abnormal odors may emanate from the ear canal.

Purulent discharge may be present in the external ear canal.

Diagnosis

A discolored and outwardly bulging tympanic membrane may be noted with otoscopic examination.

Increased density or bony changes of the bulla may be seen with skull radiographs highlighting the bulla.

Advanced imaging studies such as CT or MR **provide the best views** of the middle/inner ear.

Definitive diagnosis may be made with **myringotomy** and fluid analysis or with surgical exploration (bulla osteotomy).

Culture and sensitivity of any purulent discharge from the middle ear cavity should be performed.

Differential diagnosis

A direct otoscopic evaluation of the ear canal should reveal foreign bodies.

Tumors can result in associated local middle ear infection.

Predisposing causes of recurrent otitis externa such as allergic skin conditions, swimming, immunodeficiencies or anatomical abnormalities of the external ear canal may be evident.

Treatment

Infections from bacterial organisms should be treated with appropriate topical and systemic antibiotics based upon culture and sensitivity results. Amoxicillin/clavulanic acid (14 mg/kg PO q 12 h) in combination is a reasonable antibiotic to begin treatment with prior to receiving culture and sensitivity results.

Antifungal drugs may be used locally or systemically depending upon the offending organism (see section on antifungal therapy).

Foreign bodies should be removed with forceps or a similar instrument or during surgery.

Surgical drainage (bulla osteotomy) **is often needed** for curative treatment.

Prognosis

The prognosis for treatment of middle ear disease with either appropriate antimicrobials or surgery **is usually good.**

Surgery of the bulla may result in complications such as a head tilt and facial nerve paralysis which may be persistent.

Prevention

Early appropriate treatment of otitis externa may be helpful in preventing extension to the middle ear.

Correcting anatomical defects of the ear canal decreases the risk of otitis.

Decrease or stop activities that predispose to water or foreign material collecting in the ear.

SPASTIC PUPIL SYNDROME**

Classical signs

- Pupils are usually fixed at a midrange size and do not dilate appropriately with dark adaptation.
- Pupil diameters may alternate in size between eyes.
- Pupil movement is abnormal (inability to fully dilate in the dark; sluggish constriction to light stimulation).

Pathogenesis

Many, if not all, of these cats are positive for the **feline leukemia virus**.

A **C-type RNA virus** has been demonstrated in the short ciliary nerves and ganglion of some cats.

Additionally, **feline immunodeficiency virus** may play an associated role.

Clinical signs

The pupils are usually fixed at a midrange size and do not dilate appropriately with dark adaptation.

The pupil diameters may alternate in size between eyes, and pupil movement is abnormal. There is inability to fully dilate in the dark and sluggish constriction to light stimulation.

Diagnosis

The diagnosis is suspected in a cat with the appropriate clinical signs that is also FeLV positive.

Differential diagnosis

Rule out **primary iris movement problems such as synechia**.

Treatment

There is no specific treatment for this disease.

Prognosis

The prognosis for the pupillary abnormality is variable.

The overall prognosis will be determined by other associated FeLV-related neoplastic conditions that may arise.

Prevention

Decrease exposure to other FeLV-positive cats.

Vaccination of FeLV infection may provide some prevention.

ANTERIOR UVEITIS**

Classical signs

- Miosis is often present in association with other signs of ocular inflammation including aqueous flare, iridal edema, corneal edema, conjunctivitis, hemorrhage from the iris surface and hypopyon.
- Blepharospasm and photophobia may be seen.
- In some instances, abnormal ocular discharge is present.

See main reference, page 1303 "The Cat With Abnormal Iris Appearance" or page 1165 "The Blind Cat or Cat With Retinal Disease".

Pathogenesis

The underlying process is an **inflammation within the anterior chamber of the eye**.

The miosis may result from ocular pain mediated through a trigeminal (cranial nerve V) constrictor center (oculosensory pupillary reflex) or from **iridal vascular changes**.

Viral disease such as **feline infectious peritonitis infection** and protozoal diseases such as **toxoplasmosis** are often present.

Clinical signs

Miosis is often present in association with **other signs of ocular inflammation** including aqueous flare, iridal edema, corneal edema, conjunctivitis, hemorrhage from the iris surface and hypopyon.

Blepharospasm and **photophobia** may be seen.

In some instances, abnormal ocular discharge is present.

Diagnosis

Clinical evaluation of the anterior chamber for signs of inflammation is performed.

A fine needle aspirate of the anterior chamber may reveal inflammation. See page 1283 Infectious chorioretinitis or anterior uveitis in "The Cat With Abnormal Pupil Size, Shape or Response" for a description of the technique.

Titers for viral diseases (FeLV, FIV) and toxoplasmosis may be helpful.

Titers for feline infectious peritonitis are unreliable.

Differential diagnosis

Rule out other causes of ocular disease such as glaucoma.

Consider local infections such as herpesvirus, *Mycoplasma*, or *Chlamydia*, which cause conjunctivitis and ocular discharge.

Evaluate for systemic organ dysfunction that may accompany FIP and toxoplasmosis.

Treatment

Treatment depends upon the underlying cause. See page 1292 "The Cat With Abnormal Iris Appearance".

HEAD TRAUMA**

Classical signs

- Miosis together with superficial lacerations, bleeding or bruising may indicate a traumatic etiology.
- Trauma to the central nervous system often results in paresis, abnormal consciousness or cranial nerve abnormalities.
- Trauma to the nerves of the brachial plexus may cause lower motor neuron signs (paresis or paralysis, decreased to absent spinal reflexes, decreased to absent muscle tone) in the ipsilateral thoracic limb.

Pathogenesis

External trauma to the body may damage the ocular structures or the nerves to the eye.

Bruising and functional damage (neuropraxia) as well as anatomical disruption (axonotmesis and neurotmesis) may result.

Brachial plexus avulsion resulting in miosis is most often associated with tearing or avulsion of sympathetic nerves that arise in the T1–T3 spinal cord segments and exit the vertebral canal.

Central nervous system trauma may disrupt the sympathetic pathways in either the brain or cervical spinal cord.

Misplaced hypodermic needles in the jugular furrow during blood collection can rarely damage the sympathetic nerves to the eye.

Clinical signs

Miosis may occur with trauma due to involvement of the sympathetic system.

Superficial lacerations, bleeding or bruising may indicate a traumatic etiology.

Trauma to the central nervous system often results in paresis, abnormal consciousness or cranial nerve abnormalities as well as miosis.

Trauma to the nerves of the brachial plexus may cause lower motor neuron signs (paresis or paralysis, decreased to absent spinal reflexes, decreased to absent muscle tone) in the ipsilateral thoracic limb as well as Horner's syndrome in the ipsilateral eye.

Diagnosis

The diagnosis is supported by either a history of known trauma or superficial evidence of lacerations or bruising.

Damage to the nerves of the brachial plexus may result in signs of denervation on electromyographic studies. Abnormal potentials usually begin around 5 days after the trauma.

Advanced imaging studies (CT or MR) provide the best views of the central nervous system.

Differential diagnosis

If active bleeding or bruising is present, an evaluation for underlying clotting disorders such as coagu-

lopathies, platelet abnormalities and vasculitis should be performed.

Treatment

Standard critical care protocols for treatment of traumatized animals should be implemented as needed.

Primary treatment for nervous injury is not possible.

If it could be determined that a nerve is compressed or lacerated, surgical decompression or reconstruction is theoretically possible but is rarely performed.

Prognosis

Milder injuries usually result in a favorable prognosis.

Conversely, severe injuries may result in permanent dysfunction.

Prevention

Keep animals in controlled environments that limit access to automobiles and other traumatic potentials.

Use caution during jugular venepuncture.

TOXINS (ORGANOPHOSPHATE)**

Classical signs

- Acute onset of miosis, salivation, urination, defecation and muscle weakness.
- Rarely, lethargy, anorexia and persistent weakness without associated autonomic signs.

Pathogenesis

Organophosphate intoxication potentiates the effect of acetylcholine at the neuromuscular junction and other synapses, by binding with and inactivating acetylcholinesterase. This leads to increased acetylcholine concentrations at the neuromuscular junction, increased receptor stimulation and fatigue.

A delayed neurotoxicity in cats is reported associated with the use of **chlorpyrifos** spray for household application against fleas. There is individual variation in sensitivity to chorpyrifos, and signs of toxicity have occurred even when used according to label instructions. Toxicity has also been reported with the **flea collars** containing chlorpyrifos.

Clinical signs

Cats with organophosphate intoxication may have **acute signs including salivation, urination, defecation and muscle weakness**.

Postural reactions and spinal reflexes may be depressed in some cats, but may be normal in other cats.

The pupils may be bilaterally dilated and poorly responsive to light stimulation.

Ventroflexion of the neck and muscle tremors may be evident.

Diagnosis

History of exposure to an organophosphate.

Serum cholinesterase activity may lend support to the diagnosis, but may be non-diagnostic for chronic organophosphate toxicity. Values less than 500 IU (normal 900–1200 IU) are considered consistent with organophosphate toxicity.

Electromyographic changes are occasionally present and include fibrillation potentials, positive sharp waves and bizarre high-frequency discharges. A decremental response to repetitive nerve stimulation may be present.

Beware that edrophonium (used to test for myasthenia gravis) **will produce an acute worsening** of signs, which should be treated with atropine (0.05 mg/kg IV).

Differential diagnosis

Rule out other diffuse causes of weakness.

Treatment

Treatment includes 2-PAM (20 mg/kg q 12 h IV) and **diphehydramine** (1–2 mg/kg q 8–12 h).

Atropine (0.2–0.4 mg/kg) can be given with acute toxicity to decrease autonomic signs. Current recommendations suggest its **use only if marked bradycardia** is present as this drug may precipitate respiratory arrest.

Salivation and defecation are not life threatening and generally do not require atropine.

Diazepam should be avoided in these cats as it may result in generalized muscle tremor, hypersalivation, miotic pupils and vomiting similar to acute muscarinic signs of organophosphate toxicosis.

NEOPLASIA*

Classical signs

- Miosis with or without signs of Horner's syndrome.
- Accompanying signs depend on the location of the tumor.
- Tumors causing miosis can occur in the middle ear, ventral cervical area, cervical spinal chord and brain.
- A mass may be palpated in the ventral cervical area with neoplasia of the vagosympathetic trunk.

Pathogenesis

Neoplastic disease may **infiltrate or compress the sympathetic nerves centrally or peripherally**.

If the **middle ear** is affected, the most **common tumors are adenocarcinoma and squamous cell carcinoma**.

Diffuse neoplastic diseases such as lymphoma and leukemias may infiltrate the sympathetic nerves.
- Lymphoma can be associated with feline leukemia virus infection.

Clinical signs

Miosis may be the primary sign or it may occur with other signs of Horner's syndrome. Other neurological signs depend on the location of the tumor.

Neoplasia involving the middle ear can result in pain upon opening the mouth or during palpation around the ear, abnormal otic discharge and swelling around the ear.
- Head tilt, facial paralysis and nystagmus can also be present when both the middle and inner ear are involved.

Neoplasia of the intracranial nervous system can be associated with circling, seizures, behavioral abnormalities, paresis or cranial nerve abnormalities.

Neoplasia of the cervical spinal cord can result in tetraparesis or hemiparesis and cervical pain. If the neoplasia involves the cervical intumescence or the brachical plexus, lameness, decreased reflexes, muscle atrophy and decreased muscle tone may be present in the ipsilateral thoracic limb.

A mass may be palpated in the ventral cervical area with neoplasia of the vagosympathetic trunk.

Lymph node enlargement may be found diffusely if a systemic neoplastic disease is present or locally in the submandibular nodes if middle ear disease is present.

Diagnosis

Palpation of the mass lesion in or around the location of the sympathetic nerves is helpful for diagnosis.

FeLV-positive status may suggest the presence of associated lymphoma.

Fine-needle aspiration of a mass may reveal neoplastic cells.

CBC may reveal circulating neoplastic cells or high WBC counts.

Bone marrow analysis may show the presence of lymphoma or leukemia.

Advanced imaging studies (CT or MR) provide the best views of the nervous system.

CSF analysis may rarely show neoplastic cells.

Increased density or bony changes of the bulla may be seen with **radiographs**, however, advanced imaging studies (CT or MR) provide the best views of the middle/inner ear.

Definitive diagnosis is made with surgical biopsy of a mass.

Differential diagnosis

If a mass lesion is found, other causes of proliferative tissue such as inflammation, infection, hemorrhage and fluid should be ruled out.

Treatment

Chemotherapies are used as definitive treatment of diffuse neoplastic diseases such as lymphoma and leukemia.

Focal masses may be amenable to **surgical resection**.

Radiation therapy may help some neoplastic lesions.

Prognosis

Long-term prognosis with neoplastic conditions such as adenocarcinoma and squamous cell carcinoma involving the ear is poor.

Remission may be achieved with lymphoma following appropriate treatment.

PARASYMPATHOMIMETIC DRUGS

Classical signs

- Local instillation of parasympathomimetic drugs into the eye can cause miosis.
- Systemically administered drugs such as bethanecol result in systemic parasympathomimetic signs, salivation, urination, defecation, vomiting, diarrhea or weakness.

Pathogenesis

Drugs or toxins can stimulate parasympathetic receptors of the iris locally or of the parasympathetic system centrally.

Clinical signs

If there is only **local instillation of parasympathomimetic drugs** into the eye (e.g. pilocarpine, demecarium), **miosis** is likely to be the only clinical sign.

If systemic drug administration occurs causing diffuse parasympathetic stimulation (e.g. bethanecol) **other clinical signs** could include salivation, urination, defecation, vomiting, diarrhea and weakness.

Diagnosis

A history of instillation or administration of these drugs in most helpful.

If the drug works by inhibiting acetylcholinesterase (e.g. organophosphate or carbamate), **cholinesterase activity measured in blood** may be helpful. Values less than 500 IU (normal 900–1200 IU) are considered consistent with toxicity.

Blood cholinesterase activity, however, may not be reflective of drug exposure in all instances, especially in chronic toxicity.

Differential diagnosis

Rule out other causes of miosis.

Treatment

If the drug was administered locally in the eye, stopping additional administrations and allowing time for the drug to be metabolized is most sensible, as this is rarely life threatening for the animal.

In some instances, **local administration of a parasympatholytic drug or sympathomimetic drug** may counterbalance the effects of the parasympathomimetic.

Prognosis

The prognosis is good if the drug was only administered locally in the eye as stopping additional administrations and allowing time for the drug to be metabolized will often bring about resolution of clinical signs.

Prevention

Avoid excessive or inappropriate use of these drugs.

DISEASES CAUSING MYDRIASIS

IRIS ATROPHY***

Classical signs

- Older cats, usually > 5 years of age.
- Pupils are inappropriately dilated.
- Often the margins of the iris are irregular or have tears within.
- The pupils constrict poorly with light stimulation.
- Dyscoria may also be present.

See main reference page 1299 "The Cat With Abnormal Iris Appearance".

Pathogenesis

Iris atrophy is an age-related degeneration of the iris.

Clinical signs

Degeneration of the iris is a common cause of poor pupillary constriction in older animals.

Pupils are usually inappropriately dilated.

Often the margins of the iris are irregular or have tears within.

The **pupils constrict poorly** with light stimulation.

Dyscoria may also be present.

Diagnosis

Diagnosis is based upon the **characteristic clinical signs** consistent with iris degeneration in an aged cat.

Differential diagnosis

Rule out other causes of mydriasis.

Treatment

No treatment is necessary.

Prognosis

Iris atrophy is a non-life-threatening problem that does not result in morbidity.

HEAD TRAUMA**

Classical signs

- Mydriasis may occur secondary to caudal transtentorial brain herniation after brain trauma.
- Facial lacerations, bleeding from the nose and mouth, bruising, or hemorrhage in the external ear canals.

See main reference on page 823 (The Cat With Stupor or Coma).

Clinical signs

Signs usually begin acutely after trauma.

Intracranial signs most commonly seen include stupor and coma, paresis and gait abnormalities, and cranial nerve deficits.

With caudal transtentorial herniation, cranial nerve III is compressed and becomes dysfunctional.

This results in an **ipsilateral dilated pupil** which is poorly responsive to light stimulation.

Evidence of external trauma to the head and face such as facial lacerations, bleeding from the nose and mouth, bruising or hemorrhage in the external ear canals may be clues to the traumatic etiology.

Diagnosis

The diagnosis of trauma is usually straightforward when the trauma is witnessed.

In some instances, animals are presented with an acute onset of neurological signs and an unknown history, **examining for external signs of trauma** such as lacerations or skull fractures is important.

Evaluating the retinas and external ear canals for acute hemorrhage may also provide clues to the diagnosis.

Advanced imaging studies such as **CT or MR** imaging are useful, primarily for determining structural damage to the brain.

THIAMINE DEFICIENCY**

Classical signs

- Initially, lethargy, inappetence and ataxia.
- Later, weakness, ventral flexion of the neck, dilated pupils, stupor and coma.

See main reference on pages 848, 899 for details, "The Cat With a Head Tilt, Vestibular Ataxia or Nystagmus" and "The Cat With Neck Ventroflexion".

Clinical signs

Occurs in **anorexic cats**, or cats that are fed **all-fish diets containing thiaminase**, or cats fed **meat containing the preserver sulfur dioxide**.

Thiamine deficiency **results in polioencephalomalacia** of the oculomotor and vestibular nuclei, the caudal colliculus and the lateral geniculate body.

Early, non-specific signs are typically **lethargy and inappetence**.

The earliest localizing sign is **bilateral vestibular ataxia**, which appears as an abnormal broad-based stance, loss of balance and vertigo.

There is **weakness and an inability or reluctance to walk**. The cat sits crouched with ventral flexion of the neck.

Pupils are dilated and non-responsive or poorly responsive to light reflexes.

If untreated, signs progress to semi-coma, persistent vocalization, **opisthotonos** and death.

Episodes of spastic opisthotonos or ventroflexion of the neck and muscle spasm may occur especially when the cat is lifted or stressed. They may be interpreted as seizures, but true seizure activity rarely occurs.

Diagnosis

No antemortem diagnostic test is available.

Diagnosis is based on clinical signs and rapid response to thiamine.

Differential diagnosis

Other encephalopathies and encephalitis are differentiated on history, CSF findings and lack of response to thiamine.

Head trauma may appear similar to late signs of thiamine deficiency, but can usually be differentiated on history and evidence of trauma. Thiamine-deficient cats are lethargic and inappetent days and weeks before signs are severe.

Hydrocephalus can present with central blindness and ataxia, but there is no response to thiamine.

Dysautonomia is a consideration in countries where it occurs. The bilateral non-responsive pupils and ventroflexion of the neck may appear similar to thiamine deficiency, but there is no response to thiamine.

Hypokalemic myopathy, myasthenia gravis, polymyositis and organophosphate toxicity can all cause ventral flexion of the neck, but do not cause dilated pupils unresponsive to light.

DYSAUTONOMIA**

> ### Classical signs
>
> - Younger cats (< 3 years).
> - Acute onset of depression and anorexia.
> - Dilated pupils, xerostomia, keratoconjunctivitis sicca, prolapsed third eyelids.
> - Bradycardia.
> - Megacolon, constipation, loss of anal reflex.
> - Incontinence, dysuria or distended bladder.
> - Weakness.

See main reference on page 792, "The Constipated or Straining Cat".

Clinical signs

Disease is confined to Europe or occurs in imported cats. The prevalence has decreased markedly and it is now uncommon.

Younger cats (< 3 years) are more often affected.

Clinical signs are often acute in onset over 48 hours with all cats showing depression and anorexia.

Other signs reflect autonomic system dysfunction and include ocular, gastrointestinal and urinary tract signs.

Ocular signs include fixed, dilated pupils without blindness, prolapsed third eyelids and dry eyes (keratoconjunctivitis sicca develops).

Gastrointestinal signs include regurgitation, megaesophagus, constipation and megocolon, loss of the anal reflexes, dry mouth (xerostomia).

Bradycardia (90–120 beats/min).

Dysuria and/or distended bladder or incontinence.

Generalized weakness.

Diagnosis

Diagnosis is based primarily on clinical signs and evidence of autonomic dysfunction. The indirect-acting parasympathomimetic, **physostigmine** (0.02 mg/kg IV) produces no ocular response, but direct-acting **pilocarpine (topically)** results in immediate miosis, demonstrating post-glanglionic denervation hypersensitivity. Normal cats do not demonstrate these responses.

Differential diagnosis

Differential diagnoses are many, depending on the predominant signs. Cats may present with a history of constipation or inability to urinate or dilated pupils, suggesting disease of the colon, lower urinary tract or eyes. Typical cases which exhibit most signs are classical for dysautonomia.

Treatment

No specific treatment is available, but supportive care is important, such as **syringe or tube feeding** and maintenance of fluid and electrolyte balance.

The urinary bladder should be emptied regularly to prevent distention and urinary tract infection.

Parasympathomimetic agents may improve some clinical signs.

- **Pilocarpine ophthalmic drops** (state frequency) may result in pupillary contraction and increase salivation.
- **Bethanechol** (1.25–5 mg PO q 8–12 h) may benefit constipation and urinary retention.
- **Metoclopromide** (0.2–0.5 mg/kg PO, SC, q 8 h) may improve gastric motility.

Up to a 70% mortality rate has been reported and surviving cats may have residual dysfunction such as urinary or fecal incontinence and pupillary abnormalities.

NEOPLASIA*

> ### Classical signs
>
> - ± Mydriasis.
> - Circling, seizures, behavior abnormalities, paresis or cranial nerve abnormalities.
> - ± Discharge from the ear.

Pathogenesis

Neoplastic disease may infiltrate or compress the cranial nerve III centrally or peripherally.

Diffuse neoplastic diseases such as **lymphoma and leukemias** may infiltrate the nerves.

Lymphoma can be associated with feline leukemia virus infection.

The most common intracranial neoplasia in cats is meningioma.

Peripheral involvement of cranial nerve III, most commonly occurs in the middle ear associated with squamous cell carcinoma or adenocarcinoma.

Clinical signs

Mydriasis may occur with involvement of the parasympathetic system within cranial nerve III.

Neoplasia of the intracranial nervous system can be associated with circling, seizures, behavior abnormalities, paresis or cranial nerve abnormalities.

Lymph node enlargement may be found diffusely if a systemic neoplastic disease is present or locally in the submandibular nodes if middle ear disease or other head neoplasms are present.

Diagnosis

FeLV-positive status may suggest the presence of associated lymphoma.

CBC rarely may reveal circulating neoplastic cells or high WBC counts.

Bone marrow analysis may show the presence of lymphoma or leukemia.

Advanced imaging studies (CT or MR) provide the best views of the nervous system.

CSF analysis rarely may show neoplastic cells. The most common change is a mild increase in CSF protein and normal or slightly increased cell counts.

Definitive diagnosis of neoplasia is made with surgical biopsy of a mass.

Differential diagnosis

If a mass lesion is found, other causes of proliferative tissue such as inflammation, infection, hemorrhage and fluid should be ruled out.

Treatment

Chemotherapies are used as definitive treatment of diffuse neoplastic diseases such as lymphoma and leukemia, see page 742 "The Cat With Signs of Chronic Small Bowel Diarrhea".

Focal masses such as meningioma may be amenable to **surgical resection**.

Radiation therapy may help some neoplastic diseases.

Prognosis

Long-term prognosis for cats with meningiomas is good (~24 month median survival).

Remission may be achieved with lymphoma following appropriate treatment.

ENCEPHALITIS*

Classical signs

- Mydriasis can occur due to involvement of the oculomotor nerve.
- Neurological signs are often diffuse or multifocal, but may localize to a single area.
- Cervical pain can be present.
- Fever is an inconsistent finding.
- Chorioretinitis is often present.

See main reference on page 859 for details "The Cat With Tremor or Twitching".

Clinical signs

Infectious agents causing brain disease include **viral** (feline infectious peritonitis), **fungal** (cryptococcosis, blastomycosis, histoplasmosis, coccidioidomycosis, aspergillosis), **protozoal** (toxoplasmosis), **bacterial, rickettsial, and unclassified organisms** (prototheco-sis). Signs depend on the area of the brain affected.

Mydriasis occurs secondary to **involvement of the oculomotor nerve** via direct inflammation of the nerve or damage due to nerve compression (i.e. from cerebral swelling).

Neurological signs are often **diffuse or multifocal** but may localize to a single area.

Cervical pain can be present.

Fever is an inconsistent finding.

Fundic examination is important to look for clues of systemic inflammatory diseases, as **chorioretinitis** is often present.

Diagnosis

Complete blood cell count may show evidence of systemic inflammation (e.g. leukocytosis).

Serum biochemical analysis may show evidence of systemic abnormalities if the disease diffusely affects the body (e.g. hyperglobulinemia).

Cerebrospinal fluid (CSF) **analysis** will usually show evidence of increased nucleated cells and/or elevated protein content. Occasionally, CSF will be normal.
- Evidence of inflammation on CSF evaluation alone, however, is not specific for primary encephalitis as other CNS disease (e.g. neoplasia) may result in CSF pleocytosis and protein increases.

Evaluation of titers for specific infectious diseases, is often necessary to make a diagnosis.

With feline infectious peritonitis (FIP), cerebrospinal fluid analysis may show a pleocytosis, with either mononuclear cells or neutrophils as the predominant cell type.

With toxoplasmosis, cerebrospinal fluid frequently contains a pleocytosis, usually with mononuclear cells, and occasionally, eosinophils. An increasing IgG titer or a single positive IgM serum antibody titer is suggestive of active infection. Animals with neurologic signs and positive IgM titers warrant treatment for the disease.

With cryptococcosis, identification of the organism from cytological evaluation of samples such as CSF, nasal discharge and skin lesions support the diagnosis. A neutrophilic pleocytosis and occasionally an eosinophilic pleocytosis may be found on CSF analysis. Detection of the cryptococcal capsular antigen is possible in serum, or CSF. Tissue biopsy and fungal culture, or culture of CSF may be more definitive in the diagnosis.

With parasites such as *Cuterebra* larvae, toxocara, and aberrant heartworm migration, CSF may show inflammation with eosinophils is some instances.

Imaging studies (CT and MR) are helpful for defining structural lesions. Multifocal, contrast-enhancing lesions are usually seen. Occasionally, non-contrast-enhancing lesions are present, especially with toxoplasmosis.

TOXINS*

> ### Classical signs
>
> - Cats with organophosphate intoxication may have acute signs including miosis, salivation, urination, defecation and muscle weakness.
> - Envenomation from snakes may also cause dilated pupils. Weakness, ataxia and coagulopathy may occur.
> - Sudden onset of unresponsive, bilaterally dilated pupils occasionally occurs with fluoroquinolone.

See main reference on page 949 "The Cat With Generalized Weakness" and page 861 "The Cat With Tremor or Twitching".

Clinical signs

Cats with organophosphate intoxication may have acute signs including miosis, salivation, urination, defecation and muscle weakness or tremor.
- Occasionally the pupils have been reported to be bilaterally dilated and poorly responsive to light stimulation.

Snake envenomation may be associated with dilated pupils as well as ataxia, weakness or paralysis.

Sudden onset of bilaterally dilated pupils that are unresponsive to light occasionally occurs following **fluoroquinolone** use, especially when used at higher than recommended doses. Retinas appear normal on fundoscopy. Prognosis for return of vision is guarded unless the toxicity is recognized early and the drug stopped.

Diagnosis

Serum cholinesterase activity may lend support to the diagnosis of organophosphate toxicity, but may be non-diagnostic for chronic organophosphate toxicity. Values less than 500 IU/L (normal 900–1200 IU/L) are considered consistent with organophosphate toxicity.

Diagnosis of snake bite depends on the type of snake. Weak cats with mydriasis and evidence of rhabdomyolysis (markedly elevated creatine kinase) or coagulopathy (bleeding from venepuncture sites or increased activated clotting time) should be suspected if the snake bite is from an Elapid (cobra type) snake if in the right geographical location and season.

History of recent fluoroquinolone use, especially of doses higher than the recommended dose of 5 mg/kg q 24 h.

PARASYMPATHOLYTIC DRUGS

Classical signs

- Mydriasis with or without dry mouth, tachycardia, and ileus or constipation may be seen.

Pathogenesis

Some drugs or toxins prevent or reverse stimulation of the parasympathetic receptors. **Atropine** would be a commonly used example.

Clinical signs

If there is only local stimulation of the eye, mydriasis is likely to be the only clinical sign.

If systemic parasympathetic stimulation occurs, other clinical signs could include dry mouth, **tachycardia**, ileus or constipation.

Diagnosis

Determining a **history of instillation or administration** of these drugs is the only practical way of diagnosing this problem.

Differential diagnosis

Rule out other causes of mydriasis.

Treatment

If the drug was administered locally in the eye, stopping additional administrations and allowing time for the drug to be metabolized in most sensible as this is rarely life threatening for the animal. It may take **1–2 weeks for normal pupil responses** to return.

SPONGIFORM ENCEPHALOPATHY

Classical signs

- Dilated pupils in association with other clinical signs including muscle tremors, ataxia, jaw clamping, salivation and behavior abnormalities.

Pathogenesis

There is **vacuolation** within areas of the central nervous system.

No causative agent has been identified.

Speculation of an infectious agent (prion) as in other spongiform encephalopathies as a cause has been suggested.

Clinical signs

Dilated pupils.

Other signs include **muscle tremors, ataxia, jaw clamping, salivation and behavior abnormalities**.

Signs may progress to severe ataxia and hypermetria.

Diagnosis

Definitive diagnosis is made only at necropsy and histologic examination of the nervous system.

Differential diagnosis

Rule out other causes of mydriasis.

Treatment

No treatment has been used.

Prognosis

Affected cats have died or been euthanized.

RECOMMENDED READING

Collins BK. Disorders of the pupil. In: August JR (ed) Consultations in Feline Internal Medicine, 2nd ed. Philadelphia, WB Saunders, 1994, pp. 421–428.

Holland CT. Horner's syndrome and ipsilateral hemipelgia in three cats. J Small Anim Pract 1996, 37: 442–446.

Kern TJ, Aromando MC, Erb HN. Horner's syndrome in dogs and cats: 100 cases (1975–1985). J Am Vet Med Assoc 1989; 195: 369.

Morgan RV, Zanotti SW. Horner's syndrome in dogs and cats: 49 cases (1980–1986). J Am Vet Med Assoc 1989; 194: 1096.

Neer TM. Horner's syndrome: Anatomy, diagnosis and causes. Comp Contin Ed Pract Vet 1984; 6: 740–746.

Neer TM, Carter JD. Anisocoia in dogs and cats: Ocular and neurologic causes. Comp Contin Ed Pract Vet 1987; 9: 817–823.

Scagliotti RH. Neuro-ophthalmology. Prog Vet Neurol 1990; 1: 157.

41. The cat with neck ventroflexion

Danièlle Gunn-Moore

> **KEY SIGNS**
>
> - Ventral flexion of neck and lowered head.
> - ± Stiff stilted gait.
> - ± Muscle weakness.
> - ± Muscle pain.

MECHANISM?

- Neck ventroflexion is typically seen as part of generalized muscle weakness.

WHERE?

- The muscles, neuromuscular junction or nervous system.

WHAT?

- The most common cause of neck ventroflexion is **hypokalemic myopathy resulting from chronic renal failure**; less common causes include hyperthyroidism, hypokalemic myopathy of Burmese, myasthenia gravis, polymyositis and thiamine deficiency.

QUICK REFERENCE SUMMARY

Diseases causing neck ventroflexion

ANOMALY

● **Hypokalemic myopathy (of Burmese kittens)* (p 893)**
Burmese cats from 2–6 months of age. Generalized weakness, stiff stilted gait, muscle pain and, in severe cases, respiratory paralysis.

● Devon Rex myopathy (p 900)
Devon Rex cats from 8 weeks of age. Generalized weakness, marked neck ventroflexion and dorsal protrusion of scapulae. Exacerbated by exercise or stress.

● Congenital myasthenia gravis (p 896)
Seen in cats of less than a year old. Exercise-induced muscular weakness, progressive stiffness, and muscle tremors. Rarely, regurgitation or dyspnea.

METABOLIC

● **Chronic renal failure (hypokalemic myopathy)*** (p 893)**

Most commonly seen in older cats. Polyuria, polydipsia, weight loss, generalized weakness, stiff stilted gait, muscle pain and, in severe cases, respiratory paralysis.

● **Hypokalemic myopathy*** (p 893)**

Occurs in any age or breed of cat, but most commonly in older cats associated with chronic renal failure or hyperthyroidism. Also occurs in Burmese cats from 2–6 months of age. Generalized weakness, stiff stilted gait, muscle pain and, in severe cases, respiratory paralysis.

● **Hyperthyroidism (hypokalemic myopathy and/or thiamine deficiency)** (p 893, 899)**

Usually seen in older cats. Polyphagia, agitation, weight loss, generalized weakness, stiff stilted gait, muscle pain and, rarely, respiratory paralysis.

● **Iatrogenic** (p 893)**

Administration of inappropriate IV fluids or excessive furosemide. Generalized weakness and, rarely, respiratory paralysis.

● Hypernatremic myopathy (p 903)

Very rare cause of inappetence, muscle weakness, depression and myoglobinuria.

NEOPLASTIC

● Hyperaldosteronism (hypokalemic myopathy) (p 893)

Disease of older cats. Generalized weakness, stiff gait, muscle pain, polyuria, polydipsia and weight loss, and/or signs of systemic hypertension.

NUTRITIONAL

● **Thiamine deficiency* (p 899)**

Often with a history of fish-only diet. Anorexia and depression, followed by ataxia and vestibular signs. May progress to seizure-like episodes, stupor and death.

● Inappropriate diet (hypokalemic myopathy) (p 893)

Seen occasionally, due to inadequate potassium or over-acidification. Generalized weakness, stilted gait and muscle pain. May progress to renal failure.

INFECTIOUS

● Toxoplasmosis polymyositis (p 897)

Generalized weakness, muscle pain and reluctance to move. Often part of systemic illness. May have dysphagia, megaesophagus or pneumonia.

IMMUNE

● **Acquired myasthenia gravis* (p 896)**

Exercise-induced muscular weakness, progressive stiffness, muscle tremors, and occasionally, regurgitation and/or respiratory distress.

● Immune-mediated polymyositis (p 897)

Generalized weakness and pain. Occasionally with dysphagia or megaesophagus.

continued

continued

IDIOPATHIC

- Adult-onset motor neuron disease (p 903)

Chronic progressive generalized weakness with muscle tremors and fasciculations.

TOXIC

- Subacute organophosphate toxicity (p 901)

Generalized weakness, stiff stilted gait, muscle fasciculations or tremors. Muscarinic signs (miosis and salivation) may be absent.

INTRODUCTION

MECHANISM?

Neck ventroflexion is typically seen as part of more generalized muscle weakness. Since cats lack a nuchal ligament, muscle weakness in this species is often seen first as ventroflexion of the neck.

Affected cats often have a stilted gait and limb weakness, which may worsen on exercise.

They may also show muscle pain, dyspnea, dysphagia, or megaesophagus.

Cats with hypokalemic myopathy, polymyositis or adult-onset motor neuron disease may show evidence of muscle pain.

WHERE?

Neck ventroflexion can result from disease affecting the **muscles, the neuromuscular junction or the nervous system**.

Physical examination should look for evidence of cardiovascular disease or systemic illness. In many neuromuscular diseases generalized muscle weakness may be the only abnormality.

A complete blood count may rule out anemia or systemic infections. Serum biochemistry may indicate hypokalemia, hypernatremia, raised creatinine kinase level, renal insufficiency or hyperthyroidism.

Electromyographic studies, an intravenous edrophonium test (Tensilon test), assessment of serum anti-

acetylcholine receptor antibodies, determination of serum cholinesterase levels, serology for toxoplasmosis, FIV and FeLV, muscle and/or nerve biopsies, or a combination of these tests may be required to confirm a definitive diagnosis.

WHAT?

The **most common cause** of neck ventroflexion is **hypokalemic myopathy resulting from chronic renal failure**.

- Other causes of hypokalemic myopathy are seen less frequently. They include a hereditary defect in **Burmese kittens**, administration of inappropriate IV fluids or excessive furosemide, feeding **inappropriate diets** and, occasionally, **hyperthyroidism** or **hyperaldosteronism**.

Other causes of neck ventroflexion include primary myopathies (**immune-mediated** or **toxoplasmosis polymyositis**, **Devon Rex myopathy**), neuromuscular junction diseases (**myasthenia gravis, organophosphate toxicity**, spider bite), polyneuropathies (**adult-onset motor neuron disease**) and, very rarely, **hypernatremia**.

Although **thiamine deficiency** can cause neck ventroflexion, it usually causes an active rather than passive ventroflexion, together with excessive muscle tone, torticollis and seizure-like episodes of paddling or limb spasticity and opisthotonos.

This chapter deals with disorders that are likely to present with neck ventroflexion. While **this is mostly seen as part of generalized muscle weakness, not all cases of generalized muscle weakness present with neck ventroflexion.** Disorders that primarily cause generalized weakness, of which neck ventroflexion may merely be a factor, include polyneuropathies (long-standing diabetes mellitus, idiopathic polyradiculoneuropathy), ethylene glycol toxicosis (or primary hyperoxaluria), various electrolyte abnormalities (hypophosphatemia), and severe anemia. For discussion of these conditions please refer to the chapter on The Cat With Generalized Weakness.

DISEASES CAUSING NECK VENTROFLEXION

HYPOKALEMIC MYOPATHY*** (INCLUDING HYPOKALEMIC MYOPATHY OF BURMESE KITTENS)

> **Classical signs**
>
> - General muscle weakness, neck ventroflexion, a stiff, stilted gait and muscle pain.
> - In severe cases, respiratory paralysis.
> - Other signs relate to the underlying disease, e.g. polyuria and polydipsia in chronic renal failure.
> - May be seen with no other signs in Burmese kittens.

Pathogenesis

Hypokalemia may result from:
- **Decreased potassium intake** (incorrect diets).
- **Excessive losses** (chronic renal failure, renal tubular acidosis, **inappropriate IV fluid administration, excessive frusemide administration**, hyperaldosteronism, vomiting and diarrhea).
- **Increased potassium entry to cells** (Burmese kittens, hyperthyroidism, insulin over-dose).
- Varying combinations of all three.

Hypokalemia induces muscle weakness by causing a state of persistent depolarization and loss of excitability.
- Severe hypokalemia can result in rhabdomyolysis, however, the mechanism of action is unclear.

Hypokalemic myopathy is **most commonly associated with chronic renal failure***.

- This results from excessive urinary losses, and can be exacerbated by feeding a diet with insufficient potassium (see below).

Diets that contain insufficient potassium, particularly when high in protein, or that are acidified, have the potential to induce hypokalemia, particularly when fed to a cat with existing renal failure.
- Long-term feeding of these diets can result in renal damage.

The **administration of IV fluids with insufficient amounts of potassium**** can result in clinically significant hypokalemia. This is most likely to occur in cats that have renal failure, have post-obstructional diuresis, have not eaten recently, or have been experiencing vomiting and/or diarrhea. The administration of excessive amounts of furosemide, particularly to animals that have not eaten recently, can have a similar effect.

Congenital hypokalemic myopathy may be seen in **Burmese kittens***.
- It is similar to periodic hypokalemic paralysis in man.
- It is believed to result from a sudden shift of potassium from the extracellular to the intracellular compartment.

Hyperthyroidism** may occasionally present with hypokalemia and/or thiamine deficiency and therefore result in generalized muscle weakness.
- It has been suggested that the hyperadrenergic state of hyperthyroidism enhances insulin release, which may lead to a shift in potassium into the intracellular compartment.
- Hypokalemia most typically occurs immediately after thyroidectomy, or may be associated with the stress of handling.
- Hypokalemia and hypocalcemia may occur concurrently.
- Correction of the hypokalemia may precipitate clinical signs of hypocalcemia.
- Hyperthyroidism may also cause weakness by affecting other mechanisms of muscle or nerve function.

Hyperaldosteronism (Conn's syndrome) is being reported more frequently.
- It is caused by a functional adrenal tumor, or adenomatous hyperplasia of the adrenal glands.

- The production of aldosterone results in excessive urinary potassium losses.

Clinical signs

Hypokalemia can affect **any age, sex or breed of cat**.
- It is seen most frequently in **older cats; associated with chronic renal failure**, hyperthyroidism and, occasionally, hyperaldosteronism.
- Hypokalemia in **Burmese kittens** is usually seen in kittens, of either sex, **from 2–6 months of age.**

Clinical signs of hypokalemia often take one of **two forms**; mild and chronic, or severe and acute.
- The **mild and chronic** form produces vague signs of inappetence, gradual weight loss and reduced activity (reluctance to walk or jump). In older cats these signs are often attributed to aging.
- The **severe form presents acutely** with **general muscle weakness**, often with neck ventroflexion, a stiff, stilted gait, reluctance to walk, and **muscle pain**.
- Signs of mild hypokalemia have often been present for weeks to months before the acute crisis.
- Some cats are anorexic or dysphagic.
- Some cats develop ataxia or collapse.
- Severely affected cats may die of respiratory paralysis.
- Clinical signs may be transient, episodic or persistent.
- Postural reactions and spinal reflexes are normal.

Cats with underlying **chronic renal failure** may also show:
- Polyuria, polydipsia, progressive weight loss and an ill-kept coat.

Cats with underlying **hyperthyroidism** may also show:
- Polyphagia, hyperactivity, irritability and weight loss.
- Some cats may be episodically or consistently "apathetic".
- This may result from concurrent cardiac disease or hypokalemia.

Cats with underlying **hyperaldosteronism** may also show:
- Insidious weight loss, and signs of systemic hypertension.

Burmese cats with hypokalemic myopathy may also show:
- Clinical signs induced by exercise or stress.

- Head tremors, peculiar knuckling of the carpus, a tendency to sink on their hocks, and to sit with their stifles abducted.

Diagnosis

Signs of myopathy usually occurs when the serum potassium level falls **below 3.5 mmol (Eq)/L** (normal 4–5 mmol(Eq)/L).

Serum creatinine kinase (CK) levels are usually elevated (500–10 000 IU/L; normal 50–150 IU/L). In hypokalemic Burmese kittens CK can be very elevated (> 50 000 IU/L).

Once hypokalemic myopathy has been diagnosed it is necessary to differentiate between the various causes.
- Assessment of serum urea and creatinine levels, and urine specific gravity, will determine whether there is underlying renal disease.
- Serum thyroxine levels will be elevated in cases of hyperthyroidism.
- Cats with **hyperaldosteronism** become dehydrated, and eventually develop raised urea and creatinine levels.
  - This should not be misinterpreted as renal failure.
  - The adrenal tumor can usually be visualized by ultrasonography.
  - Plasma aldosterone levels will be moderately to markedly raised. In the case of hyperplastic change, the plasma aldosterone level may only be at the top end of the reference range, but the plasma renin activity will be mildly to moderately reduced.
- Calculating the **fractional excretion of potassium (FEK+)** can make an assessment of urinary potassium loss.
  - Collect urine and serum at the same time.

$$FE_{K^+}\% = \frac{\text{Urine potassium}}{\text{Serum potassium}} \times \frac{\text{Serum creatinine}}{\text{Urine creatinine}} \times 100$$

  - The potassium and creatinine units must be the same.
  - $FE_{K}+$ should be < 5% in potassium-depleted cats with normal renal function (e.g. Burmese).
  - **$FE_{K}+$ > 10–15% indicates significant renal loss.**

– Losses can be determined more accurately measuring 24-hour urinary potassium loss.

Electrodiagnostic testing may be normal, or may show positive sharp waves and fibrillation potentials. Nerve conduction velocities are normal.

Muscle biopsies may reveal normal muscle, or mild myofiber necrosis, with little or no evidence of inflammation.

Differential diagnosis

Myasthenia gravis, polymyositis and **organophosphate toxicity** can all cause similar clinical signs.

Since hypokalemia is so readily detected by assessment of serum biochemistry, more sophisticated diagnostics are not usually required.

- If it becomes necessary to rule out specific differentials, electromyographic studies, IV edrophonium (Tensilon test), assessment of serum anti-acetylcholine receptor antibodies and serum cholinesterase levels, toxoplasmosis serology and/or muscle biopsy may be required.

Treatment

Severely affected cases may require immediate **IV potassium infusion**.

- This requires the use of an infusion pump, constant cardiac monitoring, and repeated evaluation of serum potassium levels (every 2–4 hours until the serum level has risen to 3.5 mmol (Eq)/L).
- In severe cases, despite potassium supplementation, IV fluid administration may result in hemodilution, diuresis with exacerbation of urinary potassium loss, progressive hypokalemia, and worsening clinical signs resulting in respiratory muscle paralysis and respiratory arrest.
  - **Inappropriate fluid administration is the most common cause of death in hypokalemic cats**.
  - It is therefore essential to monitor these patients closely.
  - Respiratory muscle paralysis typically occurs when serum potassium levels fall below 2 mmol/L.
  - Ventilatory support is required to save the cat and may need to be continued for 24–48 hours.

- **Where possible, give oral potassium prior to IV fluids**.
- **Oral administration of potassium is more effective in normalizing potassium than IV administration**.
  - Only use fluids to administer potassium in the most severely affected cats.
  - When using fluids give a low volume with a high potassium concentration e.g. 160 mmol (Eq)/L at 2.0 ml/kg/h. Ideally, do not exceed 0.5 mmol (Eq)/kg/h or cardiac arrest may occur.

Oral supplementation is necessary in all cases.

- It should be started immediately, as IV administration is often not adequate to normalize potassium.
- Potassium gluconate solution (Kaon Elixir), tablets or powder (Tumil K) can be added to food (4–10 mmol (Eq)/PO q 24 h, in divided doses).
- Feeding a diet that is high in potassium can also help.
- **The level of supplementation should be adjusted** according to serum potassium levels.
- The duration of supplementation will depend on the underlying cause.
  - Cats that had been fed an unsuitable diet, given inappropriate IV fluids or excessive amounts of frusemide will cease to require additional potassium once the precipitating cause has been corrected.
  - Cats with chronic renal failure will require long-term supplementation. Maintenance doses are typically 2–5 mmol (Eq)/cat q 12–24 h.
  - Some Burmese cease to need supplementation after they are about a year old, others need life-long supplementation, with an increasing need during periods of stress.

Where possible, **treat the underlying disease** or correct the dietary or fluid imbalance.

Cats with hyperaldosteronism may benefit from spironolactone (an aldosterone antagonist; up to 50 mg/kg PO q 24 h), in addition to potassium supplementation.

Prognosis

Severely affected cats, particularly those with respiratory distress, carry a guarded short-term prognosis.

The long-term prognosis is dependent on the nature of the underlying disorder.

- Complete recovery of muscle strength can take several weeks.
- In many cases, ongoing renal disease, hyperthyroidism or hyperaldosteronism will ultimately result in the cat's death.

Hypokalemic Burmese generally have a good prognosis, although some need life-long supplementation.

Prevention

Feed diets with sufficient potassium.

Measure serum potassium in 'at-risk' cats and supplement when levels are found to be low. 'At-risk' cats include:

- Cats with chronic renal failure.
- Hospitalized anorexic cats.
- Those receiving intravenous fluid therapy, high doses of frusemide or insulin therapy.
- Those with severe vomiting and diarrhea.

In Burmese cats, **pedigree analysis and a selective breeding program** may help to remove the condition.

MYASTHENIA GRAVIS (CONGENITAL AND ACQUIRED)*

Classical signs

- Exercise-induced muscular weakness, progressive stiffness, neck ventroflexion and muscle tremors.
- Facial weakness, narrowing of the palpebral fissure and protrusion of the third eyelids.
- Occasionally, regurgitation and/or respiratory distress.

Pathogenesis

Two forms of myasthenia gravis have been reported in cats, a **congenital** and an **acquired*** form.

The congenital form may be caused by a lack of acetylcholine receptors.

The acquired form occurs when auto-antibodies are directed against acetylcholine receptors.

Clinical signs

Compared to dogs, **myasthenia gravis is relatively rare in cats**.

- The **congenital form is seen in young cats**, usually kittens of less than 6 months of age.
- The **acquired form occurs in adults**, and Abyssinian and Somali cats may be predisposed.

The clinical signs are the same in both forms of the disease.

Affected cats tend to **sleep excessively** and are **reluctant to exercise**.

- When they do exercise they develop muscular weakness, which may be seen as progressive stiffness, a crouching gait, neck ventroflexion and superimposed muscle tremors.
- They eventually collapse in sternal recumbency, often with their head to one side of their front paws.
- Weakness may involve all four limbs simultaneously, or affect the fore- or hindlimbs more severely.

Weakness of the facial muscles may result in paresis of eyelids causing narrowing of the palpebral fissure, absence of a palpebral reflex, protrusion of the third eyelids, inability to close the mouth and apparent hypersalivation.

Dysphonia may be noticed, with a low or barely audible miaow.

Megaesophagus may occur occasionally, and lead to aspiration pneumonia.

Severe weakness of the respiratory muscles can also lead to respiratory distress.

Some cases of acquired myasthenia gravis have been associated with thymic abnormalities (thymoma, cystic thymus, thymic hyperplasia), and/or immune-mediated polymyositis (see below).

- Cats with thymoma may show signs of regurgitation, and/or dyspnea.
- The latter may result from the mass within the chest, or pleural effusion.

Diagnosis

Cats with myasthenia gravis are usually of good body condition, with normal complete blood counts and serum biochemistry. Some may show slightly elevated creatinine kinase levels.

Thoracic radiography may occasionally show megaesophagus, thymic enlargement and/or aspiration pneumonia.

Tensilon test: Affected cats will usually show a brief positive response to the ultra-short-acting cholinesterase inhibitor edrophonium chloride (Tensilon: 0.2–0.5 mg/kg IV).
- Response is usually brief and may only be slight, e.g. widening of the palpebral fissure.
- Unfortunately, this test is not specific for myasthenia gravis.
- When using lower doses it is rare to produce a cholinergic crisis (bradycardia, hypersalivation, dyspnea and cyanosis). If this does occur it can be treated with atropine (0.05 mg/kg IV).

Electrodiagnostic testing will show a decremental response to **repetitive nerve stimulation.**

In the acquired form, **anti-acetylcholine receptor antibodies** can be detected in the serum and anti-receptor antibodies can be seen in muscle biopsies at the neuromuscular junction.

Differential diagnosis

Hypokalemic myopathy, polymyositis and organophosphate toxicity can all cause similar clinical signs.

The lack of changes in serum biochemistry, adequate serum cholinesterase levels, and the specific electromyographic findings will help to rule out these differentials. While cats with either myasthenia gravis or organophosphate toxicity may show a decremental response to repetitive nerve stimulation, the clinical signs will worsen if a cat with organophosphate toxicity is given IV edrophonium.

Definitive diagnosis of myasthenia gravis requires positive electromyographic studies and response to edrophonium and, in the acquired form, the presence of serum anti-acetylcholine receptor antibodies.

Treatment

Treatment usually consists of **pyridostigmine bromide** (Mestinon: 0.5–3.0 mg/kg PO q 8–12 h). The dose needs to be adjusted for each individual cat, starting from a low dose.

Neostigmine (Prostigmine; 0.01–0.1 mg/kg IV, IM, SC) can be used to treat a myasthenic crisis. For longer-term use it can be given orally (0.1–0.25 mg/kg), but its short half-life requires it to be given q 4–6 h.

Some acquired cases require the addition of **prednisolone** (1–2 mg/kg PO q 12 h). The dose of corticosteroid can usually be reduced after a few days to weeks, and discontinued after a few weeks of alternate day dosing.

Some cats may go into remission. It can therefore be useful to monitor the serum anti-acetylcholine receptor antibody titer. Once it has fallen back to zero medication may be discontinued.

Where a thymoma is present, its removal may be beneficial.

Prognosis

Prognosis is very variable. Severe cases may die from aspiration pneumonia.

Some congenital and acquired cases will maintain improvement after withdrawal of medication.

It is not uncommon for acquired cases to go into remission, and recurrences may occur.

POLYMYOSITIS (IMMUNE-MEDIATED AND TOXOPLASMOSIS)

Classical signs
- Generalized muscle weakness, neck ventroflexion and/or dysphagia.
- Megaesophagus, regurgitation and/or aspiration pneumonia.
- Muscle pain, depression and reluctance to move.
- Often part of systemic illness.

Pathogenesis

Polymyositis may be **idiopathic, immune-mediated**, or result from *Toxoplasma gondii* or **retroviral infection**.

Polymyositis may affect both skeletal and smooth muscle, resulting in generalized weakness and megaesophagus.

Immune-mediated polymyositis may be associated with thymoma. When this occurs myasthenia gravis may be seen concurrently (see above).

In cats, most *T. gondii* infections are asymptomatic. When clinical signs are seen they most frequently relate to the lungs, liver, gastrointestinal tract, eyes or brain. Signs relating to muscle involvement are rare.
- Toxoplasmosis polymyositis is seen most frequently as part of more generalized disease.
- It occurs most commonly in peri-natally infected kittens or immunosuppressed adults.

While *Neospora caninum* has been shown to cause polymyositis experimentally, natural feline neosporosis has not been detected.

FIV infection may be able to cause an inflammatory polymyositis.

Clinical signs

Polymyositis may cause **generalized muscle weakness**, including **neck ventroflexion** and/or **dysphagia**.

Muscle pain may be present, the cats are often depressed and reluctant to move.

Signs of megaesophagus may include regurgitation and/or aspiration pneumonia.

Cats with concurrent thymoma may show regurgitation and/or dyspnea. The latter may result from the mass within the chest or pleural effusion.

Toxoplasmosis polymyositis is typically seen as part of more generalized disease. Affected cats are usually systemically ill, often with signs of pneumonia.

Diagnosis

Thoracic compression may be reduced when a thymoma is present. The presence of a thymoma can usually be confirmed by assessment of pleural fluid, a fine needle aspirate of the mass, or a Tru-cut needle biopsy.

Thoracic radiography may reveal megaesophagus, pneumonia or thymoma (and possibly pleural fluid).

In all except very chronic cases, serum creatinine kinase levels (and other muscle-associated enzymes) are elevated. In most cases the levels are moderate to markedly increased.

Serum antinuclear antibody tests may be positive in immune-mediated polymyositis.

Serum toxoplasmosis IgM (and sometimes IgG) levels are likely to be elevated in cases of toxoplasmosis polymyositis. Where only IgG levels can be assessed, paired serum samples usually show a fourfold increase in titer over a 2–4-week period.

All cases of polymyositis should be assessed for FIV and FeLV infection.

Electromyographic abnormalities may include spontaneous positive waves and fibrillation potentials.

Muscle biopsies may show multifocal infiltration of muscle fascicles with lymphocytes, macrophages and, occasionally, neutrophils. In the cases of toxoplasmosis polymyositis the organisms may be detected. However, failure to detect *T. gondii* cysts does not rule out this etiology.

Differential diagnosis

While **myasthenia gravis** and **organophosphate toxicity** can cause similar clinical signs, **the most important differential is hypokalemic myopathy**.
- Polymyositis and hypokalemic myopathy can be clinically identical, and both can have moderate to markedly elevated serum creatinine kinase levels.
- The lack of other changes in serum biochemistry, adequate serum cholinesterase levels, lack of serum anti-acetylcholine receptor antibodies, and electromyographic studies, will help to rule out these differentials.

Definitive diagnosis of polymyositis requires muscle biopsy and serological testing.

Treatment

Immune-mediated myositis may respond to **prednisolone** (1.5–2 mg/kg PO q 12 h).
- The dose of steroids can usually be reduced after a few weeks as the clinical signs resolve.
- Some cases need long-term, alternate-day, medication.
- Assessment of serum creatinine kinase levels may be helpful in monitoring these cases.

If a thymoma is present it should be surgically removed.

First-line **treatment for toxoplasmosis** (or neosporosis) consists of clindamycin (12–25 mg/kg q 12 h, PO or IM). If necessary, this can be given for a number of weeks.

- Alternatively, trimethoprim/sulfadiazine (30 mg/kg PO q 12 h) may be given either alone or in combination with pyrimethamine (0.5 mg/kg PO q 24 h).
  - Unfortunately, both of these drugs are unpalatable.
  - Since cats are particularly susceptible to the toxic effects of pyrimethamine it should be given for a maximum of 2 weeks.
  - Supplementation with folate (folic acid) is recommended (1 mg/kg PO q 24 h).
- Other, more modern, drugs may also be useful. These include azithromycin (7–15 mg/kg q 24 h, PO) or clarithromycin (7.5 mg/kg q 12 h PO, combined with pyrimethamine). Prolonged treatment may be necessary.

Prognosis

Prognosis for immune-mediated myositis is fair.

Despite aggressive therapy, prognosis for toxoplasmosis myositis is generally poor.

Prevention

It is not possible to prevent immune-mediated myositis. Cats may be prevented from becoming infected with toxoplasmosis by keeping them indoors, preventing them from hunting, and by feeding well-cooked food.

THIAMINE DEFICIENCY*

Classical signs

- Anorexia and depression, followed by ataxia, neck ventroflexion, torticollis and vestibular signs.
- May progress to seizure-like muscle spasms, stupor and death.
- History of fish-only diet.

Pathogenesis

Thiamine (vitamin B_1) is essential for normal carbohydrate metabolism and gluconeogenesis.

Since the central nervous system depends almost entirely on carbohydrate metabolism for its energy, it is particularly susceptible to the effects of thiamine deficiency.

Thiamine deficiency results in a progressive polioencephalomalacia (hemorrhage and necrosis). It predominantly affects the subcortical gray matter of the brain stem nuclei, particularly the vestibular, lateral geniculate and oculomotor (pupillary constriction) nuclei.

Thiamine deficiency can effect **any age, breed or sex of cat**.

It occurs most frequently in cats that are **fed a diet of mainly fish** (usually uncooked) that contain thiaminase (e.g. cod, catfish).

It may also result from prolonged anorexia or malabsorption, or the destruction of thiamine during food preparation (over-cooking) or prolonged storage. The meat preserver, sulfur dioxide, destroys thiamine and may produce thiamine deficiency in cats fed pet mince preserved with this compound. This can occur even when the mince is mixed with other food or supplemented with vitamins or brewer's yeast.

Clinical signs

Early signs include anorexia, intermittent vomiting, depression, ataxia and pupillary dilation.

Progression may result in **central vestibular signs** (including curling up when lifted, and/or a head tilt), neck ventroflexion, torticollis, behavioural changes, mydriasis, seizure-like muscle spasms or stupor.

True seizures are rare but episodes of opisthotonic posturing with paddling, spastic neck ventroflexion, and body contortions may occur, especially if the cat is lifted. These can have a seizure-like appearance.

Further progression may lead to coma and death.

Diagnosis

Measurement of blood thiamine level is not readily available.

Diagnosis is supported by improvement within 24 hours of thiamine supplementation.

Differential diagnosis

Hypokalemic myopathy, myasthenia gravis, polymyositis and organophosphate toxicity can all cause neck ventroflexion.

However, thiamine deficiency usually causes an active rather than passive ventroflexion, together with excessive muscle tone, torticollis, and more obvious central signs, such as a head tilt, behavioral changes, or seizure-like paddling or spasticity with opisthotonos.

Other differentials can usually be excluded by performing a thorough physical and neurological examination, assessing serum biochemistry (including renal enzymes, creatinine kinase and electrolytes), and a resting thyroxine level. Occasionally it may be necessary to assess serum cholinesterase levels or look for serum anti-acetylcholine receptor antibodies.

Treatment

10–20 mg/cat of thiamine IM, q 8–12 h. For longer-term supplementation; 5–30 mg/cat PO q 24 h.

If clinical signs are severe, oxygen may be beneficial.

The underlying cause should be corrected, e.g. feed a suitable diet. Oral thiamine supplementation is usually needed for a week after the diet has been corrected.

Prognosis

The prognosis is good if the condition is recognized and treated early.

Once a cat has become semiconscious, prognosis is poor.

Some chronic cases respond to treatment, but may be left with neurological deficits.

Prevention

Feed suitable diets and supplement anorexic cats with B vitamins.

DEVON REX MYOPATHY

> **Classical signs**
>
> - Young Devon Rex cats.
> - Generalized muscle weakness, with marked ventroflexion of the head and neck, and dorsal protrusion of the scapulae.
> - Signs may become accentuated during locomotion, micturition, defecation, stress or excitement.

Pathogenesis

The disease is inherited in an **autosomal recessive** manner.

The pathology is suggestive of a **muscular dystrophy**.

Skeletal and smooth muscles are affected (neck ventroflexion, megaesophagus).

Clinical signs

The disease is sometimes termed "spasticity" by breeders. However, there are no signs of central nervous system involvement.

Disease is seen in Devon Rex cats of either sex, with signs becoming **apparent from 3 weeks to 6 months of age**.

The severity of the disease varies between cats, and may be static or slowly progressive.

Affected cats show **generalized muscle weakness**, often with very **marked ventroflexion** of the head and neck, and **dorsal protrusion of the scapulae**.
- They typically have a high-stepping forelimb gait, and tire easily, with head bobbing, progressive protrusion of the scapulae, shortening of the stride, and superimposed muscle tremors.
- They eventually collapse in sternal recumbency, usually with their head to one side of their forepaws.

Clinical signs may be exacerbated by micturition, defecation, stress, concurrent illness, cold ambient temperature or excitement.

At rest they often adopt a characteristic "dog-begging" position, with their forepaws resting on a convenient raised object.

Signs of **megaesophagus** may include regurgitation and/or aspiration pneumonia.

Difficulty in maintaining a normal head position may result in **frequent episodes of laryngospasm after obstruction of the pharynx with food**. This is the most usual cause of death in these cats.

Mild muscle atrophy may occasionally be evident.

Diagnosis

Complete blood count and serum biochemistry, including creatinine kinase and aspartate aminotransferase (AST), are usually normal.

Thoracic radiography will usually reveal a megaesophagus and/or aspiration pneumonia.

Neurological examination, muscle tone and withdrawal reflexes are normal.

Electrodiagnostic studies may show sparse fibrillation potentials, and positive sharp waves. Nerve conduction velocities are normal and there is no decremental response to repetitive nerve stimulation.

Gross post-mortem examination may reveal megaesophagus, reflux oesophagitis, aspiration pneumonia and/or gastroparesis.

Skeletal muscle appears grossly normal. Histopathological changes vary between cats, and also within different muscles of the same cat.
- Findings range from normal, to those indicative of myopathy, possibly muscular dystrophy. They include increased variability in myofiber size, individual myofiber necrosis, regeneration and fibrosis.
- The degree of change depends on the severity of disease, and the advancing age of the cat.
- The dorsal cervical and proximal forelimb muscles, especially the *m. triceps brachii*, are usually most severely affected, and are therefore recommended for biopsy.

Nerves are not affected.

Differential diagnosis

Hypokalemic myopathy, myasthenia gravis, polymyositis and **organophosphate toxicity** can all cause similar clinical signs. The most important differentials are probably hypokalemia and congenital myasthenia gravis.

Devon Rex myopathy is the most likely diagnosis in a young Devon Rex cat which is showing typical clinical signs, its serum biochemistry is normal, it lacks a decremental response to repetitive nerve stimulation, has adequate serum cholinesterase levels, and its clinical signs worsen when it is given IV edrophonium (Tensilon test). Confirmation of the diagnosis requires pedigree analysis and muscle biopsy.

Treatment

There is no treatment for this condition. Aspiration pneumonia will require antibiotics.

Prognosis

Clinical signs may deteriorate up to 6–9 months of age, after which time the disease is usually stable or only slowly progressive.

The course of the disease will depend on the severity of the myopathy, particularly the degree of pharyngeal involvement. Laryngospasm is the usual cause of death.

Prevention

Since the disease is inherited, **pedigree analysis and a selective breeding program** are being used to remove the condition from the breed.

SUBACUTE ORGANOPHOSPHATE TOXICITY

Classical signs

- Muscarinic signs (miosis and salivation) may be absent.
- Generalized muscle weakness may be seen as neck ventroflexion, and/or a stiff stilted gait.

continued

Pathogenesis

Organophosphate toxicity can affect **any age, breed or sex of cat.**

Organophosphate compounds irreversibly bind to acetylcholinesterases at cholinergic synapses, resulting in continuous stimulation.

In cats, **chronic exposure can result in peripheral neuropathies.**

Unlike other organophosphates **fenthion** toxicity produces predominantly nicotinic signs (muscle weakness), with few muscarinic signs (autonomic effects).

Clinical signs

The variety of clinical signs will depend on the degree of concurrent muscarinic involvement. In subacute or chronic cases these signs (miosis, salivation, vomiting, bradycardia) may be absent.

In chronic cases, or in fenthion toxicity, the only sign may be generalized muscle weakness, often seen as neck ventroflexion and/or a stiff stilted gait. Severe muscle weakness may cause respiratory paralysis.

Muscle fasciculations or tremors may be present.

There is no muscle pain.

Diagnosis

There is usually a history of exposure to an organophosphate, typically in the form of insecticide.

Complete blood count and serum biochemistry (including creatinine kinase) are usually normal.

A low **serum cholinesterase level** will support this diagnosis. In affected cats the levels are usually less than 500 IU (normal 900–1200 IU). However, in cases where chronic exposure has caused polyneuropathy the serum cholinesterase levels may be normal.

Electrodiagnostic testing will show a decremental response to repetitive nerve stimulation.

Tensilon test: IV edrophonium (Tensilon: 0.2–0.5 mg/kg) will usually induce a cholinergic crisis (bradycardia, hypersalivation, dyspnea and cyanosis), without a positive improvement in muscle strength. If this occurs it can be treated with IV atropine (0.05 mg/kg).

Differential diagnosis

Hypokalemic myopathy, myasthenia gravis and **polymyositis** can all cause similar clinical signs.

Lack of changes in serum biochemistry, lack of serum anti-acetylcholine receptor antibodies, and a negative response to IV edrophonium in the face of a decremental response to repetitive nerve stimulation, will help to rule out the differential diagnoses.

Diagnosis is usually confirmed on finding reduced serum cholinesterase levels, typically with a history of exposure to organophosphate.

Treatment

Supportive therapy may include use of IV fluids, nutritional support, control of body temperature and good nursing care.

Atropine (0.1–0.2 mg/kg SC, as required) may be used to chemically compete with acetylcholine binding to acetylcholine receptors.

Oximes (pralidoxime chloride; 20 mg/kg IM q 8 h) may help by releasing the inhibited cholinesterase. However, oximes are of most benefit if given within the first 24 hours of exposure.

Diphenhydramine has been used to reverse nicotinic signs in dogs with fenthion toxicity.

Prognosis

It is often not possible to save severely affected cats.

Less severely affected cats may recover, often following weeks of nursing.

Chronically affected cats may be left with permanent nerve damage.

Prevention

Prevent access to organophosphate compounds.

ADULT-ONSET MOTOR NEURON DISEASE

Classical signs

- Adult-onset, chronic, progressive disease.
- Generalized weakness, neck ventroflexion, and dysphagia.
- Muscle tremors/fasciculations (particularly of the head and tongue).
- Muscle atrophy.

Pathogenesis

The cause of this **rare disease** is unknown.

Clinical signs result from chronic degeneration and loss of motor neurons.

Clinical signs

Disease is seen in **adult cats**.

Chronically progressive signs include generalized weakness, neck ventroflexion, dysphagia and muscle atrophy.

Muscle tremors particularly affect the head.

Muscle fasciculations may be localized to the tongue.

Muscle palpation may cause pain.

Diagnosis

Complete blood count and serum biochemistry (including creatinine kinase) are usually normal.

Neurological examination reveals normal mentation, cranial nerve function and conscious proprioception.

Spinal reflexes are present initially, but are lost as disease progresses.

Electromyographic studies may reveal fibrillation potentials. Nerve conduction velocities may be normal or slightly reduced.

Muscle biopsies reveal evidence of denervation.

Histopathology of the spinal cord reveals neuron loss and gliosis in the ventral horns, and consequent atrophy of the ventral nerve rootlets.

Differential diagnosis

Hypokalemic myopathy, myasthenia gravis, polymyositis and organophosphate toxicity can all cause similar clinical signs.

Lack of changes in serum biochemistry, lack of serum anti-acetylcholine receptor antibodies, adequate serum cholinesterase levels, electromyographic studies, and slowly progressive disease all help to rule out the differential diagnoses.

Histopathology of the spinal cord is required to make a definite diagnosis.

Treatment

There is no known treatment.

Prognosis

Disease may take months to years to progress to the point where the cat requires euthanasia on humane grounds.

HYPERNATREMIC MYOPATHY

Classical signs

- Inappetence, progressive muscle weakness, and depression.
- Brown-stained urine (myoglobinuria).

Pathogenesis

This **very rare cause of myopathy** has only been documented in a single, 7-month-old, cat.

Hypernatremia resulted from "neurogenic" hypodipsia, related to hydrocephalus.

Severe hypernatremia may induce myopathy by accelerating sodium–potassium exchange in myocytes. This can cause an increase in intracellular sodium and a reduction in intracellular potassium. The clinical signs are therefore similar to those of hypokalemia.

Severe myocyte dysfunction can lead to membrane damage, myoglobinemia and myoglobinuria.

Clinical signs

The cat showed inappetence, depression and progressive muscle weakness, including neck ventroflexion.

Myoglobinuria caused the urine to be brown.

Clinical signs were transient. They resolved on correction of the hypernatremia.

Diagnosis

Serum biochemistry revealed marked hypernatremia (> 200 mmol (Eq)/L; normal 148–165 mmol (Eq)/L), and increased serum osmolality (431 mmol/kg (mOsm/L); normal 295–300 mmol/kg (mOsm/L). The serum creatinine kinase level was moderately raised.

Electromyographic abnormalities included prolonged insertional activity, fibrillation potentials, positive sharp waves and bizarre high-frequency discharges. Nerve conduction velocities were normal.

Muscle biopsies were normal.

Contrast-enhanced computer tomography revealed marked hydrocephalus.

Endocrine studies revealed hypopituitarism, with hypoadrenocorticism, hypothyroidism and a lack of luteinizing hormone. The cat was small for its age, and never showed signs of estrus.

Differential diagnosis

Hypokalemic myopathy, polymyositis, myasthenia gravis and organophosphate toxicity can all cause similar signs.

The presence of severe hypernatremia should alert the clinician to the possibility of hypernatremic myopathy. Lack of hypokalemia and resolution of clinical signs on the correction of the fluid balance, would support the diagnosis.

Treatment

To increase the cat's water consumption it was fed a low-salt diet (PVD CV or NF, Nestlé Purina; Feline H/D, Hill's Pet Foods), to which water was added in excess of maintenance needs.

Correction of fluid balance resulted in resolution of clinical signs, and restoration of the hypothalamic-pituitary-adrenal axis.

Prognosis

While correcting the serum osmolality resulted in resolution of clinical signs in this case, this may not work in future cases, since response will depend on the nature of the underlying disorder.

RECOMMENDED READING

Ash RA, Harvey AM, Tasker S. Primary hyperaldosteronism in the cat: a series of 13 cases. J Feline Med Surg 2005; 7: 173–182.

Ducote JM, Dewey CW, Coates JR. Clinical forms of aquired myasthenia gravis in cats. Compend Contin Educ Pract Vet 1999; 21(2): 440–448.

Javadi S, Djajadiningrat-Laanen SC, Kooistra HS, et al. Primary hyperaldosteronism, a mediator of progressive renal disease in cats. Domest Anim Endocrinol 2005; 28: 85–104.

Jones BR. Hypokalemic myopathy in cats. In: Bonagura JD (ed) Kirk's Current Veterinary Therapy XIII. Philadelphia, PA, W B Saunders, 2000, pp. 985–987.

Malik R, Mepstead K, Yang F, Harper C. Hereditary myopathy of Devon Rex cats. J Small Anim Prac 1993; 34: 539–546.

Nemzek JA, Kruger JM, Walshaw R, Hauptman JG. Acute onset of hypokalemia and muscular weakness in four hyperthyroid cats. J Am Vet Med Assoc 1994; 205: 65–68.

Podell M. Neurological manifestations of systemic disease, Chapter 103. In: Ettinger SJ, Feldman EC (eds) Textbook of Veterinary Internal Medicine, 5th edn., Vol 1. Philadelphia, PA, WB Saunders, 1999, pp. 548–552.

Shelton GD. Diseases of the muscle and the neuromuscular junction, Chapter 46. In: Sherding RG (ed) The Cat: Diseases and Clinical Management, 2nd edn., Vol 2. New York, Churchill Livingston, 1994, pp. 1569–1576.

Shelton GD, Hopkins AL, Ginn PE, et al. Adult-onset motor neuron disease in three cats. J Am Vet Med Assoc 1998; 212: 1271–1275.

PART 11

Cat with an abnormal gait

42. The weak and ataxic or paralyzed cat

Paul A Cuddon

KEY SIGNS

- Incoordination and decreased proprioception (misplacement or knuckling of the foot).
- Weakness of one or more limbs (feet cross or are placed too far apart).
- Complete loss of any voluntary movement (paralyzed).

MECHANISM?

- Ataxia and paresis occurs when there is **physical or functional disruption** to both the **motor and sensory pathways** of the nervous system.
- This can occur at any point along the neuraxis from the cerebrum to the peripheral nervous system.

WHERE?

- Cats solely presenting with ataxia and paresis/paralysis most commonly have **spinal cord disease**.

WHAT?

- The **most common causes** of spinal cord ataxia and paresis in cats are **infection/inflammation and trauma**.

QUICK REFERENCE SUMMARY

Diseases causing a weak and ataxic or paralyzed cat

ANOMALY

• **Congenital abnormalities of the vertebral body* (p 918)**

Tetraparesis or paraparesis and ataxia (UMN or LMN) usually in cats less than one year of age due to static or dynamic cord compression.

• **Congenital abnormalities of the spinal cord (spina bifida, etc.)* (p 918)**

LMN urinary/fecal incontinence, an easily expressible atonic bladder, megacolon and a hopping gait in young kittens at or soon after birth.

NEOPLASIA

• **Spinal lymphosarcoma*** (p 909)**

Chronic progressive ataxia, asymmetrical paraparesis and focal spinal pain in young adult cats often associated with FeLV infection.

• **Spinal meningioma** (p 914)**

Spinal pain and chronic progressive UMN or LMN tetraparesis or paraparesis in cats greater than 9 years of age.

NUTRITIONAL

• **Hypervitaminosis A* (p 921)**

Cervical pain and rigidity, thoracic limb lameness, and tetraparesis/tetraplegia in cats usually between 2–9 years of age.

INFLAMMATION (INFECTIOUS)

• **Feline infectious peritonitis*** (p 911)**

Chronic progressive tetraparesis or paraparesis in young cats less than 3 years of age, commonly accompanied by decreased mentation, seizures, intention tremor and/or central vestibular signs.

INFLAMMATION (IDIOPATHIC)

• **Feline polioencephalomyelitis* (p 917)**

A stiff, staggering gait with paraparesis and thoracolumbar spinal pain in cats of any age, often with decreased mentation and seizures.

ISCHEMIA

• **Aortic thromboembolism** (p 915)**

Acute femoral and sciatic nerve hyporeflexia, cold cyanotic pelvic limbs and painful firm gastrocnemius muscles in any aged cat.

• **Fibrocartilaginous embolism* (p 922)**

Acute, non-painful LMN paraparesis/paraplegia and urinary and fecal incontinence in any aged cat.

TRAUMA

• **Spinal cord trauma – fractures and luxations*** (p 912)**

An acute transverse myelopathy with varying degrees of UMN or LMN paresis to paralysis with spinal pain. Other signs include split nails and skin abrasions and bruising.

INTRODUCTION

MECHANISM?

Ataxia and paresis occur when there is **physical or functional disruption** to both the **motor and sensory pathways** of the nervous system.

Paresis is a deficit of voluntary movement, leading to weakness in one limb (monoparesis), both pelvic limbs (paraparesis), the limbs on one side of the body (hemiparesis), or all four limbs (tetraparesis). It is caused by disruption of the voluntary motor pathways anywhere from the cerebral cortex through the brainstem and spinal cord to the spinal cord segments and the peripheral nerves supplying muscles. Neurological testing to determine whether a cat is paretic includes gait analysis and postural reaction testing, which includes hopping, wheel-barrowing, hemi-standing/hemi-walking, and the extensor postural thrust. The term **paralysis** is reserved for the patient who has a complete loss of any voluntary movements.

Ataxia is a lack of coordination of the limbs or trunk produced by disruption of the sensory proprioceptive pathways of the spinal cord and brainstem. Lesions of the cerebellum and the vestibular system also can produce ataxia. Sensory ataxia, the disruption of sensory proprioceptive pathways, can be assessed via such tests as proprioception and tactile placing.

Most cats with **spinal cord disease** have a combination of **both ataxia and paresis**, since most myelopathies cause disruption of both the motor and sensory systems. In many circumstances, therefore, separation of ataxia and paresis becomes almost impossible on routine neurological examination.

WHERE?

Cats presenting solely with ataxia and paresis/paralysis most commonly have **spinal cord disease**.

Weakness and ataxia can also occur with cerebral and brainstem disease.
- However, cats with cerebral disease will usually show seizures, behavior change, aimless wandering, and pacing along with the ataxia and contralateral hemiparesis or tetraparesis.

- Cats with brainstem disease will demonstrate cranial nerve abnormalities as well as an ipsilateral hemiparesis or tetraparesis.

Most polyneuropathies manifest as generalized weakness **without** ataxia. In many cases of peripheral nerve disease, sensory tests such as proprioception and tactile placing will be normal despite obvious muscle weakness.

Localization of myelopathies is dependent on **determining whether the thoracic and pelvic limbs have upper (UMN) or lower motor neuron (LMN) signs**. Cats with UMN paresis will demonstrate normal to increased segmental spinal reflexes (myotatic or tendon reflexes, muscle tone and withdrawal reflexes) whereas cats with LMN paresis will show decreased to absent segmental spinal reflexes. An UMN bladder, likewise, will have increased tone and be difficult to express due to external (+/− internal) urethral sphincter hypertonia, whereas a LMN bladder will be flaccid (or atonic) and easily expressed due to external urethral sphincter hypo- to atonia.

The classic spinal cord divisions when localizing a myelopathy are as follows:
- **Cervical spinal cord (C1–C5)** – UMN tetraparesis to tetraplegia.
- **Cervical intumescence (C6–T2)** – LMN signs to thoracic limbs and UMN signs to pelvic limbs.
- **Thoracolumbar spinal cord (T3–L3)** – UMN paraparesis to paraplegia. UMN bladder dysfunction.
- **Lumbar spinal cord (L4–L6)** – mixed UMN and LMN paraparesis to paraplegia (LMN to the femoral nerve and UMN to the sciatic nerve). UMN bladder and perineal reflexes.
- **Lumbosacral spinal cord (L6–S2) or cauda equina injury** – LMN paraparesis to paraplegia associated with the sciatic nerve and LMN bladder.

WHAT?

The **most common causes** of spinal cord ataxia and paresis in cats are **infectious** (including feline infectious peritonitis virus (coronavirus)), **neoplasia** (lymphosarcoma) and **trauma**.

Primary spinal neoplasia (meningioma), inflammation (feline polioencephalomyelitis), and ischemia (aortic thromboembolism and fibrocartilaginous embolism) are less common.

Intervertebral disc disease is very rare.

DISEASES CAUSING A WEAK AND ATAXIC OR PARALYZED CAT

SPINAL LYMPHOSARCOMA***

> **Classical signs**
>
> - Chronic progressive ataxia.
> - Asymmetric paraparesis.
> - Focal areas of spinal pain.

Pathogenesis

Lymphosarcoma is the **most common feline neoplasia**.

5–15% of cats with lymphoreticular malignancies develop neurologic involvement.

88% of cats with CNS involvement show thoracic and lumbar myelopathy, although the brain may also be affected.

Spinal lymphosarcoma is often **FeLV related**.

Epidural lymph channels and extramedullary hematopoietic tissue are possible sites for development of primary spinal lymphosarcoma.

Tumor growth commonly occurs longitudinally along the spinal canal (the epidural space is a low-resistance channel).

79% of cats with spinal lymphosarcoma have solitary epidural lesions.

Multifocal lesions are also possible, as is tumor involvement of multiple nerve roots.

Clinical signs

Spinal lymphosarcoma is most commonly seen in **young cats** (≤ 3 years).

Males are more commonly affected.

Most cats present with an initial insidious course of neurologic dysfunction followed by acute deterioration.

Tumors occur **predominantly between T3–L4**.

Involvement of the brachial intumescence and plexus also can occur.

Cervical spinal cord involvement is rare.

The most common clinical signs include **progressive ataxia, asymmetric paraparesis and focal spinal pain.**

If there is involvement of the **brachial or lumbosacral intumescences**, LMN signs will occur.

Nerve root involvement may result in lameness and limb pain.

Acute exacerbation of signs is commonly associated with hemorrhage.

Weight loss is the most common extraneural sign.

The **most common extraneural tumor site** associated with spinal lymphosarcoma is the **kidney**.

Diagnosis

Complete blood count, biochemistry parameters and urinalysis are often normal, although non-regenerative anemia or leukemia may occasionally be seen.

Many cats are **seropositive for FeLV** or positive on indirect fluorescent antibody testing of bone marrow.

Cerebrospinal fluid (CSF) analysis usually shows a mixed pleocytosis (mean of 161 cells/mm^3 [161 cells/μl] with a range of 0–1625 cells/mm^3 [0–1625 cells/μl]) and a protein increase (mean of 1.34 g/L [134 mg/dl] with a range of 0.12–4.05 g/L [12–405 mg/dl]).

A **monomorphous population of neoplastic lymphocytes** will be seen in some cases.

Survey spinal radiographs are usually normal.

MRI scan or myelography shows single or multiple **asymmetric extradural spinal cord compression(s)**.

Differential diagnosis

Infectious diseases, such as feline infectious peritonitis, toxoplasmosis and cryptococcosis also may produce signs of progressive spinal cord dysfunction.

However, unlike spinal lymphosarcoma, **most infectious conditions** usually result in **multifocal neurologic**

dysfunction, with involvement of the cerebrum, brainstem and/or cerebellum.
- **Ocular manifestations** secondary to uveitis, chorioretinitis and optic neuritis are also often present **with CNS infections**.

CSF analysis often helps differentiate between **infectious diseases** and spinal lymphosarcoma.
- **Feline infectious peritonitis** usually produces a marked increase in protein (usually greater than 1 g/L [100 mg/dl] and often greater than 2 g/L [200 mg/dl]) and white blood cells (mean of 734 cells/mm^3 [734 cells/µl] with a range of 69–2000 cells/mm^3 [69–2000 cells/µl]), with a predominance of non-degenerate neutrophils (50–90%).
- CSF commonly reveals the organism in cats with **cryptococcosis**.
- *Toxoplasma gondii* usually produces a mild to moderate increase in protein (0.6–1 g/L [60–100 mg/dl]) and cell counts (30–100 cells/mm^3 [30–100 cells/µl]), with the cell distribution being a mixed mononuclear and polymorphonuclear pleocytosis +/– eosinophils).

Serologic antibody or capsular antigen assays will also help differentiate the infectious diseases.

Feline polioencephalomyelitis can produce a primary thoracolumbar myelopathy.
- Since CSF in this disease also commonly shows a mild to moderate protein elevation (mean of 0.48 g/L [48 mg/dl] with a range of 0.1–0.7 g/L [10–70 mg/dl]) and a mild mononuclear pleocytosis (mean of 19 cells/mm^3 [19 cells/µl] with a range of 0–46 cells/mm^3 [0–46 cells/µl]), differentiation from lymphosarcoma may be difficult.
- Cats with polioencephalomyelitis, however, usually are FeLV negative.

Spinal neoplasia (especially meningioma) can mimic focal spinal lymphosarcoma.
- **CSF** analysis with **meningioma** usually only demonstrates a **protein increase**.
- Cats with **neoplasia** are usually **much older** (> 9 years of age) than cats with lymphosarcoma (≤ 3 years).

Treatment

Spinal lymphosarcoma is **radiosensitive**.
- Rapid reduction in tumor volume can occur within hours of delivering a **single large palliative dose of radiation** (3–4 Gy).

Chemotherapy is **important for systemic control** of lymphosarcoma although most chemotherapeutic agents do not cross the blood–brain barrier.

Cytosine arabinoside may also help control spinal lymphosarcoma.
- This anti-metabolite drug crosses the blood–brain barrier and reaches appropriate CSF levels.
- The recommended dosage is 100 mg/m^2/day as a constant rate infusion intravenously for 4 days.
- An alternative regimen is 300 mg/m^2 subcutaneously twice daily for 2 days.
- Potential toxicity includes myelosuppression (at 5–7 days); vomiting; and anorexia.
- Tumor cells rapidly become resistant to this drug's action.

Surgical decompression of the spinal cord and/or nerve roots, and tumor resection or debulking is a potential treatment option, especially **if the tumor is localized**.

Follow-up radiation and chemotherapy is recommended.

Prognosis

Prognosis is poor for long-term survival, especially when most cats are infected with the FeLV virus.

Prevention

The only effective means of prevention is **test and removal programs** directed at **controlling the spread of FeLV**.

Routine vaccination with FeLV vaccines is recommended. However, there is the risk of development of vaccine-induced sarcomas with adjuvant killed FeLV vaccines. A new recombinant FeLV vaccine is now available.

FELINE INFECTIOUS PERITONITIS***

Classical signs

- Decreased mentation and menace.
- Central vestibular disease and facial paralysis.
- Chronic progressive tetraparesis to tetraplegia or paraparesis.
- Seizures and behavior change.
- Intention tremor.
- Systemic signs such as fever, inappetance, weight loss, dyspnea and gastrointestinal signs.

Clinical signs

Feline infectious peritonitis (FIP) may produce a **non-suppurative meningoencephalitis in 29% of infected cats**.

The CNS signs are **usually** associated with the **non-effusive ("dry") form of FIP** (cell-mediated immunity is defective but not absent)

The neurological form of FIP has no breed or sex predilection, although **most cases are < 3–4 years of age**.

In most cases, the neurological signs are **multifocal** with a predominance of **caudal fossa signs (brainstem, vestibular nuclei and cerebellum)**.

- Signs can include nystagmus (positional, non-constant, rotatory, horizontal or vertical in nature), head tilt, body lean or rolling, facial paralysis, an ipsilateral hemiparesis or tetraparesis, intention tremor, and hypermetria or dysmetria.

The spinal cord and the cerebrum also can be involved.

- **Signs of cerebral disease** can include seizures, behavior change, decreased mentation, decreased menace response, compulsive walking, ipsiversive wide circling and head pressing.
- **Spinal cord involvement** will manifest as UMN and/or LMN tetraparesis or paraparesis with ataxia. Tetraplegia or paraplegia are the most severe consequences of spinal cord involvement.

Myelopathy is seen either as the sole abnormality or as part of a multifocal distribution in **25% of cases**.

The onset of FIP can be acute, although most cats have a chronic progressive course over 1 week to 3 months.

Extraneural signs may include fever, cachexia, poor body condition, dehydration, lethargy, muscle atrophy, chorioretinitis, dyspnea and gastrointestinal/hepatic signs.

Many cats present with the neurological form of FIP without extraneural signs.

Diagnosis

The diagnosis is **best** established via **CSF analysis** – marked elevation in protein (usually greater than 1 g/L [100 mg/dl] and often greater than 2 g/L [200 mg/dl]) and white blood cells (mean of 734 cells/mm^3 [734 cells/µl] with a range of 69–2000 cells/mm^3 [69–2000 cells/µl]), with a predominance of non-degenerate neutrophils (50–90%).

The **CSF FIP viral titer** is usually **positive** if CNS signs are present. It is probable that CSF anti-FIP viral immunoglobulin G is produced within the CNS.

Serum biochemical changes often consist of an elevation in total protein and hypergammaglobulinemia.

Serum FIP antibody titers are **not reliable**, and are elevated in only 58% of cats with the neurological form of FIP and are even negative in some cats.

Differential diagnosis

Numerous other infectious and immunological diseases can produce meningitis and encephalomyelitis in cats.

FeLV-associated CNS lymphosarcoma can usually be differentiated by CSF analysis, and a positive FeLV serum titer.

Cryptococcal organisms are **usually visible in CSF** with confirmation made by a latex agglutination assay or culture.

CNS toxoplasmosis is **rare** in the cat, usually producing signs of intracranial disease rather than myelopathy. Recent or active infection is diagnosed by demonstrating a positive IgM titer, a four-fold increase or decrease in IgG serum titer, a CSF IgM antibody titer or a CSF IgG titer present at a higher CSF:serum ratio than another antibody present in serum that is not produced in CSF, e.g. calicivirus.

Feline polioencephalomyelitis usually produces only a mild to moderate increase in protein (mean of 0.48 g/L [48 mg/dl] with a range of 0.1–0.7 g/L [10–70 mg/dl]) and a mild mononuclear pleocytosis (mean of 19 cells/mm³ [19 cells/μl] with a range of 0–46 cells/mm³ [0–46 cells/μl]) on CSF. This is not typical of FIP.

Treatment

No effective therapy is known against FIP.

Immunosuppressive corticosteroid therapy **may slow** the **disease** course (1–2 mg/kg prednisone or prednisolone orally twice daily).

All cats with the neurological form of FIP will **eventually die** from their disease.

SPINAL CORD TRAUMA – FRACTURES AND LUXATIONS***

> **Classical signs**
>
> - Acute variably located spinal cord dysfunction (UMN or LMN signs).
> - Focal spinal hyperesthesia.
> - Spinal crepitus.
> - External abrasions and bruising.

Pathogenesis

External spinal trauma can result from **automobile accidents**, **gunshot injuries**, **falls** from heights and blunt trauma.

Sacrocaudal fractures most often occur when the cat's tail is **forcefully pulled** away from the body.
- This most commonly occurs when the cat's tail is trapped under the tire of an automobile. The rotating tire luxates the tail at the sacrococcygeal junction or between two coccygeal vertebrae, resulting in damage to the coccygeal, sacral and lumbar nerve roots (cauda equina).

Most spinal fractures occur **at the junction of mobile and immobile segments** of the spine, such as the thoracolumbar, lumbosacral and sacrocaudal junctions.

Traction on the cauda equina in sacrocaudal luxations can also damage the nerve cell bodies in the caudal lumbar and sacral spinal cord due to cranial transmission of the forces through the dura mater and filum terminale of the cord.

The degree of spinal cord compression; the length of time of compression; and the velocity of the initial impact injury are important contributors to the resultant spinal cord injury.

There are two forms of spinal cord injury – **mechanical (primary) injury**, consisting of physical disruption of vessels and axons **and ischemic** (secondary) **injury**.

The latter leads to energy compromise within the spinal cord, cellular accumulation of calcium and resultant intracellular stimulation of enzymes.

This leads to protein and lipid breakdown (phospholipid hydrolysis), release of arachidonic acid, free radical and eicosanoid formation, and cell death.

Gray matter hemorrhages and white matter edema occur within minutes following acute spinal cord injury, progressing rapidly over the 4–6-hour post-traumatic period.

Clinical signs

Signs depend on the injury level and the degree of physical or functional disruption of the cord.

Signs in cats with sacrocaudal injuries **range from hyperesthesia over the tail base to flaccid analgesic tails** with varying degrees of urinary reflex dyssynergia or LMN urinary/fecal incontinence.
- **Reflex dyssynergia** involves a failure of urethral relaxation when the cat attempts to urinate and the bladder undergoes contraction. This leads to the production of only very small quantities of urine. The bladder will still be large and the cat will often dribble urine in between attempts to urinate.

Many cats with sacrococcygeal trauma also show **signs of LMN paraparesis** (sciatic nerve injury), consisting of dragging of the hind paws on their dorsum and a failure to flex the pelvic limb(s) when walking or when the withdrawal reflex is performed. There will also be a hypo- to areflexia of the cranial tibial and gastrocnemius reflexes.

Palpation of the sacrocaudal area of the spine will result in crepitus and pain. The tail will often be malaligned with the sacrum and the rest of the vertebral column.

Cats with spinal trauma commonly have concurrent thoracic, abdominal or pelvic trauma.

Diagnosis

Neurological and physical examination determine the localization and severity of the cord injury.

Non-contrast spinal radiographs (lateral and across the table ventrodorsal views of the entire spine) establish the **type of vertebral disruption** (fracture vs. subluxation) and the location(s) of the vertebral trauma.

Myelography, MRI or CT scans will determine the **degree of spinal cord compression**.

Differential diagnosis

Any other cause of acute myelopathy must be considered as a differential diagnosis in cats with spinal trauma.

Most other causes can be eliminated based on history and physical examination – external abrasions, bruising, splintering of claws and spinal pain are seen with trauma.

Sacrocaudal fractures must be differentiated from **aortic thromboembolism**, which also can produce an acute onset of LMN paraparesis to paraplegia, with pain.
- However, cats with this disease **do not** have dysfunction associated with the perineum, bladder, rectum and tail.
- The **lack of femoral pulses** and the presence of **cold, cyanotic pelvic limbs** would strongly support aortic thromboembolism.

Pathologic vertebral fracture secondary to neoplasia will present as an acute, painful myelopathy, and may appear superficially similar to a traumatic fracture on non-contrast spinal radiographs. However, closer examination should reveal areas of **lysis within the involved vertebral body**.

Ischemic myelopathy secondary to **fibrocartilaginous embolism** most commonly involves the lumbosacral intumescence as is the case with sacrococcygeal trauma.
- A differentiating feature of ischemic myelopathy is the **absence of spinal pain**.

Treatment

Initial medical emergency treatment should include **intravenous methylprednisolone sodium succinate (30 mg/kg)**, administered **within 8 hours** (and **preferably** within **3 hours**) of the spinal trauma.

Continued treatment consists of a constant rate intravenous infusion of methylprednisolone at 5.4 mg/kg/hour or, if not possible, a second bolus intravenous injection (15 mg/kg) at 2 hours after the initial treatment, followed by 15 mg/kg at 6 hours and then 4 times daily for 24–48 hours.

Most cases of spinal trauma will require **emergency surgical intervention** (spinal cord decompression [laminectomy and/or hemilaminectomy] and spinal fixation).

The type of decompression and stabilization technique is determined by non-contrast and contrast spinal radiographs or CT/MRI scans.

Surgical spinal stabilization is rarely necessary in sacrocaudal fractures/luxations and, due to the often-marked separation of the involved vertebrae, is difficult to achieve.

Surgical decompression of the cauda equina in sacrocaudal trauma is also unnecessary since it is a traction, not compressive, injury.

If the cat is incontinent, attention should be paid to cleanliness, bladder and bowel management, and prevention of decubital ulcers, urine scalding, and cystitis.

If there is UMN or LMN urinary incontinence, **manual expression or indwelling catheterization** of the bladder is required.

Pharmacological management of UMN urinary incontinence or reflex dyssynergia, related to sacrocaudal trauma, consists of **phenoxybenzamine**, an alpha-adrenergic receptor antagonist, to relax the internal sphincter (5 mg orally three times daily) together with **diazepam** (1.25–2 mg/cat orally two to three times daily) to relax the external sphincter.

Bladder detrusor dysfunction can then be treated with **bethanechol**, a parasympathomimetic agent (5–10 mg orally two to three times daily).

Bethanechol may help LMN urinary incontinence (encourages detrusor muscle contraction).

Fecal retention can be treated by increasing the bulk of the feces with **bran, psyllium or canned mashed pumpkin**.

In cats with sacrocaudal injury with only tail paresis, conservative medical management will often result in return of tail function.
- If this does not occur after 4–6 months, amputation of the tail is recommended.

Prognosis

Prognosis is based on the severity of the spinal cord injury. The **milder the neurological deficits**, the **better the prognosis** for recovery.

Cats with severe myelopathy or cauda equina injury with analgesia have a very poor to hopeless prognosis since they commonly have physical or functional spinal cord or cauda equina transection.
- Only 25% or less of cats with flaccid tail, perineal analgesia and LMN urinary and fecal incontinence from a sacrocaudal injury will regain neurologic function.
- 75% of cats with only tail flaccidity can regain tail function.

Prognosis should **NEVER** be **determined based on the degree of radiographic displacement** of the involved vertebra(e).

Prevention

The only preventative measure is for cats to avoid situations where trauma is a distinct possibility.

SPINAL MENINGIOMA**

> ### Classical signs
> - Chronic, progressive UMN or LMN tetraparesis or paraparesis dependent on tumor location.
> - Focal areas of spinal pain.

Pathogenesis

Although most meningiomas are found intracranially, they may also develop along the spinal cord with an **intradural, extramedullary predilection site.**

Meningiomas arise from any cell of the meninges – blood vessels, fibroblasts or arachnoid cells.

Spinal meningiomas are **usually solitary.**

Meningiomas produce signs by compressing the adjacent spinal cord causing vasogenic edema

Occasionally, other tumors such as an astrocytoma occur.

Clinical signs

Most cats are > 9 years of age.

The nature of the ataxia and paresis (UMN versus LMN signs) depends on the tumor's location.

A focal area of spinal pain or more diffuse spinal discomfort may occur weeks prior to the development of neurological dysfunction.

Signs are **slowly progressive**.

Diagnosis

Non-contrast spinal radiographs may reveal thinning or deformation of the vertebral lamina secondary to pressure necrosis from the expanding tumor.

Lumbar **CSF** most commonly reveals **increased protein** (> 0.25 g/L [25 mg/dl]) **without** an accompanying **pleocytosis**. Tumor cells are rarely seen.

MRI scan or myelography reveals an **intradural, extramedullary mass**.

Differential diagnosis

Any cause of chronic, progressive myelopathy should be considered.

The focal nature of the myelopathy with meningioma eliminates most infectious and inflammatory myelopathies, with the exception of FeLV-associated spinal lymphosarcoma.

Ischemia and trauma produce an acute myelopathy and can usually be eliminated.

Age of disease onset for meningiomas would eliminate congenital and inherited myelopathies.

Differentiation from lymphosarcoma often is based on CSF analysis (malignant lymphocytes).

Differentiation from nerve root tumors often requires **histopathology** following surgical removal.

Treatment

Surgical removal of the tumor is the **only definitive treatment**.

Post-operative radiation therapy is recommended.

Corticosteroids only transiently improve neurological function.

Prognosis

The long-term **prognosis** is **guarded to fair** if surgical removal of the tumor appears complete. Follow-up radiation probably further improves this prognosis.

Without surgery, the long-term prognosis is poor.

Prevention

There is no known prevention of spinal meningiomas in cats.

AORTIC THROMBOEMBOLISM**

Classical signs

- Acute LMN paraplegia.
- Severe pain associated with the pelvic limb musculature.
- Vocalization and anxiety.
- Weak or absent femoral pulses.
- Cyanotic and cold nail beds and foot pads.

Pathogenesis

Aortic thromboembolism results from a **thrombus** that is **dislodged from within the left heart or aorta**, leading to **obstruction of the aortic trifurcation** and severe **ischemia** to **pelvic limb muscles and nerves**.

In cats it is most commonly **associated** with **hypertrophic, dilated and restrictive cardiomyopathy**, with **thrombus** formation in the **left atrium**. It also occurs with thyrotoxic cardiac disease.

Thrombus formation requires either damage to the endocardium as occurs in cardiomyopathy, especially the dilated left atrium; blood stasis which also occurs in the dilated left atrium; or altered blood coagulability. Disseminated intravascular coagulation (DIC) was found in 75% of cats with cardiomyopathy and was associated with consumptive or liver-mediated coagulopathy or thromboembolism.

Embolism occurs when the thrombus lodges in a blood vessel.

The thrombus most often lodges in the distal aorta at the trifurcation, leading to a saddle thrombus and occlusion of blood supply to the hindlimbs. Ischemic neuromyopathy occurs and is most severe distal to the stifle. Signs are usually asymmetrical. Occasionally the right brachial artery is occluded, resulting in lameness or paresis of the right forelimb.

Occasionally cats with thromboembolic disease do not have underlying heart disease. Thrombosis may also occur with infectious or neoplastic disease.

Clinical signs

There is no breed or age predilection (average 9 years, range 2–16 years) although **males** are twice as likely to be affected.

Aortic thromboembolism usually produces an **acute onset of LMN paraplegia and severe pain**.

The hindlimbs drag behind the cat, as the hocks cannot be flexed. Hip extension and flexion is present.

Less severe ischemia leads to mild to moderate paraparesis or pelvic limb lameness.

The **gastrocnemius muscles** usually are **firm,** but soften 1–3 days after embolization.

Femoral pulses are weak or absent and the **nail beds** and footpads are **cyanotic and cold**. The distal limbs are often swollen.

Extraneural signs include vocalization, tachypnea/dyspnea, a **cardiac murmur** and **arrhythmias.** Heart failure is present in about 50% of cats with aortic thromboembolism.

Dehydration and hypothermia are often present.

Tail movement, perineal reflexes and urinary function remain intact.

Diagnosis

Increases in serum **creatine kinase** (often 1000–10 000 IU/L [normal: 60–300 IU/L]) occur secondary to **severe muscle damage**.

Creatinine and BUN are increased in more than 50% of cats and may be prerenal or renal. In some cats, concurrent embolization of the renal artery occurs.

Thoracic **radiography** reveals **cardiomegaly** (85–90% of cats) and **pulmonary edema** and/**or pleural effusion** (66%).

Echocardiography most often reveals **hypertrophic cardiomyopathy** (± a left atrial thrombus).

Electrocardiography most commonly reveals **sinus tachycardia**. Atrial fibrillation, and supra-/ventricular arrhythmias can also be seen.

Doppler (color flow) will often demonstrate the decrease in blood flow through the site of thrombo-embolism.

MRI angiography will reveal a complete or partial blood flow obstruction at the aortic trifurcation.

Differential diagnosis

A major feature that differentiates aortic thrombo-embolism from traumatic, infectious, neoplastic and ischemic myelopathies is the presence of paraparesis to paraplegia without involvement of the perineum, tail and bladder.

Cold, cyanotic pelvic limbs without femoral pulses and firm gastrocnemius muscles also are unique.

Treatment

With current treatment modalities, the results of **pallative therapy are as good as aggressive thrombolytic therapies or physical removal of the thrombus**, and considerably less expensive.

- Physical removal is via surgery or balloon embolectomy.
- Thrombolytic agents include tissue plasminogen activator, urokinase and streptokinase.
  - Current information should be consulted on administration and monitoring of thrombolytic and intensive anti-thrombotic therapies if they are to be used.
- **Reperfusion effects are a major problem with aggressive thrombolytic therapies and physical removal**. Rapid onset of **severe hyperkalemia** associated with reperfusion is common and **often fatal. Renal hemorrhage** may also occur during thrombolysis, adversely affecting survival. **Clinical hemorrhage** may require a blood transfusion to control.

Pallative therapy consists of relieving pain, heparin to help prevent another clot forming in the left atrium, **fluid, electrolyte and nutritional support**, warmth, physiotherapy (passive massage and flexing/extending legs) and **treatment of underlying heart disease**. Potassium concentrations should be monitored carefully.

Pain control is an important part of management. Injectable analgesics and a fentenyl patch should be used to provide adequate levels of pain relief.

Excessive licking or chewing of the affected limb may occur resulting in self-mutilation. Loose bandaging of the limb or an Elizabethan collar are usually effective.

Dehydration and electrolyte imbalances, especially hyper- and hypokalaemia, need correcting. Nutritional needs should be met in anorexic cats by the placement of a nasoesophageal tube for feeding.

Treatment of the underlying cardiac disease is essential (see Chapter 25).

Acutely, heparin (400 U/kg subcutaneously followed by 200 U/kg subcutaneously three times daily) can be given to prevent further activation of the coagulation cascade, although **it will not have any effect on the formed thrombus.**

Continue palliative therapy for 5–6 days and look for rewarming of the toes and returning pulses as an initial sign of improvement. Doppler is useful for detecting blood flow. If there is no sign of reperfusion after

6 days, the prognosis is hopeless and the cat should be euthanized.

Various other treatments have been advocated but there are no studies showing increased survival. These include aspirin, periactin, acepromazine and vasodilator agents.

Aspirin may be beneficial during and after an episode of thromboembolism due to its **antiplatelet effects** and decreased production of the vasoconstrictor thromboxane A_2, as well as analgesic effects. The dosage is $1/4 \times 325$ mg adult aspirin (81 mg) every second to third day. Blockade of prostacyclin production by the endothelium with aspirin is of concern, and some advocate lower doses of aspirin more frequently (1–5 mg/cat q 24 h). Prostacyclin inhibits platelet aggregation and vasoconstriction.

Acepromazine (0.1–0.5 mg subcutaneously three times daily) can be used for **sedation** and **vasodilation**.

Vasodilation with alpha-blockers is advocated by some but unproven.

Long-term warfarin therapy may decrease the frequency of rethrombosis, but needs careful monitoring using the International Normalization Ratio (INR) for PT to achieve a INR between 2 and 3. Doses of 0.06–0.20 mg/kg PO q 24 h have been advocated. A lower dose of 0.5 mg/cat PO q 48 h has also been used.

Prognosis

Only 30–50% of cats survive the initial episodes and go home.

Most will re-embolize – **long-term prognosis is poor** (average survival is 6–11 months with therapy) with less than 50% surviving 1 year.
- 50% of cats have rethrombosis even when treated with warfarin.

Most cats that survive an initial episode will show varying degrees of **neurological recovery** to their pelvic limbs, although this often takes **weeks to months**. Rarely does the neuromuscular function fully recover.

Hypothermia and azotemia prior to therapy and hyperkalemia during thrombolysis are negatively associated with survival. Echocardiographic evidence of another thrombus in the left atrium also decreases the long-term prognosis.

Prevention

Little can be done to prevent aortic thromboembolism if the underlying cardiac disease has not been previously recognized.

If cardiac disease is diagnosed, the risk of thromboembolism may be reduced by appropriate treatment of the cardiomyopathy (see Chapter 6). Efficacy of long-term aspirin (low dose 1–5 mg/cat q 24 h or a regular dose 81 mg/cat, q 48–72 h PO) or warfarin therapy in preventing thromboembolism has not been demonstrated, and most cats rethrombose.

FELINE POLIOENCEPHALOMYELITIS*

Classical signs

- Stiff staggering gait.
- Inability to jump.
- Chronic pelvic limb ataxia and paraparesis.
- Inability to retract their claws.
- Thoracolumbar hyperesthesia.
- Thoracic limb paresis and ataxia.
- Decreased mentation and seizures.
- Fever (in 50% of cases).

Pathogenesis

Feline polioencephalomyelitis is a **chronic, progressive** disease affecting the **spinal cord and brain** of cats.

The **cause** is **unknown**, although neuropathology is suggestive of a neurotrophic virus.

Recently, specific antibodies to the **Borna disease virus** have been found in 44% of cats with feline polioencephalomyelitis in Sweden.

Feline polioencephalomyelitis is a sporadic worldwide disease.

Clinical signs

Affected cats range from **4 months to 12 years of age**.

Both male and female cats are affected.

All domestic cat breeds as well as large non-domesticated cat species can contract the disease.

Neurologic **signs** usually **develop over 2–3 months** with a subacute to chronic progressive course.

The most striking neurologic signs include a **stiff staggering gait, inability to jump, pelvic limb ataxia and paraparesis**.

- Some cats have decreased spinal reflexes and some are unable to retract their claws.

Other signs may include thoracic limb ataxia and paresis, hyperesthesia over the thoracolumbar and lumbosacral regions, decreased mentation, behavior change, decreased pupillary light reflexes, hypersensitivity to external stimuli, impaired vision, seizures, increased salivation, intention tremors and pruritis.

With disease progression, **paraplegia eventually occurs**.

A **fever** is present in approximately **50% of cats**.

Diagnosis

CSF analysis usually reveals a **non-specific** mild to moderate elevation in protein (mean of 0.48 g/L [48 mg/dl] with a range of 0.1–0.7 g/L [10–70 mg/dl]) and a mild mononuclear pleocytosis (mean of 19 cells/mm³ [19 cells/µl] with a range of 0–46 cells/mm³ [0–46 cells/µl]).

Serologic testing for FIV and FeLV antibodies is negative.

Definitive diagnosis can only be made on **necropsy**.

Histopathology reveals a **disseminated meningoencephalomyelitis** with lymphocytic perivascular cuffs that is most severe in the spinal cord (gray matter) and brainstem.

Differential diagnosis

Infectious diseases (FIP and toxoplasmosis) also may produce signs of progressive spinal cord dysfunction, making differentiation based on neurological signs difficult. Uveitis, chorioretinitis and optic neuritis are often present with CNS infections, but not with polioencephalomyelitis.

Cats with spinal **CNS lymphosarcoma** commonly are FeLV positive and may have other systemic signs of tumor involvement.

CSF analysis may help differentiate between the infectious diseases, lymphosarcoma and feline polioencephalomyelitis (see sections on lymphosarcoma and FIP), although the range of values overlap between the diseases.

Treatment

Immunosuppressive steroid therapy (**prednisone** 1–2 mg/kg BID) is the recommended treatment against this disease, although data are lacking.

This may be combined with other immunosuppressive agents such as **cytosine arabinoside.**

Aggressive and persistent therapy may result in remission and possible cure after several months.

Prognosis

Prognosis is **guarded**. The disease tends to be progressive if untreated.

Prevention

Since this disease is of unknown etiology and very sporadic, there are no recommendations for prevention.

CONGENITAL ABNORMALITIES OF THE SPINAL CORD AND VERTEBRAE*

Classical signs

- UMN or LMN paraparesis or tetraparesis dependent on the anomaly and its location.
- Scoliosis (lateral curvature of the spine), lordosis (downward arching spine), or kyphosis (upward arching spine) resulting from a hemivertebra.
- Cervical pain and UMN tetraparesis to paralysis (atlantoaxial subluxation).
- LMN paraparesis to paraplegia (spina bifida and sacrococcygeal dysgenesis).
- LMN urinary and fecal incontinence (spina bifida and sacrococcygeal dysgenesis).
- Dorsal midline spinal defects or cystic structures – may drain CSF (spina bifida).
- Abnormal hair growth direction, a dimple on the skin surface or an open tract (spina bifida).

Pathogenesis

Spinal cord and vertebral **anomalies** are **classified** into abnormalities originating in the tissues of **mesodermal origin** (vertebral body and intervertebral disc) **and** those arising from tissues of **ectodermal origin** (spinal cord and meninges).

Malformations of mesodermal origin.
- **Block vertebrae**.
  – Caused by **improper segmentation of somites**, resulting in stable vertebral fusion.
- **Butterfly vertebrae**.
  – Abnormal **persistence of** the **notochord** (the embryological precursor of intervertebral discs), producing a midline cranial to caudal cleft in the vertebral body (when viewing the vertebra from the dorsoventral direction).
- **Hemivertebrae**.
  – Produced by **fusion** of **one lateral somite to one** on the contralateral side that is **not directly opposed or** by a **lack of vascularization**, leading to a failure of ossification in part of the vertebral body. This produces a **wedge-shaped vertebra**, and scoliosis, lordosis or kyphosis.
- **Transitional vertebrae**.
  – Sacralization of the last lumbar vertebra is the most common in cats. In this condition, the last lumbar vertebra has characteristics of both lumbar vertebrae and the sacrum.
- **Atlantoaxial subluxation**.
  – Results from **hypoplasia or aplasia of the dens** with secondary atlantoaxial instability.
  – It is either caused by a **developmental failure of dens** ossification **or** an **ischemic necrosis** and partial resorption **of the dens** as a result of trauma.
  – The cranial portion of the axis is displaced into the spinal canal producing cord compression.

Malformations of ectodermal origin.
- Abnormalities of the vertebral arch and spinal cord are primarily influenced by neural tube development.
- The **most common** anomaly is **spina bifida.**
- **Spina bifida.**
  – The defects of spina bifida vary from **incomplete fusion of the vertebral arch to incomplete fusion of the neural tube**, resulting in abnormal formation and/or protrusion of the meninges and/or spinal cord.
  – Pathogenesis may involve initial failure of closure or the reopening of a previously closed neural tube.
  – Spina bifida occulta represents an incomplete closure of one or more vertebral arches without protrusion of meninges or spinal cord.
  – **Spina bifida manifesta** includes **meningocele** (meningeal herniation through the vertebral arch defect) **and meningomyelocele** (herniation of the spinal cord and meninges).
  – The meningeal and/or spinal cord herniation may or may not communicate with the environment.
- **Sacrococcygeal dysgenesis of Manx cats**.
  – An **autosomal semi-lethal dominant trait**, providing the genetic basis for the absent tail as well as numerous vertebral and spinal cord abnormalities.
  – Homozygotes usually do not survive.
  – There are four phenotypic subgroups – a complete absence of coccygeal, sacral +/– caudal lumbar vertebrae (the most severe); fused caudal vertebrae; mobile but kinked caudal vertebrae; and a normal tail.

Clinical signs

Clinical signs are dependent on the type of congenital malformation and its location.

Block vertebrae are **usually stable**.
- Occasionally they can be stenotic or angulated, causing extradural spinal cord compression.
- Disc extrusion can occur at disc spaces immediately cranial and caudal to the block vertebrae.

Butterfly vertebrae are generally **incidental** findings.

Hemivertebrae commonly lead to **scoliosis, lordosis or kyphosis**.
- Signs are due to spinal cord compression or repeated trauma associated with vertebral instability. Instability produces osseous changes that secondarily compress the spinal cord.
- Signs may be acute, chronic, progressive or intermittent, but are usually first noted within the first 1–2 years of life.
- Conformation may be visibly or palpably abnormal.

Sacralization of the caudal lumbar vertebrae can result in pain and LMN paraparesis secondary to cauda equina compression.

Atlantoaxial malformation can produce episodic **cervical pain or acute/chronic UMN tetraparesis** to tetraplegia, usually in cats less than 1 year of age.
- If spinal cord injury is severe, the cat can develop respiratory paralysis and caudal brainstem dysfunction.
- Episodic opisthotonos and rigidity occasionally occur which can be misinterpreted as seizures.

Spina bifida occulta is an incidental finding.

Spina bifida manifesta produces myelopathy dependent on the degree of incorporation of the spinal cord and/or cauda equina into the herniated meningeal sac.
- Most commonly the **caudal lumbar and sacral spine** is affected, resulting in **LMN paraparesis/plegia and urinary/fecal incontinence** in newborn kittens.
- Spina bifida can be observed at birth as **dorsal midline, open regions of the spinal canal** or cystic structures that may **drain CSF**.
- Abnormal hair growth, a skin dimple or an open tract are less severe manifestations.

Sacrococcygeal dysgenesis produces a **hopping gait**.
- More severe signs at or soon after birth include **LMN urinary/fecal incontinence, megacolon, and LMN paraparesis/paraplegia**.
- Some are normal at birth but develop progressive signs over several weeks to months as the cat matures. Damage to the spinal cord with growth occurs as a result of spinal cord tethering (fixation).

Diagnosis

Breed association (Manx cat).

Signs are most commonly observed in **immature animals** (< 6 months of age).

The cat's conformation may be visibly or palpably abnormal (scoliosis, skin dimple, etc.).

Non-contrast spinal radiography demonstrates the anomaly.
- Block vertebra – joining of two adjacent vertebral bodies.
- Butterfly vertebra – sagittal vertebral body cleft.
- Hemivertebra – abnormal vertebral wedging and shortening.
- Atlantoaxial subluxation – abnormally shaped or absent dens.
- Spina bifida – vertebral arch defect.

Myelography demonstrates cord compression or a meningocele/meningomyelocele.

MRI scan or CT myelography reveals soft tissue abnormalities associated with a spinal cord that is tethered (fixed) by either meningocutaneous attachments (spina bifida) or by a failure of the terminal cord-like attachment from the spinal cord to the dura to stretch with growth. They will also reveal cord compression.

Differential diagnosis

Major **differentials for hemivertebra** include traumatic or pathologic **fracture with secondary collapse of the vertebral body**.
- **Hemivertebrae**, however, have **smooth end plates** and well-formed adjacent disc spaces.
- Difficulty in differentiation arises when vertebral osteophytes are present.

Differential diagnoses for block vertebrae include vertebral fusion secondary to discospondylitis, vertebral fracture/luxation, collapsed disc space secondary to disc extrusion, or previous disc surgery. However, all have associated reactive bone, which is not present with block vertebrae.

Atlanto-axial subluxation and spina bifida have few rule-outs, except trauma.

Treatment

Spinal cord compression from a **hemivertebra** can be treated via **surgical decompression and stabilization** (if necessary).

Treatment for **atlantoaxial subluxation** involves **stabilization** of the atlantoaxial joint via **ventral cross-pinning or screws** (preferred) or dorsal wiring.

Specific treatment for spina bifida and sacrococcygeal dysgenesis is rarely attempted.
- If signs are associated with spinal cord tethering or there is a meningocutaneous fistula without primary spinal cord anomalies, reconstructive surgery may be possible.

Prognosis

Prognosis **depends on the type of congenital anomaly** and the degree of dysfunction.

Cats with mild signs due to a surgically treatable hemivertebra or block vertebra, have a guarded to good prognosis for improvement.

Morbidity and mortality is **high with surgical stabilization of atlantoaxial subluxation**.
- With **successful stabilization**, however, cats with initially mild to moderate neurological dysfunction have a **fair to good prognosis**.

Prognosis for cats with **spina bifida or sacrococcygeal dysgenesis with anomalies associated with the spinal cord or cauda equina**, is **grave**. These cats should be euthanized if the neurological dysfunction is incompatible with a good quality of life.

Cats with spinal cord tethering (spina bifida) have a potentially fair to good prognosis with surgery.

Prevention

Prevention of further congenital malformations is best achieved by a **spay/neuter program**.

HYPERVITAMINOSIS A*

Classical signs

- Cervical and thoracic limb hyperesthesia and rigidity.
- Thoracic limb lameness.
- Chronic progressive ataxia.
- Reluctance to move.
- Chronic tetraparesis to paralysis.

Pathogenesis

Hypervitaminosis A is a **skeletal disease**, secondary to **excessive intake of vitamin A** (liver or vitamin A supplementation (cod liver oil) (> 1000 IU/ml).

Clinical signs

Affected cats are usually 2–9 years of age.

Signs include **cervical and thoracic limb hyperesthesia and rigidity** due to extensive confluent **exostosis in the cervical and thoracic spine**, thoracic limb lameness, ataxia, reluctance to move, and tetraparesis to paralysis.

Other signs include lethargy, anorexia, constipation, weight loss and an unkempt haircoat due to an inability to groom.

Exostoses develop insidiously with the above signs occurring only after the disease is advanced.

Diagnosis

Non-contrast **spinal radiographs** show **new bone formation** involving the **cervical vertebrae**.
- The sternum, costal cartilages, and long bone metaphyses also show new bone formation.
- Joints may show arthrodesis.

Differential diagnosis

Based on the clinical and neurological examinations, other differentials include infectious meningitis and myelitis, vertebral neoplasia, mucopolysaccharidosis and discospondylitis (rare).

Non-contrast spinal radiographs eliminate all differentials with the possible exception of mucopolysaccharidosis **VI**, a rare **autosomal recessive storage disease** produced by **deficiency** of the lysosomal enzyme, **arylsulfatase B**.
- Mucopolysaccharidosis VI occurs in **4–7-month-old Siamese cats**, producing spinal cord compression secondary to **fusion of the cervical and thoracolumbar vertebrae with bony proliferation**.
- These cats also have a flat, broad face, widely spaced eyes, corneal clouding and enlarged feet.

Treatment

Remove excess vitamin A from the diet to prevent further development of exostoses.

Use a **balanced commercial cat diet**.

Skeletal improvement is monitored by radiography and neurological examinations.

Analgesics may symptomatically treat the clinical signs.

- **Aspirin** – 10 mg/kg PO q 48 h.
- Narcotic analgesics such as **morphine** (4 mg/ml) – 0.5 mg/kg PO three times to four times daily.
- Non-steroidal anti-inflammatory drugs.
- Fentanyl patch.

FIBROCARTILAGINOUS EMBOLISM

Classical signs

- Acute, non-progressive, non-painful, asymmetrical LMN paraparesis to paraplegia.
- LMN urinary and fecal incontinence.

Pathogenesis

Spinal cord infarction secondary **to fibrocartilaginous embolism** is uncommon.

The **embolus** is histochemically identical **to the fibrocartilage of the nucleus pulposus**.

It is unknown how the embolus reaches the spinal vasculature from its origin.

Embolization of arteries, veins or a combination of the two may occur.

Sudden increases in intra-abdominal pressure (hard exercise) may facilitate retrograde passage of disc material through the venous sinuses and spinal veins.

Embolism results in **segmental hemorrhagic necrosis and malacia of the spinal cord**.

Clinical signs

Clinical signs reflect the location of the lesion along the spinal cord.

In cats, the **lumbosacral intumescence** is the **most common** site of myelopathy, resulting in an **acute LMN paraparesis to paraplegia**, and **LMN urinary and fecal incontinence**.

Other findings include a **lack of spinal pain, lack of disease progression** and marked **asymmetry** of neurological dysfunction.

Diagnosis

Diagnosis is based on **exclusion of other etiologies**. History and neurological exam are important.

Survey radiographs are normal.

CSF analysis is variable, ranging from normal, hemorrhagic, or showing a mild mixed pleocytosis (6–25 cells/mm^3 [6–25 cells/µl]).

Myelography will either be normal or occasionally show cord edema.

MRI diffusion studies may reveal the ischemic area of spinal cord, if the affected area is large enough.

Definitive diagnosis can only be made at **necropsy**.

Differential diagnosis

Differential diagnosis includes any cause of acute paraparesis to paraplegia.

The unique clinical signs and usual absence of abnormalities on work-up separate fibrocartilaginous embolism from other acute myelopathies.

Treatment

Immediate treatment consists of **methylprednisolone sodium succinate** (see spinal trauma).

Embolic myelopathy is **non-surgical**.

Long-term corticosteroid therapy is not recommended.

Prognosis

Prognosis depends on density of neurological dysfunction and degree of irreversible cord damage.

Cats with **severe LMN paraplegia, absent pain** sensation and LMN urinary incontinence associated with involvement of the lumbosacral intumescence have a **poor to hopeless** prognosis.

Cats with **less severe signs** have a **guarded to favorable** prognosis for partial to full recovery.

Prevention

There are no preventive measures that can be undertaken.

RECOMMENDED READING

Baroni M, Heinold Y. A review of the clinical diagnosis of feline infectious peritonitis viral meningo-encephalomyelitis. Prog Vet Neurol 1995; 6(3): 88–94.

Fenner WR. Inflammations of the nervous system, Chapter 66. In: August JR (ed) Consultations in Feline Internal Medicine 1. W.B. Saunders Company, Philadelphia, 1991, pp. 507–517.

Fox PR. Feline cardiomyopathies, Chapter 117. In: Ettinger S, Feldman E (ed) Textbook of Veterinary Internal Medicine. W.B. Saunders Company, Philadelphia, 2000, pp. 896–923.

Kroll RA, Constantinescu GM. Congenital abnormalities of the spinal cord and vertebrae, Chapter 52. In: August JR (ed) Consultations in Feline Internal Medicine 2. W.B. Saunders Company, Philadelphia, 1994, pp. 413–420.

Lane SB, Kornegay JN. Spinal lymphosarcoma, Chapter 61. In: August JR (ed) Consultations in Feline Internal Medicine 1. W.B. Saunders Company, Philadelphia, 1991, pp. 487–490.

Lundgren A-L. Feline non-suppurative meningoencephalomyelitis. A clinical and pathological study. J Comp Pathol 1992; 107: 411–425.

Munana KR. Inflammatory disorders of the central nervous system, Chapter 54. In: August JR (ed) Consultations in Feline Internal Medicine 4. WB Saunders Company, Philadelphia, 2001, pp. 425–433.

Munana KR. Encephalitis and meningitis. In: Bagley R (ed) Veterinary Clinics of North America Small Animal Practice – Intracranial Disease. WB Saunders Company, Philadelphia, 1996, pp. 857–874.

Pion P. Feline Thrombotic Disease Veterinary Information Network. http:www.vin.com/Members/SearchDB /rounds/lc990711/lc990711.htm

Thomas WB. Vascular disorders, Chapter 52. In: August JR (ed) Consultations in Feline Internal Medicine 4. WB Saunders Company, Philadelphia, 2001, pp. 405–412.

43. The cat with ataxia without weakness

Rodney S Bagley

> **KEY SIGNS**
>
> - Falling.
> - Incoordination.
> - Swaying from side to side.
> - Goose stepping gait.

MECHANISM?

- Ataxia results from sensory proprioception dysfunction and causes falling and incoordination.

WHERE?

- Cerebellum, cerebral cortex (central controlling centers for movement), vestibular system (peripheral or central) or spinal cord (sensory spinocerebellar pathways).

WHAT?

- Diseases causing ataxia without weakness most commonly involve the cerebellum and include cerebellar hypoplasia (panleukopenia virus infection), hydrocephalus, storage disease, tumors and encephalitis.
- Diseases of the vestibular system most commonly involve the peripheral apparatus and include otitis media/interna, idiopathic vestibular disease and tumors.
- Diseases of the spinal cord rarely cause ataxia without weakness.
- Intracranial, cerebellar and vestibular causes of ataxia without weakness.

QUICK REFERENCE SUMMARY

Diseases causing ataxia without weakness

DEGENERATIVE

- **Inherited cerebellar diseases** (p 934)
  Hereditary cerebellar degeneration occurs in Japans. Clinical signs begin around 7–8 weeks of age and include ataxia, dysmetria, head tremor and intention tremor. **Inherited spongiform encephalopathy** occurs in Egyptian Mau cats in the USA resulting in ataxia and hypermetria beginning at 7 weeks of age. A different spongiform encephalopathy has been reported in older Egyptian Mau cats in the United Kingdom. Clinical signs include muscle tremors, ataxia, dilated unresponsive pupils, jaw champing, salivation and behavior abnormalities. Signs may progress to

severe ataxia and hypermetria. **Neuroaxonal dystrophy** in domestic tri-colored cats results in a head tremor beginning at 5–6 weeks of age with signs progressing to ataxia and hypermetria. Affected kittens have a lilac color, which darkens with age. A similar but separate neuroaxonal dystrophy has been described in cats of various colors. Clinical signs begin at 7–9 months of age and include ataxia with paraparesis.

● Storage diseases** (p 935)

Sphingomyelinosis (Niemann–Pick type C disease) results in ataxia and tremors beginning at less than 6 months of age. Clinical signs progress to hypermetria, absent menace responses, and occasionally positional nystagmus. Death usually occurs by 8–10 months of age. Niemann–Pick type A disease occurs in Siamese and Balinese cats. Head tremor, head bobbing and dysmetria begin at 3–4 months of age. Clinical signs progress to ataxia and paresis, worse in the pelvic limbs.

ANOMALY

● Cerebellar hypoplasia*** (p 927)

Cerebellar degeneration usually occurs in neonatal to younger animals due to congenital deformities or infectious causes (panleukopenia virus infection). Cerebellar hypoplasia results from in utero or immediately postnatal infection with the panleukopenia virus. Clinical signs are most apparent when the animal begins purposeful movement and attempts to walk. Ataxia, dysmetria, intention tremor and absent menaces responses with normal vision are common clinical signs. Clinical signs usually remain static or improve with growth. No treatment is helpful.

● Hydrocephalus** (p 932)

If hydrocephalus is congenital, cats may have an enlarged, "dome-shaped" skull. A fontanelle that persists during maturation may be palpable. Acquired hydrocephalus in adults will show no outward anatomical signs. Clinical signs include seizures, poor learning ability, behavior changes, paresis, cranial nerve deficits and changes in consciousness.

● Congenital vestibular disease** (p 933)

Congenital peripheral vestibular disease is seen in Siamese and Burmese cats. Clinical signs include head tilt, vestibular ataxia (cat leans, drifts, falls, or rolls to side of head tilt) and, in some, deafness. Signs may remain persistent throughout life or may improve spontaneously.

METABOLIC

● Vascular diseases* (p 937)

Rarely, thromboembolic disease or hemorrhage involves the cerebellum. An acute onset of cerebellar signs (incoordination, swaying from side to side, goose-stepping gait, intention tremor and reduced menace) in an older animal is most common with these types of diseases. A cat with polycythemia was presented for ataxia, possibly due to increases in serum viscosity.

NEOPLASTIC

● Cerebellar and vestibular tumor*** (p 928)

Primary or secondary neoplasia involving the cerebellum is uncommon. Intracranial tumors such as meningioma and choroid plexus tumors can affect both the cerebellum or vestibular system and result in ataxia. Other signs such as an intention tremor, goose-stepping gait, menace deficits, nystagmus and head tilt may be present. Occasionally tumors of the ear cause peripheral vestibular ataxia (cat leans, drifts, falls or rolls towards the side with a head tilt). Neoplastic disease occurs more often in older cats.

continued

continued

NUTRITIONAL

● Thiamine deficiency* (p 938)

Decreased thiamine can result in brain stem disease in cats. Clinical signs initially begin with lethargy, inappetence and reluctance to walk. Later there is vestibular ataxia and episodes of spastic ventroflexion of the neck or opisthotonos, dilated pupils, stupor and coma.

INFLAMMATORY/INFECTIOUS

● Encephalitis*** (p 930)

Neurological signs are often diffuse and may not localize to a single area within the nervous system. Fever and leukocytosis are inconsistent findings. Systemic signs of disease such as fever, coughing, vomiting and diarrhea may accompany the neurologic signs. Feline infectious peritonitis, toxoplasmosis and *Cryptococcus* are more common causes of encephalitis. Non-infectious causes are less common but include feline non-suppurative meningoencephalomyelitis ("staggering disease").

● Idiopathic encephalopathy* (p 939)

An encephalomyelopathy of young cats reported in the United Kingdom had clinical signs of ataxia, paresis and "head shaking". Cats 3–12 months old were affected, however, the disease was seen in cats up to 3 years of age. Ataxia of the pelvic limbs was the initial clinical sign noted.

● Otitis media/interna** (p 936)

Clinical signs may reflect either primary ear, vestibular, or auditory dysfunction. Head tilt is most common, but nystagmus and vestibular ataxia (leaning or falling to one side) may also be present. A painful external ear and or pain on opening the mouth is often present. The facial nerve may be involved. On otoscopic examination, the tympanic membrane is often discolored (hyperemic), opaque and bulging outward with middle ear disease.

Idiopathic:

● Idiopathic peripheral vestibular disease*** (p 931)

Acute onset of peripheral vestibular signs with nystagmus (horizontal or rotary), head tilt (toward the side of the lesion), rolling and falling. No other neurological signs are seen. Clinical signs, while initially severe, are restricted to the vestibular system. Otoscopic examination, bulla radiographs and other advanced imaging studies (computed tomography (CT), magnetic resonance (MR) imaging) are normal. Signs usually improve dramatically in 1–2 weeks regardless of treatment.

Trauma:

● Head trauma*** (p 932)

Usually associated with an acute onset of clinical signs reflective of an intracranial problem. Signs present often include alterations in consciousness, paresis and cranial nerve abnormalities. Fresh blood from lacerations on or around the head, skull fractures, blood in the ear canals, and scleral hemorrhage may be clues to a previous traumatic incident.

Toxicity:

● Toxins* (p 938)

Metronidazole at high doses has been reported to result in ataxia as the initial clinical sign. Paresis is usually present, and seizures and cortical blindness may also be noted. **Bromethalin**

toxicosis may also result in ataxia in the early stages. Signs progress to paresis, depression, tremors, seizures and decerebrate posture. **Ivermectin** toxicosis has resulted in generalized ataxia, tremor, weakness, incoordination and miosis in a kitten. **Griseofulvin** therapy resulted in ataxia in a 12-week-old kitten. **Aminoglycosides,** administered either systemically or topically, may cause vestibular signs. Streptomycin and gentamicin have the most pronounced effects on the vestibular receptors, while neomycin, kanamycin and amikacin preferentially damage auditory receptors. **Chlorhexidine** solution used to clean the external ear may result in vestibular signs.

INTRODUCTION

MECHANISM?

Ataxia is an abnormality of movement wherein the animal does not move in a straight line when walking but rather sways or falls, usually from side to side.

Ataxia indicates a problem with unconscious, sensory proprioception.

Lack of unconscious, sensory proprioceptive information can also result in **dysmetria,** including **hypermetria** ("goose-stepping"; overflexing of the limbs when walking) and **hypometria** (failure to flex and extend the limb properly) resulting in a "stiff" appearance of limb movement, and tremor.

WHERE?

Disease of the cerebellum, central controlling centers for movement, or sensory pathways traveling from the spinal cord to the cerebellum are often affected.

Disease of the vestibular system may also result in ataxia and incoordination.

Diseases of the spinal cord can result in ataxia due to involvement of the spinocerebellar pathways.

WHAT?

Diseases of the intracranial nervous system resulting in ataxia often involve the cerebellum.

These include cerebellar hypoplasia (panleukopenia virus infection), hydrocephalus, storage disease, tumors, encephalitis and vascular-based diseases.

Diseases of the vestibular system include those affecting the central vestibular areas (developmental diseases, hydrocephalus, storage disease, tumors, encephalitis and vascular-based diseases) and peripheral vestibular areas (congenital vestibular disease, trauma, otitis media/interna, idiopathic vestibular disease and tumors).

Diseases of the spinal cord include compressive, degenerative, inflammatory, vascular, neoplastic, and congenital diseases (see "The Cat With Limb Weakness").

DISEASES CAUSING ATAXIA WITHOUT WEAKNESS

CEREBELLAR HYPOPLASIA***

> **Classical signs**
>
> - Signs are present from the early prenatal period.
> - Clinical signs usually remain unchanged or may improve during life.
> - Coarse tremor that worsens when the cat moves in a goal-oriented fashion (intention tremor).
> - Other signs include ataxia, hypermetria, menace deficits, head tilt and nystagmus.

Pathogenesis

Cerebellar hypoplasia results from **in utero or immediately postnatal infection with the panleukopenia** virus (parvovirus).

Infection of the fetus may occur when a pregnant queen is **vaccinated with a modified-live** panleukopenia virus **vaccination**.

This virus **destroys the external germinal layer of the cerebellum** and prevents the formation of the granular layer.

Some affected cats have a concurrent hydrocephalus and hydranencephaly.

Clinical signs

Clinical signs are present from the early prenatal period but are most apparent when the animal begins purposeful movement and attempts to walk.

Tremor accompanying the disease usually has a **slow frequency** (2–6 times/second) and **large amplitude (course tremor)**. The tremor **worsens** (increases in frequency or amplitude), **when the cat moves** in a goal-oriented way (e.g. bends down to eat), which is termed an intention tremor.

Other signs include **ataxia** (incoordination; swaying from side to side), **hypermetria** ("goose-stepping"; overflexing of the limbs when walking), **menace deficits** (with normal vision and pupillary light reflexes), **head tilt** and **nystagmus** (combination quick followed by slow movement of the eyes).

Clinical **signs** usually **remain static** or **improve with growth** as the cat compensates, causing the tremor to become less apparent.

Diagnosis

Antemortem testing for panleukopenia often results in negative findings.

Routine laboratory investigations are normal.

Definitive diagnosis is usually only obtained at **necropsy** and histopathological examination of the nervous tissue.

In some instances of cerebellar atrophy, a **smaller than normal cerebellum** may be seen on **magnetic resonance imaging** of the intracranial nervous system. This is most readily seen on the sagittal view.

Occasionally, inflammatory cells may be present in cerebrospinal fluid examination in cats with active panleukopenia viral infection. Cerebrospinal fluid with the other degenerative cerebellar conditions and with previous panleukopenia infection is usually normal.

Differential diagnosis

In this age of cat, other inflammatory central nervous system abnormalities such as **toxoplasmosis** infection are possible.

Congenital anatomical defects of the cerebellum may cause similar signs.

Trauma occurring at a young age may permanently damage the cerebellum producing similar signs.

Treatment

No treatment is currently helpful for cats affected with this disease.

Prognosis

Clinical signs associated with previous panleukopenia virus infection of the developing cerebellum usually remain static or improve with growth, causing the tremor to become less apparent.

Prevention

Do not vaccinate queens with modified live panleukopenia virus vaccine.

CEREBELLAR OR VESTIBULAR TUMOR***

> ### Classical signs
>
> - Signs usually begin in cats 5 years of age or older.
> - Signs usually are progressive over weeks to months.
> - Occasionally, clinical signs begin acutely.
> - Intention tremor is often associated with other signs of cerebellar disease including ataxia, dysmetria, menace deficits, head tilt and nystagmus.

See main reference on page 821 for details (The Cat With Stupor or Coma).

Clinical signs

Clinical signs usually begin in **cats 5 years of age or older.**

Signs are usually **progressive over weeks to months.**

Occasionally, clinical signs begin acutely.

Intention tremor is often associated with other **signs of cerebellar disease** including ataxia (incoordination; swaying from side to side), dysmetria ("goose-stepping"; overflexing of the limbs when walking), **menace deficits** (with normal vision and pupillary light reflexes), **head tilt**, and **nystagmus** (combination quick followed by slow movement of the eyes).

Signs reflect either **primary nervous parenchymal damage** from the tumor or **secondary** pathophysiological **sequelae** such as **hemorrhage and edema**.

Meningiomas are the **most common brain tumor** in cats and are usually histologically benign.
- Less-frequent tumors arise from astrocytes, oligo-dendrogliocytes, ependymal cells and choroid plexus cells.
- Medulloblastoma is a rare primary brain tumor that involves the cerebellum.
- Neoplasia may also secondarily involve the brain via **metastasis** or via **direct extension** from extra-neural sites.

Tumors involving the inner ear may damage **the peripheral vestibular system**, resulting in **vestibular ataxia**, in which the cat leans, drifts, falls or rolls toward the side of the lesion and has a head tilt. Nystagmus may also be present. Occasionally tumors extend through the tympanic membrane and are evident during otoscopic examination, but this is rare. See page 845 "The Cat With a Head Tilt, Vestibular Ataxia or Nystagmus".

Squamous cell carcinoma and adenocarcinoma are the most common tumors affecting the peripheral vestibular system.

Diagnosis

Routine laboratory data (e.g. hematology, biochemistry, urinalysis) are normal.

Diagnosis of a structural intracranial abnormality in the brain is most readily accomplished with **magnetic resonance (MR) imaging** or **computed tomography (CT)** of the brain.
- A **broad-based**, **extra-axial** (arising outside and pushing into the parenchyma) **contrast-enhancing**

mass on CT or MR imaging is found in most **instances of meningioma**.
- The CT and MR appearance of gliomas is varied and enhancement after contrast administration may not be present. As these tumors arise from brain parenchymal cells, they are **found within the neuroaxis (intra-axial).**
- **Choroid plexus tumors** often **enhance markedly** after contrast administration because of the increased concentration of blood vessels within the tumor. Because of their association with the ventricular system, associated **hydrocephalus is common.**

Cerebrospinal fluid often has **increased protein concentration** but this finding is not pathognomonic for neoplasia.

Cerebrospinal fluid may have **evidence of inflammation** (increased nucelated cells and protein content). If CSF is the only assessment made, encephalitis may be erroneously diagnosed.

Skull radiographs or advanced imaging are necessary to **assess the middle and inner ear**. Abnormalities seen with these studies, however, are not always definitive for neoplasia, and tissue diagnosis at surgery is often necessary to accurate assessment. Destruction (lysis) of the bone of the bulla is more often associated with neoplasia as compared to inflammation.

Differential diagnosis

Congential and inherited cerebellar diseases occur in younger animals.

Cerebrovascular, traumatic and inflammatory conditions can mimic the signs of a brain tumor.

Treatment

Corticosteroids (prednisolone 1–2 mg/kg q 12 h) may reduce peritumoral edema and improve clinical signs.

Surgical removal of primary brain tumors may be accomplished, especially with meningioma.

A well-encapsulated, firm whitish mass is most often encountered at surgery in cats. Cortical parenchyma is usually not infiltrated but rather compressed in cats, leaving indentations in the nervous tissue parenchyma after resection.

Radiation therapy (45–48 Gy) may control tumor growth of some brain tumors.

Treatment options of tumors of the ear include surgical resection/debulking, radiation and chemotherapies.

ENCEPHALITIS***

> ### Classical signs
>
> - Diffuse or multifocal neurological signs.
> - Cerebellar signs such as intention tremor, ataxia, hypermetria, head tilt and nystagmus.
> - Cervical pain can be present.
> - Fever is an inconsistent finding.
> - Clues of systemic inflammatory disease such as chorioretinitis are often present.
> - Other signs of polysystemic disease such as coughing, vomiting or diarrhea may be present.

See main reference on page 859 for details (The Cat With Tremor or Twitching).

Clinical signs

Depression, inappetence or anorexia and weight loss are common.

Clinical signs often reflect multiple levels of neurological involvement. Neurological signs may indicate diffuse or multifocal disease and **often do not localize to a single area within the nervous system**.

Paresis, gait abnormalities, proprioceptive deficits, cranial nerve defects, depression and occasionally stupor or coma may occur depending on the areas of brain involved.

Signs such as intention tremor, cerebellar ataxia (incoordination and swaying from side to side), hypermetria, head tilt and nystagmus may occur with involvement of the cerebellum.

Cervical pain can be present.

Fever is an inconsistent finding.

Fundic examination is important to look for clues of systemic inflammatory disease as chorioretinitis, which is often present with diseases causing systematic infection.

Other systemic signs such as vomiting, coughing and diarrhea may be seen concurrently.

Diagnosis

Complete blood cell count may show evidence of systemic inflammation (e.g. leukocytosis).

Serum biochemical analysis may show evidence of systemic abnormalities if the disease diffusely affects the body (e.g. vasculitis) such as elevated globulin, CK, liver enzymes or creatinine.

Evaluation of titers for the infectious diseases often helps to rule in or rule out the diseases.
- Infectious agents causing brain disease include viral (**feline infectious peritonitis**), fungal (**cryptococcosis**, blastomycosis, histoplasmosis, coccidioidomycosis, aspergillosis), protozoal (**toxoplasmosis**, neosporosis), bacterial, rickettsial, and unclassified organisms (prototothecosis).
- Involvement of the intracranial nervous system can occur with parasites such as *Cuterebra* **larvae, toxocara** and aberrant **heartworm** migration.

Cerebrospinal fluid analysis (CSF) will usually show evidence of **increased nucleated cells** and/or **elevated protein content**. Occasionally, CSF will be normal.
- Evidence of inflammation on CSF evaluation alone, however, is not specific for primary encephalitis as other CNS disease (e.g. **neoplasia**) **may result in a CSF pleocytosis** and protein increases.
- With feline infectious peritonitis (FIP), cerebrospinal fluid analysis may show a pleocytosis, with either **mononuclear** or non-lytic **neutrophils** as the predominant cell type and **elevated protein** concentration, often > 1 g/L (0.1 g/dl). High serum coronavirus titers are not diagnostic.
- With **toxoplasmosis**, cerebrospinal fluid frequently contains a pleocytosis, usually with mononuclear cells, and occasionally, eosinophils. Increasing IgG or a single positive IgM serum antibody titer is suggestive of active infection. Animals with **neurologic signs and positive IgM titers warrant treatment** for the disease.

With **cryptococcosis**, identification of the organism from cytological evaluation of samples such as CSF, nasal discharge and skin lesions supports the diagnosis.

A neutrophilic pleocytosis, and occasionally an eosinophilic pleocytosis, may be found on CSF analysis. If positive, detection of the cryptococcal capsular antigen in serum is usually diagnostic. Tissue biopsy and fungal culture or fungal culture of CSF may be more definitive in the diagnosis, as occasionally the serum titer is negative.

With parasites such as *Cuterebra* larvae, toxocara and aberrant heartworm migration, CSF may show inflammation with eosinophils in some instances.

Imaging studies (CT and MR) are helpful for defining structural lesions. **Multifocal, contrast-enhancing lesions** are usually seen. Occasionally, non-contrast-enhancing lesions are present, especially with toxoplasmosis.

IDIOPATHIC PERIPHERAL VESTIBULAR DISEASE***

Classical signs

- Signs can occur in any age but are commonly young to middle-aged animals.
- Acute-onset severe head tilts and nystagmus are most common.
- Cats often cannot stand initially and will continually roll.

See main reference on page 839 for details (The Cat With a Head Tilt, Vestibular Ataxia or Nystagmus).

Clinical signs

Clinical signs are of an acute peripheral vestibular disorder with nystagmus (horizontal or rotary), head tilt (toward the side of the lesion), rolling and falling.

No other neurological signs are seen.

Often these animals are initially so incapacitated that they are misdiagnosed with cerebrovascular accidents.

Clinical signs, while initially severe, will usually improve in 3–5 days. The nystagmus is the first sign to abate.

If Horner's syndrome or facial nerve paresis are also present, other differentials should be considered.

Disease occurrence may have a seasonal bias. Cats in the northeast United States are commonly affected in late summer and early fall.

Diagnosis

Otoscopic examination, bulla radiographs, and other advanced imaging studies (computed tomography (CT), magnetic resonance (MR) imaging) are normal.

Diagnosis is based on clinical signs and lack of evidence of other causes of peripheral vestibular disease on imaging.

Differential diagnosis

Differential diagnosis of peripheral vestibular disease includes otitis interna, middle ear polyps in cats, and neoplasia (squamous cell carcinoma of the middle ear). These diseases can be differentiated from idiopathic peripheral vestibular disease because lesions are evident via otoscopic examination of the ear canal and tympanic bulla and/or with imaging studies (radiographs, CT, MRI).

Treatment

No specific treatment has been shown effective.

Antihistamines (diphenhydramine at 0.5–1 mg/kg q 8 h) may help some animals.

Prognosis

Clinical signs of idiopathic vestibular disease usually improve dramatically in 1–2 weeks regardless of treatment.

The nystagmus usually resolves quickly (within the first few days).

Improvements in posture and walking occur within 5–7 days, whereas a mild head tilt may remain persistent.

While most animals compensate well, some may have episodic ataxia when performing tasks such as jumping up on furniture.

Recurrence is possible.

HEAD TRAUMA***

Classical signs

- Acute onset of signs following a traumatic event.
- Evidence of external trauma to the head and face such as facial lacerations, bleeding from the nose and mouth, bruising, retinal hemorrhage, or hemorrhage in the external ear canals.
- Cerebellar involvement may result in intention tremor, decerebellate rigidity, ataxia, hypermetria, head tilt and nystamus.

See main reference on page 823 for details (The Cat With Stupor or Coma).

Clinical signs

Exogenous injury to the brain occurs most commonly from automobile trauma, although gunshot wounds and falls may also occur.

Cerebellar involvement may result in **intention tremor, decerebellate rigidity** (extension of all four limbs and the trunk), ataxia, hypermetria, head tilt and nystagmus.

Signs usually begin acutely after trauma.

Intracranial signs most commonly seen include **stupor and coma, paresis and gait abnormalities** and cranial nerve deficits.

Evidence of **external trauma to the head and face such as facial lacerations**, bleeding from the nose and mouth, bruising or **hemorrhage in the external ear canals** may provide clues to the traumatic etiology.

- Occasionally, some animals that are incoordinated may fall and injure themselves secondarily, but this can usually be differentiated with good history taking.

Diagnosis

The diagnosis of trauma is usually straightforward when the trauma is witnessed.

In some instances, when animals are presented with an acute onset of neurological signs and an unknown history, examining for external signs of trauma such as lacerations or skull fractures is important.

- Evaluating the retinas and external ear canals for acute hemorrhage may also provide clues to the diagnosis.

Advanced imaging studies such as CT or MR imaging are useful, primarily for determining structural damage to the brain.

HYDROCEPHALUS**

Classical signs

- Dome-shaped or bossed appearance to the head or persistent fontanelles in a young cat.
- Seizures, poor learning ability, behavior changes, paresis, cranial nerve deficits and changes in consciousness.

See main reference on page 826 for details (The Cat With Stupor or Coma).

Clinical signs

In young cats prior to ossification of the cranial sutures, hydrocephalus may contribute to abnormalities of skull development such as a thinning of the bone structure, a **dome-shaped or bossed appearance** to the head or persistent fontanelles.

Clinical signs of hydrocephalus reflect the anatomical level of disease involvement.

Supratentorial, vestibular and cerebellar signs are most common.

As the supratentorial structures are often involved with hydrocephalus, **alterations in awareness and cognition are common.**

Many animals affected congenitally may appear to be **less intelligent** than normal.

Behavioral changes, paresis, cranial nerve deficits and changes in consciousness may occur.

Circling, paresis and seizure may also be seen.

Severity of clinical signs is not dependent upon the degree of ventricular dilation, but rather on a host of concurrent abnormalities including the underlying disease process, associated intracranial pressure changes, intraventricular hemorrhage, and the acuity of ventricular obstruction.

There are no pathognomonic clinical signs for acquired hydrocephalus in adult animals.

Correlation of degree of ventricular enlargement and clinical signs is poor.

Diagnosis

Routine laboratory data (e.g. hematology, biochemistry, urinalysis) are normal.

Historical, invasive techniques for diagnosis of hydrocephalus such as pneumo- or contrast ventriculography have been replaced by non-invasive diagnostic modalities.

Survey radiographs may suggest the presence of hydrocephalus, however they are usually not helpful for definitive diagnosis. Findings associated with **congenital hydrocephalus** include loss of gyral striations, separation of cranial sutures (diastasis) and **persistent fontanelles**. If hydrocephalus is acquired **after the skull has formed, abnormalities are rarely encountered**.

Electroencephalography has been used to diagnose hydrocephalus, primarily prior to advanced imaging. Classically, **slow-frequency, high-voltage** (amplitude) activity is noted. This pattern, however, can be seen with **other encephalopathies** that destroy cortical parenchyma. Because of this, EEG is rarely used as the sole means of diagnosing hydrocephalus.

Ultrasound can be used to diagnosis hydrocephalus.
- This is most readily accomplished **when a fontanelle is present** providing an "acoustic window" as ultrasound waves do not usually penetrate the skull well enough.
- If the bone is intact, a craniotomy defect can be created.
- For imaging of the lateral and third ventricles, the bregmatic fontanelle may be used.
- Often, ultrasound can be performed in awake cats as a screening test to determine ventriculomegaly.
- Depending upon the size of the fontanelle, the **lateral and third ventricles** as well as the **mesencephalic aqueduct** are usually easily identified.

Computed tomography (CT), as a non-invasive intracranial imaging modality, is often useful in defining ventricular size.

Magnetic resonance (MR) imaging also affords evaluation of the ventricular system. This modality provides for better parenchyma resolution than CT, and is especially useful for evaluation of the infratentorial structures.

Diffuse ventricular enlargement suggests congenital ventricular dilation or obstruction at the level of the lateral apertures or foramen magnum. **Focal ventricular enlargement** suggests **focal obstruction** or **parenchymal cell loss.**

Animals with an **asymmetric appearance** of the ventricles should be critically evaluated for **focal obstruction** of the ventricular system due to **mass effect**.

CONGENITAL VESTIBULAR DISEASE**

Classical signs

- Signs are usually present from the time the animal begins to walk.
- Head tilt and cat leans, drifts, falls or rolls to side of head tilt.
- ± Deafness.

Pathogenesis

Congenital abnormality of the vestibular system usually involves the **peripheral vestibular system.**

Histologic lesions are often not found.

Clinical signs

Siamese and Burmese cats are often affected.

Clinical signs are usually present from the time the animal begins to walk or begin early in life.

Signs are usually referable to **unilateral vestibular disease**; bilateral disease is less common.

The most common clinical signs are **head tilt and vestibular ataxia** (cat leans, drifts, falls or rolls to side of head tilt).

In some cases deafness is also present.

With bilateral disease, there is no head tilt but the head moves from side to side in exaggerated motions. Normal physiological nystagmus (movement of eyes side to side with movement of head) is absent.

Clinical signs are non-progressive and usually **decrease in severity with time**, but remain life-long.

Diagnosis

Diagnosis is **based primarily upon clinical signs**.

Skull radiographs, advanced imaging studies (MR or CT), CSF analysis and otoscopic examinations are normal.

Brain stem auditory-evoked potential testing may be abnormal if there are associated problems with hearing.

Differential diagnosis

Otitis interna should be evaluated for.

Other inflammatory processes involving the vestibular receptors may produce similar signs.

Trauma to the vestibular receptors is possible.

Treatment

No treatment is helpful.

Prognosis

Clinical signs may remain persistent or improve throughout life.

INHERITED CEREBELLAR DISEASES**

> ### Classical signs
>
> - Signs usually begin or are present in cats less than 1 year of age.
> - Signs usually are slowly progressive or remain unchanged.
> - Signs include coarse tremor, hypermetria, ataxia, intention tremor and menace deficits.

Pathogenesis

Cerebellar degeneration is usually an inherited disease.

A **hereditary cerebellar degeneration** has been described in Japan in cats. An autosomal recessive mode of inheritance was presumed.

Cerebellar degeneration with neuroaxonal dystrophy has been reported in domestic tri-colored cats. This is inherited as an autosomal-recessive trait.

Clinical signs

Clinical signs usually begin between **3–12 months of age.**

Cerebellar disease usually results in a **coarse tremor** that worsens (increases in frequency or amplitude) when the animal moves in a goal-oriented fashion (intention tremor).

Other signs of cerebellar disease that accompany cerebellar tremor include **ataxia (incoordination; swaying from side to side)**, dysmetria ("**goose-stepping**"; overflexing of the limbs when walking), **menace deficits** (with normal vision and pupillary light reflexes), **head tilt**, and **nystagmus** (combination quick followed by slow movement of the eyes).

An hereditary cerebellar degeneration is described **in Japan** in cats with signs beginning around 7–8 weeks of age.
- Signs include head tremor along with ataxia, dysmetria and intention tremor. An autosomal recessive mode of inheritance was presumed.

Cerebellar degeneration with **neuroaxonal dystrophy** in domestic **tricolored cats** results in **head tremors and shaking**. Clinical signs begin at 5–6 weeks of age and **progress to ataxia** and **hypermetria**. Affected kittens have a **lilac color** that **darkens with age**.
- A similar but separate neuroaxonal dystrophy has been described in cats of various colors. Clinical signs begin at 7–9 months of age and include ataxia with paraparesis.

Spongiform encephalopathy in Egyptian Mau cats results in ataxia and hypermetria, and it is presumed inherited. Clinical signs begin at 7 weeks of age.
- Another spongiform encephalopathy has been reported in older Egyptian Mau cats in the United Kingdom. Clinical signs include muscle tremors, ataxia, dilated unresponsive pupils, jaw champing, salivation and behavior abnormalities. Signs may progress to severe ataxia and hypermetria.

Diagnosis

Antemortem testing for these diseases often results in negative or normal findings.

Routine laboratory investigations (CBC, serum biochemical analysis, urinalysis) are normal.

Definitive diagnosis is often rendered only at **necropsy** and histopathological examination of the nervous tissue.

In some instances of cerebellar atrophy, a **smaller than normal cerebellum** may be seen on **magnetic resonance imaging** of the intracranial nervous system. This is most readily seen on the sagittal view.

Cerebrospinal fluid with these degenerative cerebellar conditions is **normal.**

With hereditary cerebellar degeneration described in Japan there is marked loss of Purkinje cells on histological evaluation of the cerebellum.

Neuroaxonal dystrophy is associated with pathologic changes in the brain, brain stem, cerebellum and spinal cord.

Differential diagnosis

In this age cat, other **inflammatory** central nervous system abnormalities, such as **toxoplasmosis** infection should be considered. CSF analysis and serologic testing help to differentiate it from inherited cerebellar degeneration.

Congenital anatomical defects of the cerebellum may be present with similar signs.

Trauma occurring at a young age may permanently damage the cerebellum and result in similar signs.

Treatment

No treatment is currently helpful for affected cats.

Prognosis

Clinical signs associated with degenerative cerebellar diseases progressively worsen.

Animals are commonly euthanized due to the progressive incapacitation.

Prevention

Do not breed cats affected that have produced kittens with a presumed genetic or congenital cerebellar disease.

STORAGE DISEASES**

Classical signs

- Signs usually begin or are present in cats less than 1 year of age.
- Signs usually are slowly progressive or remain unchanged.
- Signs include coarse tremor, hypermetria, ataxia, intention tremor and menace deficits.

Pathogenesis

Storage diseases result from inherited (or less commonly, acquired) intracellular metabolic derangements that result in abnormal metabolism of cellular products.

Cellular products accumulate and afferent neuronal cells physiologically or mechanically, resulting in cellular dysfunction, and hence, clinical signs.

Although signs of storage diseases are predominately referable to the brain and especially the cerebellum, some of the storage diseases also affect the peripheral nervous system.

Examples include **gangliosidosis, sphingomyelinosis, globoid cell leukodystrophy,** and **mannosidosis**.

Clinical signs

Clinical signs usually begin between **3–12 months of age.**

Cerebellar disease usually results in a **coarse tremor** that worsens (increases in frequency or amplitude) when the animal moves in a goal-oriented fashion **(intention tremor).**

Other signs of cerebellar disease that accompany cerebellar tremor include **ataxia** (incoordination; swaying from side to side), **dysmetria** ("goose-stepping"; overflexing of the limbs when walking), **menace deficits** (with normal vision and pupillary light reflexes), **head** tilt, and **nystagmus** (combination quick followed by slow movement of the eyes).

In cats with **sphingomyelinosis (Niemann–Pick type C disease)** clinical **signs begin early in life** (< 6 months) and progress to **ataxia and hypermetria**, absent menace responses, and occasionally positional nystagmus. **Death usually occurs by 8–10 months of age**.

- Similar clinical signs have been reported in a case of **type IV glycogen storage disease** in a Norwegian Forest cat.

Niemann–Pick type A disease occurs in **Siamese and Balinese** cats. **Head tremor, head bobbing, and dysmetria** begin at 3–4 months of age. Clinical signs progress to **ataxia and paresis, worse in the pelvic limbs**.

- An associated demyelinating polyneuropathy was found in one family of affected cats.

Diagnosis

Antemortem testing for these diseases often results in negative or normal findings.

Routine laboratory investigations (CBC, serum biochemical analysis, urinalysis) are normal.

Definitive diagnosis is often only obtained at **necropsy** and histopathological examination of the nervous tissue.

In some instances of cerebellar atrophy, a **smaller than normal cerebellum** may be seen on **magnetic resonance imaging** of the intracranial nervous system. This is most readily seen on the sagittal view.

Cerebrospinal fluid with these degenerative cerebellar conditions is **normal.**

In cats with sphingomyelinosis (Niemann–Pick type C disease) cerebellar atrophy, **Purkinje cell loss,** and **neuroaxonal dystrophy** are the **predominant pathological changes.**

Differential diagnosis

In this age cat, other **inflammatory** central nervous system abnormalities, such as **toxoplasmosis** infection should be considered. CSF analysis and serologic testing help to differentiate it from inherited cerebellar degeneration.

Congenital anatomical defects of the cerebellum may be present with similar signs.

Trauma occurring at a young age may permanently damage the cerebellum and result in similar signs.

Treatment

No treatment is currently helpful for affected cats.

Prognosis

Clinical signs associated with **storage diseases usually progressively worsen**.

Animals are commonly euthanized due to the progressive incapacitation.

Prevention

Do not breed cats affected that have produced kittens with a presumed genetic or congenital cerebellar disease.

OTITIS MEDIA/INTERNA**

> ### Classical signs
>
> - Signs can occur in any age.
> - Head tilt and nystagmus are most common.
> - Discharge from the ear, abnormal odors and ear pain may be present.
> - Polyploid masses may be seen in the oropharynx or ear canal.

See main reference on page 836 for details (The Cat With a Head Tilt, Vestibular Ataxia or Nystagmus).

Clinical signs

Clinical signs may reflect either primary **ear, vestibular or auditory dysfunction**.

A **painful external ear** and/or pain on opening the mouth are often present.

Head tilt and nystagmus are the most common vestibular signs. **Vestibular ataxia** (cat leans, drifts, falls or rolls to side of head tilt) may occur in more severe cases.

The **facial nerve** may be involved concurrently resulting in abnormalities of facial expression.

Abnormal odors or discharge from the ear canal may be present.

Oropharyngeal exam occasionally reveals an ear polyp.

Diagnosis

Otoscopic examination should be used to examine the tympanic membrane. This may be difficult in animals with severe otitis externa prior to cleansing.

- The tympanic membrane is often discolored (hyperemic), opaque and bulging outward with middle ear disease. Clear to yellow fluid may be seen behind the membrane.

Diagnosis may also be supported by abnormalities on **bulla radiographs or advanced imaging studies (MRI or CT)**.

- Often the bulla are fluid filled on either skull radiographs or advanced imaging studies.

Definitive diagnosis is made through **culture of the organism** via a myringotomy or at surgical exploration.

VASCULAR DISEASES*

Classical signs

- Acute onset of cerebellar signs.
- Head tilt, nystagmus, ataxia, hypermetria, and other cerebellar signs.

Pathogenesis

Injury to cerebellar tissue can occur as a result of **thrombosis or hemorrhage.**

Diseases that predispose to **hypercoagulability or vasculitis** predispose to vascular thrombosis.

Hemorrhage can occur as a result of **thrombocytopenia or coagulation abnormalities.**

Thrombosis leads to ischemia and cellular death.

A cat with polycythemia was presented for ataxia, possibly due to increases in serum viscosity.

Clinical signs

Clinical **signs are usually acute in onset**.

Head tilt, cerebellar ataxia (incoordination, swaying from side to side), **hypermetria, intention tremor and nystagmus** are possible.

Menace deficits with normal vision and papillary light reflexes may also be present.

Diagnosis

Routine laboratory evaluations (CBC, serum biochemical analysis, urinalysis) may show abnormalities in platelets or red blood cell mass or evidence of underlying systemic disease.

Coagulation studies and bleeding time assessment are useful in determining the cat's coagulation ability.

Advanced imaging studies may show evidence of hemorrhage or infarction in the cerebellum.

CSF analysis may show evidence of hemorrhage, however, should be performed with caution or avoided in animals with coagulation or platelet problems.

Differential diagnosis

Rule out other inflammatory, neoplastic and traumatic causes of cerebellar disease.

Treatment

Treatment should be directed at the underlying coagulation or bleeding disorder abnormality.

Rarely, if a hematoma is present, surgical removal may be helpful.

Prognosis

Prognosis depends upon the ability to treat the underlying disease process and the degree of cerebellar damage.

THIAMINE DEFICIENCY*

Classical signs

- Initially, lethargy, inappetence and ataxia.
- Later signs include weakness, ventral flexion of the neck, dilated pupils, stupor and coma.

See main reference on page 848 for details (The Cat With a Head Tilt, Vestibular Ataxia or Nystagmus).

Pathogenesis

Occurs in **anorexic cats** or cats that are **fed all-fish diets** containing thiaminase.

This deficiency results in polioencephalomalacia of the oculomotor and vestibular nuclei, the caudal colliculus and the lateral geniculate body.

Clinical signs

Early non-specific signs are **typically lethargy and inappetence**.

The earliest localizing sign is **bilateral vestibular ataxia**, which appears as **an abnormal broad-based stance**, loss of balance and vertigo.

There is weakness and an **inability or reluctance to walk**. The cat sits **crouched with ventral flexion of the neck**.

Pupils are dilated and non-responsive or poorly responsive to light reflexes.

If untreated, signs **progress to semi-coma**, persistent vocalization, opisthotonos, and death.

Episodes of spastic opisthotonos or ventroflexion of the neck and generalized muscle spasm may occur especially when the cat is lifted or stressed. They may be interpreted as seizures, but true seizure activity rarely occurs.

Diagnosis

No antemortem diagnostic test is available.

Diagnosis is based on **clinical signs** and **rapid response to thiamine**.

TOXINS*

Classical signs

- Metronidazole toxicosis results in ataxia, paresis, seizures and cortical blindness.
- Bromethalin toxicosis in the early stages may also result in ataxia. Signs progress to paresis, depression, tremors, seizures and decerebrate posture.
- Ivermectin toxicosis has resulted in generalized ataxia, tremor, weakness, incoordination, and miosis in a kitten.
- Griseofulvin therapy resulted in ataxia in a 12-week-old kitten.
- Aminoglycosides, administered either systemically or topically, may cause vestibular signs including ataxia.
- Chlorhexidine solution used to clean the external ear may result in vestibular signs including ataxia.

Pathogenesis

Metronidazole toxicosis has been reported to result in ataxia in cats.

- Usually, this is associated with high doses of the drug.
- As metronidazole is metabolized by the liver, however, toxic serum levels can occur with appropriate doses in animals with liver dysfunction.

Bromethalin toxicity results in vacuolization of the nervous system, most likely due to a lack of intracellular energy.

Clinical signs

Ataxia is usually the initial clinical sign of **metronidazole toxicity.**

- **Paresis** is usually present, and **seizures** and **cortical blindness** may also be noted.
- These signs in association with metronidazole administration should raise concern for toxicity.

The early stages of **bromethalin toxicosis** may also result in ataxia.

- Signs progress to paresis, depression, tremors, seizures and decerebrate posture.

Ivermectin toxicosis has resulted in generalized ataxia, tremor, weakness, incoordination and miosis in a kitten.

Griseofulvin therapy resulted in ataxia in a 12-week-old kitten.
- Clinical signs remained static up to 4 months after the initial presentation.

Aminoglycosides, administered either systemically or topically, may cause vestibular signs including vestibular ataxia (cat leans, drifts, falls or rolls to side of the head tilt), head tilt and nystagmus.
- Streptomycin and gentamicin have the most pronounced effects on the vestibular receptors, while neomycin, kanamycin and amikacin preferentially damage auditory receptors.

Chlorhexidine solution used to clean the external ear may result in vestibular signs.

Diagnosis

Serum concentrations of metronidazole will be in the toxic range if measured soon after clinical signs begin.
- If there is a delay in collecting blood for drug concentrations after the initiation of clinical signs, serum concentrations of metronidazole may decrease into the normal range even as the clinical signs remain persistent.

Diagnosis of other toxicities is supported by a history of exposure.

Differential diagnosis

Other diseases causing signs of vestibular disease include otitis interna, middle ear polyps in cats, and neoplasia (squamous cell carcinoma of the middle ear). These can usually be differentiated from toxicity on the basis of history, otoscopic examination and imaging of the bulla.

Treatment

There is no specific treatment for metronidazole toxicity.
- Discontinuation of the drug is imperative. A complete recovery is possible.

No specific treatment is available for the other toxicities.

Prognosis

With metronidazole toxicity, a complete recovery is possible after discontinuation of the drug if the signs are not severe.

Prevention

Avoid exposure to these products.

IDIOPATHIC ENCEPHALOPATHY*

> **Classical signs**
> - Ataxia, paresis, and "head shaking" in young cats up to 3 years old in the UK.
> - Ataxia of the pelvic limbs was the initial sign.

Pathogenesis

Pathogenesis is unknown, although a viral etiology was suggested but not proven.

Wallerian degeneration was noted primarily involving the spinocerebellar pathways and the ventral funiculus of the spinal cord.

Clinical signs

An encephalomyelopathy of young cats reported in the United Kingdom had clinical signs of ataxia, paresis and "head shaking".

Cats 3–12 months old were affected, however, the disease was seen in cats up to 3 years of age.

Ataxia of the pelvic limbs was the initial clinical sign noted.

Diagnosis

Diagnosis was made at necropsy.

Differential diagnosis

Diseases causing peripheral vestibular disease should be considered including otitis interna and middle ear polyps.

Treatment

No treatment was attempted.

RECOMMENDED READING

Baroni M, Heinold Y. A review of the clinical diagnosis of feline infectious peritonitis viral meningo-encephalomyelitis. Prog Vet Neurol 1995; 6: 88.

Inada S, Mochizuki M, Izumo S, et al. Study of hereditary cerebellar degeneration in cats. AJVR 1996; 57: 296–301.

Kornegay JN. Feline infectious peritonitis: The central nervous system form. J Am Anim Hosp Assoc 1978; 14: 580.

March PA. Degenerative brain disease. Vet Clinic North Am 1996; 26: 945–971.

Nowotny N, Weissenböck H. Description of feline nonsuppurative meningoencephalomyelitis ("staggering disease") and studies of its etiology. J Clin Microbiol 1995; 33: 1668–1669.

Palmer AC, Cavanagh. Encephalomyelopathy in young cats. JSAP 1995; 36: 57–64.

Saxon B, Magne ML. Reversible central nervous system toxicosis associated with metronidazole therapy in three cats. Prog Vet Neurol 1993; 4: 25–27.

Vandevelde M, Braund KG. Polioencephalomyelitis in cats. Vet Pathol 1979; 16: 420–427.

44. The cat with generalized weakness

Rodney S Bagley, Jacquie Rand, Terry King and Fiona Campbell

KEY SIGNS

- Weakness.
- Inability or reluctance to walk or jump.
- Stiff, stilted gait.
- Ventroflexion of the neck.

MECHANISM?

- Diffuse loss of muscle strength results in generalized weakness. Diseases of the peripheral nervous system, neuromuscular junction and muscle often result in generalized weakness. Systemic diseases affecting metabolism of or perfusion to, the muscles may also result in weakness.

WHERE?

- Peripheral nervous system, neuromuscular junction and muscle.

WHAT?

- Diseases include the peripheral neuropathies, neuromuscular junctionopathies (myasthenia gravis) and myopathies. One of the most common causes of weakness is hypokalemic myopathy.

QUICK REFERENCE SUMMARY

Diseases causing generalized weakness

DEGENERATIVE

- Degenerative neuropathies (p 963)

Weakness with decreased to absent spinal reflexes. Dropped hock appearance in young Birman cats, beginning 8–10 weeks of age. Storage disease may be associated with aneuropathy. These diseases are often breed-specific with clinical signs beginning in cats less than 1 year of age.

- Degenerative motor neuronopathies (p 964)

Progressive weakness and muscle atrophy in adult cats, decreased to absent spinal reflexes, tremor especially of head and tongue, cervical ventroflexion and dysphagia.

continued

continued

● Degenerative myopathies (X-linked muscular dystrophy, hereditary myopathy, Nemaline rod myopathy) (p 964)

Any breed may be affected; inherited myopathy occurs in Devon Rex. Signs begin 2–24 months of age, weakness and reduced activity, stiff, choppy gait, increase in muscle mass and hypertrophy of the tongue (x-linked muscular dystrophy), ventral flexion of neck and dorsal protusion of scapula (hereditary myopathy of Devon Rex).

METABOLIC

● Hypokalemic myopathy*** (p 945)

Typically older cats or Burmese < 1 year of age. Signs include weakness, inability or reluctance to walk or jump, stiff, stilted gait, neck ventroflexion and sensitivity to palpation of larger muscle groups.

● Diabetic neuropathy** (p 948)

Often presents as a "dropped-hock" appearance in older cats with clinical signs of diabetes (polyuria, polydipsia, weight loss), subtle generalized weakness, reduced activity, difficulty jumping and some cats have a classic plantigrade stance.

● Primary hyperoxaluria (p 967)

Uncommon clinically in cats. Domestic short-hair cats 5–9 months old. Generalized weakness, with or without concurrent signs of renal failure.

● Polymyopathy* (p 961)

Signs include ventral flexion of the neck, apparent muscle pain, muscle weakness and a stiff gait. Age of onset varies from 3 months to 13 years and most are domestic short- or long-haired cats.

● Hyperthyroidism* (p 960)

Abnormal systemic metabolism affects muscle or nerve function. Concurrent hypokalemia is common. Signs may include weakness, ventral neck flexion and reduced physical activity. Typical signs of hyperthyroidism are weight loss, polyphagia, irritability or restlessness.

● Hyperlipidemia (p 968)

Lipid granulomas may compress the peripheral nerve. Typical signs include hyperlipidemia and lipemia retinalis in association with peripheral neuropathies involving individual peripheral, cranial or sympathetic nerves.

● Hypernatremic myopathy (p 968)

Rare disease with signs similar to hypokalemic myopathy. Ventral neck flexion, weakness, reduced physical activity and a "dropped-hock" appearance may occur.

● Hypocalcemia (p 962)

Most often occurs after thyroidectomy. Muscle weakness, tetany and tremors are typical. Preparturient hypocalcemia presents as anorexia, lethargy, trembling, muscle twitching and weakness.

● Hypoglycemia* (p 956)

Most often associated with insulin overdose in diabetic cats, but also rarely caused by an insulinoma in older cats. Signs include trembling, weakness, dilated pupils, reduced alertness, and if severe, seizures progressing to coma.

● **Reduced tissue oxygenation*** (p @)

Any cause of substantially reduced tissue oxygenation will cause weakness. Examples include severe anemia, methemoglobinemia associated with acetaminophen (paracetamol) toxicity, cardiac disease, hydrothorax including pyothorax and chylothorax, and severe bronchopulmonary disease or obstructive upper respiratory disease.

NUTRITIONAL

● **Thiamine deficiency*** (p @)

Decreased thiamine can result in brain stem disease in cats. Clinical signs initially begin with lethargy, inappetence and reluctance to walk. Later there is vestibular ataxia and episodes of spastic ventroflexion of the neck or opisthotonos, dilated pupils, stupor and coma.

INFECTIOUS

● Acute sepsis (p @)

Toxemia and reduced tissue oxygenation from acute bacterial sepsis may cause weakness and depression, resulting from bacteremias via the uterus (pyometritis), thorax (pyothorax), abdomen (peritonitis), skin (subcutaneous abscess). Pyrexia or hypothermia may be present. Signs referable to the infection site (dyspnea, vaginal discharge or uterine distention abdominal guarding, skin abscess) are often evident.

● **Toxoplasmosis*** (p @)

Protozoan organism that commonly affects the muscle or peripheral nerve. Most cats are asymptomatic. Signs are most severe in cats under 1 year of age and especially in young kittens. They include lethargy, anorexia, dyspnea, icterus, uveitis, retinal hemorrhage and central nervous system signs. Weakness or stiffness may occur with signs of spinal cord, peripheral nerve or muscle involvement.

● Feline immunodeficiency virus (p @)

A subclinical myopathy has recently been described. Diagnosis is based on a positive FIV antibody test and inflammatory changes on muscle biopsy, in the absence of *Toxoplasma gondii* organisms. Some cats had elevated CK and EMG abnormalities.

Inflammatory:

● **Myasthenia gravis*** (p @)

Typically adult cats or Siamese < 1 year of age. Signs include generalized weakness induced by movement, a stiff, stilted gait prior to collapse, ventral neck flexion and a decreased palpebral reflex.

● Polyneuritis (p @)

A rare cause of weakness with decreased spinal reflexes and conscious proprioceptive deficits.

● **Polymyositis*** (p @)

Primary inflammation of the muscles resulting in loss of muscle strength and neck ventroflexion.

Idiopathic:

● **Idiopathic peripheral neuropathy*** (p @)

A primary neuropathy without a definable cause. Signs include marked weakness with conscious proprioceptive deficits and decreased spinal reflexes. Lower motor neuron tetraparesis is the predominant sign. Signs are similar to dogs with polyradiculoneuropathy (Coon Hound paralysis).

continued

continued

- **Chronic relapsing polyneuropathy* (p 966)**

Peripheral neuropathy of cats which has no definitive cause. Marked weakness with decreased spinal reflexes and conscious proprioception. Signs similar to polyradiculitis neuropathy (Coon Hound paralysis) but cats recover then relapse months later.

- **Myotonia (p 967)**

A disease associated with excessive muscle contraction. Signs include stiffness and muscle spasm, short, stilted gait and increased muscle size.

- **Dysautonomia* (p 961)**

A disease primarily seen in younger cats (< 3 years) in Britain. Clinical signs are often acute in onset and reflect autonomic system dysfunction. They include depression, anorexia, dilated pupils, megacolon, constipation, xerostomia, keratoconjunctivitis sicca, prolapsed third eyelids, bradycardia, loss of anal reflex, incontinence and weakness.

TOXICITY

- **Organophosphate toxicity** (p 947)**

Toxicity usually occurs from misuse of flea and tick products and is associated with muscle weakness. Signs include acute onset of miosis, salivation, urination, defecation and muscle weakness. Rarely, persistent weakness occurs without associated autonomic signs. Cats may attempt to walk a few steps, then collapse in sternal recumbency mimicking cataplexy/narcolepsy.

- **Snakebite envenomation from Australian snakes** (p 950)**

Australian snake venoms are predominately neurotoxic and usually strongly coagulant. Usually there is no local reaction at the site of venom injection. Generalized muscle weakness and dilated pupils that are poorly responsive to light are features. Complete flaccid paralysis is a common finding. Vomiting and rapid respiration are present in 30% of cases. Excessive bleeding from venepuncture sites may be evident. Hypothermia is a poor prognostic sign.

- **Snakebite envenomation from USA snakes** (p 949)**

Coral snake envenomation is most often seen in the southeastern US. Clinical signs are of a progressive flaccid paralysis. Palpebral reflexes may be diminished, as is rectal temperature. Recovery rates have been good in a small number of reported cats.

- **Tick toxicity** (p 953)**

In Australia, toxin from the *Ixodes* tick affects muscle and nerve transmission and causes acute onset of flaccid paralysis, beginning in the hindlimbs and ascending and acute onset of dypsnea. In North America, *Dermacentor* and *Argas* ticks may also cause paralysis.

- **Red-back spider envenomation (*Latrodectus mactans hasselti*; Australia) (p 974)**

Envenomation occurs from the bite of the female red-back spider and often there is moderate to severe pain, erythema, edema and localized swelling at the bite site. Venom causes depletion of acetylcholine reserves at motor nerve endings, which may result in a patchy paralysis of voluntary muscle. The spider is found Australia-wide, avoiding only the hottest desert habitats and cold alpine altitudes.

- **Ciguatoxin intoxication (p 971)**

Signs begin within 3–6 hours of ingestion of a toxic meal of reef fish (toxin found in large carnivorous fish species). Toxins affect neuromuscular transmission and hindleg paresis and vomiting are the most prominent. Cardiovascular shock and/or respiratory distress may precede coma and death within 24 hours of ingestion.

● Tetrodotoxin intoxication (p 973)

Tetrodotoxin is produced by *Vibrio* bacteria in the intestines of marine fish including toadfish, pufferfish, newts and the blue-ringed octopus and accumulates in tissues. The toxins affect neuro-muscular transmission. Signs begin 10–40 minutes after ingestion. Initial signs are gastrointestinal–drooling, vomiting and diarrhea. Neuromuscular signs follow with weakness and ataxia progressing to flaccid hindlimb paralysis. Pupillary dilation is usually a feature. With severe toxicity, cardio-vascular shock and labored respiration often precede convulsions and death within hours.

INTRODUCTION

MECHANISM?

Loss of muscle strength causes generalized weakness. The gait may have a stiff, stilted appearance. Loss of cervical muscle strength results in an inability to hold the head up, which appears as ventroflexion of the neck, and is a common sign of weakness in cats.

WHERE?

Disease either of the peripheral nervous system, neuro-muscular junction and/or muscle often results in gener-alized weakness.

Systemic diseases affecting metabolism or perfusion to the muscles may also result in weakness.

WHAT?

Diseases include the peripheral neuropathies, neuro-muscular junctionopathies (myasthenia gravis) and myopathies. The most common cause of generalized weakness is hypokalemic myopathy. In some geogra-phic locations, tick toxicity and snakebite are relatively common.

Hypoglycemia from an insulin overdose is a relatively common cause of metabolic weakness. Causes of reduced muscle oxygenation include severe anemia, methemoglobinemia associated with acetaminophen (paracetamol) toxicity, cardiac disease, hydrothorax including pyothorax and chylothorax, and severe bron-chopulmonary disease or obstructive upper respiratory disease. Most of these causes of weakness have other prominent signs such as pale or cyanotic mucous mem-branes, dyspnea or heart murmur.

An evaluation for underlying metabolic disease is imperative in determining the cause of weakness.

Accurate diagnosis often requires evaluation with elec-trodiagnostics, and muscle and nerve biopsy.

Fibrillation potentials, positive sharp waves, and pro-longed insertional activity are abnormal electromyo-graphic findings, and occur when there is myocyte inflammation and abnormal membrane electrical activ-ity. This occurs when there is muscle inflammation, degeneration or denervation.

DISEASES CAUSING GENERALIZED WEAKNESS

HYPOKALEMIC MYOPATHY***

> **Classical signs**
>
> - Aged cats or Burmese < 1 year.
> - Ventral neck flexion.
> - Stiff, stilted gait.
> - Reluctance to walk or jump and physical inactivity.
> - +/– Sensitivity to palpation of larger muscle groups.

See main reference on page 893 for details (The Cat With Neck Ventroflexion).

Pathogenesis

Potassium is important in maintaining normal muscle cell membrane potentials.

Potassium depletion can result in alterations in muscle cell membrane potentials, muscle cell glycogen content and synthesis, and blood flow to muscle.

Hypokalemia results in hyperpolarization of muscle cell membranes which then require greater stimulus for depolarization, leading to generalized muscle weakness.

Hypokalemia occurs when the **dietary intake is insufficient to replace urinary and fecal loss**.

A major contributing factor to hypokalemia **in older cats** is the inability of the kidney to conserve potassium.

Acidification of diets to prevent struvite urolithias increases renal and fecal potassium loss.

Diets deficient in potassium may induce signs. Clinical signs occurred in one group of cats fed a **vegetarian diet**.

Burmese cats have an **inherited hypokalemic myopathy** producing signs of periodic muscle weakness, with signs first evident **before 12 months of age**, usually between 4–12 weeks.

Clinical signs

Signalment is typically **aged cats > 8 years** or **young Burmese** < 1 year (usually 2–6 months).

Typically there is a history of **acute onset of weakness**. However, decreased activity and inappetence are often present for weeks to months prior to presentation.

Clinical signs include **ventral neck flexion, stiff, stilted gait** and a reluctance to walk or jump. Typically, weak cats do not walk far, but soon sit or lie, flopping down, instead of carefully sitting as normal cats do. Sensitivity to palpation of larger muscle groups may be noticed.

Dyspnea occurs when the potassium is very low (2.0–2.5 mmol/L), because of weakness of the respiratory muscles. It may occur after **fluid administration** because volume dilution and increased urinary potassium loss induced by diuresis may lead to further worsening of the hypokalemia.

Young Burmese cats are susceptible to this disease, and potassium depletion may have played a role in the previously described myopathy of Burmese cats. Transient episodes of weakness may occur beginning between 2–12 months of age.

Diagnosis

Diagnosis is made by finding decreased serum potassium concentrations (usually < 3.5 mmol/L) in association with clinical signs. The severity of signs varies between cats when potassium is 2.5–3.5 mmol/L. Below 2.5 mmol/L and especially below **2.0 mmol/L, signs are life threatening**, with death occurring from **respiratory muscle failure**.

Serum creatine kinase (CK) may be elevated reflecting the mypoathy associated with hypokalemia.

Electrodiagnostic evaluation is rarely performed. Abnormalities that may be found include increased insertional activity, fibrillation potentials and positive sharp waves and some bizarre high-frequency discharges.

Muscle biopsies often have minimal change present. Mild myonecrosis is possible.

Differential diagnosis

Myasthesia gravis, polymyositis and organophosphate toxicity can all cause similar clinical signs. **Hypokalemia** is readily differentiated from these on serum potassium concentration and response to treatment.

Rarely snake bite or tick paralysis may cause weakness similar to severe acute signs of hypokalemia. Other clinical signs, history and serum potassium concentration allow differentiation. Typically, cats with bites from Brown or Tiger snakes have increased plasma (CK) activity and increased clotting times. Cats with tick bite have increased respiratory effort and a tick is usually found with careful searching.

Treatment

Supplementation with potassium is essential. **Oral supplementation is more effective** and is associated with fewer complications than intravenous administration. Concurrent and intravenous administration should be reserved for severely weak cats.

Caution should be used when administering potassium intravenously in fluids, as further decreases in serum potassium concentration may occur as a result of dilution and enhanced loss of potassium in urine.

Increased urinary potassium loss occurs secondary to renal sodium and water loss, when fluids are administered in excess of maintenance and induce diuresis. Clinical signs may then be exacerbated.

In severely weak cats, **use a low volume of fluid with a high potassium concentration** (e.g. 160 mmol (Eq)/L at 2 ml/kg/h. Do not exceed 0.5 mmol (Eq)/kg/h as cardiac arrest may occur.

If IV fluids are indicated because of dehydration, the rate of administration should not induce diuresis, as catastrophic decreases in potassium can occur. Until potassium is > 3.5 mmol (Eq)/h, maintenance fluid rates (e.g. 10 ml/cat/h) are recommended with potassium supplementation (80–160 mmol (mEq)/L of fluids) together with oral potassium supplementation (5–8 mg/cat PO q 12–24 h). Do not exceed 0.5 mmol (Eq)/kg/h of potassium in intravenous fluids.

Do not give fluids if the cat is not dehydrated or is not severely weak. Oral therapy (5 mg/cat bid to tid) is more effective.

Endotracheal intubation and ventilatory support is required if the cat is in respiratory muscle failure, and support may be required for 1–2 days.

Do not give steroids as these increase urinary potassium excretion.

Oral supplementation (potassium gluconate) is used **for long-term management.** An empirical dose of 2–6 mmol (mEq)/cat/day is usually effective. Regular monitoring of serum potassium is required to determine the effective maintenance dose for individual cats.

Prognosis

Prognosis is excellent provided respiratory paralysis does not occur.

Signs resolve in 24 hours to 3 days.

If respiratory paralysis occurs, intensive care and ventilatory support are required for survival.

Prevention

As many older cats may have underlying renal disease, periodic evaluation of renal function and serum potassium concentration is suggested.

ORGANOPHOSPHATE TOXICITY**

Classical signs

- Acute onset of miosis, salivation, urination, defecation and muscle weakness.
- Rarely, lethargy, anorexia and persistent weakness without associated autonomic signs.

Clinical signs

Organophosphate intoxication **potentiates the effect of acetylcholine** at the neuromuscular junction and other synapses, by binding with and **inactivating acetylcholinesterase**. This leads to increased acetylcholine concentrations at the neuromuscular junction, increased receptor stimulation and fatigue. **Chronic exposure** can result in **peripheral neuropathies**, as cats are one of the species most prone to delayed neurotoxicosis.

A delayed neurotoxicity in cats is reported associated with the use of **chlorpyrifos** spray for household application against fleas. There is individual variation in sensitivity to chorpyrifos, and signs of toxicity have occurred even when used according to label instructions. Toxicity has also been reported with flea collars containing chlorpyrifos.

Cats with organophosphate intoxication may have **acute signs** including **miosis, salivation, urination, defecation and muscle weakness.**

Acute signs of **fenthion toxicity** are **muscle weakness with few autonomic signs.**

A more **persistent weakness without associated autonomic signs** can occur with **chronic** organophosphate **toxicity.** Cats may attempt to walk a few steps, then collapse in sternal recumbency mimicking cataplexy/narcolepsy. Typically, they are also lethargic and inappetent.

- Postural reactions and spinal reflexes may be depressed in some cats, but may be normal in other cats.
- The pupils may be bilaterally dilated and poorly responsive to light stimulation.
- Ventroflexion of the neck and muscle tremors may be evident.

Diagnosis

A presumptive diagnosis is based on the presence of consistent signs and a history of exposure to an organophosphate.

Concentration of serum cholinesterase activity may lend support to the diagnosis, but **may be non-diagnostic** for **chronic organophosphate toxicity**. Values less than 500 IU/L (normal 900–1200 IU/L) are considered consistent with organophosphate toxicity.

Electromyographic changes are occasionally present and include fibrillation potentials, positive sharp waves and bizarre high-frequency discharges. A decremental response to repetitive nerve stimulation may be present.

Beware that edrophonium (used to test for myasthenia gravis) may produce an **acute worsening** of signs. (**Treatment with atropine** (0.05 mg/kg IV) may help the associated parasympathetic signs).

Differential diagnosis

Rule out other diffuse causes of weakness. **For the acute form**, other **acute poisonings or toxicities** such as snake bite (increased CK, prolonged clotting times) or hypoglycemia (low plasma glucose usually in an insulin-treated diabetic cat) may appear similar. **Differentials for the chronic form** include thiamine deficiency (response to therapy), polymyositis (increased CK, abnormal EMG and muscle biopsy), hypokalemic myopathy (low plasma potassium), hypernatremia (very rare, hypernatremia), polyneuropathy (abnormal EMG and decreased nerve conduction velocities), hyperthyroidism (other clinical signs and elevated plasma thyroxine), and myasthenia gravis (IV edrophonium/Tensilon test, anti-acetylcholine receptor antibodies).

Treatment

Treatment includes protopam chloride (2-PAM) (20 mg/kg q 12 h IV) which reactivates cholinesterase and **diphehydramine** (1–2 mg/kg PO q 8–12 h) which reduces muscle fasciculations.

Atropine (0.2–0.4 mg/kg) can be given with acute toxicity to decrease autonomic signs. Current recommendations are that it only be used if marked bradycardia is present, because it may **precipitate respiratory arrest**. Salivation and defecation are not life threatening and generally do not require atropine.

Diazepam should be avoided in these cats as it may result in **generalized muscle tremor**, hypersalivation, miotic pupils and vomiting **similar to acute muscarinic signs** of organophosphate toxicosis.

DIABETIC NEUROPATHY**

Classical signs

- Subtle generalized weakness and reduced activity, difficulty jumping.
- Some cats have a classic plantigrade stance in the pelvic limbs.

Pathogenesis

The cause of the peripheral neuropathy is multifactorial, including diabetes-associated metabolic changes in the nerve metabolism and/or vascular abnormalities resulting in nerve ischemia.

Clinical signs

Many diabetic cats prior to initiation of treatment, or if poorly controlled, have **subtle generalized weakness**, usually evident as **reduced activity**, reluctance to move and **difficulty jumping**.

Some affected cats have a **classic plantigrade stance** in the pelvic limbs, suggesting **sciatic (tibial) nerve dysfunction** and tarsal extensor muscle weakness.

Diagnosis

Clinical signs of **polyuria, polydipsia, and weight loss**, together with hyperglycemia (usually blood glucose is > 17 mmol/L (309 mg/dl) and glucosuria, are usually diagnostic for diabetes.

Electromyographic abnormalities include evidence of **denervation** (fibrillation potentials and positive sharp waves) and **decreases in nerve conduction velocities**.

Nerve biopsies may show axonal degeneration and/or demyelination. These changes, however, are not specific for diabetic neuropathy.

Differential diagnosis

Traumatic **rupture of the gastrocnemius tendon** may cause similar signs.

Treatment

Twice daily insulin therapy is usually required to achieve good glycemic control. See page 237 (The Cat With Polyuria and Polydipsia).

Treatment of the hyperglycemia may result in improvement of sciatic nerve function if substantial peripheral nerve damage has not occurred prior to diagnosis and therapy.

ENVENOMATION BY SNAKES FOUND IN THE USA**

Classical signs

- Clinical signs are usually rapid in onset (within 24 hours of envenomation).
- Progressive lower motor neuron (flaccid) paralysis.
- Death is usually the result of respiratory muscle paralysis.

Pathogenesis

Coral snake envenomation is most often seen in the **southeastern US**.

Envenomation from Coral snakes results in a **blockage of transmission at the neuromuscular junction**.

The exact mechanism of action of the toxin is not completely defined.

Clinical signs

Signs usually are seen within 2–4 hours following envenomation, but may be delayed for several hours.

Cats present with a **rapidly progressive lower motor neuron (flaccid) paralysis.**

Rectal body temperatures may be slightly decreased.

Cranial nerve dysfunction (**decreased palpebral reflexes**) may result.

Respiratory paralysis can occur and result in death.

Physical examination may reveal small puncture wounds or the presence of small amounts of blood on the fur.

Diagnosis

A presumptive diagnosis is based on appropriate clinical signs and is supported by finding small puncture wounds.

Serum CK is often elevated.

Electrodiagnostic studies may reveal decreased or absent motor unit potentials with electrical stimulation.

Differential diagnosis

Other toxic neuropathies and myopathies may present with similar clinical signs.

Treatment

General supportive care is important including keeping the cat in a warm, comfortable environment and managing hydration status.

In the small number of cats reported with Coral snake envenomation, **recovery rates** have been **good**, usually within 2–5 days.

If respiratory paralysis results, **mechanical ventilation** may be required.

Antivenom is available for Coral snake envenomation, however, it may not neutralize all toxin present, and is relatively expensive.

Aspiration pneumonia may be a complicating factor that will require standard treatment for aspiration pneumonia.

Prognosis

Cats reported with Coral snake envenomation have had a **reasonably good prognosis for recovery.**

Respiratory paralysis may result in death unless respirator support is available.

Aspiration pneumonia may complicate the clinical signs.

Spontaneous recovery in instances with mild clinical signs is possible.

SNAKEBITE ENVENOMATION WITH AUSTRALIAN SNAKES**

Classical signs

- Australian snake venoms are predominately neurotoxic and usually strongly coagulant.
- Usually no local reaction at the site of venom injection.
- Generalized muscle weakness and dilated pupils that are poorly responsive to light are features.
- Complete flaccid paralysis is a common finding.
- Vomiting and rapid respiration are present in 30% of cases.

Pathogenesis

Bites from **Brown snakes** (*Pseudonaja* sp.), **Tiger snakes** (*Notechnis scutatus*), **Taipan** (*Oxyuranus s. scutellatus)* and **Death Adders** (*Acanthophis antarcticus*) can cause **ataxia, paralysis and dilated pupils.**

Neurotoxins act specifically at the **neuromuscular junction** to **paralyze all skeletal voluntary muscle.**

Postsynaptic neurotoxins (tiger, brown, taipan, death adder) cause a non-depolarizing block of neuromuscular transmission by **occupying acetylcholine receptors** on the motor endplate. Flaccid paralysis ensues and death is possible from respiratory failure.

Presynaptic neurotoxins (tiger, brown, taipan) **block acetylcholine release** into the neuromuscular junction after depolarization. This action is delayed, becoming evident after 30–60 minutes.

Increased catecholamine release (stress, exercise, nerve stimulation) enhances the rate of intoxication whereas low temperatures delay this process.

Antitoxin cannot reverse presynaptic binding of toxin.

The **clotting mechanism is activated** via initiation of the conversion of prothrombin to thrombin and fibrinogen to fibrin **(tiger, brown, taipan, black)**. This causes continuous bleeding from sites including trauma sites, gastrointestinal tract, and lungs manifesting as hematemesis, hematuria, hemoptosis, etc.

- Coagulant manifestations often precede neurotoxin signs.
- Antitoxin effectively blocks the clotting mechanism activation.

Rhabdomyolysis (tiger, mulga, small-eyed) manifests as myoglobinuria.

Hemolysins (taipan, black) cause intravascular haemolysis and may manifest as jaundice, anemia, hemoglobinuria and perhaps kidney tubular necrosis.

Hyaluronidase in the venom is responsible for the rapid entry of the venom into the circulation.

The lack of local reaction at the bite site is probably due to the low quantity of proteolytic enzymes in Australian snake venom.

Clinical signs

There is marked variation in type and severity of signs but **flaccid paralysis and dilated pupils** that are poorly responsive are consistent findings, that is, neurological signs predominate.

Onset is usually sudden.

Dilated pupils, ataxia to paresis, trembling, flaccid paralysis, vomiting, diarrhea, respiratory distress, hypothermia, weakness, pallor, jaundice, dark urine and bleeding from multiple sites may all be present.

Less commonly there is a history of initial collapse followed by apparent full recovery followed by a steady progression of clinical signs over the ensuing hours, which may take from 5 minutes to 24 hours in the cat.

The bite site may not be found unless there is bleeding from the site.

Multiple bite sites usually result in the introduction of large quantities of venom.

Diagnosis

A **history of being bitten** by a snake and finding the snake greatly aids diagnosis, but more often the bite is unobserved.

Table 44.1 Comparison of main actions of snake venoms

	Neurotoxin	Coagulant	Myotoxin	Hemolytic
Tiger	+++	+++	+++	+
Death Adder	+++	+	−	+
Brown	+++	++++	−	+
Black	+	++	+++	+++
Copperhead	++	++	+++	++
Taipan	+++	++++	+++	+
Mulga	++	+++	+++	+
Small Eyed	+++			

Table 44.2 Comparative frequency of commonly observed signs of snakebites

	Snake specified–all animals				Animal specified (cats)
	Tiger	Brown	Black	Copperhead	
Sudden collapse soon after bite, temporary recovery then relapse	+	++	+		+
Neurological signs, weakness, ataxia, flaccid paralysis	++++	++++	++++	++++	++++
Excitement, trembling, salivation, vomiting, defecation, muscle spasm	+++	+++	+++	+++	++
Pupils dilated, pupillary light reflex slow or absent	++++	+++	+++	+++	++++
Local swelling	+	+	+++	++	++
Hemoglobuinuria, Myoglobinuria, or jaundice	++	+	+		+
Non clotting blood, extended coagulation time, hematemesis, hematuria	++	++	++		++

+ 1–10% of animals show these signs; ++ 11–30% of animals show these signs; +++ 31–75% of animals show these signs; ++++ 75–100% of animals show these signs.

Typically the cat is presented with signs of a **sudden onset of paralysis, mydriasis** and has evidence of **extended clotting times**.

Identification of the snake venom using a **snake venom detection kit** to test samples from swabs of bite site, urine (most reliable if clinical signs are present), or blood is useful, but adds to the cost of treating the cat. Knowledge of the test limitations is essential. Knowledge of the types of snakes found in the area aids selection of antivenom.

Table 44.3 Clinical pathology

	ACT	Fibrinogen	CPK	Hb'uria	Mb'uria
Brown	Increased	Decreased	-	-	-
Mulga	-	-	Increased	Increased	Increased
Black	-	-	Increased	Increased	Increased
Taipan	Increased	Decreased	Increased	-	Increased
Tiger	Increased	Decreased	Increased	-	Increased
Small-eyed	-	-		-	Increased
Death Adder	-	-	-	-	-

ACT - activated clotting time
CPK - creative phospholanese
Hb'uria - hemoglobinuria
Mb'uria - myoglobinuria

Increased creatine phosphokinase (tiger snake even-omation) may be found on biochemistry analyis.

Evidence of **neurological signs plus coagulant or myo-lysis or hemolysis** signs suggests snake envenomation.

Differential diagnosis

Tick paralysis may result in similar clinical signs of flaccid paralysis. Cranial nerve involvement is unusual in tick paralysis, and when present is often unilateral and associated with a tick on the head. Diagnosis is facilitated by finding a tick on the cat at the time of presentation.

Ciguatera and tetrodotoxin result in hindleg paresis and vomiting in a cat with access to reef fish or toad-fish, puffer fish, newts or blue ringed octopus.

Red-back spider bite may result in initial vomiting fol-lowed by agitation, muscle weakness and incoordina-tion. Muscular tremors and tachycardia may be present.

Thromboembolism is usually present in only one body area (either both pelvic limbs or a thoracic limb). Cats usually show clinical signs of pain. Affected muscles are usually firm and painful, with lack of evidence of perfu-sion (cold to touch, discolored, absent peripheral pulses).

Acute-onset sepsis results in profound weakness, hypothermia, tachypnea, bradycardia and hypotension evidenced as poor pulses, pale mucous membranes, increased capillary refill time.

Botulism and polyradiculoneuritis:may result in a similar progressive flaccid paralysis. Both are relatively uncommon in cats.

Organophosphorus poisoning especially in the early stages may look similar (vomiting, salivating) Muscle weakness may be a more predominant clinical presen-tation. Cats also may appear flaccid.

Treatment

Prompt administration of adequate amounts of the **appropriate antivenom** is the mainstay of treatment.

Identification of the snake is often helpful when plan-ning treatment, because both monovalent and polyva-lent antivenoms are available. Polyvalent antivenom may be necessary if the snake can not be identified.

Dosages are often standardized and dispensed as one dose. **Anaphylactic reactions** are possible, so caution should be used when administering these products.

Choice of antivenom and dosage when the snake has not been identified **varies on locations around Australia**.
- Polyvalent antivenom.
- QLD north of Rockhampton – Brown 1000 U and Death Adder 6000 U.
- QLD south of Rockhampton – Tiger 3000 U and Brown 1000 U and Death Adder 6000 U.
- Tasmania – Tiger 6000 U, Victoria – Tiger 3000 U and Brown 1000 U.
- NSW, SA, WA, NT – Tiger 3000 U and Brown 1000 U and Death Adder 6000 U.

Antivenom is given diluted in 100 ml saline slowly over 15–30 minutes after premedication with chlorpheni-ramine (1 mg/kg IM), dexamethasone (2 mg/kg IV), and epinephrine (0.05 mg/kg SC). **Wait 20 minutes after premedication** before giving antivenom.

Table 44.4 Choice of antivenom dosage when snake has been identified

	Recommended antivenom for veterinary use	Initial dose (Units)
Tiger snake	Tiger snake antivenom	3000
Death Adder	Death Adder snake antivenom	6000
Taipan	Taipan snake antivenom	12 000
Brown	Brown snake antivenom	1000
Black	Tiger snake antivenom	3000
Mulga	Tiger snake antivenom	9000

Maintenance of airway and breathing may involve intubation and mechanical ventilation if there is respiratory paralysis. Oxygen therapy is indicated if there are moderate respiratory efforts.

Packed cell volume, total protein, urea and activated clotting time are minimal diagnostic requirements.

Fluid therapy is needed for resuscitation, rehydration, and maintenance (see treatment of dehydration, page 557, in The Cat With Polycythemia). Blood and plasma products may be necessary to control coagulation.

Monitor respiration (spO$_2$), **ventilation,** (ET, CO$_2$, blood gases), and circulation (heart rate, blood pressure, pulses, capillary refill time, electrocardiogram)

Monitor blood parameters (packed cell volume, total protein, BUN, potassium, CK, creatinine).

Monitor urine output to ensure that 1–2 ml/kg/h is being produced.

Nutritional support should be provided as recovery can be slow.

Nursing includes soft bedding, warmth, bladder and bowel control, analgesia, physiotherapy, catheter care, eye care.

Anticipate respiratory failure requiring mechanical ventilation, DIC, renal failure, aspiration, corneal ulceration, sudden death as complications.

TICK TOXICITY**

Classical signs

- Acute-onset flaccid paralysis, beginning in the hindlimbs and ascending.
- Acute-onset dyspnea.

Pathogenesis

Worldwide, 43 species of ticks have been reported to cause paralysis in domestic animals.

In North America, *Dermacentor andersoni, Dermacentor variabilis,* and *Argas (Persicargas) radiatus* are the species of ticks most commonly associated with paralysis.

In Australia, the paralysis tick is *Ixodes holocyclus,* which is found along the **eastern coast of Australia.**

Ixodes holocyclus is a **three-host tick**: larvae, nymphs and adult females engorge on a host over several days before detaching to develop to the next stage in the environment.

Native hosts of *Ixodes holocyclus,* bandicoots and possums, rarely develop disease.

Ixodes holocyclus produces disease in accidental hosts, including cats and dogs.

Most cases of tick toxicity occur during spring and early summer.

Usually a **single adult female tick** will cause disease; rarely, large numbers of larvae or nymphs will cause disease.

The tick must feed on the host for at least 5 days before disease develops.

The toxin produced by the tick acts to:
- **Inhibit the release of acetylcholine from the neuromuscular junction to produce flaccid paralysis.**
- **Block potassium efflux from cardiac myocytes to produce heart failure.**

Clinical signs

Acute onset of **paresis/ataxia of the hindlimbs** is the most consistent clinical sign. This rapidly progresses over several hours to **flaccid paralysis** and **ascends to involve the forelimbs and results in lateral recumbency**.

Dyspnea accompanies paralysis, and severe **dyspnea with forced expiration and cyanosis** occurs terminally.

A **change in voice** and **inappetence** may occur early in the course of disease.

Pupils are dilated and become non-responsive to light. The nictitating membrane may protrude across the globe.

The **gag reflex is impaired** and **drooling of saliva** occurs.

Regurgitation/vomiting can occur rarely at any stage.

Death can occur within 24–48 hours of onset of signs.

Scoring systems to describe the progressive stages of paralysis and respiratory compromise are as follows:
- **Gait score system**.
  - Score 1: Can walk: able to stand from recumbency and ambulate.
  - Score 2: Cannot walk: requires aid to stand but can maintain stance.
  - Score 3: Cannot stand: unable to maintain a standing position.
  - Score 4: Cannot right: unable to maintain sternal recumbency.
- **Respiratory score system**.
  - Score A: Normal character and rate (less than 30 breaths per minute).
  - Score B: Normal character and increased rate (greater than 30 breaths per minute).
  - Score C: Altered character with expiratory sigh/grunt (undefined rate).
  - Score D: Cyanosis and severe dyspnea.

Diagnosis

Diagnosis is made when clinical signs typical of tick toxicity are observed in an animal in an area where *Ixodes holocyclus* or other paralysis ticks are endemic and either:

- **One** (or more) **adult female** *Ixodes holocyclus* tick(s) or other paralysis ticks are found on the animal.
- A **"crater"**, the feeding lesion which remains after the tick has detached, is found on the animal.
  - **Multiple larval or nymphal** *Ixodes holocyclus* ticks are found on the animal.
  - A tick or "crater" is not found but the animal responds to specific treatment for tick toxicity.

Differential diagnosis

Various snake envenomations may present similarly but are not usually associated with dyspnea.

Visualization of the *Ixodes holocyclus* tick or other paralysis ticks are diagnostic. The brown dog tick, *Rhipicephalus sanguineus,* is found in some of the same areas as *Ixodes holocyclus,* but it very rarely parasitizes cats and is not associated with paralysis.

Treatment

Treatment involves removing the tick(s), administration of specific antitoxin serum and supportive care.

With *Ixodes holocyclus* (Australia), often clinical signs will progress during the first 24 hours of treatment due to the delayed onset of the toxin's action. In USA, signs usually resolve rapidly after tick has been removed, and supportive therapy is rarely necessary.

The **tick can be removed manually** using curved forceps or a pair of partially opened scissors to lever out the tick while avoiding any pressure on the tick's body. **Search thoroughly for additional ticks**. Apply tickicides (fipronil, pyrethrins) to kill any additional unseen ticks.

Tick Antitoxin Serum (TAS) for treatment of *Ixodes Holocyclus* toxicity is manufactured from canine serum so there is a **risk of anaphylaxis** when administered to cats. TAS can also produce a **vagally mediated systemic reaction** seen clinically as bradycardia, hypotension and circulatory shock (B-J reaction). To minimize these risks give:
- **Acepromazine** (0.03 mg/kg SC or IM) to relieve anxiety and respiratory distress. Wait 20–30 minutes before giving TAS.
- **Atropine** (0.04–0.1 mg/kg SC) to block the B-J reaction, reduce salivation, and produce bronchodilation. Wait 20–30 minutes before giving TAS.

- **Prednisolone sodium succinate** (5–10 mg/ kg IV) to reduce the likelihood and severity of anaphylaxis. Wait 10–30 minutes before giving TAS.
- **Epinephrine** 1:10 000 (3 ml SC) about 5 minutes prior to administration of TAS to reduce the likelihood of anaphylaxis.
- **TAS** (0.5–1 ml/kg) diluted 50:50 with 0.9% NaCl and warmed to room temperature; either give slowly IV (over 20–30 minutes) or give IP.

Supportive care.
- **Oxygen therapy** (oxygen cage, flow-by, nasal catheter, or positive pressure ventilation) is indicated for moderate to severe dyspnea.
- **Furosemide** (2–5 mg/kg IV) should be given to reduce pulmonary edema in dyspneic animals and repeated as necessary.
- **Metoclopramide** (0.5 mg/ kg IM or IV) is indicated in vomiting animals to reduce the risk of aspiration.
- **Eye ointment** should be applied to prevent corneal desiccation.
- **Nil per os** is essential until the gag reflex returns. Then introduce oral fluids slowly.
- **Parenteral fluids are not routinely indicated and must be used with care** due to the potential worsening of pulmonary edema. Colloid or heta/penta starch fluids may be used to maintain circulating fluid volume if the hematocrit is significantly elevated. Crystalloids may be given after 24 hours at submaintanence rates if slow return of the gag reflex delays introduction of oral fluids.
- If possible animals should be **positioned sternally** to minimize pulmonary ventilation–perfusion mismatching. Laterally recumbent animal should be positioned with the **shoulders elevated** to aid pharyngeal drainage and turned every 2 hours to reduce ventilation–perfusion mismatching.
- Urine retention often occurs and **manual expression of the bladder** may be needed during recovery.
- **Stress** must be minimized.
- Provision of a **cool (not cold) environment** may alleviate signs.

Prognosis

Prognosis for gait scores 1–3 and respiratory scores A–C is good. Gait score 4 and respiratory score D confers a guarded prognosis.

Cardiac effects may persist after limb paralysis has resolved. Cats should not be stressed for 2–3 weeks after recovery from paralysis. In dogs, stress may cause sudden death up to 3 weeks after discharge from hospital.

Prevention

Check daily for ticks.

Use a preventative product (fipronil, pyrethrins).

MYASTHENIA GRAVIS*

> ### Classical signs
>
> - Adult cats or Siamese < 1 year of age.
> - Episodic muscle weakness induced by movement.
> - Ventral neck flexion.
> - Decreased palpebral reflex.

Pathogenesis

There are **two forms** of this disease; a **congenital form** that is not associated with antibody production, and an **acquired form** that is **associated with antibodies** being produced against the acetylcholine receptor.

The congenital form occurs **Siamese cats**. **Abyssinian cats** and possibly Somali's may be predisposed to the **acquired form**.

The acquired form can occur idiopathically, or **secondary to a variety of tumors** (thymoma). With thymoma, the tumor either produces excess antibody or antibody is produced against a similar antigen within the tumor and in muscle.

Clinical signs

This is a rare disease in cats. Generally a disease of **adult cats**, except for the congenital form **in Siamese** which presents at **< 6 months of age**.

Exercise intolerance and **episodic weakness induced by walking** or playing are typical signs. The cat may walk a few steps and flop down. Recovery occurs with rest.

Muscle tremors are usually episodic and occur in muscles that are being used.

A stiff, stilted gait is often noted prior to collapse.

Weakness of facial muscle may also be seen, and this is most evident as a **decrease in the palpebral reflex** and narrowing of the palpebral fissure. This appears to be a more consistent finding in cats versus dogs.

Megaesophagus is uncommon and may lead to aspiration pneumonia.

One cat has been reported with a jaw-drop and dysphagia as the only clinical signs.

Diagnosis

Diagnosis is based upon clinical signs of exercise-induced weakness that is resolved with edrophonium.

An edrophonium response test may suggest the disease if strongly positive. Edrophonium is an anticholinesterase that potentiates acetylcholine (ACH) at the neuromuscular junction. When given IV (0.1 mg/kg), this drug can reverse the clinical weakness seen with myasthenia gravis for a short period of time.

Electromyography and nerve conduction studies will be normal. A decremental response may be seen during repeated stimulation of a peripheral nerve in some, but not all cats.

Single fiber EMG is a relatively new technique that may aid diagnosis of this disease in the future.

Documentation of **antibodies to the acetylcholine receptor** in serum appears to be the most definitive diagnostic test. In congenital disease, however, these antibodies will not be present.

Differential diagnosis

Rule out other inflammatory, toxic and degenerative causes of muscle weakness and tremor.

Other causes of ventral neck flexion and generalized weakness include thiamine deficiency (response to therapy), polymyositis (increased CK, abnormal EMG and muscle biopsy), hypokalemic myopathy (low plasma potassium), hypernatremia (very rare, hypernatremia), polyneuropathy (abnormal EMG and decreased nerve conduction velocities), hyperthyroidism (other clinical signs and elevated plasma thyroxine) and

organophosphate toxicity (decreased serum cholinesterase activity).

Treatment

A long-acting anticholinesterase product (**pyridostigmine** Mestinon, 0.5–3 mg/kg PO q 8–12 hours) can be given to enhance the effect of ACH at the neuromuscular junction. Start at the lower dose and increase as required.

Cats may be more sensitive to the effect of this drug, and therefore, slightly lower dosages than those used in dogs should be used initially.

Additionally, immunosuppressive therapy with **corticosteroid** (1–2 mg/kg PO q 12 hours) or plasmapheresis may be needed to control clinical signs in acquired forms.

Prognosis

Prognosis for some animals is good, with occasional spontaneous cures or remission. Recurrences may occur.

Treatment responses may not be as dramatic in cats compared to dogs.

Complicating factors include severe weakness with respiratory compromise and aspiration pneumonia secondary to megaesophagus.

Prevention

Avoiding breeding from sires and dams known to produce congenitally affected offspring. Advise pedigree analysis to remove carriers.

HYPOGLYCEMIA*

> ### Classical signs
>
> - Trembling, weakness are most common.
> - Dilated pupils.
> - Reduced alertness or lethargy.
> - If hypoglycemia is severe, seizures and progression to coma may result.

Pathogenesis

Hypoglycemia can also occur secondary to some endocrine disorders such as hypoadrenocorticism, lack of glucose production by the liver in liver failure from lack of iron, and with some tumors (liver, spleen, GI) which may produce hypoglycemia through excess IGF-2 production.

Hypoglycemia is most often associated with **insulin overdose in diabetic cats**, but is also rarely caused by an **insulinoma** in older cats.

Because the central nervous system (CNS) requires a constant supply of glucose, clinical signs of hypoglycemia relate to **CNS dysfunction** and **activation** of the **sympathetic nervous system**.

Clinical signs

Signs include trembling, weakness, dilated pupils, reduced alertness, and if severe, seizures progressing to coma.

Insulinoma occurs in aged cats.

Diagnosis

Diagnosis of hypoglycemia is based upon finding hypoglycemia (blood glucose < 60 mg/dl: < 3.3 mmol/L) in the face of clinical signs.

Concurrent **serum insulin concentration** will help in determining the presence of an insulin-secreting tumor. Non-pancreatic tumors producing hypoglycemia are associated with low insulin concentrations.

Abdominal ultrasound may be helpful when assessing the pancreas, liver and lymph nodes for presence of tumor.

Differential diagnosis

Signs of hypoglycemia can mimic other seizure and generalized weakness disorders.

Treatment

Diabetic cats with clinical hypoglycemia are best treated with **intravenous dexdrose** (20–50%) ½–2 ml to effect. Subsequent insulin doses need to be reduced by 50%. Some cats are in remission and do not need insulin.

Surgical removal of an insulinoma will normalize serum glucose concentrations if there are no metastases, and results in a better long-term outcome than medical management. Post-operative pancreatitis may be a complication.

Medical management of insulinoma or other tumor producing hypoglycemia is only **palliative** and consists of **frequent small meals** low in carbohydrate, diazoxide (12.5 mg bid PO) and **corticosteroids** (0.5–6 mg/kg/day in divided doses, beginning at lower dose) to increase blood glucose. The somatostatin analog octreotide (10–40 µg/cat SC bid–tid), has also been used in cats. Small doses of glucagon subcutaneously may be effective.

In some instances of insulinoma, intravenous dextrose administration may actually bring about worsening signs, most likely because these tumors retain some responsiveness to serum glucose concentrations and respond by increasing insulin secretion.

Prognosis

With insulinoma and other tumors producing hypoglycemia, clinical signs may be controlled, however the long-term prognosis is poor unless the tumor can be removed by surgery.

Correction of any underlying disorders will determine the ultimate prognosis.

REDUCED TISSUE OXYGENATION*

> ### Classical signs
>
> - Palor, cyanosis, decreased capillary refill times, tachycardia and/or, hypothermia.
> - Tachycardia, gallop rhythms, murmurs, coughing and vomiting with cardiac disorders.
> - Tachypnea, panting and open-mouthed breathing with respiratory disorders.
> - Facial edema with acetaminophen toxicity.

See main reference page 118 for details (The Cyanotic Cat).

Pathogenesis

Any cause of substantially reduced tissue oxygenation will cause weakness. Examples include severe anemia, methemoglobinemia associated with acetaminophen (paracetamol) toxicity, cardiac disease, hydrothorax including pyothorax and chylothorax, and severe bronchopulmonary disease or obstructive upper respiratory disease.

Clinical signs

Signs may be generalized or localized and are most easily seen in the **mucous membranes, nail beds or conjunctiva.**

Palor, cynaosis, decreased capillary refill times, **tachycardia** and hypothermia are common associated signs.

Tachycardia, **gallop rhythms, murmurs**, coughing and vomiting may accompany cardiac disorders.

Tachypnea, panting, and open-mouthed breathing may accompany respiratory disorders.

Facial edema may be present with acetaminophen toxicity.

Diagnosis

PCVs and complete blood cell counts are used to determine the presence of anemia.

Arterial blood gas analysis is used to determine relative tissue oxygenation.

A **pulse oximeter** reading may aid in determining the degree of oxygenation.

Chest radiographs can be used to identify pulmonary and cardiac diseases.

In addition, an ECG and echocardiogram is useful when evaluating for heart disease.

Differential diagnosis

Other causes of weakness should not have cyanosis and pallor.

Treatment

Treat the underlying cause of the reduced oxygenation and provide oxygen if signs are marked.

Prognosis

Depends upon the underlying cause.

TOXOPLASMOSIS*

> ### Classical signs
>
> - Most cats are asymptomatic.
> - Signs are most severe in cats under 1 year of age and especially young kittens.
> - Lethargy, anorexia, dyspnea.
> - Uveitis, retinal hemorrhage.
> - ± Weakness.

Clinical signs

Most cats are asymptomatic.

Signs are most severe in cats under 1 year of age, especially young kittens, although any age of cat can be affected.

Lethargy, anorexia and dyspnea due to pneumonia are the most frequent signs of generalized infection.

Fever may be present.

Gastrointestinal or hepatic signs such as icterus, vomiting and diarrhea and abdominal effusion may occur as a result of diffuse organ involvement or from a granuloma.

Toxoplasma gondii can affect any area of the nervous system resulting in encephalitis, myelitis, peripheral neuropathy or myositis.

The organism damages the nerve and muscle either primarily, or secondarily through associated inflammation.

Weakness may be present if the **spinal cord, peripheral nerves or muscles** are involved.

Hyperesthesia on muscle palpation, stiff gait or shifting leg lameness suggests myositis.

Experimental innoculation with meospora coninum also causes clinical signs in cats.

Diagnosis

Diagnosis is based upon the presence of **IgM antibodies** to *Toxoplasmosa gondii*, which appear within

1–2 weeks and **persist for 3 months**, but sometimes for years, or **rising IgG titers** which appear by the fourth week of infection, increase over 2–3 weeks and persist for months or years. **Visualization** of the protozoan in **biopsy specimens** is also diagnostic.

Differential diagnosis

Rule out other myopathies (hypokalemic, polymyopathy) and inflammatory causes of muscle disease as well as other neuropathies.

Treatment

Treatment for toxoplasmosis currently is **clindamycin** (8–25 mg/kg, q 8–12 hours; do not exceed 50 mg/kg q 24 hours) for 14–28 days, however the **addition of trimethoprim sulfa drugs** PO, IM or SC may provide a better clinical response.

Newer drugs, such as **azithromycin** and **clarithromycin** (macrolides), are being tested in other species, but are unproven in cats.

Watch the literature for new recommendations.

THIAMINE DEFICIENCY*

Classical signs

- Initially, lethargy, inappetence and ataxia.
- Later, weakness, ventral flexion of the neck, dilated pupils, stupor and coma.

See main reference on page 848 for details (The Cat With a Head Tilt, Vestibular Ataxia or Nystagmus).

Clinical signs

Early non-specific signs are typically **lethargy and inappetence**.

The earliest localizing sign is **bilateral vestibular ataxia**, which appears as an **abnormal broad-based** stance, **loss of balance and vertigo**.

There is **weakness** and an **inability or reluctance to walk**. The cat sits crouched with **ventral flexion of the neck**.

Pupils are dilated and non-responsive or poorly responsive to light reflexes.

If untreated, **signs progress to semi-coma**, persistent vocalization, opisthotonos and death.

Episodes of **spastic opisthtonos or ventroflexion of the neck** and muscle spasm may occur especially when the cat is lifted or stressed. They may be interpreted as seizures, but true seizure activity rarely occurs.

Diagnosis

Diagnosis is based on **clinical signs** and **rapid response to thiamine**.

Cats that have progressed to a comatose state have a poor prognosis.

Differential diagnosis

Other encephalopathies and encephalitis are differentiated on history, CSF findings and lack of response to thiamine.

Head trauma may appear similar to late signs of thiamine deficiency, but can usually be differentiated on history and evidence of trauma. Thiamine-deficient cats are **lethargic and inappetant** days and weeks before signs are severe.

Hydrocephalus can present with central blindness and ataxia, but there is no response to thiamine.

Dysautonomia is a consideration in countries where it occurs. The bilateral non-responsive pupils and ventroflexion of the neck may appear similar to thiamine deficiency, but there is no response to thiamine.

Hypokalemic myopathy, **myasthenia gravis**, **polymyositis** and **organophosphate toxicity** can all cause ventral flexion of the neck. However, ventral neck flexion in thiamine deficiency is the result of active muscle contraction associated with increased muscle tone rather than **passive ventroflexion** from **weakness**. Thiamine deficiency responds to thiamine supplementation unless in terminal stages.

Treatment

Treatment is administration of thiamine dosed typically at 5–30 mg/cat/day per os. Maximum dose up to 50 mg/cat/day.

Severely affected cats should receive at least 1 mg parenterally.

Change the diet to one with adequate thiamine and supplement with thiamine for at least a week.

HYPERTHYROIDISM*

> ## Classical signs
>
> - Weakness and ventral neck flexion.
> - Cats may progress to collapse with minimal exercise.

See main reference page 304 for details (The Cat With Weight Loss and a Good Appetite).

Clinical signs

The metabolic effects of the hyperthyroid state may in some way affect muscle and/or nerve function. Many of these cats are **also hypokalemic**. Clinical signs of **hypokalemia may be precipitated** by **thyroidectomy** and be apparent on recovery from anesthesia.

Weakness and ventral neck flexion occurs in a few cats with hyperthyroidism.

Cats may progress to **collapse with minimal exercise**.

Other typical signs of hyperthyroidism may also be present such as weight loss, polyphagia, irritability or **restlessness**.

Some cats are lethargic.

Intermittent vomiting or diarrhea occurs in many cats.

With practice, a **palpable thyroid nodule** is detected in most cats.

Diagnosis

In some cats, electromyography shows evidence of denervation.

Diagnosis is made by demonstrating **elevated serum total thyroxine (T4)** concentrations. When total T4 concentration is at the high end of normal, but signs are consistent with hyperthyroidism, measurement of **free T4** or a **T3 suppression** test may help to confirm the diagnosis.

Differential diagnosis

Differential diagnoses include other causes of hypokalemic myopathy such as chronic renal failure, other myopathies and inflammatory causes of muscle disease.

Myasthenia gravis (positive tensilon test, anti-acetylcholine receptor antibodies), chronic organophosphate toxicity (history of exposure), and polymyositis (muscle biopsy) should be considered.

Treatment

The weakness may improve with treatment for hyperthyroidism.

Correct hypokalemia.

POLYMYOSITIS*

> ## Classical signs
>
> - Weakness and neck ventroflexion.

Clinical signs

Polymyositis may be **idiopathic, immune-mediated** or result from infections with *Toxoplasma gondii* or **feline immunodeficiency virus**.

Signs typically are of **generalized muscle weakness** and **neck ventroflexion**.

Megaesophagus may occur with smooth muscle involvement.

Thymoma may be present in some cats, and myositis may occur concurrently with myasthenia gravis.

Regurgitation and/or dyspnea may be present with megaesophagus and thymoma.

Diagnosis

Serum CK may be elevated.

Abnormal **spontaneous muscle electrical activity** consistent with myocyte inflammation and abnormal membrane electrical activity (e.g. fibrillation potentials, positive sharp waves, **complex repetitive discharges**) may be present on electromyography.

Multifocal areas containing mononuclear cell infiltrates are present in the muscle biopsy.

Differential diagnosis

Hypokalemic myopathy is differentiated on the basis of hypokalemia.

Myasthenia gravis may occur concurrently with myositis.

Chronic organophosphate toxicity is differentiated on the basis of a history of exposure and sometimes reduced cholinesterase activity.

Treatment

Corticosteroid treatment (1–2 mg/kg PO q 12 hours) may improve clinical signs.

DYSAUTONOMIA*

Classical signs

- Younger cats (< 3 years).
- Acute onset of depression and anorexia.
- Dilated pupils, xerostomia, keratoconjunctivitis sicca, prolapsed third eyelids.
- Bradycardia.
- Megacolon, constipation, loss of anal reflex.
- Incontinence, dysuria or distended bladder.
- Weakness.

See main reference page 792 for details (The Constipated or Straining Cat).

Clinical signs

Disease is confined to Europe or occurs in imported cats. The prevalence has decreased markedly and it is now uncommon.

Younger cats (< 3 years) are more often affected.

Clinical signs are often **acute in onset over 48 hours** with all cats showing **depression and anorexia**.

Other signs reflect autonomic system dysfunction and include:

- Ocular signs such as **fixed, dilated pupils without blindness**, prolapsed third eyelids and dry eyes (keratoconjunctivitis sicca develops).
- **Gastrointestinal signs** include regurgitation, megaesophagus, constipation and megacolon, loss of the anal reflexes, dry mouth (xerostomia).

- **Bradycardia** (90–120 beats/minute).
- **Dysuria** and/or **distended bladder** or incontinence with an easily expressive bladder.
- Generalized weakness.

Diagnosis

Diagnosis is based primarily on **clinical signs and evidence of autonomic dysfunction**. The indirect-acting parasympathomimetic, physostigmine (0.02 mg/kg IV) produces no ocular response, but direct-acting pilocarpine (topically) results in immediate miosis, **demonstrating post-glanglionic denervation** hypersensitivity. Normal cats do not demonstrate these responses.

Differential diagnosis

Differential diagnoses are many, depending on the predominant signs. Cats may present with a history of constipation or inability to urinate or dilated pupils, suggesting disease of the colon, lower urinary tract or eyes. Typical cases which exhibit most signs are classical for dysautonomia.

Treatment

No specific treatment is available, but supportive care is important, such as syringe or tube feeding.

Parasympathomimetic agents may improve some clinical signs.

- **Pilocarpine ophthalmic drops** (1%/1 drop q 6 h) may result in pupillary contraction and increase salivation.
- Bethanechol (1.25–5 mg PO q 8–12 h) may benefit constipation and urinary retention.
- Metoclopromide (0.2–0.5 mg/kg PO SC q 8 h) may improve gastric motility.

Up to 70% mortality rate has been reported.

POLYMYOPATHIES

Classical signs

- Ventral flexion of the neck.
- Muscle weakness.
- +/– Apparent muscle pain and a stiff gait.

Pathogenesis

Unknown.

Clinical signs

Age of onset varies from 3 months to 13 years.

Most cats were domestic short- or long-haired cats.

Ventral flexion of the neck and weakness was common.

Apparent muscle pain and a stiff gait may also be seen.

Diagnosis

Serum CK was usually elevated.

Many of these cats had low serum potassium levels and may have had **hypokalemic myopathy**. Some cats had clinical signs **resolve spontaneously**, others seemed to benefit from **corticosteroid therapy**.

Differential diagnosis

Rule out other inflammatory, toxic and degenerative causes of weakness.

Other causes of ventral neck flexion and generalized weakness include thiamine deficiency (response to therapy), polymyositis (increased CK, abnormal EMG and muscle biopsy), hypokalemic myopathy (low plasma potassium), hypernatremia (very rare, hypernatremia), polyneuropathy (abnormal EMG and decreased nerve conduction velocities), hyperthyroidism (other clinical signs and elevated plasma thyroxine), myasthenia gravis (IV edrophonium/Tensilon test, anti-acetylcholine receptor antibodies) and organophosphate toxicity (decreased serum cholinesterase activity).

Treatment

Some cats had clinical signs resolve spontaneously, others seemed to benefit from corticosteroid therapy (1–2 mg/kg PO q 12 hours).

Prognosis

Variable.

HYPOCALCEMIA

> **Classical signs**
> - Weakness, tetany and tremors.
> - Muscle fasciculation, cramping, rigidity and twitching.

Pathogenesis

Decreases in calcium **decrease the threshold** for neuronal and muscle **depolarization**.

Hypocalcemia most often results from **iatrogenic injury to the parathyroid gland** during surgical removal of thyroid tumors.

Primary hypoparathyroidism is possible but rare.

Hypocalcemia associated with **queening (eclampsia)** is rarely reported but occurs.

Clinical signs

Clinical signs include **weakness, tetany and tremors**.

Spontaneous muscle depolarization can manifest as muscle fasciculation, cramping, rigidity and twitching.

Queens with preparturient hypocalcemia present with **anorexia, lethargy, trembing, muscle twitching** and weakness. They resemble the clinical picture of hypocalcemia in cows, rather than the violent muscle tremor of eclampsia in dogs.

Diagnosis

Diagnosis is confirmed by finding decreased (usually less than < 1.5 mmol/L (6 mg/dl) serum calcium on serum biochemical analysis.

Differential diagnosis

Rule out other **inflammatory** causes of **muscle disease** and **acute organophosphate toxicity** (history of exposure, signs and low cholinesterase activity).

Treatment

Treatment involves calcium supplementation and vitamin D therapy.

If clinical signs are present, rapid institution of treatment is indicated with 0.5–1.5 ml/kg IV of 10% **calcium gluconate**. **Infuse calcium slowly over 10 minutes while monitoring heart rate**. Stop infusion if bradycardia occurs.

Short-term maintenance involves either SC calcium (1–2 ml of 10% calcium gluconate diluted 1:1 in 0.9% saline q 8 hours) or IV calcium (10–20 ml of 10% calcium gluconate in 500 ml of 0.9% saline) with rate adjusted to maintain normocalcemia. Monitor calcium 2–3 times daily initially.

Longer-term maintenance includes **oral calcium (25 mg/kg q 8–12 hours)** and **vitamin D**. The active form of endogenous vitamin D_3 (called calcitriol or 1,25 dihydroxycholecalciferol) is used at 2.5–10 ng/kg q 24 hours or synthetic vitamin D_3 (dihydrotachysterol) at 0.02–0.03 mg/kg q 24 hours for 3 days, then 0.01–0.02 mg/kg q 6–24 hours.

Calcium should be monitored carefully, as **hypercalemia is nephrotoxic**.
- Adjustments to doses should be made every 1–3 days based on calcium concentrations.

If hypocalcemia is the result of thyroidectomy, calcium and vitamin D therapy can be reduced gradually over 2–3 weeks, and stopped if calcium remains in the normal range.

Prognosis

Acute hypocalcemia following bilateral thyroidectomy can be fatal if not recognized early and appropriate therapy instituted.

Prevention

When performing bilateral thyroidectomy, allow 3–4 weeks between removal of each lobe.

DEGENERATIVE NEUROPATHIES

Classical signs

- Weakness with decreased to absent spinal reflexes.
- "Dropped-hock" gait in young Birman cats.

Pathogenesis

The cause of many degenerative neuropathies is not known.

Clinical signs

These diseases are often breed-specific with clinical signs beginning in cats less than 1 year of age.

Weakness with decreased to absent spinal reflexes are typical signs.

A degenerative polyneuropathy occurs in **young Birman cats**.

Clinical signs begin at 8–10 weeks of age.
- The gait is characterized by a "**dropped-hock**" appearance and **hypermetria** and **ataxia**.

Cats with **Neimann–Pick type-A storage disease** may have **alterations in peripheral nerves**. These diseases may have weakness as part of the clinical syndrome.

Other degenerative neuropathies may occur in a variety of breeds and at various ages.

Diagnosis

A tentative diagnosis is based on finding **signs of weakness** in a **young Birman** cat. Electrodiagnostic evaluations may reveal abnormalities such as fibrillation potentials, positive sharp waves, and decreased nerve conduction velocities depending upon the pathologic process present.
- In general, neuropathies with demyelination tend to be associated more commonly with decreased nerve conduction velocities, whereas neuropathies with predominant axonal abnormalities tend to be associated with fibrillation potentials and positive sharp waves (denervation potentials). Mild to moderate **fibrillation potentials, consistent with denervation**, or decreasing nerve conduction velocity may be found in some cases with electromyography and nerve conduction velocity testing, respectively.

Histologic lesions involving the axon or the myelin sheath may be present on peripheral nerve biopsy.

Differential diagnosis

Clinical signs may be similar to other diseases that affect the lower motor neuron including motorneuropathies, myopathies and some diseases of the neuromuscular junction.

Treatment

No effective treatment is known.

Clinical signs usually progress until euthanasia or death occurs months to years after initial onset of signs.

In rare instances, clinical signs may stabilize or even improve.

Prognosis

Many of these diseases are progressive, and treatments either have not been attempted or have not been beneficial.

DEGENERATIVE MOTORNEUROPATHIES

Classical signs

- Progressive weakness and muscle atrophy in adult cats.
- Decreased to absent spinal reflexes.
- Tremor, especially of the head and tongue.
- Cervical ventroflexion.
- Dysphagia.

See main reference on page 903 for details (The Cat With Neck Ventroflexion).

Clinical signs

Degeneration of the lower motor neuron cell bodies in the ventral horn of the spinal cord and occasionally the cranial nerve nuclei leads to chronic progressive signs.

All cats were adults.

Clinical signs included **progressive weakness and muscle atrophy**, **tremor**, especially of the **head** and tongue, ventroflexion of the neck and dysphagia.

Diagnosis

Mild to moderate **fibrillation potentials, consistent with denervation**, were found in the appendicular (limb) and paraspinal muscles with electromyography.

Histologic lesions were most severe in the ventral spinal gray matter, consisting of neuronal cell loss and gliosis. No effective treatment is known.

Differential diagnosis

Hypokalemic myopathy (low plasma potassium), chronic organophosphate toxicity (history of exposure), myasthenia gravis (tensilon test, anti-acetylcholine receptor antibodies, decreased serum cholinesterase activity).

Treatment

No effective treatment is known.

Clinical signs progress until euthanasia or death occurs months to years after initial onset of signs.

DEGENERATIVE MYOPATHIES (X-LINKED MUSCULAR DYSTROPHY, HEREDITARY MYOPATHY, NEMALINE ROD MYOPATHY)

Classical signs

- Signs begin 2–24 months of age.
- Weakness and reduced activity.
- Stiff, choppy gait.
- Increased muscle mass and hypertrophy of the tongue (X-linked muscular dystrophy).
- Ventral flexion of neck and dorsal protrusion of scapula (hereditary myopathy of Devon Rex).
- Any breed may be affected; inherited myopathy occurs in the Devon Rex.

Pathogenesis

An **X-linked muscular dystrophy** similar to Duchenne's and Golden Retriever myopathy has been described in **male cats**. A membrane-associated protein **(dystrophin) is deficient or absent**.

Cardiac muscle may also be affected.

A specific cause of the other myopathies has not been completely established.

Clinical signs

X-linked muscular dystrophy:

- The **gait is mildly stiff or stilted**, and cats tend to **bunny-hop to run**.
- Occasionally there is marked stiffness and reluctance to move.
- Cats often appear to have **increased muscle mass**, especially of the **neck** and **proximal limb** muscles, and stand with adducted hocks.
- The **tongue is hypertrophied** and may protrude partially. Excessive drooling of saliva occurs.
- **Dehydration** may be a recurring problem because the **tongue hypertrophy** makes it **difficult to drink**. Eating is also affected by the tongue hypertrophy.
- There may be a history of **gagging, regurgitation** or vomiting of food.
- Additionally, these cats may have fatal complications when undergoing **general anesthesia** or from manual restraint, as a result of **peracute rhabdomyolysis**.
- Signs generally develop **before 2 years of age**, and hypertrophy of the proximal limb muscles is evident as early as 10 weeks.

Hereditary myopathy in Devon Rex cats (see main reference page 900, The Cat With Neck Ventroflexion).
- Occurs in young (**3–23 months of age**) **Devon Rex cats**.
- Clinical signs include generalized muscle weakness, ventroflexion of the neck and **dorsal protrusion of the scapula**.
- Difficulty maintaining a normal head position when eating may result in **obstruction of the pharynx with food** and laryngospasm, which may be fatal.
- Megaesophagus may be present in some cats.

Nemaline rod myopathy:
- Weakness begins between 6–18 months of age.
- Clinical signs progress to a **choppy, hypermetric gait**.
- The patellar reflex is decreased, however flexion reflexes are present.

Diagnosis

These diseases usually require **electrodiagnostic evaluation and muscle biopsy** for definitive diagnosis.

X-linked muscular dystrophy:
- Increased serum **creatine kinase** (CK) and **complex repetitive discharges** upon electromyographic (EMG) evaluation may be clues.

- **Muscle biopsy** shows muscle fiber hypertrophy, fiber splitting, myonecrosis, calcium deposition, internalized nuclei and occasional fiber-type grouping.

Hereditary myopathy of Devon Rex cats:
- Serum CK levels are normal.
- Occasional **fibrillation potentials** and positive sharp waves are found with electromyographic examination.
- Muscle biopsies show variability in muscle fiber size, internal nuclei, myofiber necrosis, regeneration and fibrosis.

Nemaline rod myopathy:
- Nemaline rods are characteristic within muscle biopsies.

Differential diagnosis

Polymyositis (increased CK, muscle biopsy), organophosphate toxicity (history of exposure, reduced cholinesterase activity), hypokalemia (serum hypokalemia) and congenital myasthenia gravis (positive tensilon test) are all differentials for degenerative myopathies.

Treatment

No effective treatment is known.

Long-term fluid therapy (subcutaneous) may be required in cats with X-linked muscular dystrophy for them to survive, as tongue hypertrophy limits fluid intake.

Prognosis

Clinical signs are progressive until euthanasia or death.

With X-linked muscular dystrophy, subcutaneous fluid administration may be required to maintain fluid balance. With support, cats may live many years after diagnosis. Sudden death may occur in association with anesthesia.

With **hereditary myopathy** in Devon Rex cats, progression of clinical signs occurs until 6–9 months of age. Clinical signs may stabilize after this time. Four in six cats die suddenly of laryngospasm due to obstruction of the pharynx with food.

With **Nemaline rod myopathy,** signs progress slowly over the first year.

Prevention

Pedigree analysis and selected breeding are required to remove the genes from the gene pool.

IDIOPATHIC PERIPHERAL NEUROPATHY, CHRONIC RELAPSING POLYNEUROPATHY, POLYNEURITIS

Classical signs

- Lower motor neuron tetraparesis is the predominant sign.
- Marked weakness with conscious proprioceptive deficits, and decreased spinal reflexes occur.

Pathogenesis

Nine cats have been reported with a suspected **idiopathic peripheral neuropathy** similar to polyradiculoneuritis (Coon Hound paralysis) in dogs.

Additionally, a **chronic, relapsing polyneuropathy** has been reported in one cat and eluded to in other publications.

A cat has been reported with severe, acute **polyneuritis** without evidence of an infectious etiology.

Clinical signs

In cats with a suspected **idiopathic peripheral neuropathy**, clinical signs were similar to those dogs reported with polyradiculoneuropathy (Coon Hounds paralysis) with paraparesis to tetraparesis, rapid muscle atrophy and decreased to absent spinal reflexes.

In **chronic, relapsing polyneuropathy** marked lower motor neuron tetraparesis occurred, recovered spontaneously and reoccurred months later.

Conscious proprioceptive abnormalities, depressed spinal reflexes and muscle atrophy were present in the limbs.

One cat was reported with a severe, acute **polyneuritis** with weakness, conscious proprioceptive deficits and decreased spinal reflexes.

Icterus and anemia were associated abnormalities.

Diagnosis

In cats with a suspected **idiopathic peripheral neuropathy**, diagnosis is made on the clinical signs of rapid onset of tetraparesis with loss of spinal reflexes. Muscle atrophy is evident within 7–10 days. One cat was examined pathologically and had axonal degeneration, fragmentation and loss of axons, as well as demyelination and accumulation of macrophages in the ventral nerve roots.

In **chronic, relapsing polyneuropathy**, electrodiagnostic evaluation showed fibrillation potentials and positive sharp waves in the limb and paraspinal muscles, as well as decreased nerve conduction velocities.

Demyelination and remyelination were present in nerve biopsies.

In the cat with the acute, severe **polyneuritis**, pathologically there was extensive destruction of myelin associated with macrophages.

Differential diagnosis

Rule out other inflammatory, degenerative and toxic causes of muscle or neuromuscular disease.

Snake bite (appropriate geographic location, increased CK and clotting times), tick paralysis (geographic location, abnormal breathing and tick), **botulism** (gastrointestinal signs) all cause marked tetraparesis but have other differentiating signs, **disk prolapse** may cause tetraparesis but cats are not flaccid in all four limbs, **traumatic spinal cord injury**, diffuse hemorrhage in the spinal cord and around the nerve roots appear clinically similar.

Treatment

Spontaneous recovery occurs in cats with **idiopathic peripheral neuropathy**.

Good nursing care is essential to provide fluids, nutrition and to prevent urine scalding and pressure sores.

With **chronic, relapsing polyneuropathy** improvement, if not resolution of clinical signs, may occur in some cats after corticosteroid therapy.

In the cat reported with acute, severe **polyneuritis**, no treatment was attempted.

Prognosis

In cats with a suspected **idiopathic peripheral neuropathy**, seven cats **recovered spontaneously** and completely without specific treatment within 4–6 weeks.

MYOTONIA

> **Classical signs**
>
> - Stiffness and muscle spasm.
> - Short, stilted gait.
> - Increased muscle size.

Pathogenesis

Cats with myotonia have **sustained muscle contraction**, which is initiated voluntarily or with stimulation, and sustained involuntarily.

Myotonia most often occurs as a **congenital problem**.

Excessive muscle contraction is thought to be due to an **abnormal muscle cell membrane**, which supports persistent depolarization.

Clinical signs

Affected cats often have **a stiff, stilted gait** and have **large, bulky muscles on palpation**.

Muscle dimpling may occur with **direct muscle percussion**.

Diagnosis

Electromyography demonstrates the characteristic myotonic potentials, and muscle biopsies may be supportive of the diagnosis.

Differential diagnosis

Rule out other myopathies such as X-linked muscular dystrophy (increased serum creatine kinase, typical muscle biopsy findings). Myotonia has characteristic EMG findings.

Treatment

No treatment has been described in cats.

PRIMARY HYPEROXALURIA

> **Classical signs**
>
> - Domestic short-hair cats, 5–9 months old.
> - Generalized weakness, absent cutaneous trunci reflex.
> - Signs of renal disease may or may not be present.

Pathogenesis

It is suspected that the systemic **oxalosis damages the peripheral nerves**.

Clinical signs

Primary hyperoxaluria was reported in a colony of domestic short-haired cats.

Cats developed clinical signs between **5–9 months of age**.

In some instances, clinical signs of **weakness** occurred **prior** to the onset of **renal failure**.

Postural reactions were depressed.

Spinal reflexes were inconsistently affected.

The **cutaneous trunci reflex was absent** in most cats.

Other signs of renal failure such as inappetence, weight loss, polyuria, polydipsia were sometimes present.

Diagnosis

Positive sharp waves, milder fibrillation potentials, and occasional bizarre high-frequency discharges were found with electromyographic examination.

Pathologically, the neurons in the ventral gray matter of the spinal cord and their proximal axons were most affected.
- Swollen axons were present in the ventral nerve roots and dorsal root ganglion cells.

Differential diagnosis

Rule out other congenital causes of weakness such as **hypokalemic myopathy** (Burmese, low plasma potassium), **degenerative myopathies** (signs, muscle lesions on biopsy), and **myasthenia gravis** (some recovery with rest, and improvement after IV edrophonium).

Treatment

No treatment was attempted.

HYPERNATREMIC MYOPATHY

> **Classical signs**
>
> - Ventral neck flexion, muscle weakness and a "dropped-hock" gait.

Clinical signs

Rare disease with signs similar to hypokalemic myopathy.

Generalized progressive muscle weakness which may include **ventral neck flexion** and a **"dropped-hock"** appearance to the gait.

Diagnosis

Finding **elevated serum sodium** > 165 (mEq) mmol/L) in the presence of clinical signs.

Differential diagnosis

Hypokalemic myopathy (diagnosis based on finding hypokalemia i.e. plasma potassium < 3.0–3.5 (mEq) mmol/L).

Polymyositis (increased serum CK and muscle lesions on biopsy).

Myasthenia gravis (positive edrophonium tensilon test and anti-acetylcholine receptor antibodies).

Chronic organophosphate toxicity (diagnosis based on history and sometimes reduced cholinesterase activity).

Treatment

Treatment centers around decreasing serum sodium through fluid management. If the hypernatremia has evolved slowly, extreme caution should be exercised when attempting to decrease serum sodium with fluid therapy.

As a rule, slowly decreasing serum sodium concentrations over 2–3 days is safe. Serum sodium measurements should be determined frequently to avoid rapid decreases in sodium, which can result in life-threatening cerebral edema.

Long-term management is with a **low-sodium diet** (e.g. Hill's Feline H/D) with **water added in excess** of maintenance requirements.

HYPERLIPIDEMIA

> **Classical signs**
>
> - Hyperlipidemia and lipemia retinalis.
> - Peripheral neuropathies involving individual peripheral, cranial or sympathetic nerves.

Clinical signs

Hyperlipidemia in cats is usually the result of **primary idiopathic hyperlipidemia** or occurs secondary to **diabetes mellitus**.

Chronic weakness, paresis and decreased spinal reflexes may occur as a result of neuropathies secondary to hyperlipidemia.

The neuropathy results from **compression of nerves** by **lipid granulomata (xanthomas)**.

Signs depend on where the xanthomas form. Peripheral neuropathies involving individual peripheral, cranial or sympathetic nerves.

Diagnosis

Diagnosis is presumptive based on persistent fasting hyperlipidemia (present > 24 hours after feeding) in the presence of clinical signs of neuropathy and weakness.

Definitive diagnosis is on biopsy of the granuloma or autopsy.

Differential diagnosis

Diabetic neuropathy may appear similar and hyperlipidemia also occurs with diabetes. Xanthomas have been reported associated with the hyperlipidemia of diabetes, but are not thought to be the cause of most diabetic neuropathies. Persistent hyperglycaemia above 16 mmol/L (288 mg/dl) is diagnostic of diabetes.

Other neuropathies (e.g. neoplastic, idiopathic, inflammatory) are not associated with persistent fasting hyperlipidemia.

Treatment

Feeding a **low-fat diet** resulted in resolution of the neuropathy in 2–3 months in a few cats with peripheral neuropathy.

Gemfibrozil (7.5–10 mg/kg daily) is indicated if dietary therapy does not normalize triglyceride concentrations.

Marine (fish) oils rich in omega-3 fatty acids may help to decrease triglyceride concentrations.

ACUTE SEPSIS

Classical signs

- Generalized weakness or flaccid paralysis.
- Hypothermia.
- Tachypnea.
- Bradycardia.
- Hypotension (poor pulses, pale mucous membranes, increased capillary refill time).

Pathogenesis

Toxemia and reduced tissue oxygenation from acute bacterial sepsis may cause **weakness and depression**.

Toxemia may be associated with bacteremias originating in the **uterus** (pyometritis), **thorax** (pyothorax), **abdomen** (peritonitis) or **skin** (subcutaneous abscess).

Pyrexia or hypothermia may be present, and **signs referable to the infection site** are often evident including dyspnea, vaginal discharge, abdominal guarding or skin abscess.

Hypothermia weakens the immune system, depresses the myocardium, blunts the vasculature response to catecholamines and reduces cellular function.

Hypothermia may be associated with up-regulation of anti-inflammatory cytokine activity. **Cardiac insufficiency** is common, and coagulopathies often ensue.

Bradycardia is an inappropriate response to critical illness, and its mechanism is unknown. Increased vagal tone, sympathetic stimulation, and induction via hypothermia have all been postulated to be involved. It may be exacerbated by hypoglycemia or hyperkalemia which may accompany the septic state.

Depression of myocardial function is exacerbated by hypothermia, and continues after rewarming. Intracellular calcium overload contributes to **diastolic dysfunction**. **Systolic dysfunction** occurs secondary to ischemia, myocardial edema or infarction.

Cytokines increase vascular permeability and hypoalbuminemia reduces oncotic pressure. When combined with depressed myocardial function, the septic cat is **susceptible to fluid overload** during treatment for hypovolemia.

Anemia results in local hypoxia and local lactic acidosis.

Clinical signs

Depression and anorexia are typically present, and if sepsis is severe, the cat may be **profoundly weak or collapsed**.

Pyrexia or hypothermia may be present

Signs suggesting the infection site such as dyspnea, vaginal discharge or uterine distention, abdominal guarding, or skin abscess are often evident.

The classic signs of sepsis, labeled the "sepsis triad" (**fever, tachycardia, tachypnea**) or the hyperdynamic phase, are rarely recognized.

Sepsis in cats often presents as the "shock triad" (**hypotension, bradycardia, hypothermia**). Hypotension is evidenced as poor pulses, pale mucous membranes and increased capillary refill time.

Localized infection will often cause pyrexia, but sepsis often presents at a stage where fever is no longer sustained and **hypothermia** has developed.

Heart rate often follows temperature.

Diagnosis

Diagnosis is based primarily on **clinical signs and history**, especially if a site of infection is found.

Finding of the "shock triad" of **hypotension, bradycardia, and hypothermia** is highly suspicious.

White cell count alterations are common. Neutrophilic leukocytosis with left shift may be evident, but with overwhelming sepsis, **leucopenia with neutropenia or a degenerative left shift** occur. Monocytosis occurs with long-standing or deep-seated infection.

Thrombocytopenia can be seen from day 1.

Red cell count changes include **anemia** from hemolysis, or a falling PCV and schistocytes associated with DIC.

Coagulation testing (PT, APTT, ACT, FDPs) may indicate DIC.

Hypoalbuminemia is common.

Icterus is common, and usually results from hemolysis rather than cholestasis.

Differential diagnosis

Rule out other causes of acute muscle weakness such as metabolic, inflammatory or toxic causes.

Identification of a focus of infection such as peritonitis, pyothorax, pyometritis, pyelitis or subcutaneous abscess helps to differentiate sepsis from other causes of weakness.

Weakness with hypothermia, hypotension and bradycardia are pathognomonic.

Treatment

The **basis of therapy** is **v**entilation, **i**nfusion, and **p**umping (VIP), together with **early antimicrobial treatment**.

Ventilation reduces the work of breathing, and includes **oxygen, PEEP, intubation and/or mechanical ventilation** as necessary.

Infusion of fluids is essential. **Colloids** rapidly increase intravascular volume, and can be combined with **crystalloids** to support interstitial volume. Use

fresh whole blood if anemic, **plasma** if hypoalbuminemic, and give **clotting factors** via fresh whole blood or fresh frozen plasma if coagulopathic. Do not use a glucose solution unless hypoglycemic.

Cardiac pumping support via use of **positive inotropes** (dopamine, dobutamine, epinephrine) is essential.

Resuscitation goals are to **restore oxygen delivery** through correction and maintenance of arterial pressure, and adequate arterial oxygen content. The aims are to correct hypothermia, hypovolemia, bradycardia and anemia. If perfusion is still inadequate, address hypotension with inotropic and vasopressor support.

Rewarm with warm intravenous fluids, warm humidified oxygen, forced air heating, incubators and circulating water blankets. Care is necessary as active external **rewarming can cause a paradoxical decrease in core temperature, acidosis and shock**, because of the return of cold blood with lactic acid from the periphery.

Bradycardia is treated with adequate warming, fluid bolus, atropine (0.04 mg/kg IV), and a positive inotrope/chronotrope.

Hypovolemia is treated with crystalloids (55–60 ml/kg bolus rate IV) and colloids (5 ml/kg bolus rate IV). Adjust fluid rate to maintain envolemic status. Monitor respiratory rate and depth, and lung sounds carefully because pulmonary edema and pleural effusion are common.

Hypotension refractory to fluid therapy is treated with **exogenous catecholamines**, but many patients become refractory after 72–96 hours.
- **Dopamine** (5–20 μg/kg/min CRI) has positive inotropic, chronotropic and some vasoconstrictor effects, and has few adverse side effects.
- **Dobutamine** (5–20 μg/kg/min CRI) increases cardiac output and oxygen delivery. Seizures occur with continued (> 24 hours) use.
- **Epinephrine** (0.05–0.1 μg/kg/min CRI).
- Vasopressin.

Anemia requires **red cell transfusion** if the PCV is less than 20%.

Pain control helps maintain mental well-being, and is titrated to effect as responses are variable and affected by underlying hepatic and renal dysfunction:
- For **mild to moderate pain** use butorphanol (0.2–0.8 mg/kg IV q 2–6 h).

- For **severe pain** use methadone (0.2–0.4 mg/kg IM q 4–6 h), or morphine (0.1 mg/kg IM q 2–6 h or 0.12 mg/kg/h CRI) with or without diazepam (0.2 mg/kg IV).

Hypoglycemia is treated with 2½–5% dextrose added to IV fluids and/or boluses of dextrose at 0.25–0.50 g/kg increments.

Hyperglycemia is treated with low doses of regular insulin IV as CRI of 40–60 mU/kg/h.

Hyperkalemia is treated by adding 2 g potassium (26.8 mmol) per IL fluids, with a maximum CRI of 0.5 mEq/kg/h.

Hypocalcemia. If not giving blood products, use lactated Ringer's solution (Hartmann's) as the IV fluid, and give a slow IV bolus of calcium gluconate (20 mg/kg).

Hypomagnesemia. Administer Plasma-Lyte 148 which is compatible with blood.

Antimicrobial therapy. Early identification of the most likely pathogen is advantageous. Use antibiotic combinations ($\geq$ two antimicrobials is now routine) to gain synergy, spectrum and reduced emergence of resistance.
- Acceptable combinations while awaiting culture results include:
  - Ampicillin (20–50 mg/kg q 6 h), gentamicin (6 mg/kg q 24 h) and metronidazole (20–40 mg/kg q 24 h).
  - Cephazolin (20–40 mg/kg q 8 h), gentamicin (6 mg/kg q 24 h) and metronidazole (20–40 mg/kg q 24 h).
  - Enrofloxacin (5–11 mg/kg q 24 h), metronidazole (20–40 mg/kg q 24 h).
  OR
  - Ticarcillin/clavulanate (30–50 mg/kg q 8 h) ± gentamicin (6 mg/kg q 24 h)
  OR
  - Enrofloxacin (5–11 mg/kg q 24 h)
  - Ampicillin, cephazolin, or ticarcillin/clavulanate as above.
  - CAUTION: do not use gentamicin if there are signs of renal dysfunction. Enrofloxacin has been associated with blindness which is often irreversible.

Prognosis

Prognosis is guarded to poor, and a successful outcome relies on early intervention, and detection and elimination of the site of infection.

Prognosis worsens if shock signs (hypotension) do not respond to resuscitation within a few hours.

Severe hypothermia (T < 35°C), or **neutropenia** (neutrophil count < 1.0×10^9/L) are poor prognostic signs.

FELINE IMMUNODEFICIENCY VIRUS MYOPATHY

Classical signs

- Subclinical myopathy evident on muscle biopsy.

See main reference on page 339 for details (The Thin, Inappetent Cat).

Clinical signs

A **subclinical myopathy** has been shown to occur in experimentally infected FIV cats.

Diagnosis

A presumptive diagnosis is based on evidence of a subclinical myopathy in a FIV positive cat where other potential causes of myopathy have been excluded.

Some cats had **elevated CK levels and changes on EMG evaluation**.

Muscle biopsies may show inflammatory changes.
- Predominant histologic characteristics were perivascular and pericapillary lymphocytic infiltration and myofiber necrosis, phagocytosis and regeneration.

CIGUATOXIN INTOXICATION

Classical signs

- Signs begin within 3–6 hours of ingestion of a toxic meal of reef fish.
- Hindleg paresis and vomiting are the most prominent.
- Cardiovascular shock and/or respiratory distress may precede coma and death within 24 hours of ingestion.

Pathogenesis

Ciguatoxin is the main toxin that **accumulates in the flesh and viscera of large carnivorous species** of fish associated with **coral reefs** (mostly **coral trout, Spanish mackerel, barracuda**).

A marine benthic dinoflagellate, *Gambierdiscus toxicus,* is believed to produce a precursor to ciguatoxin, gambiertoxin, which undergoes biotransformation within the stomach of herbivorous fish. The resultant ciguatoxin is absorbed from the stomach and sequestered in the muscles and viscera (potency increases tenfold in the process).

Ciguatoxin is heat stable and not affected by cooking.

Ciguatoxin is **lipid soluble** and may cross the blood–brain barrier, which accounts for the CNS effects.

An associated toxin, **maitotoxin**, is water soluble and is believed to account for the **gastrointestinal effects**.

Ciguatoxin interferes with the sodium channels located on the cell membrane of neurons. In the muscle sarcolemma it **increases sodium permeability** of the cell membrane. Increased sodium permeability **enhances activation**.

Cardiac effects are the **most life threatening** and involve **arrhythmias** and **negative inotropy**. Focal myocardial necrosis is evident histologically.

Centrally mediated **interference with phrenic nerve conduction** may lead to **respiratory failure and death**.

Clinical signs

Cats fed reef fish are at risk of poisoning, as are humans, even though incidences are low. Cats fed **viscera and liver** of these fish may consume a lethal meal because ciguatoxin levels are 50 times greater than in fish flesh.

Signs begin within 3–6 hours of ingestion of a toxic meal and **may last up to 14 days**.

Neurological signs include **hindlimb paralysis** extending to forelimbs in severe cases, and **ataxia**. **Gastrointestinal signs** include **hypersalivation** and **vomiting**.

Less severe cases may have some mild gastrointestinal signs and mild paresis.

Respiratory difficulty and arrhythmias may also occur. Death from respiratory failure can occur several days later.

Cardiovascular effects are biphasic. **Low doses** of toxin tend to induce hypotension, hyperventilation, **bradycardia** and atrioventricular block. As toxin absorption increases, the **higher doses cause** hypertension, **tachycardia,** respiratory depression and perhaps cardiac arrest.

Recovery is slow and **signs may persist for 1–2 weeks**.

Diagnosis

History of access to coral reef fish.

Presence of **gastrointestinal signs along with neurological signs** is supportive.

A rapid **calorimetric immunoassay** (the "stick test") conducted on the fish flesh is inexpensive and quick and of use in ciguatera endemic regions.

Differential diagnosis

Rule out other causes of neurological signs, especially **tick paralysis** and **brown snake envenomation**. Cats with ciguatoxicity typically have gastrointestinal signs, a history of access to reef fish, **a lack of voice involvement** (typical in tick paralysis), and **no coagulation defects** (typical in brown snake).

Rule out **toadfish** (tetrodotoxin) poisoning largely via history of access as well as **pupillary dilation and voice changes** are more typical of tetrodotoxin.

Treatment

No specific treatment is available. Symptomatic and supportive measures including maintenance of body fluids and artificial respiration may be required.

Gastric lavage and/or induction of emesis in the early stages of intoxication may decrease the severity of signs.

Atropine (up to 1 mg/kg) helps control the gastrointestinal signs as well as reduces the bradycardia and hypotensive components of the cardiovascular effects.

Lignocaine by constant rate infusion (400 µg/kg/min) has been shown to **alleviate the cardiovascular effects** of ciguatoxin in the cat, probably by blocking the sodium channels.

Calcium gluconate (200 µg/kg/min CRI) infusion has been found to be of value in offsetting cardiac effects.

Proprandol (beta-blocker) at 1 mg/kg IV has been used to control severe tachycardias.

Mannitol (1 g/kg) infusions have not been shown to be successful in the cat, despite its reputation as the treatment of choice in humans, presumably through its effect as a free radical scavenger.

Current research is centered on production of an anti-toxin using monoclonal antibodies.

TETRODOTOXIN INTOXICATION

Classical signs

- Signs begin 10–40 minutes after ingestion.
- Initial signs are gastrointestinal – drooling, vomiting and diarrhea.
- Neuromuscular signs follow with weakness and ataxia progressing to flaccid hindlimb paralysis.
- Pupillary dilation is usually a feature.
- With severe toxicity, cardiovascular shock and labored respiration often precede convulsions and death within hours.

Pathogenesis

Tetrodotoxin accumulates in the flesh and viscera of toadfish (*Sphaeroides hamiltoni*) and puffer fish, newts and the blue ringed octopus. It is produced in the intestines of these species by *Vibrio* bacteria.

Tetrodotoxin is heat stable and is not affected by cooking.

Tetrodotoxin is a powerful vasopressor and neurotoxin. It exerts its action by inhibiting the excitability of neurones by blocking the sodium channels and decreases sodium permeability of the cell membrane (ciguatoxin has the opposite effect).

Tetrodotoxins function similarly to local anesthetics and prevent depolarization of excitable tissues.

Tetrodotoxin affects skeletal muscle membranes and vasomotor nerves, causing hypotension. Reduced neuromuscular junction impulse conduction manifests as flaccid paralysis especially of the hindlimbs and diaphragm.

Although cardiac muscle is less sensitive than nerve or skeletal muscle tissues, severe intoxication can cause bradycardias, heart block and asystole as well as ventricular fibrillation.

Clinical signs

Signs begin 10–40 minutes after ingestion.

Pawing at the mouth and licking of the lips probably equates to human reports of paraesthesia or numbness around the mouth and lips with a tingling (prickling) sensation.

Drooling, vomiting and diarrhea are usually followed by muscular weakness and ataxia. Voice loss and dyspnea occur once muscular weakness is evident.

Flaccid paralysis, especially of the hindlimbs, develops rapidly following initial signs of weakness and ataxia.

Bradycardia, cyanosis and hypotension are variable.

Pupillary dilation is usually a feature.

Death may ensue with terminal convulsions, labored breathing, tachycardia and hypotension evident.

Diagnosis

Diagnosis is usually based on a history of rapid onset of neurological signs after access to a toxin source.

No routine diagnostic laboratory tests are available.

Autopsy tissue samples can be tested by gas chromatography for toxin.

Differential diagnosis

Ciguatoxicosis typically causes similar signs although slower in onset and longer in duration and usually less intense and less acutely life threatening. Pupillary dilation is not a feature of ciguatoxin.

Tick paralysis signs are less intense and more slowly progressive and the presence of a tick is diagnostic.

Brown snake envenomation typically includes coagulation deficits.

Treatment

Gastric lavage and administration of activated charcoal are useful to remove unabsorbed toxin.

Airway maintenance, oxygen therapy and mechanical ventilation may be required.

Hypotension is treated with fluid resuscitation (up to 50–60 ml/kg of crystalloid replacement fluids) with or without peripheral vasoconstriction via norepinephrine (0.2 µg/kg/min) or dopamine (5–10 µg/kg/min CRI)

Etamiphylline (210 mg IM per cat), a cardiac and respiratory stimulant, has benefited some cases.

RED-BACK SPIDER ENVENOMATION (AUSTRALIA) (LATRODECTUS MACTANS HASSELTI) AND BLACK WIDOW SPIDER ENVENOMATION (USA) (LATRODECTUS MACTANS)

Classical signs

- Pain and swelling initially localized to the area of the spider bite. Pain may spread to remote areas over 30–60 minutes and may include abdominal pain.
- Vomiting is a variable sign.
- Agitation, muscle weakness, and incoordination occur later (1–24 hours).
- Muscular tremors and tachycardia.

Pathogenesis

Pain is produced at the **spider bite site and beyond** via an unknown mechanism which is presumed to be related to the presence of **algesic agents (e.g. histamine, 5-hydroxytryptamine, bradykinin)**. These act directly on nociceptors to promote the formation of prostaglandins and other inflammatory mediators which may act in synergism with the venom components to enhance pain production.

Venom is a protein (alpha-latrotoxin) of 130 000 daltons molecular weight, which is **predominantly neurotoxic in action**.

The **toxin action on the presynaptic terminal** of the **neuromuscular junctions** results in initial **outpouring of the neurotransmitters** (acetylcholine and norepinephrine) followed by depletion of acetylcholine reserves at motor nerve endings. This may result in **paralysis of voluntary muscles**.

The accompanying widespread **release of catecholamines causes hypertension**.

Clinical signs

Erythema, edema and localized swelling at the bite site occur **within seconds to minutes after the bite**. The pain increases in intensity within 5–15 minutes, causing generalized hyperaesthesia, vocalization, **chewing or licking** at the bite site and holding of the affected limb off the ground; swelling of the limb may occur.

Pain may appear widespread for example abdominal pain, causing **abnormal postures** such as hunched appearance, and may occur within 30–60 minutes of the bite.

Malaise, depression and vomiting may ensue.

Restlessness, tremors and weakness especially of the affected limb are common, and usually occur within 3 hours, but could be up to 24 hours

Tachycardia and hypertension occur in several cases.

Diagnosis

A presumptive diagnosis is based on the history of sudden onset of s**evere pain in a cat with access to spiders** or finding a **collapsed cat** with **no coagulation defects** near where red-back or black widow spiders have been found.

Differential diagnosis

Snake bite envenomation typically displays **coagulation defects** as well as flaccid paralysis **without obvious pain.** Hindleg paralysis associated with poor circulation is a feature. Cold, purple-blue skin and absent pulses are typical.

Trauma can usually be differentiated if other injuries are evident.

Polymyositis or polymyopathy tends to be more generalized and much less intense; there is less rapid progression and no localization to an area.

Acute abdomen typically is more confined to the abdomen and is not accompanied by weakness unless advanced. Diagnostic tests such as abdominal ultrasound, abdominocentesis and/or diagnostic peritoneal lavage may be necessary to help differentiate.

Treatment

Supplemental oxygen by mask, head box, or nasal tube should be administered at 100–200 ml/kg, if the cat is dyspneic or distressed.

Ice packs may aid local pain relief. Pressure bandages may enhance pain and probably do little to restrict venom movement once systemic signs are present. This is because there is usually a ½–3-hour lag between the bite and the onset of systemic signs.

Administer **red-back spider antivenom** (500 units IM or diluted 1:50 slowly IV or **black widow spider antivenom** (equine origin) used similarly. Repeat the dose if no appreciable response is observed in 1–2 hours. The efficacy may be reduced if given after paralysis occurs.

Administer **pain relief with opioids** (e.g. buprenorphine 0.1–0.5 mg/kg) each 4–8 hours as needed.

Fluid and electrolyte therapy is necessary, especially correction of **calcium and potassium** deficits. Replacement isotonic crystalloid fluids should be used and these may need to have 20–80 mEq/L potassium added, depending on the serum potassium concentration. Calcium supplementation may be necessary and if serum levels can be monitored, increments of 5–10 mg/kg of calcium gluconate may be given each hour added to IV fluids.

Rest, warmth and close observation are important.

RECOMMENDED READING

Atwell RB, Campbell FE. Reactions to tick antitoxin serum and the role of atropine in treatment of dogs and cats with tick paralysis caused by *Ixodes holocyclus*; a pilot survey. Aust Vet J 2001; 79: 394–397.

Dow SW, LeCouteur RA, Fettman MJ, Spurgeon TL. Potassium depletion in cats: Hypokalemic polymyopathy. J Am Vet Med Assoc 1987; 191: 1563–1568.

Gerritsen RJ, van Nes JJ, van Niel MHF, et al. Acute idiopathic polyneuropathy in nine cats. Vet Quart 1996; 18: 63–65.

Sharp NJH, Nash AS, Griffiths IR. Feline dysautonomia (the Key–Gaskell syndrome): A clinical and pathological study of forty cases. J Small Anim Pract 1984; 25: 599–615.

Shelton GD. Neuromuscular disorders. In: August JR (ed) Consultations in Feline Medicine, 2nd edn. Philadelphia, WB Saunders, 1994, pp. 405–412.

Shelton GD. Diseases of the muscle and neuromuscular junction. In: Sherding RG (ed) The cat diseases and management, 2nd edn. New York, Churchill Livingstone, 1994, pp. 1569–1576.

45. The cat with lameness

Maurine Thomson

KEY SIGNS
- Difficulty walking.
- Limping.
- Inability or reluctance to bear weight on limb.

MECHANISM?
- Structural or functional disorder of one or more limbs resulting in an altered gait or stance.

WHERE?
- Generally a disorder of the musculoskeletal system, occasionally neurological, metabolic or referred pain.

WHAT?
- Most lameness in cats is associated with trauma, particularly cat fight injuries or motor vehicle accidents.

QUICK REFERENCE SUMMARY
Diseases causing lameness

DEGENERATIVE

● **Degenerative joint disease* (p 981)**
Less common in the cat than dog, and often asymptomatic. Usually secondary to external joint trauma.

● **Intervertebral disc disease* (p 982)**
Rare in the cat, can cause paresis or lameness.

ANOMALY

● Hip dysplasia (p 987)
Rare in the cat compared to the dog, and occurs mainly in Persians. Usually asymptomatic in cats.

● Osteochondrosis dissecans (p 988)

Rare in the cat, reported in the shoulder joint.

● Femoral neck metaphyseal osteopathy (p 988)

Similar appearance to Legg–Calve–Perthes disease in dogs. Occurs rarely, exclusive to young male cats less than 2 years of age.

● Feline mucopolysaccharoidosis (p 988)

Rare inherited disorder of Siamese cats, which may cause a stiff gait.

● Osteogenesis imperfecta (p 989)

Rare inherited disorder of osteogenesis, which is characterized by brittle bones, which fracture readily with minor trauma.

● Scottish fold osteochondrodysplasia (p 989)

Occurs in Scottish folds resulting in periarticular exostoses and ankylosis.

● Pectus excavatum (p 989)

Congenital abnormality resulting in dorsal to ventral narrowing of the thorax. May be associated with limbs splaying laterally and impaired ambulation.

● Spina bifida (p 989)

Characterized by a closure defect in the neural arches, and is inherited with the gene for tailless-ness in Manx cats; causes variable neurological deficits.

NUTRITIONAL

● Hypervitaminosis A (p 990)

Seen occasionally in cats on all-liver diet. Causes joint ankylosis and spinal pain.

● **Nutritional hyperparathyroidism*** (p 990)

Due to diet low in calcium. Seen in young kittens on an all meat diet. Causes osteopenia and pathological fractures.

● Rickets (p 991)

Seen in young cats fed diet with calcium:phosphorus imbalance and vitamin D deficient. Causes osteopenia and thickening of physeal growth plates.

NEOPLASTIC

● Neoplasia (primary neoplasia of bone, synovium, connective tissue or spinal cord
   and secondary metastatic neoplasia to digits from lung carcinomas) (p 977)

Rare in cats. Generally occurs in older cats and may present acutely or with an insidious onset of lameness. There is usually swelling at the site of the neoplasia.

INFECTIOUS

● **Cellulitis and soft tissue abscesses***** (p 979)

One of the most common causes of lameness in the cat, secondary to cat fight wounds. Usually acute onset of lameness, with variable signs of systemic illness.

● Bacterial septic arthritis or osteomyelitis (p 983)

Usually secondary to bite wound or hematogenous spread from septic foci. See lameness and typical discharging sinus.

continued

continued

● Localized tetanus (p 985)

Occasionally causes paresis or paralysis of a solitary limb in the initial stages, but usually advances to generalized tetanus.

● Viral arthritis (p 983)

Can occur secondary to calici virus exposure or vaccination; also coronavirus.

● Fungal infections (p 984)

Histoplasmosis, Coccidiomycosis, Sporotrichosis usually cause non-healing lesions, draining sinuses or osteomyelitis.

● Toxoplasmosis (p 984)

More often causes CNS signs such as ataxia, and paresis but can cause stiff gait, shifting lameness and muscle and joint pain.

● Neospora caninum (p 985)

Causes encephalomyelitis with ataxia and paresis and polymyositis.

IMMUNE MEDIATED

● Feline progressive polyarthritis (erosive) (p 985)

Rare disease; proliferative subtype occurs as acute onset in 1–5-year-old male cats, deforming sub-type occurs as chronic onset in older cats. Usually several joints affected, most commonly carpus and tarsus. Proliferative subtype often has systemic signs of illness. Deforming subtype may be FeLV positive.

● Immune-mediated polyarthritis (non-erosive) (p 985)

Rare disease, due to deposition of immune complexes in the synovial membrane. Usually carpus and tarsus affected. May be idiopathic or associated with SLE or chronic infection.

TRAUMA

● **Fractures, luxation, muscular contusions*** (p 980)**

Very common cause of presenting lameness.

● Cruciate rupture (p 982)

Occurs much less frequently in the cat than the dog, and usually less symptomatic.

● Patellar luxation (p 983)

Occurs only rarely in the cat, predisposition in Devon Rex cats.

INTRODUCTION

MECHANISM?

Lameness can occur in any limb, and is defined as interference in the normal locomotion of the cat. It is usually pain related, and is secondary to tissue injury which has caused structural alteration, edema and inflammation.

The severity of the lameness will vary with the severity and type of the injury or insult, varying from a mild to a non-weight-bearing lameness.

Generally periosteum has the densest nerve supply of the deep tissues, and has the lowest pain threshold, followed by the joint capsule, tendon, fascia and muscle.

Mechanical lameness can result from an abnormal limb conformation such as shortening, angulation or a rotational abnormality.

Referred pain is pain felt in a part of the body other than that where the cause of pain is located.

Signs of weakness can be confused with lameness. See The Cat With Generalized Weakness (page 941). Paresis and ataxia can also be confused with lameness. The Weak and Ataxic or Paralyzed Cat See (page 908).

WHERE?

The origin of the lameness may be from bone, muscle, joint or neurological.

Diagnosis requires a good physical examination and orthopedic examination to localize the lameness in the affected limb or limbs.

WHAT?

The most common causes of lameness in the cat are cellulitis or an abscess from a cat bite injury, and motor vehicle trauma resulting in fracture or luxation.

The site of the injury is generally localized by palpation of pain and swelling at the affected site.

Cellulitis is often associated with pyrexia and lethargy.

Motor vehicle trauma is often associated with other signs of external injury such as grazes or scuffed nails, with or without dyspnea or internal injuries.

DISEASES CAUSING SIGNS OF LAMENESS

CELLULITIS/SOFT TISSUE ABSCESS***

Classical signs

- Acute lameness of affected limb.
- Pain and soft tissue swelling at site of injury.
- Often associated with pyrexia, anorexia, lethargy.
- Wounds in close proximity to a joint can cause septic arthritis.

Pathogenesis

Occurs secondary to a penetrating bite wound, and is one of the most common causes of lameness in the cat.

Many bacteria are present in the oral cavity of cats, but *Pasteurella*, *Bacteroides* and *Fusobacterium* are the most common organisms responsible for abscess formation, though a mixture of anaerobes and aerobes may also be present.

Infection may take the form of a discrete abscess or a diffuse cellulitis.

Occasionally L-forms of bacteria which lack bacterial walls are involved.

Clinical signs

Acute lameness.

Soft tissue swelling and pain at the affected site.

Often a small scab and evidence of a bite wound can identify the area of penetration.

Associated with variable signs of systemic illness, including depression, pyrexia and anorexia.

L-forms produce a syndrome of fever and persistently draining, spreading cellulitis and synovitis that often involve extremities. Lesion is unresponsive to most antibiotics except tetracycline group.

Diagnosis

History of a cat fight.

Clinical signs of penetrating injury.

Abscess formation can be demonstrated by aspiration of purulent material.

L-form bacteria produce a discharge containing predominantly macrophages and neutrophils, but organisms cannot usually be detected cytologically or grown on culture. Response of syndrome only to tetracycline group antibiotics suggests diagnosis.

Differential diagnosis

Soft tissue injury caused by another form of external injury.

Foreign body reaction.

Osteomyelitis often causes swelling and sinus formation. Rare in the cat and usually associated with an open fracture or bite wound.

Treatment

Abscess formation generally requires lancing, and flush with weak solution of chlorhexidine, followed by course of antibiotics sensitive to *Pasteurella*, i.e. amoxicillin and clavulonic acid 12 mg/kg for 5 days.

Rarely there may be extensive regions of necrosis, which may require debridement and delayed closure.

Cellulitis treated by broad-spectrum antibiotics, i.e. amoxycillin and clavulonic acid, or cephalosporins.

Osteomyelitis may be a rare secondary complication resulting in sinus formation after initial healing of the abscess.

L-form bacteria respond rapidly to tetracycline (22 mg/kg tid PO) or doxycycline (5 mg/kg bid PO).

Prognosis

Normally **excellent,** and resolves after initial treatment.

With extensive injury the prognosis is still excellent, although it may require more prolonged treatment.

With septic arthritis some degree of degenerative joint disease will occur, although cats tolerate this with less clinical symptoms than dogs.

FRACTURES, LUXATION, MUSCULAR CONTUSIONS***

Classical signs

- Acute, usually non-weight-bearing lameness of affected limb or limbs.
- Soft tissue swelling at the site of injury.
- Abnormal movement or angulation of the affected bone or joint.

Pathogenesis

Usually due to external trauma from a motor vehicle accident.

Can also occur from other external trauma such as dog attack, malicious attack or fall.

Hindlimb lameness in young cats less than 7 months of age is usually due to **disruption of the growth plate to the femoral head rather than hip luxation**.

Type and location of the fracture or luxation will depend on the type of forces that have occurred at the time the injury was sustained.

Clinical signs

Acute lameness of the affected limb.

Pain and swelling localized by physical examination.

Most common sites of fractures are femur, humerus, pelvis, tibia and radius.

Hip luxation is the most common form of joint disruption in the mature cat.

Pain localized to the hip in young cats is more likely due to separation of the femoral head.

Fracture/luxation injuries may be open or closed.

Open shearing injuries of the carpus and tarsus often occur due to the minimal degree of soft tissues covering over these regions.

Diagnosis

Usually history of trauma.

Localization by physical examination.

Radiography is normally required to demonstrate exact type and location of the fracture or luxation.

Differential diagnosis

Cellulitis can cause a similar degree of soft tissue swelling and lameness. Usually differentiated by evidence of penetrating wound and pyrexia.

Neoplasia of a bone or joint can present suddenly if associated with a pathological fracture. Very rare in the cat, and usually differentiated on radiographs.

Nutritional hyperparathyroidism in the young cat can present suddenly due to spontaneous fractures. Radiographically will see generalized osteopenia, with history of poorly balanced diet.

Treatment

Will depend on the location and extent of the injury.

Simple fractures in young animals may be amenable to external coaptation, i.e. splints or casts.

More extensive fractures generally require some form of internal fixation. See relevant textbooks dealing with orthopedic diseases and management.

Joint sprains or other soft tissue injuries usually respond well to brief periods, i.e. 2 weeks or less, of immobilization, or simple rest.

Prognosis

Depends on the location and degree of severity of the injury.

With appropriate treatment most injuries have a very good prognosis for return to normal function.

Excision arthroplasty in the cat for treatment of femoral head separation or fracture has a very good to excellent prognosis following surgery.

Cats are generally less symptomatic for osteoarthritis following joint trauma than are dogs.

DEGENERATIVE JOINT DISEASE*

Classical signs

- Chronic, insidious lameness of the affected limb.
- Lameness may be worse after sleeping, or when first rising.
- May have thickening of the affected joint, with decreased range of movement.
- Much less common in the cat than the dog.

Pathogenesis

Generally secondary to joint trauma such as open fracture, or penetrating bite wound.

Can occur secondary to joint conformational abnormality such as hip dysplasia in Persian cats, patellar luxation or cruciate rupture.

May be part of an immune mediated polyarthritis, e.g. systemic lupus erythematosus.

Can occur secondary to septic arthritis from hematogenous spread or direct contamination.

Occasionally occurs in association with acromegaly from excess growth hormone.

Clinical signs

Insidious lameness which may be exacerbated by strenuous activity.

Usually some degree of joint thickening and reduced range of motion on physical exam.

Often does not cause any clinical signs of lameness and may be incidental finding.

Diagnosis

History of insidious or vague intermittent lameness.

Radiographs demonstrate signs of osteoarthritis such as osteophytes, periosteal proliferation and periarticular joint thickening.

Differential diagnosis

Joint neoplasia, which is very rare in the cat. Usually expect more extensive swelling and consistent lameness.

Treatment

Most cats are not symptomatic for osteoarthritis, or if associated with a sudden exacerbation of the joint normally respond well to conservative management. This involves rest and short-term non-steroidal anti-inflammatory drugs, i.e. aspirin 10 mg/kg every 48 hours or corticosteroids, i.e. prednisolone 0.25 mg/kg daily, or other non-steroidal anti-inflammatory drugs, e.g. carprofen, ketofen or meloxicam depending on availability and registration for use in cats.

Encourage weight loss in fat cats.

In severe cases of osteoarthritis associated with erosive arthritis or joint instability, arthrodesis may be warranted.

Prognosis

Generally very good when single joint is involved.

With severe polyarthritis long-term prognosis is poor, with most cases relapsing after therapy.

INTERVERTEBRAL DISC DISEASE*

Classical signs

- Much rarer in the cat than the dog.
- Usually results from traumatic herniation of the disc.
- Clinical signs vary with the location of the disc herniation.
- Signs may be acute or progressive in onset.

Pathogenesis

Usually results from traumatic herniation of the disc, resulting in acute spinal cord compression.

Much rarer in the cat than the dog.

Clinical signs

Location of the site of herniation dictates type of clinical signs seen.

Usually associated with paresis of the hindlimbs. See The Weak and Ataxic or Paralyzed Cat (page 908).

Diagnosis

Lesion identified by neurological examination.

Confirmation of disc herniation by radiographs, myelography or CT imaging.

CRUCIATE RUPTURE

Classical signs

- Acute onset of hindlimb lameness.
- May have thickening of the affected joint due to synovitis, with pain evident on palpation of the stifle.
- Positive cranial drawer sign or tibial thrust.
- Much less common in the cat than the dog.

Pathogenesis

Usually due to external trauma such as a fall, hyperextension injury of the stifle, or excessive internal rotation of the tibia.

Generally causes rupture of the anterior cruciate, rarely is the caudal cruciate involved, unless there has been major stifle disruption.

Clinical signs

Acute lameness of the affected hindlimb.

Generally there will be stifle swelling and pain present on joint palpation.

A positive cranial drawer sign or tibial thrust is generally evident on palpation, though pain may prevent an adequate examination of the joint.

Chronic cases may show a mild intermittent lameness as opposed to the acute injury.

Diagnosis

By identification of a positive cranial drawer sign and pain in the stifle.

Differential diagnosis

Traumatic disruption of all stifle ligaments due to excessive trauma. Usually palpation will reveal laxity in a mediolateral direction also if the collaterals have been disrupted.

Treatment

Conservative therapy with rest and anti-inflammatories is generally sufficient for return to normal function in most cats.

Degenerative joint disease will usually occur, but this does not normally cause clinical signs of lameness.

In refractory cases the stifle can be stabilized with an extra-articular surgical technique. See relevant texts on surgical management of cruciate disease.

Prognosis

Generally the prognosis is very good to excellent with both conservative and surgical management.

PATELLAR LUXATION

Classical signs

- Can be congenital or acquired secondary to trauma.
- Much rarer in the cat than the dog, though a predisposition occurs in purebred cats such as the Devon Rex.
- Lameness may be worse after sleeping, or when first rising.
- May have thickening of the affected joint, with decreased range of movement.

Pathogenesis

The congenital form occurs secondary to malalignment of the quadriceps mechanism, generally resulting in a medial luxation of the patella.

Varying degrees of deformity of the trochlear groove and tibial tuberosity can occur depending on the severity of the luxation.

The acquired form can occur secondary to external joint trauma from a fall or motor vehicle accident.

Clinical signs

The congenital form is characterized by varying degrees of lameness depending on the severity of the condition. The lameness if often insidious and intermittent.

Usually occurs in young, purebred cats.

The acquired form can occur at any age, usually presenting with an acute lameness.

Palpation of the stifle will demonstrate luxation of the patella.

Diagnosis

Palpation of the stifle demonstrates patellar luxation, usually in a medial direction.

Lameness present in the affected limb, which varies with the severity of the underlying disease.

Treatment

In cats with clinical disease surgery is generally warranted.

Type of surgery varies with the severity of the disease, ranging from lateral imbrication, deepening of the trochlear groove and transposition of the tibial tuberosity.

Prognosis

Generally excellent, despite the progression of some degree of degenerative joint disease.

BACTERIAL SEPTIC ARTHRITIS OR OSTEOARTHRITIS

VIRAL ARTHRITIS

Classical signs

- Lameness may be of a single limb or multiple.
- If all limbs involved will be reluctant to ambulate at all.
- Can cause erosive or non-erosive signs radiographically.
- Considered rare in the cat as a cause of lameness.

Pathogenesis

Bacterial:
- Generally from a blood-borne infection that arises from a septic foci elsewhere in the body.
- Can occur from direct bite wound or open joint injury.
- Rarer in cats than dogs.
- Can occur in kittens secondary to umbilical vein infections.
- *Pasteurella* species are most commonly identified.
- Can be due to bacterial L forms, which are mutant bacteria, which have lost their cell wall.

Viral:
- **Calicivirus** polyarthritis can occur uncommonly in young kittens following natural exposure or after live attenuated vaccination.
- Lameness usually occurs 7–10 days after mild respiratory tract signs, though can occur in the absence of respiratory signs.
- **Coronavirus** has also been associated with polyarthritis.

- The effusive form of **feline infectious peritonitis** (FIP) virus occasionally causes lameness, with leakage of fluid into joint spaces.
- The granulomatous form of FIP may cause paresis or paralysis as a result of spinal cord inflammation.

Mycoplasma:
- *M. gatae* is linked to arthritis and tenosynovitis in older cats.
- Mycoplasmal infection may incite an antigenic response resulting in the formation of immune-mediated disease such as rheumatoid-like (deforming) arthritis.

Clinical signs

Acute onset of lameness in one or several limbs.

Usually associated with **systemic signs such as pyrexia, lethargy**.

May appear weak rather than lame if all four limbs involved.

Usually demonstrate joint pain on manipulation of limbs.

Diagnosis

Radiographic signs may demonstrate changes of erosion and periosteal proliferation in advanced cases, but may show no abnormalities initially.

Arthrocentesis generally required for cytology and culture and sensitivity.

Differential diagnosis

Weak or paretic cat can appear similarly. See The Weak and Ataxic or Paralyzed Cat (page 908).

Immune-mediated polyarthritis.

Treatment

Antibiotics for bacterial infection depending on results of culture and sensitivity.

L form infections respond well to 10–14-day course of tetracycline or doxycycline.

Calicivirus is often self-limiting, and cats recover well.

TOXOPLASMOSIS

Classical signs

- More commonly causes CNS signs such as ataxia and paresis.
- Can cause a stiff gait, shifting leg lameness, hyperaesthesia on muscle palpation and joint pain.

See main references on page 705 for details (The Cat With Signs of Acute Small Bowel Diarrhea) and page 958 (The Cat With Generalized Weakness).

Clinical signs

CNS signs seen most frequently, see The Paretic Cat (page 911).

May cause shifting limb lameness.

Can cause arthritis and myositis.

Diagnosis

High IgM titers suggest recent infection, but do not confirm that *T. gondii* is responsible for the clinical signs in a given cat.

The organism can sometimes be seen in a muscle biopsy or very rarely in CSF.

FUNGAL INFECTIONS

Classical signs

- Cats less commonly affected than dogs.
- Lameness due to fungal osteomyelitis.
- Can be a single bone involved, or more commonly multiple sites affected.
- Spores usually inhaled from the soil.

See main references on page 368 for details (The Pyrexic Cat) and page 401 (The Cat With Enlarged Lymph Nodes).

Clinical signs

Occurrence tends to be location dependent:
- *Coccidioides*: south-western USA, Mexico, Central and South America.

- *Blastomyces*: small area of distribution mainly in North America and near fresh water.
- *Histoplasma*: widespread in temperate and subtropical regions of the world, not Australia.
- *Cryptococcus*: worldwide distribution.
- *Sporotrichosis*: worldwide distribution.

Result in non-healing tumor-like lesion of the distal limbs and draining sinus tracts (sporothrix) or lameness due to fungal osteomyelitis.

Radiographically, see tumor-like lesions present in the bone with bone bony destruction and proliferation seen.

Diagnosis

Organism is often evident in cytological preparation of aspirates or discharge from lesion or in a biopsy section.

Positive fungal titer may aid diagnosis.

NEOSPORA CANINUM

Classical signs

- Neurological signs such as ataxia and paresis.
- Polymyositis frequently present.

Clinical signs

Polymyositis and encepalomyelitis with ataxia and paresis are seen most frequently.

Diagnosis

Serum titers and muscle biopsy results are the most common methods of diagnosis.

LOCALIZED TETANUS

Classical signs

- Retrograde axonal transport of the toxin from an infected focus.
- Can cause paralysis of single limb.
- Usually progresses to generalized tetanus.

See main references on page 1340 for details (The Cat With an Abnormal Third Eyelid).

Clinical signs

Occurs following penetrating trauma and tissue devitilization.

Retrograde axonal transport of the **Clostridium tetani neurotoxin occurs**.

Can see **paresis or paralysis of a solitary limb in the initial stages**.

Generally **advances to generalized tetanus**.

Diagnosis

History of recent wound and clinical signs.

EMG findings characteristic with persistent electrical motor unit discharges following needle insertion or tapping of muscles.

Serum antibody titer to tetanus toxin compared with control cats may aid diagnosis.

IMMUNE-MEDIATED POLYARTHRITIS (NON-EROSIVE)

Classical signs

- Are considered rare diseases in the cat.
- Can be acute or chronic onset.
- Often associated with other systemic signs such as lethargy, pyrexia and anorexia.
- Can cause erosive or non-erosive signs radiographically.

Pathogenesis

Erosive form (feline progressive polyarthritis):
- **Chronic progressive polyarthritis has proliferative and deforming subtypes**.
- **Proliferative form occurs in male cats aged 1–5 years**.
- Deforming type occurs more rarely in older cats.
- Severe subchondral bone destruction may occur, leading to joint instability and deformity.
- Radiographic signs are similar to those of rheumatoid arthritis in other species.
- Often associated with feline leukemia virus-positive cats.

- Mycoplasmal products have been postulated to chronically stimulate immune-mediated diseases such as deforming arthritis.

Non-erosive form: (immune-mediated polyarthritis).
- Can be due to systemic lupus erythematosus, chronic infection elsewhere, or idiopathic.
- Due to deposition of immune complexes in the synovial membrane which incites an inflammatory response.
- The inciting agent is usually not identified, but if the cat is on medication this may be a potential source and should be discontinued.

Clinical signs

Deforming type of progressive polyarthritis has a **chronic onset**. All other forms tend to be **acute onset of lameness and stiffness**.

Often affects **carpus and tarsus** more severely than other joints.

Diagnosis

Radiographic signs in erosive forms show marked **destruction and deformity** of the distal joints often resulting in **luxation or subluxation** but with minimal periosteal proliferation.

The proliferative form is characterized by **periarticular soft tissue swelling** in the early stages, then progressing to extensive **periarticular proliferation.** This is most frequently seen in the carpi, tarsi and smaller distal joints.

Arthrocentesis preferably done on two or more joints. Joint fluid is generally slightly increased in amount, slightly turbid, and with reduced viscosity. Cytology typically reveals a non-septic purulent inflammation, with cell counts in the range of 4000–70 000 nucleated cells/μl, and predominantly non-degenerative neutrophils. A variable number of small and large mononuclear cells may also be present.

Joint cultures are negative for bacteria and *Mycoplasma*.

Rheumatoid factor, ANA and LE cell tests are consistently negative.

Hematological parameters are generally unremarkable.

Differential diagnosis

Infectious arthritides, such as viral infections.

Causes of weakness and paresis in the cat. See The Weak and Ataxic or Paralyzed Cat (page 908).

Treatment

Remove the cause if secondary to drug administration or chronic infection.

Treatment consists of immunosuppressive doses of corticosteroids for several months, or in combination with chlorambucil at 1.0–1.25 mg/cat once daily, and prednisolone 10–20 mg twice daily until resolution of clinical signs, then slowly taper the dose of prednisolone over 2–4 months. Continue the chlorambucil at the same dose every other day. Combination of prednisolone and gold salts (aurothioglucose 1 mg/kg by injection once a week) has also been used.

Prognosis

Good initial response to drugs, but greater than 50% of cases are likely to relapse, becoming more refractory to treatment.

NEOPLASIA (PRIMARY NEOPLASIA OF BONE, SYNOVIUM, CONNECTIVE TISSUE OR SPINAL CORD AND SECONDARY METASTATIC NEOPLASIA TO DIGITS FROM LUNG CARCINOMAS)

Classical signs

- Rarer in the cat than dog.
- May be acute or insidious onset of lameness.
- Usually associated with swelling at site of neoplasia.

Pathogenesis

Primary bone tumors are rare in the cat. Osteosarcoma is the most commonly identified tumor.

Generally occurs in cats older than 10 years.

Primary bone tumors are much less metastatic in the cat than the dog.

Metastatic spread from carcinomas to bone is very rare in the cat, compared to the dog.

Can get carcinomas of the digits secondary to primary lung tumors.

Joint neoplasias are very rare in the cat, and are due to synovial cell sarcomas or other soft tissue sarcomas.

Multiple cartilaginous exostoses or feline osteochondromatosis can transform to a malignant disease in the cat.

Lameness can also occur from nerve sheath tumors of the plexus or spinal cord, but these are very rare in the cat.

Clinical signs

Can be acute or insidious onset of lameness.

Rarely can be associated with pathological fracture.

Usually thickening identified at site of disease, which may or may not be painful.

Diagnosis

Radiographically, will see bone lysis in the metaphyseal region of long bones, or joint thickening and proliferation.

Histopathology is required for definitive diagnosis.

Thoracic radiographs should be taken to demonstrate primary lung tumor if multiple digits are swollen, or prior to amputation to rule out metastatic disease.

Differential diagnosis

Osteomyelitis.

Septic arthritis.

Treatment

If no evidence of metastatic disease, amputation is the treatment of choice.

If a solitary tumor of a digit is present, often this can be removed and the limb saved.

Prognosis

If no evidence of metastatic disease, then amputation is often curative, with median survival times greater than 2 years.

Primary bone tumors in the cat are a lot less aggressive than in the dog and generally not followed with chemotherapy.

HIP DYSPLASIA

> **Classical signs**
>
> - Usually occurs in Persian and long-haired cats.
> - Usually asymptomatic in cats compared to dogs.
> - Generally requires only conservative management.

Pathogenesis

Congenital disorder of Persian and other long-haired cats.

Radiographically, see luxation of the coxofemoral joint, with varying degrees of osteoarthritis present.

Clinical signs

Usually no clinical signs of lameness are seen.

Pain may be exhibited on flexion and extension of the hip joints.

Occasionally may show signs of a stiff gait or lameness, which is exacerbated by excessive activity.

Diagnosis

Pain on manipulation of the hip joints in a long-haired cat.

Radiographic evidence of hip laxity and osteoarthritis.

Treatment

Usually conservative management consisting of rest, weight loss and intermittent anti-inflammatory drugs is all that is required in symptomatic cats.

If lameness persists femoral head and neck arthroplasty results in an excellent prognosis.

OSTEOCHONDROSIS DISSECANS

Classical signs

- Onset of forelimb lameness in the cat less than 1 year of age.

Pathogenesis

Very rare in the cat.

Has been reported as cause of shoulder lameness.

Occurs due to a defect in osteochondral ossification.

Clinical signs

Insidious forelimb lameness in cats less than 1 year of age.

Pain identified on full extension and flexion of the shoulder joint.

Diagnosis

Radiographically a thickened flap of cartilage or joint mouse can be identified in the shoulder joint.

Treatment

Surgical removal of the cartilaginous flap.

Prognosis

Excellent.

FEMORAL NECK METAPHYSEAL OSTEOPATHY

Classical signs

- Onset of hindlimb lameness in the cat less than 1 year of age.

Pathogenesis

Uncommon condition.

Reported in male cats less than 2 years of age.

Idiopathic necrosis of femoral neck.

Clinical signs

Vague, progressive hindlimb lameness.

May be bilateral.

Diagnosis

Radiographically, see radiolucency of the femoral neck and proximal femoral metaphysis.

Differential diagnosis

Traumatic fracture of the femoral neck.

Treatment

Femoral head and neck osteotomy.

Prognosis

Excellent.

FELINE MUCOPOLYSACCHARIDOSIS

Classical signs

- Rare inherited disorder in Siamese and Siamese cross cats.
- Causes a stiff gait and paraparesis.
- Cats also have a broad maxilla, corneal clouding, pectus excavatum and neurological abnormalities.

Clinical signs

Rare inherited disorder that occurs as a result of a lysosomal enzyme deficiency in Siamese and Siamese cross cats.

Usually present at less than 6 months of age.

Typically have dysmorphic facial features (a broad maxilla), plump paws (from thickened skin) and corneal clouding.

Generally exhibit a stiff gait and paraparesis with diffuse neurological signs.

Also present with a chronic mucoid ocular discharge and chronic respiratory tract infections.

Diagnosis

Constellation of clinical signs suggests the diagnosis.

Radiographs show dysplastic femoral heads and necks and subluxated hip joints.

Excessive granulation of neutrophils, and **vacuolation of lymphocytes** are suggestive.

Positive urine toluidine test for sulfated beta glycos-aminoglycans is consistent with diagnosis.

Definitive diagnosis is via enzyme assays of leukocytes and skin fibroblasts to demonstrate deficient beta glu-curonidase activity.

OSTEOGENESIS IMPERFECTA

Classical signs

- A defect in osteogenesis results in multiple spontaneous fractures.
- Present with multiple sites of bony pain due to fractures, or unwilling to ambulate.
- Lameness generally of young cats.

Clinical signs

A heritable disease with failure of osteoprogenitor cells to develop into mature osteoblasts.

Results in bones that are very brittle and fracture spontaneously.

Spontaneous fractures can occur in any bones, although the long bones are more commonly affected.

Diagnosis

Radiographically the cortical bone is very osteopenic, with multiple fractures present.

SCOTTISH FOLD OSTEOCHONDRODYSPLASIA

Classical signs

- Disease affecting cats with at least one fold-eared parent.
- Lameness generally occurs at 5–6 months of age.

Pathogenesis

Inherited disorder of fold-ear cats.

Get shortening of the coccygeal vertebrae, metacarpal and metatarsal bones and phalanges.

They may develop periarticular exostoses and joint ankylosis.

PECTUS EXCAVATUM

Classical signs

- A congenital disorder characterized by dorso-ventral flattening of the thorax.
- Kittens and cats show variations in respiratory and cardiovascular abnormalities.
- Also associated with lateral limb deviation.

Clinical signs

A deformity of the sternal and costal cartilages resulting in narrowing of the thorax.

Occurs as a congenital abnormality of cats, with the specific cause unknown.

Can be associated with the so-called "wimmer's"syndrome, in which there is lateral deviation of the limbs and impaired ambulation.

Kittens and young mature cats < 1 year of age may show respiratory and cardiovascular abnormalities associated with flattening of the thorax.

Diagnosis

Based on clinical signs and radiographic findings of dorso-ventral flattening of thorax and lateral deviation of limbs.

SPINA BIFIDA

Classical signs

- Congenital disorder caused by a closure defect of the vertebral arches.
- Inherited with the gene for taillessness in Manx cats.

(continued)

Classical signs—Cont'd
- Varying degrees of severity of the condition exist.

See main references on page 920 for details (The Weak and Ataxic or Paralyzed Cat).

Clinical signs

Improper closure of the neural tube during embryogenesis occurs, with varying severity of neurological signs seen affecting hindlimb function and urinary and fecal control.

In the Manx cat it is often associated with sacral dysgenesis.

Diagnosis

Based on clinical signs, radiographic findings.

HYPERVITAMINOSIS A

Classical signs
- Due to excessive intake of vitamin A, usually from an all-liver diet.
- Lameness occurs due to bony exostoses around the cervical vertebrae and ankylosis of joints.

Pathogenesis

Due to excessive vitamin A intake over several months, usually from an all-liver diet.

Causes bony exostoses of spine and osseous hyperplasia and proliferation at joint margins, particularly the shoulder and elbow joints.

Excess vitamin A causes increased reactivity of the periosteum, resulting in bony proliferation at sites of joint capsule and soft tissue attachments to bone.

Clinical signs

Cats are often reluctant to move around, and are very painful.

They often display an abnormal posture with a stiff neck and gait.

Diagnosis

Radiographically there is ankylosis of cervical and cranial thoracic vertebra, and new bone proliferation around shoulder and elbow joints.

History of diet almost exclusively of liver.

Treatment

Correction of the diet, ideally on a balanced commercial diet.

May require short-term analgesics.

Prognosis

Correction of the diet halts the progression of disease, and some remodeling of existing bone may occur. However, bony changes are often permanent and pain may persist.

NUTRITIONAL HYPERPARATHYROIDISM

Classical signs
- Lameness present in multiple sites in young kittens.
- Due to a diet deficient in calcium, such as an all-meat diet.

Pathogenesis

Due to increased parathyroid hormone from persistent hypocalcemia, either from an absolute dietary calcium deficiency or secondary to excessive phosphorus intake relative to calcium.

Causes generalized osteopenia.

Most commonly seen in kittens on an all-meat diet. Occurs with an all-meat diet even if the kittens have access to milk.

Clinical signs

Osteopenia can result in spontaneous fracture.

Diagnosis

History of inadequate diet.

Radiographs demonstrate diffuse osteopenia, with or without folding fractures.

Treatment

Correct the diet by adding calcium, or more appropriately, change to a balanced commercial diet formulated for kittens.

Confine if multiple folding fractures are evident.

Prognosis

Very good if fractures have not resulted in malunion.

Residual deformity of the spine and pelvis may result in chronic partial bowel obstruction with constipation.

RICKETS

Classical signs

- Lameness present in multiple sites in young kittens.
- Due to a diet deficient in vitamin D or insufficient mineral content, such as an all-meat diet.

Pathogenesis

Diet deficient in vitamin D or with insufficient mineral content causes the cartilaginous matrix of the growth plate not to calcify.

Results in osteopenia and widening of the growth plates.

Clinical signs

Osteopenia can result in spontaneous fracture.

Abnormalities of the growth plate with rickets can cause angular limb deformities.

Diagnosis

Diffuse osteopenia, and may see pathological fractures.

With rickets see widened growth plates and osteopenia.

Treatment

Correct the diet by feeding a balanced commercial diet, and adequate exposure to light.

May require confinement if multiple fractures have occurred.

Prognosis

Usually excellent prognosis if there is not abnormal limb angulation. Correction of the diet corrects the underlying osteopenia and growth plate defect.

RECOMMENDED READING

Bojrab MJ. Disease Mechanisms in Small Animal Surgery, 2nd edn. Lea and Febiger, Philadelphia, PA, 1993.
Carro T. Polyarthritis in cats. Comp Continu Edu Pract Vet 1994; 16: 1, 57–67.
Greene CE. Infectious diseases of the dog and cat, 2nd edn. Philadelphia, PA, WB Saunders, 1998.
Slatter D. Textbook of Small Animal Surgery, 3rd edn. WB Saunders, Philadelphia, PA, 2003.
Withrow SJ, MacEwen EG. Small Animal Clinical Oncology, 3rd edn. Philadelphia, WB Saunders, 2001.

PART 12

Cat with behavioral problems

46. The cat with aggression

Kersti Seksel

> **KEY SIGNS**
>
> - Body position, piloerection.
> - Hissing, spitting.
> - Spraying.
> - Scratching, biting.

MECHANISM?

- Aggression is a **threat, challenge or attack** that is directed towards one or more individuals.
- It can be intra- (members of the same species) or interspecific (members of other species).
- Aggression may be normal or abnormal depending on the context.
- Aggression can be **overt** (active, e.g. obvious distance increasing signals) or **covert** (passive, e.g. blocking access).
- Several types of aggression may occur concurrently (see list below).

WHERE?

- The **hypothalamus and amygdala** are involved in defense and aggression.
- **Monoamines and androgenic steroids act as modulators** of established offensive and defensive aggressive behaviors.

WHAT?

- Currently **11 diagnostic categories of feline aggression** are recognized and they may co-occur. The actual prevalence of each category is unknown.
- Most causes of aggression are the result of the **interplay between environmental and genetic factors,** as well as previous experiences (learning).
- Medical conditions and drugs have also been associated with feline aggression.

QUICK REFERENCE SUMMARY

Diseases causing aggression

• Play aggression** (p 995)

Aggression usually exhibited by young cats with no contact with other cats in early development. Often directed towards humans, but can be other cats or animals. May involve stalking, chasing, pouncing and biting (usually inhibited) but rarely vocalization and is directed towards moving objects.

• Redirected aggression** (p 996)

Aggression directed towards another cat or a human when the original target of the aggression is not accessible. It is of sudden onset, can be prolonged in duration and usually alters the behavior of the victim.

• Intercat, intermale aggression** (p 998)

Aggression directed by an entire male cat towards another entire male cat in response to its presence in the near proximity, and is more common during the breeding season.

• Fear aggression** (p 999)

Aggression seen in a confined or cornered animal, and it is usually preceded by attempts to escape. Cats can be fearful of people, places, other cats, or various stimuli such as noises or odors.

• Aggression when patted** (p 1000)

Exhibited towards humans after tactile stimulation of variable duration. It can occur even if the cat seeks the initial attention.

• Impulse control or status-related aggression** (p 1002)

Aggression directed towards people when the cat is actively or passively prevented from controlling an interaction or situation. The cat may even initiate contact and demand attention but then attack.

• Territorial aggression* (p 1003)

Aggression exhibited in response to an intruder, another cat or person, coming into an area in which the cat has established itself. The cat does not try to avoid encounters with the intruder.

• Pain aggression* (p 1004)

Aggression exhibited in response to a painful stimulus.

• Predatory aggression (p 1005)

Aggression exhibited in response to a natural prey object.

continued

continued

● Maternal aggression (p 1006)
Aggression exhibited in response to the proximity of any human or animal which is perceived as threatening the kittens.

● Idiopathic aggression (p 1007)
Unprovoked and unpredictable aggression. No underlying cause can be identified and diagnosis is by exclusion. Very rare in cats.

INTRODUCTION

MECHANISM?

As a behavioral event, aggression can be **both a description and a diagnosis.**

Aggression is a non-specific sign. It may be **passive (covert)** or **active (overt)** and involve a threat, challenge or an actual attack.

Signs may be **visual (changes in body posture, piloerection), auditory (hissing, spitting),** or **olfactory (spraying, scratching)** and may involve use of **teeth** and/or **claws.**

Covert or passive aggression may involve behaviors such as staring or sitting in doorways and blocking access, and as such is often missed by the owners.

Overt or active aggression may involve more obvious visual signs such as hissing, spitting growling, swatting and actual fighting.

Excitation of the ventromedial hypothalamus (VMH) and amygdala leads to a defensive response.
● The **medial amygdaloid nucleus** is involved with **intraspecies aggression**.
● Stimulation of **lateral amygdala** facilitates **predatory attack and defensiveness**. More defensive cats have less predatory aggression.

In most behavioral conditions, the underlying pathogenesis is unknown but is likely to be neurochemically complex.

WHERE?

The hypothalamus and amygdala are involved in defense and aggression.

Monoamines and androgenic steroids act as modulators of established offensive and defensive aggressive behaviors.

WHAT?

There are 11 diagnostic categories of aggression – play, redirected, intercat/intermale, fear, aggression when patted, status related, territorial, pain, predatory, maternal or idiopathic.

Most causes of aggression are the result of the **interplay between environmental and genetic factors** and previous experience (learning).

Medical conditions such as toxoplasmosis, ischemic vascular problems, hepato- encephalopathy, encephalitis, meningioma, lead poisoning, arthritis, sensory (hearing and/or sight) deficits, hyperthyroidism, epilepsy, feline lower urinary tract disease, feline immunodeficiency virus, and rabies have all been associated with feline aggression.

The use of **medications** such as **anesthetic agents and corticosteroids** has been linked with feline aggression.

Careful history taking and physical examination is essential in making a diagnosis.
● A complete description of physical location, body posture, vocal and physical signals, and the behavior sequences are essential data to make an accurate diagnosis.
● Diagnosis may involve complete blood work and radiography to rule out contributing medical factors.

Behavior-modifying drugs are increasingly being used in the treatment and management of behavior problems in cats. The rationale for using psychotropic medication is based on their purported neurochemical actions in the brain. Most drugs in common use are not registered for this purpose in cats. Drugs should always be an adjunct to behavior modification therapy not a replacement.
● **Many classes of medications** have been used in the treatment of behavior problems including antihistamines, anxiolytics, antidepressants and anti-

convulsants. Medications that may have anxiolytic actions include the benzodiazepines, tricyclic anti-depressants (TCAs), antihistamines, azaperones, barbiturates, selective serotonin re-uptake inhibitors (SSRIs) and beta blockers.

CATEGORIES OF AGGRESSION

PLAY AGGRESSION**

> **Classical signs**
>
> - Aggression involves stalking, pouncing, chasing, hiding, laying in wait but rarely vocalizing.
> - May involve biting as well as scratching.

Pathogenesis

As with most behavioral conditions the underlying pathogenesis is as yet unknown, but is likely to be neurochemically complex.

Young cats, possibly orphaned, **hand raised or early weaned** are most likely to exhibit this type of aggression due to lack of appropriate socialization. Social play is seen between 4–12 weeks of age, and by 14 weeks of age is replaced by social fighting.

It is likely to be **associated with owner-facilitated learning** (that is the owner encourages rough play or attacks) and long-term potentiation or early orphaning and the absence of appropriate stimuli during the sensitive period for modulating responses.

Clinical signs

The cat may **stalk, chase, pounce and lay in wait for people** passing by and rarely vocalizes. The cat may also bite but the bites are usually inhibited.

Targets are usually moving objects or people and may be another cat or other animal in the household, especially an older one, in the household.

Young cats, especially early weaned, are more likely to show this type of aggression and it may be normal behavior.

It is sometimes difficult to recognize play aggression as some cats play more roughly than others and do not retract their claws when they swat.

Diagnosis

Based on careful complete behavioral history and thorough physical examination. Key features include:
- **A young cat, that lacked contact with its mother** or conspecifics (other members of its own species) in the socialization period may be more likely to exhibit this type of aggression.
- The behavior occurs when **the target is moving** at the time the aggression occurs.
- **The cat does not vocalize** and the bites are usually inhibited.

Differential diagnosis

Other types of aggression need to be considered.
- **Predatory aggression** may have similar signs and vocalization rarely occurs in either type of aggression, however in cases of play aggression, the target is not normally considered prey.
- **Redirected aggression** may have some signs in common but a lack of history of precipitating events and an early environment lacking in social contact will suggest play aggression. Additionally, cats with play aggression will stalk and lay in wait for their victim whereas this is not usually seen in redirected aggression.
- **Status-related aggression** may have similar signs but this is usually seen in cats after social maturity (after 2–4 years of age).

Cats may exhibit several types of aggression concurrently.

Treatment

The cat should be provided with appropriate toys that dangle or move and can be kept at a distance from people, for example cat dancers™, cat wire toys, or cat tracks™ on which to pounce and direct these behaviors.
- The toys need to be changed at regular intervals, even daily, for the cat to maintain interest.
- The cat may need to be taught how to play, and then encouraged to play with toys.

Rough play, especially using hands or other body parts, **should be discouraged**.
- Whenever the cat plays in this manner, play should be interrupted or suspended.
- The cat's attention should be directed to appropriate toys instead.

Direct punishment, such as smacking, may actually encourage the behavior and is **generally unhelpful** and may lead to other problems, such as fear aggression.

Indirect punishment not connected with the owner, such as clapping hands, may help to distract the cat and the owner can then divert attention to a favorite toy.

Provision of a regular routine that involves interactive play time involving toys 2–3 times daily for 5–10 minutes is important to provide a natural outlet for the behavior.

A second kitten, preferably one that is not very young, may help to teach appropriate behavior.

Prognosis

Generally favorable if owners are prepared to put in the time.

Generally decreases with age.

REDIRECTED AGGRESSION**

Classical signs

- Sudden onset of aggression.
- The original target of the aggression (e.g. other animal or cat outside) is not accessible.
- The cat then directs its aggression towards an unrelated target, a person or another cat, that enters the area soon after.

Pathogenesis

As with most behavioral conditions underlying pathogenesis is unknown, but is likely to be neurochemically complex. The ventromedial **hypothalamus** likely to be involved and long-term potentiation involving excitatory amino acids and post-synaptic second messenger systems may be involved in the repeated displays.

Cats have been used as models for "kindling". Once stimulated, the cells then have a very low threshold for stimulation and cats stay reactive and aroused for up to 24 hours.

Clinical signs

The eliciting factors of the aggression are different in the initial and subsequent episodes.

The **first episode is triggered by a stimulus that the cat is thwarted** in its attempts to respond to and may be missed.

- The cat is highly aroused and directs its attention onto the next person or cat it sees. For example, a cat sees another cat through the window, it is highly aroused but is thwarted in its attempts to reach it. Another cat in the household then enters the room and the cat redirects the aggression to the second cat.

In the second, and subsequent episodes, the initial stimulus no longer has to be present to elicit the aggression, just the target of the first attack.

Additionally, the behavior of the target also changes. Often this results in a prolonged conflict, with the second cat now acting warily, running away, and showing avoidance behavior, whenever the first cat enters the room or approaches.

The cat is highly aroused and may growl, hiss, pace, lash its tail, piloerect, have dilated pupils and inflict serious bites if approached or handled.

Diagnosis

Possible history of previous encounter with another cat or thwarted access to some arousing stimuli (e.g. sight, sound or smell of another cat or animal, e.g. possum).

Sudden onset of aggression.

Physical examination reveals no evidence of problems, e.g. pain, middle cerebral artery infarct.

Differential diagnosis

Other types of aggression should be considered.
- **Intercat, intermale aggression** is usually directed between entire males in the breeding season.
- **Territorial aggression** is commonly directed towards a new cat introduced into the household or a visitor. The cat does not try to avoid the perceived intruder and may directly approach.
- **Fearfully aggressive cats** usually show classic body postures (lowered body position, piloerection, flattened ears, etc.) and will give many warning signals to try to avoid conflict.
- **Status-related aggression** is usually not of sudden onset and the cat may initiate contact or attention but then threatens or attacks.

Cats may exhibit several types of aggression concurrently.

Treatment

It is inadvisable to approach any highly aroused cat, especially to try to calm or reassure it. The cat should be left alone until it is calmer. This may be 24 hours.

If another cat is involved, then **the cats should initially be separated** regardless of whether it is the victim or the instigator (the thwarted one).

- They should be **placed in separate rooms** so that they can hear and smell each other, but no visual contact occurs.
- The cats should be **rotated around all the rooms** until they have distributed their scent in all rooms.
- While separated a **regular routine should be established** with each cat so that feeding and playing occur at a set time each day. Ideally the cats are fed 5–6 small meals each day.

Treatment then involves **slowly reintroducing the cats to each other** (the same way a new cat is introduced into the household).

- The aim is for them to have a **positive association with each other**. This essentially means that "good" things such as play or feeding only happen in the presence of the other cat.
- The cats are then slowly reintroduced. Initially they are **only in the same room during meal times and are separated at other times**. They are placed in cages (or on a cat harness and lead) at opposite ends of the room and are fed at this time. This should create a positive association with food and the presence of the other cat.
- If no hissing or spitting occurs and the cats eat the food, **the cages are gradually brought closer** and closer to each other over a period of days and meals. This may take several weeks or even months.
- Then **one cat at a time is allowed out of its cage** to explore and if no aggression occurs then both are allowed to interact under supervision.
- The re-introduction needs to be slow.

Anxiolytic medication may also be needed to treat one or both cats.

- **Tricyclic antidepressants** (TCAs) such as **amitriptyline** (0.5–1 mg/kg PO q 12–24 h, average 5–10 mg/cat PO q 24 h) or **clomipramine** (0.5 mg/kg PO q 12 h) or selective serotonin re-uptake inhibitors (SSRIs) such as **fluoxetine** (0.5 mg/kg PO q 24 h) may be useful for the aggressor.

- **Benzodiazepines**, such as diazepam (0.2–0.4 mg/kg PO q 12 h – average 1–2 mg/cat PO q 12 h), may be necessary for the victim. Care as it can lead to hyperexcitement and has been associated with hepatopathy.
- **Azaperones** – Buspirone has been reported to be helpful in some cases (0.5–1.0 mg/kg PO q 8–12 h).
- **Blood biochemistry** analysis should be done prior to medication to determine a **baseline especially for liver and kidney** parameters as all are metabolized by the liver and excreted through the renal system. These parameters should be checked every 6–12 months depending on the age and general health status of the cat.
- The cats may require medication for a prolonged period – up to 6–12 months – and then should be slowly weaned off.

The synthetic pheromone, Feliway®, can also be beneficial. It should be sprayed on 4–6 prominent objects in each room at cat nose height for a period of 30–45 days and is said to decrease anxiety. A Feliway® diffuser plugged into the room in which the cat spends most of its time can also be very helpful. Treatment should continue for at least 1 month.

If aggression is directed towards a person, the cat should be avoided in all stimulating circumstances.

- Whenever the cat is calm desensitization and counter-conditioning can be used. This means **rewarding the cat** (this may involve feeding or playing) **for being relaxed** in the person's presence and walking away if the cat starts to become aroused.
- Punishing the cat will exacerbate the problem as it may lead to even greater arousal.

Prognosis

Generally good if it is a single event and people can recognize the initiating stimuli and avoid them.

Poor if the aggression is intense, of long duration and there are multiple stimuli that cannot be identified.

Even though the aggression is of sudden onset it may take weeks, or even months, for the cats to be successfully reintroduced.

INTERCAT, INTERMALE AGGRESSION**

Classical signs

- Usually seen in entire males at around 2–4 years of age.
- May be associated with social role (status) in neutered cats and tends to appear later.

Pathogenesis

Male–male aggression involves hormonal changes associated with sexual maturity and neurochemical changes associated with social maturity. The brain is masculinized prenatally and the production of testosterone later leads to presence of male behaviors. Aggression also involves limbic system changes and changes in the serotonin system.

In entire males, intermale aggression usually starts when they reach social maturity, at **around 2–4 years of age,** but may be seen after sexual maturity at 1–3 years of age.

In neutered cats, it occurs later and is associated with their social role or status. It is less likely to occur in cats that were well socialized as kittens.

Clinical signs

Very common.

Usually seen in entire males around 2–4 years of age, but may occur as early as 1 year of age.
- Behavior may be normal male–male aggression associated with mating. It increases during breeding season and with overcrowding.
- In male–male aggression the cat flattens its ears, howls, hisses, piloerects and uses both the teeth and claws in fights.

In social aggression the signs depend on the mode and may be active (threatening) or passive (blocking access). Outright fighting is rare. Cats that have been well socialized before 12 weeks of age are less likely to fight or inflict serious damage.
- May be associated with social role (status) in neutered cats and tends to appear later.

Diagnosis

Diagnosis is based on a complete behavioral history (an entire male cat showing aggression during breeding season) and thorough physical examination to rule out any concurrent medical conditions.

Differential diagnosis

Other types of aggression need to be considered.
- **Territorial aggression** is commonly directed towards a new cat introduced into the household or a visitor and is not associated with breeding.
- **Status-related aggression** is more often displayed towards people and the cat may initiate contact and then threaten or bite if it cannot control the situation.

Need to recognize what is normal male–male aggression as this may not require treatment.

Cats may exhibit several types of aggression concurrently.

Treatment

Prepubertal and post-pubertal castration reduces or stops the frequency of fights in about 90% of cases between entire males.

Treatment may involve **changing the social environment** as well as the neurochemical one. Cats in the same household should be reintroduced slowly as described above for redirected aggression (page 997). It is important not to try to introduce them too fast or too soon.

Anxiolytic medication may also be needed to treat one or both cats to alter the neurochemical environment.
- **Tricyclic antidepressants** (TCAs) such as amitriptyline (0.5–1 mg/kg PO q 24 h, average 5–10 mg/cat PO q 24 h) or clomipramine (0.5 mg/kg PO q 24 h) or **selective serotonin re-uptake inhibitors** (SSRIs) such as fluoxetine (0.5 mg/kg PO q 24 h) may be useful for the aggressor.
- **Benzodiazepines,** such as diazepam (0.2–0.4 mg/kg PO q 12 h average of 1–2 mg/cat PO q 12 h), may be necessary for the victim. Care as it can lead to hyperexcitement and has been associated with hepatopathy.
- **Azaperones** – Buspirone has been reported to be helpful in some cases (0.5–1.0 mg/kg PO q 8–12 h).
- **Blood biochemistry analysis** should be done prior to medication to determine a baseline especially for liver and kidney parameters as all are metabolized by the liver and excreted through the renal system.

These parameters should be checked every 6–12 months depending on the age and general health status of the cat.

- The cats may require medication for a prolonged period – up to 6–12 months – and then should be slowly weaned off.

The **synthetic pheromone, Feliway**, can also be beneficial. It should be sprayed on 4–6 prominent objects in each room at cat nose height for a period of 30–45 days and is said to decrease anxiety. A Feliway® diffuser in the room where the cats spend most of their time has also proved useful.

Prognosis

Intermale aggression generally **responds well to treatment**.

Social aggression can be more difficult to treat especially if it is very long-standing and getting worse. Clients need to be able to recognize it early but this is often difficult with passive (covert) aggression where the cat just blocks access to areas.

The prognosis is relatively good with early intervention, and if the cats share the area and different times.

FEAR AGGRESSION**

Classical signs

- Cats can be fearful of people, places, other cats, or various stimuli such as noises or odors.
- The aggression exhibited may be a combination of offence and defense.

Pathogenesis

As with most behavioral conditions the underlying pathogenesis is unknown, but is likely to be neurochemically complex. **The amygdala and long-term potentiation are involved in learning fear**, while the forebrain is involved in unlearning fear. The locus ceruleus (LC), the principal norepinephric nucleus, is involved with supplying the limbic system and hence the "emotional" signs seen with fear.

Genetically two types of cat personality are recognized – either **timid and fearful cats** or **confident,** friendly cats, and is affected by the temperament of the tom. This may account for some fearful behavior seen in cats.

Inadequate or lack of socialization and handling prior to 12 weeks of age may also contribute to the cat's responses to people.

Inadequate or lack of socialization with other cats early in life may contribute to the cat's responses to other cats.

Cats learn to be fearful of certain situations, especially if they have had a bad experience with no opportunity to escape (e.g. rough handling, noises, smells at veterinary hospitals).

Inappropriate punishment can also cause fear and lead to aggression.

It may also be **exacerbated by accidental reinforcement**, that is attempting to calm an anxious cat by speaking softly or stroking and hence rewarding the fearful or aggressive behavior.

Clinical signs

Fearful cats will typically hiss, spit, growl, swat, piloerect, flatten their ears against the head and show a low, hunched or crouched body position. Additionally, they may try to flee or attack, depending on the circumstances. **Pupillary dilation** is common and the **mouth is open with teeth bared**.

Often the behavior is a combination of offence and defense.

The fearful cat generally will **initially attempt to avoid the stimulus** if that is an option and **many warning signals are given**.

Aggression is usually the last resort but is violent and may become learnt.

Diagnosis

The diagnosis is based on a complete behavioral history and a thorough physical examination to rule out medical causes.

A **history of exposure to a fear-provoking stimulus**, combined with a description of body language (ears back, "Halloween" cat) and aggression typify fear aggression.

Differential diagnosis

Other types of aggression should be considered.

- **Redirected aggression** may have some signs in common but different body language and history of fear-provoking events will suggest fear aggression.
- Although some of the signs are similar cats that exhibit **play aggression** generally have a more confident body posture and behavioral history and context of the aggression are different. There is no stalking or pouncing involved in fear aggression.
- **Territorial aggression** is usually directed towards another cat or person and the cat is confident and approaches the intruder and threatens. Fearfully aggressive cats will try to avoid contact.

Cats may exhibit several types of aggression concurrently.

Treatment

Depending of the severity of the problem the cat may need no treatment or may need behavior modification, such as desensitization and counter-conditioning, in combination with psychopharmacological intervention in severe or long-standing cases.

Behavior modification involves desensitization and counter-conditioning by slowly introducing the cat to the fearful situation in a gradual, controlled sequence.

- First, **the cat is offered a tasty treat** such as vegemite, chicken, cheese or dehydrated liver. If the cat eats then it is usually a good indication that it is not too anxious.
- Then, while the cat is eating, the **fearful stimulus**, such as a person, is **gradually introduced at a distance**. The initial distance should be great enough not to cause any fearful response from the cat.
  - If the cat continues to take food the person approaches the cat very slowly.
  - The time frame for the gradual approach may vary from **days to months** depending on the severity of the problem.
- The cat should not be forced into the fearful situation as that will exacerbate the fear.

Anxiolytic medication may also be needed to treat the cat to alter the neurochemical environment.

- **Tricyclic antidepressants** (TCAs) such as amitriptyline (0.5–1 mg/kg PO q 12–24 h, average of 5–10 mg/cat PO q 24 h) or clomipramine (0.5 mg/kg PO q 24 h) or **selective serotonin re-uptake inhibitors** (SSRIs) such as fluoxetine (0.5 mg/kg PO q 24 h) may be necessary.
- The cat may require medication for **a prolonged period (up to 6–12 months).** Attempts to wean off medication should be slow and some cats may need life-long treatment.
- **Blood biochemistry** should be done prior to medication to determine a baseline especially for liver and kidney parameters as all medications are metabolized by the liver and excreted through the renal system. If long-term or life-long medication is needed then repeat blood test should be done at 6–12-month intervals depending on the age and general health status of the cat.

The **synthetic pheromone, Feliway®,** can also be beneficial. It should be sprayed on 4–6 prominent objects in each room at cat nose height for a period of 30–45 days and is said to decrease anxiety. A Feliway® diffuser in the room in which the cat spends most of its time has also proved useful.

Punishment, or forced restraint will aggravate the situation and should be avoided. It may increase the anxiety and impede learning.

Prognosis

Prognosis is good if the behavior is of recent onset, the cat is adult and the fear-eliciting stimuli can be defined.

Prognosis worsens if the problem is of long duration or the cat stays aroused or reactive for long periods after exposure to the fear-provoking stimulus.

The prognosis may be poor if the cat is genetically timid and there has been no early exposure during the sensitive period (before 12 weeks of age).

AGGRESSION WHEN PATTED**

Classical signs

- The cat may suddenly bite or scratch people after tactile stimulation of variable duration.

Pathogenesis

As with most behavioral conditions underlying pathogenesis is unknown, but is likely to be neurochemically complex. Long-term potentiation, exitatory amino acids, "kindling", and increased arousal are all contributing factors.

Some cats have a very low tolerance to being patted or stroked. The cat may even seek out attention and jump on the owner's lap, but still not tolerate long periods of stroking.

The behavior is reported to be **more common in unneutered males** and is thought to relate to social grooming behavior.

It can be a **manifestation of status-related aggression.**

Clinical signs

The cat may swipe or bite if the petting stops, or if the stroking is carried out for a prolonged period.
- Some cats appear to be content just sitting on a lap as long as no stroking or other tactile stimulation occurs.

The cat may stiffen, or lash with the tail and may or may not give a warning bite while being patted.

Owners are most commonly bitten or scratched on the hands and arms.

Diagnosis

Based on the behavioral history of **sudden aggression during petting** with no obvious warning but the owner learns to recognize the signs of twitching and stimulation.

Thorough physical examination is essential to rule out medical causes such as pain due to **arthritis,** etc., that may cause the cat to resent being handled or **dermatological conditions** that may cause irritability or inflammation of the skin.

Differential diagnosis

Other types of aggression such as:
- Although some of the signs are similar cats that exhibit **play aggression** generally have a more confident body posture and the behavioral history and context of the aggression are different. There is

no stalking or pouncing involved and the **aggression only occurs when the cat is being petted or soon after the petting stops.**
- **Status-related aggression** has similar signs but will also be exhibited in other contexts, not just associated with petting and it may also involve passive aggression such as blocking access to rooms, etc.
- **Pain** needs to be considered as an underlying or concurrent factor. However, pain aggression may be exhibited in other contexts, not just associated with petting.

Cats may exhibit several types of aggression concurrently.

Treatment

Many of these cats can be **taught to gradually tolerate longer periods of stroking**.

Initially determine how long the cat can tolerate attention.
- If the cat usually tolerates a short period of stimulation, e.g. 3 minutes, but not 4 minutes the cat should be slowly stroked for only 2 minutes, that is the period should always be below the cat's current threshold for non-tolerance of stimulation. The cat should then be rewarded with food treats.
- The **time can be gradually increased over a period of days/weeks** until the cat tolerates longer and longer periods. Always stop the stroking prior to the cat showing signs of arousal.
- The training session should be **held at predictable times each day**.

Punishment is not effective as it tends to lead to more aggression as the cat is already aroused and overstimulated.

Anxiolytic medication may also be needed to treat the cat to alter the neurochemical environment.
- **Tricyclic antidepressants** (TCAs) such as amitriptyline (0.5–1 mg/kg PO q 12–24 h, average of 5–10 mg/cat PO q 24 h) or clomipramine (0.5 mg/kg PO q 24 h) or **selective serotonin reuptake inhibitors** (SSRIs) such as fluoxetine (0.5 mg/kg PO q 24 h) may be necessary.
- **Blood biochemistry analysis** should be done prior to medication to determine a baseline especially for liver and kidney parameters as all are metabolized by the liver and excreted through the renal system. These parameters should be checked every 6–12

months depending on the age and general health status of the cat.

- Some cats may require medication for a prolonged period (up to 6–12 months or even life-long) and then should be slowly weaned off if possible.
- Feliway® sprayed on hands before handling may also help decrease arousal.

Prognosis

Some cats never learn to like being stroked, and the safest option is to leave them alone.

Punishment tends to aggravate the situation and should be avoided.

STATUS-RELATED AGGRESSION**

Classical signs

- The cat may try to control territory or people by blocking access to an area.
- The cat may bite when approached or handled yet solicit attention and then bite if it is or is not given.
- Biting may also occur when the attention ceases.

Pathogenesis

The behavior is about the cat's need to control specific situations or interactions and may indicate an underling anxiety. It involves **overt as well as covert behaviors**. See expanded section on aggression when patted (page 1000).

As with most behavioral conditions underlying pathogenesis is unknown, but is likely to be neurochemically complex. The hypothalamus is the primary area involved with threat displays. There may be genetic as well as learnt components.

It may be associated with lack of impulse control.

Clinical signs

The cat may bite when the owner attempts to approach, lift, move or handle the cat (overt aggression).

The cat may also block access to areas for example by sitting in doorways and staring (covert aggression).

It can also involve behaviors such as **soliciting attention by biting**.

Diagnosis

Diagnosis is based on a complete behavioral history that indicates the aggression occurs in contexts where the cat is displaying assertive or controlling behaviors.

Thorough physical examination is essential to rule out medical causes such as **pain**, for example due to arthritis, or dermatological conditions that may cause irritability or inflammation of the skin that may also elicit aggression.

Differential diagnosis

Other forms of aggression including:
- **Territorial aggression** is usually seen in a different context and is directed towards another cat or person that approaches the defined territory and the cat threatens.
- **Aggression when patted may be a part of status-related aggression** however, that is the only context in which the behavior is elicited.
- Although some of the signs are similar in cats that exhibit **play aggression** the behavioral history and context of the aggression are different. Additionally in play aggression the cat is younger and there is generally stalking or pouncing involved.

Many cats can exhibit several types concurrently.

Treatment

Identify and then avoid all situations that may be provocative, e.g. approaching, stroking, handling.

Instigate a behavior-modification program where the cat is taught to earn all attention or rewards by deferring to the owner.
- It has to **come or sit at the owner's request**, prior to any interaction with the owner.
- It is **not allowed to initiate any interaction**. If the cat does solicit attention the owner should completely ignore the cat or walk away.
- **No reward/attention is given until the cat defers** and responds to the command (e.g. sit or come).

Desensitization and counter-conditioning to handling, moving, etc., can be done and the cat rewarded for appropriate acceptable behavior – see aggression when patted for details (page 1000).

- If the cat shows any sign of aggression then move away and stop all interactions.
- **Physical punishment should be avoided** as that will exacerbate the problem.
- **Anxiolytic medication** may also be needed to treat the cat to alter the neurochemical environment.
  - **Tricyclic antidepressants** (TCAs) such as amitriptyline (0.5–1 mg/kg PO q 24 h, average of 5–10 mg/cat PO q 24 h) or clomipramine (0.5 mg/kg PO q 24 h) have proven useful in some cases.
  - **Selective serotonin re-uptake inhibitors** (SSRIs) such as fluoxetine (0.5 mg/ kg PO q 24 h) have also proved useful and can be easier to administer as they are available in a liquid formulation.
  - **Benzodiazepines** are **generally not recommended** as they may disinhibit aggression.
  - Blood biochemistry analysis should be done prior to medication to determine a baseline especially for liver and kidney parameters as medications are metabolized by the liver and excreted through the renal system. These parameters should be checked every 6–12 months depending on the age and general health status of the cat.

The cat may require life-long medication or for prolonged periods of up to 6–12 months. Attempts to slowly wean off medication may be made.

Prognosis

The behavior can usually be managed, not cured, with owner education and compliance.

The prognosis is poor if the eliciting stimuli cannot be defined, the attacks are severe or people cannot read the cat's body language.

Punishment tends to aggravate the aggression and should be avoided at all times.

TERRITORIAL AGGRESSION*

Classical signs

- The aggressive behavior is directed towards intruders approaching or entering into the cat's established domain.

Pathogenesis

As with most behavioral conditions the underlying pathogenesis is unknown. There is often an underlying anxiety component.

The cat's territory may be patrolled and can be marked by rubbing, bunting and/or spraying to maintain social distance and define hierarchy.

The aggression can be intra- and interspecific (between members of the same species or between other species), including people.

Classical signs

The **cat exhibits aggression to anyone approaching or entering its territory** and may attack.

The behavior may be **more marked in entire toms in the breeding season**.

Aggression decreases with increased distance away from the territory.

It is **often seen when a new cat is introduced** into the household or the **cat returns from a visit to a cattery or veterinary hospital** and now is not recognized by the other cat.

Diagnosis

Diagnosis is based on a complete behavioral history and a thorough physical examination.

Differential diagnosis

Other types of aggression should be considered including:

- **Status-related aggression and territorial aggression may co-exist,** however, the contexts in which territorial behavior is elicited will be different.
- **Intercat intermale aggression is seen in entire males during the breeding season**, whereas territorial aggression may be seen at other times and may be exhibited by males and females.

Cats may exhibit several types of aggression concurrently.

Treatment

Avoid situations that may be provocative to avoid reinforcing the behavior.

- If directed towards another cat within the home they may **need to be separated -** see section on redirected aggression on how to reintroduce (page 997).

Anxiolytic medication may also be needed to treat the cat to alter the neurochemical environment.

- **Tricyclic antidepressants** (TCAs) such as amitriptyline (0.5–1 mg/kg PO q 12–24 h – average of 5–10 mg/cat PO q 24 h) or clomipramine (0.5 mg/kg PO q 24 h) or **selective serotonin reuptake inhibitors** (SSRIs) such as fluoxetine (0.5 mg/kg PO q 24 h) have proved useful in managing the behavior of the aggressor.
- **Benzodiazepines**, such as diazepam (0.2–0.4 mg/kg PO q 12 h – average of 1–2 mg/cat PO q 12 h), may be necessary for the victim to alter its behavior. Care with benzodiazepines as they may disinhibit aggression.
- **Blood biochemistry** should be done prior to medication to determine a baseline especially for liver and kidney parameters. The cat may require medication for a prolonged period of up to 6–12 months and then should be slowly weaned off.

The **synthetic pheromone, Feliway®**, can also be beneficial. It should be sprayed on 4–6 prominent objects in each room at cat nose height for a period of 30–45 days and is said to decrease anxiety. A Feliway® diffuser placed in the room that the cats spend most of their time has also proved helpful.

The cats may need to be permanently separated or one of the cats may have to be rehomed if the problem is very severe or long-standing.

If directed towards people deny the cat access to areas that may be guarded. If the cat shows any signs of aggression then move away and stop all interactions.

Physical punishment should be avoided as it will exacerbate the problem.

Prognosis

May be difficult to treat if long-standing or severe but it can usually be managed with environmental manipulation.

Prognosis is worse if directed towards other cats and is long-standing and severe.

PAIN AGGRESSION*

> **Classical signs**
>
> - **The cat responds to being handled or approached in an aggressive manner.**
> - **History of a painful stimulus or elicitation of pain.**

Pathogenesis

This is a defensive behavior and can become fear aggression if associated with long-term painful treatment or chronic pain.

Any source of pain or painful stimulus can lead to the cat exhibiting aggression. The stimulus may range from actual handling of a painful area to just patting, grooming or trying to medicate the cat.

As with most behavioral conditions the underlying pathogenesis is unknown. Long-term potentiation associated with true pain or circumstances in which the pain was originally elicited is likely to be involved.

Clinical signs

The cat may show signs of **offensive (distance increasing signals** or postures such as staring, swatting with the front paw, growling) or **defensive** (signals or postures such as arched back, piloerection, flattened ears, hissing) **aggression** and/or **avoidance with handling**.

The signs may be exhibited prior to any manipulation or when the cat is approached.

Diagnosis

Diagnosis is based on a complete behavioral history and a thorough physical examination.

Hematological and biochemistry analysis and imaging techniques such as X-ray may be required to make a diagnosis.

Differential diagnosis

Other types of aggression should also be considered but the diagnosis should be able to be made on physical examination and history.

- **Status-related aggression or aggression when patted** may have similar signs, however, **the history of any painful stimulus or elicitation of pain** should delineate the problem.
- **Fearful behavior or aggression may be secondary to pain**. The behavior can then become learnt.

Cats may exhibit several types of aggression concurrently.

Treatment

Relieve the source of the pain (appropriate analgesics or anti-inflammatory medication as indicated).

Treat the anxiety associated with the pain (anxiolytics, e.g. diazepam, tricyclic antidepressants, e.g. amitriptyline – see page 1001 for dose rates).

Avoid all accidental reinforcement by patting, telling the cat "it's okay" in an effort to calm, especially when the cat is aroused. This may reward aggressive behavior and may prolong the response.

Avoid all potentially painful situations.

Some learnt aggression may result. The cat has associated previous handling with pain, so **desensitization and counter-conditioning** may also be necessary so that the cat learns to relax when handled.
- Offer treats when the cat remains relaxed when approached or gently handled.
- Gradually increase the amount of time and the area that is being manipulated, rewarding for relaxed and non-aggressive responses.

Try to prevent the aggression developing by providing appropriate analgesia with all painful manipulations, especially surgery.

Avoid punishment as that may exacerbate the aggression.

Feliway® may help decrease arousal.

Prognosis

Depends on adequacy of the pain relief, as well as duration of pain and duration of the aggression but generally good.

Prevent occurrence if possible.

PREDATORY AGGRESSION

Classical signs

- The cat exhibits signs of predatory behavior such as stalking in silence, a lowered body posture, crouching and sudden lunge or pounce when target moves suddenly but it is directed towards non-prey.

Pathogenesis

Predatory aggression needs to be differentiated from predatory behavior, which is normal and instinctive. The focus of predatory aggression (e.g. non-prey item, body part) and outcome (do not eat) are different.

The cat shows all the contextual behaviors of predatory behavior, stalking in silence, lowered body posture, crouching and sudden lunge or pounce when target moves suddenly, **but it is out of context**.

There are no warning signs and may be directed towards people as well as other animals.

As with most behavioral conditions the underlying pathogenesis is unknown. The hypothalamus is involved with active biting and attack. Experimentally **stimulation** of the **lateral amygdala facilitates predatory aggression**. More defensive cats appear to show less predatory aggression.

Clinical signs

The cat stalks and may lie in wait for the "victim", then pounces when the target moves.

There are no preceding threats.

Although the behaviors are the same as predatory behavior (normal), the context in which the behaviors are exhibited make this behavior abnormal.

Diagnosis

Diagnosis is based on a behavioral history (of sudden attacks with no preceding threats, that is usually directed towards moving targets), which are not normal prey and a thorough physical examination.

Differential diagnosis

Other types of aggression such as:

- **Predatory behavior** that is directed towards prey (rodents, birds and although it may be undesirable is normal behavior and should be differentiated from predatory aggression when non-prey are the targets. It is instinctive behavior hence difficult to modify. The cat may not eat the prey item even if caught.
- **Play aggression** has many of the elements of predatory aggression but the context is different. It is also seen more in **younger cats** that are practicing their hunting skills and it is more easily redirected.
- **Status-related aggression** should also be considered however, the silent stalk and pounce is not seen with status related aggression.

Cats may exhibit several types of aggression concurrently.

Treatment

For aggression directed towards prey.
- **Avoid all potentially problematical situations**.
- Confine cat indoors or to a specific area to prevent predation.
- Confine cat outdoors in wire-mesh enclosures, runs and tunnels. These are being sold as 'modular cat parks' which are modular enclosures that can be joined together to provide extensive outdoor enclosures for the cat.
- Supervise when outside.
- **Provide appropriate toys** for mental stimulation and ability to hunt. Vary these on a daily basis.
- Put several bells at intervals on the cat's collar to provide warning to prey.

For aggression directed towards non-prey.
- Avoid all potentially problematical situations.
- Confine cat to a specific room or area to **prevent access to victim**, especially at times the cat is most likely to exhibit this behavior.
- **Put several bells on the cat's collar** at varying intervals so that the victim has warning signal of the cat's presence. This is not always successful but worth trying.
- **Redirect the pounce onto toys**. When the aggression is directed towards people, toys dangled at the end of a fishing rod, to keep the cat at a distance from the person, can be helpful.

Distracters such as loud noises can be useful when the owner sees the cat in pre-pounce mode. **They should not be used as a punishment** as that may redirect the aggression.

This can be a dangerous situation especially when the targets are children and the elderly as the cat can inflict severe damage. **Euthanasia** or **re-homing may need to be considered as options.**

Prognosis

Good if the cat can be monitored and the behavior redirected or the cat confined to prevent access to prey.

Not good if the target is a helpless individual and the cat cannot be monitored.

MATERNAL AGGRESSION

> ### Classical signs
>
> - The queen threatens when she, the kittens or the nesting are approached. She will attack if cornered.
> - It may involve aggression directed towards the kittens.

Pathogenesis

This occurs in the periparturient period and may involve protecting the nest area as well as the kittens.

This is normal behavior if the approach distance is long or generalized. It is due to hormonal influences on the hypothalamus, and associated with the presence and the proximity of the kittens.

The queen may be aggressive in the presence of male cats and this may be related to the fact that free-ranging males have been reported to commit infanticide.

The behaviors seen may also be anxiety related and hence the neuropathology is the same.

Clinical signs

Generally the queen will hiss and give other long-distance signals when she, the kittens or the nesting area is approached.

It usually involves more threats than actual attack and usually is directed toward unfamiliar individuals.

Attack tends to be a last resort and occurs if she is cornered.

Some queens may cannibalize their own kittens and this is considered to be abnormal. It may happen if the queen is stressed or malnourished and the incidence has been reported to increase if the litter is very large, it is a second pregnancy, or the kittens are ill. However, it can be normal if the queen eats stillborn or aborted fetuses. It may also occur during overzealous eating of the placenta after birth.

Diagnosis

Diagnosis is based on the behavioral **history of aggression in the presence of kittens** and thorough physical examination to exclude pain or other causes of aggression.

Differential diagnosis

Other types of aggression should be considered such as territorial, pain and status-related aggression, however this type of aggression should be easily differentiated as it occurs **only in queens with kittens in the peri-parturient period.**

Cats may exhibit several types of aggression concurrently.

Treatment

Avoid approaching the queen during this period.

Separate the queen from other cats, especially males.

Spey the queen that exhibits infanticide.

Prognosis

The aggression should resolve when the kittens are removed from the queen but may recur with the next litter.

IDIOPATHIC AGGRESSION

Classical signs

- The aggression is unprovoked and unpredictable.

Pathogenesis

This is a diagnosis of exclusion and very rare.

It is not well understood and reflects truly abnormal behavior.

As with most behavioral conditions the underlying pathogenesis is unknown, but is likely to be neuro-chemically complex. It is a very rare condition and may reflect seizure activity.

Clinical signs

Sudden mood changes and aggressive episodes with neither obvious provocation nor predictability.

It has been described as **"toggle-switch" aggression** as it may start suddenly as if a switch has been turned on. It can stop just as suddenly and the cat may appear to be unaware of any change in its behavior.

Diagnosis

Diagnosis is based on a behavioral history **of sudden episodes of unpredictable aggression** and thorough physical examination and rule out of all other causes, both medical and behavioral.

Differential diagnosis

All other types of aggression as well as **medical causes, such as seizures**, should be considered.

Treatment

It is difficult to treat using standard behavior-modification techniques because it is truly unpredictable.
- Additionally, avoiding situations that may be provocative is not possible as there is no true provocation or obvious context.

Treatment with anticonvulsants such as **diazepam or phenobarbitone** should be considered.

No physical punishment should be used.

Prognosis

Poor as the underlying cause is not known.

RECOMMENDED READING

Beaver B. Feline Behavior: A Guide for Veterinarians. Philadelphia, PA, W.B. Saunders Company, 2003.

Landsberg G, Hunthausen W, Ackerman L. Handbook of Behavior Problems of the Dog and Cat. Oxford, Butterworth-Heinemann, 2003.

Overall KL. Clinical Behavioral Medicine for Small Animals. St Louis, Missouri, Mosby, 1997.

Simpson BS, Simpson DM. Behavioral pharmacotherapy. In: Voith VL, Burchelt PL (eds) Readings in Companion Animal Behavior. Trenton, NJ, Veterinary Learning Systems, 1996, pp. 100–115.

47. The cat with anxiety-related behavior problems

Kersti Seksel

> ## KEY SIGNS
>
> - Over-grooming (including psychogenic alopecia, feline hyperesthesia and self-mutilation).
> - Pica.
> - Inappropriate vocalization.
> - Inappropriate elimination (spraying).

MECHANISM?

- Anxiety, fears, phobias, stereotypies and obsessive-compulsive disorder (OCD) are neuro-chemically related but do not have the same underlying mechanism.
- Anxiety is the anticipation of future danger or misfortune.
- Obsessive-compulsive disorders are constant and repetitive behaviors that appear to serve no obvious purpose and interfere with the animal's normal functioning.
- Stress is thought to play a key role in the development of anxiety-related conditions.

WHERE?

- The prefrontal cortex, amygdala and limbic system, and hypothalamus (hypothalamic-pituitary-adrenal axis) are involved in the regulation of fear.
- Serotonin, norepinephrine, dopamine and GABA are all involved in the development of fear and anxiety.
- The anatomical focus of OCD is believed to be the limbic system.

WHAT?

- Anxiety-related disorders include excessive self-grooming, changes in appetite and inappropriate elimination (spraying).

Diseases causing anxiety–related behavior problems

PSYCHOLOGICAL

- **Over-grooming (including psychogenic alopecia, feline hyperesthesia and self-mutilation)** (p 1015)

Alopecia diagnosed by exclusion when no underlying medical problem is evident. Hair loss and saliva discoloration are only evident on parts of the body that can be reached by the teeth and/or tongue. Plucked hair has microscopic evidence of shear.

- **Pica (eating non-food material)* (p 1018)**

Ingestion of non-nutritive substances that appear to be of no benefit to the cat.

- **Inappropriate vocalization** (p 1017)**

Vocalization that is excessive in duration, intensity or frequency that is not associated with other causes such as pain or symptoms of estrus.

- **Inappropriate elimination – spraying*** (p 1012)**

Marking of usually prominent vertical areas with or without urine, and often associated with overt or covert intercat aggression.

INTRODUCTION

MECHANISM?

Anxiety, fears, phobias, stereotypies and obsessive-compulsive disorder (OCD) are neurochemically related but probably do not have the same underlying mechanism. OCD in humans is classified as a subset of anxiety-related disorders. Anxiety is thought to be the common factor underlying stereotypic behaviors and OCD.

Anxiety is the anticipation of future danger or misfortune without any obvious cause. The threat may be real or imagined and may be normal or abnormal depending on the context.

- When it is out of context and occurs at a constant and elevated level then it is likely to become a problem.

Anxiety is usually accompanied by signs of **hypervigilance** (e.g. scanning), **autonomic hyperactivity** (e.g. gastrointestinal upsets) and **increased motor activity** (e.g. pacing).

Anxiety disorders constitute more than 75% of problems diagnosed in veterinary patients presented to behavior clinics.

Obsessive-compulsive disorders include stereotypies and self-directed behaviors.

- They are constant and repetitive in form, appear to serve no obvious purpose, and interfere with the animal's normal functioning.
- They are **often derived from otherwise normal behaviors like grooming, eating or walking** but are abnormal in that they are excessive in duration, frequency or intensity in the context in which they are performed.

Stress or anxiety in cats may be manifest as a change in appetite (e.g. a decrease in appetite or pica); grooming (e.g. increased or decreased); elimination (e.g. spraying or non-spraying marking); changes in social interactions (e.g. vocalization); and physical activity (e.g. increased or decreased).

WHERE?

Positron emission tomography scans indicate **biochemical and structural abnormalities in anxiety, panic and OCD**.

- The prefrontal cortex, central nucleus of the amygdala, limbic system and hypothalamus (hypothalamic-pituitary-adrenal axis) are involved in the regulation of fear and anxiety. Long-term potentiation of fear and anxiety is a contributing factor.

- Serotoninergic, noradrenergic, dopaminergic and GABA-ergic systems are involved in the development of fear and anxiety. The neurotransmitter **serotonin** has been identified as a **mediator of fear and anxiety**.
- The locus coeruleus, which is part of the noradrenergic system, is involved in the mediation of many of the physiologic reponses associated with anxiety such as hypervigilance.
- The anatomical focus of OCD is believed to be the limbic system. Computed tomography indicates that the basal ganglia near the caudate nucleus are involved.
- Dopaminergic, serotonergic and opioid pathways are thought to be involved in compulsive and self-injurious behaviors.
- **Aberrant serotonin metabolism and possibly endorphin metabolism** are thought to contribute. Increased dopamine in the basal ganglia and a relative increase in the serotonin metabolite 5-hydroxy indole acetic acid (5-HIAA) in the cerebrospinal fluid (CSF) have also been detected.

Stress responses are modulated through **altered cholecystokinin, opioid and dopaminergic mechanisms**.

- Physiological measurements of stress include: increased catecholamine levels and resultant tachycardia (sympathetic autonomic nervous system); increased corticosteroid levels resulting from stimulation of the pituitary-adrenal axis; decreased neutrophil/lymphocyte ratios; and altered response to adrenocorticotropic hormone (ACTH) stimulation test.

Production and release of **substance P** may also be responsible for some behavioral effects such as salivation and gastrointestinal distress.

WHAT?

Anxiety can occur after sensitization to a specific stimulus and then become generalized to other situations. It may also be non-specific in origin.

Anxious or stressed cats may exhibit a variety of non-specific signs such as **autogrooming, changed appetite or spraying.**

The following are the most common signs of anxiety exhibited by cats. The actual prevalence of anxiety-related conditions is unknown but they are probably the most common class of disorders in pet animals.

Medical conditions such as **hyperthyroidism** have been **associated with feline anxiety**, as have some medications.

The longer that these conditions are unrecognized and untreated, the more complex they become.

Diagnosis is based on a complete behavioral history and thorough physical examination. It may involve complete blood work, dermatological and neurological work up, as well as radiography to rule out contributing or concurrent medical factors.

CONDITIONS CAUSING ANXIETY-RELATED BEHAVIOR PROBLEMS

INAPPROPRIATE ELIMINATION-SPRAYING***

> ### Classical signs
>
> - Urination and/or defecation outside the litter box.

Pathogenesis

Elimination problems are the most common behavioral problem reported in cats, accounting for between **40–75% of behavioral problems**.

Both males and females, neutered and entire, present with elimination problems. They have been reported in all breeds and across all age groups.

Cats that are urinating out of the litter box usually squat, produce a **large quantity of urine**, use a horizontal surface and often scratch afterwards. In contrast to marking, urination outside of the litter box is associated with the elimination of waste.

Predisposing factors for inappropriate urination include:
- **Medical conditions** such as cystitis, diarrhea, constipation, feline lower urinary tract disease and diseases causing polyuria.
- **Litter box aversion** may be due to a new type of litter or a dirty box. Aversion can also be induced by "catching" the cat in the litter box prior to performing potentially unpleasant procedures such as medicating or grooming.
- **Litter box location preference** can develop. Many cats prefer to eliminate in quiet or safe places where

they will not be disturbed, e.g. under beds, behind furniture. They may have learnt to urinate in the location where the litter box was originally placed, even though the litter box has now been relocated.

- **Litter box location aversion** can also develop if the cat has an unpleasant experience while in the box. Cats that experience pain while urinating (e.g. with cystitis, arthritic pain) may develop an aversion to using the litter tray in that location.
- **Substrate preference**. Some cats prefer to scratch in soft textures or surfaces, others on hard.
- **Substrate aversion**. Some cats do not like getting their feet wet or dirty so they will not use soiled litter boxes. Every cat litter also has a different odor, so many cats develop a preference or aversion to a particular scent.
- **Fear and anxiety**. Separation anxiety can cause elimination problems, and this is usually seen when the owner is absent. The cat may choose to eliminate on the objects associated with the owner, e.g. clothes, bedding, briefcases, shoes. It is usually seen after separation greater than 12 hours, or immediately the owner returns. Fearful cats may eliminate where they are hiding, as often they are too frightened to go to the litter box.

Spraying is a marking behavior, often associated with anxiety. It may be territorial, sexual or agonistic. In multi-cat households it is associated with overt or covert aggression.

- **Cats that spray** usually stand, but may squat, usually produce only a **small quantity** of urine, frequently use vertical surfaces but may use horizontal surfaces and **rarely scratch** afterwards.
- It is estimated that 10% of castrated males and 5% of spayed females spray at some time in their life. Spraying appears to be more common in multi-cat households with a 100% chance of at least one cat spraying in a household with more than 10 cats. Male cats that live with a female cat are more likely to spray than those living with another male cat.
- **Predisposing factors include:**
  - **Medical conditions** ranging from those associated with the urogenital system such as renal calculi, renal failure and cystitis, as well as viral diseases such as FIV and FELV and impacted anal glands. It is reported that up to 30% of cats that present for spraying may have a concurrent medical condition.

- **Hormonal factors**. Entire cats spray more than neutered cats, and male cats spray more than female cats.
- **Territorial**, agonistic encounters or any highly arousing circumstances.
- **Environmental stimuli** such as the sight, sound or smell of another cat, within the household, as well as outside.
- Anxiety-related problems including separation anxiety, changes in routine (for example, moving house), the introduction of a new spouse, new baby or new cat in the area.

Inappropriate defecation is associated with the elimination of waste.

Predisposing factors for inappropriate defecation include:

- **Medical conditions** such as cystitis, diarrhea and constipation have been reported as associated factors.
- **Cats that experience pain** while defecating (e.g. constipation, arthritic pain) sometimes develop an aversion to using the litter box.
- Factors, which predispose to inappropriate urination also predispose to inappropriate defecation. These include **litter box aversion, litter box location preference, litter box location aversion, substrate preference, substrate aversion, fear and anxiety. Rarely defecation may be a marking behavior.**

Clinical signs

The elimination of urine or feces in an inappropriate location. The **amount and frequency may also be altered**.

Inappropriate elimination is a non-specific sign. It may be associated with a medical condition, fear or anxiety, or factors associated with the litter box.

Inappropriate urination or defecation involves the cat **passing normal amounts of urine or feces** outside the litter box.

Spraying or urine marking involves the cat passing **small amounts of urine** usually on **vertical objects,** often in response to an anxiety-provoking stimulus.

Diagnosis

Diagnosis is based on a **complete behavioral history** with a finding of inappropriate elimination. A thorough physical examination, hematological and biochemical analysis, urinalysis, even radiography may be required to exclude medical causes.

Careful questioning of the owner is important to differentiate urine marking from inappropriate urination. Medical problems need to be dealt with prior to, or at least concurrently with, any behavioral therapy that is instigated.

The treatment of a non-specific sign such as inappropriate elimination is not acceptable and will ultimately lead to treatment failures.

Differential diagnosis

Medical problems need to be dealt with prior to, or at least concurrently with, any behavioral therapy that is instigated. One or several of the following should be considered as contributing to the possible underlying causes.
- Medical conditions such as cystitis, diarrhea, constipation, feline lower urinary tract disease, diabetes, renal disease and urinary incontinence.

Treatment

Treatment of inappropriate urination and/or defecation.

After addressing any medical problem, the treatment involves: (1) Increasing the attractiveness of the area the owner wants the cat to use, and (2) Decreasing the attractiveness of the area that the cat wants to use.
- **Litter box problems.** To help make the litter box more attractive to the cat:
  - **Change the type of litter.** Alternatives include sawdust, soil, rabbit pellets, shredded newspaper (or recycled-paper litter), clumping litters, sand or other type of commercial litter. Sometimes a combination of substrates is effective. Cats appear to prefer finely textured litter that is not too heavy (fine sand consistency).
  - Try an empty litter box for those cats that prefer smooth surfaces like bath tubs and sinks.
  - Increase the frequency with which the litter box is **cleaned and changed**.
  - **Change the cleaning agent** used to clean the litter box. Do not use disinfectants, try using soapy water or water only.
  - **Increase the number of litter boxes** (a good rule of thumb is one litter box per cat and one extra).
  - Cover the litter box to make it more private for the cat. Often just putting a cardboard box, with

appropriate openings, over the litter box is helpful. Sometimes changing the type of litter box also helps, such as one with higher or lower sides.
  - **Make the location of the litter box more acceptable to the cat**. Place a litter box over the area being used by the cat. Then very gradually change the location of the litter box until it is in an area that is more socially acceptable. This may mean gradual increments as small as 5 cm daily.
  - **Decrease the attractiveness of the area** the cat prefers to use by changing its significance. Most cats will not eliminate in their feeding or play areas so try feeding the cat in this spot. Dry cat food appears to work best as it takes longer to consume. Some very determined cats will eat the food first, then eliminate in the area. Supergluing 8–10 pieces of dried cat food to an old saucer or piece of cardboard and placing it in the cat's favorite elimination spot will provide a long-term stimulus of food.
  - Leave the cat's toys or bedding in the area.
  - Confine the cat to a small area to retrain the cat. Only allow access to larger areas gradually once the cat uses the litter box consistently.
  - Make the area less accessible and less pleasant to the cat by covering the area with thick plastic, aluminum foil, double-sided sticky tape, Snappy trainers, sandpaper or place trays of marbles in the area so the cat cannot get a solid surface on which to stand.
  - If the cat persists in urinating or defecating in the bath tub sometimes leaving a few inches of water in the bottom helps to control this behavior.
- **For inappropriate elimination related to anxiety**, remove or **minimize the cause of the anxiety** if possible. Provide a **regular predictable routine**, such as feed and play at a set time each day.

Treatment of spraying.
- **Owner education** of normal cat behavior is important so that they understand that the **behavior cannot always be eliminated** but can be managed.
- Treatment of any concurrent or underlying medical problem is essential.
- Remove or **minimize the cause of the anxiety** if possible. Provide a **regular predictable routine**, such as feed and play at a set time each day.
- **Environmental manipulation:** This can often be difficult to achieve in practice, although theoretically it should work well. It is rarely possible or

practical to remove the neighbor's cat, the new baby, or new spouse, or entirely prevent other anxiety-provoking circumstances such as moving house. However, if possible:

– Decrease the number of cats in the household.
– Decrease the access to windows and doors to decrease the sight, sound and smell stimuli.
– Change the amount of time spent indoors/outdoors.
– Prevent access to arousing stimuli.
– Make the sprayed areas less attractive to the cat to spray on by making them feeding or play areas instead.
– Feliway®, the synthetic analog of the F3 fraction of the cheek gland pheromone of cats, may help if sprayed daily for 30 days onto soiled areas.
– A Feliway Diffuser® plugged into the room in which the cat(s) spend most of their time has proven to be helpful in decreasing spraying, especially if inter-cat aggression is contributing to the spraying.

Surgery for spraying cats.
● **Neutering the entire cat**. Spraying is a marking behavior and in 87% of entire male cats, castration alone solves the problem.
● **Olfactory tractotomy** is reported to be effective in about 50% of refractory cases in males and in most females. The surgical transection of the olfactory tract causes anosmia (loss of sense of smell), which is thought to be an important factor in spraying. This technique is rarely used or recommended now.

Pharmacological treatments: These treatments are generally aimed at reducing the anxiety level of the cat by altering the neurochemical environment, and should be used in conjunction with behavioral modification and environmental manipulation techniques.
● Potential side effects should be explained to the owner prior to instigating any therapy, as most of the drugs are not registered for use in animals. Hematological and biochemical analysis should be carried out prior to instigating drug therapy. Anxiolytic medication should always be gradually withdrawn, never suddenly stopped.
● Medications that influence serotonin metabolism, such as the selective serotonin reuptake inhibitors and the tricyclic antidepressants have been used in the treatment of anxiety-related disorders. Anxiolytic medication has also proved useful in some cases.

● **Tricyclic antidepressants** (TCAs) such as:
– Amitriptyline (0.5–1 mg/kg PO q 12–24 h, average of 5–10 mg/cat PO q 24 h).
– Clomipramine (0.5 mg/kg PO q 24 h).
– Nortriptyline (0.5–2.0 mg/kg PO q 12–24 h).
● **Selective serotonin re-uptake inhibitors** (SSRIs) such as:
– Fluoxetine (0.5 mg/kg PO q 24 h).
– Paroxetine (0.5 mg/kg PO q 24 h) (2.5 mg/cat) have been successful in controlling signs in some cases.
– Fluvoxamine (0.25 mg/kg PO q 12 h) – concurrent use with benzodiazepines should be avoided.
● **Benzodiazepines** such as:
– Diazepam (0.2–0.4 mg/kg PO q 12 h, average of 1–2 mg/cat PO q 12 h) They affect depth perception, so cats may fall off objects or miss objects when they jump until they learn to compensate. At therapeutic levels, there should be a calming effect but little or no effect on motor or mental functions. Cats may stagger for the first 1–2 days, but this should then spontaneously resolve. If it does not, then the dose should be decreased or withdrawn, as the potential for cumulative effects and toxicity due to the intermediate metabolite may occur. Use with caution in aggressive animals as diazepam may lead to disinhibition and potentiate aggression. Adverse effects usually disappear with a decrease or withdrawal of medication. High doses have been associated with increased liver enzymes, hepatotoxicity and convulsions, especially in overweight cats.
– Oxazepam (0.2–0.5 mg/kg PO q 12–24 h) has been successful in other cases and is useful if diazepam produces excessive sedation.
● **Azaperones**.
– Buspirone (0.5–1 mg/kg PO q 8–12 h).
● **Antihistamines**.
– Cyproheptadine (0.4–0.5 mg/kg PO q 12 h) has been reported to be successful in some cases of spraying.

Cleaning the soiled areas with non-ammonia-based products such as enzymatic washing powders is important. Products such as Anti-Icky Poo have also been advocated as successful in eliminating odors. Additionally, neutralizers such as Bac to Nature used after cleaning can be effective in removing the odor.

Punishment is not effective in changing behavior. It serves to further increase the anxiety, as well as impede learning of non-anxious behavior.

Multi-cat households: For treatment to be effective it is essential that a correct diagnosis is made and the correct cat(s) treated. One way of trying to determine which cat is spraying in a multi-cat household is to administer fluorosceine to each cat in turn. All cats should be tested, as it is not unusual for more than one cat to spray. Place five or six fluorosceine strips (or liquid) in a gelatin capsule and give once daily for 3–5 days until the cat(s) is identified. An ultraviolet light will make it easier for the owner to detect fluorosceine in urine. A washout period of 24–48 hours between each cat has been recommended. However, fluorosceine is not an infallible way of detecting urine and a study has shown that the substrate as well as an individual cat's metabolism will affect detection rates. Additionally, fluorosceine may stain the substrate.

Prognosis

The **prognosis is generally good for both inappropriate elimination and spraying.** However, it depends on owner commitment, the success in determining the underlying cause, and the ability to manage the underlying problem. Prognosis also **deteriorates with increased length of time** that the behavior is left untreated and with recidivistic events.

Owner education of normal feline behavior is essential to achieve compliance.

OVER-GROOMING (INCLUDING PSYCHOGENIC ALOPECIA, FELINE HYPERESTHESIA AND SELF-MUTILATION)**

Classical signs

- Hair loss and discoloration only on the parts of the body that can be reached by the teeth and tongue.
- Plucked hair has evidence of shearing.
- Ulceration and self-mutilation may occur.

Pathogenesis

Normal adult cats spend about 30–50% of their time awake grooming.

Grooming serves many purposes including cleaning, removal of parasites, thermoregulation and alleviation of stress (e.g. after punishment, intercat aggression).

Self-licking, biting and hair loss are non-specific signs.

As with most behavioral conditions, the exact pathogenesis is unknown but likely to be complex.

- It may be a behavioral response to environmental conditions which stress the cat and result in stereotypic or obsessive-compulsive behaviors over time.
  - There are numerous reported **causes of anxiety in cats** which include **any environmental changes** such as: moving; a new baby or spouse; separation from the owner; too many cats in the household or area; presence of new cats in the area; loss of territory; punishment from the owner; presence of attacking birds (e.g. magpies) and lack of stimulation.
- **Lowered serotonin and increased dopamine levels** are associated with some obsessive-compulsive disorders. Dopamine is also associated with stress.

Medical conditions such as flea allergy, dietary allergy, sensitivity to dust mites **can trigger** the initial grooming episodes.

Currently **feline hyperesthesia, over-grooming, self-mutilation and psychogenic alopecia** are considered to be **part of the anxiety response**.

Clinical signs

Hair can be removed by plucking, barbering or just by licking and excoriation.

Self-licking, biting and alopecia are seen **wherever the cat can reach**, especially around the sides and rump, back legs and groin. The **head and back of neck may still have a normal hair coat.**

- Usually the **alopecia is non-symmetrical** and the **skin may look normal**.
- The **hair** in the area is a **ginger or rusty brown color** due to the action of the saliva.

Microscopic examination of **plucked hair shows evidence of shear**.

In some cats, over-grooming becomes excessive and self-mutilation and ulceration occur in the affected areas. Secondary bacterial infections may then occur necessitating treatment. **Occasionally**, the over-grooming is so severe that **ulcers develop in the mouth** (tongue, pharynx and hard palate) making eating difficult or impossible. Bleeding may occur associated with hard palate ulcers.

In feline hyperesthesia syndrome, cats may become agitated and aggressive and show skin rippling and muscle spasms, usually over the lumbar area after stimulation such as stroking. They may exhibit frenzied behavior such as licking or biting at the flanks, back or tail or frantic running.

Diagnosis

Diagnosis is based on a complete behavioral history, and thorough physical examination including a complete blood count and biochemistry panel.

No evidence of dermatological causes, such as atopy, external parasites, food allergy is identified.

Microscopic examination of **plucked hair has evidence of shear**. Hair that is lost due to **endocrine conditions has telogen bulbs visible.**

Differential diagnosis

Any skin disease causing pruritus should be eliminated.
- **External parasites,** dermatitis of **fungal or bacterial origin** are differentiated on the basis of dermatological examination.
- **Food allergy** is differentiated by use of a food trial for 6–8 weeks that leads to resolution of signs when a novel protein such as venison or duck is introduced.
- **Endocrine disorders** are differentiated on the basis of **distribution of hair loss** that is usually **symmetrical**, as well as microscopic examination of hair indicating the **presence of telogen bulbs**.
- **Feline hyperesthesia syndrome** is a poorly understood condition which may be differentiated on the basis of signs of extreme sensitivity to touch on the dorsal region, skin rippling, biting or licking of the area with no obvious dermatological or neurological basis.
- **Pain** associated with any condition including trauma or infection is differentiated by response to analgesia or alleviation of pain.

Treatment

Treatment of any concurrent or underlying medical problem is essential, such as elimination of fleas, or resolution of food allergy by changing the diet.

Remove or minimize the cause of the anxiety if possible.

Provide a **regular predictable routine**, such as feed and play at a set time each day. Treatment involves altering the neurochemical as well as the physical environment. Potential side effects should be explained to the owner prior to instigating any therapy, as most of the drugs are not registered for use in animals.
- Medications that influence serotonin metabolism, such as the selective serotonin reuptake inhibitors and the tricyclic antidepressants have been used in the treatment of anxiety-related disorders. Anxiolytic medication has also proved useful in some cases. The comparative effectiveness of each medication remains to be evaluated and may depend on eliciting causes.
- **Tricyclic antidepressants** (TCAs) have proved to be effective.
  - **Amitriptyline** (0.5–1 mg/kg PO q 12–24 h, average of 5–10 mg/cat PO q 24 h). Start at the lowest dose and increase after 10 days if no response.
  - **Clomipramine** (0.5 mg/kg PO q 24 h).
- **Selective serotonin re-uptake inhibitors** (SSRIs) such as **fluoxetine** (0.5 mg/kg PO q 24 h) have been successful in controlling signs in some cases. Toxicity has been reported in humans when used with cyclosporine.
- **Benzodiazepines,** such as diazepam (0.2–0.4 mg/kg PO q 12 h – average of 1–2 mg/cat PO q 12 h) are effective in some cats. Oxazepam (0.2–0.5 mg/kg PO q 12–24 h) is useful where diazepam leads to excessive sedation.
- Blood biochemistry analysis should be done prior to medication to determine baseline concentrations especially for liver and kidney parameters. The cat may require **medication** for a **prolonged period (up to 6–12 months)** and then **slow withdrawal of medication** should be attempted. If cats require longer-term or lifetime medication, biochemistry parameters should be monitored every 6–12 months.

Punishment is not effective in changing behavior. It serves to further increase the anxiety, as well as impede learning of non-anxious behavior.

Prognosis

Prognosis is **variable** and depends on owner commitment, success in determining an underlying cause, and management of the underlying problem. Prognosis deteriorates with increased length of time the problem is left untreated.

INAPPROPRIATE VOCALIZATION**

> ### Classical signs
>
> - Vocalization of increased duration, frequency or intensity.

Pathogenesis

Excessive vocalization may be a **normal innate behavior in some breeds** such as the Siamese.

Vocalization may indicate a **need for social contact, attention or food**. This has been reported in cats that are on restricted-calorie diets.

Septal, ventral hypothalamic lesions as well as hippocampal abnormalities have been associated with excessive vocalization.

Anxiety resulting from social stressors such as the **presence of other cats**, a **change in routine**, or **after a move** has been implicated as a trigger.

Excessive vocalization may be a **function of aging,** cerebral degeneration and alteration of neurotransmitter activity. It may be seen in aged cats exhibiting other signs of senile behavior.

Clinical signs

Vocalization is a non-specific sign.

With excessive vocalization associated with anxiety, the **vocalization is of changed duration, frequency or intensity**.

It may be nocturnal, or just more noticeable at night.

It is **relatively common in older cats** with decreased perceptual and locomotor abilities. It may also be due to reduced cognitive function (senility).

Diagnosis

Diagnosis is based on a **complete behavioral history** documenting inappropriate vocalization. A thorough physical examination, and hematological and biochemical analysis must exclude medical causes.

Hyperthyroidism is excluded based on a normal thyroxine (T4) concentration.

Differential diagnosis

Estrus is a normal behavior and may be **differentiated on the basis of the presence of classical behavioral signs** of restlessness, frequent urination, spraying, rolling, lordosis, etc., during the breeding season. As the cat is seasonally polyestrus these will recur on average every 3 weeks for several months if the cat is not mated.

Oriental breeds tend to vocalize more than other breeds and this is a normal behavior that is differentiated on the basis of breed.

Vocalizations that are a normal behavioral response to physical stressors such **as cold** and **hunger** are differentiated on the basis of a thorough history and **response to removal of these stressors**.

Cognitive dysfunction (aging, senility) is differentiated on the basis of age (cats are usually **more than 12 years of age**) as well as the presence of other signs which may include changes in sleep–wake cycles, decreased social interaction with owners, disorientation, and loss of previously learnt behaviors such as toilet training. Cognitive decline is of gradual onset.

Hyperthyroidism is differentiated on the basis of **classical signs** (weight loss, increased appetite, restlessness, increased vocalization) and **elevated T4 concentration.**

Feline hyperesthesia syndrome is a poorly understood condition which may be differentiated on the basis of signs of extreme sensitivity to touch on the dorsal region, which stimulates skin rippling, biting or licking of the area and often frantic running. Diagnosis is based on signs and lack of other dermatological or neurological disease.

Pain associated with any condition including trauma or **urinary tract infection** is differentiated by response to analgesia or alleviation of pain.
- Vocalization may decrease with pain, so it is important to know what is normal for the cat.

Attention-seeking behavior is differentiated on the basis of a history that is suggestive that vocalization **only occurs in the presence of the owner** when the owner is not paying attention to the cat.

Travel can induce a panic or fear response in cats, and this can be differentiated on the basis of history that the behavior occurs only in these circumstances.

Treatment

Owner education of normal cat behavior is important so that they understand that the **behavior cannot be eliminated** but can be managed.

Treatment of any concurrent or underlying medical problem is essential.

Remove or **minimize the cause of the anxiety** if possible.

Provide a **regular predictable routine**, such as feed and play at a set time each day.

Environmental enrichment with toys that are changed daily, places to hide, and opportunities to play provides a stimulating mental and physical environment for the cat.

Treatment may also involve altering the neurochemical as well as the physical environment.
- Medications that influence serotonin metabolism, such as the selective serotonin reuptake inhibitors and the tricyclic antidepressants have been used in the treatment of anxiety-related disorders. Anxiolytic medication has also proved useful in some cases. Potential side effects should be explained to the owner prior to instigating any therapy, as most of the drugs are not registered for use in animals.
- **Tricyclic antidepressants** (TCAs) such as:
  - Amitriptyline (0.5–1 mg/kg PO q 12–24 h, average of 5–10 mg/cat PO q 24 h) or clomipramine (0.5 mg/kg PO q 24 h).
- **Selective serotonin re-uptake inhibitors** (SSRIs) such as:
  - Fluoxetine (0.5 mg/kg PO q 24 h) have been successful in controlling signs in some cases.
- **Benzodiazepines** such as:
  - Diazepam (0.2–0.4 mg/kg PO q 12 h, average of 1–2 mg/cat PO q 12 h) have been successful in others cases. However, benzodiazepines can lead to increased vocalization in some cats.
- The **monoamine oxidase inhibitor** (MAOI) **selegiline** (deprenyl) at 0.5 mg/kg PO q 24 h has been reported to be effective in some cases for cognitive dysfunction associated with senility.
- Blood biochemistry and hematology analysis should be done prior to beginning medication to determine baseline values especially for **liver and kidney parameters**. The cat may require medication for a prolonged period (up to 6–12 months). **Gradual withdrawal** of medication could be attempted by reducing the dose by half every 2–4 weeks once the symptoms have been successfully controlled for 2–3 months.

Punishment is not effective in changing behavior as it further increases anxiety and impedes learning of non-anxious behavior.

Prognosis

The **prognosis is variable**. It depends on owner commitment, the success in determining the underlying cause and the ability to manage the underlying problem. Prognosis also **deteriorates with increased length of time** that the behavior is left untreated.

Owner education of normal feline behavior is essential to achieve compliance.

PICA (EATING NON-FOOD MATERIAL)*

Classical signs

- Abnormal ingestion of non-nutritive substances.

Pathogenesis

Plant eating may be due to lack of access to grass or vegetation, or be normal investigatory behavior. Young cats especially, may chew, but not necessarily ingest, non-food substances as part of their normal exploratory behavior.

It may represent **obsessive-compulsive disorder** (OCD) with stereotypic chewing or mouth movements. The chewing is carried out differently from eating food items.

Neurochemical and neuroanatomical changes are seen on positron emission tomography scans with OCD.

Wool chewing is a ritualistic or stereotypic behavior. Generally these behaviors are more annoying than damaging, unless they start interfering with the animal's normal functioning.

- More common in **oriental breeds such as Siamese and Burmese**, although it has been reported in all breeds including crossbreeds.
- No sex predisposition for wool eating has been reported.
- Behavior is reported to begin **from 2–8 months of age up to 1–2 years of age**.
- It is reportedly more common in cats that are **entirely indoors**.
- It can be **triggered by stress**.
- **Hunger stimulates the behavior.**
- Postulated causes include:
  - **Early weaning** (at 2–4 weeks); in contrast, feral cats may suckle until 6 months of age.
  - Insufficient handling of kittens before homing.
  - Insufficient fibre in the diet.
  - Separation anxiety.
  - Having no opportunity to develop exploratory and hunting behaviors.
  - A malfunction in the neural control of appetitive behavior.
- Some cats appear to **grow out of it** and the problem resolves during early adulthood without treatment.
- Wool chewing and pica appear to be **inherited.**

Wool sucking may be different in that it **occurs in very early-weaned cats**.

Ingestion of houseplants may occur in cats confined indoors with no access to grass or vegetation. Ingestion of small amounts of grass or other vegetation is normal behavior in cats.

Clinical signs

Pica may include the ingestion of substances such as soil, rubber, paper, wood, string, houseplants, wool or fabric.

Individual cats tend to **ingest one type of substance only**.

Fabric-eating cats appear to **start by eating woollen fabrics**. They **may then proceed to other fabrics** such as cotton, silk and synthetics, but this is not always the case.

- Cats do not appear to like eating raw wool. It is postulated that they do not like the taste or texture of the lanolin.

While the cat is chewing it appears to be **totally engrossed**. They pull and tug on the wool, then grind with their molars. Note that **some cats just suck** the item, and this behavior may be of different origin.

Quite large quantities can be ingested.

- This is a problem if blankets, socks and sweaters are eaten, as there is the **potential for intestinal obstruction.**

Diagnosis

Diagnosis is based on a behavioral history of observation of the ingestion of non-food substances, and exclusion of other underlying disease. A thorough physical examination including a neurological examination should be performed.

A complete blood count, and biochemical analysis including measurement of electrolytes should be performed to exclude medical conditions.

Normal serum lead levels.

Normal thyroxine (T4) concentration.

Differential diagnosis

Hyperthyroidism is differentiated on the basis of typical signs (weight loss, increased appetite, restlessness, increased vocalization) and elevated T4 concentration.

Lead poisoning is differentiated on the basis of signs of weight loss, inappetence and elevated blood lead concentration.

Other neurological disease causing pica, such as encephalitis (e.g. feline infectious peritonitis (FIP) or neoplasia, should be excluded based on neurological examination and other ancillary tests (e.g. CSF analysis).

Dietary deficiencies are differentiated by examination of the diet.

Intestinal parasites are differentiated by presence of eggs on fecal flotation.

Normal investigative behavior is differentiated on the basis of which substances are ingested and the amount consumed. It is more common in young cats.

Lack of access to grass or vegetation resulting in ingestion of small quantities of houseplants is usually confined to indoor cats.

Treatment

Avoid allowing the cat **access** to potentially harmful ingestible materials.

Taste deterrents such as **bitter apple** or **chilli** can prove effective and may be more potent if they are paired with a **distinctive scent such as eucalyptus oil or cologne**, to provide an additional (olfactory) cue that the material is to be avoided. Thus, the cat learns to associate the smell of the oil with an unpleasant taste and eventually the scent alone is enough for the cat to avoid the material. This appears to deter some cats if the behavior is of recent origin.

Provide a regular predictable routine to minimize stress.
● Provide **set times to interact, play and feed the cat**.

Increase environmental enrichment by providing toys and mental stimulation.
● Provide an indoor garden with grass, catnip and or cat mint as a safe source of vegetation, as well as environmental enrichment.

Other suggestions reported to help are:
● Allow the cat **access to dried food all day**.
● **Increase the fiber content** of the diet by adding bran or vegetables.
● Provide **gristly meat and raw bones to chew** on to increase time spent chewing and eating.
● Give small strips of woolen fabric or sheepskin to ingest with their meal. This must ONLY be done under veterinary supervision, and the owner warned that it could lead to constipation or intestinal obstruction.

Do not use direct punishment as this may increase anxiety and exacerbate the problem.
● Environmental punishments such as double-sided sticky tape or **Snappy trainers** may help keep cats away from some areas. A Snappy trainer is a standard mousetrap with a red plastic paddle attached to the moving lever. When the lever is activated, the paddle flips over. This is designed to scare the cat but the paddle prevents injury, because the cat cannot get its paw or face caught in the trap.

Treatment with **psychotropic medication** may be needed if a diagnosis of OCD is made. Potential side effects should be explained to the owner prior to instigating any therapy, as most of the drugs are not registered for use in animals. Anxiolytic medication should always be gradually withdrawn, never suddenly stopped.
● Premedication hematology and serum biochemistry analysis is recommended to provide baseline values, which is especially important if the cat has to stay on long-term or life-time medication. These should be repeated every 6–12 months depending on the age and health status of the cat.
● **Tricyclic antidepressants** such as:
  – Amitriptyline (0.5–1 mg/kg PO q 12–24 h, average of 5–10 mg/cat PO q 24 h). Start at the lowest dose and increase if no response seen after 10 days.
  – Nortriptyline (0.5–1 mg/kg PO q 12–24 h). This is useful if cat is very sedated with amitriptyline.
  – Clomipramine (0.5 mg/kg PO q 24 h).
● **Selective serotonin re-uptake inhibitors** such as:
  – Fluoxetine (0.5 mg/kg PO q 24 h) have proved useful in some cases.
● A **minimum treatment period of 6 months** is recommended as some medications may take 6–8 weeks to reach therapeutic levels.
  – **Gradual weaning off medication** can be attempted when the behavior has been **successfully managed for 3 months.** This can be achieved by halving the dose every 2–4 weeks as long as the symptoms are still controlled.

Prognosis

Treatment takes time and patience so owner commitment is essential.

Prognosis is guarded if an inherited predisposition is suspected. However, most cases can be successfully managed.

Prognosis is good in young cats when signs constitute normal investigative behavior.

RECOMMENDED READING

Beaver B. Feline Behavior: A Guide for Veterinarians. Philadelphia, PA, W.B. Saunders Company, 2003.

Houpt KA. Domestic Animal Behavior for Veterinarians and Animal Scientists. Ames, Iowa State University Press, 1998.

Landsberg G, Hunthausen W, Ackerman L. Handbook of Behaviour Problems of the Dog and Cat. Oxford, Butterworth-Heineman, 2003.

Overall KL. Clinical Behavioral Medicine for Small Animals. St Louis, Missouri, Mosby, 1997.

Seksel K, Lindeman MJ. Use of clomipramine in the treatment of anxiety-related and obsessive-compulsive disorders in cats. Aust Vet J 1998; 76: 317–321.

Simpson BS, Simpson DM. Behavioral pharmacotherapy. In: Voith VL, Burchelt PL (eds) Readings in Companion Animal Behaviour. Trenton, NJ, Veterinary Learning Systems, 1996, pp. 100–115.

PART 13

Cat with skin problems

48. The cat with miliary dermatitis

Ruadhri Michael Seosaimh Breathnach and Mike Shipstone

KEY SIGNS

- Multiple papulocrustous skin lesions.

MECHANISM?

- Miliary dermatitis is a distinct clinical entity, consisting of the presence of multiple papulocrustous lesions affecting the skin. Pruritus contributes to lesion development. Alopecia and secondary infection are common sequelae.

WHERE?

- Skin – widespread papulocrustous lesions can develop in many sites of the body. The precise location of lesions will vary with the specific condition.

WHAT?

- Most cases of miliary dermatitis are due to hypersensitive reactions, with flea allergy being the most common. Other causes include ectoparasitism, microbial infections, neoplasia and various miscellaneous factors such as dietary imbalances, etc.

QUICK REFERENCE SUMMARY

Diseases causing miliary dermatitis

NUTRITIONAL

● Essential fatty acid or biotin deficiency (p 1041)

Widespread papulocrustous dermatitis. Dry, brittle coat in growing cats. Excess scale formation. Uncommon in cats on well-formulated diets. History of a poorly formulated diet, or poor storage conditions leading to rancidity, or prolonged antibiotic therapy.

INFECTIOUS:

Bacterial:

● Staphylococcal dermatitis (p 1041)

Erythema, scale and crustiness. Hair follicles are commonly involved. Papules are common, but not pus. Primary staphylococcal dermatitis is uncommon in cats.

Fungal:

● **Dermatophytes** (p 1032)

More common in young kittens. Erythematous plaques, alopecia and scale. Lesions may progress to larger gray areas of alopecia and hyper-keratosis.

Parasitic:

● **Flea dermatitis*** (p 1025)

Extremely common problem. Pruritus, alopecia and crustiness occur commonly on the dorsal spine and abdomen. Fleas and/or flea feces may be evident in the coat, but may require careful combing to find.

● *Otodectes cynotis* (p 1037)

Papulocrustous dermatitis, often associated with otitis externa. Pruritus, alopecia and secondary infection. Miliary dermatitis is less common than otic signs.

● *Notoedres cati* (notoedric mange) (p 1039)

Severe pruritus. Only common in certain geographical areas. Alopecia, hyperkeratosis and gray, crusty exudate. Secondary infection common.

● *Cheyletiella* species (cheyletiellosis) (p 1036)

Seborrhea and papules, most marked on dorsum. Mild to moderate pruritus. Movement of mites in heavy infestations resembles walking dandruff.

● *Neotrombicula autumnalis* (neotrombiculosis) (p 1038)

Erythema, papules and alopecia. Moderate to marked pruritus. Any contact surface on the body can be involved. Feet, head and limbs most common sites. Larval stages appear as red-orange dots to the naked eye.

● *Felicola subrostratus* (p 1035)

Pruritus, alopecia and occasional secondary infection. Lice and lice eggs may be visible. Often associated with neglect, malnutrition, matted coats, etc.

continued

continued

● Cat fur mite (*Lynxacarus radovsky*) (p 1040)

Dry, dull coat with scale and scurf. Hairs are easily epilated leading to patchy alopecia. Variable pruritus. Common sites include tail-head, perineum and thighs. Only common in limited geographic locations.

IMMUNE-MEDIATED

● Flea allergic dermatitis (FAD)*** (p 1025)

Extremely common cause of miliary dermatitis. Lesions most prevalent along dorsal spine, caudo-medial thighs and ventral abdomen. Signs may be seasonal or perennial. Pruritis is a classical feature.

● Adverse food reaction (food hypersensitivity)** (p 1029)

Probably the second most common allergic cause of miliary dermatitis. Results in moderate to marked pruritus, often involving the head and ears, which is often poorly responsive to corticosteroids. Non-seasonal and may mimic many other cutaneous disorders. Concurrent signs of gastrointestinal or respiratory involvement are usually absent. An affected cat may have been on diet for some time.

● Atopic dermatitis** (p 1030)

Variably pruritic condition which may present as miliary dermatitis, symmetrical alopecia or eosinophilic granuloma complex. Secondary infection may occur. Some animals have only alopecia, and no history of pruritus or skin lesions. Can be seasonal or perennial. Most common in young to middle-aged cats.

● Mosquito bite hypersensitivity** (p 1031)

Variable pruritus with lesions most commonly affecting hairless areas of head, nose, ears and pads. Lesions include papules, crusted papules, plaques, nodules and alopecia. Common in certain geographical locations.

● Drug reaction/hypersensitivity (p 1034)

Uncommon cause of miliary dermatitis, but can occur in any age group. Signs vary from mild erythema to urticaria to necrosis/sloughing. Variably pruritic. Often mimics many other dermatoses. Most common signs are erythema, pruritus and self-induced trauma in areas where topical medications are being applied.

● Intestinal parasite hypersensitivity (p 1035)

Multifocal or generalized papulocrustous reaction pattern. Seborrhea and pruritus. Gastrointestinal signs occasionally present. Pruritic.

● Auto-immune dermatoses (p 1042)

Primarily a pustular or erosive group of conditions resulting in scale, erosions and alopecia. Face, ears and feet are common sites. Pruritus and pain are variable.

IDIOPATHIC

● Idiopathic (p 1043)

Papulocrustous dermatitis. Pruritic. Diagnosis of exclusion when all other etiologies ruled-out.

INTRODUCTION

MECHANISM?

Miliary dermatitis is a term used to describe a cutaneous reaction pattern in cats consisting of **multiple papulocrustous lesions.** It is important to emphasize that it is a clinical, not an etiological, diagnosis. Miliary dermatitis should be suspected when a cat shows evidence of:

- **Multiple papulocrustous lesions** on the skin surface.
- Lesions which typically appear in clusters.
- Alopecia.
- Secondary bacterial infection is sometimes present. The skin/coat may feel hot and sticky.
- The **mechanism of lesion** development is often **inflammatory or immune-mediated in nature,** but can vary with the underlying etiology.
- **Pruritus** is a significant feature, which contributes to lesion development. The typical **response of cats to pruritus** is to **lick or over-groom** rather than scratch, and it is believed that the barbs on the tongue may contribute to lesion development.
- Controversy exists as to whether the term miliary dermatitis should be limited to a few distinct causes, rather than an exhaustive list of differentials.
- A definitive etiology is not always apparent, and in such cases the cat is usually treated symptomatically.

WHERE?

Skin: Widespread papulocrustous lesions can develop in many sites of the body.

- The precise location of lesions will vary with the specific condition.
- The most common sites affected include the **dorsal trunk, flanks, caudo-medial thighs and ventral abdomen.**

WHAT?

Most cases of miliary dermatitis are due to **hypersensitivity reactions.**

- **Flea allergic dermatitis** is by far the most common underlying **etiology** of this syndrome.
- **Food allergy, atopic dermatitis** and other hypersensitive disorders are less common.

- Other causes include **ectoparasitism** and microbial infections.
- Neoplasia and various miscellaneous factors such as dietary imbalances are possible causes in a small minority of cats.
- Diseases covered in The Cat With Pruritus Without Miliary Dermatitis may also present with military dermatitis and should be considered.
- Many factors including the history, age of cat, lesion distribution and even geographical location should help to limit the list of differentials in certain cases.

DISEASES CAUSING MILIARY DERMATITIS

FLEA ALLERGIC DERMATITIS (FAD)***

Classical signs

- Moderate to severe pruritus, seasonal or all year round.
- Numerous papules mainly on the dorsum and ventral abdomen.
- Self-trauma leads to alopecia, crustiness, erosions and secondary infection.
- Because cats are very efficient at grooming the fleas from the coat, fleas or flea dirt may or may not be seen.

Pathogenesis

Ctenocephalides felis is the species most frequently involved in flea allergic dermatitis on a worldwide basis. Other species of flea, including **hedgehog and rabbit fleas** may be involved.

Flea allergic dermatitis is the **most common hypersensitive skin disease** reported in cats, and has been **associated with many cutaneous reaction patterns,** such as **miliary dermatitis, symmetrical alopecia and feline eosinophilic granuloma complex.**

The hypersensitive response develops following binding of **haptens in flea saliva** to dermal collagen.

Whilst flea allergic dermatitis can represent both a type I and type IV hypersensitive reaction in dogs, only the **immediate type reaction** is currently recognized in cats.

The development of hypersensitivity is **not dependent on the number of fleas** infesting or biting the host.

It is postulated that the presence of **atopy may predispose** to the development of flea allergic dermatitis.

The clinical condition may be **seasonal or perennial** in individual animals, depending on geography and other environmental conditions.

Clinical signs

Numerous papules are principally seen on the **dorsum, caudo-medial thighs, flanks and ventral abdomen,** though individual lesions can occur in other sites.

Pruritus is a classical feature. The manifestation of which may be **biting, licking, rubbing, chewing, scratching** or any combination of these. This may be done out of the owner's view, so tufts of hair in the environment, hair caught in the teeth or within the feces are clues to pruritus. Self-trauma leads to alopecia, crustiness, erosions and secondary infection.

There may be **evidence of fleas, or flea feces** may be present within the coat.

Lesions present as a **papulocrustous dermatitis** with alopecia, and rarely, secondary infection characterized by pyotraumatic dermatitis.

Severely affected animals may be depressed and inappetent, with occasional cases showing peripheral lymphadenopathy.

Other cutaneous reaction patterns may be evident.

Some affected cats may also be infested with *Dipylidium caninum*.

Diagnosis

A tentative diagnosis is **based on the history and physical examination.** Finding fleas on the cat is not essential, although fleas and/or flea feces will be present in some cats. Cats are very efficient at grooming the fleas from the coat, and fleas or flea dirt may or may not be seen.

Using a fine flea comb is essential in cases of low levels of infestation, particularly when the coat color is dark. The comb should be brushed through the entire coat including the **perineal, inguinal and ventral chin.** The collected debris should be examined on a white piece of paper. The **flea feces** appear as fine black fragments, but can be present as fine coils. This will turn a red/brown (rust) color if water is dropped onto it, because the major component of the feces is dried blood.

An **intradermal challenge** with commercially available flea saliva antigen may be used, with the reaction being read at 15–20 minutes. The reaction is compared to a positive and negative control (histamine and phosphate-buffered saline). In practice, however, **this test may be difficult** or even impossible to interpret in cats. The presence of a positive test does not confirm flea allergic dermatitis nor does a negative test rule it out. It **merely shows sensitization to the allergen,** NOT whether or not this sensitization is significant.

Blood eosinophilia and skin biopsy may be suggestive of flea allergic dermatitis, but are not in themselves diagnostic.

Serological tests based on such techniques as ELISA are available, although their sensitivity and specificity are still under some investigation. The problem is that the incidence of sensitization in normal cats is so high, that **the positive predictive value of the test is low.**

Response to a strict insect elimination trial may prove a **more reliable means of establishing a retrospective diagnosis.** One method is to apply Fipronil spray to the whole body at 0, 2 and 4 weeks and assess the reduction in pruritus. **Greater than 80% improvement confirms the diagnosis.** An approximately **50% improvement** shows that **insects are a component** of the problem, and < 30% rules the diagnosis out. However, in practice, the percentage improvement may be difficult to gauge.

Differential diagnosis

All of the conditions included in this chapter should be considered as differential diagnoses. However, flea allergic dermatitis is by far the single most common cause of this syndrome.

Other differentials which warrant consideration include **atopic dermatitis, food allergy and various ectoparasitic and microbial skin infections.**

Response to a strict insect elimination trial as outlined is the first step in the investigative process.

Treatment

Flea control is vitally important. A wide variety of anti-flea preparations are available, for example, topical powders, sprays, spot-on formulations and collars. Active ingredients that act as adulticides include: **pyrethrins, organophosphates, fipronil, imidacloprid, nitenpyram and selamectin. Insect growth regulators (lufenuron, methoprene, pyriproxyfen)** may also be used as part of a complete control program to reduce environmental stages of the lifecycle. It is essential to treat in-contact dogs and cats because they may act as reservoirs that will contaminate an environment.

The ideal flea control program should include the **concurrent use** of an **adulticide** to eliminate adult fleas on the pet, and an **insect growth regulator** to control immature flea stages.

- The easiest adulticide to apply is a **monthly "spot on" application of either fipronil, imidacloprid or selamectin** (all have similar therapeutic claims), together with an insect growth regulator, which may be administered topically (methoprene, fenoxycarb, pyriproxyfen), orally (lufenuron) or as a depot injection (lufenuron).
- This **integrated approach** is **essential** because **no adulticide has 100% consistent activity** for the registered duration of action. This means that **viable egg production** may begin **from day 22** after application, although the application interval is 30 days. The modern adulticides (fipronil, imidacloprid and selamectin) are only available as products with a recommended dosing interval of 30 days. Thus, the **integrated approach** ensures that any **eggs laid are non-viable,** and also **delays development of resistance** to both the adulticides and the insect growth regulators. It also means that any infestation picked up through contact with untreated animals or their environment does not become established on the treated animal, or continue to contaminate its environment.

In **sick or neonatal** animals, simple **combing of the coat** with a flea comb may be sufficient to remove fleas.

Systemic corticosteroids are indicated initially, for example, prednisolone (1–2 mg/ kg q 24 h for 7–10 days), tapering over 7–14 days to 0.25–0.5 mg/kg q 48 h as required. If good flea control can be achieved, long-term cortisone use is unnecessary.

Depot corticosteroid preparations and megoestrol acetate are sometimes used when oral therapy is unable to be given, but are more likely to be associated with side effects.

Antihistamines may be useful, although they generally have a slow onset of action and so may need to be combined with prednisolone for the first week or two of therapy. Chlorpheniramine (2–4 mg q 12 h PO) or hydroxyzine (2 mg/kg q 12 h PO) are the most commonly used.

Topical or systemic antimicrobial therapy may be used if secondary bacterial infections are present.

Hyposensitization has been attempted, but to date most reported results have been disappointing. However, work is continuing with different vaccine antigens and future results may be more encouraging.

Prognosis

The **prognosis is good** but **strict flea control** must be maintained life-long or relapses will occur. To date, hyposensitization results have been disappointing.

Transmission

Fleas are transmitted principally by **contact with an infested environment,** although some direct animal-to-animal transfer is possible. The hypersensitive component is not contagious.

Prevention

Adoption of **strict flea control measures** (see flea dermatitis).

Intermittent or long-term alternate day use of prednisolone may be required to control clinical signs if the flea control is inadequate.

FLEA DERMATITIS***

> ### Classical signs
> - Lesions on dorsum and ventral abdomen.
> - Pruritus, alopecia, crust formation and secondary bacterial infection.
> - Fleas and/or flea feces may be seen but may be difficult to find.

Pathogenesis

The movement and blood-sucking activities of fleas leads to **irritation, pruritus and self-trauma.**

Many species can parasitize the cat. *Ctenocephalides felis* is the dominant species involved.

The rabbit flea, *Spilopsyllus cuniculi*, may cause pinnal dermatitis.

Adult *C. felis* begin feeding immediately on the host. If reproduction is not disturbed, the female may produce **up to 50 eggs a day (average 25)** and lay for **up to 100 days,** so the potential for environmental contamination is large, although the normal grooming habits will significantly reduce this.

The **lifecycle** is typical for insects with an egg, larvae, pupa, and adult stage, and under conditions of ideal temperature and humidity, may **occur in as little as 21 days.** However, the duration of the pupal stage is very variable and if conditions are not ideal, the flea may rest in the pupae in a dormant state for up to 180 days, extending the overall lifecycle to around 200 days.

C. felis acts as the intermediate host for *Dipylidium caninum*, so the cat may also be infected with tapeworms.

Many cases of infestation are sub-clinical, but these animals may act as the reservoir contaminating the environment for other co-habiting clinically affected animals.

Transmission is via direct contact with an **infested environment,** although some direct transfer from an infested animal may occur.

Clinical signs

Pruritus and self-trauma occur, and are expressed as **licking or over-grooming rather than scratching.** This results in alopecia, crust formation, miliary dermatitis and secondary infection.

Lesions occur mainly along the **dorsal, inguinal and ventral abdominal areas.**

Severe infestation may lead to anemia, especially in young kittens.

Occasionally, *D. caninum* segments are identified in feces.

Diagnosis

Diagnosis is based on clinical signs and **finding evidence of fleas.** The absence of fleas on examination does not rule out a diagnosis, because cats are very efficient at grooming the fleas and flea dirt from the coat.

Fleas may be detected by a methodical examination of the skin and coat, and with the use of a flea comb. Flea feces can be identified by its red-brown color when suspect material is placed onto damp white paper.

Evidence of infestation on **in-contact animals** or in the environment may be relevant.

Response to a strict insect elimination trial is a **reliable means of diagnosis.**

Flea dermatitis is the **result of flea infestation.** It does not imply or require a hypersensitivity or allergic response to be developed in the affected animal for lesions to occur. The pruritus and self-trauma are related to the **irritation of the flea feeding and moving through the coat.**

Differential diagnosis

Other ectoparasitic, hypersensitive and psychogenic skin conditions. Response to a strict insect elimination trial (outlined under flea allergic dermatitis) is the first step in investigation.

Treatment and prevention

A **wide variety of anti-flea preparations** are available. See section on flea allergic dermatitis. It is essential to treat in-contact dogs and cats, because they may act as reservoirs that will contaminate an environment.

In sick or neonatal animals, simple combing of the coat may be sufficient.

Antibiotics and glucocorticoids may be indicated.

Prognosis

Prognosis is excellent with diligent flea control. However, re-infestation is common.

Transmission

Transmission is by direct or indirect contact, but occurs largely from a **contaminated environment.**

FOOD ADVERSE REACTION (FOOD HYPERSENSITIVITY)**

Classical signs

- Moderate to marked pruritus, often involving the head and ears.
- Often poorly responsive to corticosteroids.
- Non-seasonal.
- May mimic many other cutaneous disorders.
- Concurrent signs of gastrointestinal or respiratory involvement are usually absent.

Pathogenesis

Adverse food reaction or food hypersensitivity accounts for **1–2% of feline dermatoses** seen in practice, and is probably the second most common allergic cause of miliary dermatitis.

Adverse food reactions have been reported to be associated with both **immediate and delayed hypersensitive reactions.**

Ingestion of the offending allergen may occur for months to years before there is sensitization and subsequent clinical reaction.

No sex, age or breed predisposition.

Cats may become sensitized to whatever is being fed, and so the common allergens will vary with local feeding habits of the country. However, **beef, lamb, fish, milk and chicken** are most often implicated.

Clinical signs

The dominant clinical sign is **pruritus,** the manifestation of which may vary from **licking, rubbing, biting, scratching** through to severe excoriation. Pruritus is often poorly responsive to corticosteroids.

Lesions include **erythema, papules, pustules, crusts and ulcers.**

Whilst any part of the body can be involved, the **head and ears are common sites.**

Gastrointestinal tract and respiratory signs are **occasionally present.**

Peripheral lymphadenopathy is rarely present.

Signs of adverse food reaction may mimic many other cutaneous disorders.

Diagnosis

Intradermal and scratch testing are of **no practical benefit** in establishing a diagnosis.

Serological testing is available, but has a very low predictive index and is **not recommended.**

Feeding a true elimination diet for a period of 6–13 weeks, and **demonstrating recovery,** and then **relapse on challenge** with the original diet, is the only accurate method of making a diagnosis. An accurate dietary history is essential so that the **protein selected** for the diet is one that the **cat has never been exposed to.** Depending on the local feeding history this could be goat, horse, rabbit, kangaroo, duck or venison. This diet is **fed exclusively** for the period of the feeding trial.

- If the condition then markedly improves, the diagnosis is confirmed by provocative exposure to the previously incriminated diet. If the cat is food allergic, **a flare in pruritus is expected within 7–10 days,** although most will flare within 24–48 hours of exposure.
- In practice, however, many owners are content to simply let their cat remain on the new diet. If this is done, then they must be warned that the diagnosis has not been confirmed, and that any return in the clinical signs warrants further investigation for other allergic diseases that may have been out of season at the conclusion of the food trial (e.g. atopy, flea allergic dermatitis).
- Once the diagnosis has been confirmed by provocative exposure, the cat can be left on the new diet, provided it is complete and balanced. Alternatively, a **sequential rechallenge with individual food allergens** can be done to try and identify the specific food that is causing the problem, because in over 90% of cases **only 1 or 2 allergens are involved.** All the previous diet components should be fed sequentially over a short period so that it minimizes the chance of a seasonal change occurring, causing a flare in atopic dermatitis, which may then erroneously be attributed to a specific food.

Differential diagnosis

All of the conditions included in this section can be considered as differential diagnoses. However, flea allergic dermatitis is the single most common differential for this syndrome.

Other differentials which warrant consideration, include **atopic dermatitis and various ectoparasitic and microbial skin infections.**

The **investigation must follow a step-wise process** to eliminate other diseases and confirm the diagnosis. That is, if signs still persist after a strict insect elimination trial with control of any secondary infection, a food trial is performed. If the clinical signs still persist, then other differentials including atopy must be considered.

Treatment

A nutritionally balanced elimination diet will need to be **fed long-term.**

- If home-produced diets are to be fed for maintenance, they must be properly balanced to meet the animal's long-term nutritional requirements. A home-prepared diet can be balanced using a meat protein, combined with a carbohydrate (potato, sweet potato, tomato, lentils) supplemented with a balanced calcium source (with correct calcium:phosphorus ratio), safflower, flax seed oils and a multivitamin additive.

Alternatively, commercial hypoallergenic diets are more convenient and provide a nutritionally balanced diet designed for long-term maintenance. A variety of hypoallergenic diets is available including diets using hydrolyzed protein (e.g. Hills z/d).

Prognosis

The prognosis is excellent. However, some cats may later become hypersensitive to the new diet.

ATOPIC DERMATITIS**

Classical signs

- Pruritic dermatosis presenting as miliary dermatitis, symmetrical alopecia or eosinophilic granuloma complex.

Classical signs—Cont'd

- Self-trauma, alopecia and secondary infection.
- Some animals have only alopecia and no history of pruritus or skin lesions.
- Seasonal or year round.

Pathogenesis

The precise pathogenesis of atopic dermatitis is not well understood in cats. A **genetic predisposition is suspected** but has not been proven.

Clinical signs may be **seasonal or non-seasonal depending on the allergen**(s) involved.

Most cats first develop **clinical signs before 3 years of age.**

There are no known breed or sex predilections.

The route of entry of the offending allergen(s) is not well understood, but may include both **inhalation and cutaneous absorption.**

A range of allergens including **dust mites, grass, weed and tree pollens and mold spores** have been identified as causing disease. The clinical signs are not related to the specific allergen sensitivity identified.

Clinical signs

Some cats with atopic dermatitis have **pruritus, papulocrustous lesions and/or alopecia.**

Other cats are **not seen to be pruritic** by the owner, and may have no lesions on the skin but present with a **non-inflammatory alopecia.** In these cats examination of the hairs in the affected area will show that they have been cropped and have broken ends.

Distribution of lesions is not as well defined as in dogs, although the **face and ears** are frequently involved.

Cats may present with a particular cutaneous reaction pattern, such as **eosinophilic granuloma complex, symmetrical alopecia or miliary dermatitis.**

Occasionally peripheral lymphadenopathy may be seen, particularly in cats with miliary dermatitis or eosinophilic plaques.

Some cats may present with **respiratory signs** including rhinitis, chronic cough or asthmatic wheeze.

Diagnosis

In cats with no history of pruritus, **a trichogram and possible trial therapy with an Elizabethan collar** should be considered to ensure the lesions (particularly alopecia and miliary dermatitis) are not self-induced. When questioning the owner, all manifestations of pruritus should be described including biting, rubbing, licking, biting scratching, as some owners only recognize or equate scratching with itch.

- **A trichogram is collected by plucking hairs** using mosquito forceps, padded with tape, from the affected area. The ends of the hairs are examined microscopically for signs of trauma including splitting, fractures, cropped, squared off ends, rather than a smoothly tapered end of the undamaged hair.

Histopathology is not diagnostic.

Intradermal skin testing is potentially useful using a panel of allergens based on geographical location. All tests **should include dust mites,** but the grass, weed and pollen selection will depend on the specific location. Allergen manufacturers generally have well-established recommendations for specific antigen selection in the USA and Europe. However, it should be emphasized that the results of intradermal testing can be difficult to interpret in some cats.

Serological tests (ELISA, etc.) for the detection of allergen-specific IgE are commercially available, although data to confirm the sensitivity and specificity of many of these tests are **often lacking.**

Differential diagnosis

All conditions included in this section can be considered as differential diagnoses.

- **Flea allergic dermatitis** is the single most common differential for this syndrome, and should be first ruled out by a thorough insect elimination trial.
- **Adverse food reaction** is the next most common condition, and can be eliminated on the basis of a strict food trial.
- Other differentials which warrant consideration, include various ectoparasitic and microbial skin infections.

Treatment

Prednisolone (initial dose 1–2 mg/kg/day for 7–10 days) should be used to control the clinical signs. The dose may be gradually tapered over 2–3 weeks to 0.5–1.0 mg/kg q 48 h as required to control clinical signs.

Antihistamines such as chlorpheniramine (2–4 mg/cat twice daily) may be effective.

Essential fatty acid supplements of the omega 3 and omega 6 series may help in treatment regimes, particularly if combined with prednisolone or chlorpheniramine.

Hyposensitization is often the treatment of choice, and can be expected to give some control in 60–70% of cases. An accurate diagnosis of the offending allergen(s) is essential.

In **severe, refractory cases** immunosuppressive therapy using **chlorambucil** (0.1–0.2 mg/kg q 24 h) has been reported, but should only be used where high-dose prednisolone (2–3 mg/kg q 24 h) has been unsuccessful. **Cyclosporin** (5 mg/kg q 24 h for 2–3 weeks and then reducing to 5 mg/kg q 48–72 hours) has been effective, but large-scale controlled studies have yet to be published.

Prognosis

The prognosis is good, although on-going medication or hyposensitization, will be required.

If the allergen(s) can be successfully avoided, e.g. tobacco smoke, then the prognosis is excellent.

Prevention

Future episodes may be ameliorated by appropriate medication or hyposensitization.

Whilst a specific inherited predisposition has not yet been proven in cats, judicious breeding programs may be appropriate.

MOSQUITO BITE HYPERSENSITIVITY**

> **Classical signs**
>
> - Papules, erosions, crusting and depigmentation of the nose and pinnae

> ### Classical signs—Cont'd
>
>   principally, although the preauricular skin
>   may also be affected.
> - The footpads may become swollen and
>   develop fissures and scale.
> - Pruritus is variable.

Pathogenesis

Disease is restricted geographically to **areas where
mosquitoes are endemic,** and is more common in
spring and summer in association with an increase in
mosquito breeding, and regresses through winter.

The condition is **seasonal,** and involves **cats with outdoor access.**

Some components appear to involve a **type I hypersensitive response.**

Lesions resolve spontaneously when the cat is moved
to a **mosquito-free environment.**

Clinical signs

All ages and breeds of cat are affected.

Pruritus is variable, and is not a constant feature.

Initial **papules and plaques** commonly **ulcerate and
crust** over.

Later lesions include **nodules, alopecia, excess scale
and depigmentation.**

Sites include the **bridge of the nose, ears and preauricular areas.** Other sites include the chin, lips and feet.
The **pads** are swollen with cracking and scale formation.

Pyrexia, peripheral blood eosinophilia and peripheral
lymphadenopathy may be seen.

Diagnosis

Diagnosis is based on the response to therapy, or by
maintaining the animal indoors. There is no specific
laboratory test.

Differential diagnosis

All conditions included in this section can be potentially
considered as differential diagnosis.

In mosquito bite hypersensitivity, the **presenting lesions
and restriction to the hairless areas of the head and
feet** are quite characteristic.

Flea allergic dermatitis is the most common differential
for this syndrome. Other differentials, which warrant
consideration **include food hypersensitivity, atopic
dermatitis and various ectoparasitic and microbial
skin infections.**

Treatment and prevention

Maintain the cat indoors during the mosquito season
or at times of potential mosquito feeding.

Use suitable mosquito repellents containing **dimethyl
metatolilimide (DEET)** or put **butoxypolyporpon** on
areas of the cat likely to be bitten.

Glucocorticoids can be used judiciously to ameliorate
clinical signs.

DERMATOPHYTES**

> ### Classical signs
>
> - More common in young kittens.
> - Erythematous plaques and scale.
> - Lesions progress and expand to form
>   larger grayish areas of alopecia and
>   hyperkeratosis.
> - Infection may be sub-clinical.

Pathogenesis

Dermatophyte species **parasitize the superficial keratinized layers of the skin,** hair follicles and nails.

Microsporum can is is frequently involved in the cat.

Younger or immunosuppressed cats are at particular
risk.

Dermatophytes can induce a localized inflammatory or
even a hypersensitive response.

Infection may lead to **hyperkeratosis, epithelial
hyperplasia and folliculitis.** This can result in hair
shaft breakage and alopecia.

Secondary bacterial infection may occur.

Viable dermatophyte organisms can still be isolated from lesions after clinical resolution. In the case of *M. canis*, viable **fungal elements can survive up to 18 months in the environment.**

A genetic predisposition is possible in certain breeds (e.g. Persians).

M. canis has a **high zoonotic potential,** and it has been reported in 30–70% of cases, that at least one in-contact human becomes infected in households with infected cats.

Transmission is via **direct contact** with infected animals or **indirect contact of contaminated environment or fomites** (bedding, grooming equipment, etc.). Spores have survived in the environment for over a year.

Clinical signs

The **face, head and feet** are common initial sites.

Raised, erythematous plaques and scale may be seen clinically.

Alopecia develops and lesions expand to form larger plaques, which appear grayish and hyperkeratotic.

Initial **hair loss** occurs in the **center of the lesion.** Hairs on the periphery appear discolored and brittle.

Upon regression, initial hair re-growth appears in the center of the alopecic areas.

Secondary bacterial infection is common.

Infection that involves the **whiskers or nail beds** may lead to **deformities** of these structures on resolution of the infection.

Infection of deeper tissues may result in **nodular skin lesions.**

Diagnosis

Fluorescence under ultraviolet light (Wood's lamp), may **detect approximately 30–80%** of cases of *M. canis* infections. The Wood's lamp must be turned on and warmed up for 5–10 minutes prior to use to allow the wavelength of light produced to stabilize. The affected area is exposed to the light in a dark room for 3–5 minutes. A positive result is a bright apple green **fluorescence of individual hair shafts, not the scale and sebum.**

Skin scrapings and hair plucks may allow identification of the **spores and fungal hyphae** on the **outside of the hair shaft.** Rarely, fungal hyphae can be identified on stained acetate preparations of the epidermis overlying lesional skin.

Fungal culture of scrapings, hair plucks and nail samples can identify the species of dermatophyte involved.

Biopsies of affected tissue can be collected to allow visualization of dermatophyte hyphae in the follicles or stratum corneum. This may require special stains to highlight the fungal elements.

Differential diagnosis

Dermatophytosis is a **follicular infection** and as such the major differentials also affect the follicles and include **demodicosis and staphylococcal folliculitis.**

Differentials for circular areas of alopecia with crust and inflammation include **pemphigus, flea bite hypersensitivity, food allergy and atopy.**

Treatment

A variety of agents are available for both **topical and systemic treatment** of dermatophytosis.

Topical agents include **clotrimazole, ketoconazole, enilconazole and miconazole.**

Systemic agents include **griseofulvin** (from 10–50 mg/kg/day for 4–8 weeks). As this is potentially **teratogenic,** it should not be administered to pregnant cats. Anemia, leucopenia, vomiting, diarrhea, depression, pruritus, fever and ataxia have been described. This reaction is thought to be idiosyncratic but may be more common and more severe in Persian, Himalayan, Siamese and Abyssinnians and FIV-positive cats. Thus, if it is used, bone marrow monitoring via complete blood tests must be done.

Ketoconazole (10 mg/kg bid PO) for 4 weeks is also effective. Hepatic dysfunction and pregnancy are contraindications. Although more expensive, itraconazole (2.5–5.0 mg/kg bid PO) and fluconazole (10–20 mg/kg bid PO) are highly effective and generally less toxic.

Terbinafine (30–40 mg/kg PO sid) is a newer systemic agent with relatively high efficacy, although treatment may need to be administered for up to 4 months or more.

Although fungal vaccines have not been effective as prophylactic agents in challenge exposure experiments, data are available to indicate they may be beneficial as an adjunct to conventional therapies once clinical disease has occurred.

Anecdotal reports on the efficacy of lufenuron have not been supported by corroborative data.

The **hair coat should be clipped** in affected cats. In short-coated cats, clip a **6 cm margin around all lesions.** In long-haired cats, the **body should be completely clipped** including the whiskers. The rationale is to **remove infective material** that would otherwise be shed into the environment, and **make topical treatment easier** for the owner.

Secondary bacterial infections should be treated with **appropriate antibacterial therapy.**

Prognosis

Prognosis is generally good, but if lesions persist after 8 weeks of treatment, suspect either a **resistant strain,** an **underlying systemic disorder** that is interfering with a normal immune response, or that the **genetic background of the cat** (e.g. Persians) is such that prolonged treatment may be necessary.

Prevention

New animals in catteries should be isolated until confirmed free of infection.

Isolate infected animals. **All in-contacts** should be examined and **treated prophylactically** with a systemic medication **until all cats are culture negative.** This is especially **important in large pure-bred catteries.**

Disinfect premises and **potential fomites with undiluted bleach** (5.25% sodium hypochlorite) or 1% **formalin,** or dispose of bedding, clothing, grooming combs, etc.

Immunity to dermatophyte infection is not complete at the time of clinical resolution.

DRUG REACTION/HYPERSENSITIVITY

Classical signs

- Variably pruritic affecting skin or mucous membranes.

Classical signs—Cont'd

- A wide range of skin reactions is possible, varying from urticaria, to erythema multiforme to auto-immune skin disease.
- Often mimics many other dermatoses.
- Most common signs are erythema, pruritus and self-induced trauma in areas where topical medications are being applied.

Pathogenesis

Virtually **all drugs are capable of inducing an adverse reaction.** Reactions to drugs are predictable or unpredictable. Unpredictable reactions may have an immunological or genetic basis.

- **Predictable reactions** occur when the adverse effects are **related to the drug's mode of action,** and are normally **dose-dependent.**
- **Unpredictable or idiosyncratic reactions** are normally not dose-dependent, and are related to the cat's **immunological response** to the drug, or are **the result of differences in the individual's susceptibility to the drug,** commonly because of a metabolic variation, for example an enzyme deficiency.

Predictable reactions include signs such as **alopecia due to corticosteroids** or anti-neoplastic drugs.

Immunological reactions can be types **I, II, III or IV hypersensitivity** responses.

Some cases of toxic epidermal necrolysis (TEN), erythema multiforme (EM) and systemic lupus erythematosus (SLE) may have an underlying drug etiology, but these presentations are rare in cats.

Certain drugs are over-represented in many surveys, including **sulfonamides, penicillins and cephalosporins.**

Generally, **drug reactions occur in the first few weeks of therapy,** and while the drug is still in the body. However, exposure and sensitization to the drug could have been in the preceding weeks or months. Re-exposure in these circumstances can lead to the very rapid (within hours) development of new lesions.

Clinical signs

The clinical signs can **mimic** most, if not all, **other types of skin diseases.**

Erythema, papules, plaques, vesicles/bullae and urticaria may be seen initially, and may become annular or ulcerate.

Necrosis and sloughing of affected skin is possible, particularly in more severe cases.

The most common morphologic patterns in cats are **contact dermatitis** to topical agents, and **pruritus with self-induced traumatic lesions.**

Common sites include the **mouth, face, ears, mucocutaneous junctions, groin and feet.**

Pruritus is variable, but can be severe.

The **extremities** may exhibit lesions, including annular areas of necrosis and ulceration, particularly if a vasculitis reaction is involved.

Systemic signs including inappetance and pyrexia may be present.

Diagnosis

A definitive diagnosis is often difficult to make, and may only be confirmed retrospectively. **Suggestive factors include:**
- Prior history of drug administration.
- The reaction pattern resembles one of hypersensitivity.
- The clinical signs resolve following withdrawal of the drug. Provocative exposure is theoretically possible, but not recommended.
- Histopathology is suspicious, but not diagnostic.

Differential diagnosis

All conditions included in this section can be considered as differential diagnoses.

The most common presenting pattern for a drug reaction in cats is contact dermatitis, so the index of suspicion should be increased if an animal suddenly deteriorates, and develops **erythema, pruritus and self-induced trauma in areas where topical medications are being applied.**

Treatment and prevention

Withdraw the suspect medication.

Symptomatic therapy to alleviate signs.

Do not use the offending drug or any cross-reacting drug in the future in that patient.

Prognosis

Generally good, unless lesions affect a significant area of skin, e.g. necrosis.

The prognosis is more guarded for serious systemic involvement.

INTESTINAL PARASITE HYPERSENSITIVITY

> **Classical signs**
> - Multifocal or generalized papulocrustous reaction pattern.
> - Pruritus.
> - Seborrhea and urticaria.
> - GI tract signs sometimes exhibited.

Clinical signs

No age, breed or sex predilection is reported.

Pruritus and a papulocrustous reaction pattern, either **multifocal or generalized** is reported.

Seborrheic dermatitis with erythema, grease and scale may be present. Urticarial lesions may be present.

Gastrointestinal tract signs may be present.

Diagnosis

Confirm the presence of intestinal parasites with **fecal tests. Ascarids, hookworms, tapeworms and coccidia** have all been reported causing the disease.

A **tentative diagnosis** is possible based on **resolution of skin signs** with appropriate anthelminthic therapy.

FELICOLA SUBROSTRATUS

> **Classical signs**
> - Pruritus, alopecia and occasional secondary infection.
> - Lice and lice eggs may be evident on visual inspection.
> - Cat may be immunosuppressed or have intercurrent disease.

Pathogenesis

Felicola subrostratus is a **biting louse.** The adults feed on epithelial debris and hair.

Pruritus develops as a result of the movement and feeding behavior of the louse.

Infestation is commonly a disease of **poor hygiene, immunosuppression or over-crowding.**

Cats with **matted coats** are more at risk.

Disease is more common in **colder months** of the year.

Transmission is via **direct contact** with an infested animal or with **contaminated bedding** or **grooming equipment.** They do not survive for more than a few days off the host.

Clinical signs

Infestation may be sub-clinical, but in most cases **pruritus** is reported. **Alopecia, seborrhea and secondary infection** can develop subsequent to the lice infestation.

Common sites include **body apertures** (mouth, anus, vulva) and **under long, matted hair.**

The cat may exhibit signs of intercurrent disease.

Diagnosis

Diagnosis is based on finding lice by **gross visual inspection.** Both the adults and eggs are visible. A hand-held magnifying lens may aid this exercise.

Clear acetate tape can be used to trap and immobilize adults for identification microscopically. The lice are stuck to the acetate tape, which is then adhered to a glass microscope slide for examination.

Differential diagnosis

All conditions included in this section can be considered as differential diagnoses.

Flea allergic dermatitis is the single most common differential for miliary dermatitis and should be ruled out with a strict insect elimination trial.

Other differentials which warrant consideration include **food hypersensitivity, atopic dermatitis and various ectoparasitic and microbial skin infections.**

Treatment and prevention

Pyrethrins are commonly used. **Ivermectin and fipronil** are not licensed for this particular indication, yet appear to have good efficacy. Organophosphates are less popular and have a much lower safety index. **Selemectin** is registered for use on cats and should be effective.

Repeat treatment is indicated to kill newly hatched eggs.

Grooming equipment and **in-contact animals** should be treated also.

Predisposing factors should be addressed. Grooming of the coat is important.

Prognosis

Excellent, if predisposing factors are addressed.

CHEYLETIELLA SPECIES (CHEYLETIELLOSIS)

> **Classical signs**
> - Pruritus.
> - Seborrhea and papules. Often referred to as "walking dandruff".
> - Most common in young animals.

Pathogenesis

Cheyletiella mites are **superficial, surface dwellers** that feed on skin debris and are quite mobile.

Cheyletiella blakei is the most common species in cats.

The entire life cycle is completed on the host in as little as 21–35 days.

The feeding behavior leads to **pruritus and self-trauma.**

A hypersensitive response may develop.

Most common in young animals.

Mites are contagious.

These mites are **zoonotic** and may cause a pruritic, papular rash on in-contact people.

Clinical signs

Initially, a **fine dry scale with minimal pruritus** may be seen along the backline, but with time the **pruritus may become extreme** along with an increase in the severity of the scale formation.

Some cats will develop a **widespread papulocrustous reaction.**

The mites are large (~400 µm) and visible to the naked eye. In heavy infection, movement of mites through the coat may resemble the appearance of **"walking dandruff".**

Diagnosis

Diagnosis is based on **clinical signs** and **finding the mites.** Mites and mite eggs may be visible on the skin or hair coat with a magnifying glass.

If mite numbers are low, the chance of success is increased by **combing the coat with a fine comb.** The collected debris is then examined microscopically for the presence of mites.

Occasionally, mites have been detected via fecal floatation techniques as a result of grooming.

Differential diagnosis

The differential diagnoses for the early lesions of **mild scale** include **ectoparasitism, poor nutrition, diabetes or hepatic disease.**

With more severe pruritus and a papulocrustous eruption, all the differentials for miliary dermatitis need to be considered. Combing with a fine comb and examination of the debris microscopically will facilitate a diagnosis.

Treatment and prevention

Pyrethrins are effective. Other effective agents include **sulfur preparations and ivermectin** (not licensed). **Selamectin** is registered for cats and should be effective. Organophosphates are more toxic and should be used with great care, if at all.

In-contact animals should also be treated.

Prognosis

Prognosis is excellent with appropriate treatment.

Transmission

Transmission is via **direct contact** with an infested animal or with **contaminated bedding** or **grooming equipment.** The immature stages do not survive for more than a few days off the host, but the **adult female may survive up to 10 days.**

OTODECTES CYNOTIS

> **Classical signs**
>
> - Signs of miliary dermatitis may be accompanied by an exudative otitis externa.
> - Pruritus, alopecia and secondary infection.
> - Lesions around head and neck.

Pathogenesis

Otodectes mites cause **irritation** because of their **movement** and **feeding habits.** They **feed on** the **epithelium and tissue fluid** from the superficial epidermis. The resultant inflammation leads to pruritus and self-trauma.

The primary site of infestation is the **external ear canal,** although ectopic infestations may also be found on other areas including the **abdomen, neck, rump and tail.**

Papules and secondary staphylococcal dermatitis develop on the skin.

The life cycle typically takes **3 weeks.** Eggs are laid, and after 4 days hatch to produce a larva which feeds for 3–10 days. The larva then molts to form a protonymph, and after a short resting phase, the protonymph molts to form a deutonymph. Adults are produced once the deutonymph molts and can survive for approximately 2 months.

Sub-clinical infection is common.

Most cats acquire the infestation as kittens from a **carrier queen.** An entire litter may be affected.

Clinical signs

Many cases present with a **waxy otitis externa** and **head-shaking** due to irritation generated by the mites feeding. Classically the debris has a **brown "coffee ground"** appearance. However, the amount of debris can range from minimal to near complete obstruction of the canal.

The **ectopic infestations** can cause **pruritus, alopecia, miliary dermatitis and secondary infection** which resembles other allergic disease, but is less common than otic signs.

Diagnosis

Diagnosis is based on clinical signs and **finding the mites.** Mites are often visible on otoscopic examination.

- Samples of exudate can be examined using magnifying glasses, or microscopically on slides to identify mites.

Ectopic infestations may not be identified on cytology, rather a presumptive diagnosis is made on **response to systemic miticide therapy.**

Differential diagnosis

The aural manifestation of mites is quite distinct, but **other infectious causes of otitis (including bacteria and *malassezia*)** need to be ruled out.

The ectopic infestation may cause a pruritic dermatitis that can resemble **flea allergic dermatitis, food hypersensitivity, atopic dermatitis** and **various ectoparasitic and microbial skin infections.**

Treatment

Otitis externa may be treated with **drops containing agents such as milbemycin, pyrethrins/piperonyl butoxide, thiabendazole or lindane. Fipronil** and **imidacloprid** have also been reported as effective topical therapies. If the discharge is marked, the ears may need to be cleaned with a **ceruminolytic first** to allow adequate penetration and dispersion of the miticide.

Systemic medications that are effective include selemectin and ivermectin (200 µg/kg subcutaneously or orally, repeated 2 weeks later). However, ivermectin is not licensed for this purpose. The systemic medication is essential in cases (or suspected cases) of ectopic infestation, and because of the highly contagious nature of mites, all in-contact animals should also be treated.

Antibacterial treatment, with or without corticosteroids, may be indicated to alliviate severe self-trauma.

Prognosis

Prognosis is excellent with appropriate treatment.

Prevention

Repeat treatment of the affected cat and all in-contact animals is required to prevent reinfection.

Transmission

Transmission occurs via **direct spread** from one cat to another in most cases, but mites may survive off host for a short period.

NEOTROMBICULA AUTUMNALIS (NEOTROMBICULOSIS)

Classical signs

- Pruritus.
- Erythema, papules and alopecia.
- Feet, head and limbs commonly involved.
- Larval stages appear as orange-red dots with the naked eye.

Pathogenesis

There are over 700 species of harvest mites, although only approximately 20 have been identified as causing animal disease.

The adult stages are not parasitic and are free living, feeding on decaying vegetable matter. The six-legged **larval stages** of the mites are **parasitic** of animals and feed on surface debris.

The resultant reaction may give rise to significant **self-trauma** and in some cases a **hypersensitivity** response may develop.

More common in **summer** and **autumn,** particularly in **grassy areas or hedgerows.**

Larval stages are **contracted** from **gardens, hedges,** etc, and are not normally spread from cat to cat.

Clinical signs

Pruritus occurs, and in some cases is extreme, and **self-trauma.**

Papules, crusted papules, alopecia are common and secondary infections of the affected areas may also develop.

The most common areas affected are in contact with the vegetation, so **feet, lower limbs, ventrum and the head are common sites.**

Infestation seems to be more common around the **head and ears** of cats, but this can be differentiated from *Otodectes* by the bright red/orange color of the larvae.

Diagnosis

Diagnosis is based on clinical signs and finding the mite. Larval stages are the **size of a pin-head,** and are a characteristic bright orange-red color, tightly adhered to the skin.

The mites may be collected via mild **superficial scrapes** or adhering the mites to acetate tape and transferring this to a glass microscope slide for examination.

Differential diagnosis

All conditions included in this section can be considered as differential diagnoses.

Allergies (flea, food and atopy) are the most common, and can be differentiated by identification of the characteristic mites on the skin and at the sites of the papulocrustous eruptions.

Treatment

Sulfur-containing products are effective. Non-licensed agents include **fipronil** and **ivermectin. Selemectin** is registered for use on cats, has a similar mode of action as ivermectin and should be effective, although no efficacy data have been published for this indication. Organophosphates are less popular because of their toxicity and low safety index, and should be used with care.

Corticosteroids may be indicated to relieve pruritus.

Prognosis

Prognosis is excellent with appropriate treatment. However, **re-infestation is common** if the cat has continued access to the infested vegetation.

Prevention

Repeat courses of treatment are required to combat re-infestation.

Keep cats away from contaminated grass and hedgerows during summer and autumn.

NOTOEDRES CATI (NOTOEDRIC MANGE)

Classical signs

- Severe pruritus, with marked secondary changes.
- Ears, neck, face and occasionally paws.
- Alopecia, hyperkeratosis and gray, crusty exudate.
- Secondary bacterial infection.

Pathogenesis

The **burrowing activity** of *Notoedres cati* produces mechanical irritation, with resultant inflammation.

A hypersensitive response may develop.

The **mites feed on skin debris.**

N. cati has been reported virtually worldwide in the past. However, its occurrence today seems to be very **localized or sporadic.**

Infestation is generally spread via **direct contact,** and is **highly contagious,** so that entire litters may be affected.

Clinical signs

Initial lesions usually appear on the **tips and edge of the ears,** and then spread over the face and neck.

The mites **burrow through the superficial epidermis** and this leads initially to the production of **very small papules.** With time the **skin thickens** and **marked hyperkeratosis** develops, which is seen grossly as **thick scale** and **crust formation.** This may develop a yellow to gray color.

Pruritus is marked which may lead to **self-inflicted trauma** and quite severe excoriation which may then become **secondarily infected.**

Less commonly the **feet** may also be involved.

Diagnosis

Diagnosis is based on clinical signs and finding the mites. The mites are found in burrows in the superficial epidermis. **Superficial skin scrapes** should be collected: use a blunt scapel blade to remove the surface scale and crust. This material is transferred to a microscope slide for examination.

Biopsy of affected skin may reveal mites or eggs along with non-specific superficial perivascular inflammation.

Differential diagnosis

All conditions included in this section can be considered as differential diagnoses.

Flea allergic dermatitis is the single most common differential for miliary dermatitis.

Other differentials which warrant consideration include **food hypersensitivity, atopic dermatitis and various ectoparasitic and microbial skin infections.**

Treatment and prevention

Lime-sulfur dips or shampoos (2.5%) are highly effective. Treatment should be repeated every 10–20 days. **Malathion** dips (0.25–1.25%) and **amitraz** washes (0.025%) are also effective.

Ivermectin (usually at dose levels of 200–300 µg/kg SC although occasionally at dose levels as high as 1000 µg/kg SC for 2–3 treatments) has been successfully used, but is not licensed.

Antibacterial cover and corticosteroids may be indicated.

In-contact animals should be treated if appropriate.

Prognosis

Prognosis is excellent with appropriate treatment. In some cases, an immune response may develop leading to resolution of infection, even without treatment.

CAT FUR MITE (*LYNXACARUS RADOVSKY*)

Classical signs

- Dry, dull coat with hairs easily epilated.
- Excess scale and scurf.
- Tail-head, perineum and thighs affected.
- Variable pruritus.

Pathogenesis

Lynxacarus radovsky is reported in northern Australia, USA and certain other tropical regions.

All stages of the life cycle are found on the cat.

Adult and larval stages **feed on skin debris and secretions.**

The mites generally do not burrow. Hence, **lesions are mainly found on the coat.**

Immunosuppression may be a factor.

Transmission is via **direct contact,** but the contagious nature of the mite is variable.

Clinical signs

Typically there is **scurfiness of the coat.** The **mites appear as white flecks** on the hairs, towards the tips and are best visualized on cats with dark coat colors.

The **coat is dull and dirty,** and the hairs are frail and easily epilated leading to **patchy alopecia.** In more severe cases, a **generalized maculopapular to exfoliative dermatitis** may develop.

Lesions common along the **lower back and perineal/thigh areas.**

Pruritus is mild to absent, unless lesions develop on the skin.

Diagnosis

Diagnosis is based on clinical signs and finding the mites. Examination of affected hairs under the **microscope** reveals **adult mites attached to the hair.**

Differential diagnosis

All conditions included in this section can be considered as differential diagnoses.

Flea allergic dermatitis is the single most common differential for this syndrome.

Other differentials, which warrant consideration, include **food hypersensitivity, atopic dermatitis and various ectoparasitic and microbial skin infections.**

Treatment and prevention

Lime-sulfur dips are effective, although several dips may be required. Other routine agents are also effective.

Selemectin may be effective and **ivermectin,** whilst not registered for this use, has been reported as effective.

In-contact animals may require treatment. Not all in-contact animals will be infested.

Assess for underlying immunosuppressive diseases.

Prognosis

Prognosis is excellent, provided there is no underlying immunosuppressive disorder.

STAPHYLOCOCCAL DERMATITIS

Classical signs

- Erythema and scale/crustiness.
- Hair follicles often involved.
- Lesions may progress to papules, but pus is rare.

Clinical signs

Primary staphylococcal dermatitis is rare in cats. Consequently, there may be signs of an underlying immunosuppressive disease which allows the infection to develop.

There may be erythema and scale/crustiness.

The **hair follicles are usually involved,** which commonly leads to **papule formation centered on the follicle,** so a miliary dermatitis pattern may develop.

Frank purulent material or pustules are rarely present.

Staphylococcal infection may present as **abscesses** or infections of the **ears or conjunctiva.** Generally the **infections are superficial,** involving the epidermis to superficial dermis, and deeper infections are infrequent.

Diagnosis

Cytological examination of either acetate preparations or impression smears of the lesions (papules) may show the presence of activated (multi-nucleated) **neutrophils,** along with **cocci** either extra- or intracellularly. This is the fastest method and may easily be performed in the consultation room.

Culture from infected lesions may be helpful. Care is required, as most normal cats possess coagulase-positive staphylococci on their skin.

Biopsy may show evidence of bacterial folliculitis, pyoderma or deeper infection.

ESSENTIAL FATTY ACID OR BIOTIN DEFICIENCY

Classical signs

- Widespread papulocrustous dermatitis.
- Dry, brittle coat, with excess scale.

Pathogenesis

Deficiencies of essential fatty acids (EFA) are **uncommon.** They are reported in animals fed dry **diets** that are **poorly formulated or inappropriately stored,** homemade recipes, and diets that are poorly preserved. Cats require **arachidonic acid and linoleic acid** in the diet.

Rancidity may lead to a deficiency of essential fatty acids, as can a **deficiency of antioxidants.**

Essential fatty acid deficiency leads to **abnormal keratinization, hyperplasia and hyperkeratosis.** Clinical signs only develop after several months.

Biotin deficiency can arise from **diets rich in uncooked eggs or prolonged antibiotic therapy.**

Clinical signs

Papulocrustous lesions can be seen particularly with **biotin deficiency.**

Excess scaling, alopecia and a poor hair coat occur in cats with essential fatty acid deficiency.

The skin becomes **thick and greasy.** Affected sites include the **ears, feet and various skin folds.**

Pruritus and secondary infection occur.

Diagnosis

Diagnosis is based on **clinical signs** and a **detailed dietary history** or **food analysis** demonstrating deficiency of the appropriate dietary component.

Biopsy is non-specific.

Differential diagnosis

All conditions included in this section can be considered as differential diagnoses.

Flea allergic dermatitis is the single most common differential for this syndrome.

Other differentials which warrant consideration include **food hypersensitivity, atopic dermatitis and various ectoparasitic and microbial skin infections.**

Treatment

Rectify the dietary imbalances present, using commercial diets where appropriate.

Change any feeding practices which predispose to biotin or essential fatty acid deficiencies.

Prognosis

Prognosis is excellent with correction of the diet.

Prevention

Feed a well-balanced diet that meets current international standards for feline diets. **Store food at appropriate temperatures** and **use before expiry date.**

Anticipate possible biotin deficiency **if the cat requires prolonged antibiotic therapy** and prevent by **supplementing with a B-group multivitamin including biotin**.

AUTOIMMUNE DERMATOSES

Classical signs

- Vesico-bullous, pustular or erosive lesions.
- Erythema, pustules, scale, erosions and alopecia in pemphigus foliaceus.
- Common sites include the face, ears, feet, footpads, groin and nipples.

Classical signs—Cont'd

- In SLE and discoid lupus erythematosus, lesions consist of exfoliative erythroderma, seborrhea, scale, crusts and alopecia. The face and ears are commonly involved.

Pathogenesis

The pathogenesis varies dependent on the form of autoimmune disease present. Many accepted theories may not be relevant to cats.

Pemphigus foliaceus is the **most common clinical form** of autoimmune disease in cats.

- Tissue is damaged from a **type II hypersensitivity reaction** where IgG or IgM antibody binds to cellular antigens, resulting in destruction of the cells. In pemphigus, **antibodies** are directed against **intercellular space substances** and parts of the **epidermal cell wall.** This leads to release of enzymes causing degeneration of intercellular space substances and destruction of the intercellular bridges. The result is loss of intercellular adhesion, and break down of the cohesion between neighboring cells, called acantholysis. Separation of epithelial cells occurs causing bullae, erythema, scaling, crusting, ulceration and tissue proliferation.

In **systemic lupus erythematosus** (SLE), tissue is damaged by a **type III hypersensitivity** reaction. **Circulating immune complexes** composed of IgG or IgM antibodies bound to antigens diffuse through the vascular endothelium into the tissues and **activate the complement cascade**. This stimulates migration of mononuclear cells and neutrophils into the area, producing vasculitis and tissue destruction.

- In SLE, damage to keratinocytes by **ultraviolet light** is thought to predispose to antibody formation.
- Damaged keratinocytes release various mediators, which potentiate the inflammatory response.

Clinical signs

Pruritus and pain are variable. Many cats with pemphigus or discoid lupus erythematosus (DLE) are otherwise healthy.

Pemphigus foliaceus presents as **erythematous macules or pustules.** The pustules are quite fragile and may be quite transient and develop to form **scale, crusts, erosions, epidermal collarettes** and later **alopecia**. Occasionally a positive Nikolsky sign may be present. This is considered positive if, when the edge of the lesion is rubbed, the skin is easily peeled/pushed off the underlying dermis.

Lesions are common on the **face, ears, feet, groin and nipples**, but may become generalized. Often the **feet lesions** present as a characteristic, **thick creamy/ cheesy exudate around the nail beds.**

Mucocutaneous and oral involvement are rare.

In **SLE,** lesions are extremely variable but may include **exfoliative erythroderma** (generalized **erythematous hue to the skin** along with generalized scale), **crusts and alopecia**. The **face, pinnae and feet** are commonly involved.

Lesions in **discoid lupus erythematosus** are similar to SLE, with the **face and pinnae** most commonly affected. Pedal involvement is uncommon.

Diagnosis

Cytology of pustular lesions of pemphigus may show **non-degenerate neutrophils** along with **rafts of acantholytic keratinocytes** (rounded up with a viable nucleus).

Histopathology is the procedure of choice for the diagnosis of pemphigus, however, it is not always diagnostic. Classically, lesions of **pemphigus foliaceus** will show **subcorneal pustules** with large numbers of **acantholytic keratinocytes,** and may be associated with non-degenerate neutrophils. **Discoid lupus erythematosus** classically shows a **superficial lichenoid inflammatory** infiltrate (lymphocytes, plasma cells), along with hydropic degeneration of the basal epithelial layer. **SLE** has a similar histopathologic picture as discoid lupus, except that the predominate inflammatory cell are **lymphocytes,** there may be **thickening of the basement membrane and vasculitis** may be associated with the inflammation.

Tests for **antinuclear antibody titers** in serum are recommended for diagnosing SLE. However, most published data relates to the dog and man.

Differential diagnosis

Differentials for **pemphigus** include **bacterial folliculitis, dermatophytosis, demodicosis** which are common, and discoid lupus and SLE which are much rarer.

Treatment and management

Immunosuppressive doses of prednisolone (2.2–4.4 mg/kg orally per day) until complete resolution is achieved. The dose may then be **gradually tapered,** reducing the dose by 25% per fortnight in a step-wise process. Cats that fail to respond to prednisolone may respond to **dexamethasone** (0.2–0.4 mg/kg q 24 h).

Chlorambucil (0.1–0.2 mg/kg q 24–48 h) has been additionally employed in difficult cases.

Gold therapy may be useful for refractory cases of pemphigus (aurothioglucose 1 mg/kg IM weekly until remission). After remission, the dose is reduced to q 14 days for 28 days and then to q 28 days for 3 months. Both chlorambucil and aurothioglucose may cause **bone marrow suppression,** and so **complete blood counts** should be **performed weekly** during the induction, then monthly whilst on therapy.

Insufficient data are currently available to make any recommendation on the use of cyclosporin in the management of feline pemphigus complex.

Cats with **discoid lupus erythematosus** may respond to **avoiding sunlight,** and application of **sun-screens or topical glucocorticoids.** If this is unsuccessful, **systemic medication** may be required. **Niacinamide** (nicotinamide or vitamin B3) in combination with **doxycycline** has been used in dogs (but not cats) with variable efficacy. Other alternatives are prednisolone, chlorambucil or aurothioglucose.

Cats with **SLE** require **systemic immunosuppressive therapy** (prednisolone, chlorambucil).

Prognosis

The long-term **prognosis for pemphigus complex and discoid lupus is generally good.**

The prognosis for **SLE** depends on the extent of other organ system involvement.

IDIOPATHIC MILIARY DERMATITIS

Classical signs

- Papulocrustous dermatitis.
- Pruritus.

Clinical signs

Pruritus and self-trauma occur, and are expressed as **licking or over-grooming rather than scratching**. This

results in alopecia, crust formation, miliary dermatitis and secondary infection.

Lesions occur mainly along the **dorsal, inguinal and ventral abdominal areas**.

Diagnosis

Diagnosis is based on clinical signs and exclusion of all other etiologies after extensive diagnostic work-up.

RECOMMENDED READING

Baker KP, Thomsett LR. Disorders associated with pathogens. In: Canine and Feline Dermatology. Oxford, UK, Blackwell Scientific Publications, 1990, pp. 95–171.

Foil CS. Dermatophytosis. In: Griffen CE, Kwochka KW, McDonald JM (eds) Current Veterinary Dermatology. Missouri, Mosby, 1993, pp. 22–33.

Gauguere E, Prelaud P. A Practical Guide to Feline Dermatology. Paris, Merial, 2001.

Moriello K, Mason I. Pruritus in cats. In: Handbook of Small Animal Dermatology. Oxford, Pergamon, 1995, pp. 153–162.

Pedersen NC. Viral diseases. Parasitic diseases. In: Feline Infectious Diseases. Goleta, CA., American Veterinary Publications Inc., 1988, pp. 11–15, 347–366.

Quinn PJ, Donnelly W, Carter ME, et al. Diseases of the skin. In: Microbial and Parasitic Diseases of the Dog and Cat. Philadelphia, PA, W.B. Saunders, 1997, pp. 292–340.

Rosenkrantz WS. Immune-mediated dermatoses. In: Griffen CE, Kwochka KW, McDonald JM (eds) Current Veterinary Dermatology. Missouri, Mosby, 1993, pp. 141–166.

Scott DW, Miller WH, Griffen CE. Immunologic skin diseases. In: Muller and Kirk's Small Animal Dermatology, 6th edn. Philadelphia, PA, W.B. Saunders, 2001.

49. The cat with pruritus without miliary dermatitis

*Ruadhri Michael Seosaimh Breathnach
and Mike Shipstone*

KEY SIGNS

- Licking or over-grooming.
- Alopecia, erythema.
- + Papules, plaques.

MECHANISM?

- Pruritus in cats usually manifests as licking or over-grooming, rather than scratching or self-trauma obvious to the owner. In many instances, owners are not aware that the cat is pruritic.

WHERE?

- Skin.

WHAT?

- Diseases presenting with pruritus without miliary dermatitis are most commonly eosinophilic plaques, poxvirus and neoplasia. However, all the differentials covered in Chapter 48 (The Cat With Miliary Dermatitis) should be considered for a cat that presents with pruritus, even if no miliary dermatitis pattern is evident.

QUICK REFERENCE SUMMARY

Diseases causing pruritus without miliary dermatitis

INFECTIOUS

Viral:

- **Feline orthopoxvirus infection** (p 1047)

Initial solitary lesion is commonly present on the head or neck. Numerous papules develop later. Ulceration and scab formation occurs. Alopecia and scarring are evident when the scabs fall off. Pruritic.

Parasitic:

- Demodicosis (p 1047)

Localized or generalized alopecia of the face and trunk. Erythema and scale. Periocular and nasal involvement is common. Most cases are non-pruritic.

continued

continued

Neoplastic:

● Cutaneous lymphoma (p 1049)

Presentation varies. Multiple erythematous nodules, ulcers or proliferative lesions. Exfoliative erythroderma with general flushing and scaling of skin. Lymphadenopathy and systemic illness may be present. Uncommon.

● Mast cell tumor (p 1050)

Single or multiple lesions which are usually benign. Papules and plaques are common. Poorly circumscribed dermal masses are possible. Head and neck are common sites. A papular form occurs in young Siamese on the head and ears and may spontaneously regress.

Miscellaneous:

● Contact dermatitis (p 1048)

Erythema and papules on affected surfaces. Pruritus leads to skin thickening and hyperpigmentation.

● **Eosinophilic plaques** (p 1046)**

Well-circumscribed plaques, which often ulcerate. Common on the abdomen and medial thighs. Very pruritic.

INTRODUCTION

MECHANISM?

Pruritus is not as common a presentation in feline practice as compared to the situation in the dog. That is not to say that the problem is unusual, rather it points to the fact that feline pruritus may manifest in ways other than scratching, or self-trauma, which is immediately obvious to the owner. In many instances, owners are not aware that the cat is pruritic. The cat may be presented with a complaint of excessive licking, alopecia or miliary dermatitis.

WHERE?

Skin.

WHAT?

The list of differential diagnoses for pruritus in cats is long. Most cases are due to **infectious agents** such as microbes and ectoparasites, or **hypersensitivities**. As miliary dermatitis is frequently associated with pruritus, all of the differentials covered in Chapter 48 (The Cat With Miliary Dermatitis) should be considered for the animal that presents with pruritus, even if no miliary dermatitis pattern is clinically evident. This chapter lists some additional conditions, which may also present with pruritus and are less likely to have miliary dermatitis.

DISEASES CAUSING PRURITUS WITHOUT MILIARY DERMATITIS

EOSINOPHILIC PLAQUES**

> **Classical signs**
>
> ● Raised "glistening" plaques, well circumscribed and often ulcerative.
> ● Pruritus.
> ● Regional lymphadenopathy possible.

Clinical signs

Eosinophilic plaques are usually multiple, raised, round to oval lesions, often several centimeters in diameter. Common sites include the **abdomen, medial thighs and mucocutaneous junctions**.

Frequently there is ulceration and serum oozing from the lesion, which may give the classic "**glistening**" **appearance to the lesion.**

The lesions are generally **markedly pruritic**, evidenced by **licking and trauma** to the area.

Regional lymphadenopathy and **secondary infection** are sometimes present.

Affected cats may also exhibit **indolent ulcers, eosinophilic granulomas or ocular lesions**.

Diagnosis

Diagnosis is via biopsy and demonstration of the **characteristic histopathology** consisting of markedly **thickened epidermis with spongiosis and eosinophil infiltration**, which may also extend to affect the follicular epithelium. Erosions may be present.

Peripheral blood eosinophilia may be present.

Intercellular immunoglobulin is frequently found within the epidermis; however, this should not be mistaken for an autoimmune skin disease.

FELINE ORTHOPOXVIRUS INFECTION**

Classical signs

- Initial single lesion around head or neck.
- Numerous papules develop later, and frequently erode or ulcerate.
- Scab formation. When scabs fall off, alopecia and scarring evident.
- Pruritus and secondary infection.

Clinical signs

Orthopox virus is more common in **young to middle-aged cats.**

The **initial lesion** is a **macular eruption** (5 mm diameter), which rapidly progresses to a **non-healing ulcer** with a raised indurated border on the head, neck or forelimbs.

Eroded or ulcerated papules, which **scab** over, **appear in several sites.**

When the scabs fall off, areas of **alopecia and scarring** are evident. These lesions gradually heal. As some lesions heal, new lesions may also develop.

Pruritus is variable, but may be present at all stages.

New hair growth takes 6–8 weeks.

Secondary infection, abscesses or cellulitis are possible.

Vesicular to ulceroproliferative **lesions may develop in the mouth, pharynx, conjunctiva and on the muzzle.**

Many cats are **systemically ill** with mild pyrexia, inappetence and depression, particularly during the viremic stage.

Diagnosis

Diagnosis is based on biopsy demonstrating **intracytoplasmic inclusion bodies** (types A or B). Healing lesions may be negative for inclusion bodies.

Electron microscopic examination of an unfixed scab or biopsy material can identify orthopoxvirus particles. Immunohistochemical techniques can also be performed on skin biopsies.

Viral isolation techniques are available in specialist laboratories.

Serological tests are available at certain laboratories.

DEMODICOSIS

Classical signs

- Localized/generalized alopecia of face and body trunk.
- Erythema and scaliness. Secondary infection.
- Periocular and nasal involvement is particularly common.

Pathogenesis

Whilst **most normal animals** have a **low mite burden** probably derived from maternal transmission, cats with clinical demodicosis have a **proliferation in mite numbers.**

Immunosuppression appears to be an **important factor,** and has been associated with diabetes mellitus, FeLV and FIV infections, hyperadrenocorticism and systemic lupus erythematosus.

A genetic predisposition has not been reported in cats.

In cats, there are two species of democid mites that are recognized to cause disease.

Demodex cati inhabits **hair follicles and sebaceous glands.** *Demodex gatoi* appears to replicate within pits of the **stratum corneum**. The clinical significance of a third, as yet unnamed species, is currently unknown.

The **proliferation of mites** leads to damage to hair shafts, folliculitis and **follicular disruption.**

Clinical signs

D. cati causes disease which is **variably pruritic,** consisting of **patchy erythema, scale, crust** and **alopecia,** more commonly seen affecting the **eyelids, periocular area, head and neck** although generalized disease may also develop.

Pruritus is not a dominant feature in most cases.

Secondary infection is possible, particularly if there is significant self-trauma.

D. gatoi causes signs that are more consistent with **allergic skin disease,** including **severe pruritus, alopecia, scale, crust and excoriation,** particularly on the **head, neck and elbows.** Some cats may develop more generalized disease.

Diagnosis

Diagnosis is based on clinical signs and **demonstration of the mites via skin scrapes.** Superficial scrapes are sufficient for *D. gatoi*; however *D. cati* requires deeper scrapings. Squeeze the affected area, apply a small amount of mineral oil to the skin and scrape using a blunt scalpel blade until capillary oozing is present.

Biopsy may also be used to demonstrate mites.

Differential diagnosis

Differential diagnoses which should be considered for *D. gatoi* include **hypersensitivities (atopy, food, flea), contact dermatitis and psychogenic causes**. Careful skin scrapings should be performed, followed by therapeutic trial (e.g. lime-sulfur weekly for 4–8 weeks). If there is no response to a treatment trial, then a food elimination trial and other diagnostic tests should be performed.

Treatment

Lime-sulfur baths (once/week for 4–8 weeks) are safe and effective. This agent has sometimes been combined with **phosmet.**

Amitraz (0.0125–0.0250%) applied topically once a week for 6–8 weeks is effective, although clinicians should beware of toxicity.

Efficacy of ivermectin in feline demodicosis is unclear.

D. gatoi is contagious, so **all in-contact cats should be treated simultaneously**.

Address any underlying immunosuppressive disease.

Prognosis

Spontaneous remission is possible in **some younger animals** after weeks to months.

However, in many cats signs persist and may worsen over time. The prognosis is affected by underlying disease conditions that cannot be rectified, e.g. FIV or FeLV infection.

Prevention

Avoid stress and treat potentially immunosuppressive diseases (diabetes mellitus, hyperadrenocortism).

There is no evidence to currently support the exclusion of clinically affected animals from a breeding program, although such an approach may be judicious.

CONTACT DERMATITIS

> **Classical signs**
> - Erythema and papules on contact surfaces.
> - Pruritus and secondary infection.
> - Skin thickening and hyperpigmentation.
> - Severe cases may develop ulceration.

Pathogenesis

Irritant contact dermatitis is more common than contact allergic dermatitis.

Primary irritant contact dermatitis causes an inflammatory response in the majority of exposed cats. No prior sensitization is required.

Allergic contact dermatitis is an **immunologic response** to a hapten. Haptens are small chemically reactive compounds that must bind to a protein before becoming a complete antigen. The initial phase of the hypersensitivity is the afferent phase during which time the immune system is sensitized. Experimentally this may be as little as 3–5 weeks, although it is much longer in naturally occurring cases (> 2 years in > 70% of cases). Subsequent exposure in a sensitized animal leads to the development of the efferent (or elicitation) phase, during which time a gross clinical lesion develops.

Whilst a delayed-type hypersensitive reaction has traditionally been suspected, recent studies have shown this may not be the case.

Clinical signs

Initial lesions may present as **erythema, macules and papules**. Chronically, alopecia, hyperpigmentation, lichenification, excoriation may develop.

Lesions are initially confined to the **hairless (or sparsely haired) contact areas** including **ventral abdomen, thorax, scrotum, lips, point of chin, concave aspect of pinnae.** However, the lesions may be widespread for an agent applied over most of the body, e.g. shampoo.

Irritant contact dermatitis may occur as a **single episode**, whereas **contact allergic dermatitis** often has repeat episodes.

Diagnosis

Irritant contact dermatitis is often initially suspected on the basis of **clinical signs and history** of acute exposure to an irritant compound.

Response to symptomatic therapy and avoidance is helpful in supporting the diagnosis.

Provocative exposure is possible, but often unnecessary.

In the case of contact allergic dermatitis, the diagnosis may be confirmed by **provocative exposure or patch testing.**

Close patch testing may be performed by applying the suspected allergen(s) to the skin, and then applying a body bandage to secure the site. This is removed after 48 hours and the site examined for the presence of erythema and edema at 72 and 96 hours.

Biopsy is non-specific.

Differential diagnosis

Other hypersensitive, ectoparasitic and psychogenic skin conditions should be considered.

Whilst the lesions and clinical signs may be similar, generally it is possible to differentiate on the basis of the **lesion distribution** limited to hairless areas, **history of exposure** and **response to provocative exposure and patch testing.**

Treatment

Treatment involves **avoiding the suspect irritant or allergen**. If this is not possible, some form of symptomatic therapy will be required as long as exposure to the irritant/ allergen continues.

Glucocorticoids (topical or systemic). In some instances **topical cortisone** creams may be sufficient. If not, then **oral prednisolone** may be used (2 mg/kg q 24 h for 5 days, then 1 mg/kg q 48 h as required).

Symptomatic therapy, if appropriate.

Mild, non-medicated cleansing shampoos may be used to remove irritant chemicals.

Prognosis

Prognosis is excellent, if avoidance possible.

If not, then judicious glucocorticoid medication is indicated.

Prevention

Try to avoid any offending irritants or allergens.

CUTANEOUS LYMPHOMA

Classical signs

- Presentation varies with tumor type.
- Non-epitheliotropic forms exhibit multiple erythematous nodules, with occasional exfoliative erythroderma.
- Epitheliotropic forms exhibit exfoliative erythroderma, plaques/nodules, ulcers or proliferative lesions.
- Lymphadenopathy occurs in epitheliotropic cases.

Clinical signs

Clinical signs vary markedly.

Non-epitheliotropic forms commonly present as **multiple, solid erythematous nodules**, dermal or subcutaneous in position.

Exfoliative erythroderma seen as **generalized flushing** of the skin with excess scale formation. **Arciform (semicircular) or solitary lesions** are less common.

Epitheliotropic forms commonly present in the later stages as one or a combination of the following: exfoliative erythroderma, ulcers and depigmentation at mucocutaneous sites, multiple plaques or nodules.

Ulcerative or proliferative **oral lesions** are possible.

Generalized lymphadenopathy may be present in many epitheliotropic cases.

Earlier lesions include focal alopecia, erythroderma and scale.

Signs of systemic illness may be present, and include **inappetence, lethargy and depression**.

Diagnosis

Diagnosis is based on **characteristic histopathology**.

Direct immunofluorescence testing may reveal deposition of immunoglobulin in the affected cells. This should not be mistaken for a diagnosis of pemphigus complex.

MAST CELL TUMOR

Classical signs

- Lesions are very variable from single or multiple lesions, well-circumscribed papules and plaques to poorly circumscribed multiple dermal masses.
- Head and neck common sites.

Clinical signs

Lesions are most commonly reported around the **head and neck.**

Four different presentations are recognized:
- **Multiple poorly demarcated masses** (up to 5 cm in diameter), which are often edematous and fixed to the skin.
- **Smaller (2–10 mm) multiple, well-circumscribed papules** which are solid and light in color.
- A **plaque-type form** (1–7 cm), which is erythematous, firm, raised and well circumscribed. These plaques are **generally pruritic** and may **ulcerate**.
- Solitary, often alopecic, well-circumscribed, variably sized (3–30 mm), **dermal nodules** are occasionally seen.
  - A **papular form** on the **head and ears** of **young Siamese cats** (6 weeks to 4 years) which may spontaneously regress.

Diagnosis

Diagnosis is based on **characteristic histopathology**.

Stained impression smears and tissue aspirates are often diagnostic.

Electron microscopy is often required for rarer forms.

Treatment

Surgical excision is the treatment of choice for **solitary lesions** that cause difficulties.

In **disseminated forms, prednisolone** (0.5 mg/kg sid) may be used.

The majority of these tumors in the cat are **not malignant,** and so chemotherapeutic and radiotherapeutic measures are often unnecessary. However, a metastatic rate of up to 22% has been reported in one study.

The rare papular form in Siamese cats often spontaneously regresses.

RECOMMENDED READING

Baker KP, Thomsett LR. Disorders associated with pathogens. In: Canine and Feline Dermatology. Oxford, GB, Blackwell Scientific Publications, 1990, pp. 95–171.

Moriello K, Mason I. Pruritus in cats. In: Handbook of Small Animal Dermatology: Oxford, GB, Pergamon, 1995, pp. 153–162.

Pedersen NC. Viral diseases. Parasitic diseases. In: Feline Infectious Diseases. Goleta, CA., American Veterinary Publications Inc., 1988, pp. 11–15, 347–366.

Quinn PJ, Donnelly W, Carter ME, et al. Diseases of the skin. In: Microbial and Parasitic Diseases of the Dog and Cat. Philadelphia, PA, W.B. Saunders, 1997, pp. 292–340.

Scott DW, Miller WH, Griffen CE. Immunologic skin diseases. In: Muller and Kirk's Small Animal Dermatology, 6th edn. Philadelphia, PA, W.B. Saunders, 2001.

50. The cat with alopecia

Ruadhri Michael Seosaimh Breathnach and Mike Shipstone

KEY SIGNS

- Partial or complete loss of hair.

MECHANISM?

- Alopecia is the loss or absence of hairs from areas of the body that would normally possess hairs.
- The most common mechanism is the excessive loss from over-grooming because of pruritus. The characteristic feature of this mechanism is the presence of damaged/fractured ends to the remaining hair shafts in the area of alopecia.

WHERE?

- Skin.

WHAT?

- Numerous pruritic conditions, most commonly allergic in origin, lead to alopecia from self-trauma. Occasionally self-trauma can also arise for psychogenic reasons. Non-pruritic causes may be congenital or hormonal in etiology, with hyperthyroidism and diabetes mellitus most common. Folliculitis is seen with microbial or ectoparasitic infections, leading to non-pruritic loss of hair.

QUICK REFERENCE SUMMARY
Diseases causing alopecia

PRURITIC CAUSES OF ALOPECIA

INFLAMMATORY

- Allergic (p 1030)

If fractured or cropped hairs are present in the affected areas, pruritus is the most likely cause. See Chapter 48 (The Cat With Miliary Dermatitis or Pruritus).

NON-PRURITIC CAUSES OF ALOPECIA

FAILURE OF NORMAL HAIR PRODUCTION

ANOMALY

● **Congenital/genetic alopecia** (p 1055)**

Focal or generalized alopecia seen at birth or in first months of life. Alopecia may be pathologic, or result from an intentional breeding program where it is not viewed as abnormal, for example perauricular alopecia in some Siamese cats and generalized alopecia of Sphinx cats.

● Pili torti (p 1062)

Generalized alopecia which can also involve the feet and eye regions resulting in pedal dermatitis and paronychia. Many affected kittens die.

LOSS OF EXISTING HAIRS

METABOLIC

● Hyperadrenocorticism (p 1063)

Alopecia and an unkempt coat. Thin and fragile skin. Secondary infection and comedones possible. Systemic signs often present.

● **Hyperthyroidism** (p 1058)**

Systemic signs are present in most cats and include polyphagia, weight loss, restlessness, tachycardia and/or intermittent vomiting or diarrhea. Cutaneous signs occur in 30% of cats and include dry or greasy seborrhea, matting of the coat, focal or regional alopecia and thinning of the skin. Symmetrical alopecia is occasionally seen.

● **Diabetes mellitus** (p 1059)**

Polydipsia, polyuria, weight loss and polyphagia or inappetence are typically present. A poorly groomed seborrheic coat is common with generalized fine dry scale, and thinning of the skin. Symmetrical alopecia on abdomen, perineum or groin regions may be present. Secondary bacterial or fungal infections are sometimes present.

● Telogen defluxion (p 1062)

Gradual alopecia affecting part or all of the body several months after a stressful event. Rest of skin appears normal.

NUTRITION

● Dietary alopecia (p 1065)

Patchy or generalized alopecia. Seborrhea and poor coat quality. Secondary infections are possible.

NEOPLASTIC

● Alopecia mucinosa (p 1065)

Alopecia and excess scale of the head, neck and ears. Plaque-type lesions may develop later and have histological findings consistent with lymphoma or mycosis fungoides. Very rare disease.

PSYCHOLOGIC

● **Psychogenic** (p 1056)**

Loss of hair from excessive grooming commonly affects the abdomen, thighs, inguinal region, forelegs or dorsal spinal region. Hairs appear broken and uneven, and the coat can feel rough.

continued

continued

Affected skin may become thickened and hyperpigmented. An environmental stressor may be identified in the history.

INFLAMMATION/INFECTION:

Bacterial:

● **Staphylococcal dermatitis* (p 1064)**
Primary staphylococcal dermatitis is uncommon in cats, and an underlying disease process should be suspected. Typically there is erythema, scale and crustiness. Hair follicles are commonly involved. Papules are common, but rarely is pus present.

Fungal:

● **Dermatophytosis** (p 1060)**
More common in young kittens. Erythematous plaques, alopecia and scale. Lesions may progress to larger gray areas of alopecia and hyperkeratosis.

Parasitic:

● **Demodicosis* (p 1061)**
Localized or generalized alopecia of face and trunk. Periocular and nasal involvement are most common. Lesions have erythema and scale. Most cases are non-pruritic.

Immune:

● Alopecia areata (p 1066)
Focal or multi-focal alopecia which is gradual in onset, and not symmetrical. The skin is not inflamed and there is no pruritus. Hyperpigmentation may occur chronically. Rare.

Toxic/drug

● **Drug reaction* (p 1061)**
Usually associated with immunosuppressive or anti-neoplastic agents. Alopecia is most common on the body trunk, but can affect other sites. Secondary infection is often present. Glucocorticoids may produce cutaneous signs of hyperadrenocorticism.

INTRODUCTION

MECHANISM?

Alopecia is the loss or absence of hairs from areas of the cat's body that would normally possess hairs.

● This phenomenon can result either from a **failure to grow hair** or as a consequence of the **abnormal loss** of hairs.

Some causes of alopecia are **genetically programmed**. **Acquired cases** may arise because of **hormonal** influences that interfere with hair growth, or as a result of **folliculitis.** Hairs may also be lost as a direct result of **self-trauma** for a variety of reasons.

● Failure to grow hair **may be a life-long problem**, as occurs in congenital or genetically programmed alopecias.

Abnormal hair loss has a wide variety of causes, and is **normally divided** clinically into those cases which are accompanied by pruritus and those which are not. The majority of cases seen in feline practice are due to self-trauma as a consequence of pruritus.

The **breakage of hair shafts** may occur in dermatophytosis and psychogenic dermatoses.

Cessation of hair growth may arise due to endocrinopathies, telogen defluxion and drug reactions.

Hairs may also be shed following an episode of folliculitis.

Rare causes of feline alopecia include pancreatic neoplasia.

Some conditions give rise to specific **focal alopecia**, often in association with underlying skin pathology, such as injection reactions, solar dermatitis or squamous cell carcinoma.

The term **feline symmetrical alopecia** (FSA) represents a cutaneous reaction pattern, rather than a distinct syndrome.
- It is characterized by a seemingly **non-pruritic, symmetrical alopecia affecting the abdomen, caudo-medial thighs, proximal tail and perineum.** Affected hairs are easily epilated and no inflammatory changes are usually present in the skin.
- Most, if not all, such cases are the result of **pruritus or self-trauma due to an underlying problem**, and are not related to sex steroids or other hormones.
- Feline symmetrical alopecia is not included as a distinct condition in this chapter. Rather the clinician is encouraged to investigate such cases to see if an underlying etiology such as **flea allergic dermatitis or psychogenic factors** can be identified.
- If no such cause can be found, then the term idiopathic feline symmetrical alopecia may be used.

The histologic appearance of the hair follicle varies with the stage of the follicle's growth cycle. **Anagen** is the active growth phase and is characterized by a well-developed hair follicle bulb. **Catagen** is a transition period between the active growth and resting stage. **Telogen** is the resting stage, characterized by a small dermal papilla, separate from the bulb, absence of an inner root sheath and a club or brush-like hair.

WHERE?

The abnormal organ is **skin**, but it may be affected secondarily by disease of other body systems.

Alopecia can affect any part of the body, although certain conditions tend to cause hair loss in characteristic areas.

The hair loss may be **partial or complete, focal or generalized.**

WHAT?

Numerous pruritic conditions lead to **alopecia from self-trauma. Allergic diseases** are the most common and are covered in the chapters on Miliary dermatitis and Pruritus.
- Self-trauma can also arise for **psychogenic reasons**.
- Folliculitis is seen with **microbial or ectoparasitic infections.**

Non-pruritic alopecia can be **congenital or acquired**.
- Congenital alopecia often arises because of intentional breeding programs and is considered normal for the breed.
- **Hormonal causes** of acquired alopecia include **diabetes mellitus, hyperthyroidism and hyperadrenocorticism.**

DISEASES CAUSING NON-PRURITIC ALOPECIA

CONGENITAL/GENETIC ALOPECIA**

Classical signs
- Focal or generalized alopecia or thin hair coat present at birth.
- Further hair loss may occur in the first few months of life.
- Excessive sebum or wrinkling of the skin.
- Often breed specific and considered normal.

Pathogenesis

Congenital alopecia has been reported in Sphinx cats with affected individuals being the result of an intentional breeding program involving cats with a spontaneous mutation.

Animals born with congenital alopecias may possess additional ectodermal defects.

The mode of inheritance involves a monogenic recessive trait. However, in Russian hairless cats, the alopecia is determined by a semi-dominant gene with the participation of other genes.

Congenital hypotrichosis has been reported in several breeds including Burmese, Devon Rex, Cornish Rex, Siamese and Birman cats. The condition is inherited as an autosomal recessive trait in Birman and Siamese cats.

Although several kittens in the one litter may be affected, no sex predisposition has been reported.

Skin pathology can vary from hypoplasia to complete absence of hair follicles and related adnexal structures.

Clinical signs

Clinical signs vary with the specific condition and the breed involved. Alopecia or thin hair coat is **present at birth. Further hair loss** may occur in the **first few months of life.**

Depending on the syndrome, there may be an absence of primary hairs.

Congenital alopecia may be **pathologic**, but is more often the **result of an intentional breeding program**, and is not viewed as abnormal by the owner.

Alopecia may be regional or focal, for example preauricular alopecia seen in some Siamese cats.

A more **generalized alopecia** known as feline alopecia universalis is seen in Sphinx cats. These cats have no primary hairs and no whiskers.

- **Excess sebum** is commonly present on the skin due to an abnormal opening of the sebaceous glands onto the skin surface.
- Poor grooming habits frequently lead to poor skin hygiene.

Devon and Cornish Rex cats, Siamese, Burmese and Birmans can exhibit **hypotrichosis.** The hair coat appears to be quite sparse so that the underlying skin is more visible. This is the result of selective breeding. Many kittens in a litter can be involved.

- The hair coat can be deficient or totally absent at birth. Any hair initially present can be lost in the first months of life.
- Excessive wrinkling of the skin occurs in these kittens.
- Affected Burmese kittens also lack whiskers and claws.

Diagnosis

Diagnosis is often possible on the basis of the breeding history and clinical signs.

Histopathology of affected skin can provide additional diagnostic information.

Treatment

Mild anti-seborrheic shampoos (containing sulfur, salicylic acid) may be required intermittently in Sphinx cats to remove the excess sebum accumulation.

Owners should also be warned to minimize UV exposure in cats with non-pigmented skin, so that cumulative actinic damage is avoided later in life.

PSYCHOGENIC**

> ### Classical signs
>
> - Loss of hair commonly affecting the abdomen, thighs, inguinal region, forelegs or dorsal spinal region.
> - Hairs appear broken and uneven and the coat can feel rough.
> - Affected skin may become thickened and hyperpigmented.

Pathogenesis

The main reason for the alopecia is **excessive or inappropriate grooming behavior**.

Most cases are presumed to have an **underlying psychological component**.

Various stressful factors can be involved including a new pet, change of home or routine, or competition from a dominant animal.

The action of licking/chewing is postulated to stimulate release of ACTH and MSH. This in turn can lead to an increase in endorphin production.

- Endorphins help to reduce stress, but may reinforce the behavior pattern.

Some cats concentrate on a particular area, and lick or chew incessantly at that site. This can lead to significant lesion development.

Other cats may have milder signs or the excessive licking/chewing may be concentrated over a much wider area.

Excessive grooming, etc. may not actually be noticed by the owner, as many cats are secret groomers.

Clinical signs

Hair loss is typically concentrated on the areas of the body where the cat can access to lick or chew.

The ventral abdomen, inguinal region, inner thighs and inner aspects of the forelegs are common sites.

Some cats concentrate on the dorsal spinal region, particularly in the lumbar and sacral/tail areas.

The licking/chewing behavior leads to fracture of the hair shafts, roughening of the coat and alopecia.

Some cats develop an inflammatory pattern, characterized by red plaques.

The alopecia may be symmetrical in some cases.

Long-standing cases develop thickening and hyperpigmentation of the affected sites.

Diagnosis

A tentative diagnosis is based on clinical signs and excluding other causes of alopecia. A definitive diagnosis is rarely possible.

A detailed history should be taken to try and elucidate any cause of stress or anxiety. If one cannot be identified, it does not rule out a diagnosis of psychogenic alopecia.

Even if the owner has not noticed excessive grooming behaviour, facts such as tufts of hair in the animal's bed or the vomiting up of hairballs are suspicious. Videotaping of cats in the cattery may reveal evidence of self-grooming.

Clinical examination reveals short, broken hairs, often with roughened ends. The hairs are not easily epilated.

- A trichogram reveals broken tips to the hairs and may also demonstrate that some of the hairs were in anagen.

All the other differentials for alopecia need to be ruled out. Thus a basic work-up consisting of skin scrapings, fungal culture etc. is normally warranted. Flea dermatitis and flea allergic dermatitis are particularly important differentials.

Biopsy is non-diagnostic, but may help to rule-out many other differentials.

Placing an Elizabethan collar on the cat for a period of weeks will often lead to a significant re-growth of hair in affected areas.

Differential diagnosis

Alopecia can be caused by all the conditions listed in this chapter. Exogenous administration of progestogens or glucocorticoids should also be excluded, as should dietary causes. Ectoparasites also need to be excluded, particularly fleas. Diabetes mellitus, hyperadrenocorticism and hyperthyroidism can produce similar alopecia but systemic signs are present.

Treatment

Try to remove or ameliorate any stressful factors that may be acting as the underlying cause.

An Elizabethan collar will often give a clinical improvement. However, it does not properly address the issue and is resented by many cats.

In cases that warrant such an approach, medical therapy may be attempted. Phenobarbitone (2–6 mg/kg orally bid) and diazepam (1–2 mg/cat orally sid or bid) have both been employed.

Naloxone, an endorphin blocker, has been used successfully at a dosage rate of 1 mg/kg subcutaneously every few weeks.

Clomipramine and various progestogens have also been reported to be somewhat effective.

Some of the above medications are not licensed for use in cats in many countries.

Prognosis

The prognosis depends totally on **whether the inciting cause can be identified and resolved**.

If not, then long-term management, sometimes involving drug therapy is generally required.

HYPERTHYROIDISM**

> **Classical signs**
>
> - Systemic signs including polyphagia, weight loss, restlessness, tachycardia.
> - Dry, greasy, seborrheic or matted coat.
> - Focal or regional alopecia or shedding of the coat.
> - Overgrown nails.

See main reference on page 304 (The Cat With Weight Loss and a Good Appetite).

Clinical signs

Hyperthyroidism occurs mainly in **older cats** (> 8 years of age).

The majority of cats have **systemic signs including polyphagia, weight loss, restlessness, tachycardia and/or intermittent vomiting or diarrhea.**

Approximately **30%** of cats with hyperthyroidism **exhibit cutaneous manifestations.**

Often there is excessive matting of the hair coat, and the cat may groom excessively.

A dry coat, or dry or greasy seborrhea may be present.

Alopecia, when present, may be patchy, regional or generalized, and in some cases may appear symmetrical.
- The major site affected by alopecia is the **body trunk.**

Thinning of the skin (or loss of skin elasticity) is a common finding.

Excessive rates of nail growth may give rise to **overgrown claws**.

Diagnosis

A tentative diagnosis is based on **age, history and clinical signs**.

An **enlarged gland or thyroid nodule** may be palpable.

Various abnormalities may be encountered on routine hematological and biochemical analysis.
- These commonly include increases in serum ALP, AST, LDH and blood urea concentrations.
- Changes on hematology are variable and unreliable.
- A mature neutrophilia, or an eosinophilia, are sometimes present.

Cardiac abnormalities may be detected on ECG and echocardiography.

A definitive diagnosis is based on finding an increased basal thyroxine (**TT4**) concentration in blood.

As not all hyperthyroid cats will exhibit elevated values for basal thyroxine, measurement of free thyroxine, a triiodothyronine (T3) suppression test or TRH stimulation test may be necessary. Further testing should only be performed if signs are consistent with hyperthyroidism, and thyroxine concentration is in the top half of the reference range.
- **Free thyroxine** must be measured with a validated feline assay using equilibrium dialysis, and if available, is the easiest test to use in cats with clinical signs consistent with hyperthyroidism but thyroxine concentration does not exceed the upper limit of the reference range.
- In the **T3 suppression test**, thyroxine and T3 concentration are measured before and 3 hours after the administration of seven doses of 20 µg of liothyronine sodium (T3) at intervals of 8 hours. Euthyroid cats will exhibit a significant drop in thyroxine concentration (approximately 50%) after T3 administration, and a significant rise in total T3 concentration. Hyperthyroid cats will have no significant inhibition.
- In the **TRH stimulation test,** thyroxine concentration is measured before and approximately 4 hours after the intravenous administration of 0.1 mg/kg of TRH. Hyperthyroid cats exhibit no significant stimulation of thyroxine concentration

(< 50% increase in concentration) following TRH administration, whereas euthyroid cats or cats with non-thyroidal illness show a more significant increase (>60%).

Radionuclide thyroid scanning is available in certain specialist referral centers.

Differential diagnosis

Alopecia can be caused by all the conditions listed in this chapter. However, as most cats presenting with this complaint will have a combination of systemic and cutaneous signs, the major differentials would be **hyperadrenocorticism and diabetes mellitus**. Exogenous administration of progestogens or glucocorticoids should also be excluded.

Treatment

Medical treatment may be attempted using either carbimazole or its metabolite, methimazole. Carbimazole is generally given at a dosage rate of 5 mg/cat q 8 h until the cat is euthyroid. Once euthyroid, the frequency of administration may be reduced to twice daily. Carbimazole has also been used prior to surgery.

Surgery can be performed in many cases **to remove the hyperplastic or neoplastic tissue.** The effects of hyperthyroidism on other tissues increase the anesthetic risk.

- If a nodule can be felt on one side of the gland only, some veterinarians prefer to remove just that one lobe. Others choose to remove the gland in its entirety and may supplement the cat with exogenous thyroid hormones. If all four parathyroid glands are also removed, supplementation with calcium and vitamin D is required. Severe life-threatening hypocalcemia can occur rapidly after surgery and needs intensive monitoring and treatment.

Radioactive iodine therapy can be employed in certain referral establishments. The hyperfunctional thyroid cells concentrate the radioactive iodine, whilst surrounding normal tissue receives a much smaller dose. This technique is simple and effective in many cats.

DIABETES MELLITUS**

> ### Classical signs
>
> - Polydipsia, polyuria, weight loss and polyphagia or inappetence.
> - Plantigrade stance.
> - Scurfy seborrheic haircoat.
> - Symmetrical alopecia of the groin, perineum, abdomen and hindlimbs.

Clinical signs

Polydipsia, polyuria, weight loss and polyphagia or inappetence are typically present. Cutaneous manifestations are less obvious.

A **poorly groomed seborrheic** coat is commonly present. It is most commonly a **dry scurfy seborrhea.**

Alopecia involving the **groin, perineum, lateral abdomen and hindlimbs** is occasionally present, and may or may not be symmetrical.

A few cats with diabetes mellitus also have underlying hyperadrenocorticism, which may be responsible for some of the cutaneous signs.

The **skin appears thin and hypotonic**, which may be from hyperadrenocorticism or protein catabolism as a result of the failure to properly utilize glucose.

Secondary bacterial and fungal skin infections may occur because the immune system is compromised.
- Staphylococcal dermatitis, *Candida* spp. infections and dermatophytosis have all been reported.

A rare skin manifestation is the presence of **xanthomas.** These are benign, granulomatous lesions associated with abnormal lipid metabolism.

Diagnosis

A tentative diagnosis is based on **history, clinical signs and glycosuria,** with or without ketonuria.

Definitive diagnosis is confirmed by documenting **persistent fasting hyperglycemia** (blood glucose > 12 mmol/L).

Routine biochemical analysis may demonstrate increased hepatic enzymes, cholesterol and triglyceride concentrations. Electrolyte abnormalities (sodium and potassium) may also be present.

Radiology and ultrasonography usually reveal **hepatomegaly**.

Demonstrating **increased fructosamine** concentration is useful to confirm that hyperglycemia is persistent and not transient. The normal fructosamine concentration in the cat is 175–400 µmol/L.

DERMATOPHYTOSIS**

Classical signs

- More often in young kittens, rather than adults.
- Erythematous plaques, alopecia and scale.
- Lesions progress to larger grayish areas of alopecia and hyperkeratosis.

Pathogenesis

In cats, **94–98% of cases are caused by *Microsporum canis*.** Occasionally lesions are caused by *Trichophyton mentagrophytes* or *Trichophyton terrestre*, but *Microsporum gypseum* is rare.

The prevalence of dermatophytosis **varies with the climate and the natural reservoirs**. In a hot, humid climate, a higher incidence is observed than in a cold, dry climate. The mere presence of a dermatophyte spore is generally insufficient to cause infection and clinical disease. Transmission occurs via contact with an infected particle. In the case of **M. canis,** this occurs via contact with an **infected animal or environment.** Infection with *M. gypseum* is via exposure to **spores in soil**, and *Trichophyton* infection occurs via contact with rodents (usually asymptomatic carriers), horses, cattle or a contaminated environment.

A **minimum number of spores** is required for infection along with **other factors** that allow an infection to develop.

These factors include: **grooming behavior** (provides mechanical removal of the spores), presence of **microtrauma on the skin** which allows invasion, increased **hydration and maceration** of the skin also increases probability of infection establishing. The **immune competence** of the host is extremely important.

Recovery from infection requires a strong cell-mediated immune response. Anti-dermatophyte antibodies do not provide protection, and a failure to form a strong cellular response may be the cause of chronic infection or tolerance in some cats. Concurrent **immunosuppressive drug therapy**, **compromised immune status**, poor nutrition, stress and the presence of intercurrent disease, e.g. multiple-cat environment with poor health care (strays) with endemic infections (FIV/FeLV) may facilitate transmission.

Clinical signs

Skin fungal infections are more commonly seen in **young kittens, rather than adults.**

Initial lesions are commonly present on the face, head and feet. Large areas of the body can be involved.

Raised, erythematous plaques may develop, and are accompanied by scaling.

Alopecia develops and lesions expand to form larger plaques, which appear grayish and hyperkeratotic. Erythema may still be a feature.

Initial hair loss tends to be in the **center of the lesion**. Hairs on the periphery appear discolored and brittle. As lesions regress, initial hair re-growth appears in the center of the alopecic areas.

Secondary bacterial infection is commonly seen. Infection may involve the whiskers or nail beds, with resultant deformities.

Infection of deeper tissues may result in **nodular skin lesions.**

Infection may be sub-clinical or mild, and easily overlooked.

Diagnosis

A **tentative diagnosis** is based on **clinical signs. Definitive diagnosis** is based on **skin scrapings, hair plucks and fungal culture**.

Fluorescence under ultraviolet light (Wood's lamp), may detect approximately half the cases of *M. canis* infections in cats.

Skin scrapings and hair plucks may be examined microscopically for the presence of spores or hyphae.

Fungal culture of scrapings, hair plucks and nail samples can identify the precise species of dermatophyte involved, but is time-consuming.

Biopsy of affected tissue may confirm a diagnosis. Special stains may be required.

DEMODICOSIS*

Classical signs

- Non-pruritic alopecia typically periocular and nasal.
- Erythema and scaliness are often present.

Clinical signs

Most cases exhibit **focal, partial alopecia particularly in the region of the eyes, nose and ears.** Lesions may also develop on the chin, thorax, abdomen, inner thighs, flanks and perineum.

Mild erythema, scale and occasional papules.

The alopecia may become more generalized in some cases.

Hyperpigmentation and bilaterally symmetrical alopecia may develop.

Secondary infection and a crusting dermatitis may be seen. Pruritus is not a dominant feature in the majority of cases.

Diagnosis

A **definitive diagnosis** is based on identifying *Demodex* **species mites** in skin scrapings. Superficial scrapes are normally sufficient for detecting *D. gatoi* and the other unnamed species in the epidermis. *D. cati*, on the other hand, requires deeper scrapings.

Mites may also be detected on biopsy.

Attention should be paid to identifying any underlying cause of immunosuppression.

DRUG REACTION*

Classical signs

- Alopecia primarily of the body trunk.
- Bacterial, and less commonly, fungal skin infections.

Classical signs—Cont'd

- Ulceration or necrosis on trunk, limbs or mucocutaneous junctions may be evident.
- History of treatment with immunosuppressive or anti-neoplastic drugs.

Pathogenesis

Most of the drugs implicated in cutaneous drug reactions are **immunosuppressive or anti-neoplastic agents.** The reaction pattern varies with the specific drug.

Drugs such as **glucocorticoids and anti-neoplastic agents** can often **interfere with hair follicle activity,** resulting in alopecia.

Clinical signs

Drugs such as **glucocorticoids and anti-neoplastic agents** may produce **alopecia**, primarily affecting the body trunk.

- The **skin** may become **thin and hypotonic**, particularly with glucocorticoid medication.
- The classical cutaneous changes of hyperadrenocorticism may develop.
- Secondary bacterial or fungal infection is not uncommon.

When the reaction mimics a **hypersensitive response**, the signs may be more severe and involve **ulceration or necrosis**. The **extremities and mucocutaneous junctions or trunk** may be affected (see page 1034, The Cat With Miliary Dermatitis).

Diagnosis

Diagnosis can be difficult in some cases, because the drug reaction may cause cutaneous or systemic signs similar to the disease for which the cat was initially placed on that medication.

A **tentative diagnosis is based on history and clinical signs**. As alopecia is well recognized as a complication of treatment with glucocorticoids and anti-neoplastic agents, use of these drugs should always be ascertained from the history.

Withdrawal of the drug usually leads to a **gradual resolution** of the alopecia, although this is not true in all cats. If the cutaneous changes are not interfering with the quality of life, drug withdrawal may not be appropriate, depending on the underlying condition for which the drug was prescribed.

If drug hypersensitivity is suspected, see page 1034, The Cat With Miliary Dermatitis, for details of diagnosis.

Differential diagnosis

Alopecia can be caused by all the conditions listed in this chapter. However, the major differentials would be **diabetes mellitus, hyperadrenocorticism and hyperthyroidism.** Dietary causes should also be excluded.

Treatment

If appropriate, the offending medication should be withdrawn.

Treat any secondary infection, and crusted or ulcerated areas with appropriate antimicrobial agents and symptomatic therapy as indicated.

PILI TORTI

> ### Classical signs
>
> - Generalized alopecia by 10 days of age.
> - Pedal dermatitis and nail-bed infections.
> - Affected kittens normally die or require euthanasia.

Pathogenesis

The pathogenesis is unknown.

Curvature of the hair follicle results in flattening and rotation of hair shafts.

This leads to a generalized alopecia in young kittens, with **virtually all secondary hairs** becoming involved. Primary hairs are not usually affected.

Pili torti is usually an inherited disorder in man, with affected individuals having additional systemic and skin abnormalities.

Acquired syndromes similar to pili torti are additionally reported following various physical and chemical insults in man.

Both autosomal dominant and recessive inheritance patterns have been reported in human patients with a combination of pili torti and varying degrees of hearing loss. Other ectodermal defects are also documented in affected individuals.

A localized form of disease may occur secondary to follicular inflammation.

Clinical signs

Appears as **generalized alopecia** in young kittens affecting secondary but not primary hairs. Most affected kittens have marked alopecia by 10 days of age.

Periocular and pedal involvement are commonly present. Affected kittens thus commonly present with **pedal dermatitis and paronychia.**

Affected kittens usually **die or are euthanized.**

Diagnosis

A **tentative diagnosis** is based on the **history and clinical signs**.

A **definitive diagnosis** is possible with **skin biopsy** of affected areas and examination of affected secondary hairs.

Electron microscopy of these secondary hairs can provide additional diagnostic information.

Treatment

No treatment is available.

TELOGEN DEFLUXION

> ### Classical signs
>
> - Alopecia affecting any or most parts of the body.
> - Gradual shedding of telogen hairs, usually 1–3 months after a stressful event.
> - Skin is clinically normal.

Clinical signs

Telogen defluxion normally results from the **premature cessation of hair growth** in anagen follicles because of a stressful factor, e.g. pregnancy, internal disease, etc.

Signs compatible with the underlying problem may be present or have been present in the past.

Telogen defluxion results in **widespread loss of hairs** from many or most parts of the body.

The hair loss normally **occurs 1–3 months** following the stressful event.

The skin is clinically normal.

The hairs themselves often appear normal. They are not fractured or broken.

Diagnosis

A **tentative diagnosis** is based on the combination of **history and clinical signs**. Often, the history or signs would indicate a stressful event such as pregnancy or internal disease within the last 1–3 months.

Examination of hair samples microscopically reveals the typical features of telogen hairs. These include uniform shaft diameter, as well as slightly clubbed and non-pigmented roots.
- There is no evidence of dysplastic changes or fracturing of the hair shaft.

Skin biopsy is of little additional benefit, because it simply reveals that all the hair follicles are in telogen.

Re-growth of the coat within a few months if the stress factor is removed or managed successfully can be used to confirm the diagnosis retrospectively.

HYPERADRENOCORTICISM

Classical signs

- Polyuria, polydipsia and polyphagia.
- Abdominal distention and pot-bellied appearance.
- Alopecia of the trunk, lateral thighs and ventrum, and unkempt hair coat.
- Thin, fragile skin.
- Bruising and tearing of the skin with mild trauma.
- Secondary bacterial skin infections and poor wound healing.

See main reference on page 251 (The Cat With Polyuria and Polydipsia).

Clinical signs

The majority of cats with hyperadrenocorticism have **systemic signs including polyuria, polydipsia and polyphagia**. Intermittent inappetence or anorexia may be present.

Many cases have **concomitant diabetes mellitus.**

Abdominal distention, giving a pot-bellied appearance is commonly seen.

Muscle wastage is a prominent feature.

Affected cats exhibit **alopecia and an unkempt hair coat**. Hair loss is commonly seen on the **trunk, flanks and ventrum**.

Hyperpigmentation occurs in a small number of cases. Secondary bacterial dermatitis may be a feature. Abscessation is occasionally present.

The **skin is thin and very fragile** in many cases. This leads to bruising and tearing with mild trauma.

Affected cats have **poor wound healing ability**. Comedone formation is also present in some cases.

In many cases, the disease is iatrogenic and there is a long history of depot glucocorticoid or progestagen use.

Diagnosis

Routine hematology and biochemistry values are not as markedly affected by hyperadrenocorticism in cats as they are in the dog. Consequently, many of the changes seen in the dog are inconsistently found in the cat.
- When present, such changes are frequently attributable to secondary diabetes mellitus, e.g. **hyperglycaemia, hypercholesterolaemia.**

The cat does not have a glucocorticoid-induced isoenzyme of alkaline phosphatase.

Urine specific gravity may on occasions be reduced to isosthenuric levels, except in cats with secondary diabetes mellitus, where glycosuria will affect the specific gravity value.

Adrenal function tests are not as well established in cats compared to dogs.

A normal **urine cortisol:creatinine ratio** is useful for **excluding hyperadrenocorticism**, but lacks specificity for diagnosis.

The **low-dose dexamethasone suppression (LDDS) test using 0.1 mg/kg** is the screening test of choice for feline hyperadrenocorticism. Cats with pituitary-dependent hyperadrenocorticism may fail to suppress, or exhibit suppression at 3 or 4 hours followed by "escape" of suppression at 8 hours. The latter pattern is diagnostic for pituitary-dependent disease, and makes further testing unnecessary.

The **corticotropin (ACTH) stimulation test** is best used to differentiate endogenous from iatrogenic hyperadrenocorticism, rather than as a diagnostic test for hyperadrenocorticism, because 15–30% of cats with hyperadrenocorticism have a normal response.

The **combined dexamethasone suppression/ACTH stimulation test** has been used successfully to diagnose hyperadrenocorticism in cats. The combined test does not appear to be more advantageous than either the ACTH stimulation or dexamethasone suppression test evaluated separately.

Measurement of endogenous ACTH concentrations is useful in differentiating pituitary-dependent from adrenal hyperadrenocorticism. Normal to increased ACTH concentrations support a diagnosis of pituitary-dependent disease. Low concentrations support adrenal disease. This test must only be used after hyperadrenocorticism is confirmed by other tests.

Abdominal ultrasonography may provide evidence of unilateral or bilateral adrenal enlargement.

Exogenous administration of progestogens or glucocorticoids should also be excluded.

Differential diagnosis

Hyperthyroidism and diabetes mellitus are the major differential diagnoses as most cats presenting with hyperadrenocorticism will have a combination of systemic and cutaneous signs.

Treatment

The **success rates** reported with drugs including **mitotane, ketoconazole and metyrapone have been poor to moderate.**
- Whilst successful management is possible in individual cases, the overall results are not as encouraging as in the dog.

- Metyrapone has been used successfully prior to **adrenalectomy** in some cats.

Adrenalectomy is favored by many authors as the **current treatment of choice**. This procedure can result in a significant survival time and a reduced insulin requirement.
- **Unilateral adrenalectomy** is performed in cases of an **adrenal tumor. Bilateral removal** is performed for **pituitary-dependent** hyperadrenocorticism.
- **Mortality rates higher than 25%** have been reported post-operatively, especially where diabetes mellitus is present.
- **Post-operative complications** include electrolyte imbalances, pancreatitis, thrombosis and sepsis. Glucocorticoids and mineralocorticoids are required peri- and post-operatively. Following successful control of the hyperadrenocorticism, the requirement for insulin therapy in diabetic cats may be reduced or abolished altogether.

STAPHYLOCOCCAL DERMATITIS*

Classical signs

- Erythema and scale/crustiness.
- Hair follicles are often involved.
- Lesions may progress to papules, but pus is rare.

Clinical signs

Primary staphylococcal dermatitis is rare in cats. Consequently, there may be signs evident which relate to an **underlying disease condition** e.g. diabetes mellitus or FeLV/FIV.

Erythema and scale/crustiness are seen clinically.

The hair follicles are usually involved. Lesions may progress to appear as **papules**, and thus take on a **miliary pattern.**

Affected cats may exhibit **alopecia** over the **head and neck.** Other common sites affected include the **feet, ears and dorsum.**

It is rare for purulent material to be present in or on the lesions.

Staphylococcal infection in the cat is more commonly seen as abscesses or infections of the ears and conjunctiva. Deeper infections, such as granulomas with fistulation, are infrequent.

Diagnosis

A tentative diagnosis is based on **clinical signs.**

Staphylococci can be readily cultured from infected lesions. Care must be exercised in interpretation of culture results, however, as most normal cats possess coagulase-positive staphylococci on their skin.

Biopsy of affected tissue may show evidence of **bacterial folliculitis, pyoderma or deeper infection.**

DIETARY ALOPECIA

> ### Classical signs
>
> - Patchy or generalized alopecia.
> - Seborrhea and poor coat quality.
> - +/– Secondary skin infection.

Clinical signs

This syndrome is not commonly seen in practice, except where economic conditions are poor or cats are fed on **improperly balanced diets**, for example, vegetarian diets, or diets low in vitamin A.

Alopecia may be patchy or generalized.

Seborrhea and **poor coat quality** are sometimes seen.

Hairs may be brittle and easily broken.

Poor skin hygiene and immune function may predispose to secondary skin infections.

Diagnosis

A tentative diagnosis is based on clinical signs and a detailed dietary history.

Other causes of alopecia need to be ruled out.

Differential diagnosis

Alopecia can be caused by all the conditions listed in this chapter. However, the major differentials would be **diabetes mellitus, hyperadrenocorticism and hyperthyroidism.** Exogenous administration of **progestagens or glucocorticoids** should also be excluded.

Treatment

Correct the underlying dietary imbalance.

Often, simply feeding a well-balanced commercial formulation appropriate to the cat's requirements, will be sufficient to give an overall improvement within weeks to months.

ALOPECIA MUCINOSA

> ### Classical signs
>
> - Alopecia and scaling of affected skin on the ears, head and neck.
> - Plaque-type lesions may develop at lesion site at a later date.

Clinical signs

Alopecia mucinosa is a **very rare** syndrome in cats, which is suspected of being a **precursor lesion** for **cutaneous lymphoma**.

Typically there is **alopecia**, which affects the **head, ears and neck**, and **fine scaling** of the affected skin. Pruritus is not a feature initially.

Within months, plaques may develop at the lesion site. Biopsy of these plaques has yielded results compatible with **cutaneous lymphoma or mycosis fungoides** in the two cats reported in the literature.

Diagnosis

Diagnosis is based on **biopsy of the affected skin**. Initial histopathology reveals **mucinosis of the epidermis** and of the outer root sheath of the hair follicles.

Later, biopsy specimens of plaque-type lesions may reveal findings consistent with cutaneous lymphoma or mycosis fungoides.

Treatment

No effective treatment is currently available. Treatment as for cutaneous lymphoma could be attempted if the biopsy results were suggestive of this. There are too few case reports to make any prescriptive treatment recommendations.

The prognosis is therefore poor.

ALOPECIA AREATA

> **Classical signs**
>
> - Gradual onset of focal or multi-focal areas of alopecia.
> - Non-pruritic.
> - The skin is non-inflamed and appears otherwise normal.
> - Long-standing lesions may become hyperpigmented.

Pathogenesis

In humans, an **immune-mediated basis** is suggested by:
- Accumulations of lymphoid cells around hair bulbs during the active phase of the disease.
- Occasional association of alopecia areata with other immune-mediated diseases.
- Increased incidence of various autoantibodies in alopecia areata.
- Decreased numbers of circulating T-cells.
- Deposition of C3 or IgG or IgM at the basement membrane zone of hair follicles.

Clinical signs

Rare condition in cats.

Typically there are **single or multiple sites of alopecia**, which are generally **well-demarcated** and usually **non-symmetrical.** Hair loss is gradual.

The most common locations affected include the **head, neck and trunk**.

The affected skin appears otherwise normal. There is **no inflammation evident** grossly and pruritus is not a feature.

Chronic lesions may develop **hyperpigmentation.**

Diagnosis

A tentative diagnosis is based on the history of gradual hair loss, and the **clinical signs** of well-demarcated alopecia, without any significant inflammation.

Biopsy of early skin lesions reveals a **mononuclear inflammatory cell infiltrate** both surrounding and within the **hair follicles.**

At later stages, the inflammation is largely absent. Catagen and telogen hair follicles predominate at this timepoint. Follicular atrophy is also evident. In some biopsy specimens, there is complete absence of follicles.

Treatment

There may be **spontaneous re-growth** of hair **in some cats** after a variable period of time.

Glucocorticoids have been employed by a variety of routes. However, no data are available to support the use of glucocorticoid medication in the treatment of this disease.

RECOMMENDED READING

Baker KP, Thomsett LR. Heritable defects. In: Canine and Feline Dermatology. Blackwell Scientific Publications, 1990, pp. 63–75.

Mooney CT. Unusual endocrine disorders in the cat. In *Practice* 1998; 20(7): 345–349.

Moriello K, Mason I. Alopecia in cats. In: Handbook of Small Animal Dermatology. Pergamon, 1995, pp. 163–168.

Scott DW, Miller WH, Griffen CE. Acquired alopecias. Congenital and hereditary defects. Psychogenic skin diseases. In: Muller and Kirk's Small Animal Dermatology, 5th edn. Philadelphia, PA, W.B. Saunders, 1995, pp. 720–735, 736–805, 845–858.

51. The cat with skin lumps and bumps

Rodney Clement Straw

KEY SIGNS

- Soft or firm masses on the skin or under the skin.

MECHANISM?

- Masses are usually inflammatory and infectious in nature.
- Neoplasia is less common and may be caused by cumulative solar irradiation (SCC), viruses (fibrosarcoma), as a sequel to vaccination (sarcoma) or have an unknown etiology.

WHERE?

- Skin, subcutaneous tissue and superficial, palpable anatomical structures.

WHAT?

- Most cats with skin lumps and bumps have inflammatory lesions such as abscesses; neoplasia is less common.

QUICK REFERENCE SUMMARY

Diseases causing skin lumps and bumps

ANOMALY

- Multiple cartilaginous exostosis (p 1079)

Young cat (less than 2 years old) with hard masses fixed to underlying bone on extremities or skull, scapula, ribs, pelvis or multiple sites. These are progressive and painful swellings.

MECHANICAL

- **Foreign body* (p 1073)**

Typically vegetable material such as a grass seed or awn is involved. Relatively acute onset of swelling, often with draining tracts. Can become chronic discharging sinus and location of swelling may move in position on the body.

continued

continued

NEOPLASTIC

- **Squamous cell carcinoma** (p 1069)**

Usually occurs in older cats and appears as a crusty or ulcerated lesion in poorly pigmented and sparsely haired regions of skin.

- **Basal cell tumor* (p 1070)**

Solitary cutaneous lesion in an older cat usually on the dorsum.

- **Fibrosarcoma* (p 1071)**

Soft, subcutaneous mass with poorly defined margins; 50% occur on the limbs and 25% on the head and neck.

- Fibroma (p 1077)

Small, solitary, non-invasive mass in the skin or subcutaneous tissue.

- **Mast cell tumor* (p 1074)**

Solitary or multiple cutaneous masses especially on the head and neck of oriental breeds. Usually firm, raised, well-circumscribed, hairless dermal nodules between 0.5–3 cm in diameter. Intermittently pruritic and occasionally ulcerated (especially histiocytic form). If disseminated, there may be signs of systemic illness including weight loss, anemia, vomiting and anorexia.

- Sweat gland neoplasia (p 1077)

Subcutaneous masses often around the base of the ear and ear canal.

- **Hemangioma and hemangiosarcoma* (p 1075)**

Appear as dark-red, cutaneous nodule or nodules. In the subcutaneous and muscular tissue appear as a soft mass, and there may be a zone of echymosis surrounding the mass. May also appear as an ulcerated lesion on the nose.

- Cutaneous lymphosarcoma (p 1078)

Very rare tumors in cats. Appear as solitary or multiple skin or subcutaneous masses varying from a few millimeters to over a centimeter in diameter. Can be moist and erythematous or dry and flaky. Mucocutaneous junctions may be involved with areas of superficial ulceration. Lesions may consist of plaques, papules, nodules and areas of erythema, focal alopecia with crusting and ulceration.

- Melanoma (p 1079)

The majority appears as dark-pigmented nodules in the skin of the head, and very rarely on the extremities. Ocular melanomas may occur and very rarely melanoma involves the oral cavity.

- **Mammary gland tumors* (p 1076)**

Nodule or nodules in the mammary chain, on average 3 cm in diameter. Often multiple, and may involve both mammary chains. May be ulcerated.

INFECTION

- **Catfight abscess*** (p 1079)**

Painful subcutaneous mass, usually febrile.

- Fungal (p 1080)

Variably ulcerated, cutaneous or subcutaneous mass. (e.g. *Cryptococcus* sp.)

TRAUMA

- Hematoma **(p 1080)**

Subcutaneous mass, acute onset, painful.

INTRODUCTION

MECHANISM?

Masses seen on the skin, or palpable masses on or under the skin are usually inflammatory, or less commonly neoplastic in origin.

Neoplasia may be caused by cumulative solar irradiation (SCC), viruses (fibrosarcoma), as a sequel to vaccination (sarcoma) or have an unknown etiology.

Multiple cartilaginous exostosis is probably of viral etiology.

WHERE?

Skin, subcutaneous tissue and superficial, palpable anatomical structures.

WHAT?

Most cats with skin lumps and bumps have inflammatory lesions such as **abscesses**; **neoplasia** is less common and often more serious, requiring early diagnosis and prompt appropriate treatment.

DISEASES CAUSING LUMPS AND BUMPS ON THE SKIN

CATFIGHT ABSCESS***

> **Classical signs**
> - Painful subcutaneous mass, usually febrile.

See main references on page 390 (The Pyrexic Cat) and page 401 (The Cat With Enlarged Lymph Nodes).

Clinical signs

There is a sudden onset of swelling under the skin often with a discharging sinus.

Many cats are depressed, febrile and/or anorexic.

Diagnosis

Purulent exudate or sheets of neutrophils with intra- and extracellular bacteria are evident on cytology.

SQUAMOUS CELL CARCINOMA**

> **Classical signs**
> - Reddened flaky skin on sparsely haired, non-pigmented skin.
> - Non-healing ulcer on predisposed areas of head.

Pathogenesis

Chronic exposure to **UV light** may lead to the development of **dysplasia of epithelial cells** in **poorly pigmented and sparsely haired skin**. The effect of UV irradiation is **cumulative**, and the dysplastic cells may undergo neoplastic change, with development of carcinoma in situ. This lesion will progress to **invasive squamous cell carcinoma.**

Clinical signs

Most squamous cell carcinomas occur on the **head of older cats.**
- Predisposed sites include **non-pigmented areas** of the nasal planum, eyelids (including the third eyelid) and periorbital skin, infra-auricular skin and pinnae.

Lesions vary from small areas of **reddened and flaky skin,** to **deep ulcers** with peripheral zones of swelling and proliferation.
- Characteristically cats are presented because of **chronic non-healing ulcers**. There can be considerable necrosis and odor with advanced lesions.

Squamous cell carcinoma occasionally involves the **ear canal**.
- In advanced lesions there can be **extension** to the **osseous bullae**, and **vestibular signs** may be present.

Bone lysis accompanies advanced-stage lesions, particularly those located in the **periorbital area or ear canal**.

Diagnosis

A **tentative diagnosis** is based on the history and typical lesions located on poorly pigmented and sparsely haired regions.

Definitive diagnosis depends on histopathological evaluation of a biopsy specimen.

Radiological studies are rarely useful unless there is considerable extension to underlying bone.

Cytology may be helpful.

Cytological evaluation of any enlarged **regional lymph node** can be very useful for **staging**.

Differential diagnosis

The main differential diagnosis is **eosinophilic granulomas** of the lips, which can appear similar to squamous cell carcinoma lesions on the nasal planum.
- Eosinophilic granuloma lesions are usually **confined to the lips** and are often quite symmetrical.
- Diagnosis is based on histopathology or perhaps cytology. Classical cytological appearance is of sheets of well-differentiated eosinophils.

Treatment

The treatment of choice is **ablative surgery with wide margins**.
- This may involve such procedures as removal of pinnae, nasal planectomy, full-thickness eyelid resection, enucleation with partial orbitectomy and reconstructive procedures such as caudal auricular artery axial pattern flap.

Resected specimens should be evaluated histopathologically for completeness of resection. Incomplete resection is associated with very high rates of tumor recurrence.

Cryosurgery may be useful for carcinoma in situ, or early stages of invasive squamous cell carcinoma, and is particularly useful for small lesions of the eyelids.
- At least two freeze–thaw cycles (rapid freeze and slow thaw) should be used.
- The lesion and a cuff of normal-appearing surrounding tissue should be frozen to –25°C or colder.
- Unfortunately recurrence rates are high.
- **Radiation therapy** can be used, and generally is most effective for carcinoma in situ or early stages of invasive squamous cell carcinoma. Radiation therapy includes:

- Soft external beam therapy delivered by ortho-voltage machines.
- Electron beam treatment from a linear accelerator.
- Brachytherapy using radioactive implants.

Prognosis

Prognosis varies with the stage of disease, but is usually good.

Squamous cell carcinomas of the skin are generally very **slow to develop and progress**.
- However, cats with late stages of disease seem to deteriorate quickly.

Metastasis to regional lymph nodes occurs late in the course of the disease.

The major debilitating signs are associated with the local tumor.
- Pulmonary metastases are rare for solar-induced cutaneous squamous cell carcinoma.

With **complete surgical excision**, the prognosis is very good, and **80–100%** control rates can be achieved.

New lesions can develop as a consequence of continued exposure to the sun.

Prevention

Prevent exposure of high-risk cats to UV irradiation by **keeping them indoors** during high-risk times of the day.
- It is very difficult to prevent sun exposure in climates where UV irradiation is high.

In geographic regions where there is a high risk of UV irradiation, **breeding cats with pigmented skin** would decrease the incidence of tumors.

Tattooing non-pigmented skin does not prevent the development of squamous cell carcinoma.

BASEL CELL TUMORS*

Classical signs
- Skin nodule often on the dorsum.
- May have intact epithelium or variably ulcerated.
- Often chronic history.

Pathogenesis

Basal cell tumors result from **malignant transformation of the basal cells** of the skin.

The etiology of these tumors is unknown, but they tend to affect **older cats**.

Clinical signs

Basal cell tumors are a **common** skin tumor in **older cats**.

These tumors develop in the basal epithelium of the skin.

The tumors are **usually solitary**.
- They usually occur on the skin on the dorsum of the head, neck, thorax and lumbar area.

Diagnosis

Cytological examination of a fine-needle aspirate may be suggestive, but definitive diagnosis requires **histopathological evaluation** of a biopsy specimen.

Differential diagnosis

Diagnosis cannot be necessarily made by the gross appearance, and basal cell tumors need to be differentiated from other skin neoplasms such as **squamous cell carcinoma** and **mast cell tumors** by histopathology.

Treatment

Nearly all basal cell tumors can be permanently **controlled by complete surgical excision,** although the histological appearance of these tumors would tend to imply an aggressive natural behavior.
- Margins of about 5–10 mm are appropriate.

Prognosis

The **prognosis is very good** if these tumors are removed completely.
- Only rarely have metastases been reported.

Prevention

Since the etiology is unknown, preventative measures cannot be recommended.

FIBROSARCOMA*

Classical signs
- Soft, subcutaneous mass with poorly defined margins.
- Slowly growing.
- Not painful.

Pathogenesis

Fibrosarcomas are non-encapsulated tumors of malignant **mesenchymal cells** with potential for **local tissue invasion**.

Feline sarcoma virus, which is a retrovirus that depends on feline leukemia virus for replication, causes **multicentric fibrosarcomas** in young cats.

The cause of solitary fibrosarcomas in older cats is usually unknown.

There is a form of fibrosarcoma that grows in vaccination sites that is thought to be associated with post-vaccination inflammation (**vaccine-associated sarcoma**, VAS).
- Killed vaccines with aluminum salt adjuvant have been implicated as causative agents, but the true etiology, pathogenesis and epidemiology are still unknown.
- Rabies vaccines have been implicated, but other vaccines may also play a role.
- Frequency of occurrence varies worldwide.
- There is a low incidence in some countries such as Australia, perhaps because rabies vaccine is not used.

Solitary fibrosarcomas in adult, FeLV-negative cats are **locally invasive** and have a **low metastatic rate** (approximately 10% of cats will develop distant metastasis).

Clinical signs

Typical signs are a **solitary, soft, subcutaneous mass** growing larger and firmer over a period of months. With increasing size, the mass may **ulcerate** and become secondarily infected.

The **multicentric form** occurs in cats generally **less than 5 years of age**.

Vaccine-associated sarcoma arises in the area of vaccination, usually in the **interscapular space** in the dorsal subcutaneous tissue.

Fibrosarcomas are usually **not painful.**

Tumors may occur anywhere on the body, with **50% occurring on limbs** and **25% on the head and neck**.

Diagnosis

Cytological examination of **fine-needle aspirates** demonstrates **mesenchymal cells** with malignant characteristics. This suggests fibrosarcoma.

Definitive diagnosis requires **histopathological evaluation** of properly acquired biopsy material.
- Care must be taken to perform the biopsy, so the entire biopsy site may be removed with the tumor at the time of resection.

There is usually an inflammatory component to the histology of vaccine-associated sarcoma, with predominantly lymphocyte and macrophage populations.

Histological grading including determining the **mitotic index**, derived from evaluating ten high-power fields, may add prognostic information.

Regional radiography may help determine the local tumor stage and direct surgical planning.

Thoracic radiography and **regional lymph node cytology** are required for staging although metastasis is rare for cats with solitary fibrosarcoma.

Cats with viral multicentric fibrosarcoma will be FeLV positive.

Differential diagnosis

Fibromas and old wounds with abundant fibroplasia can have similar cytological appearance on fine-needle aspirates.

Other names are given to these soft tissue sarcomas such as spindle cell tumors, neurofibrosarcomas or nerve sheath tumors.

Treatment

Wide surgical excision is the treatment of choice.
- **Tumor margins** should be evaluated histologically for completeness of resection.

- Adjuvant chemotherapy has been recommended but has not been shown to be beneficial.

Cats with **multicentric fibrosarcomas** can only experience **temporary palliation**.
- Surgery cannot be expected to cure these cats.

Cats with vaccine-associated sarcoma are also more difficult to treat.
- Recurrence and metastasis has been reported after surgery.
- Combinations of **surgery, external beam radiation and chemotherapy** show promise in controlling these very aggressive tumors.

Prognosis

The **prognosis is good** for **solitary fibrosarcomas** in adult cats where complete surgical excision has been performed.
- The ability to completely excise the mass depends on the tumor location, tumor size and expertise of the surgeon.

Histological grade including mitotic index may help predict survival following surgery, and cats with high-grade tumors should be followed more closely or may be given adjuvant therapy.

The **prognosis is poor** with **multicentric fibrosarcomas.**

Vaccine-associated sarcoma is associated with a **variable prognosis** with often disappointing outcomes even with wide excision.

Prevention

The Vaccine-Associated Feline Sarcoma Task Force (VAFSTF) was formed to address this evolving and important issue and can be found at http://www.avma.org/vafstf/default.htm on the Internet.

The VAFSTF has made a number of recommendations:
- Cats should not be vaccinated unnecessarily.
  - Rabies vaccines licensed for every 3 years should not be given yearly and strictly indoor cats should not be vaccinated for FeLV.
- Vaccines should not be given in the interscapular space.
  - It is suggested that the **rabies vaccines** are given on the **right hindlimb** and the FeLV be given on the left hindlimb.

- It is recommended that these vaccines be given in a distal location when possible, so that the limb may be amputated if a sarcoma develops, thus sparing the cat's life.
  - Other vaccines should be given over the lateral shoulders away from the interscapular site.
- Single-dose vial usage is recommended.
  - **Multi-vaccine products should be avoided**.
- When giving booster vaccinations, **previous vaccine sites** should be **avoided**.
- In the past, it has been suggested that IM administration be performed instead of SQ injection. This may only result in more difficult detection, reducing the chance of early detection and surgical cure.
- Monitoring for masses occurring in common vaccination sites should be performed by owners and reported to the veterinarian.
  - **Vaccine-associated granulomas are common**. A recent study evaluated cats receiving rabies vaccines from four different manufacturers, and found that 100% of the cats developed local reactions. Reactions often occurred within a few weeks, and resolved by 1–2 months later.
- Do not vaccinate cats that have had a prior history of a vaccine-associated sarcoma.

GUIDELINES FOR RECORDING SUSPECTED CASES OF VACCINE-ASSOCIATED SARCOMA

The location, vaccine type, manufacturer, serial numbers of the vaccine should be recorded in each patient's record.

All other medications administered subcutaneously or intramuscularly should be recorded as well.

Any vaccine response, whether inflammatory or neoplastic, should be reported to the vaccine manufacturer.
- Also report outcome of the case as it becomes known.

MANAGEMENT OF VACCINE-ASSOCIATED SARCOMA IN CATS

If a **mass** in a vaccine site **persists for longer than 1 month**, or if it exhibits rapid growth, a Tru-cut®, wedge or **excisional biopsy** should be performed.
- If a granuloma is identified, a conservative resection may be planned, if excision was not already performed.

- If a sarcoma is identified, then **wide or radical surgical excision** should be performed.

Test for FeLV to reduce the suspicion of FeSV-related sarcoma.

Although the rate of distant metastasis is low, it is recommended that thoracic radiographs be performed prior to excisional surgery.

Wide surgical excision with margins of up to 5 cm has been recommended. Margins should be evaluated via histology.

Wide surgical excision with less than 5 cm performed at the first occurrence with adjuvant external beam radiation therapy has a good chance of long term control of this cancer.

Recurrent tumors are always more difficult to manage than the initial tumor with adjustments external been radiation thoraphy.

FOREIGN BODY*

> ### Classical signs
> - Mass under the skin, often with a discharging sinus.
> - Swelling may "come and go" and may be chronic.

Pathogenesis

Any foreign body under the skin may result in an **abscess or chronically draining lesion**. The foreign body is usually of plant origin such as a grass seed or awn, but may even be a tooth broken off during a cat fight.

Clinical signs

Typically there is an acute onset of a **soft tissue swelling** under the skin, which can occur anywhere on the body.

The swelling may be acute or chronic.

Purulent material sometimes drains from a sinus in the mass.

The swelling is variably painful, and is often less painful if chronic.

The owner may describe the lesion as "moving", because it may appear in slightly different locations if the foreign body is migrating. Alternatively it may appear to "come and go".

The mass is persistent, and wound drainage is only **partially responsive to antibiotics**.

Diagnosis

Definitive diagnosis requires identification of the foreign body.

Fine-needle aspirate cytology is consistent with granulomatous inflammation and contains neutrophils and macrophages.

The foreign body is usually discovered at surgery, and rarely by radiography or ultrasonography.

Treatment

Treatment involves **surgical removal of the foreign body**, and drainage or removal of the sinus tract.

Perioperative antibiotics are indicated.

Prognosis

Prognosis is **excellent** with surgical removal of the foreign body, but the foreign body can be hard to find.

MAST CELL TUMORS*

Classical signs

- Solitary or multiple cutaneous masses.
- Usually on the head and neck.
- Usually firm, raised, well-circumscribed, hairless dermal nodules between 0.5–3 cm in diameter.
- Intermittently pruritic and occasionally ulcerated (especially histiocytic form).
- If disseminated, there may be signs of systemic illness.
- Weight loss, anemia, vomiting and anorexia.

Pathogenesis

Mast cell tumors are comprised of **anaplastic mast cells** and **histiocytic cells**.

There is no known etiology for feline mast cell tumors.

Siamese cats appear to be predisposed.

Clinical signs

Mast cell tumors typically appear as firm, raised, well-circumscribed, hairless **dermal nodules** varying in size from 0.5 cm. They are **often multiple**; 20% were multiple in one report and the majority in another.

The **head and neck** are more commonly affected than the trunk or limbs.

Tumors are usually **not painful**, but may be **itchy**. Occasionally the tumors may become **ulcerated**, especially the histiocytic form.

Mast cell tumors can have visceral involvement, but the **visceral form** usually occurs as a **separate entity** (see systemic mastocytosis, page 689).

Lesions may become **erythematous and edematous after manipulation** (Darier's sign).

Cats with **systemic involvement** are **usually sick**, with weight loss, anorexia, vomiting, diarrhea (variably with bloody stools), anemia and even shock.
- Usually, however, cats with cutaneous mast cell tumors are otherwise healthy.

There are **two major forms** of cutaneous mast cell tumors in cats, **mastocytic and histiocytic**.
- **Mastocytic** mast cell tumors occur typically in **middle- to old-aged cats**.
- Most mastocytic tumors are the compact form with a fairly benign behavior.
  - A few are the **diffuse form**, which are more **anaplastic and malignant**.
- **Histiocytic** mast cells tumors are **uncommon**, occur in cats **less than 4 years of age** (mean age 2.4 years) and **Siamese are predisposed**.
- Histiocytic tumors usually occur as multiple cutaneous nodules around the head.
  - These lesions are of **low grade** and may even spontaneously regress.

Diagnosis

Fine-needle aspirate cytology is **often diagnostic** showing round cells with metachromatic granules. **Histopathology** is usually necessary to **diagnose the histicytic form** where granules are not prominent.

Extension to regional lymph nodes is not common, but any enlarged node should be evaluated at least by fine-needle aspirate.

In cats where **disseminated disease** (spleen or intestinal forms) is suspected, tests such as hematology, serum biochemistry, buffy coat smear or bone marrow aspirate, coagulation studies, thoracic and abdominal radiography and abdominal ultrasonography should be considered.

Differential diagnosis

Other cutaneous neoplasms should be considered as differential diagnoses. Differentiation is based on fine-needle cytology or histological examination.

Treatment

For the mastocytic form, surgery is the preferred treatment. Surgical margins need not be as wide as for canine mast cell tumors (3 cm), since most have a relatively benign biological behavior. **Wider margins** are necessary in the case of **diffuse mastocytic forms**. Conservative resection is appropriate for the histiocytic form.

Cats with the splenic form benefit from **splenectomy**, even though tumor cells may be disseminated.

Little is know of the efficacy of adjuvant therapy for mast cell tumors in cats.

Prognosis

In general, the prognosis for most cats with mast cell tumors is very good.

Most cats experience **long-term control** after complete surgical excision.

Local recurrence rates for the mastocytic form following surgery **vary up to 24%**.
- If the tumor recurs, it usually does so within 6 months of surgery.

The metastatic rate has been reported to be as high as 22%.

Some cats do acquire new primaries.

HEMANGIOMA AND HEMANGIOSARCOMA*

Classical signs
- Dark red cutaneous nodule.

Pathogenesis

Hemangiomas are benign tumors of vascular endothelium. The **malignant, anaplastic** counterpart is **hemangiosarcoma**.

Hemangiosarcomas of the nasal planum and eyelid may be solar induced.

Clinical signs

Hemaniomas and hemangiosarcomas are **very rare in cats**.

In the skin, they usually appear as **red to dark-red nodules of varying size**.
- **Spontaneous hemorrhage** from the lesions may be a feature.

They may also appear as an **ulcerated lesion on the nose**.

Hemangiosarcoma can occur in the **subcutaneous and muscular tissue as a soft mass**, and there may be a **zone of echymosis** surrounding the mass.

Hemangiosarcoma can also occur in **visceral organs**, and rarely the skin lesions may be secondaries to primary disease in the viscera.

Diagnosis

Cytological examination may be unrewarding because the cells do not exfoliate well.
- Malignant mesenchymal cells may be found at the feathered edge of cytology slides.

Definitive diagnosis requires histological examination.

Treatment

Surgical resection is the treatment of choice, and for hemangiosarcomas, as wide a margin as possible should be taken, preferably greater than 10 mm.

Prognosis

Hemangiomas are benign.

Cutaneous and subcutaneous hemangiosarcomas appear to be **locally invasive** only, and metastases are not common.

Hemangiosarcomas have a high metastatic potential when intra-abdominal or intrathoracic organs are involved.

However, **hemangiosarcomas involving muscles** also appear to have a high incidence of **metastasis**.

MAMMARY GLAND TUMORS*

Classical signs

- Nodule or nodules in the mammary chain, on average 3 cm in diameter.
- Often multiple, and may involve both mammary chains.

Pathogenesis

There is a **seven-fold greater risk** of mammary carcinoma in **intact cats** compared to spayed cats.
- Unlike in dogs, ovariohysterectomy before the first estrus does not eliminate the possibility of mammary tumor, but appears to have some sparing effect.

It has been observed that **long-term progesterone therapy** in cats is associated with an increased incidence of mammary tumors and dysplasias.

Mammary tumors are the **third most common tumor** in cats.
- The overall risk is 25.4/100 000 female cats.
- Age range is 2.5–19 years with **70% between 9–13 years,** and an average of 10.8 years.
- There is no breed predilection.

The majority of mammary gland tumors are **malignant (86%).**
- Of the malignant tumors, **adenocarcinoma** is the predominant type.
- Mammary neoplasia can further be evaluated based on (1) cellular differentiation and the degree of tubule formation, (2) nuclear pleomorphism, and (3) the frequency of mitosis.

- Adenocarcinomas may further be divided into tubular, papillary and solid carcinomas.

Clinical signs

The tumors usually lie in the **subcutaneous tissue adjacent to the nipple**, and adhere to the overlying skin.
- The size of tumor is variable, with a mean size of **3 cm** and rarely exceeding 9 cm in diameter.

About 15–25% are ulcerated at the time of diagnosis.

Local invasion into underlying musculature and cutaneous ulceration is **common**.

Feline mammary tumors **grow rapidly**.
- The average duration of the history at the time of diagnosis is 5 months.

About **66%** of feline mammary tumors will be **multiple,** and about **35% involve both chains** of mammae.

Regional lymph nodes are involved early.

Some cats with tumors that have been present for a long time may present with signs referable to **metastasis**, including **weight loss, dyspnea and coughing**.

Differential diagnosis

Benign lesions such **as adenomas, focal mammary dysplasia and fibromas** can mimic the gross appearance of mammary gland tumors, and can be differentiated on histopathology.

Diagnosis

Presumptive diagnosis of a mammary gland tumor can be made on the presence of a mass in the breast tissue.

Cytological examination of a fine-needle aspirate may reveal malignant cells, but false-negative cytology is possible.

Definitive diagnosis can only be made by a surgical biopsy and **histological examination**.

Due to the high metastatic potential of female mammary gland tumors, **chest radiography** should be performed **before any surgical procedure**.

Treatment

The treatment of choice is **radical mastectomy of all glands on the affected side,** because of the high local recurrence rate, high rate of malignancy and the frequent multicentric origin of feline mammary gland tumors.

- The **opposite side should be removed in 2–4 weeks**, or a bilateral mastectomy performed if possible.
- All **regional lymph nodes** should be palpated and removed if enlarged.
- In cases of local recurrence, a second surgery is often possible and may be indicated to prolong survival.

Doxorubicin alone (1 mg/kg IV every 21 days for 4–5 treatments), or **doxorubicin and cyclophosphamide** (200 mg/m² IV or orally) combination chemotherapy may help as adjuvant therapy to prolong the disease-free survival.

Prognosis

The prognosis in **general is poor.**
- The **median survival time** of cats treated with surgery alone is **10–14 months**.

Tumor volume has a significant effect on postoperative survival time.
- Cats with a total tumor volume of < 9 cm³ can be expected to survive greater than 18 months, cats with a total tumor volume of 10–27 cm³ can be expected to survive 12 months, and cats with a tumor volume greater than 27 cm can be expected to survive 7 months.

Cats with **well-differentiated tumors** appear to survive longer than those with poorly differentiated tumors.

FIBROMA

Classical signs

- Solitary cutaneous or subcutaneous mass usually not greater than 10 mm in diameter.

Pathogenesis

Fibroma is caused by **benign hyperplasia of fibrocytes**. The cause not known.

Clinical signs

Fibromas are either **slow growing** or have a long history of stable size.

Typically they appear as a **non-painful small cutaneous or subcutaneous mass**, usually less than 10 mm diameter, which is generally not ulcerated.

Tumors are **mobile**, and **not invasive** to adjacent structures.

Diagnosis

On fine-needle aspirate, not many cells exfoliate and the cells do not have characteristics of malignancy. The cells are elongated with small nuclei.

A fibrous and tough texture is often noticed when performing needle aspirates.

No bone lysis is evident in adjacent skeletal structures.

Definitive diagnosis requires **histopathological examination** of an excised specimen.

Treatment

Excisional biopsy is diagnostic and curative.

Prognosis

Prognosis is excellent.

SWEAT GLAND NEOPLASIA

Classical signs

- Masses of the head and neck, especially around the external and middle ear canal.

Pathogenesis

Sweat gland tumors arise from **apocrine or ceruminous gland cells**. Most commonly they arise around the external and middle ear canal.

The etiology of sweat gland tumors is unknown.

Most of these adnexal tumors are **malignant (carcinomas)**, and are **locally invasive** with a **variable metastatic potential**.

Extension to regional lymph nodes and later to the lung can be seen.

Clinical signs

Ceruminous and apocrine gland neoplasms are **relatively common** in cats, however perianal tumors are rare.

Cats usually present because of a **mass** often around the base of the ear and ear canal, or for **signs of otitis externa**.

Regional lymph nodes may be enlarged.

Diagnosis

Cytological examination and demonstration of **typical polyhedral cells in rafts with nuclear pleomorphism** and other malignant characteristics may be helpful as a screening test, but **definitive diagnosis** requires **histological evaluation** of a biopsy.

Regional lymph nodes, particularly cranial cervical nodes, need to be evaluated by cytology, histology or both, and **pulmonary radiography** should be performed for staging.

- Palpate the neck carefully and perform **fine-needle aspirate cytology on any enlarged nodes**, or remove or perform Trucut needle biopsy on such nodes for histopathology.
- Take thoracic radiographs in both lateral projections and ventrodorsal or dorsoventral projections.

Treatment

Wide surgical excision including total ear ablation for external ear canal ceruminous carcinomas is the treatment of choice.

Adjuvant radiation and chemotherapy have been described, however many lesions will progress despite extensive treatment.

Prognosis

Long-term remission is possible where clean surgical margins are attained in cats with no metastatic disease.

Overall a fair prognosis must be given.

CUTANEOUS LYMPHOSARCOMA

Classical signs

- Solitary or multiple skin or subcutaneous masses varying from a few millimeters to over a centimeter in diameter.
- Can be moist and erythematous or dry and flaky.
- Mucocutaneous junctions may be involved with areas of superficial ulceration.

Pathogenesis

Cutaneous lymphosarcoma lesions are comprised of **diffuse infiltrates of malignant, poorly differentiated lymphoid cells (B-lymphocytes)**. A **T-cell form (mycosis fungoides)** has been described.

Since affected cats are usually older and FeLV negative, the cause of this disease is not well understood.

Clinical signs

These tumors are **very rare** in cats.

Appear as **solitary or multiple skin** or **subcutaneous masses** varying from a few millimeters to over a centimeter in diameter.

- Can be **moist and erythematous or dry and flaky**.
- **Mucocutaneous junctions** may be involved with areas of superficial ulceration.

Lesions may consist of **plaques, papules, nodules, and areas of erythema, focal alopecia with crusting and ulceration**.

Usually there is **no systemic involvement**, and there are minimal abnormalities on hematology or serum biochemistry.

Diagnosis

Cytological examination showing **abundant malignant round cells** is useful to establish a presumptive diagnosis.

Definitive diagnosis requires **histopathology**.

Treatment

For **solitary lesions, excisional surgery may be curative**.

Small lesions may respond well to **superficial radiation therapy**.

Single or multimodal chemotherapy may be used, but the response to therapy is often disappointing. **Mycosis fungoides** may be treated with **retinoides** such as isotretinoin.

Prognosis

The prognosis for cats with **widespread disease is poor**.

Cats with small solitary lesions may do well initially with surgical excision, but **generalized disease is likely to occur within 12 months**.

MELANOMA

Classical signs

- Black pigmented cutaneous lesion.

Pathogenesis

- Melanoma can be induced experimentally with feline sarcoma virus, but this is not thought to be involved in the pathogenesis of the clinical disease.

Clinical signs

Melanoma is **very rare** in cats and can be **benign or malignant**.

The majority appears as **dark-pigmented nodules in the skin of the head**, and very rarely on the extremities.

Very rarely melanoma involves the oral cavity.

Ocular melanomas usually affect the **intraocular structures or the eyelid**, and may occur in the uveal tract.

Diagnosis

Cytological examination showing **heavily pigmented large solitary cells or lightly grouped cells** varying from round to spindloid in shape is highly suggestive,

but a definitive diagnosis should be obtained by histopathology.

Treatment

Treatment of choice is **surgical excision**, preferably with margins of 10 mm or greater. **Cryosurgery** is an alternative for small lesions or eyelid tumors.

Prognosis

The prognosis for non-ocular dermal melanomas is fair; reported metastatic rates are 5–25%.

MULTIPLE CARTILAGENOUS EXOSTOSIS

Classical signs

- Multiple firm masses palpable mostly over the ribs, scapulae, pelvis, the skull and possibly some long bones in a young, skeletally mature cat.
- Swellings are progressive and painful.

Pathogenesis

Multiple cartilaginous exostosis is thought to have a **viral etiology** because virtually all cats are **FeLV positive.** It does not appear to have a familial basis as it does in dogs.

There is **continuous bone growth** from **ectopic cartilage caps** particularly on flat bones, and at sites such as the scapulae, vertebrae, mandible and skull.

Lesions **progress after skeletal maturity**, unlike the static character of solitary cartilaginous exostoses in mature dogs.

Exostoses may undergo **malignant transformation**.

Clinical signs

Multiple firm masses occur which are palpable mostly over the ribs, scapulae, pelvis, the skull and possibly some long bones in a **young, skeletally mature cat.**

Rapid progression may occur over just a few weeks to months, resulting in prominent hard swellings causing pain, lameness and loss of function.

Occur in young cats, less than 2 years old.

Differential diagnosis

The main differential diagnosis is **osteosarcoma** which usually only affects one bone at presentation.

Diagnosis

Diagnosis is based on clinical signs, radiographic findings and biopsy results.

Radiographic appearance is of **multiple, focal exostoses** that blend with normal underlying bone.

Most cats are **FeLV positive**.

Definitive diagnosis relies on histopathology.

Treatment

Lesions can be excised for palliation, but there is no effective cure.

Prognosis

Prognosis is extremely poor, because the lesions are usually progressive, and recurrence following surgery is common. The disease is painful and debilitating.

Fungal

> **Classical signs**
>
> - Variably ulcerated, cutaneous or subcutaneous mass. (e.g. *Cryptococcus* sp.).

Clinical signs

There are often ulcerated skin lesions which do not respond to antibiotics.

Numerous common and less common fungi are capable of producing cutaneous masses in cats including *Cryptococcus, Sporothrix* and *Coccidiodides*.

Systemic signs such as inappetence, weight loss and fever may be present. Dyspnea or CNS signs may be present in some cats.

Diagnosis

The diagnosis is made by demonstrating the organisms on cytology, histology, fungal culture or serology.

HEMATOMA

> **Classical signs**
>
> - Subcutaneous mass, acute onset, painful.

Clinical signs

Hematomas may occur as solitary or multiple subcutaneous swellings. Purple dicoloration of the overlying non-pigmented skin may be evident. There may be a history of trauma or coagulopathy.

Diagnosis

A presumptive diagnosis is based on ruling out other disorders by fine-needle cytology (peripheral blood, macrophages and other inflammatory cells may be identified), combined with a history of trauma or identification of a coagulopathy.

RECOMMENDED READING

Withrow SJ, MacEwen EG (eds) Small Animal Clinical Oncology, 3rd edn. WB Saunders Co., Philadelphia, 2001.

52.   The cat with non-healing wounds

Gregory Burton

KEY SIGNS

- Erosion, ulceration.
- Nodules or plaques with ulceration or fistulae.
- Serosanguineous to purulent exudate +/− tissue grains.
- Subcutaneous fibrosis.
- Extracutaneous symptoms may be present.

MECHANISM

- Non-healing wounds occur where there is a failure of re-epithelialization, dermal fibroplasia and or angiogensis.

WHERE?

- Skin (diseases involving the epidermis, dermis, panniculus and cutaneous blood vessels) and mucocutaneous junctions.

WHAT?

- Most cats with non-healing skin wounds have infections (mycobacteria, aerobic and/or anaerobic bacteria, or fungi). Neoplasia, allergies, immune-mediated and metabolic diseases are less common.

QUICK REFERENCE SUMMARY
Diseases causing non-healing wounds

ANOMALY

- Cutaneous asthenia (p 1100 - 1101)

Congenital disease resulting in hyperextensibility and fragility of the skin. Kittens present with spontaneous tears or necrotic, slow-healing crusted ulcerations.

- Epidermolysis bullosa (p 1101)

Congenital epidermal basement membrane disease with signs evident shortly after birth. Skin, foot pad and mouth ulcers particularly at frictional areas. Nail shedding is common.

continued

continued

METABOLIC

● Acquired cutaneous fragility syndrome (p 1098)

Thin, fragile skin which is not hyperextensibile, and which tears easily. Secondary to metabolic conditions such as hyperadrenocorticoidism (endogenous or iatrogenic) or diabetes.

● Xanthoma (p 1099)

Plaques or nodules with a yellowish-white appearance which often ulcerate and occur mostly over bony protuberances (areas of incidental trauma). Most common in cats associated with hyperlipidemia.

● Metabolic epidermal necrosis (MEN) (p 1099)

Crusting lesions at mucocutaneous junctions and pressure points in an unwell cat. Skin lesions are secondary to pancreatic or hepatic disorders.

NEOPLASIA

● **Squamous cell carcinoma** (p 1089)**

Occurs in old cats (average age 9 years). Multiple or single lesions occur on the pinnae, philtrum, nares, forehead and palpebrae, in non-pigmented, thinly haired areas. Lesions may be proliferative or ulcerative, and are slow to metastasize.

● Multicentric squamous cell carcinoma in situ (p 1089)

Occurs in older cats (> 10 years). Multifocal lesions occur over the head, neck, shoulders and forelimbs on pigmented, thickly haired skin. Begin as hyperkeratotic macules and evolve to thick-crusted, ulcerated plaques. Progress slowly, with waxing and waning signs.

● Melanoma (p 1097)

Occurs in older cats (average age 10 years) as solitary lesions on the head or neck. Size and shape are variable ranging from a dome, to a plaque or polypoid shape, and ulceration is frequent.

● Basal cell carcinoma (BCC) (p 1097)

Frequently pigmented and/or cystic tumors of the head, neck, thorax, nasal planum and eyelids of older cats. Usually solitary and frequently ulcerated.

● **Mast cell tumor* (p 1092)**

Occur as single to multiple tumors on the head of older cats. Tumors may "enlarge" and become erythematous after palpation or aspiration. Rarely young Siamese cats have multiple nodules around the head.

● Cutaneous lymphoma (p 1097)

Very rare tumors in cats. Signs of T cell tumors (mycosis fungoides) include "non-inflammatory" alopecia, scaling, erythroderma (diffuse reddening of the skin), hypopigmentation of hair or skin, ulceration, plagues and nodules. B cell neoplasia produces dermal nodules with or without ulceration. Systemic signs of weight loss, diarrhea and respiratory distress may be present.

NUTRITIONAL

● Pansteatitis/vitamin E deficiency (p 1104)

Cats eating diets high in oils, especially fish oils may develop fever, lethargy, painful skin, generalized firm feel to the subcutaneous fat, and skin sinuses with gelatinous exudate.

INFLAMMATORY/INFECTIOUS

Viral:

● Pox virus (feline cowpox)* (p 1091)

Caused by orthopoxvirus, which is not uncommon in Western Europe. Transmission is via direct contact with rodents, mostly in male free-roaming adult cats. Focal ulcer or abscess is followed 7–10 days later by generalized small (0.5–1 cm) crusted ulcers. Concurrent pneumonia is a poor prognostic sign.

● Herpesvirus 1* (p 1092)

Cutaneous manifestation of feline rhinotracheitis infection produces ulcerative lesions seen mostly on the nasal planum. There may or may not be concurrent ocular or respiratory disease.

Bacterial:

● Bacterial infections*** (p 1086)

Usually preceded by history of skin penetration, e.g. cat fight. Actinomycotic mycetoma are characterized by the triad of tumefaction, sinus tract formation and tissue grains within the exudate. Other bacterial infections include *Nocardia*, *Staphylococcus*, L forms, and *Yersina pestis*. *Staphylococcus* produces a firm subcutaneous to dermal nodule, which may be alopecic, ulcerated, abscessed with or without numerous draining tracts. *Yersina pestis* (plague) infection commonly results in submandibular lymphadenopathy, fever and subcutaneous abcessation. L forms produce cellulitis 4–5 days after injury. The cellulitis spreads rapidly with the development of multiple fistulae and febrile response. Septic arthritis is a common sequel, and affected joints ulcerate producing a grayish mucinous exudate.

Mycobacterial:

● Atypical mycobacterial infections*** (p 1085)

Occur secondary to skin penetration, for example, the cat bite abscess that does not heal. Insidious progression from circumscribed plague or nodule to multiple sinuses with seropurulent exudate, board-like fibrosis and pain on palpation. Occur mostly on the tail-base and ventral abdomen.

● Feline leprosy* (p 1090)

Mostly young cats (1–3 years). Non-painful, ulcerated nodules on the limbs and head.

● Cutaneous tuberculosis (p 1093)

Mostly caused by *M. bovis* from ingestion of unpasteurized milk. Abscesses, nodules, ulcers and plaques develop with thick green or yellow exudates. Many cats have other organ involvement including GIT, CNS or respiratory signs.

Fungal:

● Sporotrichosis (p 1095)

Traumatic implantation of fungi occur via vegetable foreign bodies, or secondary to a cat fight. Sporotrichosis is an important zoonosis. The cutaneolymphatic form is most common. It appears as a wound on a limb, with a tract of nodules which may ulcerate, extending along the local lymphatics.

● Eumycotic mycetoma (p 1093)

Occurs in geographic areas along the Tropic of Cancer. Infection occurs via wound contamination. Ulcerated papules or nodules on the limbs or face, which develop draining sinus tracts. Black or

continued

continued

white grains are evident in the mycetoma from the fungal hyphae. Black-grained – *Curvularia geniculata* and *Madurella grisea*. White-grained – *Pseudoallescheria boydii* and *Acremonium hyalinum*.

● Pseudomycetoma (p 1094)

Occurs exclusively in Persian cats. Subcutaneous nodules form mainly on the dorsum and may ulcerate. They represent granulomas from *Microsporum canis* infection. More typical signs of superficial dermatophytosis may be evident.

● **Cryptococcosis* (p 1089)**

Skin lesions occur as multiple or single papules and nodules, which often ulcerate. They may or may not occur with CNS, respiratory or ophthalmic signs. Most common sign is a firm swelling over the bridge of the nose or planum nasale, or a polyp-like mass in the nasal opening.

● Pheohypomycosis (p 1095)

Occurs as a solitary nodule, usually on the paw, nose, limb or trunk. The lesion may ulcerate with sinus formation. Dissemination is rare.

● **Histoplasmosis, blastomycosis and coccidiomycosis* (p 1090)**

Chronically draining lesions together with dyspnea and weight loss. Blastomyces and coccidioidomyces are very rare in cats. Histoplasmosis is most frequent along Ohio, Missouri and Mississippi river valleys in the US.

Immune-mediated:

● **Feline eosinophilic granuloma complex*** (p 1088)**

Brightly erythemic plague associated with incessant grooming of the site, or appears as an indolent ulceration of the upper lip adjacent the nasal philtrum. Oral ulcerations and nodules may be present.

● Vasculitis and miscellaneous ulcerative dermatoses (p 1103)

Ulcerations of extremities (nose, ear tips, tail tip and foot-pads). In some cats is associated with neoplasia or a drug reaction.

● Erythema multiforme/toxic epidermal necrolysis (p 1105)

Multifocal (erythema multiforme) or confluent (toxic epidermal necrolysis) ulceration and crusting of skin and mucous membranes.

Idiopathic:

● Idiopathic feline ulcerative dermatosis (p 1103)

Sudden appearance then insidious course of ulceration and crusting of the dorsal cervical area. Pruritus is variable but may be intense and not glucocorticoid responsive.

Toxic/drug:

● Chemical dermatitis (p 1102)

Hair loss, ulcers or crust-covered erosions on contact sites. Oral ulceration and ptylism may result from ingestion of the chemical during grooming.

Trauma:

● Traumatic panniculitis (p 1104)

Non-antibiotic responsive, discharging wound in inguinal or dorsolumbar area which presents 2–3 weeks after blunt trauma at that site.

INTRODUCTION

MECHANISM?

Wound healing is characterized by chronologically overlapping phases of inflammation, proliferation (epithelial regeneration and fibroplasia), angiogenesis and tissue remodeling.

Wound healing is prolonged or prevented if there is **prolongation of inflammation** (e.g. because of infectious agents), or **proliferation is inhibited** (e.g. from ischemia, ongoing cellular injury, anti-mitotic drugs), or there is **inhibition of angiogenesis or altered tissue remodeling** (e.g. from increased tissue protease activity).

Each stage of wound healing is intrinsically interdependent. Interference at any stage can lead to a failure of wound healing.

Wounds that have **not resolved within 3 weeks** should be considered non-healing wounds.

WHERE?

Epidermis, dermis, panniculus and cutaneous blood vessels.

WHAT?

Non-healing wounds involving the **epidermis** are most commonly: neoplasia, viral, chemical toxicity, immune-mediated diseases and congenital abnormalities.

Non-healing wounds involving the **dermis** are most commonly: infectious agents, hypersensitivy diseases, neoplasia.

Non-healing wounds involving the **panniculus** are most commonly: infectious agents, traumatic ischemia.

Non-healing wounds involving **blood vessels** are most commonly: immune-mediated disease.

DISEASES CAUSING NON-HEALING WOUNDS

ATYPICAL MYCOBACTERIAL INFECTIONS***

Classical signs

- Alopecic plaques with multiple fistulae.
- Chronic serosanguineous exudate.
- Progressive subcutaneous fibrosis.
- Discomfort on palpation of skin.

Pathogenesis

Mycobacteria organisms are ubiquitous within the environment in soil and water. They enter the body via **penetrating wounds** including cat fights, vegetable foreign body and abrasions.

Organisms most frequently isolated include *Mycobacterium smegmatis, M. fortuitum, M. chelonae, M. thermoresistible, M. xenopi, M. phlei*. They are selective for the panniculus because of their triglyceride requirement and the immunological advantage. The **complex cell wall structure allows mycobacteria to survive intracellularly**.

Clinical signs

Initially there is a **circumscribed plaque or nodule** that progresses to **alopecic areas** with **numerous fistulae**.

Serosanguineous exudates are typical.

Board-like thickening of the skin and **pain** is evident on palpation. Lesions occur most commonly on the **ventral abdomen and lateral flanks**.

There may be a **history** of trauma to skin.

Diagnosis

Diagnosis is based on **demonstration** of the **organism** in the exudate or in biopsied tissue.

Cytological examination of material obtained from the sinus tracts reveals **pyogranulomatous inflammation.** Ziehl–Neelsen (ZN) stain may show acid-fast bacilli.

Histopathological examination requires **deep biopsy** to include subcutaneous fat. Take a wedge section avoiding the sinuses. This is submitted in formalin for routine H&E stains, Gram stain for bacteria, Gomori methanine silver stain for fungi and ZN stain for mycobacteria. Histopathology reveals pyogranulomatous to granulomatous panniculitis with neutrophil-rimmed lipocysts. With ZN stain low numbers of **acid-fast bacilli** may be seen **within the lipocysts (extracellular)**.

Culture additional wedges biopsies collected. Sterilely trim off the epidermis, and submit the remaining tissue in a sterile, saline-moistened guaze swab for culture. Specifically request mycobacterial culture if suspected. Aspiration of wound fluid and rapid innoculation of a culture medium may be better than a deep tissue sample, if you have ready access to a laboratory that specializes in mycobacterial culture and identification.

PCR confirmation of mycobacteriosis and species identification is available at some laboratories.

Differential diagnosis

Differential diagnoses include **bacterial mycetoma, subcutaneous mycosis, sterile panniculitides.** Clinical signs can be indistinguishable if tissue grains are not evident. Special stains of histological sections and anaerobic, aerobic, fungal and mycobacterial culture allow for differentiation.

Treatment

Treatment involves **prolonged antibiotic therapy** (months) to reduce the size of the lesion **combined with surgical excision**.

Where possible, choice of antibiotic should be based on in-vitro sensitivities.

Commonly used drugs for atypical mycobacteria include **doxycycline** 5 mg/kg/day, **fluoroquinolones** 5 mg/kg/day, **clofazamine** 2–8 mg/kg/day and **clarithromycin** 10 mg/kg bid. **Combinations** may be considered where sensitivities are not known.

Surgery requires a wide excision. Extensive reconstruction may be required following excision of affected tissue.

Antimicrobial drugs should be continued for several months post-operatively.

Prognosis

Prognosis is guarded where extensive disease exists at the time of presentation. Early diagnosis, including identification of the organism, and aggressive surgical and antimicrobial treatment offers a more favorable outcome.

BACTERIAL INFECTIONS***

> ### Classical signs
>
> - Nodules, plaques or abscesses.
> - Fistula formation.
> - Serosanguineous to purulent to "tomato soup" exudate +/– tissue grains.

Pathogenesis

Infections usually involve **commensal mouth organisms** or **ubiquitous environmental organisms** introduced to the skin through traumatic implantation via claw wounds, bites, vegetable, foreign bodies, etc.

Organisms include:
- **Actinomyces** from oral and bowel flora.
- **Nocardia**, a soil saprophyte.
- *Staphylococcus* from the oral cavity.
- *Yersinia pestis* (plague) from a lagomorph or rodent reservoir and transmission via inhalation, ingestion or arthropod vector.
- **L forms** which are mutated from the parent organism.

Clinical signs

Actinomyces and *Nocardia* have **several different presentations** but dissemination is rare.
- **Cutaneous form** is associated with firm **subcutaneous to dermal nodules** which frequently are ulcerated, abscessed or contain numerous drainage tracts.
  - Head, neck, flank, thoracic and abdominal wall are the most common sites.

- The exudate often appears as "**tomato soup with sulfur granules**".
- Regional lymph nodes are enlarged.
- Actinomycotic mycetoma are characterized by the triad of tumefaction, sinus tract formation and tissue grains within the exudate.
- **Effusive form** occurs in the chest or abdomen. Signs include fever and depression as well as respiratory distress or abdominal enlargement.
- Osteomyelitis form presents with lameness, fever and hyperesthesia.

Staphylococcus (**botryomycosis**) produces a firm subcutaneous to dermal nodule that may be alopecic, ulcerated, abscessed, with or without numerous draining sinuses.

- Visceral forms have been reported with symptoms varying dependent on organ involved.

Yersina pestis (**plague**) infection commonly results in submandibular lymphadenopathy, fever and subcutaneous abcessation.

- Septicemia has also been reported and mortality rates are up to 33%.

L forms produce **cellulitis** 4–5 days after injury. The cellulitis spreads rapidly with the development of **multiple fistulae** and febrile response.

- Lameness from septic arthritis is a common sequel. Joints are affected by hematogenous spread, and may be distant to the initial site. Lower limbs, especially the tarsus and carpus, are the most commonly affected.
- Most affected joints ulcerate producing a grayish mucinous exudate.
- There is no systemic spread of lesions throughout the body.

Diagnosis

Diagnosis is based on clinical signs and identification of the organism.

Cytological examination of exudates or a **squash preparation** of the "**sulfur granules**" may reveal the organism.

Biopsy and histological examination is often required to demonstrate organisms. **Special stains should be requested**, for example, Gomorri Methanine Silver or Ziehl-Neelson (ZN) stains because organisms such as acid-fast bacilli, are not always visible on routine H&E.

Culture of deep tissue is required for successful diagnosis. A large tissue sample is best, for example, a cubic centimeter of tissue. Prepare the biopsy site as for sterile surgery, remove an elliptical biopsy which must include the subcutaneous fat, and avoid sampling sinuses because of surface contamination. Trim the epidermis and submit the remaining tissue in a sterile moistened swab within an air-tight sterile specimen container for culture.

- Request aerobic, anaerobic, fungal and mycobacterial culture.
- If copious exudate is present, aspirate the exudate into a sterile syringe, cap the syringe and submit for culture.

For plague, culture is a public health risk.

Indirect fluorescent antibody testing of a fine-needle aspirate, or of tissue collected by biopsy gives the fastest diagnosis for plague. False negatives can occur.

Serology for plague requires two blood samples to demonstrate an increasing titer. Maximum titer occurs at day 12 after infection, therefore the first sample for serology must be collected early to be useful.

L forms are **not visible in tissue samples** even with special stains, and **do not grow on culture**. On electromicroscopy, organisms are visible **intracellularly within phagocytes**. Diagnosis is often made by response to tetracyclines as a therapeutic trial.

Differential diagnosis

Differential diagnoses that should be considered include atypical mycobacteriosis, cutaneous tuberculosis, dermatomycoses, foreign bodies, sterile and nutritional paniculitides and neoplasia.

Treatment

Treatment differs depending on the organism

Nocardia: treatment involves lavage, drainage and debridement combined with long-term antimicrobial therapy (enrofloxacin 5 mg/kg). Treatment should continue for several months after all lesions resolve.

Actinomyces: Penicillin is the drug of choice (e.g. amoxycillin 12 mg/kg twice daily). This should be combined with **en bloc excision of lesions**, and careful search for foreign bodies. Treatment course should be prolonged for 3–4 months.

Botryomycosis: **En bloc excision** combined with long duration anti-staphylococcal **antimicrobials** (e.g. cephalexins 22 mg/kg twice daily).

Plague: **aminoglycosides, tetracyclines and trimethoprim-sulfur** are effective, but penicillins are not.

L forms: are exquisitely sensitive to **tetracyclines** (e.g. doxycycline 5 mg/kg/day).

Prognosis

Prognosis varies from fair to good depending on the practicality of surgical excision, and presence or absence of dissemination.

Prevention

For plague, strict flea control in endemic areas is indicated.

Zoonotic potential

Plague (*Yersinia pestis***) is an important zoonotic organism,** and great care should be taken so that human infection does not occur from suspect cats. The relevant authorities should be notified.

FELINE EOSINOPHILIC GRANULOMA COMPLEX ***

> ### Classical signs
>
> - Glistening, erythemic plaque (eosinophilic plaque).
> - Ulceration of the upper lip adjacent the philtrum (indolent ulcer).

Pathogenesis

Eosinophilic plaque and **indolent ulceration** are cutaneous reaction patterns in cats associated with allergic skin disease.

Clinical signs

Eosinophilic plaque presents as variably sized, alopecic, glistening, red plaques most commonly found on the **ventral abdomen and medial thighs**.

Indolent ulceration presents as a progressive erosion on the **upper lip and/or nasal philtrum** region.

Diagnosis

Diagnosis is based on clinical and histological appearance.

Histopathology of eosinophilic plaque shows severe spongioisis, and intense neutrophilic and eosinophilic dermal infiltration. Peripheral blood eosinophilia is often present.

Indolent ulceration has a very characteristic clinical appearance. Histopathology is non-specific but rules out neoplasia. Blood eosinophilia is absent.

It is important to note that **indolent ulcer and eosinophilic plaque are clinical symptoms,** and are not a diagnosis. **The underlying allergy needs to be determined.**
- **Allergy investigation** involves a flea elimination trial, a food allergy trial using a novel protein for 6–12 weeks, and intradermal skin testing for atopy.

Differential diagnoses

Differential diagnoses which should be considered for **eosinophilic plaque** include pyoderma, lymphoma and mast cell tumor.

The **differential diagnosis** to consider for **indolent ulcer** is neoplasia.

Treatment

Specific treatment involves treating the underlying cause using flea control, dietary allergen avoidance or hyposensitization for aeroallergies.

Non-specific treatment to reduce inflammation involves use of **corticosteroids** (2–4 mg/kg daily) until signs are controlled, and then reducing dose to low-dose alternative day therapy.
- **Chlorambucil, aurothioglucose and progestagens** may be indicated if specific therapy and corticosteroids are not effective. Use of progestagens is discouraged because of the high incidence of drug-induced complications.
- **Cyclosporin 5 mg/kg/d (not registered for use in cats).**

Prognosis

Prognosis is good if the allergy is identified, and signs can be controlled with specific therapy.

SQUAMOUS CELL CARCINOMA (SCC)**

> **Classical signs**
>
> - Proliferative and/or ulcerative lesions on non-pigmented facial extremities.

See main references on page 1069 for details (The Cat With Skin Lumps and Bumps).

Clinical signs

Squamous cell carcinoma affects **any gender or breed of cat**, and the **average age** of affected cats **is 9 years.**

The **pinnae, philtrum, nares, forehead and palpebrae** are the most affected sites, especially in non-pigmented, thinly haired areas.

Lesions are multiple in 45% of affected cats.

Lesions may be **proliferative or ulcerative**, and occasionally cutaneous horns are seen.

SCC tends to be **locally invasive** and **slow to metastasize**.

Nail-bed SCC behave more aggressively.

Diagnosis

Diagnosis is based on histopathology of the lesion which shows **irregular cords of keratinocytes** which breach the dermo–epidermal junction and invade the dermis. Cellular atypia, dyskeratosis, loss of cellular orientation with or without solar elastosis may be evident.

CRYPTOCOCCOSIS*

> **Classical signs**
>
> - Soft tissue swelling over the bridge of the nose (Roman nose) or polyp in nasal opening.
> - Single or multiple papules or nodules in the skin which may ulcerate.

See main references on page 25 for details (The Cat With Signs of Chronic Nasal Disease) and page 847 (The Cat With a Head Tilt, Vestibular Ataxia or Nystagmus).

Clinical signs

Typically there is a **firm swelling over the bridge of the nose** or planum nasale giving the appearance of a Roman nose, or there is a **polyp-like mass visible in the nasal opening**.

Cutaneous lesions occur in up to 40% of cases, and consist of **papules or nodules** varying from 0.1–1 cm in diameter.

Lesions may ulcerate and exude serous fluid, or remain as intact nodules.

Skin lesions may be **single or multiple**, and occur alone, or with involvement of other organs.

Lesions favor **face, pinnae and paws**, and can occur with or without co-existent respiratory, CNS or ophthalmic signs.

Diagnosis

Diagnosis is based on clinical signs and **demonstration of the organism** in association with the lesion.

Cytological examination of fluid draining from a skin lesion, nasal exudate, a fine-needle aspirate of a skin nodule, spinal fluid, vitreal or aqueous paracentesis stained with **new methylene blue** (NMB) and Gram stains usually demonstrates the organism. Organism is **yeast-like** (5–15 μm) and is surrounded by a **wide, clear capsule.**

Serology to detect cryptococcal capsular antigen in blood, CSF or urine is useful if positive. Note that this test may be negative when the disease is localized to the skin.

Tissue biopsy can be used to identify the **pleomorphic yeast-like organisms with a refractile halo** (mucinous capsule). PAS and methanamine silver stains make the organisms more readily detectable.

Differential diagnosis

Differential diagnoses that should be considered for the cutaneous form of cryptococcosus include feline leprosy, atypical mycobacteria, bacterial granuloma, other fungal granulomas, xanthoma and neoplasia.

FELINE LEPROSY*

> **Classical signs**
>
> - Young cats in coastal locations.
> - Painless, ulcerated nodules on head and/or limbs.

Pathogenesis

The causative agent of feline leprosy is thought to be *Mycobacterium lepraemurium.*

Infection is probably acquired from cats **contacting rodents**. Cat-to-cat transmission has not been reported.

The incubation period is **2–12 months**. Immuno-deficiency is not needed for infection to occur.

Clinical signs

Typically occurs in young cats in coastal locations.

Multiple or single cutaneous nodules mostly on the **head and limbs.**

Lesions are **painless, and often ulcerated,** but rarely fistulated or exudative.

Local lymphadenopathy may be seen but visceral dissemination is rare.

Diagnosis

Diagnosis is based on clinical signs and demonstration of the organism.

Cytological examination demonstrates **pyogranulomatous inflammation with intracellular acid-fast bacilli.**

Histopathology shows **tuberculoid or lepromatous forms** of the organism.

Culture is rarely used in diagnosis because the organism has fastidious growth requirements.

PCR where available.

Treatment

Treatment is best accomplished via a **wide surgical excision**.

Spontaneous remission has been reported.

The organism has been reported to respond to **fluoroquinolones and clofazamine**. Dose of clofazamine is 2–8 mg/kg daily then twice weekly for 1–2 months. Reversible pinkish-orange discoloration of the skin and elevated liver enzyme (alanine transferase) have been reported.

Zoonotic potential.

There is no zoonotic potential.

HISTOPLASMOSIS, BLASTOMYCOSIS AND COCCIDIOMYCOSIS*

> **Classical signs**
>
> - Dyspnea.
> - Weight loss.
> - Chronically draining skin lesions.

See main references on pages 371, 387 for details (The Pyrexic Cat) and page 755 details (The Cat With Signs of Chronic Small Bowel Diarrhea).

Clinical signs

Histoplasmosis is most frequent along Ohio, Missouri and Mississippi river valleys in the US. Blastomyces and coccidiomyces are very rare in cats.

Clinical signs are often non-specific and include fever, anorexia and weight loss.

Dyspnea and harsh lung sounds without coughing is common in histoplasmosis and bastomycosis, but occurs in only 25% of cats with coccidiomycosis.

Solitary, regional or generalized peripheral and visceral **lymphadenopathies** are frequently present.

Pale mucous membranes, icterus, hepatomegaly or splenomegaly may be evident, most often with histoplasmosis.

Chronically draining skin lesions are the most frequent sign of infection in cats with coccidiomycosis, and were reported in 56% of cats in one study.

- Lesions begin as small bumps and progress to abscesses, ulcers or draining tracts.

- **Draining skin lesions** may occur in blastomycosis and are usually a manifestation of systemic disease rather than local disease.
- Skin lesions may occur with histoplasmosis.

Ocular signs are common with blastomycosis, but infrequent with histoplasmosis and coccidiomycosis, and may include conjunctivitis, anterior uveitis, retinal detachment or chorioretinitis.

Gastrointestinal signs may occur infrequently with histoplasmosis, and include chronic diarrhea and mesenteric lymphadenopathy.

Osseous lesions produce soft tissue swelling and lameness.

Diagnosis

Diagnosis is based on the history of travel to endemic area, clinical signs and **identification of the organism** in cytological or histological samples.

Serology may be useful for diagnosis of blastomycosis and coccidiomycosis, but is unreliable for histoplasmosis.

Culture for histoplasmosis is not recommended in a veterinary practice because the organism is a dangerous zoonotic.

Direct animal-to-animal, or animal-to-human transmission has not been reported, and infection occurs from a common environmental source.

Differential diagnoses

Differential diagnoses that should be considered include disseminated mycobacteriosis, feline plague and neoplasia.

POX VIRUS (FELINE COWPOX)*

Classical signs

- Focal ulcer, or large abscess with cellitus.
- Followed 7–10 days later by generalized small (0.5–1 cm) crusted ulcers.
- Occurs in roaming adult male cats.

See main references on page 1113 for details (The Cat With Paw or Pad Problems).

Pathogenesis

Orthopoxvirus infection causing **feline cowpox is not uncommon in Western Europe**.

Transmission is via **direct contact** with **rodents**, usually through a bite or already broken skin. The oronasal route of transmission may also be possible.

Disease occurs mostly in **male free-roaming adult cats**.

The viremic stage virus is transported via monocytes.

Clinical signs

Primary lesions vary from a **small ulcer on the head or limbs**, to a **large abscess with cellulitis**. Secondary lesions appear 7–10 days later as generalized small (0.5–1 cm) crusted ulcers.

Mild **lethargy, anorexia** and **coryza** occur.

With immunosuppression, for example with concomitant FIV, **pneumonia and non-healing wounds** may occur.

Pneumonia is a poor prognostic sign.

In immunocompetent cats, host **healing occurs within 4–6 weeks.**

Diagnosis

Diagnosis is based on finding **characteristic histopathological changes**, consisting of typical ballooning degeneration and viral inclusion bodies within the epidermis.

Viral culture can be used for definitive diagnosis of the virus.

Differential diagnoses

The **differential diagnosis** which should be considered for the primary lesions is a cat bite abscess; for secondary lesions, causes of miliary dermatitis should be considered. In immunocompromised cats, bacterial and fungal granulomas, systemic mycoses, tuberculosis and neoplasia are differentials.

Treatment

No specific treatment is available.

Antibiotics and symptomatic treatment should be used where indicated.

Corticosteroids are contra-indicated.

Prognosis

Prognosis is good in an immunocompetent cat and spontaneous resolution occurs in 4–6 weeks.

Transmission

Scabs shed virus, which survives in cool dry environs for **months to years**.

Cats represent a common **zoonotic threat** to people. Normal hygiene measures generally suffice for prevention.

FELINE HERPES VIRUS*

> **Classical signs**
>
> - **Non-healing ulceration of the dorsal nasal bridge or nasal planum.**

See main references on page 7 (The Cat With Acute Sneezing or Nasal Discharge) and page 1212 and page 1208 (The Cat With Ocular Discharge or Changed Conjunctival Appearance).

Pathogenesis

Feline rhinotracheitis is an α herpesvirus.

Trauma may initiate nasal lesions.

Clinical signs

Chronic non-healing ulceration or erosion on the **nasal planum or dorsal nasal bridge** may occur with herpesvirus infection.

Ulceration can also occur elsewhere, including on the paws.

The cat may or may not have signs of concurrent ocular or respiratory disease.

Diagnosis

Histopathological examination of a biopsy shows **eosinophilic dermal inflammation**. In acute lesions, basophilic, intranuclear **inclusion bodies** may be evident within the epithelium at the margin of the ulcer.

Demonstration of feline herpesvirus 1 in tissue from the ulcer by **PCR** is available from some laboratories.

Virus culture is available from some laboratories.

Virus can be demonstrated in lesional tissue with **electromicroscopy**, but this is not routinely available.

Differential diagnosis

Chronic non-healing erosions on the nasal planum or bridge of the nose may occur with mosquito bite hypersensitivity, squamous cell carcinoma and eosinophilic granuloma complex. Differentiation is based on appearance of the lesion and any other associated lesions, and biopsy with histopathology.

Treatment

Lysine supplementation (250 mg PO daily).

Prognosis

Based on reports in the literature, it suggests a guarded prognosis. However in the author's experience, lysine therapy has resulted in resolution of the ulcer.

MAST CELL TUMOR*

> **Classical signs**
>
> - **Single to multiple tumors on the head of older cats.**
> - **Tumors may "enlarge" after palpation or aspiration.**
> - **Rarely young Siamese cats have multiple nodules around the head.**

See main references on page 1074 for details (The Cat With Skin Lumps and Bumps).

Clinical signs

The average age of cats with mast cell tumors is **10 years**, and there is no sex or breed predisposition.

Tumors may occur at any site, but the **head is most frequently affected.**

Appearance varies from a **discrete solitary nodule** to **multiple papulonodular tumors** to a **plaque-like mass.**

Skin tumors may "enlarge" and become erythematous after palpation or aspiration.

Paraneoplastic syndromes may be evident including gastrointestinal tract ulceration, delayed wound healing, hypotension, cutaneous flushing, local ulceration and swelling and coagulation abnormalities.

Histiocytic mast cells tumors are uncommon, occur as multiple skin nodules around the head of cats less than 4 years of age (mean age 2.4 years) and Siamese are predisposed.

Diagnosis

Diagnosis is based on demonstration of characteristic mast cells associated with a skin mass. Fine-needle aspirate shows **round cells with granules**, which stain well with Wright's stain.

Histopathological examination shows a **round cell tumor with variable pleomorphism** and granule formation, which is dependent on the grade of the tumor.

Abdominal radiology, ultrasound and laparotomy may be useful for staging the tumor.

CUTANEOUS TUBERCULOSIS

Classical signs

- Yellow/green thick purulent exudate from skin lesions.
- Lymphadenopathy.
- GIT, respiratory, CNS or ophthalmic signs.

Pathogenesis

Mycobacterium bovis is the causative agent in 96% of cases. *M. tuberculosis*, *M. avium* and *M. microti* have also been reported.

The reservoir of *M. bovis* is **infected cattle**.

Cats are infected via ingestion of **unpasteurized milk** or **eating contaminated meat** or **offal**.

M. tuberculosis is a reverse zoonosis.

The method of transmission with *M. avium* and *M. microti* is unknown. It may involve the cat's natural predation of rodents and birds.

Incubation period in natural infections is **months** to greater than **one year.**

A breed susceptibility for *M. avium* infections has been reported in the **Siamese** cat.

Clinical signs

Skin lesions are usually part of a more generalized disease, evident in 56% of cases.

Single or multiple **ulcers**, **abscesses**, **plaques** or **nodules** with thick green or yellow **purulent exudate**.

Additional signs vary with route of entry and degree of dissemination of the organism, and may include **GIT, respiratory, CNS or ophthalmic signs.**

Diagnosis

Diagnosis is based on clinical signs and **identification** of the **organism**.

History, physical examination, radiography, urinalysis and blood testing (hematology and biochemistry) are important in the diagnostic work-up.

Cytological examination may reveal **acid-fast bacilli** in **skin aspirates or biopsies**, or in **urine**.

On microbiological culture the organisms are **slow to grow**, and require **special media**.

Intradermal skin testing with BCG or purified protein derivative (PPD) is not reliable.

Serological testing is unreliable in cats.

EUMYCOTIC MYCETOMA

Classical signs

- Papules or nodules on the limbs and face.
- Sinus formation.
- White or black tissue grains in the mycetoma.

Pathogenesis

Eumycotic mycetomas are **subcutaneous fungal infections**.

Organisms are ubiquitous in soil. **Infection occurs via wound contamination**.

Most frequently occurs in geographic areas along the Tropic of Cancer.

Black-grained mycetomas are produced by *Curvularia geniculata* and *Madurella grisea*.

White-grained mycetomas are produced by *Pseudoallescheria boydii* and *Acremonium hyalinum*.

Clinical signs

Solitary papules occur on the **limbs and face**, and evolve to painful nodules and fistulae, resulting in sinus tracts.

White or black tissue grains are evident in the mycetoma, which represent the fungal hyphae.

Infection may involve the underlying deeper structures.

Diagnosis

Diagnosis is based on clinical signs and **demonstration of the organism**.

For **cytological examination**, make a squash preparation of the tissue grains. Gritty grains may need 10% KOH digestion first. Fungal hyphae are visible microscopically.

Histopathological examination reveals **granulomatous to pyogranulomatous inflammation** and **tissue grains of fungal hyphae**.

Culture requires special media using SDA.

Immunodiffusion is available in some laboratories. Some fungi can be diagnosed by serum testing for specific antibodies with agar immunodiffusion. Tissue samples may also be stained with fluorescein conjugated with specific antibodies.

Differential diagnosis

Differential diagnoses that should be considered include mycobacterial infections, neoplasia, actinomycotic mycetoma, pseudomycetoma, botryomycosis, foreign bodies and chronic bacterial abscesses.

Treatment

Wide surgical excision is the treatment of choice, which may require limb amputation to remove sufficient tissue.

Antifungal therapy is often ineffective. The imidazoles are worth trying where in vitro sensitivites are not available, for example itraconazole (10 mg/kg twice daily). Anorexia and elevated liver enzymes are the most frequently encountered adverse effects.

Prognosis

Cutaneous mycetomas are not life threatening, but **can be difficult to resolve if wide surgical excision** is not possible.

PSEUDOMYCETOMAS

> **Classical signs**
>
> - Exclusively Persian cats.
> - Subcutaneous nodules often together with superficial dermatophytosis.

Pathogenesis

Pseudomycetomas represent **subcutaneous infection caused by the dermatophyte, *Microsporum canis***.

They occur **exclusively in Persian** cats and immune incompetence has been suggested.

Clinical signs

Non-painful subcutaneous nodules that may **ulcerate and drain**.

Most occur on the dorsum.

The nodules may or may not be associated with obvious superficial dermatophyte infection.

Diagnosis

Diagnosis is based on signalment (Persian cats), signs and demonstration of organism.

On **histopathological examination** a Splendori-Hoeppli reaction is evident, which consists of **fungal hyphae surrounded by amorphous eosinophilic material**, which represent antibody–antigen complexes. PAS stains show up the fungal hyphae.

Examine coat for signs of superficial infection using a Wood's lamp, and sterile coat collection using the toothbrush technique and **culture for *M. canis***.

Assess the immune status of the cat and determine if intercurrent disease is present using hematological, biochemistry, urinalysis, FeLV and FIV testing.

Differential diagnosis

Differential diagnoses that should be considered include bacterial, fungal and mycobacterial granulomas and neoplasia.

Treatment

If there is a single lesion, **surgical excision** is the treatment of choice.

Medical treatment using **itraconazole** (20 mg/kg daily) for several months may be effective. Anorexia may occur and reflect hepatopathy and require cessation of therapy.

SPOROTRICHOSIS

Classical signs

- Chain of subcutaneous nodules following the lymphatic tract, and extending away from primary wound.

Pathogenesis

Sporothrix schenckii is the causative organism, and is ubiquitous in **soil and organic debris**, especially in humid environs.

Infection occurs via **traumatic inoculation** via a **vegetable foreign body, cat claw**, or via wound contamination.

Clinical signs

The **cutaneous form** looks similar to a **cat bite abscess**.

The **cutaneolymphatic form** has corded **lymphatics with secondary ulcerations** occurring **along the lymph pathway**, extending away from the primary wound.

The disseminated form is rare.

Diagnosis

Diagnosis is based on identification of the organism.

Cytological examination shows numerous **pleomorphic yeasts**, which may be intra- or extracellular.

Histopathological examination reveals **oval, round or cigar-shaped organisms**. PAS and GMS stains facilitate identification.

Immunoperoxidase or fluorescent antibody techniques are useful if tissue numbers are low. This is usually not required in cats.

Culture from a **deep sinus tract swab or tissue biopsy** for definitive identification of organism.

Differential diagnosis

Differential diagnoses that should be considered include bacterial, mycobacterial, fungal granulomas, neoplasia, sterile panniculitis.

Treatment

Traditional therapy involved use of a saturated solution of **potassium iodide** (SSKI; 20 mg/kg PO q 12–24 h) administered for 30 days beyond clinical cure. Cats are **susceptible to iodism**, and many develop signs including anorexia, vomiting, depression, twitching, hypothermia and cardiovascular failure.

Ketaconazole (5–10 mg/kg twice daily) either singly or together with potassium iodide has been used successfully. Gastrointestinal, neurological signs and jaundice are reported associated with ketaconazole use.

Newer **imidazoles** may be useful, such as itraconazole (10 mg/kg/day PO).

Surgical excision is useful for the cutaneous form, where wide excision is possible.

Prognosis

Prognosis is guarded for all but the localized cutaneous forms.

Sporothrix is a serious zoonosis. In households with young children or immunosuppressed adults, it may be unwise to treat the cat because of the risk of infection.

Prevention

To prevent zoonotic infections, all discharging non-healing wounds in cats, especially where lymphatic cording is present, should be handled with great caution using gloves, careful cleaning after handling, etc.

PHEOHYPHOMYOCOSIS

> **Classical signs**
>
> - Ulcerated nodule on the nose or limb.

Pathogenesis

Fungi reported in cats associated with pheochromocytosis include *Dresclera spicifera*, *Curvularia lunata* and *Exophiala jeanselmei*.

These are **saprophytic** fungi that produce dermataceous (dark) hyphal elements in tissues. They occur most commonly in **tropical or subtropical areas.**

Infection is by **traumatic implantation** via cat claw wounds or a plant foreign body.

Immunosuppression increases susceptibility.

Clinical signs

Pheohypomycosis occurs as a **solitary nodule**, usually on the **paw, nose, limb or trunk**.

The lesion may **ulcerate with sinus formation**.

Dissemination is rare.

Diagnosis

Diagnosis is based on **identification of the organism** associated with the lesion.

Cytological or histological examination can be used to identify **pigmented fungal element**s.

Definitive diagnosis is based on **culture** on SDA at 25–35°C, and identification of the organism.

Assess for concurrent immunosuppressive disease by testing for FIV and FeLV.

Differential diagnosis

Differential diagnoses that should be considered include bacterial, fungal and mycobacterial granulomas and neoplasia.

Treatment

Treatment of choice for the cutaneous form is **wide surgical excision**. Where wide surgical excision is not possible, amphotericin B combined with an imidazole such as itraconazole, and/or cryotherapy may be tried, although relapse is common.

Prognosis

Prognosis is good if surgical excision is possible, although relapse may occur. The disseminated form has a grave prognosis.

MULTICENTRIC SQUAMOUS CELL CARCINOMA IN SITU

> **Classical signs**
>
> - Multifocal, hyperkeratotic or ulcerated plaques.
> - Occur on pigmented, thickly haired skin of older cats.

Pathogenesis

Papilloma virus antigen has been detected in some lesions.

Ultraviolet radiation and arsenicals are not thought to play a role.

Clinical signs

Lesions are found in **older cats** (> 10 years usually).

Multifocal lesions occur over the **head, neck, shoulders and forelimbs** on **pigmented, thickly haired skin.**

Begin as hyperkeratotic macules and evolve to **thick-crusted, ulcerated plaques**.

The neoplasia often have a long course **over a couple of years**, with **waxing and waning signs.**

Diagnosis

Diagnosis is based on **histopathological findings**.

Excise the lesion and submit for histopathology. Histologically, there is abrupt transition from normal to atypical epithelium. The **dermo–epidermal junction is not breached**.

Differential diagnosis

Differential diagnoses which should be considered include mycobacterial, fungal and bacterial granulomas and other neoplasia.

Treatment

Treatment of choice for **thin lesions** is **beta radiation**. Treatment does not prevent new lesions.

Etretinate and isoretinoin can be used in thicker lesions, but the response is variable.

Prognosis

Cats are often euthanized for cosmetic reasons and owner frustration at poor response to therapy.

Metastases have **not been reported**.

MELANOMA

Classical signs

- Ulcerated, pigmented nodule on head or neck.

See main references on page 1079 for details (The Cat With Skin Lumps and Bumps).

Clinical signs

Melanoma typically occurs in **older cats of any breed** (average age is 10 years).

Tumors usually occur as **solitary lesions** on the **head or neck**.

Size and shape are variable ranging from a **dome**, to a **plaque or polypoid shape,** and ulceration is frequent.

Diagnosis

Diagnosis is based on histopathological examination of an excisional biopsy. Characteristic findings are **atypical melanocytes in nests, sheets and cords.** Cells may exhibit epithelioid or spindle morphology or a combination of both.

BASAL CELL CARCINOMA (BCC)

Classical signs

- Pigmented, cystic tumor on head or neck of older cats.

See main references on page 1070 for details (The Cat With Skin Lumps and Bumps).

Clinical signs

Basal cell carcinoma occurs frequently as a **pigmented and/or cystic tumor of the head, neck, thorax, nasal planum or eyelids in older cats**.

Usually occur as a **solitary tumor** and are **frequently ulcerated**.

Diagnosis

Diagnosis is based on histopathology.

CUTANEOUS LYMPHOMA

Classical signs

- Alopecia and scale.
- Erythroderma.
- Hypopigmentation of hair or skin and mucocutaneous junctions.
- Nodules or plaques which often ulcerate.

See main references on page 1078 for details (The Cat With Skin Lumps and Bumps).

PATHOGENESIS

Cutaneous lymphoma is a **very rare tumor** in cats, and results when **malignant T or B lymphocytes infiltrate** the skin.

Most cases are **FeLV negative**.

Clinical signs

Signs of **epitheliotropic T cell tumors** (mycosis fungoides) include "non-inflammatory" alopecia, scaling, erythroderma (diffuse reddening of the skin), hypopigmentation of hair or skin, ulceration, plaques and nodules.

B cell neoplasia shows **dermal nodules** with or without ulceration, and with or without lymphadenopathy.

Systemic signs of weight loss, diarrhea and respiratory distress may be present.

Diagnosis

Diagnosis is based on clinical signs and histological examination of biopsied tissue.

Fine-needle aspirate and cytological identification of abundant malignant round cells is useful to establish a presumptive diagnosis.

Histopathological examination is required for a definitive diagnosis to demonstrate diffuse infiltrates of malignant, poorly differentiated lymphoid cells. The epetheliotropic form has Pautrier's microabscesses, which are focal aggregates of neoplastic T cells in the epidermis.

Blood evaluation, radiographs, ultrasound, lymph node aspirates and bone marrow biopsy are important for clinical staging.

Differential diagnosis

Differential diagnoses for the **epitheliotrophic form** include systemic lupus erythematosus, dermatophytosis, demodecosis, cutaneous flushing syndromes, drug eruption and hypersensitivities.

Differential diagnoses for the **nodular forms** include bacterial and fungal granulomas and other neoplasia.

Treatment

Retinoides (vitamin A analogs), such as isotretinoin (Accutane) or acitretin (Soriatane) can be used for palliative treatment of the epitheliotropic form (**mycosis fungoides**).

B cell lymphoma is treated with excision of solitary lesions and standard lymphoma protocols. Excisional surgery may be curative for solitary lesions. Small lesions may respond well to superficial radiation therapy. Results of chemotherapy for multiple lesions are often disappointing.

Prognosis

Prognosis is poor.

Cats with small solitary lesions may do well initially with surgical excision, but generalized disease is likely to occur within 12 months.

The epidermotropic form often has an insidious progression.

ACQUIRED CUTANEOUS FRAGILITY SYNDROME

> **Classical signs**
> - Large tears in paper-thin skin.
> - Evidence of underlying disease, e.g. hyperadrenocorticoidism.

Pathogenesis

Dermal and epithelial atrophy occurs secondary to **hyperadrenocorticoidism, progestagen** administration or metabolic conditions and diseases such as **starvation, neoplastic cachexia, diabetes**, etc.

Clinical signs

Skin is **thin** (atrophic) and mechanically weak, and may **spontaneously tear**.

Skin is **fragile but not hyper-extensible**.

Diagnosis

Cutaneous signs are very characteristic.

Histopathological examination reveals **epidermal and dermal atrophy**.

Identification of the underlying pathology may require hematological and serum biochemistry examination, urinalysis, radiology, ultrasound and specific endocrine testing.

Differential diagnosis

The main differential diagnosis is **cutaneous asthenia**.

Treatment

Correct the underlying pathology.

Avoid trauma to the skin, or exerting tension on the skin while restraining the cat.

Prognosis

Prognosis is variable, and is dependent on the initiating cause.

XANTHOMA

Classical signs

- Yellowish, ulcerated nodules or plaques over bony points.
- Associated with hyperlipidemia.

See main references on page 570 for details (The Cat With Hyperlipidemia).

Clinical signs

Xanthoma appear as **alopecic nodules and plaques** which are **often ulcerated** on foot pads, lateral hocks, elbows, oral cavity or at sites of injury.

They often have a **whitish** or yellowish **waxy appearance**.

Cutaneous xanthomatosis has been described in cats with diabetes mellitus and is associated with hyperlipidemia.

Most common in cats associated with hyperlipidemia.

Diagnosis

Definitive diagnosis is based on histopathological evidence of **Touton giant cells**, which are considered pathognomonic.

History taking including drug history, physical examination and blood testing is required to differentiate primary and secondary hyperlipidemia.

Differential diagnosis

Differential diagnoses which should be considered include eosinophilic granuloma complex, bacterial and fungal granulomas and neoplasia.

METABOLIC EPIDERMAL NECROSIS (MEN)

Classical signs

- Crusting, erosions and erythema of mucocutaneous junctions and bony protuberances.
- Pad hyperkeratosis.

Pathogenesis

Metabolic epidermal necrosis is the **cutaneous manifestation of hepatic** and occasionally **pancreatic disease**.
- Other terms include superficial necrolytic dermatitis, necrolytic migratory erythema (NME) and hepatocutaneous syndrome.

Metabolic epidermal necrosis has been associated with **hepatic and pancreatic disease** in cats, but is poorly understood. It is possible that the pathological process causing the skin lesions is triggered by a variety of systemic metabolic derangements.
- Deficiencies in certain nutrients such as amino acids, zinc, essential fatty acids and biotin may cause keratinocyte degeneration.
- Because low plasma amino acid concentrations were found in dogs and high-quality protein diets or supplementation with egg leads to resolution of signs in some animals, it has been postulated to be associated with an **amino acid deficiency.**

In dogs and people it is associated with **glucagon-secreting tumors** and a variety of other diseases not associated with a hyperglucogonemia, especially hepatic disease. The role of glucagon is not understood, but it is postulated to affect catabolism of amino acids to glucose.

In cats it has been reported with pancreatic carcinoma, chronic hepatopathy and thymic amyloidiosis.

Clinical signs

Alopecia, erythema, crusts, erosions and ulceration of the skin most frequently seen at mucocutaneous junctions and frictional areas of the skin. The skin can be thickened and may become fissured.
- The skin lesions are often **secondarily infected** with bacteria or yeast.

Footpads show marked hyperkeratosis and fissuring.

Diagnosis

Diagnosis is based on **histopathological examination** of the skin lesions and demonstration of **diffuse parakeratosis**, which includes follicles, epidermal pallor, basal cell hyperplasia (red, white and blue effect).

Measurement of **plasma glucagon** concentration is indicated to rule out a glucagonoma.

Diagnosis of the hepatic or pancreatic disease requires **serum biochemistry analysis** to demonstrate increased liver enzymes, and **ultrasound** to demonstrate liver or pancreas pathology.

Hepatic or pancreatic biopsy via ultrasound guidance or exploratory laparotomy is usually needed for definitive diagnosis of the underlying condition.

Differential diagnosis

Differential diagnoses include bacterial and fungal infections, neoplasia and pemphigus foliaceous.

Treatment

Treatment should be directed at controlling the underlying disease and nutritional support.

Amino acid supplements can be given by feeding a cooked egg yolk daily, and/or feeding a commercial recovery diet containing high-quality protein and increased levels of amino acids.
- A slow IV **infusion of an amino acid** formulation designed for parenteral administration has been used successfully in some patients.

Supplementation with **zinc and essential fatty acids** may help some patients.

Anti-malassezial shampoos (miconazole containing) may help control the skin lesions.

Surgical resection of glucogonoma is indicated if present.

Prognosis

Prognosis is poor for long-term survival.

CUTANEOUS ASTHENIA

> ### Classical signs
> - Fragile, hyperextensible skin which tears easily.
> - Focal necrosis and paperaceous scars.
> - Patchy alopecia.

Pathogenesis

Cutaneous asthenia results from a **congenital defect of collagen I synthesis**.

Clinical signs

Cutaneous asthenia appears as **hyperextensible skin and/or "spontaneous" tearing of the skin**.

Focal necrosis of the skin (necrotic eschars), particularly involving the dorsal neck, may occur.

Numerous **paperaceous scars** and patchy alopecia may be evident.

Hematomas may occur.

Occasionally joint laxity and/or ophthalmic opacities are seen.

Diagnosis

Diagnosis is based on **clinical appearance** and **increased extensibility index** of the skin. An extensibility index of greater than 19% is considered abnormal.

- The extensibility index is measured by stretching the skin dorsally within pain limits. The vertical height of this skin fold is expressed as a percentage of the crown to rump length.

Histopathological examination with routine H&E is **not diagnostic**. Masson's trichrome stain, which is designed to stain dysplastic collagen red and normal collagen blue, has been reported to be a sensitive indicator of this disease. However, the author has not found this stain to be helpful in Burmese cats.

Electron microscopy is the definitive test and shows **irregular orientation of collagen fibrils.**

Differential diagnosis

The differential diagnosis which should be considered is acquired cutaneous fragility secondary to hyperadrenocorticoidism, progestagen administration, or other metabolic conditions. Importantly, the **skin is fragile but not hyperextensible** in acquired cutaneous fragility.

Treatment

Management involves **avoiding injury** by keeping the cat indoors, and taking care when handling the cat not to exert tension on the skin.

Suture tears rapidly to prevent further tearing.

Prognosis

Most cats can have a good-quality life if trauma is minimized.

EPIDEMOLYSIS BULLOSA

Classical signs

- Ulcerative lesions in young kittens.
- Nail shedding.

Pathogenesis

Epidermolysis bullosa results from a **congenital defect of the dermo–epidermal junction** of the skin.

The disease is classified as epidermolysis bullosa simplex, junctional epidermolysis bullosa and dystrophic epidermolysis bullosa, depending on the ultrastructural defect.

Clinical signs

Signs appear in **kittens often by 5–12 weeks of age**, at the time of increased activity and mechanical stress on the skin.

Signs include **nail shedding, foot pad ulceration, hard palate ulceration** or **skin ulceration** in frictional sites.

Diagnosis

Clinical signs in a young kitten are highly suggestive.

Histopathological examination of skin shows **dermo–epidermal separation** (cleft formation) without inflammation.

Electro microscopy together with immunolabeling is necessary to identify the ultrastructural level of the split, and the nature of the defect at that level, that is, the specific element that is missing.

Differential diagnoses

Differential diagnoses that should be considered include thermal injuries, chemical burns and vasculitis.

Treatment

There is **no specific treatment** for epidermolysis bullosa.

Avoid trauma and provide symptomatic wound care.

Onycectomy can be performed for pain relief, if the major sign is nail shedding.

Prognosis

Prognosis is guarded. Euthanasia is an option if the quality of life is not adequate.

CHEMICAL DERMATITIS

> **Classical signs**
> - Ulcers or crust-covered erosions at contact sites.
> - Ptalism.

Pathogenesis

Strong alkalis, acids or cationic detergents can cause a chemical dermatitis if they are in contact with the skin.

Clinical signs

Ulceration or crust-covered erosions develop at contact sites.

Oral ulceration and ptalism may result from ingesting the chemicals while grooming.

Diagnosis

A tentative diagnosis is based on **clinical signs** consistent with chemical dermatitis, together with a **history** of possible exposure to irritant chemicals.

Differential diagnoses

Differential diagnoses that should be considered include thermal injuries, trauma and calicivirus infection.

Treatment

Remove chemical from skin using copious, gentle irrigation with saline or 0.05% chlorhexidine.

Use **prophylactic antibiotic** cover to minimize secondary bacterial infection.

Feed soft foods, or if oral ulceration is severe, use nasogastric or esophageal tubes for feeding.

Intravenous fluids may be required, so monitor carefully for dehydration and protein loss through the skin.

Wound care may require judicious debridement, and use of non-adherent bandages changed daily until the lesions re-epithelialize.

Prognosis

Prognosis is good if there is not extensive skin involvement.

TRAUMATIC PANNICULITIS

> **Classical signs**
> - Multiple fistulae with serosanguineous to gelatinous exudates.
> - Inguinal or dorsolumbar area.
> - History of prior blunt trauma to site.

Pathogenesis

Ischemia of individual lipocytes may occur following **trauma,** and the resultant release of triglycerides **induces inflammation.**

Clinical signs

Blunt trauma may cause **panniculitis**, which **presents 2–3 weeks later** with signs.

Lesions are most common in the **inguinal or dorsolumbar** areas. There is **alopecia** of the **overlying skin**.

Sinus tracts or fistulae may form, with a resultant **serosanguineous to gelatinous exudate**.

Subcutaneous fibrosis occurs with healing.

Diagnosis

A **tentative diagnosis** is based clinical signs and a history of trauma.

No organisms are detected on cytology, biopsy or culture.

There is no response to antimicrobial therapy.

Differential diagnoses

Differential diagnoses that should be considered include infectious, immune-mediated and nutritional panniculitis.

Treatment

Treatment involves **surgical excision** of the involved fat pad.

Glucocorticoids (prednisolone at anti-inflammatory doses of 0.5–1 mg/kg q 24–48 h for 4–6 weeks) help reduce inflammation.

Vitamin E 200 IU/cat/day may help reduce inflammation.

Prognosis

Traumatic panniculitis is often frustrating to treat if surgical excision is not possible.

Prevention

Oxypentoxifylline (10 mg/kg q 12 h) and **vitamin E** (200 IU/cat q 24 h) immediately following trauma may help to improve tissue perfusion and stabilise cell membranes.

Early debridement of **necrotic fat** following trauma is indicated to reduce inflammation.

VASCULITITIS AND MISCELLANEOUS ULCERATIVE DERMATOSES

Classical signs

- Ulcers and crusts (skin and/or mucocutaneous junctions).

Pathogenesis

Immune-mediated ulcerative dermatoses represent a heterogeneous group of diseases in which the primary lesion is cutaneous ulceration.

Vasculitis resulting in skin lesions is rare in cats. It may be associated with immune complexes secondary to infectious or neoplastic disease, drugs and as part of autoimmune syndromes, such as SLE or be idiopathic.
- Predisposed sites have minimal collateral circulation such as the pinnae, paws and tail tip.
- Ulceration and necrosis are typical.

Cold agglutinin disease is a rare disease where cold-reacting IgM erythrocyte antibodies cause autoagglutination in the cooler peripheral vasculature of the extremities resulting in ischemic necrosis of the ear and tail tips and foot pads.

Clinical signs

Typically there is **cutaneous ulceration**, which may be crust-covered.

Lesions often involve the **muco-cutaneous junctions, foot pads, nail–skin junction, oral cavity, inguinal and axillary** areas and extremities (ear and tail tips).

Vasculitis may be associated with **necrosis** particularly of pinnae, foot pads and tip of the tail.

Systemic signs such as fever and lethargy are not uncommon.

Diagnosis

Diagnosis is based on clinical signs and histological findings.

Early and late lesions should be examined **histopathologically**. For small ulcers, excise the entire ulcer together with the marginal skin. For large ulcers, an elliptical biopsy should be collected extending from grossly normal skin through the edge of the ulcer to the ulcerated skin.

An accurate drug history is important.

Diagnostic tests should be performed to rule-out concomitant neoplasia.

Differential diagnosis

Differential diagnoses which should be considered include bullous pemphigoid, systemic lupus erythematosus (SLE), discoid lupus erythematosus (DLE), vasculitis, cold agglutinin disease, erythema multiforme (EM), toxic epidermal necrolysis (TEN).

Treatment

Treat the underlying disease if possible, and stop drug treatment or change to a different class of drug if signs appeared during drug treatment.

Where an underlying trigger (drug or neoplasia) cannot be found, immunomodulation is recommended rather than immunosuppression.

Drugs commonly used include **pentoxifylline** (10 mg/kg q 12 h) which is a gastrointestinal tract irritant so should be given with food, **prednisolone** (2–4 mg/kg q 24 h or divided into twice daily and taper to response), chlorambucil or aurothioglucose.

Prognosis

Prognosis is guarded if the trigger cannot be found and resolved.

PANSTEATITIS/VITAMIN E DEFICIENCY

> ### Classical signs
>
> - Fever, lethargy and pain on cutaneous palpation.
> - Cutaneous ulcerations with gelatinous exudate.

Pathogenesis

Vitamin E is an important natural antioxidant. A relative or absolute deficiency of vitamin E can result in peroxidation of bonds in unsaturated fat. This may occur with diets containing large amounts of **unsaturated fish oils**.

The unsaturated oils undergo oxidation, and release **reactive peroxides** in the body fat of the cat, causing painful inflammation of fat (pansteatitis).

Signs have been reported in cats that were fed mainly **oily fish such as red tuna.** Cats fed diets supplemented with cod-liver oil deficient in vitamin E are also at risk.

Clinical signs

Classical signs are lethargy, inappetence, fever, reluctance to move and pain on **cutaneous palpation**.

Subcutaneous fat has a generalized firm feeling on palpation.

Cutaneous ulcerations may form with a gelatinous exudate.

Diagnosis

Diagnosis is based on clinical signs and histological examination of biopsied fat.
- **Grossly**, affected fat may have a **brownish discolorization**.
- **Histopathological examination** shows **lobar and septal panniculitis** with characteristic ceroid deposition.

Differential diagnosis

Differential diagnoses which should be considered include infectious panniculitides, traumatic panniculitis and immune-mediated panniculitis.

Treatment

Treatment involves dietary correction and use of anti-inflammatory drugs such as prednisolone (1 mg/kg/day).

Prognosis

Prognosis is guarded to poor.

IDIOPATHIC FELINE ULCERATIVE DERMATOSIS

> ### Classical signs
>
> - Dorsal neck ulceration.

Pathogenesis

Pathogenesis is unknown and may be multifactorial.

Ulceration has been associated with use of **topical spot-on insecticidal agents** as an idiosyncratic reaction.

There is often a **history of vaccination** at the site within the last 12 weeks. This is a common site for vaccination, therefore a positive history does not equal causative role.

It has been associated with a variety of **allergies** including food allergy, and especially flea allergy, ectoparasites (demodex, notoedres, otodectes) and dermatophytosis.

Clinical signs

Chronic ulceration is usually present on the **dorsal neck area,** but may involve the face and base of ears.

Ulceration appears rapidly, and then follows a very insidious course.

The lesion **may spontaneously resolve** over 8–12 weeks **or persist**.

Pruritus varies from intensely itchy to not at all.

Diagnosis

Clinical signs are classical.

Check history of injections or application of insecticidal agents at the site.

Histological examination of a deep elliptical biopsy including the area affected with panniculus may show lymphocytic vasculitis/panniculitis, faded follicles and **linear subepidermal fibrosis**.

Differential diagnosis

Differential diagnoses that should be considered include trauma, cutaneous asthenia, necrotizing envenomation and thermal injury.

Treatment

Response to use of **glucocorticoids** is often **disappointing** because the pruritus is often steroid resistant.

A small number of cases treated by the author have responded (or spontaneously resolved) while on **pentoxifylline** (10 mg/kg twice daily).

Keeping the **lesion wrapped** until it is completely healed, and using **Soft Paws** (Soft Paws Inc., Lafayette, LA, USA) on the hind feet may be successful in some cats. Soft Paws are vinyl caps that glue to the cat's claws and protect against skin damage from scratching.

A **hypoallergenic diet** may help some cats and a lime-sulfur dip every 5 days for 5–7 treatments has been suggested to rule out *Demodex gatoi*.

Wide surgical excision of the lesion and the use of Soft Paws on the claws of the hind feet are curative in some cats.

In cats resistant to treatment or where there is reoccurrence of the lesion after surgical excision, **declawing of the hind feet** has led to successful resolution of the lesion. However, Soft Paws should be trialed first and declawing used only as a last resort.

ERYTHEMA MULTIFORME (EM) AND TOXIC EPIDERMAL NECROLYSIS (TEN)

Classical signs

- Multifocal to confluent cutaneous ulceration.
- Muco-cutaneous junction ulceration.

Pathogenesis

Erythema multiforme and toxic epidermal necrolysis involve a **cytotoxic CD8+ T-cell response** against keratinocytes, which can be activated by drugs, viruses, neoplasia and foods.

Erythema multiforme is an **acute eruption of the skin and mucous membranes** and is most commonly associated with a drug sensitivity. Penicillin and aurothioglucose have been associated with erythema multiforme in cats.

Toxic epidermal necrolysis is an **acute disseminated disease** involving the mucous membranes and skin, and is associated with **systemic signs**.

- There is intracellular edema in the dermis and separation of the dermo–epidermal layers.

Clinical signs

Typically, onset of signs is **acute**.

In both conditions, lesions consist of **erythematous macules** (flat circumscribed red areas of skin ≤ 1 cm) and **ulceration,** which may be annular, arciform or serpiginous (snake-like).

Vesicles, blisters or bullae may be observed which ulcerate, ooze and crust over.

The ventral abdomen, peri-mammary area, ear pinae, perioral and perineal areas are often affected.

Erosion or ulcers may be present on the **oral mucosa.**

Toxic epidermal necrolysis is associated with **systemic signs including pyrexia, depression,** anorexia.

Diagnosis

A presumptive diagnosis is based on the **clinical appearance of an acute ulcerative condition** involving the skin and mucous membranes, which is associated with a recent history of drug administration. Other differential diagnoses need to be excluded.

Histopathological examination of erythematous macules or ulcer margins reveals epidermal changes including hydropic degeneration, prominent single cell to apoptosis, lymphocyte and macrophage satellitosis and variable dermal edema (EM) to full thickness epidermal necrosis (TEN). Inflammatory changes in the dermis are mild to marked in EM but often absent in TEN.

Differential diagnosis

Other vesicular and pustular disorders, e.g. bacterial infections, pemphigus foliaceous, burns, chemical dermatitis need to be ruled out.

Treatment

Cyclosporin 5 mg/kg PO q 24 h. Not registered for use in cats.

Remove drug or diet triggers if identified.

Supportive treatment (intravenous fluids, warmth, avoidance of sepsis) needed where large amounts of epithelium are lost.

Prognosis

Prognosis is good if the trigger can be removed and the area affected is small, but is poor where large areas of epidermis have been lost.

RECOMMENDED READING

Baldwin CJ, Panciera RJ, Morton RJ, Cowell AK, Waurzyniak BJ. Acute tularaemia in three domestic cats. J Am Vet Med Assoc 1991; 199: 1602–1605.

Dillberger JE, Homer B, Daubert D, Altman NH. Prototheccosis in two cats. J Am Vet Med Assoc 1988; 192: 1557–1559.

Dunstan RW, Credille KV, Walder EJ. The light and the skin. Kwochka K, Willemse T, von Tscharner C (eds) Advances in Veterinary Dermatology, Vol 3. Blackwell, Cornwall, UK. 1998, pp. 3–37.

Eidson M, Thilsted JP, Rollag OJ. Clinical, clinicopathological, and pathological features of plague in cats: 119 cases (1977–1988). J Am Vet Med Assoc 1991; 99: 1191–1196.

Gunn-Moore D, Shaw S. Mycobacterial diseases in the cat. In Practice 1997; 493–500.

Jacobs GJ, Medleau L, Calvert C, Brown J. Cryptococcal infection in cats: Factors influencing treatment outcome, and results of sequential serum antigen titers in 35 cats. J Vet Int Med 1997; 11: 1–4.

Lemarie RJ, Lemarie SL, Hedlund CS. Mast cell tumors: Clinical management. Compendium 1995; 17: 1085–1099.

Malik R, Martin P, Love DN. Localised *Corynebacterium pseudotuberculosis* infection in a cat. Aust Vet Pract 1996; 26: 27–31.

Ruslander D, Kaser-Hotz B, Sardinas JC. Cutaneous squamous cell carcinoma in cats. Compendium 1997; 19: 1119–1127.

Theon AP, VanVechten MK, Madewell BR. Intratumoral administration of carboplatin for treatment of squamous cell carcinomas of the nasal plane of cats. Am J Vet Res 1996; 57: 205–209.

Werner AH, Werner BE. Feline sporotrichosis. Compendium 1993; 15: 1189–1197.

53. The cat with paw or pad problems

Isobel Phebe Johnstone

KEY SIGNS

- Erythema, scaling, crusting, and/or pruritic lesions.
- Nodules, draining tracts, ulcers and/or abscesses.
- Distortion of the nails or deformity of the foot.

MECHANISM?

- A wide variety of diseases can have paw or pad problems as part of more generalized signs, or the lesions can be confined solely to the foot.

WHERE?

- Disease of the feet includes the paw, pads, digits and nails. Interdigital spaces are seldom affected in cats.
- It is rare for the disease to be confined solely to the feet. Usually the feet are affected in conjunction with other areas of the skin.

WHAT?

The most common problems seen in the paw are:
- Bacterial paronychia from a variety of causes.
- Immune-mediated diseases.
- Nodules or ulceration due to infections or neoplasia.

QUICK REFERENCE SUMMARY

Diseases causing paw or pad problems

ANOMALY

- **Variation in number of the digits* (p 1118)**
Hereditary variations in the number of digits, generally six toes, occur most commonly on the front feet.

- Hypomelanosis (vitiligo) (p 1122)
Loss of epidermal melanin is evidenced by non-pigmented patches in otherwise pigmented areas such as the nose, lips, mouth and paw pads.

continued

continued

● **Hyperpigmentation (lentigo simplex)** (p 1113)**

Dark pigmented patches ("freckles") occur in the non-haired areas of orange cats older than 1 year of age.

● Epidermolysis bullosa (p 1123)

A hereditary claw-shedding disease seen in Siamese kittens causes the claws to shed easily with minor trauma.

METABOLIC

● Hypothyroidism (p 1121)

Erythematous, scaling lesions of the footpads occasionally occur with hypothyroidism. Seborrhea sicca and a dry lusterless hair coat, which is easily epilated, and has poor regrowth after clipping may be evident. It is very rare in cats, and occurs most commonly after bilateral thyroidectomy.

● **Hyperthyroidism** (p 1113)**

Unkempt hair coat and overgrown claws are commonly seen. Systemic signs include weight loss, polyphagia, polydypsia/polyuria and nervous/hyperactive temperament. Usually seen in cats older than 8 years.

● Hyperadrenocorticism (p 1121)

Rare condition in cats that results in very thin and easily torn skin, especially on the digits. Other systemic signs include polyphagia, polydypsia/polyuria, abdominal enlargement and skin infections.

● Diabetes mellitus (p 1122)

Whitish, waxy nodules in the paws are a rare complication of diabetes mellitis. Other systemic signs include polyuria/polydypsia, weight loss and polyphagia or anorexia.

● Calcinosis cutis (p 1123)

Metastatic calcification occasionally occurs in the pads of the feet secondary to renal failure. Affected pads are enlarged, firm and painful. A chalky white-to-pink material may be visible through the intact epidermis. Pads may ulcerate and exude a chalky, white, pasty material.

MECHANICAL

● Foreign bodies (p 1120)

Foreign bodies may result in nodules, abscesses or draining tracts in the interdigital web. Foreign bodies are much rarer in cats than dogs.

NEOPLASTIC

● Primary and secondary neoplasia (p 1116)

Neoplasia may cause swollen painful pads or digits that become ulcerated. Various neoplasms have been recorded as having a predilection for the feet; squamous cell carcinoma, metastatic ungual carcinoma, fibrosarcoma and malignant fibrous histiocytoma have been more commonly reported.

● Cutaneous horns (p 1122)

Cones of hard keratin growing out from the skin occasionally occur on the feet.

PHYSICAL

● Irritant contact dermatitis or chemical burns* (p 1119)

Erythema and ulceration of the footpads often occur together with salivation, mouth ulcers and anorexia.

● Burns (thermal)* (p 1119)

Superficial to deep ulceration on the footpads occurs, depending on the severity of the burn.

● Frostbite (p 1120)

Frostbite may result in erythema, edema, necrosis and sloughing of extremities.

INFECTIOUS (VIRAL)

● Feline pox virus infection** (p 1113)

Multiple papules, vesicles, plaques or crusts and ulcers may occur on the face, ears, limbs and paws associated with pox virus. Paronychia and sloughing of footpads may occur.

● Infectious pododermatitis*** (p 1111)

Viral, bacterial (most common), fungal and parasitic agents may cause pad and paw disease. Bacterial: Paronychia involving one or more claws, and more rarely pyoderma or fistulated inter-digital abscesses are usually caused by the more common opportunistic bacterial infections such as *S. intermedius* and more rarely by the yeast *M. pachydermatitis*. Fungal: Single or multiple ulcerated nodules, or draining fistulated areas are usually associated with the rare opportunistic bacterial and fungal infections. Pheomycotic lesions are very darkly (black) pigmented. Non-pruritic, erythematous scaling, alopecic lesions are associated with dermatophytes and usually there are lesions elsewhere on the body as well. Kerion (nodular furunculosis) formation and onychomycosis (fungal claw infection) are rare. *Malassezia* causes brown staining at the base of the nails only, or a more generalized scaly erythematous dermatitis. Viral: Calici virus may pro-duce footpad ulceration in association with oral ulceration, usually without the more classical respiratory signs of sneezing and nasal discharge. Parasitic: Erythematous, alopecic lesions may occur with *Demodex cati* infections, or pruritic crusting lesions with *Notoedres cati*. Usually there are lesions on other parts of the body.

INFLAMMATION (IMMUNE-MEDIATED)

● Pemphigus* (p 1117)

Pemphigus foliaceus is most common. A symmetrical pattern of lesions occurs on the face, ears, trunk, feet and mucocutaneous junctions consisting of erythema, oozing, crust, scales and alope-cia. Some cats may present with only foot lesions.

● Systemic lupus erythematosus (p 1121)

SLE is a multi-systemic disease, which may involve the skin with ulcerative lesions of the feet and paronychia.

● Plasma cell pododermatitis* (p 1115)

Plasma cell pododermatitis results in swollen and very soft ("mushy") footpads with normal pad symmetry. Normally it is non-painful, but the pads may become ulcerated.

● Insect bite hypersensitivity** (p 1114)

Symmetrical pattern of erythematous papules, ulcers and crusts occur on thinly haired areas, especially the bridge of the nose and/or ear tips. Sometimes the footpads are also affected. Lesions have a seasonal occurrence.

continued

continued

ALLERGY

● **Atopy and adverse food reaction*** (p 1116)

Atopy or adverse food reaction may just involve the feet with nail biting and chewing. More typically it manifests as skin lesions affecting the head, face, ears and inner thigh. These include non-inflammatory alopecia, miliary dermatitis and granulomatous ulcerated skin from licking and scratching, particularly of the face and neck.

TOXIC

● Thallium poisoning (p 1124)

Thallium-containing rodenticide toxicity results in hyperkeratosis and scaling of the footpads, as well as similar lesions elsewhere on the body.

TRAUMA

● **Shredded nail tips or avulsed nails (trauma)*** (p 1111)

Shredded nail tips or avulsed nails are typically evident in cats involved in road accidents.

● Declawing complications (p 1120)

Deformed claws, keratinaceous foreign bodies at the ends of the digits or draining tracts may result from imperfectly completed declawing procedures.

● Arteriovenous fistulae (p 1124)

An arteriovenous fistula is a very rare condition resulting in local edema and distinct, tortuous, pulsating blood vessels near the area.

INTRODUCTION

MECHANISM?

Foot problems are less commonly seen in cats as a presenting complaint than in dogs.

The feet of cats can be affected, along with other areas of the body, in numerous feline dermatoses and systemic diseases.

Lesions confined primarily to the paw or pads are rarely seen.

Three categories of lesions are seen:
● **Scaling, crusting and pruritic** lesions, which usually result from immune-mediated and allergic diseases or infectious causes such as viral, fungal and parasitic.
● **Nodules, draining tracts, ulcers and abscesses**, which usually result from the more unusual bacterial and fungal infections or neoplasia.

● **Disorders of the claws and paronychia**, which usually result from trauma, bacterial paronychia or neoplasia.

WHERE?

Disorders of the feet including paws, pads, claws and ungual folds.

Careful history taking and a thorough physical examination are very important in establishing a list of differential diagnoses and for selection of appropriate laboratory tests.

For many of the diseases, definitive diagnosis is by histological evaluation of biopsy specimens.

WHAT?

The most common causes of foot problems are infectious agents, especially bacterial and fungal, and trauma.

Less common causes are tumors, immune-mediated diseases and endocrinopathies.

DISEASES CAUSING PAD OR PAW PROBLEMS

SHREDDED NAIL TIPS OR AVULSED NAILS (TRAUMA)***

Classical signs

- Broken or torn claws.
- Feathered ends to claws.

Clinical signs

Broken or torn claws.

Feathered ends to claws are classically seen in cats involved in a **road accident**, and result from dragging of the claws on the rough road surface.
- If the history of an injured cat is unknown, then feathered claw tips can be a clue to road trauma.

Diagnosis

Diagnosis is based on history and physical examination.

INFECTIOUS PODODERMATITIS***

Classical signs

- Paronychia involving one or more claws.
- Ulcerated nodules or fistulated areas.
- Non-pruritic, erythematous, scaling, alopecic lesions.

Pathogenesis

Common cause of foot problems in cats and is often **secondary** to factors such as **trauma or immune suppression** (FeLV, FIV, systemic disease).

Infectious agents can be bacterial, fungal or viral.

Bacterial.
- Various **opportunistic bacteria** have been reported, most commonly *Staphylococcus inter-*

medius, *Escherichia coli*, *Pseudomonas* sp., *Proteus* sp. or *Pasteurella* sp.
- More rarely other bacteria reported are *Mycobacterium* sp., *Listeria monocytogenes*, *Dermatophilus congolensis*, *Nocardia asteroides*.

Fungal.
- **Dermatophytes**, primarily *Microsporum canis, M. gypseum* and *Trichophyton mentagrophytes*, can be found on the paws but would rarely be found there as the only site on the body.
- Rare cases of **opportunistic saprophytic fungal infections** have been reported including:
  - Pheohyphomycosis caused by *Exophiala jeanselmei, Moniliella sauveolens, Cladosporium* sp., *Stemphyllium* sp. and *Scolecobasidium humicola*.
  - *Paecilomyces fumosoroseus* and *Sporothrix schenckii*.
- **Yeast infections** with *Cryptococcus neoformans, Rhodotorula mucilaginosa* and *Malassezia pachydermatis* usually also involve other areas of the body.

Viral.
- **Pox virus** causes foot lesions and is covered separately (see page 1113).
- Occasionally *Calici virus* may cause footpad ulceration, in addition to the more common clinical signs in other organs.

Parasitic.
- **Demodicosis** is reported to be a rare cause of claw disease.
- An opportunistic infection with *Leishmania braziliensis* has been reported causing a large vegetative lesion in the interdigital area.

Clinical signs

Bacterial.
- **Paronychia** involving one or more claws, and more rarely pyoderma or fistulated interdigital abscesses are usually caused by the more common opportunistic bacterial infections such as *S. intermedius*.
- **Single or multiple ulcerated nodules, or draining fistulated areas** are usually associated with the rare **opportunistic bacterial** (including *Nocardia, Listeria monocytogenes Dermatophilus congolensis*) **and fungal infections**.

Fungal.
- A variety of saprophytic fungi produce **draining tracts, ulcerated nodules and chronic non-healing wounds.** Pheomycotic lesions are very darkly (black) pigmented.
- Kerion (nodular furunculosis) formation and onychomycosis (fungal claw infection) are rare.
- *Malassezia pachydermatitis* is a yeast which is a secondary infectious agent, causing **brown staining at the base of the nails** only, or a more generalized scaly erythematous dermatitis. Rarely it causes paronychia involving one or more claws.
- Infection by **dermatophytes** causes hair loss and rarely infection of the nails (onychomycosis). Other areas of the body are usually also involved with irregular or circular alopecic patches, with or without scale, that are **non-pruritic and may be erythematous.**

Viral.
- **Pox virus** produces **multiple papules, vesicles, plaques or crusts** and ulcers, which may occur on the face, ears, limbs and paws. Paronychia and sloughing of footpads may occur.
- **Calici virus** infection may produce **footpad ulceration** in association with oral ulceration, usually without the more classical respiratory signs of sneezing and nasal discharge.

Parasitic.
- **Erythematous, alopecic** lesions may occur with *Demodex cati* infections, or pruritic crusting lesions with *Notoedres cati.* Usually there are lesions on other parts of the body.

Diagnosis

Wood's lamp examination or direct examination of hair and scales mounted in paraffin oil or KOH may detect dermatophytes.

Cytological examination of smears of the **exudate** from moist lesions, stained with Diff-Qik may reveal the primary organism present including *Malassezia, Cryptococcus* or bacteria.

Culture exudate to identify the organism, and obtain sensitivity for antibiotic treatment if bacterial.

Biopsy nodular or fistulous areas for histopathology, and culture tissue to identify the rarer opportunistic infections.

Serology to detect cryptococcal antibody is usually positive in cats with cryptococcosis.

Hair pluck/skin scrape to detect Demodex.

Differential diagnosis

Symmetrical bacterial paronychia can appear similar to **immune-mediated** disease such as pemphigus foliaceus.

Nodules and ulcerated areas can appear similar to **neoplastic lesions.**

Treatment

Bacterial infections.
- Use **appropriate antibiotics** selected based on culture and sensitivity.
- Treatment for several weeks may be necessary for deep infections.
- If lesion recurs, **check immune status** (FeLV, FIV, systemic disease).

Fungal infections.
- **Griseofulvin** (50–100 mg/kg PO q 24 h, preferably with a fatty meal) is effective only for dermatophytes. Beware of adverse drug reactions including teratogenicity, gastrointestinal upsets and bone marrow suppression.
- **Ketoconazole** (5–10 mg/kg PO q 24 h) has been effective for most fungal and yeast infections but has more side effects than itraconazole. Adverse reactions include anorexia, fever, depression, vomiting, diarrhea and neurologic abnormalities. Lower doses or alternate day therapy may be necessary if reactions occur.
- **Itraconazole** (5–10 mg/kg PO q 24 h) may work better than ketoconazole, and has fewer side effects, but is more expensive.

Parasitic infections.

Demodex.
- Feline demodicosis has responded to simple treatments such as three dips of **malathion or lime-sulfur** at weekly intervals.
- **Ivermectin** is very effective against mites, although its use in cats is off-label. For demodectic mange the dose rate is 0.6 mg/kg daily orally continued

for up to 30 days after negative skin scrapings. Stopping too early results in relapses.

- Similarly **Doramectin** at 0.6 mg/kg sc weekly can be used.

Leishmania.

- Successful treatment in cats has not been reported.

Prognosis

Prognosis varies depending on the type of infection and the underlying cause. The recurrence rate is high for bacterial paronychia if there is an underlying immune deficiency.

The prognosis is more guarded for the rarer opportunistic bacterial and fungal infections. Cures are reported with the use of the imidazole drugs (ketoconazole and itraconazole).

HYPERPIGMENTATION (LENTIGO SIMPLEX)**

Classical signs

- Black asymptomatic spots that gradually enlarge and become more numerous.
- Occur in cats with orange coat color.

Clinical signs

Hyperpigmented areas ("freckles") in orange (ginger) cats are termed lentigo simplex.

Freckles usually appear **before 1 year of age** and increase in number with age.

There are multiple hypermelanotic macular lesions on the **nose**, **lips**, **eyelids** and **footpads**.

Lesions are **asymptomatic** and do not develop into melanomas.

Diagnosis

Diagnosis is based on the history of asymptomatic black spots developing in the poorly haired areas of cats with a ginger coat color.

HYPERTHYROIDISM**

Classical signs

- Weight loss with polyphagia.
- Unkempt hair coat.
- Nervous, hyperactive.

See main reference on page 304 for details (The Cat With Weight Loss and a Good Appetitie).

Clinical signs

Most commonly there is **weight loss despite a ravenous appetite**. More rarely is appetite depressed.

Other signs may include tachycardia, polydipsia/polyuria, vomiting or diarrhea, and a heart murmur.

A **palpable thyroid nodule** in the neck is present in the majority of cats.

Restlessness and hyperexcitability are often evident.

An unkempt haircoat and **overgrown claws** are typical.
- The overlong claws catch in floor coverings or click on bare floors as the cat walks.

Usually occurs in cats older than 8 years of age.

Diagnosis

A tentative diagnosis is based on **history and physical examination**.

Increased total thyroxine (T_4) levels confirm the diagnosis. Cats with a high normal T4 concentration and signs consistent with hyperthyroidism should either be retested several weeks later, or free T4 concentration be measured by equilibrium dialysis, or a T3 suppression test performed. Concurrent disease can decrease a high T_4 into the normal range.

FELINE POX VIRUS INFECTION**

Classical signs

- Multiple nodules, papules, crusts, and ulcerative plaques.
- Commonly on the face, limbs and paws.
- Pruritis, pain, fever, conjunctivitis and dyspnea may be present.

Pathogenesis

Infection is caused by a virus from the **orthopoxvirus** genus. The origin of the virus is unclear. It was attributed to the cow-pox virus, but now it is thought there could be a **feline pox virus.**

Reported infections are from **England and Europe**.

Clinical signs

Skin lesions occur on the **face**, **ears**, **limbs** and **paws** with **multiple papules, vesicles, plaques or crusts and ulcers**.

On the feet there can be **paronychia and sloughing of the footpads**.

Diagnosis

Biopsy and histologic examination of the crust or affected skin demonstrates **eosinophilic intracytoplasmic inclusion bodies** within keratinocytes.

Specialist tests that may be available also include a serologic test for virus-neutralizing antibodies, electron microscopy of crusts or affected skin to detect the virus, and virus isolation. **Virus isolation** is currently the only method for making a precise diagnosis.

Differential diagnosis

Bacterial and fungal infections, eosinophilic granuloma and neoplasia may all cause similar lesions but can be differentiated on biopsy and histological examination.

Treatment

Treatment is not thought to affect the outcome of the disease, and is not regarded as necessary as most cats **recover spontaneously within 1–2 months.**

Secondary bacterial infection should be treated with antibiotics.

Glucocorticoids are contraindicated.

Prognosis

Prognosis is good as cats recover spontaneously, however, there may be permanent scarring.

Transmission

The natural reservoir for infection is not known, but is thought to be **small wild animals** and the cat is infected whilst hunting them.

Transmission of cow pox virus from infected milk has also been blamed.

The pox virus can be **transmitted to in-contact cats, dogs and humans;** immunocompromised individuals are more at risk. Warn in-contact people of the **zoonotic potential.**

The virus is killed by most disinfectants, particularly chlorine-based ones.

Prevention

Prevent the cat from hunting or contact with an infected cat.

INSECT BITE HYPERSENSITIVITY**

> ### Classical signs
>
> - Erythematous, crusted, pruritic lesions.
> - Symmetric lesions on ear tips, face, nose and footpads.

Pathogenesis

Hypersensitivity resulting in skin lesions is associated with **flying and biting insects.**

It is most often seen in cats that go **outdoors** when **mosquitoes or midges** (*Lasiohelia townsvillensis*) are present.

Clinical signs

Thinly haired areas are most commonly affected, especially the **bridge of the nose, ear tips and the junction of haired skin and the footpad ("ears, nose and toes syndrome").**

Lesions have a symmetrical pattern, and begin with **erythematous papules to plaques**.

Lesions are pruritic, and the cat traumatizes itself, so that the affected areas become **ulcerated and crusted**.

Chronic lesions develop **nodules, pigment changes (dark or pale patches), and alopecia**.

Footpads may be affected with swelling, scales or crusts, hyperkeratosis, fissures and pigment changes.

Diagnosis

Seasonal occurrence is evident coinciding with mosquito or midge season in cats allowed outdoors.

Tentative diagnosis can be confirmed by **keeping the cat indoors or hospitalized for 5 days** and demonstrating great improvement of lesions.

Biopsy and obtain small specimens (4-mm biopsy punch) carefully, as the **ears and nose bleed easily** and readily show scars. Histopathological changes are similar to those of cats with atopy, food and flea bite hypersensitivity.

Differential diagnosis

Food allergy commonly results in pruritis of the face, head, pinnae and neck, in contrast to just the nose and/or ears affected with insect hypersensitivity. Lesions are usually asymmetrical and very excoriated. Non-seasonal occurrence, and does not respond to the indoor confinement trial, but responds to an elimination dietary trial.

Autoimmune diseases such as pemphigus foliaceus/erythematosus and discoid lupus erythematosus typically also have a symmetric pattern, but usually there is extensive crusting and exudation of head and body. Depression and anorexia are often present. Pruritis is variable.

Treatment

Keep the cat indoors at the times of greatest insect activity, usually early morning and dusk.

Topical insect repellents applied to the affected area. Try a variety, as not many are well tolerated by cats; ointments or creams are best tolerated.

Petroleum jelly smeared on the ear tips and nose has also been used successfully.

Oral prednisolone (0.5–2 mg/kg on alternate days) or injectable glucocorticoids (repositol methyl prednisolone acetate, 20–40 mg/cat subcutaneously).

Prognosis and prevention

Good control of the problem is possible if the cat can be kept away from biting insects, or will tolerate insect repellent.

However, lesions may increase with severity over the years if exposure cannot be controlled.

PLASMA CELL PODODERMATITIS*

> **Classical signs**
> - Swollen, very soft footpads, generally non-painful.
> - Normal pad symmetry.

Pathogenesis

Plasma cell pododermatitis is a **rare skin disease** affecting the footpads.

The cause is unknown, but is thought to be **immune-mediated or allergic**.

One study found 50% of cases to be feline immunodeficiency virus-positive.

Clinical signs

Typically, the **footpads are swollen, very soft and fluctuant (mushy).** Usually the larger metacarpal and metatarsal pads are the ones affected.

Normal pad symmetry is not disturbed by the swelling, but the stretching of the skin over the swollen pad results in a **white, silvery, cross-hatched appearance.**

Lesions involve one or more feet.

Normally, the **lesions are non-painful** and the cat is not lame, although cases of cats limping on the affected feet have been reported.

The pad may become **ulcerated,** and drain hemorrhagic fluid.

Some cats also have plasma cell stomatitis, immune-mediated glomerulonephritis or renal amyloidosis.

Diagnosis

Fine-needle aspirate of the lesion contains large numbers of uniform plasma cells with a few neutrophils and lymphocytes.

Deep wedge biopsy from a footpad near the pad margin is diagnostic. A punch biopsy may not go deep enough to be diagnostic.

- If a number of pads are affected choose a more mildly affected one to biopsy as a severely affected one may not heal well.

Differential diagnosis

Undifferentiated sarcoma may appear very similar and needs a biopsy to differentiate.

Treatment

This is not necessary if the cat is asymptomatic, as the disease may **spontaneously regress.**

Immunosuppressive doses of **prednisolone** (up to 4 mg/kg/day) have been recommended, but may not be effective.

Chrysotherapy (aurothioglucose; Solganol; 1–2 mg/kg IM weekly) may be effective.

Surgical excision of the footpad. A new footpad grows back. Reported to be the best therapy at present.

Prognosis

Prognosis is guarded as the recurrence rate is high, usually within 4–6 months.

ATOPY AND ADVERSE FOOD REACTION*

Classical signs

- Pruritis, which is manifested as scratching, licking or chewing.
- Skin lesions varying in severity from alopecia to miliary dermatitis to ulcerated plaques or granulomas.

Clinical signs

Atopy and adverse food reactions result in various **other dermatological manifestations** such as ulcerated plaques, miliary dermatitis, symmetrical alopecia and pruritis of the **face and neck**.

Pruritis is present but may not be obvious to the owner.

- Over-grooming results in non-inflammatory alopecia ("fur mowing").

Foot or claw chewing may initially be the only presenting clinical sign.

- The cat drags the claws through the teeth with loud clicking noises, which brings the problem to the attention of the owner.
- **One or more ulcerated areas of the paws** (digits, periungual areas or interdigital spaces) may be present.
- Histologically these lesions are typical of eosinophilic granuloma complex.

Diagnosis

Rule out other causes of claw problems, especially **infectious pododermatitis and neoplasia.**

Control external parasites. A good choice is fipronil as this controls fleas, and anecdotally mites (*Cheyletiella*, *Sarcoptes*, *Otodectes* and *Notoedres*) and provides partial control of ticks.

Try a dietary trial using a food source that the cat has not been exposed to before. It may take ingenuity to find a new food that the cat is willing to eat. Duck, venison or rabbit (2/3 cup) with cooked rice or pasta (1/3 cup) are often tolerated. A trial period of a minimum of 9 weeks has been advocated for cats and up to 16 weeks preferably. Re-challenge the cat with the old diet to confirm the diagnosis, although owners may be unwilling to risk signs recurring.

Intradermal skin testing to test for atopy. This is technically more difficult in cats than dogs, as reactions are less intense and more transient.

PRIMARY AND SECONDARY NEOPLASIA*

Classical signs

- Swollen, painful digit(s) and/or paronychia.
- Ulcerative destructive lesion of the paw and digits.

Pathogenesis

Neoplasia involving the foot is rare in cats and is usually seen in older cats. The neoplasia may be primary or secondary. Secondary neoplasia results from metastasis of primary neoplasia in other organs.

Squamous cell carcinoma.
- Rare primary tumor arising from the nail bed epithelium.
- Appears to be more aggressive than squamous cell carcinomas in other parts of the body.
- On clinical examination it may be mistaken for paronychia or pyoderma.

Metastatic digital (ungual) carcinoma.
- Usually presents as lameness associated with multicentric digital carcinoma.
- Seen in aged cats (average age 13 years) with asymptomatic bronchogenic carcinoma or squamous cell carcinoma of the lung.
- Lesions can involve a number of digits and more than one paw. Typically there is swelling of the digit, ulceration of the skin or purulent discharge, and either fixed exsheathment, deviation or loss of the nail.

Fibrosarcoma.
- Seen in older cats and is not associated with feline sarcoma virus.
- Lesions are usually solitary and can involve the digits.
- The area is alopecic, ulcerated and the tumor has rapid infiltrative growth.

Undifferentiated sarcoma.
- Seen in older cats and involves the footpads of one or more feet.
- Affected pads are soft, mushy, painful and maybe ulcerated.

Malignant fibrous histiocytoma.
- Seen in older cats.
- The lesions are solitary, firm, poorly circumscribed, variable in size and shape and locally invasive.
- Legs, especially the paw, and shoulders are the most common sites.

Diagnosis

Biopsy of representative areas and histopathology.

Differential diagnosis

Plasma cell pododermatitis also has swollen mushy pads, which may be ulcerated.

Bacterial or fungal infections, especially the rarer opportunistic ones, can look very similar. Biopsy for histopathology and culture will distinguish between these.

Treatment

Radical surgical excision is the treatment of choice for tumors without evidence of metastasis.

Mean survival for metastatic digital carcinoma was 67 days.

PEMPHIGUS*

Classical signs
- Crust, scales, alopecia in a symmetrical pattern.
- Areas usually involved are face, ears, trunk, feet and mucocutaneous junctions.
- Occasionally have only foot lesions.

Pathogenesis

Pemphigus is an **immune-mediated disease**, with auto-antibodies directed against intercellular cement in the epidermis causing **loss of cohesion between keratinocytes** and resulting in the formation of bullae.
- Bullae are very transient in cat skin due to the thin epidermis, and may not be observed.

What initiates the auto-antibodies is unknown, but **drugs and chronic skin disease** have been implicated in some cases.

Different types of autoimmune dermatitis may involve cats' paws but the **most common** is *Pemphigus foliaceus*.

Clinical signs

Erythema, oozing, crusts, scales and alopecia occur with a **symmetrical pattern on the face, ears, trunk, feet and mucocutaneous junctions**.

Lesions commonly involve the **feet and footpads**, causing **hyperkeratosis and ulceration**. Some cats are presented with only footpad lesions and sometimes lameness.

Paronychia and **involvement of the nipples** are commonly seen in cats.

Diagnosis

Direct smears from intact vesicles or pustules may show numerous **acantholytic keratinocytes**; these are strongly suggestive of pemphigus.

Biopsy of primary lesions or at the periphery of the most recent lesions shows **subcorneal pustules** consisting of acantholytic keratinocytes and neutrophils.

Direct immunofluorescence of biopsies shows diffuse intercellular fluorescence.

Differential diagnosis

Systemic lupus erythematosus is rare and usually also has systemic signs.

Insect hypersensitivity is common, but lesions are usually confined to the bridge of the nose, tips of the ears, and occasionally footpads. Seasonal occurrence and history of biting insects being observed around the cat helps differentiate this from pemphigus.

Treatment

Therapy is often difficult as side effects from the drugs are common.

High doses of glucocorticoids (4–8 mg/kg daily) will induce remission in most cases (about 2 weeks). Once in remission, reduce to alternate day therapy and to the minimum dose which maintains remission.

Chlorambucil (0.1–0.2 mg/kg every 24–48 hours) can be added if glucocorticoids are insufficiently effective.

Chrysotherapy (gold salts; aurothioglucose: Solganal; Schering) has been useful in cats when other treatments have failed. Begin with 1 mg/kg IM weekly until remission, which may take up to 12 weeks to occur. If no response is evident after 12 weeks of therapy, increase dose to 1.5–2 mg/kg. Once the cat responds, give the dose every 2 weeks and then monthly for several months. Alternatively the dose can be started at 0.25 mg/kg IM for the first week, 0.5 mg/kg the second week, then 1 mg/kg weekly until remission and then a gradually decreasing dosage.

Prognosis

Prognosis is guarded, because the inciting cause is usually unknown, and the side effects of the therapy are often severe.

VARIATION IN NUMBER OF DIGITS*

Classical signs

- Abnormal number of toes (six most common).
- Agenesis or fusion of digits.

Clinical signs

Variation in the normal number of digits is present from birth.

Ectrodactyly is **agenesis** of all or part of a digit and is an inherited defect involving the fore-paws.

Polydactyly refers to **extra toes**.
- The mode of inheritance is dominant.
- There is considerable variation from animal to animal with the number of extra toes and how perfectly formed they are.
- Usually there are **six toes on each front foot,** but sometimes there can be seven toes on the front feet and six on the hind feet. The hind feet are not affected unless the front feet are involved.
- The **incidence varies** with it being common in some countries and not seen in others.

Syndactyly refers to **fusion of the digits**. It is also called "split-foot" or "lobster-claw".
- Typically it manifests as a **central cleft** of either one or both front feet. However, there may be fusion of the bones of the foot to produce double claws.
- The evidence is for **dominant heredity**, possibly with variable expression, as the number of affected animals is less than expected, with some genetically affected animals appearing normal. The right side tends to be more severely affected than the left.

IRRITANT CONTACT DERMATITIS OR CHEMICAL BURNS*

Classical signs

- Variable erythema, ulceration, necrosis of the contact areas.
- Hyperkeratosis and scaling.
- Salivation and saliva staining around the mouth and paws with chemical burns.

Pathogenesis

Irritant contact dermatitis or chemical burns are commonly caused by chemicals used in the environment such as **herbicides, garden fertilizers, fuel oil** and other common household or cattery cleaning products and disinfectants including chlorine bleach (sodium hyperchlorite), strong alkalis, strong acids, pine oils, phenolic compounds and quaternary ammonium compounds.

Chemical burns with ulceration may occur if the product is incorrectly diluted.

- Typically this occurs if the product is applied undiluted and then water is used to dilute and wash the chemical away. Highly concentrated product may remain in less accessible areas, causing chemical burns to the feet and mouth.
- Signs develop when the cat inadvertently walks on them.

Most common in cats living outdoors.

Clinical signs

Typically, there is **erythema and ulceration of the footpads, interdigital spaces and around the nails**. Usually more than one paw is affected.

Pain and pruritis are sometimes evident.

Oral ulcers and salivation are often present, and result from the cat licking its feet. Regurgitation may result from chemical esophagitis.

Less toxic chemicals or concentrations may cause erythema, and excessive licking of the feet rather than ulceration.

Diagnosis

Diagnosis is based on history and physical examination.

Treatment

Bathe to remove traces of offending chemical.

Corticosteroids (prednisolone, 0.5–1 mg/kg PO q 24 h) to reduce inflammation.

Non-steroidal antiinflammatory drugs can be given for pain relief and to reduce inflammation. Ketoprofen is registered for use in cats (2 mg/kg SC or PO initially then 1 mg/kg PO daily). Meloxicam (0.2 mg/kg SC or PO initially then 0.025 mg/kg PO 2–3 times/week).

Antibiotics, if there is secondary infection.

Protective dressings may be necessary if ulceration is severe to promote healing.

BURNS (THERMAL)*

Classical signs

- Initially the skin may be dry and hard.
- Necrotic skin sloughs leaving large raw areas.
- Purulent discharge when secondarily infected.

Pathogenesis

Burns occur when cats walk or jump onto hot surfaces such as **barbecues or stove hot plates,** usually with the intent of stealing food.

More generalized burns occur in **cats trapped in house fires.**

Clinical signs

Signs depend on the severity of the burn, and include superficial to deep ulceration and sloughing of the burnt area.

Initially the skin may be dry and hard. Necrotic skin sloughs leaving **large raw areas**.

Purulent discharge occurs when the burnt area becomes secondarily infected.

Treatment

Silver sulfadiazine cream or **aloe vera gel** applied under a non-adherent dressing are excellent topical treatments for burns.

Burn healing is slow, taking weeks to months of treatment.

Very extensive or deep burns may heal with scarring that interferes with function, necessitating reconstructive surgical procedures.

DECLAWING COMPLICATIONS

Classical signs

- Claw deformity or keratinaceous growths at the end of the digits.
- Swollen ends of digits and draining tracts.

Clinical signs

Regrowth of claws may result from persistent germinative epithelium after incomplete removal during declawing.

Regrowth can vary from **deformed claws to keratinaceous foreign bodies** at the ends of the digits.

Swollen ends of digits and draining tracts may develop.

Diagnosis

A history of a declawing procedure having been performed.

Excisional biopsy of deformed ends of the digits is diagnostic and curative.

FROSTBITE

Classical signs

- Frozen skin is pale and cool to the touch.
- Mild erythema, edema and pain after thawing.
- Necrosis and sloughing in severe cases.

Clinical signs

Frostbite typically affects the **tips of the ears and the digits**, areas that are not well insulated.

Whilst frozen, the skin appears pale and cool to touch, and has decreased sensation.

After thawing, there may be **mild erythema, edema and pain.**

In severe cases, the skin becomes necrotic and sloughs.

Treatment

Rapidly thaw frozen area by the gentle application of warm (42–44°C) water.

Handle tissues gently to prevent further damage and pain.

Aloe vera gel applied topically helps to prevent vasoconstriction and tissue hypoxia.

Any resulting necrotic areas may need surgical debriding.

Antibiotics may be needed to control secondary infection, in cases where there is extensive tissue damage.

FOREIGN BODIES

Classical signs

- Nodules, abscess and draining tracts.

Clinical signs

Objects such as **plant awns, thorns** can become embedded in the interdigital space. This is much rarer in cats than in dogs.

Nodules, abscesses and draining tracts result.

Treatment

Surgical debridement and removal of foreign body.

Use antibiotics if secondary infection develops.

SYSTEMIC LUPUS ERYTHEMATOSUS

Classical signs

- Multi-systemic disease including the skin.
- Generaliszd or localized erythematous, scaly or crusted skin lesions.

Clinical signs

Dermatological signs occur in 20–30% of cases.
- Typically, there are generalized or localized **scaly or crusted lesions** on the face, ears and eyelids. Alternatively, **ulcerative lesions** may be present on the face, trunk and feet. Periocular leukotrichia may be evident.
- **Paronychia** and **oily seborrhea** may occur.

Systemic signs include intermittent pyrexia, anorexia, depression and weight loss.

Involvement of other organs may result in **immune-mediated anemia, thrombocytopenia, glomerulonephritis** and **polyarthritis**.

Diagnosis

Definitive diagnosis is very challenging, as the disease is so variable in its clinical presentation.

Skin biopsies show hydropic interface dermatitis.

A high positive **ANA titer** may occur in some cats.

Laboratory results demonstrating **multi-systemic disease** suggest a tentative diagnosis of SLE.

HYPOTHYROIDISM

Classical signs

- Lethargy, inappetence, obesity.
- Seborrhea sicca and a dry, lusterless hair coat, easily epilated with poor regrowth.

Clinical signs

Hypothyroidism may result in **erythematous, scaling and papular lesions**, which affect the **forehead, abdomen, tail and footpads**.

Often there is seborrhea sicca and a dry, lusterless hair coat, which is easily epilated, and has poor regrowth after clipping. The skin may be myxoedematous and thickened.

Other signs of hypothyroidism may be present including lethargy, inappetence, obesity, hypothermia and bradycardia.

Most commonly **occurs after bilateral thyroidectomy** for hyperthyroidism. Spontaneous hypothyroidism is very rare.

Diagnosis

If available, the **thyroid stimulation test** shows minimal to no stimulation.

Free T_4 or **free T_4 by equilibrium dialysis** are below the normal values for the laboratory.

Response to **trial therapy with thyroxine** (0.05–0.1 mg once daily) for 4 weeks results in improved clinical signs.

HYPERADRENOCORTICISM

Classical signs

- Pot-bellied appearance and muscle wasting.
- Unkempt hair coat with thin, easily torn skin.
- Polydypsia/polyuria and often associated diabetes mellitus (80% of cases).

See main reference on page 251 for details (The Cat With Polyuria and Polydipsia).

Clinical signs

Bilaterally symmetrical alopecia involving the face, flanks and limbs.

The **skin is often very thin** and **easily torn** especially **on the digits.**

Systemic signs of polydypsia, polyuria and weight loss are usually associated with diabetes mellitus.

Diagnosis

Low-dose dexamethasone test (0.1 mg/kg) or ACTH stimulation test is used for diagnosis.

Imaging the adrenals by abdominal ultrasound helps differentiate pituitary from adrenal-dependent hyperadrenocorticism.

DIABETES MELLITUS

> **Classical signs**
>
> - Polydypsia, polyuria, polyphagia and weight loss.

See main reference on page 236 for details (The Cat With Polyuria and Polydipsia).

Clinical signs

Cutaneous xanthomatosis has been described in cats with diabetes mellitus.

This may present as **whitish, waxy nodules in the paws.**

Typical signs include polydypsia, polyuria, polyphagia and weight loss.

Diagnosis

A tentative diagnosis is based on a history of polydypsia and polyuria with weight loss.

A definitive diagnosis is based on demonstrating **persistent hyperglycemia** > 12 mmol/L (> 216 mg/dl).

HYPOMELANOSIS (VITILIGO)

> **Classical signs**
>
> - Patches of complete lack of pigment.

Clinical signs

Loss of epidermal pigmentation (hypomelanosis) can be **primary** as with **vitiligo,** or **secondary** as in post-inflammatory change.

Vitiligo is a **hereditary lack of pigment** in the skin, and may have an autoimmune pathogenesis.

- Three affected Siamese cats had antimelanocyte antibodies, whereas four normal Siamese cats did not.
- There can be **symmetric macular depigmentation,** especially of the nose, lips, buccal mucosa and facial skin, also footpads and claws.
- Lesions are most noticeable in the dark coat colors where the normally dark footpads have pink patches.
- Onset of the condition is usually in young adulthood.

Diagnosis

Diagnosis is based on the history of a young age with patches of unpigmented skin in normally dark-pigmented areas.

In vitiligo there is no history of trauma or inflammation that could have damaged melanocytes.

CUTANEOUS HORNS

> **Classical signs**
>
> - Firm, horn-like protuberance on the skin.

Pathogenesis

The term cutaneous horn is used to describe a **keratotic mass** that is generally higher than it is wide, usually several millimeters in diameter and 1–2 cm high.

Cutaneous horn of the footpads in cats is a rare disorder. Affected cats have been **positive for FeLV** and the virus has been isolated from the horn material.

The viral-affected horns occur on the **footpads only**.

Clinical signs

Single or multiple firm horn-like formations arising from any area of skin. **Footpads** seem to be predisposed sites.

Diagnosis

Diagnosis is based on the typical clinical appearance and **histopathology** of dense laminated hyperkeratosis.

Biopsy may be necessary to **check for squamous cell carcinoma at the base**.

Check FeLV status.

Treatment

Surgical excision is the treatment of choice. Recurrences are frequent.

CALCINOSIS CUTIS

Classical signs

- Enlarged, painful and firm pads.
- The pads may be ulcerated and exuding a white paste of gritty material.
- Signs of chronic renal disease.

See main reference on page 245 (The Cat With Polyuria and Polydipsia).

Clinical signs

Calcinosis cutis is a rare complication of chronic renal disease.

Affected pads are **enlarged, firm and painful**.

A **chalky white-to-pink material** with feathery margins may be seen through the intact epidermis of non-ulcerated lesions.

Older lesions **may ulcerate** and extrude a chalky, white, pasty to gritty material.

Other signs associated with **chronic renal disease** such as polyuria/polydypsia, and weight loss.

Diagnosis

A **definitive diagnosis** is based on **biopsy** of the lesion that demonstrates metastatic calcium deposition in the tissues.

Clinical and laboratory findings are consistent with chronic renal failure.

EPIDERMOLYSIS BULLOSA

Classical signs

- Uncommon congenital disorder.
- Avulsion of the claws with minor trauma.
- Erosive lesions on the hard palate.

Pathogenesis

Separation of epidermal tissues from the dermis occurs after minor trauma because of **defective adherence** of the dermo–epidermal junction.

Epidermolysis bullosa is an uncommon congenital disorder, that has been reported in a line of Siamese cats.

Clinical signs

Nails are shed after minor trauma. The **entire claw is avulsed**, leaving the corium quick exposed. Regrown claws may be **deformed.**

There may also be **ulcers** on the **footpads and hard palate**.

The onset is noticed when kittens become ambulatory and start climbing.

Lesions may have secondary bacterial infection.

Diagnosis

A definitive diagnosis is based on histopathology of an amputated P3 which demonstrates dermo–epidermal separation without inflammation or basal cell injury.

Differential diagnosis

Bacterial paronychia can be very similar, but the history and histopathology will differentiate.

Immune-mediated disease affecting the claws, but generally there are severe dermatological signs elsewhere on the body.

Treatment

Curative treatment is not available, but **amputation of P3 of affected digits** will prevent recurrent claw loss with associated pain and infection.

Secondary infection should be managed with suitable antibiotics.

Avoid trauma.

ARTERIOVENOUS FISTULAE

Classical signs

- Localized persistent or recurrent edema.
- Distinct and tortuous blood vessels near the area.

Pathogenesis

Arteriovenous fistulae are **traumatically induced** from penetrating wounds, blunt trauma or post-surgical complications of onychectomy.

Clinical signs

Arteriovenous fistulae may be associated with **persistent or recurrent edema and bacterial paronychia** of one paw.

Pulsating blood vessels, palpable thrills and continuous machinery murmurs are present in the area of the fistula.

Diagnosis

A tentative diagnosis is based on the **clinical signs.**

Definitive diagnosis is by demonstration of the fistula by contrast radiography.

Treatment

Surgical removal of the fistula or amputation of the affected part.

THALLIUM POISONING

Classical signs

- Easily epilated hair.
- Cutaneous erythema, erosions, crusts, necrosis and alopecia.
- Lesions on ears, nose, abdomen.
- Marked redness of mucous membranes.

Pathogenesis

Thallium is a **cumulative rodenticide** rapidly absorbed through the mucosae and skin. Its use is now banned in many countries.

Clinical signs

Skin lesions are seen in association with chronic toxicity, and are characterized by **chronic dermatitis**. There is **severe redness of mucous membranes, cutaneous erythema, erosions, crusts, necrosis and alopecia**.

Lesions are usually present around **body orifices** and on the **nose, ears, abdomen** and **feet**. The footpads become hyperkeratotic and ulcerated.

Hair is easily epilated.

Diagnosis

Diagnosis is based on a **history of exposure** to thallium and **positive test for thallium in the urine**.

Skin biopsies demonstrate dermatitis consistent with thallium poisoning.

Differential diagnosis

A number of diseases can have a similar crusted and ulcerated appearance, and distribution to thallium toxicosis, and skin biopsies are needed to differentiate. These include:
- **Autoimmune disorders**.
- **Drug eruptions**.
- **Erythema multiforme and toxic epidermal necrolysis**.
- **Lymphoreticular neoplasia**.

Treatment

Prussian blue (100 mg/kg IV) given daily until urinary tests for thallium are negative has been used to treat thallium toxicosis, but is relatively ineffective when clinical signs are already present.

The recommendation at present is combination treatment with **charcoal for gastrointestinal trapping** of thallium and **potassium chloride supplementation** (1–2 g q 8–12 h) to **promote renal excretion of thallium**.

Supportive care such as intravenous fluids and antibiotics for secondary infection.

Prognosis

Prognosis is very guarded, and **most cases die**.

RECOMMENDED READING

Bertazzolo W, Toscani L, Calcaterra S, Crippa L, Caniatti M, Bonfanti U. Clinicopathological findings in five cats with paw calcification J Feline Med Surg 2003; 5: 11–17.

Dias-Pereira P; Faustino A. Feline plasma cell pododermatitis: a study of 8 cases. Vet Dermatol 2003; 14: 333–337.

Foil CS. Facial, pedal, and other regional dermatoses. Vet Clin North Am Small Anim Pract 1995; 25: 923–944.

Guaguere E, Hubert B, DeLabre C. Feline dermatoses. Vet Derm 1992; 3: 1–12.

Scott DW, Miller WH Jr, Disorders of the claw and clawbeds in cats. Comp Cont Educ 1992; 14: 449–455.

Scott DW, Miller WH Jr, Griffin CE. Muller and Kirk's Small Animal Dermatology, 5th edn. 1995.

PART 14

Queen and kitten with problems

54. The fading kitten

Julie Levy

> **KEY SIGNS**
> - Crying.
> - Ineffective nursing.
> - Weakness and inactivity.
> - Hypothermia.

MECHANISM?

- **Kittens appear healthy and vigorous at birth**. The fading syndrome develops when an underlying medical problem results in poor nursing, hypoglycemia and hypothermia.
  Signs of the fading syndrome include:
- Loss of suckling reflex.
- Weight loss.
- Weakness and inactivity.
- Bloated abdomen.
- Hypothermia.
- Crying.

WHERE?

- Polysystemic effects lead to generalized weakness, ineffective nursing and inactivity.

WHAT?

- Fading and death may result from the primary condition or from the debilitation that follows.

QUICK REFERENCE SUMMARY

Diseases causing a fading kitten and neonate

ANOMALY

● Congenital defects* (p 1138)

Most common life-threatening congenital anomalies are cleft palate (nasal reflux, sneezing and dyspnea), portosystemic vascular shunt (stunted growth, neurological signs), cardiac (heart murmur, cyanosis, dyspnea, palpable thrill and stunted growth), gastrointestinal defects including mega-esophagus (regurgitation), blind intestinal loops (vomiting) and atresia ani (abdominal distention).

METABOLIC

● Neonatal isoerythrolysis (NI)** (p 1134)

Acute hemolytic anemia in the first 2 days of life in kittens with blood type A who nurse on type B queens. Signs range from acute death on the first day of life to a fading syndrome over several days. Hemoglobinuria and anemia are highly suggestive.

● Hypoglycemia*** (p 1133)

Life-threatening complication of other conditions, including sepsis, malnutrition, hypothermia, parasitism. Signs usually occur in kittens up to 6 weeks of age, and include weakness and cessation of nursing or eating, ataxia, disorientation, agitation and in severe cases seizures, blindness, coma and death.

● Prematurity* (p 1141)

Respiratory distress due to immature pulmonary development is life threatening. Kittens also have no hair on ventrum or paws, ineffective sucking and MCV > 90 fl.

NUTRITIONAL

● Nursing failure** (p 1135)

May result from inadequate maternal milk supply due to agalactia or mastitis. Also ineffective nursing occurs due to weakness, competition or congenital anomaly. Occasionally, inappropriate milk replacer or feeding techniques are the problem. Signs usually occur in the first week of life and include weight loss, weakness and ineffective nursing.

● Weaning stress* (p 1127)

Transition to solid food may be affected by delayed physical development of unthrifty kittens or attachment to bottle feeding in hand-reared kittens. Kittens (6–8 weeks old) are reluctant to accept solid food but suckle well.

PSYCHOLOGICAL

● Maternal neglect* (p 1135)

Inexperienced queens, maternal illness or a distracting environment may cause queens to neglect their kittens. Queens may actively reject or attack sick kittens. Kittens may be agitated and crying or be small, weak and have little suckling activity. Usually occurs in the first week of life.

continued

continued

PHYSICAL

● **Hypothermia*** (p 1131)**

Hypothermia develops rapidly in neonatal kittens deprived of an external heat source or secondary to many other diseases. Hypothermia leads to gastrointestinal stasis, bradycardia, hypoglycemia and dehydration. Usually occurs in kittens <3 weeks of age but occurs as a secondary problem up to 6 weeks of age. Signs include cessation of nursing, inactivity and the kittens are cold to touch.

INFLAMMATION/INFECTIOUS

Viral:

● Feline leukemia virus infection (FeLV) (p 1142)

Systemic viral infections such as FeLV may cause fetal losses, fading neonates or illness of weanling kittens, but disease is most common in kittens 8 weeks and older. Likely to affect most or all of the litter.

● Feline infectious peritonitis infection (FIP) (p 1143)

FIP may cause fetal losses, fading neonates, or illness of weanling kittens, but disease is most common in kittens 8 weeks and older. Weight loss, ascites and cycles of unexplained fever may occur in kittens older than 8 weeks.

● Panleukopenia virus infection (p 1142)

Typically causes severe vomiting, diarrhea, dehydration and panleukopenia, most commonly in kittens older than 6 weeks of age. May cause peracute deaths without typical signs. Intrauterine infection may cause an intention tremor apparent when the kittens begin to walk.

● **Upper respiratory infection (herpes virus**, calcivirus**) (p 1137)**

Herpes and calicivirus typically cause upper respiratory infections from 2 weeks and older. Infected kittens are inactive, crying and have a poor appetite, lose weight and may be hypothermic or pyrexic. Sneezing, nasal discharge, oral ulcers, corneal ulcers, conjunctivitis are common.

BACTERIAL

● **Bacterial sepsis*** (p 1128)**

This is the most common cause of death in 1–6-week-old kittens. Pathogens are most likely to be acquired from the normal flora of the queen and the environment. Signs range from sudden death to a fading syndrome lasting a few hours to a few days. Signs include inactivity, weakness, crying and ineffective nursing. Abdominal bloating and dyspnea may also occur.

PARASITIC

● **Intestinal parasitic infection (ascarids*, coccidia*, giardia, toxoplasmosis) (p 1141)**

Diarrhea, dehydration and cachexia due to coccidia (common) and giardia (uncommon) occurs in kittens 5 weeks and older. Ascaridiasis (very common) causes weight loss, diarrhea, and intestinal obstruction in 8-week and older kittens if severe. Toxoplasmosis (uncommon) causes systemic illness in kittens of all ages.

● **Flea anemia* (p 1140)**

Severe anemia due to heavy flea infestation is common in all ages of kittens.

INTRODUCTION

MECHANISM?

Kittens appear **healthy and vigorous at birth**.

Infectious diseases, inadequate nutrition, congenital conditions or environmental extremes debilitate kittens.

The fading syndrome develops when the primary condition leads to poor nursing, hypoglycemia and hypothermia.

WHERE?

Regardless of the cause of illness, fading kittens frequently have a similar appearance: **generalized weakness, ineffective nursing, hypothermia and inactivity.**

The primary condition produces adverse effects on multiple organs, resulting in fading kitten syndrome.

WHAT?

The cause of fading kitten syndrome is frequently related to the age of the kitten.

Neonates succumb to **congenital defects, maternal neglect, nursing failure, neonatal isoerythrolysis and environmental stresses**.

Bacterial sepsis is the biggest threat to 1–6-week-old kittens.

Viruses, parasites, and weaning stress are more common in 4–8-week-old kittens.

Hypoglycemia occurs most commonly up to 6 weeks of age.

Hypothermia occurs most commonly up to 6 weeks of age.

DISEASES CAUSING THE FADING KITTEN OR NEONATE

BACTERIAL SEPSIS***

Classical signs

- Loss of suckling reflex.
- Hypothermia.

Classical signs—Cont'd

- Crying.
- Gastrointestinal stasis and bloating.
- Inactivity.
- Dyspnea.
- Kittens 1–6 weeks of age.

Pathogenesis

Sepsis is the leading cause of death in neonatal kittens in the 1–6-week age range.

In most cases, septic kittens have become systemically infected with organisms that are found among the normal cutaneous and intestinal flora of cats and not from exotic pathogens.

Kittens are born with an immature immune system and are largely dependent on passive immunity acquired from maternal colostrum to prevent bacterial infection.

- **Failure of passive transfer is an important cause of sepsis in kittens**.
- Other contributing factors are poor nutrition, environmental stress and concurrent debilitating illness.

Bacterial sepsis frequently affects entire litters, with kittens falling ill and perishing within a few hours or days of each other.

Clinical signs

Clinical **signs range from sudden death to a fading syndrome** that lasts a few hours to a few days.

Neonatal sepsis is **characterized by rapid deterioration and lack of response to therapy** in kittens that appeared to be healthy a few hours earlier.

Dyspnea may develop in the presence of bronchopneumonia.

External abscessation, particularly of the umbilical stump, may be present.

Hypothermia is common. Young kittens are unable to mount a febrile response to infection, so fevers are not present even in severe systemic infections.

Abdominal distension due to gastrointestinal stasis leading to gas accumulation is common.

Diagnosis

Sepsis is difficult to differentiate from other causes of fading kitten syndrome because there are rarely specific findings such as external abscesses.

Hypoglycemia is common.

Complete blood count often reveals leukocytosis with left shift and toxic changes. Leukopenia is a particularly grave finding.

Bacterial culture and sensitivity may be performed on blood, urine and exudates.

Complete necropsies with microbial culture and sensitivity of kittens that succumb to fading kitten syndrome are essential to prevent deaths of remaining littermates and to resolve recurrent problems in breeding programs and facilities that house kittens.

Necropsies often reveal widespread visceral abscessation in kittens that appeared to be thriving only hours before death.

Differential diagnosis

Hypoglycemia, hypothermia, and most causes of fading kitten syndrome mimic the clinical signs of bacterial sepsis.

Inflammatory leukogram changes in combination with clinical signs are highly suggestive of sepsis.

Because sepsis is so common in kittens aged 1–6 weeks, it should be the leading differential for fading kittens in this age group.

Treatment

Treatment for sepsis should begin as soon as the condition is suspected and should not be delayed for confirmation of the diagnosis.

Parenteral administration of fluids, medications and blood products can be challenging in neonatal kittens due to their small size.

- **Intravenous (IV) access can be achieved via the jugular vein** with a short 24- or 22-gauge catheter, even in very young kittens.
- If venous catheterization is not feasible, **the intraosseous (IO) route** may be used. After preparing the site aseptically, a 22-gauge hypodermic or spinal needle is inserted in the proximal humerus or femur and can be bandaged in place for repeated or long-term use. Most fluids, medications and transfusions administered IV can also be given IO.
- **The peritoneum** provides a large surface area for absorption of fluids, blood products and drugs, but systemic blood levels following intraperitoneal (IP) administration may be delayed compared to IV and IO routes.
- The small muscle mass of neonatal kittens makes repeated intramuscular (IM) administration of medications impractical.
- Fluids and medications can also be administered subcutaneously (SC), although absorption may be poor if peripheral vasoconstriction is present.

Antibiotic therapy should cover the spectrum of the most commonly isolated agents of neonatal sepsis. These include *Streptococcus*, *Staphylococcus*, and **Gram-negative enteropathogens.** *Bordetella bronchiseptica* may cause life-threatening bronchopneumonia. Dose adjustments of antibiotics may be appropriate in neonatal kittens, but guidelines are largely empirical and based on other species.

- **Enrofloxacin** (5 mg/kg once daily, SC; current data suggest that absorption of enrofloxacin following oral dosing may be poor in neonatal kittens). Dose reduction of enrofloxacin is not required in kittens. It is effective against many agents of neonatal septicemia, but has poor activity against streptococcal species and anaerobes.
  - SC administration of enrofloxacin may result in permanent alopecia at the site of injection.
  - Cartilage erosions have not been reported in kittens treated with clinically relevant dosages.
  - Blindness due to retinal degeneration has been reported in adult cats, especially at higher doses.
- **Broad-spectrum parentally administered antibiotics** (e.g. enrofloxacin 5 mg/kg IV or SC q 24 h plus ampicillin 22 mg/kg IV or SC tid).
- **Amoxicillin-clavulanate** (22 mg/kg PO bid) provides extended coverage for kittens that do not require parenteral administration.
- **Initially, antibiotics are administered parenterally** to assure reliable absorption and adequate blood levels. As the kitten returns to health, oral administration may replace injection, although disruption of the normal intestinal flora and diarrhea may result.
- Treatment duration should be a minimum of 2 weeks.

Because **passive immunity is believed to be critical for protecting the neonate against bacterial pathogens**, it is essential to assure that affected kittens have adequate levels of immunoglobulin. This may be **confirmed by measuring serum IgG levels**. The delay in waiting for test results may put at-risk kittens in danger of illness however, so it may be warranted to **administer serum** empirically to provide protection for kittens at risk for septicemia. See page 1137 (maternal neglect and nursing failure) for details of serum administration.

Nutritional support is usually required because septic kittens fail to nurse. Even brief lapses in food intake can lead to hypoglycemia, immunosuppression and villus atrophy of the intestines, resulting in decreased defenses against pathogens. Some form of assistedfeeding is usually required. Nasogastric intubation (indwelling 3.5 or 5 French catheter) is a convenient route for feeding without the stress of forced hand-feeding or repeated orogastric intubation. Use a formula suitable for orphan kittens such as KMR (Kitten Milk Replacer). The recommended volume is 25 ml/100 g BW per day. Newborn kittens do not tolerate more than 2 ml at a feeding for the first 1–2 days, and should be fed every 2–4 hours. Thereafter, feeding volumes can be gradually increased to 5 ml/feed the first week, 10 ml/feed the second week, and 15 ml/feed the third week. After the first few days the kitten can be fed 4–6 times per 24 h. Weak kittens may not tolerate volumes this large without regurgitating and need to be fed smaller volumes more frequently.

Prognosis

Survival is low in kittens that are showing clinical signs of sepsis, particularly if dyspnea is present.

Prognosis for littermates that appear healthy at the time therapy is initiated is good.

Kittens from *Streptococcus canis*-infected queens that are treated empirically at birth have an excellent prognosis.

Transmission

Most bloodstream infections are acquired from the normal flora of the queen or from the environment. They invade the bloodstream via the umbilicus or from colonization of the gastrointestinal, respiratory or urinary tracts.

***S. canis* is acquired from the vaginal mucosa of carrier queens during birth**. The organism is believed to invade via the umbilicus and the oronasal passages.

Prevention

***S. canis* transmission from carrier queens can be prevented** by routine use of penicillin at the time of birth. The queen is given a 1-ml SC injection of a product containing 150 000 IU benzathine penicillin and 150 000 IU procaine penicillin per ml. At birth, each newborn kitten receives 0.25 ml SC of a 1:6 dilution of the same product, and their navels are dipped in a 2% solution of tincture of iodine.

Passive transfer of maternal antibodies represents the strongest protection against bacterial sepsis. If there is any question about adequate colostrum intake by kittens, a serum IgG level can be determined. Alternatively, serum may be administered empirically as a source of immunoglobulin to kittens at risk for failure of passive transfer.

Because entire litters frequently succumb to bacterial infections, **littermates of kittens that have died of sepsis should be treated with antibiotics**.

If sepsis or failure of passive transfer is documented in one kitten of a litter, it is wise to prophylactically provide serum for the remaining kittens.

HYPOTHERMIA***

Classical signs
- Inactivity.
- Bradycardia.
- Respiratory depression.
- Intestinal gas accumulation.
- Kittens less than 6 weeks of age, but mostly less than 3 weeks.

Pathogenesis

During the first two weeks of life, normal body temperature is 35°C.

Neonatal kittens lack a shiver reflex and are **unable to raise their body temperature more than 7°C above ambient temperature**.

- **Separation from the queen or littermates may result in rapid loss of body heat**.

If the core temperature drops below 32°C, **the digestive tract becomes non-functional and nursing ceases**.

Severe hypothermia **depresses heart rate, respiration and metabolic functions**.

Although kittens living outdoors may develop primary hypothermia from environmental exposure, **most hypothermic kittens presented for veterinary care have a predisposing medical condition**.

Hypothermia is an almost universal sequella of all causes of fading kitten syndrome. **Concurrent hypoglycemia is very common**.

Primary **hypothermia due solely to exposure is most common up to 3 weeks of age, whereas hypothermia secondary to other stressors** such as cachexia, systemic illness and hypoglycemia **may be seen in kittens as old as 6 weeks or more**.

Clinical signs

Cessation of nursing.

Inactivity.

Cold to touch.

Diagnosis

Subnormal rectal body temperature.

- < 35°C in kittens under 2 weeks of age.
- < 37°C in kittens greater than 2 weeks of age.

Differential diagnosis

Any cause of fading kitten syndrome may result in hypothermia.

Treatment

First efforts should be directed at correcting hypothermia and hypoglycemia, if present.

Mildly hypothermic kittens can be rewarmed by external heat sources such as heating blankets, warm water bottles and heat lamps.

- Care should be taken to assure that recumbent kittens are not over-warmed or burned if they are too weak to move away from the heat source.

Severely hypothermic kittens (< 32.5°C) should by warmed at the core before surface warming is attempted. Heating the skin first causes peripheral vasodilation before the cardiopulmonary system is capable of supporting non-critical tissues.

- Core warming can be accomplished by administering **fluids warmed to 37°C (IV, IO or IP), warm water enemas, and heated inspired air**.
- Care should be taken not to warm the kitten too fast to avoid overtaxing the depressed cardiopulmonary system.

Simultaneously, blood glucose should be measured. If measurement is not available, the kitten should be **presumed to be hypoglycemic and treated empirically with dextrose** (see Hypoglycemia for details).

- If the body temperature is below 32°C, dextrose must be administered parentally since gastrointestinal dysfunction may prevent absorption of oral sugar solutions.

Once body temperature and blood glucose have been corrected, a search for a predisposing cause should be initiated if environmental conditions do not explain the hypothermia.

Debilitated kittens frequently relapse with hypothermia and hypoglycemia, so careful monitoring and preventive measures are important.

Prognosis

Prognosis for a full recovery is good if hypothermia and hypoglycemia were not too prolonged and if primary predisposing causes are correctable.

Prevention

Healthy kittens should thrive if they have access to the queen and littermates for warmth.

Neonatal kittens without a queen should be kept in warm quarters (≥ 27°C) or have **access to a heat source** such as a lamp or heating pad. To avoid overheating, kittens should be able to move to an unheated area of the nest.

HYPOGLYCEMIA***

Classical signs

- Weakness.
- Seizures.
- Blindness.
- Coma.
- Kittens up to 6 weeks of age, occasionally older.

Pathogenesis

Regardless of the cause of illness, sick neonates frequently stop nursing, dehydrate and become hypothermic, all of which contribute to hypoglycemia.

Neonates are especially susceptible to hypoglycemia because **energy requirements of neonates are 2–3 times higher than adults. Limited fat and glycogen stores** further predispose neonates to hypoglycemia if nutrition is inadequate.

Hypothermia is a common sequella to many diseases in neonates and contributes to hypoglycemia by several mechanisms:

- Mild to moderate hypothermia (< 34.5°C) suppresses nursing behavior.
- Severe hypothermia (< 32°C) results in gastrointestinal stasis and prevents absorption of glucose and other nutrients.
- Hypothermia reduces metabolic activity, including gluconeogenesis.

Parasitism and other intestinal diseases may disrupt nutrient absorption, leading to malnutrition and hypoglycemia.

Infection, inflammatory processes and stress increase utilization of glucose that may exceed the neonate's ability to replace it.

Hypoglycemia results in decreased metabolic functions, especially in the central nervous system.

- **Neurologic signs of hypoglycemia progress from weakness, lethargy and mental dullness to seizures, coma and death** if not corrected in time.

Clinical signs

Early signs of hypoglycemia are **weakness and cessation of nursing or eating**.

Neonatal kittens become **inactive**, whereas kittens older than 3 weeks may be **ataxic and appear disoriented or agitated**.

Severe hypoglycemia may **result in seizures, blindness, coma and death**.

Diagnosis

Hypoglycemia should be suspected in all fading kittens.

Home glucometers can be used to measure glucose quickly with a drop of blood.

Laboratory glucose results are the most accurate, but may take longer.

Blood glucose < 3.3 mmol/L (60 mg/dl) is consistent with clinical hypoglycemia.

If blood glucose measurement is not available, **response to treatment with IV dextrose or oral sugar solutions supports a diagnosis of hypoglycemia**.

Since hypoglycemia is frequently secondary to another medical condition, a thorough evaluation for a predisposing problem should be performed.

Differential diagnosis

Any cause of fading kitten syndrome may resemble hypoglycemia. **Although a low blood glucose level confirms hypoglycemia, concurrent conditions are also common**.

A normal blood glucose test differentiates hypoglycemia from **other causes of neurologic signs** such as head trauma, encephalitis, primary seizure disorder, portosystemic vascular shunt and inborn errors of metabolism.

Treatment

Emergency treatment for life-threatening hypoglycemia is **25% dextrose (1–2 ml/kg slowly IV).** If venous access is not available, 10% dextrose may be administered IP or IO. Oral sugar solutions (e.g. 50% dextrose, corn syrup) can be given if body temperature is normal, but effect is slower and less predictable.

Clinical **response to glucose replacement should be rapid**. Delayed or partial response may occur if prolonged, severe hypoglycemia is present.

Continuous infusion of 5–10% dextrose or repeated bolus q 2–6 h may be required to maintain euglycemia until the underlying cause can be eliminated.

Hypothermia must be corrected before feeding is attempted.

Frequent small meals of high-protein diet supplemented with dextrose are given until euglycemia is maintained.
- Nasogastric or orogastric tube feeding may be required for neonatal or weak kittens with hypoglycemia.

Prognosis

If the underlying condition can be corrected, prognosis for full recovery is excellent.

In some cases, neurologic damage such as blindness from hypoglyemia may be irreversible.

Prevention

Good husbandry should assure against most causes of hypoglycemia.
- Neonates should be kept warm and be evaluated for nursing effectiveness.
- Older kittens should receive adequate high-quality nutrition and be free of parasites and gastrointestinal diseases.

Kittens should be evaluated daily for adequate food intake, weight gain and body composition.

NEONATAL ISOERYTHROLYSIS (NI)**

Classical signs

- Hemoglobinuria.
- Anemia.
- Acute death on first day of life or gradual decline over several days.

Pathogenesis

At this time, the blood group system in cats is known to include: type A, type B and type AB, but additional blood groups may emerge as more cats studied.

Type B cats produce natural anti-A antibodies, even prior to first transfusion or pregnancy. Type B queens pass these antibodies to the newborn kittens in the colostrum.

When type A kittens (blood type inherited from type A stud) absorb the anti-A antibodies from the type B queen, the kittens' own red blood cells are lysed (neonatal isoerythrolysis), leading to acute anemia, hemoglobinuria and organ failure.

Because most mixed breed cats are type A, neonatal isoerythrolysis is uncommon.
- In the US, more than 95% of mixed breed cats are type A, < 5% are B, and AB is very rare.
- In other continents, B is more common in domestic shorthair cats. For example, in Australia 73% are type A, 26% are type B and AB < 1%.

Some breeds have up to 50% type B cats and are at high risk for neonatal isoerythrolysis. The breeds with the highest percentage of type B cats are Devon Rex, British shorthair, Cornish Rex, exotic shorthair, Sphinx, Scottish fold, Somali, Persian, Japanese bobtail, Birman and Abyssinian.

Clinical signs

Kittens are born healthy and nurse vigorously.

Dark red-brown urine (hemoglobinuria) appears soon after colostrum is ingested.

A fading syndrome develops in first few days of life. Death may also occur acutely without any prodromal signs.

Tail tip necrosis may occur in milder cases.

Diagnosis

The clinical history suggests kittens were healthy until colostrum was ingested.

Urinalysis and PCV reveal hemoglobinuria and hemolytic anemia.

Blood typing confirms incompatible parental blood types (type A stud, type B queen).

Differential diagnosis

Hemoglobinuria differentiates neonatal isoerythrolysis from other causes of early fading kitten syndrome.

Treatment

Remove kittens from queen during first day of life to prevent further colostrum ingestion.

If a transfusion is required in the first days of life, administer **washed type B red blood cells (available from the queen)** to the kitten.

- 3–5 ml donor blood is collected in CPD-A (citrate-phosphate-dextrose-adenine). A heparinized syringe can be used to collect donor blood in emergencies if CPD-A is not available.
- The blood is centrifuged for 10 minutes at 1500 rpm. The plasma (containing anti-A alloantibodies) is discarded. The red blood cells are reconstituted with saline (volume equal to discarded plasma), recentrifuged, and the saline discarded. A second saline wash is performed, and then the saline is discarded. A volume equal to half of the discarded plasma is added, yielding washed packed red blood cells ready for transfusion.
- Administer the packed red blood cells IV, IO or IP.
  - Avoid volume overload when using IV or IO routes.
  - Approximately 70% of RBCs administered IP reach the circulation by 72 h.

If transfusions are required **after 2 weeks of age, red blood cells of the kitten's own type A can be transfused**. However, **a major cross match** (donor cells + recipient plasma) **should be performed** to assure the period of incompatibility has passed).

Routine supportive care is essential during the hemolytic phase of neonatal isoerythrolysis.

Prognosis

Acute death without prodromal signs occurs in some severe cases.

Early recognition and treatment is expected to save many kittens with neonatal isoerythrolysis.

Some mildly affected kittens have only laboratory evidence of disease without clinical signs.

Kittens that survive the acute crisis generally recover to full health.

Prevention

Avoid incompatible breedings (type A stud, type B queen).

Breeders may choose to eliminate type B cats from the breeding pool entirely.

If incompatible breeding is unavoidable, **prevent nursing on maternal queen for the first 2 days of life**. Foster the litter on a type A queen or bottle feed during this time. **Administer serum from type A donor for passive immunity** in place of colostrum. Kittens can be returned to queen on day 3 because antibody absorption is complete by that time.

Rapid in-clinic blood typing of kittens by card test can be used to identify and segregate kittens at risk for neonatal isoerythrolysis.

NURSING FAILURE** AND MATERNAL NEGLECT*

> **Classical signs**
>
> - Ineffective nursing efforts.
> - Crying.
> - Loss of suckling reflex.
> - Weight loss.
> - Weakness.
> - Usually present in first week of life.

Pathogenesis

Inadequate milk supply.

- Absent or inadequate milk production may be caused by premature delivery, delayed milk letdown, or maternal illness or malnutrition. Primiparous queens are more likely to have poor milk production.
- **Mastitis may result in milk that is toxic** or contains microbial pathogens. Uncomfortable queens may reject nursing attempts.
- **Large litters may overwhelm the queen's ability to produce enough milk**. Less-vigorous kittens may not compete well for access to nipples.
- **Poor maternal behavior** may result from difficult delivery that causes illness or exhaustion in the queen. Some queens simply fail to bond to their kittens and make no attempt to care for them.

Ineffective suckling.

- **Premature kittens** commonly lack a suckle reflex.
- **Hypothermia, hypoglycemia and weakness due to other illnesses may abolish the suckle reflex**.
- **Congenital anomalies** (e.g. cleft palate, mega-esophagus) may prevent effective suckling.

Failure of passive transfer.

- Colostrum is produced during the first 1–5 days of lactation. Colostrum has increased IgG, IgM and IgA compared to milk.
- **Kittens absorb virtually all of their maternal antibody from colostral milk in first day of life**. Less than 10% of antibodies are acquired before birth.
- **Failure to absorb adequate immunoglobulin leaves kittens susceptible to infection**. Kittens at the highest risk of failure of passive transfer are orphans, those with delayed nursing after birth (e.g. cesarean section delivery), and kittens nursing queens with poor colostrum quality.

Clinical signs

Inadequate milk supply.

- Kittens are vigorous and show strong interest in suckling. **Hungry kittens are agitated and cry continuously**. Eventually, kittens may become weak from dehydration and malnutrition.

Ineffective suckling.

- Kittens may be **small, weak, inactive and show little suckling activity** in response to oral stimulation.
- Milk may leak from the nostrils (cleft palate, regurgitation).

Maternal neglect.

- **Queen is distracted and inattentive to kittens**. **Overt aggression** toward kittens is sometimes observed.
- Kittens are alert and agitated, crying and attempting to nurse.
- Some queens may not care for any kittens until the entire litter is delivered. First-born kittens may suffer from neglect during this time. Maternal neglect is **most common with inexperienced queens**.

Diagnosis

Examine the queen for general condition, mammary gland health and milk supply.

Observe maternal behavior.

Examine the kittens for congenital anomaly, general vigor, stomach fullness and suckling responses.

Failure of passive transfer is diagnosed by serum IgG concentration (normal >1000 mg/dl the day after colostrum ingestion).

Healthy kittens weigh approximately 100 g at birth and **should gain 10% body weight daily during the first week of life. Daily weight checks provide early detection of kittens that fail to thrive.**

Differential diagnosis

Any cause of fading kitten syndrome may lead to weakness and failure to nurse.

Queens that appear to be displaying poor or aggressive maternal behavior may be culling kittens with subclinical illnesses.

Treatment

Correct primary medical conditions of the queen or kittens that prevent effective nursing if possible.

Poor maternal behavior can often be corrected by **reducing stress and distraction in a quiet, safe environment free of human interference.**

- If the queen still neglects the litter, she should be **confined to a small space with kittens**. Resting benches and other alternatives to the nest box should be removed.
- If necessary, **the queen may be restrained to allow the kittens to nurse**. Queens often accept their litter after several nursing sessions.
- If the queen is highly distracted or agitated, **mild sedation may encourage maternal behavior**. Sedated queens should be monitored continuously for aberrant behavior.
- **Hand-rearing or transfer to a foster queen** may be required if bonding is unsuccessful.

Because inanition occurs quickly in undernourished kittens, **prompt nutritional intervention** is indicated for kittens with nursing failure.

- Feed kitten milk replacer by bottle or syringe if kitten will nurse.
- Transient forced feeding may be achieved by repeated orogastric intubation. **Prolonged feeding is less stressful if an indwelling nasogastric (3.5**

French catheter) tube is placed. See page 1131 (Bacterial sepis) for details.

- If the **queen or a foster cat has good maternal behavior, she can be allowed to care for the kittens even if she is not lactating or if milk quality is poor**, as long as nutritional supplementation is provided. Kittens raised by queens frequently have better social development than hand-reared kittens.

- If kittens are to be reared completely by hand, **urination and defecation must be stimulated** by rubbing the perineum with a damp cotton ball. **Kittens develop the ability to urinate and defecate on their own by 3–4 weeks of age.**

Documented or suspected hypoglobulinemia due to **failure of passive transfer can be corrected by administration of donor serum**.

- The **best donor is a healthy, blood type A, vaccinated cat** free of FeLV, FIV and other infections. Cats that share the same environment as the kittens are most likely to have antibodies against pathogens the kittens may encounter. However, since most infections in kittens are due to ubiquitous normal flora and common feline viral pathogens, serum from any healthy, vaccinated cat is likely to be protective.

- **Serum is administered at a dose of 15 ml/100 g** body weight **SC or IP to achieve normal IgG concentration.**
  - The serum administration is divided into **3 doses of 5 ml** each administered **every 12 h** to avoid volume overload.
  - Catteries and facilities caring for large numbers of young kittens can prepare single-dose aliquots of donor serum for future use. Serum stored at –20°C remains adequate for immunoglobulin supplementation for more than a year after collection.

Prognosis

Prognosis is excellent when the underlying cause of nursing failure can be corrected.

Foster-rearing is time consuming, but can be performed by most pet owners. Healthy kittens that are free of underlying disease have an excellent prognosis if hand-reared.

Septicemia due to failure of passive transfer is one of the leading causes of death in neonatal kittens.

- Once signs of sepsis appear, prognosis for survival is poor. Administration of serum after clinical signs appear is less likely to affect outcome.
- Serum administered prior to the development of disease offers protection against sepsis.

Prevention

Breeding queens should be well-nourished and free of infectious disease. Vaccinations should be complete prior to breeding. **Queens with poor maternal behavior should be eliminated from breeding programs.**

Kittens should be kept warm and well-nourished.

Maternal behavior should be observed to ensure adequate access to milk by the kittens.

Queens and their litters should be kept in private, quiet quarters to avoid distracting or stressing the queen.

If ingestion of colostrum is uncertain, serum should be provided. Serum IgG can be measured in the kittens, but it is often more practical to administer serum empirically.

If sepsis or failure of passive transfer is documented in one kitten of a litter, it is wise to prophylactically provide serum and antibiotics for the remaining kittens.

UPPER RESPIRATORY INFECTION (HERPES VIRUS**, CALICIVIRUS*)

Classical signs

- Nasal discharge.
- Sneezing.
- Conjunctivitis.
- Oral ulceration.
- Corneal ulceration.
- Dyspnea.
- Kittens 2 weeks and older.

See main reference on page 7 for details (The Cat With Acute Sneezing).

Clinical signs

There is much overlap between the clinical signs caused by herpes- and calicivirus, so it is impossible to definitively distinguish between the two viruses based on clinical signs alone. **Mixed infections are common**.

Neonatal kittens may develop severe viral respiratory disease as early as 2 weeks of age.
- At this age, kittens have nasal and ocular discharge and may become severely dyspneic.
- Conjunctivitis neonatorum may accompany upper respiratory infections in neonatal kittens that have not yet opened their eyes.
  - The eyelids are greatly distended by accumulation of fluid and purulent material in the conjunctival space behind the sealed lids. (See page 1212, The Cat With Ocular Discharge or Changed Conjunctival apperance).

Kittens (> 6 weeks) are less likely to become severely dyspneic.
- Kittens with calicivirus or herpes virus may have **oral ulcerations** that lead to salivation and refusal to eat.
- Older kittens with herpes virus may develop **corneal ulcers**.
- Some older kittens develop "febrile limping kitten syndrome" following natural exposure or vaccination with calicivirus.
  - High fevers (> 40°C) and severe joint pain are present.
  - Classical signs of upper respiratory infection may be absent.
  - The syndrome spontaneously resolves within a week with or without treatment.

Upper respiratory infection with *Bordetella bronchiseptica* may be complicated by dyspnea due to bronchopneumonia.

Diagnosis

Clinical signs are classical. In addition, there may be a history of upper respiratory infections in other household cats.

Viral culture of pharyngeal swabs can be used to differentiate herpes and calicivirus.

B. bronchiseptica is diagnosed by bacterial culture of pharyngeal swabs or tracheal wash specimens.

Bulging eyelids (conjunctivitis neonatorum) may occur in kittens prior to natural separation of the lids.

Thoracic radiography may reveal pneumonia.

Differential diagnosis

Bronchopneumonia, heart failure and oral ulceration due to caustic substances or electric shock can be differentiated from upper respiratory infection by careful physical examination ± thoracic radiography.

Treatment

Safe and effective systemic antiviral agents for herpes- and caliciviruses are not available.

Therapy is limited to **supportive care** including **fluid replacement, nutritional support** and **prevention of secondary bacterial infection** (amoxicillin/clavulanate 10–20 mg/kg PO bid, doxycycline 10 mg/kg PO q 24 h, or azithromycin 5–10 mg/kg PO q 24 h for 5–7 days).

Conjunctivitis and corneal ulceration are treated with topical antibiotic ointment (without corticosteroids).
- Severe ocular herpes infection may benefit from topical antiviral compounds.
- Lysine has been shown to inhibit herpes virus in cats at 100 mg/kg orally once daily.

Although *B. bronchiseptica* may be susceptible to amoxicillin/clavulanate, some strains are resistant to penicillins and cephalosporins. Fluoroquinolones, doxycycline, and azithromycin are effective against most isolates.

In kittens with **conjunctivitis neonatorum, the eyelids should be gently separated** and the **purulent material flushed out,** followed by topical antibiotics and frequent cleansing of the eyes.
- Despite a dramatic clinical appearance at the time of diagnosis, most kittens fully recover with normal vision.

Intranasal vaccination against viral upper respiratory infection (**not** panleukopenia virus) beginning **as early as 3–4 weeks of age has ameliorated upper respiratory outbreaks** in some catteries with endemic infections.

CONGENITAL DEFECTS*

Classical signs

- Cleft palate: milk from nostrils during nursing.
- Cardiac defect: heart murmur, dyspnea, cyanosis.

- Gastrointestinal defect: vomiting, regurgitation, constipation.
- Portosystemic vascular shunt: salivation, neurologic signs.

Pathogenesis

Drug administration (e.g. cleft palate from griseofulvin), vaccination (e.g. cerebellar hypoplasia from modified live virus panleukopenia), and infection (e.g. thymic atrophy from FeLV) during pregnancy may cause congenital defects.

Genetic predisposition for specific deformities occurs in some breeds (e.g. cleft palate in Siamese, craniofacial deformity in Burmese).

Spontaneous defects are the most common.

Clinical signs

Signs are dependent on type of defect.
- In **cleft palate, milk leaks from nostrils during nursing**. Rhinitis, sneezing and dyspnea may be present.
- **Cardiac defects** may be accompanied by heart murmur, cyanosis, dyspnea, palpable thrill and stunted growth. Many kittens may be asymptomatic until they are older.
- Kittens with **megaesophagus** (primary or secondary to vascular ring anomaly) have regurgitation from the time of birth. Other gastrointestinal defects such as blind intestinal loops, motility disorders and atresia ani also have signs from the time of birth including vomiting, abdominal distension, crying and constipation.
- **Signs in kittens with portosystemic vascular shunt (PSS) are usually delayed** until weaning or later.
  - Intermittent salivation and neurologic signs (ataxia, seizures, disorientation, blindness) are common and **may** be associated with meals.
  - Signs of cystitis may occur if urate calculi form in bladder.
- Cerebellar hypoplasia is accompanied by intention tremor and ataxia, which is observed when kittens begin to walk.

Diagnosis

Thorough physical examination (cleft palate, cardiac defect, atresia ani) is essential.

Radiography ± contrast and ultrasonography (cardiac defect, megaesophagus, intestinal defect, PSS) may characterize the specific anatomic defect.

Post-prandial bile acids or plasma ammonia are elevated in kittens with PSS.

Nuclear scintigraphy is helpful for confirming diagnosis of PSS.

Differential diagnosis

Transient innocent murmurs are common during the first weeks of life but **usually cease by 8 weeks of age**. A patent ductus arteriosus (PDA) may close spontaneously during the perinatal period.

Anemic kittens may develop a flow murmur that resolves with correction of the anemia.

Treatment

Surgical correction is often the ideal treatment (cleft palate, vascular ring anomaly, patent ductus arteriosis, PSS).

Affected neonates may require aggressive nutritional support via nasogastric or esophagostomy tube feeding until they are large enough for surgical correction.

Prognosis

Prognosis is good to excellent for surgically correctable defects (e.g. PDA, PSS).

Cleft palate repair is often **complicated by postoperative healing problems and may require multiple surgeries**.

Early correction of vascular ring anomalies usually improves regurgitation, but not all cases return to normal.

Megaesophagus may occasionally resolve spontaneously. Aspiration pneumonia is a common complication of megaesophagus and may lead to euthanasia.

Cardiac defects in some cats may remain asymptomatic for years without treatment (e.g. ventricular septal defect, tetrology of Fallot).

Congenital gastrointestinal defects carry a poor prognosis for normal function following surgery.

Prevention

Avoid drug administration, especially known teratogens, during pregnancy.

Avoid modified live virus vaccination during pregnancy.

Select breeding stock that is free of inherited diseases.

WEANING STRESS*

> ### Classical signs
>
> - Reluctance to accept solid food in kittens 6–8 weeks old.
> - Crying, agitation.

Clinical signs

Reluctance to accept solid food in kittens 6–8 weeks old. **Kittens suckle well on queen or bottle**.

Inability to compete with larger littermates around the food bowl.

Kittens may have a withdrawn or anxious personality.

Crying, agitation.

Diagnosis

Good suckle reflex.

Thrives with queen or littermates of similar size and maturity.

Differential diagnosis

Medical causes of failure to thrive can appear similiar.

Excessive competition from littermates.

Treatment

Extend nursing or hand-rearing of kittens with delayed maturation.

Hand-feed gruel (food–milk mixture) to assist transition to solid food.

House with other kittens of similar maturity.

Hand-reared **kittens with "bottle addiction"** may require **increasing time intervals between feedings and formula offered in a dish** before they will accept solid food.

FLEA ANEMIA*

> ### Classical signs
>
> - Inactivity.
> - Inappetence.
> - Pale mucous membranes.
> - Heavy flea infestation.
> - Kittens 2–8 weeks old.

Clinical signs

Progressive weakness and inactivity.

Pale or white mucous membranes.

Heavy flea infestation or marked accumulation of flea feces in hair-coat.

May develop systolic heart murmur secondary to anemia.

Affects entire groups of cats with young kittens developing the most severe anemia.

Diagnosis

Clinical signs are classic.

CBC reveals anemia and hypoproteinemia due to blood loss. The anemia is usually regenerative unless concurrent iron deficiency develops.

Differential diagnosis

Anemia secondary to hookworm infection is differentiated by fecal examination.

Severe anemia secondary to FeLV infection is uncommon in young kittens and is excluded by testing for the virus.

Severe anemia in mixed breed, Burmese and Siamese kittens associated with transient hyperlipidemia at 4–5 weeks of age is eliminated based on lack of severely lipemic plasma found in hyperlipidemia.

Treatment

Remove fleas with a kitten-safe flea adulticide (imidacloprid, fipronil). Treat the other household pets and the environment to prevent reinfestation. Selamectin can be used from 6 weeks of age, but debilitated kittens may have adverse reactions.

If anemia is severe, **whole blood or packed red blood cell transfusion** may be required. If intravenous catheterization is not possible, blood may be administered IO or IP. Approximately **70% of red blood cells administered IP reach the circulation within 72 hours.**

INTESTINAL PARASITIC INFECTION (ASCARIDS*, COCCIDIA*, GIARDIA, TOXOPLASMOSIS)

Classical signs

- Weight loss.
- Diarrhea.
- Dehydration.
- Abdominal distention.
- Kittens 4 weeks and older.

Clinical signs

Diarrhea, weight loss and abdominal distention are common findings of intestinal parasitism.

Severe coccidial diarrhea may cause dehydration and hypoglycemia.

Vomiting occurs uncommonly.

Diagnosis

Fecal flotation and direct smear.

Response to treatment.

Differential diagnosis

Bacterial or viral gastroenteritis and malnutrition cause similar signs and may occur concurrently with intestinal parasitism.

Treatment

Supportive care (e.g. fluid replacement, nutritional supplementation) as needed.

Coccidia: sulfadimethoxine (50 mg/kg PO first day, then 25 mg/kg PO q day for 10–20 days until asymptomatic and fecal flotation negative). All exposed kittens should be treated, and environmental contamination should be controlled. Some kittens may have persistent or recurrent infections.

Ascaridiasis: pyrantel pamoate (10 mg/kg PO, repeat in 2–4 weeks) or selemectin (administered topically to the skin can be used monthly for fleas and ascarids from 6 weeks of age). Because ascaridiasis is very common, all kittens should be routinely treated regardless of fecal test results.

Giardia: fenbendazole (50 mg/kg PO q day for 5 days).

PREMATURITY*

Classical signs

- Incomplete hair-coat.
- Low birth weight.
- Ineffective suckling reflex.
- Dyspnea.
- Kittens in first days of life.

Clinical signs

Lack of hair on ventrum and paws.

Low birth weight (< 80 g).

Absent or ineffective suckling efforts.

Dyspnea if pulmonary development is inadequate.

Diagnosis

Physical examination.

Breeding date known.

Immature fetal hematology (mean corpuscular volume > 90 fl, increased nucleated red blood cells).

Differential diagnosis

None.

Treatment

Tube feeding.

Oxygen supplementation.

If dyspneic or more than a few days premature, prognosis for survival is poor.

FELINE LEUKEMIA VIRUS (FELV) INFECTION

Classical signs

- Loss of suckling reflex or appetite.
- Weight loss.
- Hypothermia.
- Inactivity.
- Crying.
- Kittens 4 weeks and older.

Clinical signs

Perinatal infection may result in abortions, stillbirths, and fading kittens, although **most clinical illness is seen in weaned kittens and adolescents**.

Poor appetite.

Weight loss.

Hypothermia if kittens are less than 6 weeks old.

Crying and inactivity.

Perinatal FeLV is likely to affect most or all of the litter.

Abortions and stillbirths.

Kittens in apparently healthy litters individually fade and die over several weeks to months.

Some infected kittens are long-term survivors.

Diagnosis

Test queen and each kitten for FeLV antigen.

It is **common for infected kittens to have delayed seroconversion for FeLV antigen for several weeks to**

months, leading to **false-negative tests** in litters of fading kittens at the time of initial testing.

Delayed seroconversion and inconsistent infection within litters makes it inappropriate to test only representative littermates.

- **All kittens should be tested**, and **serial testing may be required** to confirm infection status.
- **The probability that an infected queen will transmit FeLV to her kittens is high**.

Some individuals in an affected litter may escape infection.

DIFFERENTIAL DIAGNOSIS

Any cause of fading kitten syndrome may mimic FeLV infection. Losses from FeLV occur more commonly in older kittens (> 4 weeks) than in neonates.

Treatment

Treatment is largely supportive, although specific antiviral therapy may have added benefit by reducing viral burden. **Claims for clinical benefits of immune modulator therapy have not yet been substantiated** in controlled clinical trials.

Recombinant feline interferon omega (antiviral dose: 1 MU/kg SC × 5 days at day 0, day 14, day 60).

AZT (antiviral dose: 5–15 mg/kg PO or SC bid). Treated cats had improved one-year survival compared to cats receiving placebo.

Recombinant human interferon alpha (antiviral dose: 100 000–1000 000 IU/kg SC q day).

Recombinant human interferon alpha (immune modulator dose: 30 IU/cat PO q 24 h alternate weeks).

Staphylococcus protein A (immune modulator dose: 10 μg/kg IP twice weekly).

Provide supportive care with fluid replacement, antibiotics and blood products if indicated.

Although aggressive therapy may improve the condition of clinically ill kittens, **seroconversion to negative status is uncommon**.

PANLEUKOPENIA VIRUS INFECTION

Classical signs

- Intention tremor (evident about 5 weeks of age).

- Severe vomiting and diarrhea (usually ≥ 7 weeks old).
- Hypothermia or fever.
- Severe dehydration.

Clinical signs

Intrauterine infection may result in intention tremor (cerebellar hypoplasia), which becomes apparent when kittens begin to walk. This condition is **non-progressive** and does not affect health unless tremor severity prevents adequate food intake or leads to injury.

Postnatal infection causes necrosis of intestinal mucosa and hematopoietic progenitor cells resulting in **severe vomiting, diarrhea, dehydration and panleukopenia**.

- Most common in kittens ≥ 7 weeks old when protection from maternal antibodies is lost.

Hypothermia occurs in **kittens < 6 weeks old** or older kittens in endotoxic shock. **Fever** is common in **kittens > 7 weeks old**.

Panleukopenia commonly affects entire litters, but some kittens may escape infection if passive immunity is protective.

Peracute deaths may occur without typical signs in some kittens.

Diagnosis

Clinical signs of gastroenteritis in the presence of severe panleukopenia are classical findings.

Non-regenerative anemia and hypoproteinemia are common.

Detection of parvovirus antigen in feces by point-of-care tests for canine parvovirus appears to be useful, although the test accuracy of these tests in cats is unknown. Cats recently vaccinated against panleukopenia may also shed virus and test positive.

Necropsy and histopathology findings are diagnostic.

Differential diagnosis

Panleukopenia virus can be differentiated from other causes of gastroenteritis such as sepsis, FeLV and enteric bacterial infections by identifying parvovirus in the feces. In addition, the degree of leukopenia is usually much more severe in panleukopenia virus infection.

Treatment

Aggressive intravenous fluid replacement is essential. IO fluid administration may substitute if venous access is limited. IP SC or oral fluid administration is less likely to provide adequate fluid support for the duration of illness (5–10 days). Fluids should be supplemented with potassium, dextrose and water-soluble vitamins as needed.

Parenteral broad spectrum antibiotics (e.g. enrofloxacin 5 mg/kg IV or SC q 24 h plus ampicillin 22 mg/kg IV or SC tid) are administered due to the severity of the leukopenia. Anti-emetics may be required if nausea is severe.

Blood transfusions may be required to treat anemia, hypoproteinemia and to provide passive humoral immunity.

Nothing is offered orally until vomiting has ceased.

Mortality is high in untreated kittens, but most aggressively treated patients should survive.

FELINE INFECTIOUS PERITINITIS VIRUS (FIP) INFECTION

- Abortions, stillbirths, fading kittens.
- Recurrent fever.
- Weight loss.
- Ascites.
- Kittens 4 weeks and older.

Clinical signs

Perinatal infection may result in abortions, stillbirths and fading kittens, although **most clinical illness is seen in weaned kittens and young adults**.

Cycles of unexplained fever and weight loss are common in older kittens (> 8 weeks).

Ascites, pleural effusion or uveitis may be present in older kittens (> 8 weeks).

FIP is **more likely to affect individual kittens** or litters than to cause widespread outbreaks of disease.

Diagnosis

Biopsy and necropsy tissues contain **pyogranulomatous inflammation and vasculitis**.

Serum coronavirus antibody titers are unreliable for diagnosis of FIP, but very high titers tend to correlate with clinical FIP.
- Although a high percentage of kittens within the household are likely to have positive coronavirus titers, only a few are expected to develop the disease.

Coronavirus PCR is unreliable for confirmation of FIP.

Hyperproteinemia (polyclonal gammopathy), often accompanied by non-regenerative anemia and lymphopenia, is consistent with FIP.

High-protein, pyogranulomatous effusion in the peritoneal, thoracic or pericardial cavity is highly suggestive of FIP.

The Rivalta test on serum or effusions may be the most reliable diagnostic test for FIP.

Differential diagnosis

FIP can be difficult to differentiate from other causes of fading kitten syndrome. Cyclic fevers and modified transudates are strong evidence for FIP.

Treatment

Medical treatment is usually ineffective for FIP, especially for fading kittens. Transient palliation of clinical signs may sometimes be possible with corticosteroid treatment.

RECOMMENDED READING

Hoskins JD (ed). Veterinary Pediatrics: Dogs and Cats from Birth to Six Months, 2nd edn. WB Saunders Co., Philadelphia, 1995.
Lawler DF. Causes and management of wasting syndromes in kittens. In: August JR (ed) Consultations in Feline Medicine 2. WB Saunders Co., Philadelphia, 1994, pp. 645–652.
Murtaugh RJ. Pediatrics: the kitten from birth to eight weeks. In: Scherding RG (ed) The Cat: Diseases and Clinical Management, 2nd edn. Churchill Livingstone, New York, 1994, pp. 1877–1891.

55. The infertile queen

Isobel Phebe Johnstone

> **KEY SIGNS**
> - Normal estrus cycles and failure to produce a litter.
> - Failure to cycle.
> - Prolonged interestrous intervals.

MECHANISM?

- Infertility is the failure of a queen to produce a litter. It is the result of abnormalities in the **female** (e.g. infection, congenital abnormalities) or **male** or **environmental management practices** which prevent successful mating and pregnancy.
  Signs of infertility include:
- Normal estrus cycles and failure to produce a litter.
- Failure to cycle.
- Prolonged interestrous intervals.

WHERE?

- **Reproductive tract** (ovaries, uterus, vagina and vulva).

WHAT?

- The **most common problems** associated with infertility are:
- **Environmental** and **management** practices.
- **Viral** or **bacterial** infections.

QUICK REFERENCE SUMMARY

Diseases causing an infertile queen

ANOMALY

- Congenital abnormalities (p 1156)

The queen appears physically normal but there is a structural abnormality in the reproductive tract that is a barrier to intromission or to the movement of sperm. Chromosomal abnormalities can present as phenotypically normal females that do not exhibit estrus.

continued

continued

METABOLIC

● Ovarian cysts (cystic follicles)** (p 1151)

Either prolonged anestrus or persistent estrus if the cysts are hormonally active. A possible problem in queens held back from breeding or the use of progestogen contraception products.

● Cystic endometrial hyperplasia** (p 1152)

Failure to produce kittens despite normal mating. Usually seen when queens have many estrus cycles without being mated or after the use of progestogen contraception products.

NUTRITIONAL

● Hypovitaminosis A (p 1158)

Anorexia, weight loss, hyperkeratosis, corneal infections, night blindness and reproductive problems of anestrus, fetal resorption, abortion or kittens with birth defects. Can be a problem in queens fed poor-quality food.

● Taurine deficiency (p 1159)

Retinal degeneration, cardiomyopathy and reproductive problems such as fetal resorption, stillborn kittens or live kittens of low birth weight with brain and limb deformities. Rare now that the problem has been recognized and commercial diets are appropriately supplemented.

NEOPLASTIC

● Neoplasia (p 1157)

Maybe a palpable abdominal mass (unusual) or ascites from metastases. Irregular estrus cycles occur with hormonally active ovarian tumors. Usually seen in older queens (9 years and over).

PHYSICAL/ENVIRONMENTAL

● Physical and environmental factors (female/queen)*** (p 1148)

A diverse range of causes producing signs ranging from anestrus, to prolonged interestrous intervals to normal estrus but refusal to mate to normal mating but no pregnancy.

● Physical and environmental factors (male/tom)** (p 1150)

A variety of problems that can prevent successful mating or male infertility which will present as normal mating but no ensuing pregnancy.

● Inadequate photoperiod* (p 1153)

The queen fails to exhibit estrus behavior and is housed in an area with inadequate lighting.

INFLAMMATION/INFECTIOUS

Viral:

● Feline panleukopenia (p 1154)

Fetal death, mummified fetuses or kittens born with neurological signs. The natural infection is now rare, but vaccination of a pregnant queen with live virus vaccines can produce the same problems.

● Feline leukemia virus* (p 1153)

Reproductive failure due to resorption or abortion. A common cause of reproductive failure in some countries unless vaccination programs are in place.

- **Feline herpes virus** (p 1154)

Pregnant queens may abort after a severe bout of respiratory disease. Now a much rarer cause of reproductive failure due to effective vaccines.

BACTERIAL/RICKETTSIAL

- *Bartonella henselae* (p 1155)

Infection has resulted in reproductive failure in experimentally infected cats.

- *Chlamydophila felis* (p 1155)

Causes acute respiratory disease and sometimes fatal pneumonia in 6–12-week-old kittens. It is poorly documented whether it is a cause of poor reproductive performance, especially abortion in cats.

INTRODUCTION

MECHANISM?

Infertility can be defined as the **failure from any cause, of a female cat (queen) to produce a litter**. It is not a specific diagnosis but **a sign of a problem**. The problems encountered that can result in infertility can be subdivided into three categories.

Normal estrus cycle but failure to produce a litter.
- Evaluate the **general health of the queen**.
  - A queen may be infertile due to dysfunction of other organ systems such as the kidneys or liver.
  - Ensure the queen is vaccinated and free of diseases known to affect fertility, such as feline leukemia virus and *Chlamydophila felis*.
- **Problems within the reproductive tract** can cause infertility.
  - Developmental defects or neoplastic masses can block the passage of sperm.
  - There can be implantation failure or abortion of fetuses due to problems with the uterine wall such as cystic endometrial hyperplasia or neoplasia.
- Evaluate the **fertility of the male cat** (tom).
  - Review the breeding history of the male, particularly his ability to sire litters in the previous 6–12 months.
  - Use a proven sire who works well with any queen.
- Review breeding **management practices**.
  - Ensure the queen is allowed adequate time with the male for sufficient matings to stimulate ovulation.

  - She should be housed with the male for as long as she is in estrus as the queen is an induced ovulator and needs a number of matings to stimulate a sufficient hormonal surge for ovulation.
  - The stud cat owner should observe matings to ensure that normal matings and mating behavior are happening.

Failure to cycle.
- Previous ovariohysterectomy should be ruled out.
- The **general health of the queen** may be compromised to such an extent that her estrus cycles cease.
  - Factors such as poor nutrition, overcrowding, stress of cat shows and debilitating illness can suppress estrus cycles.
- **Inadequate photoperiod.**
  - **Adequate light exposure** is essential for normal polyestrus cycles.
  - Cats are seasonally polyestrus, commencing estrus cycles with increasing day length.
  - At least 12–14 hours of light per day are necessary for normal estrus cycles.
- **Disorders of sexual development.**
  - Chromosomal abnormalities can result in a lack of fully functional ovaries and/or interfere with the normal development of the reproductive tract.

Prolonged interestrous intervals.
- **Pseudopregnancy** produced by **spontaneous ovulation** will produce a prolonged interestrous interval.
- **Hormonal dysfunction of the ovaries**.
  - **Polycystic ovaries** or **ovarian neoplasia** can halt the normal functioning of the ovaries.

WHERE?

Ovaries, uterus, vagina and vulva.

WHAT?

Environmental and management practices are a common cause of infertility in the cat.

In the cat there are **many infectious diseases** that can cause infertility.

DISEASES CAUSING SIGNS OF INFERTILITY IN THE QUEEN

PHYSICAL AND ENVIRONMENTAL FACTORS (FEMALE/QUEEN)***

Classical signs

- Failure to exhibit estrus behavior.
- Failure to permit breeding.
- Normal mating but no pregnancy.
- Prolonged interestrous intervals.

Pathogenesis

Age of puberty varies markedly between breeds.
- It may be as early as **4.5 months of age in Burmese and Siamese** to as long as **18 months of age in Persians**.
- Failure to exhibit estrus can be as simple as insufficient time to reach puberty.

Cats **need to reach a body weight of 2.3–2.5 kg** before normal estrus cycling commences. Although a cat may be of a sufficiently mature age it may be underweight.

Previous ovariohysterectomy. A new owner may be unaware of the previous history of the queen.

Environmental stress such as the show circuit, overcrowding, travel or unfamiliar locations can suppress estrus cycles or estrus behavior (silent heat).

Male preference; the queen may aggressively reject a certain male.

Spontaneous ovulation.
- Cats are **normally induced ovulators** but it is now known that spontaneous ovulation in cats is more frequent than once thought.
- If the queen has already ovulated then she may not permit mating.
- Pseudopregnancies from serial spontaneous ovulations, especially if the queen is a quiet caller, may be interpreted as pathological prolonged interestrous intervals.

Insufficient matings to induce ovulation. A certain level of luteinizing hormone is required to trigger ovulation. Normally this is only attained after several matings over a number of days.

Clinical signs

An apparently normal, healthy cat with a history of failing to show estrus.

An **underweight** cat.

A **nervous, highly strung** cat.

Normal matings but failure to become pregnant.

Diagnosis

History, especially of the cattery environment and management practices such as:
- **Cattery mating practices** and observations of mating behavior.
  - Inexperienced queens and studs should be paired with experienced ones.
  - The stud owner should remain in attendance during mating as foreplay, mating and separation can be quite violent. Some studs can become very rough and frighten a queen, especially an inexperienced one, and she may refuse to mate. Conversely a queen can be too aggressive for the stud and mating may be unsuccessful.
  - The stud owner needs to watch closely to ensure that successful mating has actually taken place.
  - A queen should be allowed at least three observed matings and the queen and stud should run together for at least 2 days, mating at will.
  - A queen usually needs 4–12 matings before there is a sufficient luteinizing hormone (LH)

surge for ovulation. The more matings the higher the LH surge.
- **Quality and quantity of the food being fed**. Poor-quality, incomplete diets or insufficient food can cause reproductive failure.
- The **housing with respect to the amount of light**, overcrowding and other possible "stresses".
- The **show history of the queen**, for example, if she was held back from breeding for a show career.

● **Physical examination**, noting weight and condition of the cat as well as general health, especially the condition of the teeth is important for detecting physical causes of infertility.
● Severe dental disease is debilitating to general health.
- The cat may be reluctant to eat and be below minimum weight for estrus cycles.
- Circulating bacteria and toxins can damage other organs such as the heart, liver and kidneys, which in turn affect the health of the cat.

Vaginal smears obtained once or twice per week for 1–2 months during the breeding season **can reveal if the queen is silently calling**.
● Cornified epithelial cells (superficial and anuclear) predominate during the follicular phase and estrus coincides with the end of the follicular phase.

Progesterone levels measured 1–2 weeks after suspected estrus, detected either by vaginal cytology or behavior, will diagnose pseudopregnancy. A level > 6.36 nmol/L (2 ng/ml) indicates ovulation has occurred and by 1–2 weeks the level has risen to between 31.8–63.6 nmol/L (10–20 ng/ml) whether pregnant or pseudopregnant.

Differential diagnosis

If mating occurred but there is failure to produce a litter, or there is failure to cycle, or prolonged interestrus intervals are occurring, see other causes of female infertility in this chapter.

Chromosomal abnormalities can produce a small, non-cycling queen. Karyotyping is necessary to definitively distinguish this from a problem due to poor nutrition. However, ensuring proper feeding practices will solve the latter problem in time.

Treatment

Correct housing conditions and management problems such that the queen is living in the least stressful environment that can be devised.

Ensure **good nutrition** and that the **cat is actually eating** the food.

For a **queen that is aggressive** towards a male:
● Try a **more gentle introduction** such as removing the male from his pen and housing the queen there for a few days to get used to the smell and new surroundings and then reintroduce the male.
● Select a **different, experienced male** and see if the queen will accept him, if not try another.
- Some queens are aggressive to all males despite being on full call, this is very unusual and it is possible that these have a subtle hormonal problem affecting their mating behavior.

For a **queen that spontaneously ovulates, house her long-term with a male** so that he can mate her immediately he detects she is in estrus so that sperm are there ready to fertilize the eggs.

For queens that appear healthy and no problem can be found to account for the lack of estrus, try **housing these with calling queens and/or close to a tom cat**, so that pheromones may stimulate ovarian activity.

Anestrus queens with normal ovaries can be induced to cycle by **exogenous hormones**.
● 2 mg follicle-stimulating hormone (FSH) IM once daily until onset of estrus (3–7 days).
● Then follow with either natural mating or 250 IU of human chorionic gonadotropin (hCG) to induce ovulation.

Prognosis

The prognosis is good for problems that can be solved by adjusting cattery conditions and practices.

Prevention

Ensure cattery conditions and management are always of the highest standard.

Do not breed from a line of cats if breeding problems are encountered in more than one female from that line.

PHYSICAL AND ENVIRONMENTAL FACTORS (MALE/TOM)**

Classical signs

- No mating behavior.
- Inability to mate.
- Unsuccessful mating (copulation failure).

Pathogenesis

Physical problems with the male such as:
- Congenital or acquired phimosis or bands of tissue connecting the penis to the prepuce.
  - There will be an inability to extrude the penis properly.
- **Preputial hair ring**.
  - A matte of hair becomes wrapped around the shaft of the penis, particularly long-haired cats, interfering with penile penetration.
- **Dental disease**.
  - Tooth pain or lack of teeth can prevent the male from making the important neck grip during mating, and he cannot keep the female still and remain mounted for intromission.

Behavioral and psychological problems with the male.
- He may be **timid and submissive**.
  - This could be a basic genetic behavioral trait or be due to insufficient testosterone.
- The male has **not reached puberty yet**.
  - Age at which males show mating behavior varies markedly. Some have been known to sire litters at 7 months of age, others do not start working until about 2 years of age.
  - Spraying behavior can start months before mating behavior.
- The male may have started working but is **still very inexperienced** and may not be able to manage certain queens.

Mismatched body size.
- The male and female must be of similar body size/length as the male has to have a firm neck grip at the front and yet be able to reach the vulva with his penis at the rear.

Changes to the male's territory may interrupt his mating behavior.
- Tom cats are very territorial and usually will only mate successfully in their own familiar territory.

- Normally the tom is housed in a stud cage, around which he sprays frequently to make it his territory, and the queens are brought to him.
- New housing or too vigorous cleaning of his cage will interfere with his familiarity with his territory.

Male infertility. Lack of sperm, abnormal sperm or retrograde ejaculation into the bladder cause male infertility.

Clinical signs

Disinclination to mate or aggressive behavior towards the queen.

Attempts to mate are unsuccessful.

Normal mating but the queen does not become pregnant.

Diagnosis

Ask questions regarding the **housing of the tom and mating practices** at the stud cat's establishment.
- Are the stud quarters adequate for introducing the queen, and for mating behavior?
- Are the stud and queen allowed to live together for unlimited matings?

Ask questions regarding the **mating behavior and ability of the tom**.
- Are normal matings observed?
- Are the tom and queen evenly matched in size?

Physical examination of the tom for general health and especially:
- The presence of two apparently normal testes.
- Check teeth for dental problems.
- Extrude penis and examine for problems that would prevent intromission.
- **Measure serum testosterone to check for inadequate production**. Normal levels range from nondetectable to 17.3 nmol/L (5 ng/ml) or more and so a stimulation test is necessary to document adequate testosterone production.
  - Give 25 µg GnRH IM and measure serum testosterone 1 h later; normal range 17.3–41.6 nmol/L (5–12 ng/ml).
  - Or give 250 IU hCG and measure serum testosterone 4 h later; normal range 10.4–31.2 nmol/L (3–9 ng/ml).

- **Assess if the tom is fertile**.
  - Find out the reproductive success of queens mated at around the same time as the queen in question.
  - Swab the vagina of the mated queen to look for sperm.
  - Check the urine of the tom after mating for evidence of sperm. Their presence will at least confirm production of sperm, however, the infertility problem may be retrograde ejaculation into the bladder.
  - Electro-ejaculation of the tom to assess sperm quality. This technique is likely to be only available in specialist practices.
  - Tom cats can be trained to an artificial vagina but this takes time and patience.

Treatment

Ensure adequate tom cat housing and allow the tom to mark his territory adequately so that he is happy to work there.

- The stud quarters should be of a sufficient size to allow free movement for mating, at least 2.5×1.8 m (8×6 ft), with sleeping quarters and shelves for observation, exercise and escape from the queen.

Ensure the health of the tom including provision of **adequate nutrition**, especially vitamin A for functioning testes and maintenance of dental health.

Remove physical obstructions to normal penile function.

Allow adequate time for puberty, and **match an inexperienced tom with an experienced queen**.

Timid or submissive males could be given testosterone (50–150 mg SC or IM monthly) to see if this improves their performance, however, it may be inadvisable to persevere with them in case there is a hereditary basis to their inadequacy.

Prognosis

Problems that can be solved by adjusting management practices or attending to physical problems such as dental disease or preputial hair rings hold a good prognosis for future successful matings.

However, if there is male infertility, insurmountable psychological problems or other unsolvable problems, then it is best to choose a new stud.

- If a pregnancy is desired from this particular stud then artificial insemination (AI) is successful in cats.
  - Either train the male to use an artificial vagina or find a specialist center with electro-ejaculation facilities.
  - Allow the queen to come into a natural estrus preferably, or estrus can be induced as per above (page 1149), then give 500 IU of hCG IM at the time of AI to induce ovulation.

OVARIAN CYSTS (CYSTIC FOLLICLES)**

Classical signs

- Prolonged estrus behavior.
- Alternatively, prolonged interestrous interval or anestrus.

Pathogenesis

Cystic follicles may be hormonally active producing estrogen and hence persistent estrus.

Non-functional follicles can interfere with normal ovarian function and produce prolonged interestrous intervals or anestrus.

Clinical signs

Prolonged estrus behavior.

Alternatively, prolonged interestrous intervals or anestrus.

Diagnosis

Abdominal ultrasonography is a reliable means of **identifying cystic structures**.

Persistently **increased plasma estrogen levels** (> 20 pg/ml; 73 pmol/L) supports a diagnosis of cystic ovaries.

Exploratory laparotomy and visualizing the ovaries. This allows surgical treatment if the diagnosis is confirmed.

Differential diagnosis

Ovarian granulosa cell tumors can be hormonally active and also result in persistent estrus. These are usually seen in cats older than 5 years and are rare.

Treatment

Mate the queen to see if breeding can ovulate the cysts.

Try to **induce follicular rupture with hCG** (predominantly LH); 250 IU IM daily for 2 days.

Surgical removal of the cyst(s). Cysts can be ruptured mechanically, or if only one ovary is involved then remove the ovary if the cyst is large.

Prognosis

Prognosis is good for future pregnancies if the cysts can be ruptured by one of the methods above.

Prevention

Do not allow a young queen frequent estrus cycles without mating. Breed queens frequently, long periods of estrus without mating are conducive to the formation of cystic ovaries. The statement "Queens should be pregnant, lactating or both" is often quoted as being the ideal for good reproductive health.

CYSTIC ENDOMETRIAL HYPERPLASIA**

Classical signs

- Normal estrus cycles and mating but failure to produce a litter.

Pathogenesis

Cystic endometrial hyperplasia involves chronic hyperplasia and cystic glandular development of the endometrium.

In the dog, these changes have been produced by prolonged exposure to progesterone.

This mechanism may be possible in those cats that undergo serial spontaneous ovulations and hence prolonged exposure of the uterus to progesterone. However, spontaneous ovulation is an uncommon occurrence in cats.

Usually intact non-pregnant females undergo waves of follicular development and then atresia. Therefore, in cats the changes in the endometrium are likely caused by estrogens.

Cystic endometrial hyperplasia is associated with **infertility from implantation failure or early embryonic death**.

The incidence of cystic endometrial hyperplasia increases with age. It can be seen as early as 5–6 years but is more likely from 10 years of age. It is more common in nulliparous queens than in multiparous queens.

Clinical signs

The queen is apparently healthy, with normal estrus cycles. Mating behavior is normal but no litter eventuates.

Diagnosis

Abdominal ultrasound may be able to visualize the cysts in the uterine wall and is a non-invasive way of detecting the condition.

Exploratory laparotomy and biopsy of the uterus provide a definitive diagnosis.

Differential diagnosis

Other causes of normal mating but failure to produce a litter.
- Poor general health of the queen. A history and physical examination should detect any problems.
- Fertility and mating problems of the male cat. A history of recently siring litters and observations of normal mating are reassuring of fertility of the stud.
- Management practices should be checked to ensure that they allow an adequate number of matings to produce ovulation.
- Reproductive tract abnormalities. Ultrasonography may reveal neoplasia. An exploratory laparotomy will be necessary to detect developmental abnormalities, and biopsy of the uterus to detect abnormal conditions such as cystic endometrial hyperplasia or neoplasia. Cystic endometrial hyperplasia is a relatively common cause of the problem.

Treatment

Once the endometrium has undergone cystic change, there does not seem to be a treatment that reverses the changes.

Prognosis

Prognosis for producing a litter is poor, as the cystic endometrium interferes with implantation.

Prevention

Pregnancy protects the queen against pathologic changes in the uterus that interfere with fertility.

INADEQUATE PHOTOPERIOD*

Classical signs

- Failure to exhibit estrus behavior.

Pathogenesis

Cats are seasonal breeders, commencing estrus cycles with increasing day length.

A **day length (photoperiod) of 14–16 hours of bright light per day** is necessary for normal estrus cycling.

Clinical signs

A queen of apparently good health, normal body weight and not "stressed" that **fails to commence estrus cycles in the breeding season**.

Diagnosis

History and clinical examination to ensure a normal healthy cat.

Question the owner on housing arrangements and access to light.

Differential diagnosis

Other causes of anestrus.
- Poor nutrition. These cats have poor body condition and are below the minimum weight of 2.3–2.5 kg for commencing estrus cycles.
- Overcrowding. There is a history of a number of queens living together in small quarters and poor cattery conditions.
  - Each adult cat should have a minimum of 2.5 square feet of floor space and no more than 12 adult cats should be housed in the same pen.

- Stress of the show circuit. Obtain a history of the frequency of showing, the amount of travel and the cat's reaction to showing.
- Poor health of the queen. A history and physical examination should detect this problem.
- Disorders of sexual development. These are detected by karyotyping for chromosomal abnormalities and exploratory laparotomy for physical defects of the reproductive tract.

History and physical examination will help to rank the possible causes into order of likelihood for the particular case.

Treatment

Ensure access to adequate environmental light in the breeding season.
- Maintain cats with a minimum of 12 hours of artificial light per day equivalent to a 100 watt bulb in a 4×4 meter room.

In the non-breeding season altering the hours of light can be used to induce estrus.
- If the hours of exposure to light can be controlled, then house the queen for 2 months at short days of 9 h of light followed by 1 month of 14 h days of light. There is a stimulant effect on estrus within 10 days.

Prognosis

Prognosis is excellent for normal reproductive function once an appropriate photoperiod is arranged.

Prevention

House cats with good access to natural lighting, either via windows or housed in outside catteries.
- If lighting in the cattery can be controlled, then the largest number of litters produced per year is when a regular 12 h light/dark cycle is maintained.

FELINE LEUKEMIA VIRUS*

Classical signs

- Fever, malaise, generalized lymphadenopathy.

continued

Classical signs—Cont'd

- Leukopenia, thrombocytopenia and anemia.
- FeLV-related disease such as lymphoid and myeloid neoplasms and reproductive failure.

See main reference on page 540 for details.

Clinical signs

Reproductive signs associated with FeLV infection may include effects on the fetus or uterus.

- Fetal effects include:
  - Unobserved **early embryonal deaths**.
  - **Resorption** of fetuses.
  - **Abortion** of normal-appearing fetuses.
  - Live-born **kittens who then fail to nurse**, become dehydrated and die in the first few weeks of life.
- **Possibly pyometra** due to immunosuppression, with consequent affect on fertility.

Diagnosis

Diagnosis is by demonstrating a positive **viral antigen test**; a variety of commercial test kits are available. See page 543 for details.

Viral isolation in the laboratory.

FELINE HERPES VIRUS

Classical signs

- Acute and chronic respiratory disease.
- Abortion and neonatal mortality.

See main reference on page 583 for details.

Clinical signs

Acute upper respiratory tract signs with **paroxysms of sneezing** and **mucopurulent oculonasal discharge**, or chronic conjunctivitis and sinusitis.

Abortion occurs in infected queens, either as a direct effect of the virus on the placenta, or due to the debilitating effects of the disease on the queen.

- Now a much rarer cause of reproductive failure due to effective vaccines.

Diagnosis

Diagnosis is based on **history and physical examination** with signs typical of herpes virus infection.

Virus isolation in tissue culture from nasal, conjunctival or oropharyngeal swabs is available at some laboratories.

Herpes virus intranuclear inclusion bodies in hematoxylin and eosin-stained sections of inflamed mucous membranes.

DNA probes with **PCR** (polymerase chain reaction) **amplification is a very sensitive test** for detecting herpes virus infections and this is now the preferred test in a clinical situation.

- Moisten well a clean dry bacteriology swab with tears or exudate, place the swab in a sterile container (no transport medium) and refrigerate at 4°C until submission. Local anesthetic may be used in the eye before firmly swabbing the conjunctival sac.

FELINE PANLEUKOPENIA

Classical signs

- Peracute disease characterized by sudden death.
- Subacute disease manifested by mild depression and diarrhea.
- Fetal infection resulting in fetal death or live kittens with neurological problems.

See main reference on page 650 for details.

Clinical signs

Signs of fetal infection depend on the gestational age of the fetus at the time of exposure.

- There may be **infertility** due to **inapparent loss of embryos**.
- There may be **abortion of mummified or macerated fetuses**.
- Kittens born alive often have **cerebellar hypoplasia** with consequent ataxia, and they may also be blind due to **retinal degeneration**.

Diagnosis

In the cat with reproductive failure but without illness, diagnosis of panleukopenia as being the cause is difficult.

Vaccination produces strong immunity and a history of regular vaccination generally rules out natural infection. However, vaccination of a pregnant queen with live virus can produce the same signs in the fetus as natural infection.

BARTONELLA HENSELAE

Classical signs

- Cats have shown fever, mild neurologic signs and reproductive disorders.

See main reference on page 390 (The Pyrexic Cat) for further details.

Clinical signs

Bartonella spp. are emerging **vector-borne pathogens** that cause persistent, often asymptomatic, bacteremia in their natural hosts.

Chronic infection may predispose the host to mild insidious non-specific manifestations.

Cats have shown fever, mild neurologic signs and **reproductive disorders**.

Bartonella henselae infection in experimentally inoculated cats resulted in **reproductive failure**, with females either **not becoming pregnant despite repeated breedings or only becoming pregnant after repeated breedings**.

It is not transmitted transplacentally, in colostrum or milk, or venereally.

Male cats bred with infected cats did not become infected.

Diagnosis

Diagnosis is based on detection of *Bartonella* in **whole blood by culture or PCR**.

Detection of *Bartonella* antibodies in serum can be used, but there is poor correlation with blood culture and PCR.

Treatment

Treatment involves use of **antibiotics** active against *Bartonella*.

To date no optimal protocol has been established. Suggested antibiotics for bartonellosis in the cat are:
- Azithromycin 10 mg/kg PO q 24 h for 4 weeks. Dose rate in cats is currently empiric.
- Doxycycline 10 mg/kg PO q 12 h for 2–4 weeks.
- Enrofloxacin 22.7 mg total PO q 12 h for 2–4 weeks. Retinal pathology may be induced at this high dose.
- Rifampin 10 mg/kg PO q 24 h for 2 weeks is effective alone, but should be given in combination with doxycycline to reduce bacterial resistance.

It is likely **prolonged administration may be necessary** to eliminate infection. Dosing for 4 weeks appears more efficacious than 2 weeks.

Post-treatment serology may be useful to determine elimination of *Bartonella* infection.

Prevention

With **rigorous flea and tick control measures** it is highly probable that transmission of *Bartonella* species will be greatly reduced or eliminated.

Zoonosis

Bartonella species are associated with several clinical syndromes in people. Immunocompromised people are particularly at risk.

CHLAMYDOPHILA FELIS

Classical signs

- Acute and chronic respiratory disease.
- Ophthalmitis, conjunctivitis and pneumonia in kittens.
- Possible infertility.

See main reference on page 13 for details.

Clinical signs

Chlamydophila felis causes **neonatal conjunctivitis and conjunctivitis** of 6–12 week-old kittens, and sometimes fatal neonatal pneumonia.

It is currently poorly understood whether *Chlamydophila* causes abortion, stillbirths and infertility.

- **Abortion** has been associated with outbreaks of *Chlamydophila* conjunctivitis in catteries, however it has not been well documented that it was the cause of the abortion.
- The mechanism by which *Chlamydophila* could cause abortion or infertility in cats is not known. It may be similar to that in people and some livestock species, or it could be secondary to systemic inflammation and pyrexia.

Diagnosis

Diagnosis is based on history and physical examination with **signs typical of *Chlamydophila* infection**.

The **PCR test** is a very sensitive test for detecting *Chlamydophila felis* infection and is now the preferred test in the clinical situation. The method of specimen collections is described above for herpes virus.

CONGENITAL ABNORMALITIES

> ### Classical signs
>
> - Failure to exhibit estrus behavior.
> - Failure to permit mating.
> - Normal mating but no pregnancy.

Pathogenesis

A variety of congenital abnormalities, resulting in different signs, can result in infertility.

A **structural abnormality** of the female reproductive tract **may prevent normal intromission**.

Structural abnormalities may result in a **barrier to the movement of sperm up the tract,** although there is normal mating.

- Missing or non-patent portions of the tract have been reported.

Chromosomal abnormalities such as X-monosomy (37,XO), which has been associated with small stature and small non-functional ovaries (ovarian dysgenesis) and 38,XX/57,XXY, which has produced hermaphroditism.

Clinical signs

A **failure to exhibit estrus** behavior despite all circumstances appearing to be normal. Stature of the queen may be small.

Normal estrus behavior but the **queen will not permit intromission**.

Normal estrus and mating behavior but there is **no resulting pregnancy**.

Diagnosis

Diagnosis is based on history, especially regarding signs of estrus and attempts at mating, and physical examination to determine if there is a barrier to intromission.

Contrast radiography of the reproductive tract.
- This is **best done at estrus** as at this time the cervix is open and the contrast is able to travel up the uterine **horns to test their patency.**

Karyotyping to check for chromosomal abnormalities. Usually 10 ml of heparinized blood at room temperature sent within 24 hours of collection is required, but check with the nearest cytogenetics laboratory for their sample requirements.

A **laparotomy to examine the reproductive tract may be required**. It is useful to take biopsies of the ovaries and uterus at this time.

Differential diagnosis

Causes of anestrus such as:
- Inadequate photoperiod. See if the queen comes into estrus after ensuring at least 14 hours of bright light per day. The queen should start estrus cycles after about 1–2 months.
- Environmental stress-induced suppression of estrus. Over-crowding causes a higher frequency of aberrant social behavior, lowers resistance to disease and there may be poor nutrition resulting from food competition. If such problems are suspected, plus there is anestrus, then check conditions at the cattery.

Treatment

Chromosomal abnormalities are not treatable.

Laparotomy and inspection of the reproductive tract would indicate if the abnormalities could be corrected surgically. However, as the abnormalities may be heritable, it would be unwise to breed from the queen.

Prognosis

Chromosomal abnormalities causing bilateral ovarian dysgenesis would not be fertile.
- Cases of chromosomal abnormalities and only unilateral ovarian dysgenesis have been reported with successful pregnancies.

Very rarely is there a structural abnormality that could be surgically corrected, so that the reproductive tract could carry a litter to term.

Prevention

Chromosomal and structural abnormalities are usually unfortunate congenital defects of development, and it is not known how to prevent them.
- If they frequently happen in a line of cats then do not breed from that line.

NEOPLASIA

> ### Classical signs
> - Irregular estrus cycles and/or aggressive behavior.
> - Swollen abdomen, and possibly a palpable abdominal mass.
> - Cystic endometrial hyperplasia and pyometra may occur.

Pathogenesis

Neoplasia involving the reproductive tract in the female cat is uncommon, and is usually seen in older cats.
- **Ovarian neoplasia**.
  - **Granulosa cell tumors** account for about half of the ovarian tumors.
  - In the queen, these are usually malignant tumors.

- They may be hormonally functional, producing either androgenic or estrogenic hormones.
- Cystic endometrial hyperplasia and pyometra may occur secondary to hormonally active tumors.
- Reported age range is 6 months to 20 years, with an average of 9 years.

Adenoma and adenocarcinoma are seen less commonly.
- They are frequently bilateral.
- The malignant form may spread to the peritoneal cavity.
- **Fibroma/sarcoma, leiomyosarcoma, teratoma and dysgerminoma** are rare.
- **Uterine and vaginal neoplasia** is extremely rare in cats.
- **Leiomyoma** and **fibroma** are the commonest types of tumor.
  - The tumors may be single or multiple and are usually in the body of the uterus.
  - Usually the cats are 9 years of age or older.
  - These tumors may be hormonally influenced, and are most likely to be seen in association with ovarian cysts or cystic endometrial hyperplasia.
- **Adenocarcinomas** are even less common and are malignant.
- **Lymphoma** has been described in association with multicentric disease.
- Vaginal tumors are less common than uterine tumors but are of the same types.

Clinical signs

The tumors may be large enough to present as a palpable abdominal mass, especially granulosa cell tumors and dysgerminomas.

If **granulosa cell tumors** are hormonally functional there may be:
- **Irregular estrus**.
- **Cystic endometrial hyperplasia and pyometra**.
- Gynecomastia and bilateral alopecia.
- Abnormal aggressive behavior.

Ovarian adenocarcinoma may metastasize to the abdominal cavity, producing an effusion, and **present as ascites**.

Uterine leiomyomas may develop rapidly following estrus, the mass **may block the uterine lumen**, and the queen may present with dystocia or pyometra.

Diagnosis

Ovarian tumors may be large enough to be seen on plain radiographs. They displace coils of the small intestine in the cranial and mid-abdomen. Retrograde vaginography using a positive contrast agent may be used to demonstrate vaginal masses. At estrus the cervix will be open and allow the contrast agent into lumen of the uterus and this may demonstrate uterine neoplasia.

Abdominal ultrasound and biopsy are invaluable to diagnose the primary tumor and detect metastases to abdominal organs.

As some tumors have been reported to metastasize to the lungs, **thoracic radiographs** should be done prior to treatment.
- Exploratory surgery and biopsy or tumor removal provide a definitive diagnosis, and are the best method of checking for metastases.

Differential diagnosis

Ovarian cysts can appear very similar to ovarian tumors.
- They occur frequently in older queens.
- **Ultrasound may be able to differentiate these**.
  - Ovarian cysts have thin walls with anechoic contents. Acoustic enhancement is a feature.
  - Ovarian neoplasia can be recognized as a mass lesion of varying size and echo-texture, maybe multicystic, but usually with irregular margins and irregular septae.
- Surgical removal and **histopathology give a definitive diagnosis**.

Treatment

Surgical removal of the ovary(ies) affected by tumor.
- A complete ovariohysterectomy is the treatment of choice as there may be uterine pathology associated with hormonally active tumors. Only leave the uterus if one ovary is unaffected and there is to be an attempt at gaining a litter from an important queen.
- Chemotherapy treatment for these tumors has not been reported. Cisplatin has been used in human and canine ovarian carcinomatosis, but this drug is contraindicated in cats.

Ovariohysterectomy should be curative for benign tumors.

Prognosis

Prognosis is guarded for **ovarian tumors** in cats, as **most are malignant**, and they are the most common type of tumor to metastasize.

Uterine tumors have a much better prognosis as the **most common types are benign**.

Prevention

Ovariohysterectomy at a young age eliminates the chance of these tumors occurring. In a queen required for breeding this is not an option. However, she should undergo ovariohysterectomy as soon as she is no longer required for breeding.

HYPOVITAMINOSIS A

> ### Classical signs
>
> - Weight loss, anorexia, hyperkeratosis of epithelial tissues, failure of glandular secretions, corneal infections, night blindness and retinal atrophy.
> - Lack of estrus cycles.
> - Fetal resorption or abortion.
> - A high proportion of the kittens with defects.

Pathogenesis

Inadequate vitamin A in the diet. **Cats require preformed vitamin A in the diet** as they are unable to process carotene into vitamin A.
- With the ready availability of good-quality commercial diets, a deficiency should be a rare occurrence.
  - There is a possibility of deficiency where a **poor-quality commercial diet** or **inadequate home-prepared food** is fed.

Clinical signs

Failure of implantation may occur. This presents as a queen with normal mating but fails to produce kittens.

There is a high proportion of kittens with **cleft palates, spina bifida, hydrocephaly and defects of the diaphragm**.

Diagnosis

Measure the vitamin A levels of the queen. Normal plasma vitamin A levels are 2866 ± 2390 IU (960 ± 770 mg/ml).

Differential diagnosis

Any of the causes of anestrus, fetal resorption or abortion.

Treatment

Feed a **good-quality commercial diet**.

Feed liver (good source of vitamin A) no more than once a week if the cat is on an inbalanced diet and the owner does not want to change to a balanced commercial diet. If liver is fed too frequently, cats can become addicted to liver and refuse to eat anything else.

Vitamin A supplementation. The amount needed for normal reproduction has been reported to be at least 2000 IU/day (670 µg/day). The NRC recommended daily requirement for cats is 5000 IU/kg.

Beware of over-dosing with vitamin A and producing skeletal exostoses.

Prognosis

Prognosis is excellent for normal reproduction once the deficiency has been rectified and the diet continues to be adequate in vitamin A.

Prevention

The best prevention is to **feed a good-quality commercial diet.** If the owner wishes to feed home-prepared food, then give good nutritional counseling so that the fundamentals of cat nutrition are understood.

TAURINE DEFICIENCY

> **Classical signs**
> - Central retinal degeneration.
> - Cardiomyopathy.
> - Reproductive failure.

See main reference on page 1181 for details.

Clinical signs

Taurine-deprived queens maintain normal weight and appetite and come into estrus, however, they commonly **reabsorb fetuses, or produce stillborn or low-birth-weight kittens**.
- Kittens may be born with **brain deformities, limb deformities, and grow slowly**.

Diagnosis

Measure plasma taurine levels. Whole blood levels of 250 nmol/ml have been suggested as representing a satisfactory taurine status.

Treatment

A requirement of 400 mg of taurine for growth, and 500 mg for reproduction, per kilogram (5000 kcal) of diet has been suggested by the National Research Council. This means approximately 25 mg of taurine per day.

RECOMMENDED READING

Feldman EC, Nelson RW. Canine and Feline Endocrinology and Reproduction, 3rd edn. WB Saunders, Philadelphia, PA, 2004.

Guptill L, Slater LN, Wu CC, Lin TL, Glickman LT, Welch DF, Tobolski J, HogenEsch H. Evidence of reproductive failure and lack of perinatal transmission of *Bartonella henselae* in experimentally infected cats. Vet Immunol Immunopathol 1998; 65: 177–189.

Hurni H. Daylength and breeding in the domestic cat. Lab Anim 1981; 15: 229–233.

Johnston SD, Root MV. Managing infertility in purebred catteries. In: August JR (ed) Consultations in Feline Internal Medicine, 3. Philadelphia, PA, WB Saunders, 1997, pp. 581–586.

Pedersen NC. Feline Husbandry: Diseases and Management in the Multiple Cat Environment. Goleta, CA, American Veterinary Publications, 1991.

Sherding RG. The Cat: Diseases and Clinical Management, 2nd edn. Churchill Livingstone, New York, 1994.

56. The cat with vaginal discharge

Isobel Phebe Johnstone

> **KEY SIGNS**
>
> ● Vaginal discharge ± systemic signs.

MECHANISM?

- Bacterial invasion of the uterus via the vagina.

WHERE?

- Uterus, vagina and vulva.

WHAT?

- Most cats with a vaginal discharge have pyometra.

QUICK REFERENCE SUMMARY

Diseases causing vaginal discharge

INFLAMMATION/INFECTIOUS

Bacterial:

● **Metritis* (p 1162)**

Causes fever, septicemia, shock and a vaginal discharge.

● **Cystic endometrial hyperplasia/pyometra complex*** (p 1161)**

Causes nephrogenic diabetes insipidus, vaginal discharge, inappetence, weight loss.

INTRODUCTION

MECHANISM?

Metritis and pyometra are caused by **opportunistic bacterial invasion of the uterus via the vagina** whilst the cervix is open. The bacteria are able to colonize in the uterus when the endometrium or uterine contents are abnormal.

- **Acute bacterial infection** can follow queening (kittening), if there has been **trauma to the reproductive tract**, and especially **if there has been abortion or retained fetuses or placental tissue**.
- **Chronic bacterial infection** is usually **a sequel of cystic endometrial hyperplasia** where, under the influence of excessive hormonal stimulation, there is endometrial growth and excessive glandular secre-

tions, which are an excellent medium for bacterial growth.

WHERE?

Uterus, vagina and vulva.

WHAT?

Most cats with a vaginal discharge have bacterial infection of the uterus.

DISEASES CAUSING VAGINAL DISCHARGE

CHRONIC CYSTIC ENDOMETRIAL HYPERPLASIA/PYOMETRA COMPLEX***

Classical signs

- Low-grade inappetence and lethargy.
- Vaginal discharge, or distended uterus palpable.
- Fever.
- Polyuria, polydypsia.

Pathogenesis

Chronic cystic endometrial hyperplasia/pyometra complex presents with **vaginal discharge**, and cats may have **polyuria and polydypsia** as a presenting sign. **Pyrexia is rare**.

Chronic cystic endometrial hyperplasia/pyometra complex occurs in intact cats of **any age**, **regardless of whether they have previously had kittens**.

Cystic endometrial hyperplasia (CEH) is thought to occur from an exaggerated and abnormal response to chronic and **repeated progesterone stimulation**.
- Use of progestagen products to prevent estrus has resulted in CEH.

CEH predisposes the uterus to develop infection.
- *E. coli* is the most common bacterium causing the infection, although numerous other bacteria have been isolated.

In cats, **susceptibility to overgrowth of bacteria** causing pyometra is increased when the uterus is under both **progesterone (diestrus) and estrogen (estrous)** influence. This situation occurs **after coital stimulation** causing ovulation and formation of corpora lutea, or after spontaneous ovulation, which can occur in cats.

Increased **uterine secretion during diestrus is an excellent medium for bacterial overgrowth**.

Stump pyometra can occur if the uterine body is not totally removed at ovariohysterectomy, but this is very rare.

It is a possibility with long-term use of progestogen products because of their potential to produce CEH.
- If remnant ovarian tissue is left, allowing ovarian cycles, then CEH can develop.
- The caudal position of the site allows easy colonization by ascending infection from the vagina.

Clinical signs

Copious vaginal discharge (**serosanguineous to mucopurulent**) is most common.

Closed-cervix pyometra with no discharge is less common; these cats often have significant **uterine distention,** which may cause abdominal enlargement.

Low-grade inappetence that may be present for weeks or months.

Weight loss.

Depression, listlessness, ± dehydration.

Usually not pyrexic.

Unkempt appearance.

Polyuria, polydypsia.

Diagnosis

Clinical signs (vaginal discharge, listlessness) plus **distended uterus on radiograph** (can only be distinguished from pregnant uterus after 47 days when calcification of fetal skeleton is visible).

Ultrasonography readily distinguishes between pregnancy and pyometra 21 days after the last breeding date.

Increased white cell count and/or left shift is found in most, but not all cats with pyometra.

Differential diagnosis

Pregnancy. Some cases of pyometra palpate as separate uterine swellings, very similar to a 3–4-week pregnancy.

A **uterine tumor** may block the lumen, producing a build up of uterine secretions and a distended uterus, similar to pyometra. The contents may be sterile (mucometra) or become infected, which will then become a pyometra. Ultrasound may reveal the tumor.

Other causes of chronically sick, inappetent cat (see page 330).

Treatment

Antibiotics should be selected on the results of culture and sensitivity. Whilst awaiting the results start the cat on a broad-spectrum antibiotic with activity against *E. coli*, as this is likely to be the pathogen.

● Penicillins, cephalosporins or quinolones are good first-choice antibiotics whilst awaiting culture and sensitivity results.
  – Amoxycillin (4–11 mg/kg 12 h PO, IV); amoxycillin-clavulanate (12.5 mg/kg 12 h PO, 24 h SC).
  – Cephalosporins (15 mg/kg 12 h PO, 6–8 h IV).
  – Enrofloxacin (5 mg/kg 24 h PO, SC); orbifloxacin (2.5 mg/kg 24 h PO).
● Antibiotics alone are unlikely to be successful in clearing the uterus of infection, and prostaglandin adjunct therapy is usually needed. Continue antibiotics for 14 days after the prostaglandin treatment.

Prostaglandin therapy.
● This is usually only used in queens required for future breeding and, combined with antibiotics, **is very successful in treating pyometra** by physically expelling the uterine contents.
● Warn the owner that there is likely to be underlying uterine pathology, and the prognosis for a future successful pregnancy is guarded.
  – Give the prostaglandin F2α, dinoprost tromethamine (Lutalyse; 0.1 mg/kg SC q 12 h) for 5 days.

  – Recheck 1 and 2 weeks after the last injection; a clear serous vagina discharge at this time suggests successful treatment of the pyometra.
  – If a purulent vaginal discharge is present, then consider a second 5-day course of injection.
  – Breed the queen on the first estrus post-treatment.

Ovariohysterectomy is the treatment of choice, especially if the queen is not required for future breeding, or if there is evidence of peritonitis.

Fluid therapy is necessary to support a sick queen.

Prognosis

With early institution of appropriate treatment (antibiotics, fluid and electrolyte support) and ovariohysterectomy **the prognosis for full recovery is good**.

The **prognosis for future fertility is not good**, as there is usually underlying uterine pathology that will interfere with carrying a litter to term.

Prevention

If a female cat is not required for breeding, then **ovariohysterectomy at a young age** will eliminate the possibility of pyometra.

A breeding queen having frequent litters is unlikely to develop cystic endometrial hyperplasia.

Queens that are held back from breeding, and allowed frequent cycles without pregnancy have an increased likelihood of cystic endometrial hyperplasia.

Be aware that the long-term use of **progestagen products** to prevent estrus **can result in cystic endometrial hyperplasia/pyometra**, and so minimize the use of these products.

METRITIS*

Classical signs

● Fever, anorexia and vaginal discharge.
● Septicemia and shock.
● Neglected, distressed, crying kittens.

See main reference on page 269 for details of acute pyometra/metritis (The Cat With Depression, Anorexia or Dehydration).

Pathogenesis

Metritis is an **acute bacterial infection** of the post-partum uterus.

- It may follow normal parturition, but especially **after abortion, dystocia and retention of placental or fetal tissues**.

Bacteria invade the uterus from the vagina and are able to establish in the uterine contents.

- Bacteria commonly involved include *E. coli*, beta-hemolytic streptococci, staphylococci, *Pasteurella* spp. and various species of anaerobic bacteria.

Clinical signs

The queen has a **fever**, **anorexia** and a purulent, **usually foul-smelling, vulvar discharge**.

Dehydration, septicemia, endotoxemia and/or shock can follow.

The owner may first be alerted to a problem by **neglected, distressed, crying kittens**.

Diagnosis

The diagnosis is based on a **history of recent parturition or litter loss**, and physical examination.

Abdominal ultrasound is useful to assess the uterine contents, especially for evidence of retained fetus(es) or fetal membranes.

Differential diagnosis

Bacterial infection of the uterus is the only likely cause of these clinical signs.

Treatment

Bacterial culture and sensitivity of the discharge is important to ensure appropriate antibiotic therapy. Type of antibiotic must be carefully chosen to avoid effects on any suckling kittens.

- Penicillins and cephalosporins are good choices until culture and sensitivity results are known, because these antibiotics are considered safe for neonates.
  - Amoxycillin (10–20 mg/kg 12 h PO, 5–10 mg/kg 12 h IV), amoxycillin-clavulanate (12.5 mg/kg PO 12 h, SC 24 h), cephalosporins (15 mg/kg 12 h PO, 6–8 h IV).
- Do not use chloramphenicol (may adversely affect bone marrow), tetracyclines (may cause bone and teeth defects) or quinolones (may affect developing cartilage).

Intravenous fluids for circulatory support. Feline plasma, if available, is useful for treating toxic shock.

- Consider using subcutaneous fluids if kittens are suckling, as an IV line may unduly distress the queen as she tries to suckle the kittens and the kittens may become entangled in it as the queen moves around.

Ovariohysterectomy should be performed if the queen is no longer required for breeding, and especially if there is evidence of uterine rupture or peritonitis.

Ecbolic agents to promote expulsion of the uterine contents are useful, especially if the queen is required for future breeding.

- **Oxytocin** (5 units IM q 12–24 h) for several days, but this is only useful in the very early post-partum period, as the uterus is only sensitized to it for about 2 days post-partum.
- **Prostaglandin PGF$_{2a}$** (Lutalyse; 0.1 mg/kg SC twice daily) for several (3–5) days.

Prognosis

With aggressive initial therapy, the prognosis is good for recovery of the queen, and for the continued nursing of any live kittens.

Prostaglandin therapy, combined with antibiotic therapy, is usually successful in clearing the uterus and the prognosis is good for a future successful pregnancy.

Prevention

Cleanliness of the queen and her surroundings will reduce bacterial contamination of the perineum. However, bacteria are always present in the vagina and can gain entry via an open cervix, and so metritis is always a possibility.

If there is evidence a queen has aborted, then **prompt investigation to check for retained fetus(es) or fetal membranes** is advised, and their removal via ecbolic agents or surgery so that they are not niduses for infection is recommended.

RECOMMENDED READING

Feldman EC, Nelson RW. Canine and Feline Endocrinology and Reproduction, 3rd edn. WB Saunders, Philadelphia, PA, 2004.

Sherding RG. The Cat: Diseases and Clinical Management, 2nd edn. Churchill Livingstone, New York, 1994.

PART 15

Cat with eye problems

57. The blind cat or cat with retinal disease

Richard IE Smith

MECHANISM?

- Blindness may be caused by a change in transparency of the ocular media (cornea, anterior chamber, lens and vitreous), inflammation of the uvea (uveitis) causing retinal detachment, retinal disease or problems that affect the central visual system. Sudden loss of vision is usually caused by retinal detachment or a central visual disturbance.

WHERE?

Structures in the visual system that may be involved in blindness include:
- The ocular media (cornea, anterior chamber, lens and vitreous).
- Retina.
- Optic nerve.
- Midbrain.
- Visual cortex.

continued

continued

WHAT?

- Blindness caused by opacity of the ocular media is discussed in the chapters headed "The Cat With a Cloudy Eye" and "The Cat With a Red Eye".
- Blindness in cats usually occurs secondary to systemic disease. Toxoplasmosis, cryptococcosis and systemic hypertension are the most common causes. Less common causes include glaucoma, taurine deficiency and central nervous disease.

QUICK REFERENCE SUMMARY

Diseases causing retinal disease

WHERE?

RETINA

DEGENERATIVE

- Hereditary retinal degeneration in Abyssinian cats (p 1183)

This is a genetically determined progressive retinal degeneration that is rare in other breeds of cats. Young cats (< 4 years) present with loss of vision. Fundoscopy reveals a hyper-reflective tapetum and attenuated retinal blood vessels.

- Feline central retinal degeneration (p 1181)

This is likely to be an early stage of taurine deficiency retinopathy. See Taurine deficiency below.

METABOLIC

- **Hypertensive retinopathy*** (p 1171)**

Relatively common in older cats. Cats present with sudden blindness, and may have a dilated pupil(s) (usually bilateral) with a red vitreous, resulting from retinal hemorrhage. Retinal detachment is common. Early cases may show hemorrhage along the larger retinal blood vessels. Check renal function, thyroid function and the heart for cardiomegaly.

- Anemic retinopathy (p 1186)

Loss of pupil light reflexes and pale retinal vessels and small hemorrhages throughout the retina. Occurs in severely anemic cats with PCV < 10% or hemaglobin levels below 5 g/dl. Other signs of severe anemia are present.

- Hyperviscosity syndrome (p 1186)

Cats with marked hyperproteinemia may show retinal hemorrhage, optic disc swelling and partial retinal detachment secondary to retinal hypoxia. Most commonly occurs associated with multiple myeloma.

- Lipemia retinalis (p 1185)

Rare in cats. Retinal blood vessels appear enlarged, with a yellow to orange hue. Although most are idiopathic, it is also seen in cats with diabetes mellitus, inherited hyperchylomicronemia and following high doses of corticosteroid administration.

MECHANICAL

- Glaucoma causing retinal degeneration (p 1178)

Cats that have advanced glaucomatous retinal changes usually have buphthalmos (enlarged globe). There is a high intra-ocular pressure above 30 mmHg. The retina may be hyper-reflective with attenuated retinal blood vessels and optic disc cupping. There may be evidence of the primary cause, e.g. chronic uveitis or neoplasia.

NEOPLASTIC

● Metastatic intra-retinal neoplasia (p 1184)

Adenocarcinoma and lymphosarcoma are the most reported metastatic neoplasias in the eye. They usually present as uveitis, but choroidal lesions can be seen causing swelling underneath the retina, which has a brownish appearance or retinal detachment.

● Trauma-associated ocular sarcoma (p 1184)

Affected cats range from 7–15 years of age, and have a history of prior ocular trauma. Cats present with signs of anterior uveitis, and may show glaucoma, and white to pink masses in the vitreous, if it can be visualized.

Nutritional

● Taurine deficiency retinopathy (feline central retinal degeneration – FRCD) (p 1181)

Usually seen in cats that are fed dog food or vegetarian diets. Early appearance is of a focal hyper-reflective area in the area centralis. As the disease progresses, this coalesces to form a broad hyper-reflective band superior to the disc. Eventually there is irreversible blindness, with a hyper-reflective tapetum and attenuated retinal blood vessels.

INFLAMMATION/INFECTIOUS

Viral:

● Feline leukemia virus (p 1179)

More commonly presents as a uveitis with changes to the iris appearance, and abnormal pupil size and shape. Retinal detachment may occur if the neoplasia involves the choroid.

● Feline infectious peritonitis virus (FIP) (p 1179)

Cats with ocular signs are typically less than 1 year of age, and initially do not have systemic signs of FIP. Ocular disease usually presents as anterior uveitis and hypopyon. Advanced cases show serous retinal detachment and may have neurological signs. Other systemic signs develop as the disease becomes chronic.

Fungal:

● Chorioretinitis caused by other fungi (p 1176)

Blastomyces dermatitidis, Coccidoides immitis, Histoplasma capsulatum. Usually presents as anterior uveitis. Examination of the retina shows focal granulomas with a cloudy vitreous. Blindness occurs in advanced cases.

● *Cryptococcus neoformans** (p 1174)

Presenting ocular signs are usually anterior uveitis. Examination of the retina shows focal granulomas, with a cloudy vitreous. Blindness occurs in advanced cases. Mucopurulent nasal discharge and nasal swelling, or skin nodules may be present.

Protozoal:

● **Chorioretinitis caused by *Toxoplasma gondii*** (p 1172)

The most common ocular presentation is anterior uveitis. The retinal change is chorioretinitis. Blindness occurs in cats with retinal detachment and optic neuritis. Other systemic signs of

continued

continued

toxoplasmosis may or may not be present, and include fever, inappetence, lethargy, dyspnea, muscle pain, CNS signs, and jaundice or increased liver enzymes.

Parasitic:

● Fly larval migration (ophthalmomyiasis) (p 1182)

Typically presents with a unilateral blindness. Examination of the fundus shows a cloudy vitreous, and linear track marks in the retina, which appear as linear areas of pigment change, and hemorrhage in early cases.

Toxic:

● Toxic retinal degeneration (p 1185)

Sudden blindness after drug administration. Fluoroquinolones, particularly enrofloxacin, may rarely cause blindness, especially at high doses. This syndrome has also been described after concurrent administration of methylnitrosurea and ketamine hydrochloride. Cortical blindness can occur following hypoxia associated with anesthesia.

Trauma:

● Traumatic retinal detachment (p 1177)

There will be a history of trauma. Usually presents acutely as a painful, red eye caused by intra-ocular hemorrhage (hyphema), and usually unilateral. Scleral and conjunctival hemorrhage may also be present. Ocular ultrasound is very useful to assess the state of the retina, lens and posterior sclera.

WHERE?
OPTIC NERVE
ANOMALY

● Optic nerve coloboma (p 1187)

Rare in cats. It may be present in cats with eyelid coloboma (agenesis). Optic disc has dark, hollow appearance (inverted funnel shape).

WHERE?
MIDBRAIN AND VISUAL CORTEX
ACCIDENT

● Ischemic encephalopathy (p 1188)

Ischemic encephalopathy results from several disease processes including embolism (feline ischemic encephalopathy), and hypotension, which is usually associated with anesthesia. Hypoxia during anesthesia may result in cortical blindness. It most often occurs after resuscitation from cardiac arrest, or following an anesthetic protocol that predisposes to hypoxia. Feline ischemic encephalopathy presents as sudden onset of unilateral thalamocortical neurological signs including mental depression and confusion, compulsive circling, and hemiparesis and rarely, severe cluster seizures or status epilepticus. Occasionally, it is bilateral and associated with blindness.

NEOPLASTIC

● Intracranial neoplasia (p 1189)

Blindness is associated with neurological signs. Blindness is caused by lesions affecting the optic chiasm (dilated pupils) or cerebral cortex (slow to normal pupils). The retina appears normal.

INFLAMMATION/INFECTIOUS:

Viral:

- Feline infectious peritonitis virus (p 1179)

Typically presents as young cats (7–9 months) with anterior uveitis. It may progress to blindness with retinal detachment and/or central blindness and neurological signs. Other systemic signs develop as the disease becomes chronic, such as weight loss, inappetence, lethargy and fever.

Fungal:

- *Cryptococcus neoformans** (p 1174)

Blindness may be central in origin or caused by extensive chorioretinitis and retinal detachment. Cats with this presentation usually have multi-organ disease.

Protozoal:

- *Toxoplasma gondii** (p 1172)

These cats may have anterior uveitis, chorioretinitis and optic neuritis. Cats with CNS disease may have central blindness and neurological signs.

INTRODUCTION

MECHANISM?

The ocular media are the transparent parts of the eye, through which light passes to the retina. They consist of the cornea, anterior chamber, lens and vitreous. Any mechanism that causes loss of clarity in these media will cause loss of vision.

- **Corneal diseases that cause loss of transparency** will affect vision, and are described in the chapter "The Cat With Diseases Confined to the Cornea" (page 1233).
- **A cloudy anterior chamber** may affect vision. This is usually seen in cases that have uveitis (inflammation of the vascular coat of the eye). Problems that cause a cloudy anterior chamber are discussed in the chapter "The Cat With a Cloudy Eye" (page 1254).
- **Hemorrhage in the anterior chamber** will cause vision loss. This is called hyphema and is discussed in the chapter "The Cat With a Red Eye" (page 1196).
- **A cloudy lens** is called a **cataract** and will cause vision loss. See the chapter "The Cat With a Cloudy Eye" (page 1254).
- **Inflammation or hemorrhage** in the vitreous will cause a vision defect. See the chapter "The Cat With a Cloudy Eye" (page 1254) or "The Cat With a Red Eye" (page 1191).

The retina is complex neural tissue that **transforms photic energy into electrical energy**. This energy transformation occurs in cells known as rods and cones. These cells form the outer layer of the neural retina.

The **cones are used for day vision and color**, and the **rods for night vision and movement**. Cats have rod-dominated retinas. The rods and cones are supported metabolically by the **retinal pigment epithelium**, which lies internally to the choroid (vascular tunic of the eye).

The rods and cones communicate with bipolar, horizontal, amacrine and Mueller cells in the inner nuclear layer of the retina. These **cells modify and integrate the stimulus** produced in the rods and cones and transfer this information to the ganglion cells, which lie in the inner retina. **Axons from ganglion cells join to form the optic nerve**.

Information from the rods and cones is thus passed via the inner nuclear layer cells and ganglion cells, to the visual cortex, where it is processed as vision.

The most common cause of blindness in cats is secondary to problems associated with this complex tissue and includes:

- **Genetic disorders** that effect metabolism of the rods and cones such as progressive retinal atrophy in the Abyssinian cat.
- **Metabolic toxins and deficiencies** may cause retinal cell death. Examples include toxic retinal degeneration, and taurine deficiency retinopathy.
- **Systemic fungal, protozoal, viral, bacterial and neoplastic conditions** pass through the retinal pigment

epithelium from the rich vascular supply of the choroid, to cause retinitis and retinal detachment.

- **Systemic conditions that affect the vascular system** can cause changes in the retina. Systemic hypertension causes inner retinal hemorrhage and detachment. Anemia, polycythemia vera and hyperviscocity syndromes can cause vision problems.
- **Glaucoma** (increased intra-ocular pressure) causes retinal degeneration by complex mechanisms that are not well understood, but include retinal vascular ischemia, and pressure-related changes in the axoplasmic flow of optic nerve fibers.

The **optic nerve connects the eye to the midbrain**. Inflammation of the optic nerve and conditions that affect the anterior brain and/or midbrain will cause vision loss, by preventing stimuli from the ganglion cells from reaching the central processing area of the visual cortex. Efferent nerve fibers controlling pupil function will usually be affected causing **changes in pupillary light reflexes**. See the main references on page 1279 "The Cat With Abnormal Pupil Size, Shape or Response" and optic neuritis is a rare condition in the cat. Causes of optic nerve disease in cats are usually confined to:

- **Inflammation or neoplasia affecting the optic chiasm**.
- **Inflammation or neoplasia of the mid-brain**.

Midbrain and visual cortex lesions can present with **blindness and normal-appearing eyes**.

Sometimes ocular lesions are present, but do not account for the blindness.

Pupil size and pupillary light reflexes help **localize the site of the lesion causing blindness.**

- If the lesion is at the **cortical level**, there will usually be a normal to slow pupil light reflex.
- If the lesion is anterior and involves the **optic chiasm**, there will be a loss of pupillary light reflex.
- If the lesion is in the **mid-brain**, there will be anisocoria (uneven-sized pupils).

The **visual cortex** occupies approximately one third of the cerebrum. Vision is an extremely complex process that is not fully understood. The ocular structures may be perfectly normal, but if the brain cannot process the information sent from the eye, the animal will appear to be blind. **Animals with central blindness generally have normal pupil reflexes**, although they may be slow.

Conditions that affect the visual cortex include:

- **Ischemia** from oxygen starvation or trauma.
- **Vascular accidents** causing ischemia.
- **Inflammation** of brain or meninges.
- **Neoplasia** of cerebral or meningeal tissue, causing pressure-related cell degeneration.

Usually other neurological signs are present suggesting there is a central lesion such as seizures, proprioceptive deficits, ataxia and weakness.

WHERE?

Structures that may be involved in blindness include:

- **The ocular media** (cornea, anterior chamber, lens and vitreous).
- **Retina**.
- **Optic nerve**.
- **Mid-brain**.
- **Visual cerebral cortex**.

WHAT?

Changes to the ocular media appear as a cloudy eye. See the main reference on pages 1254, 1233 "The Cat With a Cloudy Eye" and "The Cat With Abnormalities Confined to the Cornea".

Most cats with sudden blindness have a retinal detachment caused by infectious agents or hypertension.

Cats that have blindness associated with **abnormal pupil reflexes** and normal retinas generally have **optic nerve or mid-brain** disease.

Blind cats with normal retinas and normal pupil reflexes usually have central blindness, with lesions involving the **visual cortex**.

Pupillary light reflexes form an important part of eye examinations, and help determine the part of the visual system that is causing blindness.

The summation of retinal electrical responses to light can be measured electrophysiologically using a procedure known as **electroretinography (ERG)**.

DISEASES CAUSING A BLIND CAT OR CAT WITH RETINAL DISEASE AND BLINDNESS ASSOCIATED WITH RETINAL PROBLEMS

HYPERTENSIVE RETINOPATHY***

Classical signs

- Acute onset of vision loss in an old cat, usually bilateral.
- Dilated pupils, non-responsive or poorly responsive to light.
- Cloudy vitreous with red areas of hemorrhage.

Pathogenesis

Hypertension causes **vasoconstriction of pre-capillary retinal arterioles. Hypoxia** of the arteriole causes smooth muscle necrosis, which leads to **vascular dilatation**, and leakage of serum and blood.

Leakage from vessels causes **serous retinal detachment**, and subretinal, intra-retinal or preretinal **hemorrhage**.

Retinal blood vessels may rupture, causing hemorrhage into the vitreous.

Hypertensive retinopathy occurs most commonly secondary to **chronic renal disease, hyperthyroidism** and **cardiac disease**.

Clinical signs

Classical signs are **acute onset of vision loss** in an **old cat**, which is **usually bilateral**. The cat suddenly starts to bump into things, appears to be lost, and has very cautious movements.

The **pupils** are usually **dilated**, and non-responsive or **poorly responsive to light**.

Affected **eyes appear slightly cloudy**, and there may be focal red areas visible through the pupil, as a result of retinal hemorrhage. The vitreous may appear red. Early cases may show hemorrhage along the larger retinal blood vessels.

Hyphema may be seen in the anterior chamber.

It is difficult to visualize the **retina** on fundoscopic examination, as it **appears out of focus**. This is caused by retinal detachment, with the retina ballooning into the vitreous, **and appears as a thin veil of pale tissue**.

These cats may have **cardiomegaly**, and left ventricular hypertrophy.

There may be other signs suggestive of hypertension, for example, a **bounding cardiac apex beat**.

Systolic arterial blood pressure is usually **greater than 160 mmHg**.

Other signs suggestive of renal and/or thyroid disease, such as progressive weight loss, polydypsia, polyuria and azotemia may be present.

Diagnosis

Clinicians should suspect this problem in any old cat that has suddenly gone blind.

Ophthalmoscopy will demonstrate **vitreal hemorrhage**. The retina will appear out of focus, and hemorrhage adjacent to the major retinal blood vessels is visible.

Complete retinal detachment is common.

Blood pressure is most commonly measured in the cat using Doppler technology. Arterial blood pressure greater than 160 mmHg confirms a diagnosis of hypertensive retinopathy. Most cats with clinical signs have a blood pressure of **greater than 200 mmHg**.

BUN, creatinine and urine protein:creatinine ratios are useful clinical pathology parameters to check renal function.

Thyroid function should be checked by measuring **plasma thyroxine (T4) concentration**.

Further useful procedures include **cardiac ultrasound**, and in some cases, imaging of the thyroid with radio-isotopes.

Treatment

Amlodipine (Norvasc, Pfizer) is a **calcium channel blocker**, which has a greater effect on vascular smooth muscle cells than on cardiac muscle cells. The dose is approximately 0.625 mg/cat per day, i.e. 1/4 of a 2.5 mg tablet (USA) or 1/8 of a 5 mg tablet (Australia).

The use of corticosteroids is controversial.

If hypertension is associated with **hypertrophic cardio-myopathy**, then calcium channel blockers such as **diltiazem** may be used. For more detail see main reference on page 130 for details (The Cat With Abnormal Heart Sounds and/or an Enlarged Heart).

β-blockers such as propranolol (Inderal) can also be used in the management of the cardiac disease at 1/4 of a 10 mg tablet q 8 h.

Hyperthyroidism when present, should be treated using surgery, radioactive iodine (131-I) or anti-thyroid drugs such as carbimazole or methimazole. For more detail see main reference on page 306 (The Cat With Weight Loss and a Good Appetite).

Cats with renal disease should be placed on appropriate medical and dietary management. For more details see the main reference on page 337 (The Thin, Inappetent Cat).

CHORIORETINITIS CAUSED BY *TOXOPLASMA GONDII***

Classical signs

- Anterior uveitis (cloudy eye) is the most common sign.
- +/– Lymphocytic plasmacytic uveitis – gray to tan-colored nodules on the iris surface.
- Chorioretinitis and optic neuritis that may cause blindness.
- Rarely, systemic signs may be seen concurrently with ocular signs. These include fever, weight loss, +/– muscular pain, +/– signs of respiratory or neurological disease.

See the main reference on page 375 (The Pyrexic Cat).

Pathogenesis

Infection with *Toxoplasma gondii* occurs by three mechanisms.

- **Ingestion of tissue cysts (bradyzoites)** from an intermediate host such as cockroaches, earthworms, rodents, reptiles and birds (most common) is the common route of infection in cats, and occurs in kittens once they start to hunt. Infection may occur from eating uncooked meat from cattle, sheep, chickens and pigs, which consumed food or water contaminated by cat feces.
- **Ingestion of sporulated oocysts** from food or water contaminated by cat feces (far less common).
- **Transplacental transmission** occurs, but is less common.

After ingestion, a **gut replication cycle occurs**. The cat is the definitive host and is the only species in which this occurs. This results in the production of **unsporulated (non-infective) oocysts**, which are passed in feces. These become infective after 1–5 days, by sporulation (this requires aeration) in the environment. The spores formed are called sporocysts, and are filled with sporozoites.

The **extra-intestinal** development of *T. gondii* is similar in all species. Upon ingestion, sporozoites and bradyzoites transform into **tachyzoites**, which is the rapidly multiplying form of *T. gondii*. These may replicate in any cell type, and are disseminated to various organs in the body. Tachyzoites multiply intracellularly for a period of time, and then become **tissue cysts containing numerous bradyzoites**, which is the slowly replicating form of *T. gondii*. Release of bradyzoites from these cysts restarts the intracellular replication in cells.

Cysts may develop in the **CNS, muscles, visceral organs (particularly lungs and liver) and ocular tissues**. They may persist in a dormant state for life. Biologically they are a resting state, waiting for ingestion by a predator. Following ingestion by a mammal or bird they form tachyzoites.

Activation of bradyzoites in tissue cysts may occur associated with other disease states, such as FIV, FeLV, hemobartonellosis and FIP, which act as stressors or immunosuppressors. High-dose corticosteroid use has been known to activate dormant *T. gondii* infections.

When **bradyzoites are activated**, they undergo **rapid replication, causing destruction of tissue**. This incites an inflammatory response in various tissues, notably the **central nervous system, uveal tract of the eye, muscle, liver and lungs**. This also causes a host of immune responses, including hypersensitivity, antibody and immune-complex reactions.

It is unclear whether the inflammation in ocular toxoplasmosis is caused by cellular destruction, and the resultant local hypersensitivity, antibody, and immune-complex reactions, or whether the eye is secondarily involved from reactions occurring in tissues outside the eye.

Ocular toxoplasmosis in humans causes a posterior uveitis, with a necrotizing chorio-retinitis. In cats, the most common presenting sign is **anterior uveitis**, and in cases with disseminated disease, **chorioretinitis and optic neuritis** may be seen.

Histologically, ocular lesions in cats appear as granulomatous to lymphocytic/plasmocytic, multifocal chorioretinitis and/or iridocyclitis.

Clinical signs

The **most common ocular presenting sign is anterior uveitis, appearing as a cloudy eye**. This may be **unilateral or bilateral**.
- Affected eyes appear cloudy in acute cases, and may show **hypopyon** (pus in the anterior chamber) and **keratic precipitates**, which are focal accumulations of protein, and white blood cells on the corneal endothelium.

Cats that present with **lymphocytic, plasmocytic nodules on the iris**, seen as **diffuse focal grayish nodules** protruding from the anterior iris surface, may have ocular toxoplasmosis.

Blind cats with toxoplasmosis have **chorioretinitis**. This is seen as **small, multifocal, raised areas in the retina** that have pigment changes. These cats may also have **optic neuritis**, with an inflamed optic disc that is hyperemic and raised.

Systemic signs of toxoplasmosis in cats include:
- Fever, weight loss and muscle pain.
- Respiratory disease, especially pneumonia.
- Multifocal neurologic disease.
- Liver disease.
- Systemic signs of toxoplasmosis are very rare in adult cats. They are most common in perinatal kittens.

Diagnosis

It is very difficult to make a definitive diagnosis with demonstration of the organism in cases with *T. gondii* infection. A tentative diagnosis is usually made based on the clinical signs, supported with laboratory tests.

The classical ocular sign suggesting toxoplasmosis is anterior uveitis. The eye(s) may appear cloudy with hypopyon and keratic precipitates, or have evidence of mild uveitis with lymphocytic/plasmocytic nodules in the iris.

Serological tests have varying degrees of sensitivity and specificity:
- Measurement of antibodies may be via indirect fluorescent antibody tests (**IFA**), indirect hemagglutination tests (**IHA**), or enzyme-linked immunosorbent assay (**ELISA**). The ELISA test is available in kit form, which is a quantitative test and does not yield a titer.
- **Demonstration of a rise in IgM titers** (often measured by IFA) from paired samples taken 2–4 weeks apart, indicates a recent active infection. However, some cats do not develop detectable IgM titers, and in other cats, positive IgM titers can persist for months to years after infection.

Polymerase chain reaction (**PCR**) testing for parasite DNA in tissue or fluid samples. The specificity for active infection is improved when combined with the IgM titer.

Comparison of levels of aqueous humor *T. gondii* antibody levels with serum levels (Goldman–Witmer coefficient or C-value) has been advocated to determine that anterior uveitis has been caused by *T. gondii*, although the use of C-values is still controversial. The Goldman–Witmer coefficient compares the *T. gondii*-specific immunoglobulin concentration with the total immunoglobulin concentration in serum and aqueous humor. A *T. gondii*-specific antibody C-value > 1 in aqueous humor indicates possible local production, rather than leakage from the serum through a faulty blood–ocular barrier. *T. gondii*-**specific C values > 3 are advocated as criteria for evidence of local antibody production**.

Differential diagnosis

Differential diagnoses include other conditions that present as anterior uveitis.
- Cats with **FIP** present with **anterior uveitis (hypopyon and keratic precipitates)**. This is not as common in many geographical areas, and most commonly occurs in young cats from 6 months to 1 year of age. Currently, there is no definitive test

for FIP. Serology is confused by intestinal coronavirus infections. Cats with FIP often have increased total protein and IgG concentrations in response to viral antigen, and also from cell damage resulting from the intense tissue inflammation. It is not pathognomonic for FIP, and reflects the chronic inflammatory nature of the disease.

- **FIV uveitis** can cause a mild anterior uveitis, and anterior chamber flare. The condition can be diagnosed with serology using an ELISA test.
- **FeLV uveitis** can cause signs similar to acute *T. gondii* infection, with an inflamed swollen iris and hypopyon. The retina may be infiltrated with tumor cells, and the retina may occasionally be detached from neoplasia infiltrating the choroid.

Other inflammatory conditions that present with chorioretinitis include:

- **Fungal diseases** especially **cryptococcosis, blastomycosis, histoplasmosis, candidiasis and coccidioidomycosis**. These diseases present with signs of uveitis and multifocal granulomatous chorioretinitis that appears as small brownish nodules in the retina, and may cause blindness. Systemic signs of fever, inappetence, weight loss and dyspnea are often present. Serological tests are available to differentiate these infections.

Treatment

A combination of drugs that inhibit the production of folinic acid necessary for *T. gondii* proliferation has been the mainstay of treatment in people. The most common combination is pyrimethamine, a dihydrofolate reductase inhibitor, and a sulfonamide, which inhibits production of folic acid. Unfortunately, cats do not tolerate sulfa drugs as well as people, and often develop gastrointestinal side effects.

Trimethoprim/sulfadiazine (30 mg/kg PO q 12 h) may be given alone, or with pyrimethamine (0.5 mg/kg PO q 24 h). Supplement with folinic acid (1 mg/kg PO q 24 h).

Other antimicrobial drugs that are used to control *T. gondii* infection include **tetracyclines, clindamycin, clarithromycin and atovoquone**.

Clindamycin (Antirobe, Upjohn) at a dose rate of 12.5 mg/kg q 12 h for 3–4 weeks is the most common treatment used in cats.

Concurrent anti-inflammatory therapy for anterior uveitis, e.g. **topical 0.5% prednisolone** acetate drops applied q 6–12 h are used to suppress the inflammation associated with the infection, and prevent secondary complications such as glaucoma.

*CRYPTOCOCCUS NEOFORMANS**

Classical signs

- Sudden blindness with retinal detachment. Vitreous flare may be present making the retina difficult to examine.
- Anterior uveitis (anterior chamber flare, miosis, inflamed discolored iris).
- Exophthalmos (eye bulging forward).
- +/– mucopurulent discharge with sneezing and a swollen nose.
- Neurological signs.
- Chronic skin granulomas.

See the main references on page 25 (The Cat With Signs of Chronic Nasal Disease).

Pathogenesis

Cryptococcosis is the most common fungal infection affecting cats which **occurs throughout the world**.

Cryptococcus neoformans is a budding, capsulated yeast-like fungus found in **soil or in avian excreta**. In Australia, there is an association of the organism *C. neoformans* var. *gatti* with the **bark of a Eucalypt tree**, the River Red Gum (River and Forest varieties), which has been **exported world wide** as a timber tree.

In general, all deep fungal infections enter the body by the inhalation of aerosolized spores leading to either fungal rhinitis (e.g. *Cryptococcus*) or pneumonia (e.g. blastomycosis, histoplasmosis), with subsequent dissemination to other parts of the body, including the eye, by hematogenous or lymphatic spread.

The initial ocular site for establishment of infection is usually the **choroid**, and the **anterior uveal tract** is often involved later in the course of the infection.

Clinical signs

Cats may present with **sudden blindness** caused by **multifocal granulomatous chorioretinitis** with varying degrees of **retinal detachment**.

- **Vitreous flare** (**cloudy vitreous**) is present, and makes the retina difficult to examine in cases with severe inflammation.
- If the retina can be visualized, the granulomas appear as small **swollen brownish discolored areas** in the tapetal and non-tapetal retina.

There is usually **anterior uveitis with corneal edema, anterior chamber flare** (with or without hypopyon and keratic precipitates), **swollen iris with varying degrees of posterior synechia** causing a **distorted pupil**, and in chronic cases, new vascular growth on the anterior surface of the iris (pre-iridal fibrovascular membrane formation).

Complications include **secondary cataract and glaucoma**.

Some cats present with **exophthalmos** (eye bulging forward), where there has been an extension of the disease from the sinuses and nasal cavity into the orbital tissues.

In cases with nasal infection, there may be a **mucopurulent discharge with sneezing. Distortion and swelling** over the **bridge of the nose**, or a **polyp-like mass** projecting from the nasal cavity are present in 70% of cats with the respiratory form.

Chronic skin granulomas may be present. Skin lesions consist of **papules or nodules** varying from 0.1–1 cm in diameter. Lesions may **ulcerate and exude serous fluid, or remain as intact nodules.**

Cats with disseminated disease may show neurological signs.

Cats may **present** with **chronic nasal or skin disease**, and the ocular involvement is identified secondarily on physical examination. Cats may also be presented **primarily for the ocular signs**, where the owner has seen the development of a cloudy eye and the cat has gone blind.

Diagnosis

A tentative diagnosis is based on typical clinical signs of nasal or skin disease and concurrent ocular signs. The presence of small swollen brownish discolored areas in the retina suggests fungal disease. The frequency of occurrence of individual fungal diseases in the geographical area helps establish a tentative diagnosis.

Cytology can be very useful in the diagnosis of *C. neoformans*. Demonstration of the organism can be made via **anterior chamber centesis** or by fine-needle biopsy (using a 25 gauge needle) taken from the sub-retinal space. The sample is best stained with **new methylene blue, Indian ink or Diff-Quick**.

Serology to detect **capsule antigen** is sensitive using serum, CSF fluid or urine.

Histopathology from tissue biopsies demonstrates the organism.

Radiology of the nasal cavity, sinuses and chest may be useful in cases that do not demonstrate nasal or skin signs.

Ocular ultrasound can be used to **detect retinal detachment** when anterior chamber flare, cataract or vitreal flare prevents ophthalmoscopic examination of the fundus. It is also used in cases of exophthalmos to examine, and do ultrasound-guided biopsies of the orbital tissue.

Differential diagnosis

Other fungal diseases such **as blastomycosis, histoplasmosis, candidiasis and coccidioidomycosis** can cause similar signs. They also present with signs of uveitis and multifocal granulomatous chorioretinitis that appear as small brownish nodules in the retina, and may cause blindness. Consideration of individual fungal diseases as differential diagnoses will depend on which diseases are found in the geographical region. Serological tests are available to differentiate these infections.

Ocular toxoplasmosis. Cats present with similar signs of anterior uveitis, blindness and chorioretinitis, although the ocular inflammation is not usually as severe. Laboratory tests may be needed to differentiate these diseases. Tests for toxoplasmosis can be confusing to interpret, but serological tests for *Cryptococcus* antigen are sensitive and specific.

Ocular manifestations of FIV, FIP and FeLV are usually signs of anterior uveitis, rather than sudden blindness from retinal involvement. However, retinal disease and sudden blindness can be an uncommon presenting sign with these viruses. FIP is difficult to confirm with diagnostic tests, and is diagnosed by a process of elimination. FIV and FeLV can be diagnosed with serological tests, although these diseases can occur concurrently with cryptococcosis.

Treatment

See the main reference on page 26 (The Cat With Signs of Chronic Nasal Disease).

Cats with multifocal chorioretinitis usually have disseminated cryptococcosis, and have a very poor prognosis for treatment.

Prolonged treatment with constant monitoring of antigen titers and renal function is required.

Combinations of anti-fungal drugs appear to give the best results and include:
- **Amphotericin B**. Drug can be given IV (see standard texts) or SC (0.5–0.8 mg/kg) in 400 ml of 0.45% saline containing 2.5% dextrose. Administer subcutaneously two or three times a week for 1–3 months, until a total cumulative dose of 8–26 mg/kg is reached. Monitor serum creatinine, urea (more sensitive, but influenced by many non-renal factors) and urine specific gravity and sediment for casts. If azotemia develops, discontinue amphotericin until it resolves and reduce dose.
- 5-fluorocytosine 50 mg/kg q 8 h PO used combined with amphotericin.
- **Fluconazole** 2.5–10 mg/kg PO q 12 h may be the best of the imadazole drugs for CNS and ocular cryptococcosis, and is used after the course of amphotericin for as long as 2 years.

CHORIORETINITIS CAUSED BY OTHER FUNGI

> **Classical signs**
>
> - Chorioretinitis progressing to anterior uveitis (cloudy eye) and endophthalmitis, in a geographical area where fungal infections occur.

> **Classical signs—Cont'd**
>
> - Vision loss and reduced pupil light reflexes.
> - Other organ system disease, e.g. renal, CNS, nasal cavity.

See main references on page 25 for details (The Cat With Signs of Chronic Nasal Disease) for cryptococcosis and pages 387, 379, 371 (The Pyrexic Cat) for other fungi.

Pathogenesis

Other fungi that cause intra-ocular infections vary in their geographical distribution:
- **Blastomycosis** is a dimorphic fungus, which grows as a yeast in mammalian tissue, and as a mycelial form in the environment. It is found in the USA in the midwestern and southeastern states along the Mississipi, Ohio and Missouri Rivers and occasionally mid-Atlantic states, and in Central America, parts of Asia, Africa, Europe and Israel. Close proximity to water is a factor in its distribution.
- **Histoplasmosis** is a dimorphic fungus, which exists as a free-living mycelial form, and yeast-like organisms in mammalian tissues. It is found in central USA, especially in the Ohio, Mississipi and Missouri River basins, and in Central and South America. There is an association with moist humid conditions and nitrogen-rich soils, bat and bird excrement.
- **Coccidioidomycosis** a soil mycelial organism with a natural reservoir in desert soils, and around animal burrows. It is found in southwestern USA, Mexico, Central and South America. Animal infection occurs by inhalation of arthrospores, which can transform into spherules and then endospores in lung tissue.

Clinical signs

Most intra-ocular fungal infections cause similar ocular signs.
- **Choroidal granulomas** are the most characteristic sign on fundoscopy, and appear as a raised area of tapetal hyporeflectivity, or small swollen brownish discolored areas in the retina.
- A **generalized chorioretinitis** and **secondary retinal detachments**, with ballooning of the retina into the vitreous.

- **Optic neuritis** may be present, seen as a red, swollen optic nerve that is hyperemic.
- **Anterior uveitis** seen as cloudy, red eye with corneal edema, hypopyon and inflamed conjunctiva.

Affected cats show **varying degrees of blindness**, depending on the severity of the ocular infection.

Systemic signs can involve many other organs, especially the lungs, brain, nasal cavity, as well as the peri-orbital tissues, lymph nodes, bones, toenails and skin.

Diagnosis

A tentative diagnosis is based on the presenting signs of a cat with rapidly progressive, usually bilateral **chorioretinitis, progressing to anterior uveitis**, with signs of other systemic disease, and occurring in a geographic area where such fungal disease is known to occur.

Imaging techniques can be used to obtain more supportive evidence of a deep fungal infection:
- Thoracic radiography to demonstrate pulmonary granulomas.
- Nasal cavity radiography.
- Ocular ultrasound; signs of retinal detachment.

Confirmation of the diagnosis is based on the **demonstration of the respective organism** in:
- Cerebrospinal fluid.
- Samples taken by centesis of vitreous or subretinal exudate.
- Histopathology of enucleated globes.
- Bone marrow biopsy samples (histoplasmosis).

Serological tests can be performed, looking for elevated antibodies (blastomycosis, histoplasmosis, coccidiodomycosis).

Treatment

Antifungal medications are the cornerstone of therapy. Drugs chosen should be based on results of fungal culture and sensitivity, where possible. Treatment may need to be prolonged, depending on response.

Itraconazole 100 mg PO q 24 h with food, or 10 mg/kg q 24 h, or 5 mg/kg q 12 h PO.

Fluconazole 50 mg PO q 8 h.

Amphotericin B. This drug can be administered in a subcutaneous infusion of glucose and sodium chloride to reduce the renal toxicity (see The Cat With Signs of Chronic Nasal Discharge, page 26).

Avoid use of systemic corticosteroids.

Topical steroids or NSAIDs may be used to control the anterior uveitis.

Supportive therapy such as fluids and nutritional support.

Enucleation of the eye is recommended if endophthalmitis and/or secondary glaucoma develop.

Prognosis

Prognosis is guarded to grave in most cases where there is systemic involvement.

TRAUMATIC RETINAL DETACHMENT

Classical signs

- Acutely painful eye with hyphema.
- +/− Scleral and conjunctival hemorrhage.
- Usually unilateral.

See the main reference on page 1200 (The Cat With a Red Coloration of the globe).

Clinical signs

The typical presentation of **traumatic retinal detachment** is an **acutely painful eye**, which is usually **unilateral**.

Exophthalmos may be present from retrobulbar hemorrhage and swelling.

Most traumatic eye injuries will exhibit **some degree of ocular hemorrhage**. This may present as:
- Scleral and/or subconjunctival hemorrhage.
- A red eye with hyphema. The anterior chamber may be filled with blood, or there may be a loose clot.
- If the vitreous is visible, there may be focal areas of hemorrhage, or the vitreous may be filled with blood.

Try to visualize the pupil and pupillary light reflex. A blind eye will usually have a dilated pupil.

The retina may not be visible due to the hyphema. If there is hemorrhage in the inter-retinal space between the retinal pigment epithelium and the rods and cones, the retina will bulge forward with a red appearance.

Loss of vision may be caused by **trauma to the optic nerve**. It is not possible to visualize this part of the nerve, but hemorrhages may be present on the optic disc.

Beware of **secondary glaucoma**. Initially, traumatized eyes are very soft. Glaucoma may follow acutely from obstruction of the iridocorneal angle by hemorrhage, lens luxation or rupture, and inflammation. Cases with chronic retinal detachment may form vascular membranes, which obstruct the drainage angle.

Diagnosis

Diagnosis is based on clinical signs of a cat presented with an acutely painful, red eye. **Carefully examine the eye to determine the extent of the injury**. If the fundus is visible ophthalmoscopically, the retina will be able to be examined, and areas with hemorrhage and detachment will be visible.

Ocular ultrasound using a 10-megahertz stand-off probe, is a very useful diagnostic tool when the fundus cannot be visualized because of severe hyphema. Retinal detachment will show as a bulging hypoechoic line. Pay particular attention to the shape of the globe, as severely traumatized eyes may also have a rupture of the sclera posteriorly, and this will have a very poor prognosis. Try to visualize the muscle cone and optic nerve for swelling.

Use **tonometry** to monitor intra-ocular pressure.

Treatment

Treatment is usually conservative, and includes antibiotics and anti-inflammatory drugs.
- **Systemic broad-spectrum antibiotic** cover to prevent hematogenous infection.
- **Systemic anti-inflammatory drugs** to reduce inflammation and prevent secondary complications in the eye, such as prednisolone 1 mg/kg bid or a NSAID like ketaprofen, cartrophen or metacam.

In cases with exophthalmos, do a **temporary tarsorrhaphy** to protect the cornea.

GLAUCOMA CAUSING RETINAL DEGENERATION

Classical signs

- Buphthalmos (an enlarged globe).
- Increased intra-ocular pressure.
- Dilated pupil, poorly or non-responsive to light.
- Hyper-reflective tapetum.
- Luxated lens or cataract.

See the main reference on page 1232 (The Cat With Ocular Discharge or Changed Conjunctival Appearance).

Clinical signs

Cats blinded from glaucoma will have an **enlarged globe** (**buphthalmos**), and the condition will be chronic.

Deep episcleral vessel injection is seen in eyes with a high intra-ocular pressure (above 30 mmHg). Compared to superficial episcleral vessels, the **deep vessels** are usually **straighter and larger**, do not move when the overlying bulbar conjunctiva is moved, and do not blanch with the topical application of 1:1000 epinephrine.

The **pupil is dilated or semidilated**, with either absent or poor pupillary light reflex.

There may be signs of chronic anterior uveitis, especially abnormalities in the appearance of the iris surface for example:
- **Pinkish discoloration** associated with **fibrovascular membrane formation**.
- **Grayish nodules** on the iris surface.

There may be **signs of lens instability** including:
- An aphakic crescent (crescent shape produced by the clear space between the edge of the displaced lens and the adjacent pupillary margin).
- Anterior or posterior luxation (dislocation).
- Iridodonesis (wobbling of the iris).

There may be signs of **intra-ocular neoplasia**.

Prolonged increased intra-ocular pressure results in **collapse of the cribriform plate**. This causes obstruction to retinal vascular flow at the level of the optic disc, and obstruction to the axoplasmic flow in the optic nerves fibers. The resulting **retinal degeneration** results in the following ophthalmoscopic signs:

- A hyper-reflective tapetum.
- Attenuation (thinning) of the retinal blood vessels.
- Optic disc cupping (the optic disc is pushed backward).

Diagnosis

Diagnosis is based on the clinical appearance of buphthalmos, with any or all of the other related signs of glaucoma, such as chronic anterior uveitis and lens instability.

- Tonometry is used to measure intra-ocular pressure (IOP). Normal range for IOP in the cat is 15–25 mmHg. Readings **over 30 mmHg are supportive of a diagnosis of glaucoma**.

FELINE LEUKEMIA VIRUS

Classical signs

- Discrete iris or ciliary body masses (FeLV-associated lymphosarcoma).
- Anterior uveitis.
- Intermittent asymmetric changes in pupil size, shape or response.
- Other FeLV-associated signs, e.g. anemia.
- Retinal detachment.

See the main reference on page 1300 (The Cat With Abnormal Iris Appearance).

Clinical signs

FeLV may cause **ocular lymphosarcoma**, which appears as **discrete iris or ciliary body masses**, usually bilateral, which may cause gross distortion of the iris structure.

FeLV more commonly presents as a uveitis, with changes to iris appearance, and abnormal pupil size and shape. The **anterior chamber** may contain **fibrin and/or blood**. Anterior uveitis may occur in the absence of discernible intra-ocular neoplasia.

Some cats develop **spastic pupil syndrome**, which presents as otherwise unexplainable intermittent

asymmetric **changes in pupil size, shape or response**. For more detail see main reference on page 1278 (The Cat With Abnormal Pupil Size, Shape or Response).

It is possible to see **retinal detachment** when the neoplastic process involves the choroid.

There may be other signs of FeLV-associated disease, e.g. anemia or multicentric lymphosarcoma.

Diagnosis

Diagnosis is based on the clinical signs observed in the eye, in association with other signs suggestive of FeLV, e.g. multicentric lymphoma, FeLV-associated anemia.

Diagnosis is confirmed on **clinical pathology**, for example on cytology of lymph nodes or aqueous centesis samples, or occasionally on hematology.

A positive serological test using an **antigen-based test for FeLV** is supportive evidence of the disease. For more detail see main reference on page 543 (The Anemic Cat).

Treatment

For more detail see main reference on pages 1292 and 544 (The Cat With Abnormal Iris Appearance and The Anemic Cat).

Treatment of the ocular condition, in conjunction with systemic chemotherapy, might include **topical corticosteroids** such as 0.5% prednisolone acetate drops given q 6–12 h.

Prognosis for the eye will be poor to guarded, if secondary glaucoma has occurred.

FELINE INFECTIOUS PERITONITIS VIRUS

Classical signs

- Young cats 6–12 months of age.
- Anterior uveitis with large fibrin clots (hypopyon).
- Keratic precipitates ("mutton fat deposits") on the cornea.
- Chorioretinitis causing variable vision loss and/or abnormal pupil reflexes.

(continued)

See the main reference on page 372 (The Pyrexic Cat).

Pathogenesis

FIP is caused by a coronavirus that causes a **disseminated, pyogranulomatous vasculitis**. There are two forms of the disease that are recognized:

● An **effusive (wet) form**, that causes a fibrin-rich exudation in the peritoneal cavity.
● A **non-effusive (dry) form**, that usually manifests with ocular and neurological signs including anterior uveitis, chorioretinitis and meningitis, respectively.

There is evidence to suggest that FIP is caused by a mutation of enteric coronavirus (FECV) which occurs within about 18 months of infection.

Clinical signs

The **ocular form of the disease** is usually seen in **young cats from 6 months to a year of age**.

The main presenting sign is uveitis. Large fibrin clots mixed with exudated white and red blood cells form a **hypopyon** (cloudy eye). **Keratic precipitates** are common, and appear as large pinkish, brown spots ("mutton fat deposits") on the inferior endothelial surface of the cornea.

The **vitreous may be hazy**, because of similar exudation of cells from the ciliary body.

The retina may show a focal or total exudative **retinal detachment**. It is common to see an inflammatory exudate sheathing the major retinal blood vessels, which appears as a **cloudy sheath around the vessels**.

Blindness may be seen with **abnormal pupil reflexes** (miotic in the early stages with uveitis, followed by a dilated pupil in blind cats), and **abnormal pupil size** (**anisocoria**).

Cats with ocular signs frequently **develop neurological signs weeks or months later**, and are euthanized or die because of **meningoencephalitis**, and its associated signs, such as seizures. Most common signs in addition to seizures, are **central vestibular signs**, which include head tilt, loss of balance, nystagmus, mental depression, and postural reaction deficits, and **cerebellar signs** such as intentional tremors, and hypermetria. Behavioral changes often occur.

Cats with ocular signs of FIP rarely show systemic signs of illness such as fever, inappetence and weight loss **at initial presentation**. As the disease becomes chronic, weight loss and neurological signs develop (seizures are most common).

Diagnosis

There is no definitive diagnostic test for the FIP virus.

A tentative diagnosis is initially based on the suspicious clinical signs of a young cat with uveitis showing hypopyon and keratic precipitates.

Serology is usually regarded as being of dubious benefit in the diagnosis, as the FIP organism cross-reacts with enteric forms of coronavirus.

Diagnosis can only be confirmed on characteristic histopathology of affected tissues on biopsy or necropsy examination. The typical change is described as a **pyogranulomatous vasculitis**. Necrosis and a fibrinoid response are seen in some cases. The ocular cellular response includes neutrophils, lymphocytes, plasma cells, macrophages and large, spindle-shaped histiocytes.

Cats often have **a large increase in plasma total protein, globulin** and IgG concentration, because of the chronic nature of the inflammatory disease process. The polyclonal increase in gammaglobulins is caused by virus antigen and cell destruction from the intense inflammation associated with the infection.

Differential diagnosis

Toxoplasmosis is the main differential diagnosis. Toxoplasmosis occurs in cats of all ages. The exudative response in the eye is not usually as pronounced. Laboratory tests can be used to differentiate (see above).

All other **ocular diseases that cause anterior uveitis and chorioretinitis** should be excluded with diagnostic tests, particularly fungal infections such as cryptococcosis (see page 1268).

Treatment

There is no specific treatment for FIP, and once signs develop the disease is almost uniformly fatal.

Topical and systemic corticosteroids will initially reduce the signs of uveitis and chorioretinitis, but recurrence is common.

Supportive medical management including fluids and nutrition can be attempted. Interferon-alpha and cyclophosphamide or chlorambucil may temporarily reduce clinical signs.

Cats which are anorexic and depressed, and do not respond to supportive therapy, should be euthanized.

TAURINE DEFICIENCY RETINOPATHY (INCLUDING FELINE CENTRAL RETINAL DEGENERATION – FRCD)

Classical signs

- Vision loss in advanced cases.
- Hyper-reflective tapetal retina, beginning as an elliptical lesion in the area centralis and progressing to include the entire retina.
- Attenuated (thin) retinal blood vessels in advanced cases.
- History of inadequate diet especially cats fed commercial dog foods.
- All breeds at any age.
- Affected cats may have a cardiomyopathy.

Pathogenesis

The syndromes feline central retinal degeneration (FCRD) and taurine deficiency retinopathy are regarded by many authors as being the **same disease**. The disease is still occasionally seen in cats that appear to have adequate levels of dietary taurine, but the overall incidence of the disease throughout the world appears to have declined as the taurine content of commercial diets has been increased.

Taurine is a sulfur-containing amino acid, which is metabolized in the liver from cysteine. **Cats are** **deficient in the enzyme** cysteinesulfinic acid decarboxylase that is **necessary for the production of taurine**, and therefore need diets that contain a high level of taurine.

In cats, taurine is used almost exclusively for **bile acid conjugation**.

Taurine is dissolved in the cytosolic fluids of cells, particularly in excitable tissues. It is found in high concentrations in the retina, heart, central nervous system and skeletal muscle.

Taurine is essential for photoreceptor survival, and is found in high concentrations in inner and outer segments. It is thought to **protect the retina from light and chemical damage, regulate calcium ion transport and regulate signal transduction**.

Taurine deficiency causes a loss of photoreceptor outer segment and photoreceptor nuclei, and underlying hypertrophy and disorganization of the underlying retinal pigment epithelial cells. It is not clear why the area centralis is affected more than the outer retina, but it may be associated with increased cone density and higher levels of rhodopsin pigment in cone cells in this area. Cone cells are affected more than rods.

Ophthalmoscopically the initial lesion develops in the area centralis. **The area centralis (temporal to the optic disc) at first develops a granular appearance, then becomes hyper-reflective**. As the degeneration advances, a second hyper-reflective lesion develops nasal to the optic disc, which eventually coalesces with the area centralis lesion to form a broad hyper-reflective band, dorsal to the optic disc. Finally, generalized retinal degeneration develops, with generalized tapetal hyper-reflectivity, and retinal vessel attenuation.

Taurine deficiency also causes dilated cardiomyopathy. See main references on page 151 for details (The Cat With Abnormal Heart Sounds and/or an Enlarged Heart).

Clinical signs

Taurine deficiency may be seen in all breeds of cats, at any age, although it is less common now that functional taurine is in all commercial cat food. It is most commonly seen in cats fed **dog food or vegetarian diets**.

Initially, cats are presented with **vision loss**. In later stages, this is associated with **poor pupillary light reflexes**.

There are **five stages of the disease** described on clinical ophthalmoscopy:

- Stage 1. There is an increased granularity of the area centralis, adjacent to the optic disc. Cats are visual at this stage.
- Stage 2. The area centralis develops an ellipsoidal hyper-reflective appearance. Vision is starting to deteriorate.
- Stage 3. A second hyper-reflective lesion develops nasal to the optic disc. Vision deteriorates further.
- Stage 4. The two hyper-reflective lesions join to form a broad band of hyper-reflective tapetum. Vision is noticeably poor at this stage.
- Stage 5. There is generalized retinal degeneration, with severely attenuated retinal blood vessels. The cat is blind.

Diagnosis

Diagnosis is based on clinical signs, in particular observation of the typical retinal lesions, and a **history of inappropriate diet**.

Electroretinography (ERG) can be performed to identify altered photoreceptor function. **Cones appear to be affected more than rods**, so these cats will have reduced b waves in photopic (light) conditions, and better responses in scotopic (dark adapted) conditions.

Measurement of plasma taurine levels is the best way to diagnose the condition. Cats with plasma taurine levels below 40 nmol/ml are regarded as deficient.

Treatment

Provide taurine supplementation.
- 250–500 mg PO q 12 h.
- In the early stages, retinal damage can be reversed, but ophthalmoscopic signs remain unchanged.
- The effects of prolonged deficiency are only partially reversible.
- The ERG signs associated with rod degeneration may reverse, but **cone degeneration never totally recovers**.

Advanced cases will remain **irreversibly blind**, despite treatment.

FLY LARVAL MIGRATION (OPHTHALMOMYIASIS)

Classical signs

- Vision loss, usually unilateral.
- Cloudy posterior segment with linear track-like lesions on fundoscopy.
- Anterior uveitis associated with larva in the anterior chamber.
- Rare condition.

Clinical signs

Larval migration of the *Cuterebra* **fly** causes vision loss, usually unilateral, associated with chorioretinitis. Typically the cat is presented with a cloudy painful eye.

There are usually **poor pupillary light reflexes** in that eye, and **anisocoria**, if the condition is unilateral.

The characteristic fundoscopy signs are linear **hyper-reflective "tracks" in the tapetal fundus**, and linear light gray areas of reduced pigmentation in the non-tapetum. Hemorrhage may be evident in the early stages. Sometimes the white **body of a fly larva** is seen associated with one of the tracks.

Rarely, the larva is seen in the anterior chamber, with associated signs of anterior uveitis.

Diagnosis

Diagnosis is based on appearance of the fundoscopic lesions, or observation of the parasite in the anterior chamber and associated uveitis.

Treatment

There is no specific treatment.

Do not kill the parasite, as this may cause a severe immune reaction to the parasite proteins.

Topical and systemic corticosteroid therapy is used to minimize the inflammation in the affected eye.

A free-moving parasite in the anterior chamber or vitreous should be surgically removed.

HEREDITARY RETINAL DEGENERATION IN ABYSSINIAN CATS

Classical signs

- Progressive loss of vision occurs in young Abyssinian cats.
- Loss of pupil light reflexes in advanced cases.
- Tapetal hyper-reflectivity and retinal vessel attenuation.
- Relatively rare disease.

Pathogenesis

Two forms of hereditary retinal degeneration have been described in Abyssinian cats.

- **Rod–cone dysplasia.**
  - Inheritance is **autosomal dominant**.
  - Rods and cones degenerate at the same rate.
  - Degeneration begins centrally, with progressive loss of the photoreceptor layer.
  - The photoreceptor inner segments remain rudimentary, and the outer segments fail to elongate.
- **Rod–cone degeneration.**
  - Inheritance is **autosomal recessive**.
  - Rods degenerate rapidly, but cones are spared until the late stage of the disease.
  - Degeneration begins in the mid-peripheral regions of the retina.
  - Histological changes begin at approximately 35 days post-natally, with immature rod outer segment discs. The cones appear normal at this stage. The rod outer segments begin to form vacuoles, and the disc material clumps with subsequent drop out of the cells. Two to three years later, the cones start to degenerate and drop out. Rhodopsin levels are reduced in affected cats. Cats may also have plasma lipid abnormalities.

Clinical signs

Inherited retinal degeneration is a **rare disease** causing blindness in **young** (≤ 4 years) **Abyssinian cats**. It occurs very rarely in other breeds of cats.

Rod–cone dysplasia.
- Retinal degeneration begins at 4 weeks of age, and cats are blind by 1 year of age. The typical history is of a **young cat that goes rapidly blind**.

- Nystagmus may be present.
- Loss of vision occurs rapidly, and **mydriasis, hyper-reflective tapetum** and **attenuated retinal blood vessels** are evident.
- There is loss of pupillary light reflexes in advanced cases.

Rod–cone degeneration.
- Retinal degeneration does not begin until 1.5–2 years of age, and blindness follows over the next 2–4 years. The typical history is of **older cats that go slowly blind**.
- The **retina** on either side of the optic disc begins to develop a **subtle gray discoloration**. A more diffuse grayness of the tapetal area follows. The tapetal area then becomes **hyper-reflective** and the retinal blood vessels attenuate.
- The non-tapetal fundus may show pale areas mixed with heavily pigmented areas.
- There is loss of pupillary light reflexes in advanced cases.
- **Electroretinography (ERG)** shows a progressive reduction of the B-wave amplitude which correlates to the loss of rhodopsin.

Diagnosis

Initially, diagnosis is made on the breed and age of the cat, and the clinical presentation of vision loss. Pupils may become dilated, and the tapetum will be hyper-reflective in the advanced stage of the disease.

Histopathology will help to confirm the disease if cats can be sacrificed.

ERG with reduced B-wave amplitude is useful in the early stages of the disease.

Differential diagnosis

Taurine deficiency will present with loss of papillary light reflexes, hyper-reflective tapetum and retinal vessel attenuation. This may affect cats of all ages and all breeds. Dietary history and plasma taurine levels should help to differentiate this disease.

Hypertensive retinopathy usually occurs in older cats. There is always hemorrhage present around retinal blood vessels, or there is focal areas of hemorrhage present in the vitreous. There will be varying degrees of retinal detachment. Check these cats for renal disease and hyper-thyroidism.

Inflammatory chorioretinitis is always appears as cloudy eyes that have uveitis. Laboratory tests are useful to confirm diagnoses.

Treatment

There is **no treatment** for this form of retinal degeneration. Breeders need to be made aware of the mode of inheritance.

TRAUMA-ASSOCIATED OCULAR SARCOMA

Classical signs

- Rare, primary neoplasia that occurs in older cats (7–15 years).
- History of previous severe trauma to eye.
- Anterior uveitis, keratitis (corneal edema and pigmentation) and glaucoma.
- White to pinkish masses may be visible in the vitreous.

Clinical signs

Trauma-associated ocular sarcoma is a rare primary neoplasia reported only in cats.

It occurs in older cats, typically **7–15 years of age** that have had a history of **ocular trauma 3–10 years previously**.

Signs of anterior **uveitis and keratitis** may be evident, as edema and pigmentation of the cornea, and a cloudy eye. These changes may prevent visualization of the intra-ocular structures.

Secondary glaucoma is common at this stage of the disease. The eye will show buphthalmos (enlarged globe) with engorged scleral vessels.

If the posterior segment can be visualized, **white to pink masses** may be seen.

The condition is thought to occur **after lens trauma**, which triggers the **lens epithelial cells** to undergo **metaplasia**.

The neoplasia rapidly extends through the choroid, and infiltrates the optic nerve. Metastasis has been reported.

Survival rate is very low.

Diagnosis

Old cats that have a prior history of trauma, and present with glaucoma and signs of uveitis and keratitis, are candidates for this rare condition.

Fine-needle biopsy may be done, but may not yield a diagnostic sample if the tumor contains fibrous and cartilagenous tissue.

Histopathology of enucleated globes provides a definitive diagnosis, and will show changes that may include granulation tissue, fibrosarcoma, osteosarcoma and anaplastic spindle cell sarcoma.

Treatment

All blind globes with chronic uveitis should be watched for the development of this condition.

Early enucleation with histopathology should be done on all globes where there is a **prior history of trauma**, and there are **changes in the size and shape of the globe**, or **changes in the anterior chamber** and cornea, that are indicative of intra-ocular disease.

Severely traumatized blind eyes in cats should be enucleated, to prevent the occurrence of this condition, particularly if there has been lens rupture.

In confirmed cases, check for metastases to regional lymph nodes, and other organs such as lungs and liver.

METASTATIC INTRA-RETINAL NEOPLASIA

Classical signs

- Rare in cats.
- Uveitis with corneal edema, cloudy aqueous and distorted pupil.
- Swelling and pigment changes in the retina.

Clinical signs

This is a rare condition in cats.

Most cases present as **anterior uveitis with corneal edema and a cloudy aqueous**, and have some form of **swelling seen in the iris**, which may cause distortion of the pupil (dyscoria).

Fundoscopy may show a **bulging of the retina, and some pigment change** such as a **brownish appearance. Retinal detachment** may occur as the neoplasia extends through the choroid into the intra-retinal space.

The most common metastatic neoplasia in the eye include **lymphosarcoma, and adenocarcinoma from lung, uterus and undetermined origin**.

Diagnosis

An initial tentative diagnosis is based on the most common presentation of iris swelling, distortion of the retina and signs of uveitis.

Fine-needle biopsies may help to obtain a diagnosis.

Chest and abdominal radiology should be done to find primary adenocarcinomas.

Examination of the buffy coat for abnormal lymphocytes can be done in cases with lymphosarcoma.

Fine-needle biopsies of enlarged lymph nodes may be diagnostic.

TOXIC RETINAL DEGENERATION

Classical signs

- Rapid loss of vision within 5 days with dilated pupils.
- History of administration of methylnitrosurea in combination with ketamine hydrochloride.
- High doses of fluoroquinalones, particularly enrofloxacin, may cause blindness in cats.

Clinical signs

There are **few cases reported** of toxic retinal degeneration in the cat.

There is **rapid loss of vision** over **approximately 5 days**, usually in cats that have been administered specific drugs. This syndrome is associated with **high doses of fluoroquinalones**, particularly enrofloxacin, although it has also occurred as an idiosyncratic reaction in cats given less than the recommended dose of 5 mg/kg q 24 h. Methylnitrosurea, in combination with

ketamine hydrochloride, has also been associated with this syndrome.

- **Ketamine** also increases cerebral oxygen demand, and the visual cortex is the most sensitive area of the brain to hypoxia. Hypotension associated with acepromazine especially intravenous administration, and high doses of isoflurane, or other anesthetic agents, and mask delivery of anesthetic agents all exacerbate the hypoxia. Hypoxia of the visual cortex can result in cortical blindness following anesthesia.

Pupils become **dilated and unresponsive to light**.

Pathology is characterized by photoreceptor and outer nuclear layer degeneration.

Diagnosis

A tentative diagnosis is **based on clinical signs and history** of either:
- Sudden blindness after administration of methylnitrosourea and ketamine.
- Sudden blindness after administration of enrofloxacin, especially at a higher dose (20 mg/kg q 24 h) than the recommended rate of 5 mg/kg q 24 h.

LIPEMIA RETINALIS

Classical signs

- Retinal blood vessels appear enlarged, and may have a yellow to orange hue.
- Rare in cats.

See main reference on page 569 (The Cat With Hyperlipidemia).

Clinical signs

Cats **do not show visual impairment** with lipemia retinalis, so this condition is usually seen as an incidental finding.

Ophthalmosopic examination reveals **enlarged retinal blood vessels**, which have a **yellow to orange coloration**. There may be some haziness surrounding the major vessels from lipid leakage, and this may cause a local inflammation.

Lipemia retinalis is seen in cats that have **increased fasting triglycerides**, which is most commonly idiopathic in origin, but may be associated with **diabetes mellitus or hereditary hyperchylomicronemia**. Post-prandial lipidemia may be seen in normal cats, especially after a high-fat diet, and obese cats. It can occur after administration of corticosteroids.

Diagnosis

The **clinical signs** of large retinal blood vessels that have a yellow to orange hue should alert the clinician to lipidemia. Blood cholesterol and triglyceride levels should be checked.

Diagnosis is based on clinical signs and **increased plasma triglycerides**.

Blood glucose levels should be checked for diabetes mellitus.

There may be a history of corticosteroid use, particularly megesterol acetate.

ANEMIC RETINOPATHY

Classical signs

- Blind, weak cat with profound anaemia (PCV < 10% or hemaglobin < 5 g/dl).
- Retinal hemorrhages and attenuated, pale retinal vessels.
- Partial to complete loss of pupillary light reflex.

Clinical signs

Typically the cat presents as **blind and weak, with profound anemia** (PCV < 10%). The severe anemia is thought to cause a **hypoxic retinopathy**.

On fundoscopy there are **focal retinal hemorrhages** associated with anoxia of the retinal blood vessel cell wall. The **vessels** appear **pale and are attenuated** (thinned).

Partial to complete loss of the pupillary light reflex is present as a result of retinal hypoxia.

Other signs of severe anemia are present including pale mucous membranes, increased respiratory rate, lethargy and weakness.

Diagnosis

Diagnosis is based **initially on the clinical signs** of a severely anemic cat with poor pupillary light reflexes and multiple small retinal hemorrhages.

Diagnosis is confirmed on **hematology**, and **ruling out coagulopathy** as a cause of retinal hemorrhage. Anemia must be **profound** for this syndrome to occur, i.e. usually the PCV is less than 10% or hemoglobin less than 5 g/dl.

The cause of the anemia should be identified. Common causes of profound anemia are chronic and include FeLV-associated anemia or *Mycoplasma hemofelis* (*Hemobartonella felis*) infection. FeLV-associated anemia may also be accompanied by thrombocytopenia, which may contribute to the retinal hemorrhages.

HYPERVISCOSITY SYNDROME

Classical signs

- Blindness and loss of pupil reflexes.
- Dilated tortuous retinal vessels, retinal hemorrhages, retinal detachment.
- Monoclonal globulin spike on plasma electrophoresis.

Clinical signs

Severe plasma hyperviscosity causes **blindness and loss of pupillary reflexes**.

Markedly increased plasma proteins cause increased viscosity of blood. This results in sluggish blood flow to the retina and retinal **hypoxia**.

On fundoscopy, there are **extremely dilated, tortuous retinal vessels, retinal hemorrhages, retinal detachment**, perivascular effusion and optic disc edema may be evident.

A **variety of other clinical signs** may be present associated with the primary disease causing the hyperproteinemia, including lethargy, pale mucous membranes, neurologic signs and lameness.

Diagnosis

Diagnosis is initially based on the suspicious signs seen on fundoscopy, especially the presence of **bizarre dilated, tortuous retinal vessels**.

Diagnosis is confirmed by demonstration of a monoclonal globulin spike on protein electrophoresis of plasma.

Multiple myeloma is the most frequent cause of a monoclonal globulin spike.

BLINDNESS CAUSED BY OPTIC NERVE PROBLEMS

OPTIC NERVE COLOBOMA

Classical signs

- Rare condition that occasionally affects vision.
- Inverted funnel or black hole appearance in optic disc.
- Associated with eyelid agenesis.
- Retinal dysplasia also occurs (dark lines on tapetal fundus).

Clinical signs

Optic nerve coloboma is a **rare lesion** in cats.

It is usually seen as an **incidental finding** on ophthalmoscopic examination of cats with **eyelid agenesis (coloboma)**.

Both **hereditary and in utero infections** have been suggested as causes.

The coloboma appears as a **dark area associated with the optic disc**, and has the **appearance of an inverted funnel or black hole**.

Vision is rarely affected.

Retinal dysplasia may occur concurrently, and appears as a dark streak or depigmented rosette in the tapetal fundus.

Diagnosis

Diagnosis is based on the fundiscopic findings of an optic disc with a dark hollow appearance. Retinal dysplasia appears as dark lines in the tapetal fundus.

BLINDNESS ASSOCIATED WITH MIDBRAIN AND VISUAL CORTEX PROBLEMS

*TOXOPLASMA GONDII**

Classical signs

- Blindness with a normal PLR.
- Anterior uveitis and chorioretinitis.
- Other neurological signs of CNS involvement.

See the main reference on page 375 (The Pyrexic Cat).

Clinical signs

Cats with CNS involvement may show blindness, with normal to slow pupillary light reflexes, if the lesions involve the cerebral visual cortex.

Uveitis and chorioretinitis may be present. See above (page 1173).

Blindness may be caused by extensive chorioretinitis and/or CNS disease involving the visual cortex.

Diagnosis

See the main reference above under chorioretinitis (page 1173).

*CRYPTOCOCCUS NEOFORMANS**

Classical signs

- Cats of all ages.
- Uveitis with hypopyon and keratic precipitates.
- Blindness with or without CNS signs.

See the main reference on page 25 (The Cat With Signs of Chronic Nasal Disease).

Clinical signs

Cryptococcosis affects cats of all ages.

Blindness may occur with or without CNS signs. **Blindness may be central** or associated with **retinal**

detachment and optic neuritis. Cats with CNS signs may show seizures, ataxia and/or depression.

Uveitis with hypopyon and keratic precipitates is a common presenting sign.

Affected cats often show **other signs** that may include one or all of the following: **chronic nasal discharge** with swollen bridge of the nose or polyp-like mass protruding from nostril, skin lesions, swollen lymph nodes, anorexia and weight loss.

Treatment of the ocular disease may alleviate signs, only to be followed by **blindness with or without CNS signs** such as seizure and ataxia.

Diagnosis

CSF tap may confirm the presence of typical yeast-like organisms visible either directly, or found on culture.

Serology may support the diagnosis.

ISCHEMIC ENCEPHALOPATHY

Classical signs

- Young adult to middle-aged cats.
- Sudden-onset blindness.
- Normal, slow or absent papillary light reflexes.
- Seizures, ataxia and/or motor defects.

See the main reference on page 800 (The Cat With Seizures, Circling and/or Changed Behavior).

Clinical signs

Ischemic encephalopathy can result from several disease processes including embolism (feline ischemic encephalopathy), and hypotension, which is usually associated with anesthesia.

Feline ischemic encephalopathy is a syndrome more common in **young adult to middle-aged cats**. The pathogenesis is unknown, but is thought to be an associated embolic event resulting in cerebral ischemia.

- In contrast, cerebrovascular accidents resulting in hemorrhage into the brain, are rare in cats, and older animals are more at risk, especially if hypertensive from renal failure or hyperthyroidism.

Ischemic encephalopathy may also occur as a **complication of anesthesia**, particularly in cats resuscitated after cardiac arrest. The **visual cortex is the most sensitive area of the brain to hypoxia**. Hypoxia of the visual cortex can result in cortical blindness.

- **Hypotension** associated with **acepromazine**, especially intravenous administration, and **high doses of isoflurane, or other anesthetic agents**, and **mask delivery** of anesthetic agents (which combines high doses of inhalant agents and poor airway maintenance), all exacerbate anesthesia-associated hypoxia. **Ketamine** also increases cerebral oxygen demand and has been associated with cortical blindness.
- Cortical blindness associated with anesthesia is evident once the cat wakes up. Other neurological signs may be evident such as paresis, ataxia, proprioceptive deficits, circling and seizures.
- Typically, there is **blindness** with dilated pupils, and normal to slow pupillary light reflexes.

In **feline ischemic encephalopathy** typically there is a **peracute onset of unilateral forebrain signs (mental** depression and confusion, compulsive circling, hemiparesis and ataxia) and rarely, severe cluster seizures or status epilepticus. Vision defects including **loss of menace response** may be present. Blindness does not occur unless the infarction involves both hemispheres, which is uncommon.

Diagnosis

A tentative diagnosis is based on clinical signs of a sudden onset of neurological problems in an adult cat unassociated with anesthesia (feline ischemic encephalopathy), or on recovery from anesthesia.

CT scan or MRI using dyes may help to localize and diagnose the problem, if feline ischemic encephalopathy is suspected. A CSF tap may show red blood cells, or hemosiderin in more chronic cases.

FELINE INFECTIOUS PERITONITIS VIRUS (FIP)

Classical signs

- Typically, young cats 6–12 months of age.
- Central blindness with normal PLR or anisocoria.
- Central vestibular and cerebellar signs.

See the main reference on page 372 (The Pyrexic Cat).

Clinical signs

Feline infectious peritonitis is an infrequent disease causing **central blindness**, and most often occurs in young cats that were in **multi-cat households or obtained from breeders** within the previous 18 months.

Cats with central blindness have the **dry form of FIP**, and usually have a history of **uveitis and the classical signs of hypopyon and keratic precipitates**.

The choroid of the eye is homologous embryologically with the meninges, so cases with meningitis often also show chorioretinitis.

Central blindness is associated with **normal to slow pupillary light reflexes** for cortical lesions, or anisocoria if the midbrain is involved. Concurrent involvement of the eyes may result in abnormal reflexes.

FIP is usually a protracted disease, often with **vague systemic signs such as inappetence, weight loss, lethargy** and pyrexia.

Central vestibular and cerebellar signs may be seen. Affected cats often develop seizures.

Ocular disease may initially respond to corticosteroid therapy, with the cat then developing CNS signs and blindness weeks or months later.

Diagnosis

There is **no definitive diagnosis for FIP**.

Diagnosis is initially based on the suspicious **clinical signs of a young cat with uveitis**, showing hypopyon and keratic precipitates, **followed up to months later with neurological signs**.

Serology is usually regarded as being of dubious benefit in the diagnosis, as the FIP organism cross-reacts with enteric forms of coronavirus.

Diagnosis can only be confirmed on characteristic histopathology of affected tissues on biopsy or necropsy. The typical change is described as a **pyogranulomatous vasculitis**. Necrosis and a fibrinoid response are seen in some cases. The ocular cellular response includes neu-trophils, lymphocytes, plasma cells, macrophages and large, spindle-shaped histiocytes.

Cases usually show a large increase in IgG due to the chronic nature of the disease, seen as **increased plasma total protein and globulin concentration**. There is a polyclonal increase in gammaglobulins caused by virus antigen, and cell destruction from the intense inflammation associated with the infection.

INTRACRANIAL NEOPLASIA

Classical signs

- Slowly progressive unilateral or bilateral vision loss.
- Older cats.
- Normal pupillary light reflex or anisocoria.
- May show neurological signs.

See the main reference on page 881 (The Cat With Anisocoria or Abnormally Dialated or Constricted Pupils).

Clinical signs

Intracranial neoplasia causing blindness usually presents as an **older cat with a loss of vision**, which may be unilateral or bilateral.

- If the lesion affects the **optic chiasm**, the **pupils will be dilated and non-resposive to light**. Meningiomas and pituitary tumors have been reported in this area.

Mid-brain masses may cause anisocoria, but vision defects will not be as apparent. Meningioma has been reported in this area.

Meningiomas in the region of the **visual cortex** may cause blindness. The pupil should have a **normal to slow response to light**.

Diagnosis

The **clinical presentation** of vision loss in an older cat with a normal fundus and abnormal PLRs increases the index of suspicion for an intracranial mass.

CT scan and MRI are useful tools to diagnose and localize the lesion.

RECOMMENDED READING

Barnett KC. A Color Atlas of Veterinary Ophthalmology. Wolfe Publishing Ltd, London, 1990.

Gelatt Kirk N (ed). Veterinary Ophthalmology, 2nd edn. Lea & Febiger, Philadelphia, 1991.

Gelatt Kirk N. Veterinary Ophthalmology, 3rd edn. Lippincott, Williams and Wilkins, Philadelphia, 1998.

Gelatt Kirk N. Essentials of Veterinary Ophthalmology. Lippincott Williams and Wilkins, Philadelphia, 2000.

Gelatt Kirk N. Color Atlas of Veterinary Ophthalmology. Lippincott Williams and Wilkins, Philadelphia, 2001.

Gelatt Kirk N, Gelatt JP. Handbook of Small Animal Ophthalmic Surgery, Vol. 1 Extraocular Procedures. Permagon Veterinary Handbook Series, Florida, 1994.

Gelatt Kirk N, Gelatt JP. Handbook of Small Animal Ophthalmic Surgery, Vol 2. Intra-ocular Procedures. Permagon Veterinary Handbook Series, Florida, 1995.

Ketring KL, Glaze MB. Atlas of Feline Ophthalmology. Trenton, NJ, Veterinary Learning Systems, 1994.

Peiffer RL, Petersen-Jones S. Small Animal Ophthalmology, A Problem Oriented Approach, 3rd edn. Saunders, Philadelphia, 2001.

58. The cat with a red coloration of the globe

Richard IE Smith

> **KEY SIGNS**
>
> - Hemorrhage in any part of the eye.
> - Engorged scleral vessels.
> - Erythema of conjunctiva.
> - Red appearance through pupil.

MECHANISM?

- In this chapter, the globe refers to the eyeball, and does not include the supporting structures such as eyelids, third eyelid and orbital structures.
- The globe appears red on the exterior when the conjunctival vessels are inflamed, or the scleral vessels are engorged, or there is diffuse conjunctival hemorrhage.
- The interior of the globe appears red due to hemorrhage in the anterior chamber, vitreous or retina.
- In animals with color-diluted genes, the fundus (that part of the retina that can be examined through the pupil) may have a red reflection from the so-called "tigroid retina".

WHERE?

- Conjunctiva, choroid.
- Iris.
- Anterior chamber.
- Vitreous.
- Retina.

WHAT?

- Trauma is a common cause of a red globe and this involves hemorrhage in the conjunctiva, sclera, anterior chamber (hyphema) or vitreous.
- Inflammation of the iris and ciliary body (anterior uveitis) may cause hyphema.
- Retinal hemorrhage from trauma, inflammation or hypertension may cause hemorrhage in the vitreous.

QUICK REFERENCE SUMMARY

Diseases causing a red coloration of the globe

WHERE?

BULBAR CONJUNCTIVA (THE CONJUNCTIVA COVERING THE GLOBE)

METABOLIC

● Hemorrhage associated with bleeding disorders (p 1197)

Bleeding disorders can cause echymoses in the conjunctiva, and in severe cases hyphema. Other signs such as oral hemorrhages, skin hemorrhages and malena may be present.

INFLAMMATION

● **Uveitis*** (p 1198)**

Appears uni- or bilaterally as a cloudy eye with a red appearance from inflamed, congested conjunctiva. Signs of inflammation are present within the eye, including hypopyon (cloudy anterior chamber), and swelling and color change of the iris. Pupils will be miotic, and the eye is soft. Sometimes there is anisocoria (unequal-sized pupils) and dyscoria (abnormal-shaped pupil).

● **Glaucoma* (p 1199)**

A red globe caused by engorged episcleral vessels. In chronic cases the globe is enlarged (buphthalmos). Other changes may be present in the eye such as cloudy cornea, uveitis and cataract formation.

INFECTIOUS

● **Acute infectious conjunctivitis*** (p 1197)**

Occurs most frequently in young cats. Herpesvirus and *Chlamydophila felis* may cause unilateral or bilateral signs, with chemotic (edema) and red (hyperemic) conjunctiva. Ocular discharge is first serous then rapidly mucopurulent. In *Chlamydophila felis* infection, the redness (hyperemia) is not as intense and the respiratory signs milder than in herpetic conjunctivitis. Mycoplasma produces mild inflammation and serous discharge, and is readily responsive to most antibiotics topically.

TRAUMA

● **Hemorrhage associated with trauma*** (p 1197)**

Ocular trauma frequently results in conjunctival, subconjunctival or retrobulbar hemorrhage. There is usually a history of trauma to the head or eye. Focal or diffuse hemorrhage may be evident between the conjunctiva and sclera (subconjunctival).

WHERE?

ANTERIOR CHAMBER

INFLAMMATION

● **Hyphema associated with inflammation* (p 1200)**

Hemorrhage in the anterior chamber may occur secondary to trauma, anterior uveitis, neoplasia or bleeding disorders. Usually accumulations of blood and protein occur within the anterior chamber, and may be attached to the iris or free within the aqueous.

TRAUMA

● Hyphema associated with trauma* (p 1200)

Anterior chamber may be filled with blood so the eye appears completely red. Owners often describe the eye as "black" in color. May be hemorrhage in the conjunctiva as well.

WHERE?

IRIS

NEOPLASTIC

● Iris neoplasia* (p 1202)

Lymphosarcoma infiltrating the iris causes iris swelling, distortion, a "creamy" color change and hemorrhage on the anterior iris surface. The pupil may be distorted (dyscoria). Hyphema and hypopyon are present in varying degrees.

INFLAMMATION/INFECTIOUS

● Uveitis*** (p 1201)

FIV, FeLV, FIP, *Blastomyces dermatitidis, Candida albicans, Coccidioides immitis, Cryptococcus neoformans, Histoplasma capsulatum* are all associated with uveitis, which may result in a pink- or red-appearing iris or hemorrhage into the anterior chamber. Systemic signs associated with the agent are usually present. Anterior uveitis with pre-iridal fibrovascular membranes (PFIM) are the main presenting signs in chronic uveitis. Hemorrhage is associated with the PFIMs. Retinal hemorrhage is seen occasionally in areas of granuloma formation. Often there is no obvious cause and the uveitis is idiopathic.

IMMUNE

● Pre-iridal fibrovascular membranes (PIFMs)* (p 1201)

New blood vessel growth seen on the anterior surface of the iris that gives the iris an injected pink discoloration. Vessels are fragile and easily hemorrhage into the anterior chamber, causing hyphema. Usually seen in eyes with chronic inflammatory disease, total retinal detachment or neoplasia.

TRAUMA

● Trauma, blunt or penetrating* (p 1299)

Bleeding into the eye is caused by an injury to the iris root or ciliary body. In penetrating injuries, especially from cat claws, hemorrhage is directly associated with an injury to the iris.

WHERE?

VITREOUS

METABOLIC

● Hypertensive retinopathy*** (p 1202)

Typically presents as an older cat with a history of sudden blindness. Usually bilateral, affected eyes appear cloudy, and the vitreous has focal red areas visible through the pupil. The retina appears out of focus. Common secondary to chronic renal disease or hyperthyroidism and cardiomyopathy.

continued

continued

TRAUMA

- ### ● Traumatic hyphema* (p 1203)

  Blunt or penetrating trauma to the head and eye or may cause hemorrhage in the vitreous. The eye appears red through the pupil. There may or may not be hemorrhage in the anterior chamber or conjunctival hemorrhage.

WHERE?

RETINA

ANOMALY

- ### ● Tigroid fundus*** (p 1204)

  The appearance of a red fundus reflection can be normal in color-dilute cats such as Siamese and Color Points. This is due to lack of pigment in the retinal pigment epithelium and consequent red reflection from choroidal blood vessels (tigroid fundus). Where there is no tapetum the whole of the fundus will appear red. Where there is a tapetum, then only the non-tapetum will appear red.

METABOLIC

- ### ● Hypertensive retinopathy*** (p 1204)

  Usually occurs in older cats with a history of sudden blindness. The eye seen through the pupil may appear red from hemorrhages in the pre-retina. Focal hemorrhages are seen along the major blood vessels. The retina may look cloudy and is difficult to focus with an ophthalmoscope because of retinal detachment.

INFLAMMATION/INFECTIOUS

- ### ● Inflammatory retinal disease* (p 1205)

  Inflammatory retinal disease, especially caused by fungal infections or ocular visceral larva migrans, may cause retinal hemorrhage. Fungal infections cause anterior uveitis with inflamed conjunctiva, pre-iridal fibrovascular membranes and occasional hemorrhage in the anterior chamber (hyphema). Less commonly, hemorrhagic lesions are seen in the retina. Rarely, retinal hemorrhage is caused by larvae migrating along blood vessels causing localized damage to the retina and hemorrhage from injuries to the blood vessel they are migrating in or move through.

TRAUMA

- ### ● Blunt or penetrating trauma* (p 1206)

  The eye appears red through the pupil if there is retinal hemorrhage. Hemorrhage may be focal or diffuse depending on the degree of trauma. If the retina is not visible, ocular ultrasound will be needed to assess the posterior eye for retinal detachment or scleral rupture. Other parts of the eye may also have hemorrhage.

INTRODUCTION

MECHANISM?

Any mechanism that gives the appearance of a red globe is included in this chapter. This may involve trauma or a disease process. Single or multiple ocular tissues may be involved. Diseases primarily affecting supporting structures such as eyelids, third eyelid and orbital structures are not included in the chapter, and the reader is referred to those specific chapters.

Conjunctivitis

In conjunctivitis, the **soft tissues surrounding the eye may be red and/or swollen** (chemosis). This usually involves trauma or diseases of the conjunctiva and nictitating membrane.

Diseases of the conjunctiva are usually seen in young animals.

Cases with a red swollen conjunctiva and exophthalmos usually have **orbital inflammation** (see "The Cat With Abnormal Globe Position or Size", page 1309).

Trauma is common in all ages, and usually shows focal or diffuse hemorrhage in the bulbar conjunctiva.

Cats with **bleeding disorders** may show echymoses of the conjunctiva (see "The Bleeding Cat, page 481).

Uveitis

Uveitis is a common cause of a red eye.

In **anterior uveitis**, the conjunctiva, anterior uvea (iris and ciliary body), and the appearance of the anterior chamber will be altered, which may give the **appearance of a cloudy and red eye**.

The conjunctiva will usually be inflamed. The redness is caused by **hyperemia of the conjunctival blood vessels**.

There may be a **diffuse corneal edema** caused by disruption to the endothelium and leakage of plasma, which occurs secondary to inflammation associated with the uveal tract.

Keratic precipitates (KPs) may be visible through the cornea. They appear as gray to tan, dot-like or sometimes coalescing opacities on the endothelial surface of the cornea, and represent focal accumulations of white blood cells and protein on the lower surface of the endothelium.

The **anterior chamber** will show **flare** which is a diffuse cloudiness caused by protein and white blood cells floating in the aqueous humor, and there may be **hypopyon** (a dense accumulation of protein and blood cells within the anterior chamber).

The **intra-ocular pressure (IOP) is low** (usually below 10 mmHg – normal 12– 25 mmHg). When the ciliary body is inflamed, the production of aqueous is reduced.

In chronic uveitis, the **iris may show new blood vessel growth** on the surface. These are called pre-iridal fibrovascular membranes (PIFMs). This also occurs in cases that have ciliary body neoplasia, and in chronic retinal disease.

The **pupil is usually miotic** (constricted) and **may be distorted** from adhesion onto the anterior lens capsule (posterior synechia).

The **lens may have an altered appearance** with iris pigment and protein on the anterior lens capsule. The lens fibers may be cloudy from cataract formation.

In cases of **posterior uveitis** (inflammation of the choroid), the **vitreous may be cloudy** due to the presence of white blood cells and protein dispersed within the vitreous. This is caused by leakage of protein and cells from the ciliary body and choroidal blood vessels. If the retina is visible there may be changes in its appearance. A serous detachment occurs when protein and blood cells leak from the choroidal vessels and push the retina forward, off the retinal pigment epithelium. This may be seen as a **fold in the retina** or it may be difficult to focus on the retina with an ophthalmoscope. Focal areas of inflammation appear as color changes in the tapetal and non-tapetal retina. There may be decrease or increase in the appearance of the pigment.

Glaucoma

In glaucoma, the conjunctival vessels have mild inflammation. **The redness is caused by the deeper, engorged, episcleral vessels** resulting from interrupted venous drainage. Engorgement is much more subtle than occurs in dogs.

The **intra-ocular pressure** is **increased** above 25 mmHg.

The cornea may show **mild diffuse (blotchy) edema** from disruption to the endothelial physiology.

The globe may be enlarged **(buphthalmos)** due to stretching of the sclera.

The **lens may be subluxated or luxated,** because the zonules rupture when the sclera stretches.

The **retinal blood vessels may be thinned** (attenuated), caused by increased pressure at the cribriform plate when it collapses.

The optic disc may be pushed inwards (**optic disc cupping**). It appears deeper and darker, and the blood vessels curve over the outer rim and plunge deeply into the depressed disc. This happens because the cribriform plate is the weakest point in the sclera.

Blindness is a sequela, as the nerve bundles in the optic nerve become damaged by the disruption to their axoplasmic flow when the disc collapses. There are likely to be other adverse effects on nerves at a cellular level, but they are not well defined at present.

Hyphema

Hyphema is **hemorrhage within the eye**.

When **diffuse** in the anterior chamber, the iris and pupil will not be visible.

There may be **focal areas of blood**, seen as free accumulations of redness in the anterior chamber or overlying the iris.

If the anterior chamber is clear, and the iris is visible but the eye appears red through the pupil space, this will be due to either **hemorrhage in the vitreous or retina**, or a **normal red reflection seen in the color-diluted fundus**.

The appearance of a **red fundus reflection** can be **normal in a color-dilute cat**. This is due to lack of pigment in the retinal pigment epithelium and consequent red reflection from choroidal blood vessels (tigroid fundus). Where there is no tapetum, the whole of the fundus will appear red. Where there is a tapetum, then only the non-tapetum will appear red.

Neoplasia

Lymphosarcoma occasionally occurs as a secondary infiltration of the conjunctiva with neoplastic lymphoid cells. The **conjunctiva** appears **swollen and thickened with a pink appearance**, which may be confused with chemosis and inflammation, because it looks like an inflammatory conjunctivitis. The surface usually appears to be dry, and may be covered with a dry mucoid discharge. It is not a common disease.

WHERE?

The most common areas of the eye that appear as a red eye include:
● The conjunctiva and nictitating membrane in cats with **conjunctivitis**.
● The conjunctiva, cornea, anterior chamber, iris and vitreous where there is **anterior uveitis**.
● The conjunctiva and scleral blood vessels in cats with **glaucoma.**
● The conjunctiva, nictitating membrane, cornea, anterior chamber, iris, lens, vitreous and retina in eyes that have had **trauma.**

One or more of these processes may be involved in a cat with red eye.
● For example, an eye with **uveitis** may have **secondary glaucoma** caused by a disruption to the outflow of aqueous humor, occurring somewhere between the ciliary body, the pupil and the drainage mechanism in the irido-corneal angle.

WHAT?

Most processes involving reddening of the ocular structures are **inflammatory or traumatic**, and involve either **frank hemorrhage, hyperemia or vascular infiltration of tissue**.

Vascular neoplasia and immune-mediated diseases can cause hemorrhage.

Determine which ocular tissue is affected and, initially go to that chapter in the book for more detailed information.

DISEASES CAUSING A RED GLOBE: THE RED BULBAR CONJUNCTIVA

ACUTE INFECTIOUS CONJUNCTIVITIS***

Classical signs

- Usually occurs in young animals.
- Intense inflammation and chemosis with mucopurulent discharge (*Chlamydophila felis* infection).
- Less intense inflammation but very injected vessels and serous discharge (herpesvirus conjunctivitis).
- Mild inflammation and serous to mucoid discharge (*Mycoplasma* infection).

See the main reference on page 1212 for details (The Cat With Ocular Discharge or Changed Conjunctival Appearance) and page 13 (The Cat With Acute Sneezing or Nasal Discharge).

Clinical signs

Young cats with *Chlamydophila felis* conjunctivitis show **intense chemosis and redness of the conjunctiva**, and a mucopurulent discharge usually develops. There may be **signs of respiratory disease,** with sneezing and nasal discharge.

The inflammation in **herpesvirus (FHV-1) infection** is less intense, but the conjunctiva can become quite red. Respiratory signs are more marked. Discharge is usually serous.

A mild inflammation is seen with *Mycoplasma* conjunctivitis, and the discharge is more serous to mucoid in nature.

Diagnosis

For more details on diagnosis of conjunctival infections see page 1213 (The Cat With Ocular Discharge or Changed Conjunctival Appearance).

Chlamydophila felis conjunctivitis.
- Commonly occurs **initially as unilateral** signs, followed days later as bilateral disease.

- **Serous to mucopurulent discharge**, which may be more copious than FHV-1 conjunctivitis.
- **Conjunctival follicles** form in chronic cases.
- **Conjunctival swabs or scrapings** taken with a spatula may be positive on a fluorescent antibody test.
- **Cytology specimens** may demonstrate the presence of intracytoplasmic inclusion bodies, which are present in the first 2 weeks of infection.
- **Culture is very difficult** and requires the use of specific growth media sent to specialized laboratories.

Herpes conjunctivitis.
- The **conjunctiva is less inflamed** in acute FHV-1 infections compared to *Chlamydophila felis* infection.
- **Respiratory signs** are more pronounced with sneezing, serous discharge, anorexia, pyrexia and depression.
- Young cats are more commonly infected with acute signs.
- Severe cases may form a pseudomembrane, and later develop conjunctival adhesions (symblepharon).
- **Laboratory diagnosis** is based on PCR, virus isolation or fluorescent antibody may be supportive.

Mycoplasma felis and *M. gatae.*
- Mycoplasma usually causes a **mild form of conjunctivitis**
- Ocular discharge remains **serous**.
- A **conjunctival pseudomembrane** occasionally forms with a thick white discharge.
- **Cytology** may reveal small basophylic inclusion bodies at the level of the basement membrane.
- The organism can be **readily cultured.**

HEMORRHAGE ASSOCIATED WITH TRAUMA*** OR BLEEDING DISORDERS

Classical signs

- Bright red sclera (diffuse hemorrhage) and a history of blunt trauma.
- Conjunctiva may be swollen and bulging, and the eye may be prominent.
- Ecchymoses (small areas of hemorrhage) or petechia in bleeding states, and no history of trauma.

See the main reference on page 1223 for details (The Cat With Ocular Discharge or Changed Conjunctival Appearance).

Clinical signs

Sub-conjunctival hemorrhage is common after blunt trauma to the eye, especially from motor vehicle accidents.

The most common presentation is a **diffuse reddening of the conjunctiva** over the sclera, with very little swelling. This may be **focal or diffuse** over the entire sclera.

In severe cases, there may be **frank hemorrhage** with swelling of the conjunctiva. This may be present after orbital trauma, and frank orbital hemorrhage may cause severe bulging of the conjunctiva around the globe, and bulging of the eye forward (exophthalmos).

The hemorrhage may be seen as a **diffuse redness between the conjunctiva and sclera**, or as a **frank bleed** under the conjunctiva.

Petechia (multiple small red spots) or ecchymotic hemorrhage (larger patches of red color) may be seen in blood clotting disorders, e.g. rodenticide toxicity and thrombocytopenia.

Diagnosis

The **clinical signs** of diffuse or focal redness with a **history** of trauma are diagnostic. There is frequently no other associated problem.

If in doubt, **fine-needle aspirates** may be beneficial.

It is important to differentiate between hemorrhage caused by trauma and bleeding disorders (See "The Bleeding page 485).

If there is no history of trauma, laboratory tests should be done to check for **clotting or platelet disorders** (page 488).

Orbital radiology may be needed in cats with severe peri-orbital trauma to check for orbital fractures.

Orbital ultrasound (10-MHz probe) is useful to check the posterior sclera, optic nerve and the muscle cone.

UVEITIS***

Classical signs

- Any age of cat.
- Usually seen as a cloudy, red eye.

Classical signs—Cont'd

- The cornea is cloudy.
- The eye is obviously painful with blepharospasm (closed eyelids) and photophobia (squinting).
- Usually is unilateral, and may become bilateral.

See the main reference on page 1294 for details (The Cat With Abnormal Iris Appearance).

Clinical signs

Any age of cat may be affected.

Uveitis is **commonly seen unilaterally,** but may become bilateral.

The **bulbar conjunctiva can appear very red** with uveitis. This is caused by **congestion of the deep episcleral and conjunctival vessels** secondary to inflammation within the eye.

There may be hemorrhage in the anterior chamber **(hyphema),** with bleeding originating from inflammation in the iris and ciliary body.

The eye has a **cloudy appearance** (anterior chamber flare) from the accumulation of protein and white blood cells that leak from the inflamed iris and ciliary body blood vessels (hypopyon).

The inferior surface of the cornea may show **keratic precipitates,** commonly called "mutton fat deposits". They are accumulations of protein and white blood cells that have adhered to the endothelium in focal spots. The **cornea may be edematous**. Corneal changes also cause a cloudy appearance to the eye.

The **pupil is miotic (constricted)** because the iris sphincter muscles are stimulated by a prostaglandin-induced inflammation. Sometimes there is anisocoria (unequal-sized pupils) and dyscoria (abnormal-shaped pupil). There is often **swelling and color change of the iris.**

Cats with uveitis **show pain by keeping the eye closed** (blepharospasm), and it is very sensitive to light (photophobia).

Cats may be **anorexic and lethargic,** as it is usually secondary to systemic disease.

Affected eyes are hypotonic (**low intra-ocular pressure – below 100 mmHg**), because inflammation in the ciliary body reduces aqueous humor production.

Diagnosis

Diagnosis is based on clinical signs. Congested, red conjunctiva with a cloudy anterior chamber, miotic pupil, and very soft eye are almost pathognomonic for uveitis.

All cases should have a thorough clinical examination, and a minimum data base obtained through laboratory tests.

Common causes of uveitis which need to be ruled out based on diagnostic tests are FIV, FeLV, FIP, cryptococcosis, other fungal infections and toxoplasmosis.

Candida albicans is a rare cause of uveitis in cats. Ocular lesions consist of conjunctival hyperemia and chemosis, fibrin and flocculent material in all ocular chambers, and small nodular lesions in the fundus. On histological examination, organisms are evident that are free and phagocytized in the vitreal and retinal exudates.

Any problem causing a bacteremia may cause uveitis.

Many cases of uveitis are idiopathic, and no obvious cause is found.

GLAUCOMA*

Classical signs

- Red eye caused by deep episceral vessel injection.
- Increased IOP above 25 mmHg.
- ± Enlarged globe (buphthalmos).
- Cornea may be cloudy.
- Pupil mid-dilated to dilated and poorly responsive to light.
- ± Signs of chronic uveitis (changes in the appearance of the iris surface).
- ± Uveal neoplasia (change in iris color, size, shape and/or thickness).
- ± Lens instability or dislocation.

See the main reference on page 1312 for details (The Cat With Abnormal Globe Position or Size).

Clinical signs

Glaucoma causes **deep episcleral vessel injection.** Deep vessels are usually straighter and larger, do not move when the overlying bulbar conjunctiva is moved, and do not blanch with the topical application of 1:1000 epinephrine. The signs of glaucoma are more subtle in cats than in dogs.

The intra-ocular pressure (IOP) is high. In most cats with signs of glaucoma the **IOP will be above 30 mmHg** (normal 10–25 mmHg).

An **enlarged globe (buphthalmos)** may or may not be present, depending on the chronicity of the increased IOP.

The **pupil will be dilated or semi-dilated,** with either absent or poor pupillary light reflexes. The increased IOP causes paralysis of the iris sphincter muscle, retinal damage, and often blindness within days.

The **cornea may be slightly cloudy** because of pressure changes in the endothelium. The cloudiness may have a mottled appearance.

Signs of chronic anterior uveitis may be present, especially abnormalities in the appearance of the iris surface including pinkish discoloration associated with fibrovascular membranes, or grayish discoloration of the iris surface with iris melanoma.

Signs of **lens instability** may be present including:
- Aphakic crescent (crescent shape produced by the clear space between the edge of the displaced lens and the adjacent pupillary margin).
- Anterior or posterior luxation (dislocation).
- Iridonesis (wobbling of the iris).

Signs of **intra-ocular neoplasia** are occasionally present, seen as a change in the shape, thickness, color and/or contour of the iris. Diffuse black irises may be seen in older cats with melanosis and iris melanoma.

Diagnosis

Initial diagnosis is based on the appearance of buphthalmos with any or all of the other related signs of glaucoma, chronic anterior uveitis and lens instability.

Measurement of intra-ocular pressure (IOP) with tonometry. Normal range for IOP in the cat is 10–25 mmHg. **Readings over 30 mmHg are supportive of a diagnosis of glaucoma.**

DISEASES CAUSING A RED GLOBE: THE RED ANTERIOR CHAMBER

HYPHEMA ASSOCIATED WITH TRAUMA* OR INFLAMMATION*

Classical signs

- The anterior chamber may be full of blood and bright red in color.
- The eye may appear black, if bleeding is very severe.
- Signs of trauma with scleral and subconjunctival hemorrhage may be present.
- Bleeding disorders may have signs of hemorrhage on mucous membranes and skin.

Pathogenesis

Hyphema (blood in the anterior chamber) occurs because of **trauma to the iris and/or ciliary body.**

The blood may be **diffuse, filling the anterior chamber**, which appears **bright red**, or consist of a **focal** accumulation of red cells. If focal, the eye may also appear cloudy because of leakage of protein and white cells (hypopyon).

Any inflammatory disease of the iris can cause leakage of blood products into the anterior chamber. This can range from fibrin without significant numbers of accompanying red cells, to frank hemorrhage (hyphema).

Hyphema may also occur secondary to **chronic uveitis**, when **pre-iridal fibrovascular membranes (new blood vessels)** develop on the iris surface. These are **fragile and may hemorrhage**.

Hyphema may occasionally occur **secondary to systemic neoplasia**, particularly lymphosarcoma, as the blood vessel endothelial walls are disrupted.

In **bleeding states** such as rodenticide poisoning or thrombocytopenia, the anterior chamber may fill with blood.

Clinical signs

Hyphema may appear as a **focal accumulation of red cells** attached to the iris or free within the aqueous.

Protein and white cells (**hypopyon**) may also be present in the anterior chamber.

Hyphema may appear as a **diffuse reddish discoloration** of the anterior chamber from free red cells. **Fibrin** may be present as a result of hemorrhage, resulting in straw-colored strands or masses in the anterior chamber, or there may be a combination of free red cells and fibrin.

The anterior chamber may **appear black** when there has been a **severe bleed**.

The **adnexa may show signs of trauma**, including scleral and sub-conjunctival hemorrhage.

If bleeding disorders are present, mucous membranes and skin may have small hemorrhages (petchia) or blotchy hemorrhages (echymoses).

Diagnosis

Diagnosis is based on the appearance of the anterior chamber.

Ocular ultrasound is useful as an adjunct where the anterior chamber cannot be visualized. Check that the spatial arrangements within the eye are normal, such as depth of the anterior chamber, position and thickness of the iris, position and density of the lens, density of the vitreous. Also check for signs of retinal detachment and the integrity of the scleral wall.

If there are no signs of trauma, uveitis or neoplasia, assess **platelet number and function, and clotting times**.

Treatment

In severe cases of hemorrhage, some veterinary ophthalmologists inject **tissue plasminogen activator** (TPA 0.1 mg usually diluted in 0.3 ml of diluent) into the anterior chamber, as it breaks down fibrin which helps to disperse the clot. Its use is controversial, and should not be used where there is trauma to the iris root, as this may cause a re-bleed.

Topical 1% prednisolone acetate drops (q 8 h) are used to reduce inflammation and minimize iris adhesions (synechia).

Systemic corticosteroids such as prednisolone (1 mg/kg q 12–24 h), are also used to minimize inflammation and adhesion formation, particularly in cases with uveitis.

In acute cases, **systemic NSAIDs** at recommended doses are used to reduce prostaglandin-induced inflammation. Do not use in combination with corticosteroids.

The use of **drugs to manipulate the pupil** is commonly recommended in the older texts, but this is now **controversial.** Dilating the pupil with atropine reduces the iris surface area, which decreases absorption and may also predispose to glaucoma by compromising the drainage angle. Constricting the pupil with pilocarpine increases the chance of synechia formation, which may lead to iris bombé and secondary glaucoma. Manipulating the iris may also cause further bleeding.

THE RED EYE CAUSED BY CHANGES IN THE IRIS

UVEITIS***

> ### Classical signs
>
> - Red blood cells may be free floating (hyphema) or adhered to the anterior surface of the iris.
> - Other signs of uveitis such as red conjunctiva, ocular pain, miotic pupil.
> - Color change in iris (lighter or darker) and be thickened.

See the main reference on page 1294 for details (The Cat With Abnormal Iris Appearance).

Clinical signs

Uveitis is associated with changes of iris color. Darker irises may become lighter in color during the inflammatory change, but in chronic cases they often become darker with a blotchy appearance. In lighter irises, the color change is more subtle. If **pre-iridal fibrovascular membranes** form, the iris may take on **a congested, pink appearance**. The iris surface may show **areas of red,** with blood cells attached to the anterior surface, or free in the anterior chamber. Compare the abnormal iris to the opposite eye.

Changes in iris contour also occur with uveitis. The iris may appear **thickened and distorted** when it is infiltrated with a lot of inflammatory cells, and the surface may become uneven.

Red congested conjunctiva, miotic pupil, ocular pain, and a soft eye are other signs that will be present in uveitis.

Retinal hemorrhage is seen occasionally in areas of fungal granuloma formation, giving the pupil a red appearance.

FIV, FeLV, FIP, *Blastomyces dermatitidis, Candida albicans, Coccidioides immitis, Cryptococcus neoformans, Histoplasma capsulatum* are all associated with uveitis, and systemic signs associated with the agent are usually present. Often no cause is found and it is classed as idiopathic uveitis.

Diagnosis

Clinical signs of a red conjunctiva with cloudy anterior chamber, miotic pupil and very soft eye are almost pathognomonic for uveitis.

All cases should have a thorough clinical examination, and a minimum data base obtained through laboratory tests.

Common causes of uveitis are **FIV, FeLV, FIP, toxoplasmosis, cryptococcosis and other fungal infections,** and these should to be ruled out using appropriate diagnostic tests.

Any problem causing a bacteremia may cause uveitis.

Many cases of uveitis are idiopathic with no obvious cause.

PRE-IRIDAL FIBROVASCULAR MEMBRANES ("PIFMS")*

> ### Classical signs
>
> - Iris has a pink injected appearance from new vessels growing across the anterior surface.
> - Intra-ocular neoplasm or a detached retina may be evident.
> - Secondary hyphema or glaucoma may occur.

See the main reference on page 1303 for details (The Cat With Abnormal Iris Appearance).

Clinical signs

New blood vessels growing across the **anterior surface of the iris** give the **iris an injected pink discoloration**.

The vessels are fragile, and are often associated with **hyphema**.

Pre-iridal fibrovascular membrane (PIFM) formation is associated with angiogenic factors released by proliferating intra-ocular neoplasms, retinal hypoxia associated with retinal detachment, or chronic ocular inflammation. These abnormalities may be evident on careful examination of the eye.

Secondary glaucoma may occur.

Diagnosis

Diagnosis is based on the characteristic appearance of the fibrovascular membranes on the anterior stromal surface of the iris.

Occasionally an underlying cause may be apparent, such as a **ciliary body epithelial tumor** at the pupil space, or a **total retinal detachment.**

IRIS NEOPLASIA*

Classical signs

- Iris tinged with blood +/– free red cells in the anterior chamber.
- Iris is pale and thickened.
- Pupil may be distorted.

See the main reference on page 1297 for details (The Cat With Abnormal Iris Appearance and The Cat With Abnormal Pupil Size, Shape or Response).

Clinical signs

Ocular neoplasia causing **hemorrhage** is **usually associated with lymphosarcoma**. It is rare for other forms of neoplasia such as melanoma to cause hemorrhage in the eye.

Lymphosarcoma may be associated with **FeLV infection**, although often it occurs in negative cats.

The iris is infiltrated with neoplastic cells, and appears **thickened with a pale fleshy color change**.

The **iris may have red cells on the surface** mixed with protein and white blood cells. Leakage of cells and protein occurs because of disruption of the endothelial cells on the blood vessel walls, and results in **varying degrees of hyphema and hypopyon**. Lymphosarcoma does not usually cause frank hemorrhage.

The **pupil will be distorted (dyscoria)** if the iris is grossly distorted with infiltrated cells.

Glaucoma is often an associated complication.

Regional lymph nodes may be enlarged, or other signs of multicentric lymphosarcoma present.

Diagnosis

A tentative diagnosis is based on the **appearance of the iris,** which is typically thickened, with a fleshy color change, and may have focal hemorrhage on the surface.

Serology for FeLV may support the diagnosis.

White blood cell cytology looking for abnormal plump-shaped lymphocytes with large prominent nucleoli in the peripheral blood is useful in cases with lymphosarcoma.

Biopsy of regional lymph nodes is indicated if there is lymphomegaly. Fine-needle biopsy of the liver or spleen should be performed if there is organomegaly.

An **anterior chamber paracentesis** using cytology to demonstrate neoplastic lymphocytes can be done, but is not usually necessary, as the above tests usually will confirm the diagnosis.

THE RED VITREOUS

HYPERTENSIVE RETINOPATHY***

Classical signs

- Acute onset of vision loss in an old cat, usually bilateral.
- Dilated pupils, non-responsive or poorly responsive to light.
- Cloudy vitreous with red areas of hemorrhage.

See the main reference on page 1171 for details (The Blind Cat or Cat With Retinal Disease).

Clinical signs

Hypertension causes leakage of fluid and red blood cells into the retina, and rupture of retinal blood vessels.

Vitreal hemorrhage caused by **hypertensive retinopathy** appears as **acute-onset vision loss** in an old cat, and is usually bilateral. The cat suddenly starts to bump into things, appears to be lost, and has very cautious movements.

The **pupils are usually dilated**, and non-responsive or poorly responsive to light.

Affected eyes appear **slightly cloudy**, and there may be **focal red areas visible through the pupil**.

It is **difficult to visualize the retina** on fundoscopic examination, as it appears out of focus. This is caused by **retinal detachment** and the retina ballooning into the vitreous.

Hypertensive cats may have **cardiomegaly and left ventricular hypertrophy**. There may be other signs suggestive of hypertension such as a **bounding cardiac apex beat.**

Systolic arterial blood pressure is usually greater than 160 mmHg.

Other signs suggestive of **chronic renal failure or hyperthyroidism** may be present, such as progressive weight loss, polydipsia, polyuria, azotemia, inappetence or polyphasia, or a palpable thyroid nodule.

Diagnosis

Clinicians should suspect this problem in any **old cat that has suddenly gone blind.**

Ophthalmoscopy will demonstrate **vitreal hemorrhage.** The retina will be hard to focus showing hemorrhage adjacent to the major retinal blood vessels.

Blood pressure is most commonly measured in cats using Doppler technology. Arterial blood pressure **greater than 160 mmHg confirms a diagnosis of hypertension**. Most cats with clinical signs of retinopathy have a blood pressure of greater than 200 mmHg.

Blood urea nitrogen (BUN), creatinine and a urine protein:creatinine ratio are useful clinical pathology parameters to **check renal function.**

Thyroid function should be checked using thyroxine (T4) concentrations. (See page 301, The Cat With Weight Loss and a Good appetite, for details of diagnosis).

Cardiac ultrasound may be used to confirm thyrotoxic cardiac hypertrophy.

TRAUMATIC HYPHEMA*

Classical signs

- Uniform red color is seen through the pupil.
- Pupil may be dilated.
- ± Hemorrhage in the anterior chamber.
- Signs of trauma such as sub-conjunctival hemorrhage and adnexal injuries.

Clinical signs

Blunt or penetrating trauma may cause hemorrhage into the vitreous.

Hemorrhage in the vitreous appears as a **uniform red color visible through the pupil**. The eye may have a red glow caused by free red blood cells in the vitreous. Hemorrhage may also be present in the anterior chamber.

The pupil may be dilated.

On ophthalmoscopic examination, **no detail will be visible in the fundus.** The retina will not be able to be visualized because of the intense red color of the vitreous infiltrated with red blood cells.

Other **signs of trauma to the eye,** such as conjunctival and sub-conjunctival injury and hemorrhage, and adnexal injuries may be present, or there is a history of trauma.

Diagnosis

Diagnosis is based on the clinical signs of a red color visible through the pupil, and the reflection of the retina and tapetal is obscured. There is usually a history of trauma.

Ocular ultrasound using a 10-Hz probe is a very useful adjunct to diagnosis. This will show problems associated with the retina such as detachment, and rupture of the sclera, as well as hemorrhage in the orbit.

Radiology may be useful to check the orbital bones for signs of fracture.

THE RED EYE CAUSED BY RED REFLECTION FROM THE RETINA

THE TIGROID FUNDUS***

Classical signs

- A red fundus reflex is seen frequently in color-diluted cats.
- Seen in cats with a blue iris such as Siamese and Color Points.

Clinical signs

The red reflex is often seen by owners using flash photography as a "red eye".

In cats the red reflex is frequently **misdiagnosed as retinal hemorrhage**.

The appearance of a red fundus reflection can be normal in a color-dilute cat. Cats with **color dilution have no pigment in the retinal pigment epithelial cells**. As a result, the blood vessels of the choroid are seen clearly against the white background of the sclera. The blood vessels appear in a tigroid pattern (**called tigroid fundus**), and can give a striking red reflex when seen through the pupil in certain light. Where there is no tapetum, the whole of the fundus will appear red. Where there is a tapetum, then only the non-tapetum will appear red.

Occurs in **cats with a blue iris such as Siamese and Color Points**.

Diagnosis

Diagnosis is based on signs. On ophthalmic examination the eyes are normal, with the typical tigroid vascular pattern. The **breed and blue iris color** are indicators of a tigroid fundus.

HYPERTENSIVE RETINOPATHY***

Classical signs

- Sudden blindness in an old cat.
- Dilated pupils, non-responsive or poorly responsive to light.
- Retinal hemorrhages mainly along the major blood vessels with hemorrhage in the vitreous.
- The retina may be detached and difficult to visualize clearly.

See the main reference on page 1171 for details (The Blind Cat or Cat With Retinal Disease) and also page 1202 (The red vitreous).

Clinical signs

Typically appears as **acute-onset vision loss in an old cat**.

Pupils are dilated, and non-responsive or **poorly responsive to light**. Signs are usually bilateral.

Affected eyes appear slightly cloudy and focal red areas of hemorrhage are visible through the pupils.

Retinal hemorrhages occur mainly along the major blood vessels, with hemorrhage in the vitreous.

When the retina is detached, the **retinal blood vessels are not clearly in focus** with an ophthalmoscope. The retina can be seen ballooning into the vitreous, and appears as a thin veil of pale tissue.

Diagnosis

Diagnosis is based on the clinical presentation of **acute vision loss in an older cat**, the finding of **hemorrhage** adjacent to major vessels in the retina, and **systolic blood pressure > 160 mmHg**.

Blind cats usually have a total retinal detachment in both eyes. The retina cannot be visualized through the pupil with an ophthalmoscope, and a thin veil of pale tissue can be seen bulging into the vitreous.

Hyperthyroidism and chronic renal disease need to be ruled out with diagnostic tests, and thoracic radiographs or cardiac ultrasound may be useful to detect cardio-megaly.

INFLAMMATORY RETINAL DISEASE*

Classical signs

- Main sign is uveitis (red conjunctiva, cloudy aqueous, swollen iris and corneal edema in acute cases).
- Focal red areas may be seen through the pupil.
- Retina may be out of focus, or have small focal brownish-colored areas within the tapetum when looked at with an ophthalmoscope.
- Small hemorrhages may be seen along the major retinal blood vessels.

See the main reference on page 1167 for details (The Blind Cat or Cat With Retinal Disease).

Clinical signs

Any inflammatory disease of the retina may cause **pre-retinal or retinal hemorrhage.**

Hemorrhage is rarely obvious to the naked eye, but is seen on ophthalmoscopic examination in an eye that shows signs of uveitis.

In cases with **systemic fungal infection** (*Blastomyces dermatitidis, Candida albicans, Coccidioides immitis, Cryptococcus neoformans, Histoplasma capsulatum*), the eye or eyes are usually inflamed with signs of uveitis including red conjunctiva, cloudy aqueous from hypopyon, corneal edema, swollen iris, iris hemorrhage from pre-iridal fibrovascular membranes and miotic pupils.

The hemorrhage is usually related to **changes in retinal appearance** such as focal changes in tapetal or non-tapetal color. Usually there is **hyper-reflectivity in the tapetum**, and loss of black coloration in the non-tapetum.

The retina may show signs of **focal granulomas**, which appear as raised areas with a muddy brown color. These areas may have small foci of hemorrhage on the surface.

The major retinal blood vessels may have small hemorrhages close to the arteries.

There may be hemorrhage in the vitreous if there is pre-retinal hemorrhage.

Rarely, retinal hemorrhage is caused by larva (*Cuterebra* or *Metastrongylid*) migrating along blood vessels causing localized damage to the retina and hemorrhage from injuries to the blood vessel they are migrating in or move through.

In cases with **ocular larval migrans**, the characteristic fundoscopy signs are **linear hyper-reflective "tracks"** in the tapetal fundus, and linear light-gray areas of reduced pigmentation in the non-tapetum. Sometimes the white body of a fly larva might be seen associated with one of the tracks. Hemorrhage may be seen in these tracks.

Rarely, the larva might be seen in the anterior chamber with associated signs of anterior uveitis.

Diagnosis

Ocular fungi

Diagnosis is initially based on the presentation of a cat with a **rapidly progressive, usually bilateral chorioretinitis progressing to anterior uveitis**, with **signs of other systemic disease**, occurring in a geographic area where such fungal disease is known to occur.

Imaging techniques can be used to obtain more supportive evidence of a deep fungal infection:
- **Thoracic radiography** to demonstrate pulmonary granulomas.
- **Nasal cavity radiography** to demonstrate a soft tissue density and bone lysis consistent with fungal rhinitis.
- **Ocular ultrasound** to look for signs of retinal detachment when the fundus cannot be clearly visualized through the pupil.

Serological tests can be performed, looking for increased serum antibodies (cryptococcosis, blastomycosis, histoplasmosis, coccidiodomycosis).

Confirmation of the diagnosis is based on the **demonstration of the causative organism** in:
- Nasal swabs or biopsy.
- Cerebrospinal fluid.
- Samples taken by centesis of vitreous or subretinal exudate.
- Histopathology of enucleated globes.
- Bone marrow biopsy samples (histoplasmosis).
- Fine-needle aspirates of lung lesions.

Ocular larval migrans

Diagnosis is based on appearance of the suspicious fundoscopic lesions, or by observation of the parasite in the anterior chamber.

BLUNT OR PENETRATING TRAUMA*

Classical signs

- History of trauma to the head and/or eye.
- A focal or diffuse red coloration seen through the pupil.
- Varying degrees of vision loss will occur depending on the severity of the injury.
- The conjunctiva and adnexal tissue may show hemorrhage.

Clinical signs

When **blunt or penetrating trauma causes retinal hemorrhage**, there is usually a history of trauma to the head or eye, and a red appearance behind the pupil. The conjunctiva and adnexal tissue may show hemorrhage.

There may be **hyphema** causing diffuse redness of the anterior chamber, **vitreal hemorrhage** or **retinal hemorrhage** seen as a red eye through the pupil. The red color through the pupil may be diffuse through the posterior chamber (vitreal hemorrhage) or seen as retinal hemorrhage. When the red color is obvious, it is usually caused by hemorrhage from the retina into the vitreous.

The **degree of hemorrhage varies** from focal areas of blood in the vitreous or on the retina, to frank bleeding throughout the vitreous and retina.

Severe cases may have a dilated pupil.

Vision loss will be determined by the extent of the injury and the degree of hemorrhage within the eye.

Diagnosis

Diagnosis is based on a history of trauma, and **signs** of hemorrhage in the eye.

It is important to try to visualize the fundus, to determine if there is detachment or tears of the retina.

Ocular ultrasound is a very useful tool to determine the state of the retina when it cannot be visualized through the pupil. Retinal detachments are seen as a bulging line away from the sclera. The integrity of the scleral coat can be checked, and also the state of the orbit behind the globe. In some cases the sclera may be ruptured, and if this is the case, this will give a grave prognosis for vision in an affected eye.

In severe ocular trauma, **radiology of the orbit** is indicated to check for fractures.

CT scan and MRI are other tools that may be useful in difficult cases. The shape, size and position of the globe within the orbit can be compared to the other eye. Orbital fractures can be demonstrated.

RECOMMENDED READING

Barnett KC. A Colour Atlas of Veterinary Ophthalmology. Wolfe Publishing Ltd, London, 1990.
Gelatt Kirk N (ed). Veterinary Ophthalmology, 2nd edn. Lea & Febiger, Philadelphia, 1991.
Gelatt Kirk N. Veterinary Ophthalmology, 3rd edn. Lippincott, Williams and Wilkins, Philadelphia, 1998.
Gelatt Kirk N. Essentials of Veterinary Ophthalmology. Lippincott Williams and Wilkins, Philadelphia, 2000.
Gelatt Kirk N. Colour Atlas of Veterinary Ophthalmology. Lippincott Williams and Wilkins, Philadelphia, 2001.
Gelatt Kirk N, Gelatt JP. Handbook of Small Animal Ophthalmic Surgery, Vol. 1 Extraocular Procedures. Permagon Veterinary Handbook Series, Florida, 1994.
Gelatt Kirk N, Gelatt JP. Handbook of Small Animal Ophthalmic Surgery, Vol. 2. Intra-ocular Procedures. Permagon Veterinary Handbook Series, Florida, 1995.
Ketring KL, Glaze MB. Atlas of Feline Ophthalmology. Trenton, NJ, Veterinary Learning Systems, 1994.
Peiffer RL, Petersen-Jones S. Small Animal Ophthalmology, A Problem Oriented Approach, 3rd edn. Saunders, Philadelphia, 2001.

59. The cat with ocular discharge or changed conjunctival appearance

Richard IE Smith

KEY SIGNS

- Serous to mucopurulent ocular discharge.
- Chemosis, hyperema.
- Follicles.
- Diffuse or focal mass.

MECHANISM

Basic pathophysiological mechanisms of ocular discharge can include:
- Reflex lacrimation due to irritation of the corneal surface.
- Effects of infectious micro-organisms on conjunctival tissues.
- Allergic conditions causing increased tearing.
- Effects of inflammatory conditions of the orbit and adnexal tissues on conjunctival tissues.
- Reduced drainage of the tear film.

Ocular discharges can be serous, mucoid or mucopurulent.

WHERE?

A changed conjunctival appearance with ocular discharge may result from diseases of:
- Eyelid.
- Conjunctiva.
- Cornea.
- Orbit.
- Tear duct.

WHAT?

- Infectious causes of conjunctivitis such as *Chlamydophila felis* and feline herpesvirus-1 are the most common cause of increased ocular discharge in cats.

QUICK REFERENCE SUMMARY

Diseases causing ocular discharge or changed conjunctival appearance

WHERE?

CONJUNCTIVA

NEOPLASTIC

● **Squamous cell carcinoma*** (p 1217)**
Occurs in cats with non-pigmented eyelids. The conjunctival neoplasia is seen as an extension of the eyelid lesion, which will appear red and ulcerated.

● Conjunctival hemangiosarcoma/hemangioma (p 1225)
Rare in cats. Seen occasionally as a red raised lesion at the lateral limbal conjunctiva and on the leading edge of the third eyelid conjunctiva.

● Conjunctival lymphosarcoma (p 1224)
A rare condition seen as focal or diffuse swelling of the conjunctiva. Usually occurs as an extension of orbital lymphosarcoma, and secondary to systemic lymphosarcoma.

INFLAMMATION/INFECTIOUS

Viral:

● **Herpes virus conjunctivitis*** (p 1212)**
Acute conjunctivitis with hyperemia, chemosis and initially a serous discharge. Rapid progression to a mucopurulent discharge, which is usually bilateral. In young cats, respiratory signs, including paroxysms of sneezing occur. Severe cases form symblepharon (conjunctival adhesions), which can occlude tear duct puncta producing chronic epiphora. Chronic serous ocular discharge can occur in older cats.

Bacterial:

● *Chlamydophila (Chlamydia)* **keratoconjunctivitis*** (p 1215)**
In acute cases in young cats, there is conjunctival chemosis (edema) and intense hyperemia, with a serous to mucopurulent discharge. Often begins unilaterally and progresses to bilateral.
Respiratory signs such as sneezing tend to be mild or absent. Chronic cases develop follicular conjunctivitis accompanied by a serous discharge.

Protozoal:

● **Mycoplasma conjunctivitis** (p 1218)**
A mild conjunctivitis with serous discharge, unilateral or bilateral. A serous nasal discharge may be present.

INFLAMMATION/NON-INFECTIOUS

● Chemosis and/or hyperemia secondary to orbital disease (p 1211)
The globe will show exophthalmos (bulging forward) and the conjunctiva will be swollen with a mucopurulent discharge. The third eyelid may be prominent and inflamed. The cat may have dental disease or sneezing with nasal discharge.

Immune-mediated:

● **Eosinophilic keratoconjunctivitis* (p 1221)**
Proliferative white/pink plaques appear on the conjunctiva and/or cornea. The conjunctiva is inflamed with a mucopurulent discharge. The cornea may be intensely vascularized.

● **Allergic conjunctivitis* (p 1222)**

A **serous ocular discharge** with **very little inflammation** of the conjunctiva is seen in cats with allergic disorders. May be associated with atopy, food allergy or insect bites.

Trauma:

● **Trauma of conjunctival and peri-adnexial tissue** (p 1220)**

Conjunctival wounds from trauma, plant thorns and cat fights may result in conjunctival tears, chemosis, hyperemia, hemorrhage and mucopurulent discharges.

● **Sub-conjunctival hemorrhage* (p 1223)**

Blunt trauma may result in focal or diffuse subconjunctival hemorrhage, with no associated inflammation or discharge. Retrobulbar trauma may result in exophthalmos with swollen conjunctiva. There may be superficial hemorrhage on the conjunctiva, or subconjunctival hemorrhage.

WHERE?

EYELID

ANOMALY

● Eyelid agenesis (coloboma) (p 1227)

Usually the upper lateral eyelid margin is missing (abnormal) causing exposure of the conjunctiva and trichiasis (normal eyelid hair rubbing on the cornea). This results in chronic conjunctivitis, keratitis and chronic serous or mucoud discharge.

MECHANICAL

● Lower lid entropion (p 1228)

Rare in cats but seen in cases with enophthalmos (globe shrunken into the orbit), which causes the lower lid to turn inwards. The trichiasis that results may cause a chronic mucopurulent discharge and corneal ulceration. Surgical correction can be frustrating.

● Symblepharon occluding the lower nasolacrimal puncta (p 1213)

Seen as a tearing down the medial canthus and nose. Tear staining is present. Check to see if the lower puncta is present and patent. Conjunctiva appears abnormally thickened and distorted. The cornea may appear cloudy and covered by a thin membrane. There is a history of cat flu as a kitten.

NEOPLASTIC

● **Squamous cell carcinoma*** (p 1217)**

Common in white cats and cats with non-pigmented eyelids. The area is red and ulcerated.

● Meibomian gland adenocarcinoma (p 1229)

Rare in cats. The eyelid margin has a **raised rough area often in the form of a papilla**. The conjunctival surface will be swollen and discolored over the area of the meibomian gland in the tarsal plate.

INFLAMMATION/INFECTIOUS:

● **Meibomian gland inflammation** (p 1225)**

The cat presents with a history of irritated eyes, and a mucoid to mucopurulent discharge. Under the eyelid is a row of red inflamed meibomian glands. Inspissated pus and lipid material can accumulate in the glands, and is seen as raised whitish lesions. The condition can cause a lot of discomfort, seen as blepharospasm and rubbing.

continued

continued

Trauma:

● Eyelid trauma** (p 1226)

Trauma may result in lacerations, hemorrhage and a mucoid to mucopurulent discharge as the lesion heals. The wound should be obvious. Healed eyelid wounds may result in cicatricial distortion of the lids, and trichiasis or ectropian.

WHERE?

CORNEA

DEGENERATIVE

● Corneal sequestrum** (p 1231)

There may be a serous or mucopurulent discharge, with a brown or black stained area on the cornea. Ulceration and corneal vascularization may or may not be present.

MECHANICAL

● Ulcerative keratitis** (p 1230)

Causes a serous ocular discharge with blepharospasm and photophobia. Corneal cloudiness is present, and corneal erosion is evident on close examination, or with fluorescein stain.

INFLAMMATORY/INFECTIOUS

● Herpetic keratitis*** (p 1229)

Early cases seen as dendritic lesions (faint linear changes). Chronic cases develop geographic keratitis (irregular-shaped lesions) associated with superficial ulceration and scarring. All have a serous ocular discharge. History of prior cat flu with signs consistent with feline herpes virus-1 infection.

Inflammatory/immune-mediated:

● Eosinophilic keratoconjunctivitis* (p 1221)

A mucopurulent discharge with proliferative inflammatory lesion of the cornea and conjunctiva. Associated with allergic conditions.

Trauma:

● Corneal trauma*** (p 1230)

Serous to mucopurulent discharge is commonly seen in corneal injury. Fibrin tags or clots may be seen attached to the injured area of the cornea. If the cornea has been penetrated, a continuous clear discharge may be present caused by leakage of aqueous humor. The cat will show severe ocular pain, guarding the eye, blepharospasm and photophobia.

WHERE?

ORBIT

INFLAMMATORY

● Retrobulbar infection (p 1231)

Retrobulbar infection may result in exophthalmos, and swollen conjunctiva with injected blood vessels, and a mucopurulent discharge. The third eyelid may be prominent, and there may be pain on opening the mouth. Rare.

INTRODUCTION

MECHANISM?

Ocular discharge is a sign that the **eye is irritated, inflamed** or there is an **obstruction to tear drainage.** Ocular discharges vary in type.

- **A serous (watery) discharge** is present when there is excess tear stimulation. Excessive tearing is known as "epiphora".
- **A mucoid (jelly-like) discharge** is seen when the conjunctiva is inflamed and the conjunctival goblet cells produce excess mucus secretion.
- **A mucopurulent (pus) discharge** is found when the conjunctiva is inflamed, and there is a mixture of mucus secretion and inflammatory cells.

Common causes of ocular discharge include diseases affecting the **conjunctiva, cornea, eyelid, orbit or tear duct.**

- Diseases affecting the **conjunctiva** include:
  - Infectious diseases are the most common causes of ocular discharge.
  - Allergic conditions.
- Problems associated with the **cornea** include:
  - Ulcerative keratitis (inflammation of the cornea).
  - Infectious agents causing keratitis.
  - Traumatic keratitis.
- **Obstruction to tear drainage.**
  - In cats **symblepharon** (adhesion of conjunctiva to conjunctiva or conjunctiva to cornea) is the most common cause of puncta occlusion.
- **Eyelid problems** causing **irritation of the cornea** include:
  - Eyelid **agenesis** (coloboma) is the term used when there is a congenital absence of all or part of the normal eyelid margin. It causes **trichiasis** (normal eyelid or facial hair irritating the conjunctiva or cornea) and exposure and drying of the adjacent conjunctiva and cornea.
  - Eyelid **trauma** may cause trichiasis because the eyelid margin is damaged or missing.
  - Eyelid **neoplasia** may cause irritation of the corneal surface.
- **Orbital inflammation** (retrobulbar disease) may cause **chemosis** (conjunctival edema) and ocular discharge. The eye may show **exophthalmos** (bulging outwards).

  - **Dental disease** is the most common cause of orbital inflammation.
  - **Orbital neoplasia,** particularly lymphosarcoma, is another disease that may cause exophthalmos and chemosis.
  - Orbital disease may also be caused by an extension of **chronic sinus and nasal inflammation or neoplasia,** where the bony orbit has been breached adjacent to the frontal sinus or posterior nasal cavity.

Changed appearance of the conjunctiva is seen clinically as:

- **Ocular discharge,** which may be serous, mucoid or mucopurulent.
- **Chemosis** (edema), which causes the conjunctiva to swell and bulge under the eyelids.
- **Hyperemia** (redness) can be intense as the conjunctiva has a rich blood supply.
- **Follicle formation** occurs because the conjunctiva is very rich in lymphoid tissue. Antigenic stimulation in chronic inflammation or allergic states is the most common cause of follicle formation.
- **Hemorrhage.**
  - **Echymoses** (focal hemorrhage) and **petechia** (pin point hemorrhages) may be a sign of a bleeding disorder associated with a systemic disease causing thrombo-cytopenia.
  - **Coagulopathies** may show signs of conjunctival hemorrhage.
  - Sub-conjunctival hemorrhage is seen in cases of trauma.
- **Peri-ocular pruritis** (skin irritation) may be a sign of underlying conjunctival irritation.45
- **Emphysema** (accumulation of air within tissue) of the conjunctiva may be seen as a rare entity after facial trauma, when air leaks under the skin and conjunctiva to produce swelling that may be confused with chemosis. Crepitus (a crackling feeling of the tissue) will be present to help differentiate this from chemosis.

WHERE?

History and physical examination will help determine the cause of ocular discharge, and changed conjunctival appearance. It is important to determine whether it is an **acute or chronic problem.**

Look at the **conjunctiva** for changed appearance.

Examine the associated tissues as problems may arise from the **eyelids, cornea, orbit or teeth.**

Check the summary table for diseases arising from these tissues.

WHAT?

The appearance of the discharge will help localize the problem.

Serous discharge is usually associated with eyelid agenesis, corneal disease, allergic conditions or blocked tear ducts.

Mucoid and mucopurulent discharge is more common with infections of the conjunctiva, eyelid or orbit.

Infectious diseases are the most common cause of ocular discharge and changed conjunctival appearance.

Diagnosis is based on the history, clinical examination, cytology, biopsy, laboratory tests for infectious diseases and radiology of teeth, sinuses and nasal cavity in cases with orbital disease.

DISEASES CAUSING OCULAR DISCHARGE OR CHANGED CONJUNCTIVAL APPEARANCE: CONJUNCTIVAL CAUSES OF OCULAR DISCHARGE AND CHANGED CONJUNCTIVAL APPEARANCE

HERPES VIRUS CONJUNCTIVITIS***

Classical signs

- Paroxysms of sneezing or salivation.
- Hyperemia and chemosis of the conjunctiva, usually bilateral.
- Serous to mucopurulent ocular and nasal discharge.
- Conjunctival adhesions obstructing puncta of tear duct.

See main reference on pages 7, 1237 for details (The Cat With Acute Sneezing or Nasal Discharge and The Cat With Abnormalities Confined to the Cornea).

Pathogenesis

Herpesvirus is one of the most common causes of acute and chronic ocular discharge in cats.

Infection is caused by **feline herpes virus-1 (FHV-1),** a member of the subfamily Alphaherpesviridae. Serologically distinct varieties have been isolated from non-domestic cats. The virus is also commonly called **feline rhinotracheitis virus (FVR).**

The disease is **more frequent in kittens,** particularly those from **catteries with carrier cats, pet shops and shelters.**

The course of the disease is usually 10–14 days.

Histologically, **complete epithelial necrosis occurs**, accompanied by a polymorphonuclear cell infiltrate.

A chronic carrier state may persist in older cats and recurrence of viral shedding and/or signs is common. This may be because the FHV-1 virus does not stimulate effective local immunity.

Clinical signs

The earliest sign of classical herpesvirus infection is **paroxysms of sneezing or salivation.** This is usually seen in kittens and cats that have not been immunized.

In young cats, **systemic signs of upper respiratory disease** with **anorexia, pyrexia and depression** are common.

Tracheal and bronchial inflammation may result in coughing and dyspnea, and occasionally bacterial pneumonia occurs in kittens.

Acute conjunctivitis manifested by hyperemia and chemosis is seen at the same time as the respiratory signs.

Prolapse of the third eyelid may occur as part of the inflammatory process in the eye.

Serous ocular discharge is seen in the acute phase and this **rapidly progresses to a seromucous and mucopurulent discharge**.

In young cats, **ulceration** may occur in the buccal mucosa and on the tongue.

The ocular changes are usually **bilateral**, but may be unilateral initially or in older cats.

In severe cases, **symblepharon** is a complication (adhesion of conjunctiva to conjunctiva or conjunctiva to cornea), and the **puncta may be occluded** causing chronic epiphora.

In severe infections, the conjunctiva may be covered in a **gray pseudomembrane (diphtheritic)**.

In older cats with a **carrier status**, **mild signs of herpesvirus infection** may be seen after some form of stress. In these cases, the inflammation is less intense and often only a serous discharge is present. These cats may have a history of respiratory infection as a kitten.

Chronic serous ocular discharge can occur in older cats.

Corneal involvement (keratitis) may occur 1–2 weeks after initial signs. Keratitis is visible as **corneal cloudiness** (edema and inflammation), and **punctate or branching ulcers,** which may **coalesce to large ulcers**.

- Corneal perforation and secondary bacterial infection may result in destruction of the eye; this occurs more often in young kittens (ophthalmia neonatorum).
- **Herpesvirus keratitis often occurs in the absence of active upper respiratory infection**.

Diagnosis

Acute ocular and respiratory signs in a young cat suggest an infection with herpesvirus or calicivirus infection. **Herpesvirus** tends to produce **more severe conjunctivitis and mucopurulent ocular discharge** than calicivirus.

Diagnosis is usually based on clinical signs, as it is often not cost effective to establish a definitive diagnosis. Obtaining a definitive diagnosis is useful in chronic cases, or when there is a persistent cattery problem.

Definitive diagnosis is based on a variety of techniques, of which polymerase chain reaction is the most sensitive.

- **Cytology.** Intranuclear inclusions in epithelial cells can be demonstrated with immunoperoxidase stains in some acute primary infections. This is not very reliable or cost effective.
- **Immunofluorescence.** Direct or indirect fluorescent-antibody techniques can be applied to corneal or conjunctival smears or tissue sections, but it has poor sensitivity.
- **Virus isolation** by demonstration of **cytopathic effects in cell culture**. This is the gold standard for

detection of herpesvirus, but is not often used because of logistical difficulties in getting rapid results.

- **Serology** is of limited usefulness. Antibody titers tend to be of low magnitude after primary infection, sometimes reaching only 1:64 at 60 days after infection. High titers are rarely seen after recrudescent infection.
- **Polymerase chain reaction (PCR)** testing: DNA amplification of an amino acid sequence of the thymidine kinase gene is perhaps the most sensitive test available. Theoretically, the test could pick up one strand of viral DNA. The high sensitivity of nested PCR tests may reduce specificity, because non-viral DNA contaminants may be detected.
  - Conjunctival swabs and/or biopsies are used for laboratory diagnosis using PCR or virus isolation. Not all laboratories are equipped to do this work. Check with your laboratory, as you may have to send samples interstate or overseas for results.

Differential diagnosis

Calicivirus.
- Tends to produce milder respiratory signs and less severe conjunctivitis and mucopurulent ocular discharge. Ulceration of the tongue is classical.

Chlamydophila felis **conjunctivitis**.
- Commonly only unilateral, followed days later as bilateral disease.
- Serous to mucopurulent discharge, which may be more copious than FHV-1 conjunctivitis.
- Conjunctival follicles form in chronic cases.
- Conjunctival swabs or scrapings taken with a spatula may be positive to a fluorescent antibody test.
- Cytology specimens may demonstrate the presence of intracytoplasmic inclusion bodies, which are present in the first 2 weeks of infection.
- Culture is very difficult, and requires the use of specific growth media sent to specialized laboratories.

Mycoplasma felis **and** *M. gatae.*
- It usually causes a mild form of conjunctivitis
- Ocular discharge remains serous in nature.
- It has been reported to occasionally form a conjunctival pseudomembrane with a thick white discharge.

- Cytology may reveal small basophylic inclusion bodies at the level of the basement membrane.
- The organism can be readily cultured.

Neoplasia.

- Squamous cell carcinoma, particularly of the lower lid in depigmented eyelids, may present with swollen red eyelids and a mucopurulent discharge.
- Cytology or fine-needle biopsy will confirm this condition.
- Lesions are frequently ulcerated.

Bacterial conjunctivitis.

- Not common as a primary ocular disease, but is seen secondary to viral infection.
- The inflammation is less intense than the acute herpesvirus presentation, but in chronic herpesvirus cases, bacterial infection is frequently misdiagnosed as the cause of conjunctivitis and ocular discharge.
- Bacterial conjunctivitis causes a mucopurulent discharge.

Hemorrhage.

- Hemorrhage may be seen as a diffuse or focal area of redness, but there is usually little hyperemia or no inflammation.
- It is not common to have an ocular discharge with conjunctival hemorrhage.

Treatment

Topical and probably systemic **corticosteroids are contraindicated** in all cases of ocular herpesvirus infections. The effect of topical NSAIDs has produced equivocal results experimentally.

A variety of topical ocular antiviral agents are available. However, not all treatments are commercially available worldwide.

- **Idoxuridine** inhibits DNA synthesis by competing with thymidine for incorporation into viral DNA. It is no longer in production, but has been the most commonly used topical agent for treating FHV-1 infection. **Check with your "compounding pharmacist"**, as topical drops are frequently made to order. **Idoxuridine 0.1% drops most commonly used,** and produce excellent results. Drops need to be used at least three to four times daily.
- **Vidarabine** (adenine arabinoside. Vira-A, Parke-Davis) interferes with DNA polymerase and may be effective in cases that are resistant to idoxuridine. Use q 6–8 h.

- **Trifluorothymidine** (Viroptic, Glaxo Wellcome) has the best in vitro effect of all available topical agents. Use q 6–8 h.
- **Acyclovir** (Zovirax ophthalmic ointment, GlaxoSmithKline) may be the only commercially available drug in some countries. The efficacy against FHV-1 has been reported as poor. Use q 6–8 h.
- **Dilute povidine iodine** (diluted 50% in saline) has been used, but there is only anecdotal evidence of its efficacy in clinical situations, and at this strength can be very irritating to eyes.

Oral antiviral agents include:

- **Acyclovir** (Zovirax) appears very effective, even at doses far below the in vitro ED_{50}. The usual dose is 50 mg/kg q 6–12 h, but watch for toxic signs of bone marrow suppression even at this dose. Often used in conjunction with oral α interferon, and the resulting synergism significantly reduces ED_{50} of acyclovir.
- **Valacyclovir** (Valtrex, GlaxoSmithKline) is an acyclovir prodrug but rapid absorption of this drug in cats appears to make it more readily able to cause toxicity, especially in sick, acutely infected cats.
- **Interferon** α: α interferon is a cytokine produced naturally by leukocytes. It may prevent spread if given in the very early stages of infection in acutely infected cats. There are no specific dosage recommendations but commonly used dosage is 30 IU daily. This dose is made up in 1ml syringes and frozen. Each day, one syringe is thawed and two drops placed topically in the eye, the remainder given orally for absorption across oronasal mucus membranes. The dose is commonly given for 7 days on 7 days off.

Other therapies that are used include:

- **Oral lysine**: Lysine has been used in human medicine to suppress clinical signs of herpes simplex infections. Lysine competes with arginine for incorporation in the viral genome. Arginine is necessary for the replication of the FHV-1 virus, and incorporation of lysine produces a non-infective virus particle. It may be more effective in cats with corneal disease than those with conjunctivitis alone. The recommended dose is 250 mg daily.
- **Topical and/or systemic tetracycline** antibacterials are commonly used because of their specific effect on *Chlamydophila felis* and *Mycoplasma* organisms, which may be present together with herpesvirus infections.
  - **Tetracyclines have a mild anti-inflammatory** effect on ocular tissue. They suppress antibody

production and chemotaxis of neutrophils, and inhibit lipases, collagenases and prostaglandin synthesis. Research also shows that tetracyclines exert other pleiotrophic properties independent of their antimicrobial activity, which include inhibition of metalloproteases, blockade of nitrous oxide synthetase (a potent mediator of inflammatory activity), suppression of tumor progression, bone resorption and angiogenesis.

Improving **ocular hygiene** is beneficial.
- Regular cleaning of infected eyes with polyionic eye wash solutions will make the cat feel more comfortable, and suppress secondary bacterial infection.

Prognosis

The prognosis for a full and uneventful recovery in young cats is **very good**.

In young cats with very severe inflammation, symblepharon formation will create chronic eye problems that may include:
- Poor eyelid and nictitating membrane function caused by **conjunctival adhesions.**
- Disruption to the corneal limbal stem cells, which may result in permanent **scarring and abnormality of the cornea.**
- **Epiphora** results from scarring and occlusion of the puncta.
- **Keratoconjunctivitis sicca** (KCS) may be seen on rare occasions.

In adult cats, a chronic recurrent state may develop, and in these cases the prognosis for permanent recovery is guarded.

Virus replication occurs in the cornea, and although not clinically obvious at the time of infection, this will manifest in older cats as a chronic dendritic (geographic) keratitis, sometimes years after the initial infection. See The Cat With Eye Problems Confined to the Cornea (page 1238).

Transmission

FHV-1 is a ubiquitous viral organism found all over the world and is highly infectious.

Infection of kittens may occur through direct contact with a carrier queen. Virus is shed 4–6 weeks after queening.

Infection is via contamination of mucous membranes (ocular, oral or inhalation of virus).

Prevention

Vaccination with live modified or killed vaccines (see page 10, The Cat With Acute Sneezing or Nasal Discharge).

Elimination of carrier cats from catteries. Remove queens that repeatedly have infected litters, or wean kittens early.

CHLAMYDOPHILA (CHLAMYDIAL) KERATOCONJUNCTIVITIS***

Classical signs

- In kittens, intense hyperemia and chemosis, usually unilateral, followed by bilateral conjunctivitis.
- Serous ocular discharge changing to a copious mucopurulent discharge after a few days.
- Mild respiratory signs with sneezing and a seromucoid nasal discharge.
- Diffuse conjunctival follicle formation with serous discharge in older cats with chronic infection.

See main reference on page 13 for details (The Cat With Acute Sneezing or Nasal Discharge).

Pathogenesis

Chlamydophila felis psittaci is responsible for disease in about **20% of cats with respiratory tract signs**. Sneezing with a seromucoid nasal discharge may be seen.

Chlamydophila felis psittaci infections in cats **primarily affect the conjunctiva**. The organism can be found experimentally in other tissues of the urogenital and gastrointestinal tract.

The **course of the disease is 7–21 days.**

Conjunctival epithelial cells are infected, and have intracytoplasmic inclusion bodies typical of this organism.

Histologically, neutrophils predominate early, followed by infiltration with macrophages, lymphocytes and plasma cells.

Recently a new chlamydial agent, *Neochlamydia hartmannellae*, an amebic endosymbiont, has been identified in cats. In a study of 226 samples from cats with keratitis or conjunctivitis and 30 healthy cats, 12% were found to have *Chlamydophila felis* (*Chlamydia psittaci*) and 39% *N. hartmannellae*. Both organisms were found to be significantly associated with disease.

Clinical signs

Initially, there is unilateral conjunctivitis, with the signs spreading to involve the other eye several days later.

Acute infections have **intense conjunctival hyperemia,** with **chemosis** and a serous ocular discharge. This progresses to a copious purulent discharge over a few days.

Chemosis can be so severe that the cornea and intraocular structures are difficult to examine. Signs tend to be more severe in kittens than adult cats.

Conjunctival lymphoid follicles are often seen in chronic cases of the disease, and older cats. The surface of the conjunctiva may have a few, or be covered with lymphoid follicles, and this is accompanied by a serous discharge.

Respiratory signs such as sneezing are absent, or very minor compared to ocular signs.

Chlamydial keratoconjunctivitis occurs in cats of all ages.

Diagnosis

Typically, there is a history of **acute conjunctivitis**, which may be accompanied by sneezing and a mild nasal discharge. The conjunctivitis can be quite dramatic, with an intensely red swollen conjunctiva in acute cases. Chronic cases may have an obvious follicular conjunctivitis.

Conjunctival cytology may show presence of **intracytoplasmic inclusion bodies**. These are seen as **pale pink granular clusters** that may indent the nucleus.

There are **ELISA and latex agglutination tests** available to support a diagnosis. Discharges should be cleaned from the eye, and then a **dry swab or scraping** used to obtain conjunctival cells for the tests. False-

positive results occur in the presence of secondary bacterial infections.

Fluorescent antibody tests can also be done on conjunctival scrapings.

Culture is very difficult and requires specific growth media (usually embryonated eggs), and specialized laboratories.

Differential diagnosis

Herpes conjunctivitis.
- The conjunctiva is less inflamed in acute FHV-1 infections.
- Chronic cases have a serous ocular discharge with hardly any sign of conjunctivitis.
- In the acute form, respiratory signs are more pronounced, with sneezing, serous discharge progressing to mucopurulence, anorexia, pyrexia and depression.
- Young cats are more commonly infected with acute signs.
- Laboratory diagnosis based on PCR, virus isolation or fluorescent antibody may be supportive.

Mycoplasma conjunctivitis.
- A mild disease with serous discharge.
- Mild respiratory signs, unless co-infected with FHV-1.
- A pseudomembrane may develop composed of a thick white exudate.
- It responds rapidly to a wide range of antibiotics.
- Cytology may reveal small basophylic inclusion bodies, which are coccoid or coccobacillary, and are seen in the periphery of the cytoplasm of the epithelial cells.
- Culture of organism can be done in most laboratories.

Neoplasia: squamous cell carcinoma.
- Typically involves lower lid in depigmented eyelids.
- Cytology and fine-needle biopsy should confirm this diagnosis.
- Lesions are usually red, raised and ulcerated.

Primary bacterial conjunctivitis.
- This is not common in cats.
- There will be less inflammation and discharge compared to *Chlamydophila felis* and FHV-1 conjunctivitis.
- The discharge is more likely to be mucopurulent.

Hemorrhage.

- There may be diffuse or focal areas of redness, usually with little hyperemia or inflammation.
- There will be very little discharge associated with the hemorrhage.

Treatment

Topical **tetracycline** ointment applied four times daily. (may no longer be available)

Topical fluoroquinolone (particularly oflaxacin) seems to have very good results in this author's experience using tid/qid.

Oral tetracycline, for example, doxycycline 5 mg/kg PO q 12 h for 3–4 weeks.

Oral **Azithromycin (Zithromax, Pfizer)** 5 mg/kg q 24 h PO for 14 days as an alternative treatment to tetracycline.

Some chronic cases may require long-term systemic therapy.

Prognosis

Generally prognosis is very favorable with few damaging sequelae.

Recurrent infections and latent carrier state are believed to occur.

Transmission

Transmission is thought to occur by **direct contact** of susceptible cats with ocular and nasal secretions from affected cats. A chronic latent carrier state probably occurs.

Prevention

Vaccination has produced conflicting results and is not widely used.

SQUAMOUS CELL CARCINOMA OF THE EYELID AND CONJUNCTIVA***

Classical signs

- Red, slightly swollen eyelid margin with inflamed adjacent conjunctiva (early lesion).

Classical signs—Cont'd

- Red and ulcered lesion with dry crusty surface (later).
- Deep erosions may develop at medial canthus.
- Eyelid and conjunctiva eroded away (advanced lesion).

See the main reference on pages 1321, 1334, 1069, 1089 for details (The Cat With Abnormal Eyelid Appearance or The Cat With an Abnormal Third Eyelid, The Cat With Skin Lumps and Bumps and The Cat With Non-healing Wounds).

Clinical signs

Squamous cell carcinoma usually **secondarily involves the conjunctiva** from a primary eyelid lesion.

Redness and mild swelling of the eyelid is seen in the **pre-cancerous stage**. The affected area may be small initially, but later spreads to include the entire eyelid margin. It is more common on the medial part of the lower eyelid. The **adjacent conjunctiva is inflamed**.

In advanced cases, **the epithelial surface erodes to form an ulcer that may have a dry crusty surface**. **The adjacent conjunctiva may become ulcerated and red**, and can have a crusty mucopurulent discharge.

The entire lid margin including conjunctiva, can be eroded away in advanced cases.

Deep erosions may develop in the medial canthus. When lesions occur at the medial canthus, the normal canthal contour is missing. In advanced cases, it is common for **secondary bone involvement of orbital and nasal bones**.

Usually seen in cats with **non-pigmented eyelids, and is usually on the lower lid**, as this is more exposed to sunlight and ultraviolet light damage.

Diagnosis

The **lesion is fairly typical**, and consists of an ulcerated area, usually involving the lower eyelid and conjunctiva, on a poorly pigmented eyelid.

Cytology is very useful, as samples can easily be taken with a little local anesthetic. The surface of the lesion should be cleaned with saline, or an irrigating eye wash. A small scalpel blade or spatula is then used to scrape the surface of the lesion. Carefully wipe the tissue on the blade over a glass microscope slide, and stain with a cellular stain. **Neoplastic epithelial cells are large and often clumped**, with **large dark staining nuclei** and prominent nucleoli with **very small cytoplasm**. Normal epithelial cells have a large amount of pink cytoplasm, and a central small round nucleus.

Fine-needle biopsy will demonstrate similar pathology to cytology specimens. Use a 22-gauge hypodermic needle and a 5-ml syringe. Push the needle into the lesion, and suck hard on the syringe. Let the plunger go, and remove the needle from the lesion. Remove the needle from the syringe, and pull the plunger back so that the syringe is full of air. Replace the needle on the syringe, and blow the needle contents onto a microscope slide. Spread this carefully with another slide, and stain with a cellular stain. A similar pattern of cells will be seen as in the cytology sample.

Histopathology is more definitive but requires more invasive surgical techniques to remove a block of affected tissue. Place tissue in 10% buffered formalin, and send to a laboratory for sectioning and examination.

Radiology of adjacent bones is important in cases involving the medial canthal tissue and skin over the nose. Any secondary involvement of bony tissue gives a very poor prognosis.

Differential diagnosis

Granulating wounds can have a similar appearance. Use cytology and fine-needle biopsy to differentiate if needed. Granulating wounds appear healthy, with uniform redness and a smooth, moist cellular surface.

Treatment

The lesion may be excised if it is in a small focal area. If the lesion is in the medial canthus, care should be taken to try to preserve the lower puncta and nasolacrimal duct.

Radiation therapy, either with direct beta-radiation, or radioactive gold implants.

Cryosurgery is the **most common** method of treatment. There are many types of cryogens that are used.

Two or three freeze–thaw cycles using liquid nitrogen will produce the best results. The eyelid and conjunctiva has a very rich blood supply, and heals rapidly after cryo-destruction of tissue. Supportive therapy using broad-spectrum ointments or drops, and regular, gentle cleaning helps the healing process, by preventing secondary bacterial infection. (See page 1070, The Cat With Lumps and Bumps.)

Intralesional chemotherapy using cisplatin in oil adjuvant, or in plastic rods, has been used with some success. Refer such cases to a trained oncologist. (See page 1346).

MYCOPLASMA CONJUNCTIVITIS**

Classical signs

- Usually mild conjunctivitis, unilateral or bilateral.
- Serous ocular discharge becoming mucopurulent.
- Mild respiratory signs such as mild serous nasal discharge.
- Occasionally, thick white discharge across conjuntiva (pseudomembrane).

See the main reference on page 14 for details (The Cat With Acute Sneezing or Nasal Discharge).

Pathogenesis

Mycoplasma felis and *Mycoplasma gatae* are thought to cause conjunctivitis in cats.

They may only be pathogenic when **potentiated by other organisms**, for example *Chlamydophila felis,* and viruses such as herpes or calicivirus.

Infection causes a polymorphonuclear leukocyte response in the conjunctiva.

Cytology may reveal **small basophylic inclusion bodies**, which are coccoid or coccobacillary, and are seen in the periphery of the cytoplasm of the epithelial cells.

Mycoplasma organisms can be cultured in the laboratory.

Clinical signs

Usually, there is a **unilateral or bilateral conjunctivitis**, with a **serous discharge becoming mucopurulent**.

The conjunctiva may appear normal, or there may be a mild hyperemia and chemosis.

In more chronic cases, the **conjunctiva may be thickened with the formation of follicles**, which develop from focal areas of lymphoid cell stimulation.

Rarely, a **pseudomembrane** is formed, which consists of a thick white exudate covering the conjunctiva.

Respiratory signs consist of sneezing with a serous nasal discharge.

Diagnosis

Initial diagnosis is usually based on typical clinical signs of mild sneezing, with serous nasal, and mild serous ocular discharge. Chronic cases develop conjunctival follicles and on rare occasions a thick tenacious white pseudomembrane forms.

Cytology may reveal **small basophilic inclusion bodies,** which are coccoid or coccobacillary, and are seen in the periphery of the cytoplasm of the epithelial cells. There is a predominantly polymorphonuclear cell response.

Isolation of the organism can be done in most laboratories from clean conjunctival swabs. It is important to remove the discharges from the eye with sterile normal saline solution or eye washes, prior to taking the sample, as this reduces the contamination from secondary bacterial infections.

Differential diagnosis

Allergic conjunctivitis will have a similar appearance to mild cases of mycoplasma infection. There is usually a poor response to antibiotic treatments. Most cases have an allergy to insect bites, food, or the cats are atopic. The best approach for control of the ocular signs is by referral to a dermatologist or medical internist, so that the cause of the allergy can be established and the correct management instigated.

Herpetic keratitis usually presents with acute respiratory signs, including sneezing, nasal discharge, pyrexia, depression and anorexia. The conjunctiva shows chemosis and hyperemia, and the ocular discharge is more pronounced. Viral isolation and PCR tests may be helpful to differentiate herpesvirus from mycoplasma infection, and there is usually an equivocal response to antibiotic treatment.

Chlamydial conjunctivitis shows mild respiratory signs of sneezing and nasal discharge. In acute cases, the conjunctiva may show severe chemosis and hyperemia, with a serous discharge rapidly changing to a mucopurulent discharge. Chronic cases show follicle formation in the conjunctiva. Cytology, fluorescent antibody, and ELISA tests can be used to differentiate chlamydial infections from mycoplasma.

Eosinophylic keratoconjunctivitis presents with a mucopurulent discharge, and there is a proliferative inflammatory response of the conjunctiva and cornea. The presence of eosinophils in a cytological preparation of the conjunctiva and cornea is supportive for this diagnosis. The condition responds to topical and systemic corticosteroids.

Treatment

Mycoplasma conjunctivitis **responds rapidly to a wide range of antibiotics particularly tetracycline and chloramphenicol**. Tetracycline is more commonly used because this organism is frequently seen in association with *Chlamydophila felis* infection.

Respiratory and ocular signs will be suppressed by topical and systemic corticosteroids, but are not indicated for treatment.

Prognosis

The prognosis is good as complications are rare. Cases that are complicated by concomitant infection with *Chlamydophila felis* or viruses may have a complicated prognosis.

Transmission

Direct contact with affected animals. Infection is more prevalent in catteries and pet shops.

Airborne transmission occurs in confined spaces such as catteries and pet shops.

Prevention

There is no effective vaccine.

Good hygiene and separation of animals at risk from infected animals will reduce the incidence of infection.

TRAUMA OF CONJUNCTIVITIS AND PERIADNEXIAL TISSUE**

Classical signs

- Small to large conjunctival tears.
- Seromucoid or mucopurulent discharge.
- Chemosis with hemorrhage in acute cases.
- Blepharospasm, photophobia and ocular guarding reflecting ocular pain.

Clinical signs

Conjunctival wounds may present as **small to large tears**. Common causes are **cat claw wounds, plant injuries** from **thorns**, or associated with other blunt ocular trauma, commonly from **motor vehicle accidents**.

In acute cases, there is chemosis (edema) of affected conjunctiva with hemorrhage.

Ocular discharge may be serous when there are small scratches, to mucoid or purulent when large infected wounds are present in the conjunctive or peri-adnexial tissue.

There may be hemorrhage and evidence of trauma in surrounding tissue.

Ocular pain is frequently present, manifested by **blepharospasm**, photophobia and ocular guarding.

Diagnosis

If the eye is very painful, **apply a little topical anesthesia**. Proxymetacaine products are less irritating to the tissues). The cat may then open the eye making it easier to visualize the conjunctival surfaces and cornea.

Close examination should reveal any conjunctival wounds, but may be difficult in cases with chemosis.

Check for foreign bodies such as grass seeds, which may be lodged under the third eyelid, or in the upper or lower conjunctival fornix.

Differential diagnosis

Chronic cases may show healing by granulation, and have a mucopurulent discharge similar in appearance to **eosinophilic keratoconjunctivitis.** Differentiate using a **conjunctival smear**, which should have eosinophils present in eosinophilic conjunctivitis, and in a healing wound, will show predominantly neutrophils. Eosinophilic conjunctivitis usually has a history of a chronic condition that has not responded to antibiotic treatment.

Cats with **orbital cellulitis** will often have an inflamed conjunctiva, chemosis and a mucopurulent discharge. This condition may occur secondary to a conjunctival wound deep in the fornix, which has become infected with bacteria. Ocular ultrasound may be very helpful to diagnose orbital disease, where conjunctival injuries have been complicated with secondary orbital infections.

Malar abscesses caused by periodontal disease may cause chronic discharging sinuses in the lower conjunctival fornix. Check the mouth when chronic mucopurulent discharges are seen, and there is no history of ocular trauma. Dental radiology will be helpful to diagnose this condition.

Treatment

It may be necessary to use a local anesthetic and heavy sedation to **clean the eye.** Use normal saline (0.9%) or ocular irrigating solutions to gently remove discharges. Discharges are very uncomfortable for the cat, and harbor unwanted bacteria.

If the wound in the conjunctiva is very large, **suture it with fine absorbable sutures**, preferably buried underneath the conjunctiva. Sutures should be made from polygacton or polyglycolic acid using 6/0 to 8/0 sizes.

If the wound is infected, treat with **broad-spectrum topical antibiotic** drops or ointment. Common antibacterials include triple sulfonamides, neomycin/bacitracin, fucidic acid, chloramphenicol, gentamycin and framycetin. It may be prudent to take a clean swab for bacterial isolation and sensitivity, prior to starting antibiotic therapy.

Systemic drugs may be used in conjunction with topical medications, because the conjunctiva has a very rich blood supply.

EOSINOPHILIC KERATOCONJUNCTIVITIS*

Classical signs

- Proliferative white to pink inflammatory tissue on cornea with adjacent conjunctiva sometimes involved.
- The cornea may be intensely vascularized.
- Mucopurulent discharge is usually present.
- Eosinophils in cytology of affected cornea and/or conjunctiva are diagnostic.

See the main reference on page 1245 for details (The Cat With Abnormalities Confined to the Cornea).

Pathogenesis

The disease is thought to be **immune-mediated** or an allergic response.

Histologically, there is a **granulomatous response**, with a mixed population of leukocytes including lymphocytes, plasma cells, eosinophils and occasional mast cells and histiocytes. The presence of eosinophils is regarded as diagnostic.

Peripheral eosinophilia is present in about 15% of cases.

Insect bites and food allergies have been documented as causes of this condition. It has also been suggested that this response may be an ocular form of the feline eosinophilic granuloma complex, particularly the linear granuloma response. (See The Cat With a Cloudy Eye, page 1262).

Clinical signs

Signs **begin unilaterally**, but may become bilateral.

Eosinophilic keratoconjunctivitis is a **proliferative** (not ulcerative) **lesion producing plaque-like white to pink tissue**, that may be covered by a thick white discharge.

The cornea is involved primarily, and the adjacent conjunctiva is sometimes involved secondary to corneal involvement.

The **cornea may be ulcerated,** and have intense neovascularization in chronic cases.

The third eyelid may also show proliferative lesions.

Mucopurulent discharge is usually present.

Frequently, there is a history of poor response to antibiotic treatment.

Diagnosis

Initial diagnosis is based on a history of poor response to antibiotic treatment, together with signs of a **proliferative keratitis** and/or conjunctivitis, and a mucopurulent discharge.

Cytology or histopathology that demonstrates eosinophils is regarded as diagnostic.

Affected animals may have signs of skin disease or a history of digestive problems.

In tropical climates, check the ears for signs of insect bites (mosquitoes and midges).

Differential diagnosis

Chronic chlamydial conjunctivitis may look similar when there is inflamed conjunctiva and follicle formation. Differentiate with histology or cytology, and look for the presence of eosinophils typically seen in eosinophilic keratoconjunctivitis.

Treatment

The condition will rapidly respond to **systemic corticosteroids** dosed at 1 mg/kg daily. Once the inflammatory response is controlled, then alternate day therapy at 0.5 mg/kg can be used until all signs have disappeared.

Topical corticosteroids alone, using 1% **prednisolone acetate drops or dexamethasone** 0.1% drops q 8 h will control some cases, or be useful as a maintenance treatment for long-term control.

If the tips of the ears show alopecia, pruritis and crusting, the condition may be caused by biting insects. Such cases have been documented in Queensland, Australia. In such cases, the cats must be housed in conditions that are insect free for long-term resolution.

Allergic states caused by diet have been implicated. Dietary exclusion tests may be useful to eliminate this as a cause. (See The Cat With Miliary Dermatitis, page 1029).

ALLERGIC CONJUNCTIVITIS*

Classical signs

- Mild serous discharge that may be intermittent and seasonal.
- Very little pathology is evident in the conjunctiva.
- Cats may sneeze.

See the main reference on page 17 for details (The Cat With Acute Sneezing or Nasal Discharge).

Pathogenesis

Allergic conjunctivitis is an uncommon problem in cats, and may be associated with an **insect bite allergy** (fleas and biting insects such as mosquitoes and midges), **food allergy** or **atopy** (usually caused by pollens).

Clinical signs

Signs may be intermittent and seasonal, depending on the allergen.

There is a **mild serous discharge**, and the cat may show signs of irritation by rubbing its eyes.

There is usually very little conjunctival inflammation associated with this condition.

The may be concurrent sneezing, dermatitis and/or gastrointestinal signs.

Diagnosis

There are **no specific diagnostic tests** for allergic conjunctivitis. It is usually diagnosed by eliminating other causes of conjunctivitis, and on the presence of a mild serous discharge with very little inflammation in the conjunctiva.

Allergy testing done by a dermatologist may help identify the allergen in cases with atopy. (See The Cat With Miliary Dermatitis, page 1031.)

An **elimination diet** that changes the source of protein may identify a food allergy. Protein sources such as venison, duck, turkey, rabbit, kangaroo mixed with carbohydrate (rice, potato or pasta) are frequently used for periods of up to 1 month for diagnosis of food allergy, but a balanced commercial hypoallergenic diet is best for maintenance. WARNING: **Vegetarian diets will rapidly cause blindness** by depleting taurine, and should never be used in cats. They cause retinal degeneration and blindness as well cardiac problems (see The Cat With Signs Of Large Bowel Disease, page 766).

Differential diagnosis

Mycoplasma conjunctivitis can produce mild inflammation with serous discharge. However, it usually responds very well to a wide variety of antibiotics, compared with a poor response in allergic conjunctivitis.

Chronic feline herpes virus-1 conjunctivitis may produce chronic serous discharge with very little conjunctival inflammation similar to allergic conjunctivitis. Use laboratory tests to differentiate, particularly PCR or virus isolation.

Treatment

Topical corticosteroid drops used twice daily will usually control most cases with allergic conjunctivitis. The range of drops used can vary according to the severity of the signs. Very mild cases will respond to 0.1% **hydrocortisone drops**, while more acute cases will respond better to drops containing 0.5–1% **prednisolone** acetate.

If a food allergy is diagnosed based on response to an elimination diet, and reoccurrence of signs when challenged with the original diet, the cat should be transitioned from the homemade elimination diet to a **complete commercial hypoallergenic diet for maintenance.** Most homemade single protein and carbohydrate source diets are not balanced, and are suitable only for a limited diagnostic trial, and not for maintenance. Vegetarian diets will rapidly cause blindness by depleting taurine and should never be used in cats.

Where there is a confirmed allergy caused by atopy, food allergy or insect bites, exposure to allergens needs to be controlled as much as practicable. **Prevent insect**

bites by housing affected cats in insect-free conditions, for example, by confining inside.

Densensitisation for some forms of atopy may be possible when the cat has a positive skin test (see The Cat With Miliary Dermatitis, page 1031).

Prognosis

Prognosis is excellent if there is a confirmed allergy caused by atopy, food allergy or insect bites, and exposure to allergens can be controlled.

Typically this is a chronic condition that requires intermittent treatment with **topical corticosteroids** when epiphora is present.

SUB-CONJUNCTIVAL HEMORRHAGE*

Classical signs

- Mild cases of trauma show focal red areas of bleeding under the conjunctiva.
- Severe cases of trauma show diffuse reddening of the conjunctiva which may be quite swollen.
- Petechial to echymoses hemorrhages may be seen in bleeding states.

Clinical signs

Sub-conjunctival hemorrhage is common after blunt trauma to the eye, especially from motor vehicle accidents.

The most common presentation is **diffuse reddening of the conjunctiva** over the sclera, with very little swelling. This may be focal, or diffuse over the entire sclera.

In severe cases, there may be frank hemorrhage with swelling of the conjunctiva. This may be present after orbital trauma results in frank orbital hemorrhage, causing severe bulging of the conjunctiva around the globe.

Retrobulbar trauma may result in exophthalmos with swollen conjunctiva. There may be superficial hemorrhage on the conjunctiva, or subconjunctival hemorrhage.

Ecchymotic hemorrhage may be seen with blood clotting disorders, e.g. rodenticide toxicity. **Petechia and ecchymotic hemorrhages (larger areas of hemorrhage)** may be seen with thrombocytopenia. In these cases there is no history of trauma.

Diagnosis

The **clinical signs** of diffuse or focal redness with a **history** of trauma are diagnostic. There is frequently no other associated problem.

If in doubt, fine-needle aspirates of the abnormal area may be beneficial.

If there is no history of trauma, laboratory tests should be done to check for clotting or platelet disorders. (See The Bleeding Cat, page 488).

Orbital radiology, CT scan and ocular ultrasound may be needed in cases with severe peri-orbital trauma. Look for interruption of the normal scleral contour for signs of a ruptured globe using ultrasound. Check for the state of the bony orbit with radiology and CT scan.

Differential diagnosis

It is important to differentiate between hemorrhage caused by trauma and bleeding disorders (see The Bleeding Cat, page 485).

Treatment

In cases of trauma, treatment is palliative. Irrigation, hot and cold compresses, and corneal lubrication are important if swelling is present.

If swelling prevents a normal blink, and the cornea is exposed, the eyelids should be closed with a temporary **tarsorrhaphy or third eyelid flap,** otherwise corneal ulceration will rapidly develop. A temporary tarsorrhaphy is done using 4/0 or 5/0 monofilament nylon in a mattress pattern through the midpoint of the eyelid margins.

Treat bleeding disorders with appropriate drugs, and blood transfusions if needed (see The Bleeding Cat, pages 502, 511, 513, 514).

CONJUNCTIVAL LYMPHOSARCOMA

Classical signs

- Swollen, thickened conjunctiva covered with dry crusty discharge.
- Very little redness (hyperemia).
- Globe may be prominent caused by involvement of orbital tissue.
- Third eyelid may be swollen and prominent.

See the main reference on pages 1078, 1311 (The Cat With Lumps and Bumps and The Cat With Abnormal Globe Position or Size).

Pathogenesis

The conjunctiva has a rich supply of lymphoid tissue, but it usually becomes affected **secondary to orbital or systemic lymphosarcoma.**

The condition may **appear acutely**, and frequently the cat will show no other systemic signs such as swollen lymph nodes or enlarged spleen.

Focal and diffuse lesions have been reported. Infiltration of the conjunctiva with neoplastic cells causes **swelling**.

There may be a mild mucopurulent discharge. The discharge crusts on the conjunctival surface as it becomes dry and inflamed, which results from lack of tear lubrication caused by the swelling and poor ability to blink.

Clinical signs

This is a rare condition in cats.

Focal or diffuse swelling of the conjunctiva is seen. The **swelling has the same appearance as chemosis**, however, the conjunctiva is not edematous, but infiltrated by neoplastic lymphoid cells. There is **very little redness (hyperemia)** present.

The **swollen conjunctiva may be dry**, and have a **crusty mucopurulent discharge** on the surface, because the eyelids cannot close, and the tear film cannot cover the surface.

The third eyelid may be involved. **Swelling and partial prolapse** may result in abnormal prominence of the third eyelid.

There may be involvement of the orbital tissues. This will cause swelling of the conjunctiva and a prominent globe (exophthalmos).

Diagnosis

Cytology from a **fine-needle biopsy** should reveal large numbers of **plump lymphoid cells** with a large dark staining nucleus, and prominent nucleoli.

Fine-needle aspirates from enlarged lymph nodes will help to support a diagnosis. (See page 1075.)

Histopathology will show a similar infiltration of neoplastic cells in the conjunctiva.

Serology for FeLV is positive in many cases. (See page 1142.)

Hematology may be useful to support a diagnosis. Occasionally neoplastic lymphoid cells are prominent in the blood smear, especially if there are greatly increased numbers of lymphocytes.

Ocular ultrasound using a 10-MHz probe will help identify focal lesions in the orbit. Ultrasound-guided biopsies can be done by guiding a Tru-cut biopsy probe into the affected area.

Treatment

Eye lubricants and artificial tears are required to lubricate swollen and dry conjunctiva, and help to prevent secondary complications such a corneal ulceration.

Topical corticosteroid drops may be indicated as an adjunct to systemic therapy. Prednisolone acetate 1% or dexamethasone 0.1% drops instilled into the eye three to four times a day will help reduce swelling associated with neoplastic infiltration.

Chemotherapy may be effective in achieving remission in some cats. (See The Cat With Signs of Chronic Small Bowel Diarrhea, page 742.)

CONJUNCTIVAL HEMANGIOMA/HEMANGIOSARCOMA

Classical signs

- Focal raised red lesion in the lateral conjunctiva or on the outer surface of the third eyelid.
- Often described by the owner as a small blood blister on the eye.
- Red cornea adjacent to lateral conjunctival lesions in advanced cases.

See the main reference on page 1075 for details (The Cat With Skin Lumps and Bumps).

Pathogenesis

Lesions in this area are usually primary, and probably caused by UV radiation. However, it is prudent to check for systemic signs of hemangiosarcoma.

This is a rare condition in cats.

Clinical signs

Conjunctival hemangioma or hemangiosarcoma appears as a **small raised red area**, most commonly in the conjunctiva at the **lateral limbus**.

The **cornea** may become **infiltrated** with bright red tissue in chronic cases. An intense red infiltration will appear extending from the lateral limbus adjacent to the conjunctival lesion.

Hemangioma or hemangiosarcoma may also occur on the conjunctival surface at the **leading edge of the third eyelid**. A red raised focal lesion on the leading surface of the third eyelid can occur as a separate problem, not associated with lesions near the limbus.

Very little change occurs in the surrounding tissue.

Diagnosis

Biopsy is essential to differentiate hemangioma from hemangiosarcoma.

Differential diagnosis

Healing wounds with granulating tissue have a very similar appearance to hemangiosarcoma. A history of trauma may help to differentiate granulation tissue from neoplasia, but a biopsy may be required for differentiation.

Treatment

Wide surgical excision with cryosurgery of the base of the wound will usually be curative. Regular checks need to be made for regrowth.

Beta radiation may be used if available.

EYELID CONDITIONS CAUSING OCULAR DISCHARGE

MEIBOMIAN GLAND INFLAMMATION**

Classical signs

- Serous ocular discharge.
- Blepharospasm and rubbing of eyes with front paws.
- Inner surface of eyelids are bright red.
- Raised cream-colored lesions on the eyelid margin.

See the main reference on page 1324 for details. (The Cat With Abnormal Eyelid Appearance).

Pathogenesis

Meibomian gland inflammation may be caused by an infection of the glands, usually with *Staphylococcus* or *Streptococcus* **spp**.

In some cases, the infectious agent may cause a hypersensitivity reaction. This is more common with *Staphylococcus* spp.

The inflammation and hypersensitivity reaction may **change the ocular pH** on the eyelid surface, which further exacerbates the problem.

Individual glands swell with **inspissated lipid secretions**.

Clinical signs

The cat presents with a history of **irritated eyes**, and has a **serous to mucopurulent discharge** around the eyelid margins.

The condition can cause a lot of discomfort, seen as **blepharospasm and rubbing**. Ocular pain with squinting may or may not be present.

If the inner surface of the eyelids is examined, there will be an obvious redness and swelling of the meibomian glands within the tarsal plate.

There may be redness of the eyelid and conjunctiva. The inner surface of eyelids is often bright red.

It is usually a **chronic condition**, and can be frustrating to manage.

Raised cream-colored lesions with cheesy appearance represent inspissated cells swollen with accumulated lipid material, which is highly inflammatory to surrounding tissue.

Diagnosis

Careful examination of inner lid margins will show a very red inflamed row of glands.

There is usually a mucopurulent discharge.

Culture and sensitivity of meibomian secretions may be helpful. Sensitivity will often show resistance to a wide variety of antibacterial agents.

Several small punch biopsies, 2 mm in size, with histopathology, culture and sensitivity may help identify the cause.

Differential diagnosis

Eosinophilic conjunctivitis may appear similar, but has eosinophils present on cytology.

Peri-ocular skin conditions causing blepharitis such as malassezia, ringworm and immune-mediated conditions like pemphigeus foliacious.

Treatment

Hygiene is very important in these cases, and **regular cleansing and massage** of the eyelid margins is beneficial, if the cat is amenable.

Topical anti-inflammatory drugs are useful in chronic cases. **Prednisolone acetate** 0.5% instilled into the eyes two to three times daily is sufficient.

Topical antibiotics are indicated, particularly those that will treat *Staphylococcus* and *Streptococcus* spp.

Systemic tetracyclines, particularly doxycycline, have been widely used to suppress similar inflammation in human medicine. In cats, use an oral dose of 5 mg/kg PO q 24 h for 1–3 months. **Tetracyclines have a mild anti-inflammatory effect** on ocular tissue. They suppress antibody production and chemotaxis of neutrophils, and inhibit lipases, collagenases and prostaglandin synthesis. Research also shows that tetracyclines exert other pleiotrophic properties independent of their antimicrobial activity which include inhibition of metalloproteases, blockade of nitrous oxide synthetase (a potent mediator of inflammatory activity), suppression of tumor progression, bone resorption and angiogenesis.

EYELID TRAUMA**

Classical signs

- Small wounds present as tears on the margin of the eyelid or skin surface.
- Lacerated margins cause distortion with globe more prominent.

See the main reference on page 1326 for details (The Cat With Abnormal Eyelid Appearance).

Clinical signs

Eyelid lacerations are common following fights. They present with a typical wound through the eyelid margin. In severe cases, the wounds gape open exposing the globe.

Healed eyelid wounds may result in cicatricial distortion of the lids, that leads to trichiasis. Hair from the surrounding eyelid skin may rub on the eye (trichiasis), causing epiphora and keratitis.

If the eyelid margins are not apposed correctly, the lid will be distorted and chronic conjunctivitis and keratitis are common sequelae. This will result in a mucoid to mucopurulent discharge.

Cicatricial ectropion, when the lower eyelid hangs open exposing the conjunctiva, is the most common complication after lower eyelid wounds.

If the wound occurs in the area of the lower puncta, scarring may result in epiphora, as tear drainage is affected.

Diagnosis

Eyelid wounds are obvious on clinical examination. There will usually be a history of trauma.

EYELID AGENESIS (COLOBOMA)

> **Classical signs**
>
> - Unilateral or bilateral abnormality of upper outer lid margin.
> - Seromucoid ocular discharge.
> - Vascularized adjacent upper cornea with or without ulceration.
> - Most common in Persians but any breed can be affected.

See main reference on page 1323 for details. (The Cat With Abnormal Eyelid Appearance).

Pathogenesis

Eyelid agenesis is a **congenital anomaly**, and strictly speaking is a coloboma of the eyelid. The eyes should be checked for other signs of defects, as some cases also have a coloboma of the optic disc.

Clinical signs

Occurs in **all breeds of cats** including domestic shorthair cats, but is more common in **Persians.**

The agenesis is **usually bilateral,** but may be unilateral.

It mainly affects the upper eyelid, and the lateral half to one third of the eyelid margin is missing or abnormal.

Where the eyelid margin is missing, the eyelid hair directly rubs on the cornea, causing **trichiasis, keratitis and tearing.**

The conjunctiva is exposed adjacent to the area of the agenesis, causing desiccation and mucoid discharge.

Most cases present with **tearing, corneal vascularization and ulceration as kittens.**

Diagnosis

There will be a history of **chronic epiphora** with keratitis and obvious ocular irritation.

Careful examination will show that a portion of the upper eyelid margin is missing or abnormal.

Differential diagnosis

Eyelid wounds that have healed with a section of lid margin missing appear similar. Age and a history of trauma usually differentiate.

Treatment

Surgical correction is the only curative solution. There are many surgical techniques that involve **rotational or advancement flaps.** For details the reader should go to texts that have details of ophthalmic surgical techniques or refer the cat to an ophthalmologist.

SYMBLEPHARON OCCLUDING THE LOWER NASOLACRIMAL PUNCTA

> **Classical signs**
>
> - Chronic epiphora with tearing down the face causing brown staining. Unilateral or bilateral.
> - History of cat flu as a kitten.
> - Abnormal appearance of conjunctiva, and occasionally a cloudy cornea.

See the main reference on page 1212 for details (Herpesvirus conjunctivitis).

Pathogenesis

Symblepharon is the **adhesion of any part of the conjunctiva to itself or to the cornea**. It includes:
- Adhesion of conjunctiva from bulbar conjunctiva to eyelid conjunctiva.
- Adhesion of bulbar conjunctiva to cornea.
- Adhesion between third eyelid conjunctiva and eyelid or bulbar conjunctiva.

Symblepharon **occurs after severe inflammation**, following destruction of large portions of the conjunctival epithelium.

The entire corneal surface may be reduced to a thin conjunctival membrane, when the infection is so severe that it destroys the corneal stem cells at the level of the limbus. The normal corneal epithelium is absent, and is replaced with a thin conjunctival membrane.

It is seen most commonly **after acute herpesvirus-1 infection** in kittens.

Clinical signs

The **conjunctiva can be distorted, thickened**, and cover part or all of the cornea. Symblepharon may be **unilateral or bilateral**.

The eyelids may be distorted in severe cases, and the adhesion between bulbar and lid conjunctiva may cause poor eyelid function.

The **third eyelid may be thickened and distorted**, and have poor movement across the globe.

Poor eyelid function and puncta occlusion cause **chronic ocular discharges**. If the puncta is occluded, the discharges will be serous, but when the condition is severe and eyelid function is disturbed, the discharges may become mucopurulent. The chronic epiphora with tearing down the face may cause **brown staining of the fur**.

The **entire cornea may appear cloudy**, covered by a thin vascular membrane. Surprisingly, some of these cats have limited vision.

Diagnosis

There is usually a **history of acute respiratory disease as a kitten**, followed by chronic ocular inflammation and discharge.

Close examination will reveal an abnormal conjunctiva with adhesion to eyelids, cornea and/or third eyelid.

Examine the eyelid with magnification to see if the puncta has been occluded causing epiphora.

Differential diagnosis

Healed wounds with eyelid damage around the puncta area may appear similar, but there is no history of acute inflammation or respiratory disease.

Healed wounds of the third eyelid usually have some form of deformity to the contour of the margin, and the third eyelid is rarely adhered to surrounding tissues.

In **ulcerative keratitis** with a large corneal deficit, conjunctiva or third eyelid conjunctiva may have adhered to the healing cornea, but this will usually occur near the limbus, and not centrally over the entire cornea.

Treatment

The need for treatment depends on the severity of the condition.

Specialized surgical techniques to reposition the conjunctiva are required, but even in experienced hands the results are not rewarding, as the adhesions invariably reform.

Surgery to re-establish tear drainage is rarely successful because of severe damage to the nasolacrimal ducts, and occlusion of the puncta.

Conjunctivo-rhinostomy techniques have been described to establish tear drainage to the nose.

Prevention

Try to prevent formation of symblepharon in kittens with acute conjunctival inflammation using appropriate treatment.

- Treat kittens with severe ocular inflammation with **broad-spectrum antibiotics and anti-viral** agents (see Herpes conjunctivitis, page 1214). **Tetracycline** antibiotic ointment is best, because *Chlamydophila felis* or mycoplasma infection may complicate herpesvirus infection.
- **Hourly lubrication with artificial tears** appears to be very beneficial.

LOWER LID ENTROPION**

Classical signs

- Lower eyelid is curled inwards.
- Chronic ulcerative keratitis caused by eyelid hair rubbing on the cornea.
- Mucoid to mucopurulent discharge.

See main reference on page 1320 for details (The Cat With Abnormal Eyelid Appearance).

Clinical signs

Usually the central portion of the lower eyelid margin rolls inwards towards the globe. **Lid hair adjacent to the margin may appear moist or be coated in conjunctival mucus**.

Enophthalmos is often present as the underlying cause, or chronic blepharospasm **caused by painful corneal diseases**.

Corneal surface disease **is present from the eyelid hair rubbing on the cornea. This can include superficial ulceration, sequestrum formation, and a vascular response from the limbus adjacent to the area of lid irritation**.

Chronic discharge occurs **ranging from mucoid to mucopurulent**.

Diagnosis

Diagnosis is based on the characteristic sign of an inward rolling eyelid margin with secondary corneal changes and chronic ocular discharge.

MEIBOMIAN GLAND ADENOCARCINOMA

Classical signs

- Localized or diffuse eyelid swelling.
- ± Surface ulceration.

See main reference on page 1324 for details. (The Cat With Abnormal Eyelid Appearance).

Clinical signs

Meibomian gland adenomas or carcinomas are seen as a **nodular or diffuse mass causing localized thickening of the eyelid**. The tumor may have an ulcerated surface.

Diagnosis

Tentative diagnosis is based on the appearance of the eyelid lesion.

Exfoliative cytology is useful in some cases that show ulceration.

Fine-needle biopsy can be useful in cases where there is discreet swelling.

Definitive diagnosis is based on histopathological examination of affected tissue.

CORNEAL DISEASE CAUSING OCULAR DISCHARGE

HERPETIC KERATITIS***

Classical signs

- Ocular pain seen as blepharospasm and photophobia.
- Mild serous ocular discharge. Superficial corneal ulceration in a dendritic or geographic distribution.
- Superficial vascularization and scarring, if chronic.

See main reference on page 1237 (The Cat With Abnormalities Confined to the Cornea).

Clinical signs

Cats present with signs of ocular pain, seen as blepharospasm and photophobia.

A **mild serous discharge** is common.

Superficial ulceration in an irregular (geographic) or linear (dendritic) pattern is seen when the cornea is examined under magnification, or with a slit lamp biomicroscope. The corneal lesion is in the epithelium or superficial stroma.

There may be varying degrees of **superficial vascularization and scarring**.

There is often a history of **quiescent phases, followed by recurrence** of serous discharge, and eye discomfort after stress.

A history of prior cat flu, often as a kitten, with signs consistent with feline herpesvirus-1 infection, may be present. **Corneal involvement** (keratitis) may first occur 1–2 weeks after upper respiratory signs, or may be unassociated with respiratory signs.

Diagnosis

A **history** of respiratory infection as a kitten, followed by chronic episodes of ocular discharge and pain, indicates a tentative diagnosis of herpetic keratitis. **Close examination** will show dendritic lesions or geographical ulceration.

Laboratory tests such as PCR may support a diagnosis of FHV-1 infection. See Herpetic conjunctivitis, page 1213.

CORNEAL TRAUMA***

> ### Classical signs
>
> - Blepharospasm and photophobia with ocular guarding.
> - Initially a serous ocular discharge becoming mucopurulent.
> - +/– Copious watery discharge from constant leakage of aqueous humor if cornea is perforated.
> - Blue or cloudy cornea.
> - Retention of fluorescein stain.
> - Black appearance to the corneal deficit, if iris is prolapsed through wound.

See main reference on page 1249 (The Cat With Abnormalities Confined to the Cornea).

Clinical signs

Ocular pain is evident as **blepharospasm and photophobia**.

There will be an **ocular discharge**, which is serous at first and becomes mucopurulent.

In cases where the **cornea is perforated**, there may be a copious watery discharge from constant leakage of aqueous humor out of the wound.

The surrounding cornea will have **corneal edema** seen as a blue or cloudy eye.

There will be **retention of fluorescein** stain where there is a large deficit of epithelium. If the wound is leaking aqueous, the fluorescein will wash off the cornea away from the perforation.

Fibrin tags or clots may be seen attached to the injured area of the cornea, plugging the wound.

In large perforations, **iris tissue may be prolapsed** (iris prolapse) through the wound giving a black appearance to the corneal deficit.

Diagnosis

Diagnosis is based on the clinical signs of severe ocular pain with a serous discharge, and evidence of corneal trauma, such as a tear in the cornea, which may be plugged with fibrin, or have an iris prolapse.

Ocular discharge which will vary from serous to very watery, if aqueous is leaking.

ULCERATIVE KERATITIS**

> ### Classical signs
>
> - Painful closed eye with a serous discharge.
> - Focal or diffuse corneal cloudiness.
> - Conjunctival inflammation.
> - Corneal erosion.
> - Positive green stain with fluorescein dye.
> - Red appearance of cornea in chronic cases.

See main reference on page 1246 for details. (The Cat With Abnormalities Confined to the Cornea).

Clinical signs

Serous ocular discharge is often the presenting sign.

Signs of ocular pain with **blepharospasm (resulting in a closed eye), and photophobia** are present.

Focal or diffuse corneal edema (cloudiness) occurs, depending on the amount of epithelial loss.

Erosion of epithelium and stroma is present, depending on severity of the ulceration.

There will be **retention of fluorescein stain** by the exposed corneal stroma.

Chronic cases may show **varying degrees of vascularization.**

Large ulcers usually develop **corneal vascularization**, which may be superficial or deep, and result in a red appearance of the cornea. This depends on how long the ulcer has been present, and what the cause is.

The eye may be red because of conjunctival inflammation.

Diagnosis

Diagnosis is based on **signs of ocular pain** with a serous discharge, and the presence a **corneal deficit** on examination of the cornea.

The ulcerated area of cornea will retain fluorescein dye (staining yellow-green).

CORNEAL SEQUESTRUM**

> ### Classical signs
>
> - A serous or mucopurulent ocular discharge.
> - Brown staining of the cornea.
> - +/– Signs of ocular discomfort.

See main reference on page 1233 for details (The Cat With Abnormalities Confined to the Cornea).

Clinical signs

Corneal sequestrum is more common in **brachycephalic breeds** such as Persians and color-points, but can occur in any breed.

The classical presentation is an area of **brown or black staining of the cornea**, which may be superficial, or involve deep layers of the stroma. The lesion rarely absorbs fluorescein dye, except in cases where the periphery is ulcerated.

A **serous ocular discharge** is present in non-ulcerated cases.

Chronic cases may have **ulceration around the diseased area of cornea.** These often have secondary bacterial infection, and a mucopurulent ocular discharge.

Cats may or may not show signs of ocular discomfort.

There may be a **history of herpesvirus infection** as a kitten. However, there are probably other causes, such as **medial entropion** in brachycephalic cats and **corneal ulceration**.

Diagnosis

Clinical signs of ocular discharge associated with brown staining of the cornea.

Sequestrum may be associated with FHV-1 infection, which can be confirmed with laboratory tests.

ORBITAL DISEASE CAUSING OCULAR DISCHARGE AND CHANGED CONJUNCTIVAL APPEARANCE

RETROBULBAR INFECTION

> ### Classical signs
>
> - Prominent globe (exophthalmos).
> - Chemosis of the conjunctiva, with injected blood vessels and a mucopurulent discharge.
> - The third eyelid may be prominent or swollen.
> - Pain and reluctance to open the mouth.
> - Rare.

See main reference on page 1310 (The Cat With an Abnormal Globe Position or Size).

Clinical signs

Cats will have **varying degrees of exophthalmos**, depending on the extent of the orbital inflammation.

In acute cases, there is usually a **mucopurulent discharge,** that may be copious if there is orbital cellulitis.

The **conjunctiva may be red** with injected blood vessels, and show chemosis (edema).

The **third eyelid is prominent and may be swollen**, when the swelling is outside the muscle cone in the orbit.

Acute cases show severe pain, and **resist opening the mouth**.

It may be difficult to retropulse the globe into the orbit.

Retrobulbar infection may be **hematogenous**, associated with **foreign body penetration**, or from extension of **dental or sinus disease**. Check the cat for signs of dental disease, especially molar root disease, or nasal discharge.

It is **rare** in cats compared to dogs.

Diagnosis

Initial diagnosis is based on the classical signs of exophthalmos, with chemosis and inflammation of the conjunctiva, and a mucopurulent discharge. Pain when the mouth is opened supports the diagnosis.

Check the teeth for dental disease, and the nose for nasal discharges suggesting sinus problems.

Ocular ultrasound is very useful. The orbit is examined for changes in echodensity. **Abscesses** appear as **focal hyper-echoic areas**. If the inflammation is diffuse, the normal muscular cone will be hard to visualize.

Dental radiology is used to check the roots of the molar teeth for periodontal disease.

Radiology of the orbit and sinuses is useful if one suspects the infection has extended from these areas. The orbital rim is examined for signs of erosion adjacent to the frontal and nasal sinus.

CT or MRI of the nose and sinuses is used to rule out an extension of disease from these areas to the orbit. There will usually be an erosion of the bony orbit, and signs of disease in the nose or sinuses.

RECOMMENDED READING

Barnett KC. A Colour Atlas of Veterinary Ophthalmology. Wolfe Publishing Ltd, London, 1990.

Gelatt Kirk N (ed). Veterinary Ophthalmology, 2nd edn. Lea & Febiger, Philadelphia, 1991.

Gelatt Kirk N. Veterinary Ophthalmology, 3rd edn. Lippincott, Williams and Wilkins, Philadelphia, 1998.

Gelatt Kirk N. Essentials of Veterinary Ophthalmology. Lippincott Williams and Wilkins, Philadelphia, 2000.

Gelatt Kirk N. Colour Atlas of Veterinary Ophthalmology. Lippincott Williams and Wilkins, Philadelphia, 2001.

Gelatt Kirk N, Gelatt JP. Handbook of Small Animal Ophthalmic Surgery, Vol. 1. Extraocular Procedures. Permagon Veterinary Handbook Series, Florida, 1994.

Gelatt Kirk N, Gelatt JP. Handbook of Small Animal Ophthalmic Surgery, Vol. 2. Intra-ocular Procedures. Permagon Veterinary Handbook Series, Florida, .

Ketring KL, Glaze MB. Atlas of Feline Ophthalmology. Trenton, NJ, Veterinary Learning Systems, 1994.

Peiffer RL, Petersen-Jones S. Small Animal Ophthalmology, A Problem Oriented Approach, 3rd edn. Saunders, Philadelphia, 2001.

60. The cat with abnormalities confined to the cornea

Richard IE Smith

KEY SIGNS

- Cloudy cornea.
- Redness from vascularization.
- Pink or white plaque.
- Coffee to black staining lesion.
- Ocular pain (blepharospasm, photophobia).

MECHANISM?

- Superficial damage to the epithelial surface causes an erosion (superficial ulcer). Loss of epithelium and stromal tissue results in a deep ulcer with a loss of transparency of the cornea because of edema of the stromal tissue.
- Cats with uveitis secondary to systemic disease may show changes in the inner endothelial cell layer. This will be seen as corneal edema (diffuse grayish appearance) and there may be "keratic precipitates" (focal deposits consisting of white blood cells and fibrin) present on the endothelium.
- The cat has some unique degenerative and immune-mediated corneal diseases.

WHERE?

- Cornea (epithelium, stroma, endothelium).

WHAT?

- Trauma and infectious diseases affecting the upper respiratory system are the main causes of corneal disease in cats.
- The cat cornea develops a unique degenerative disease, which forms a corneal sequestrum.
- An immune-mediated disease called eosinophylic keratitis is seen associated with allergic states.
- Corneal edema and keratitic precipitates are seen in cats with uveitis, usually secondary to systemic disease.

QUICK REFERENCE SUMMARY

Diseases causing abnormalities confined to the cornea

DEGENERATIVE

- Calcific degeneration (p 1252)

Rare in cats. Seen as a band of gritty white material in the anterior stroma, usually secondary to chronic herpetic keratitis. Known as a band keratopathy.

- **Corneal sequestrum (feline keratitis nigrum)** (p 1241)

Presents with an axial (central) area of staining (light brown to black) in the cornea, usually unilateral. Most common in brachycephalic breeds such as Persians and Himalayans. Approximately 80% are associated with herpetic keratitis. In the early stages there is no ulceration, but chronic lesions may have ulcerated borders, and there may be intense deep stromal vascularization associated with these ulcerated lesions. It is a focal area of stromal degeneration surrounded by an inflammatory zone.

ANOMALY

- Stromal dystrophy of Manx cats (p 1252)

A rare condition in young Manx cats that starts with axial stromal edema and progresses to a diffuse corneal edema with a thickened stroma full of bullae (fluid-filled vesicles). A blinding corneal disease with no treatment possible.

- Endothelial dystrophy (p 1252)

Seen in Domestic Short Hair cats. A very rare condition seen in young cats evident as a cloudy blue cornea caused by diffuse corneal edema secondary to an endothelial dystrophy. There is no specific cause, and no treatment is possible.

METABOLIC

- Lysosomal storage diseases with ophthalmic manifestations (p 1253)

GM 1 gangliosidosis, GM 2 gangliosidosis, mannosidosis, mucopolysaccharidosis 1 (MPS1). Mucopolysaccharidosis 2 (MPS2) may be associated with corneal changes. The cornea shows opacity caused by vacuoles in the keratocytes and endothelial cells. Seen in young animals that also have neurologic signs of ataxia, muscular tremors and paralysis.

INFLAMMATION/INFECTIOUS

- **Feline herpes virus 1 (FHV-1) keratitis** (p 1237)

Cats may have a history of FHV-1 infection as kittens, with acute upper respiratory tract signs, salivation, sneezing, pyrexia, lethargy and anorexia. Often appears as a unilateral disease in older cats. The epithelium may show dendritic lesions (finger-like projections of thickened epithelium that stain with rose bengal stain) in early cases. Chronic cases show irregular (geographic) ulceration to the level of the superficial stroma. Scarring and vascularization of the cornea follows after repeated inflammatory episodes.

- **Bacterial ulcerative keratitis** (p 1248)

Usually secondary to corneal trauma. Ulcers stain positive with fluorescein dye. There is a variable presentation depending on the depth of the ulcer and the type of infection. *Pseudomonas* infection may cause a "melting ulcer" (keratomalacia) with digestion of stromal tissue by bacteria and cellular enzymes.

● Florida keratopathy ("Florida spots")/mycobacterial keratitis (p 1251)

Focal grayish opacities seen in the stroma caused by a mycobacterium. Only seen in the southeast USA.

Inflammation:

● **Keratitis secondary to uveitis** (p 1251)

Usually seen as a diffuse blue eye caused by corneal edema from a compromised corneal endothelium. The eye may have an associated red injected conjunctiva. The anterior chamber may have a hypopyon (accumulation of protein and white blood cells) and the inferior endothelium may have keratic precipitates (focal accumulations of white blood cells and protein). Frequently associated with systemic diseases such as cryptococcosis, toxoplasmosis, FeLV, FIV, FIP (young cats) and systemic mycoses (USA).

Immune-mediated:

● **Eosinophilic keratitis*** (p 1245)

Seen as a cloudy, red cornea, sometimes with a muco-purulent discharge. A proliferative white to pinkish plaque develops on the cornea, with superficial and in chronic cases, deep vascularization. Usually a history of poor response to antibiotic therapy. Eosinophils demonstrated on cytology from corneal scrapings are diagnostic.

Trauma:

● Neurotropic keratitis (p 1250)

Ulcerative keratitis results from denervation of the cornea or paralysis of the eyelids. The cornea has a dry lusterless appearance, often with superficial ulceration and vascularization. The cat cannot blink the eye, or there is no corneal reflex when the cornea is touched with a thread. Usually seen after accidents that affect the facial and/or trigeminal nerve.

● **Ulcerative keratitis (not associated with specific corneal disease or corneal perforation)*** (p 1246)

Appears as a very painful, cloudy eye with serous discharge. Edema, blepharospasm and ulceration, or a penetrating wound are typical. Usually occur secondary to corneal trauma. Foreign bodies such as grass seeds and thorns or blunt trauma from motor vehicle accidents are the most common causes of corneal trauma. Trauma may cause a superficial ulcer, deep ulcer or penetrating wound. Melting ulcers appear as a very cloudy cornea with a soft gelatinous appearance. A black area within the ulcer and a thin bulging membrane indicate a descemetocele.

● **Ulcerative keratitis caused by corneal perforation (cat fight wounds)** (p 1242)

Very painful, closed eye with serous discharge and sometimes bleeding. Anterior chamber may be full of blood and protein. Cats commonly attack their opponent's eyes, usually causing a penetrating corneal wound with a claw. An iris prolapse is a common complication, and is seen as a light to dark brown bulge in the center of the corneal wound (and distorted pupil if visible). Lens rupture is a devastating complication that causes an acute uveitis, glaucoma and blindness.

● **Blunt trauma*** (p 1249)

Painful, cloudy and red eye. Cornea may have superficial ulcer or be ruptured (usually around the limbus). The anterior chamber may be filled with blood (hyphema). Conjunctiva may be red from subconjunctival hemorrhage. Eye may be bulging (exophthalmos) from edema and hemorrhage in the orbit.

INTRODUCTION

MECHANISM?

The main supportive tissue of the cornea is the **stroma,** which consists of cells that stretch from one side to the other, known as **keratocytes**, and an intercellular matrix that contains collagen fibers and glycosaminoglycans. The outer surface is covered by an **epithelial layer**, about six cells deep, that has a very thin basement membrane. The inner surface has a cell monolayer called the **endothelium,** which has a very thick basement membrane called **Descemet's membrane**.

The **cornea is transparent** because it does not have a blood supply, contains no pigmented cells, the collagen fibers are laid down in very specific planes and the hydration of the intercellular matrix is controlled.

The epithelium and endothelium have properties that prevent fluid from entering the stroma. If the epithelium is eroded, the stromal matrix will absorb fluid, swell and become cloudy. This is known as **corneal edema**. Similarly, if the endothelium is compromised, aqueous humor will enter the stroma and cause corneal edema.

Very simply, the cornea is kept alive by the tear film, which provides nutrients for the cells and immune mechanisms to protect the eye from disease. **Oxygen enters the cornea by diffusion through the tear film**.

The cornea is the main refractive tissue for the optical mechanism of the eye.

Diseases of the cornea in cats are generally confined to the outer epithelium and the supportive stromal tissue.

The cat cornea heals very well with limited scarring and melanin pigment deposition compared to other species.

Inflammation of the cornea is known as "keratitis". Keratitis may be acute or chronic, and ulcerative or infectious. Inflammation is associated with erosions and edema.

When the epithelium is damaged, a corneal ulcer develops. The ulcer may be **superficial** if only the epithelium is missing, or **deep** if the epithelium and stroma are eroded. When the epithelium and entire stroma are eroded as far as Descemet's membrane, the condition is called a **Descemetocele**. Descemet's membrane is very elastic in the cat. When there is a large stromal deficit, the Descemetocele will be seen as a large bulge of transparent tissue.

The integrity of the epithelium is tested with a water-soluble dye called fluoresein. The epithelium prevents water-soluble substances from entering the stroma. If the epithelium is disrupted, the dye will be absorbed by the stroma and remain temporarily as a yellow green stain. The dye coloration can be enhanced by using ultraviolet light (the blue filter on direct and indirect ophthalmoscopes). **Rose bengal** is another stain that is used to show minor changes in the epithelial layer. It may be useful to show the dendritic lesions seen in feline herpesvirus-1 keratitis.

Corneal ulcers may be caused by trauma, infectious diseases, immune processes that affect the epithelium and stroma, and by any mechanism that prevents the normal tear film from covering the eye.

Endothelial disruption may be caused by trauma or inflammation within the eye, usually secondary to uveitis (an inflammation of the vascular tissue in the eye). An inherited form of endothelial dystrophy has been described in the Manx cat.

The cornea has a very rich nerve supply emanating from the trigeminal nerve. Nerve endings are found throughout the cornea up to the level of the basal epithelial cells. Any disruption of the epithelium causes severe ocular pain, which is manifested by blepharospasm (eyelid spasm), photophobia (pain from light) and ocular guarding. The pain will stimulate excessive tear production causing a serous ocular discharge.

The cat cornea has some unique diseases caused by degeneration of the stroma, and proliferative lesions, which develop from immune mechanisms associated with systemic reactions to allergic disease.

Chronic superficial corneal disease will stimulate vascular in-growth from the limbus (the area where the cornea merges with the sclera) known as **corneal**

vascularization. Superficial blood vessels grow in a branching pattern and may bring melanin cells with them, causing pigmentation and loss of transparency.

Acute inflammation within the eye (uveitis) will cause an intense, deep stromal vascular infiltration around the periphery (limbus) known as a **"brush border"**. Corneal edema and keratic precipitates are seen in eyes that have uveitis. The epithelium is usually intact, but the endothelium is disrupted.

Corneal pigmentation develops secondary to corneal vascularization as melanin cells from the limbal melanocytes are dragged into the stroma with the blood vessels. This is not as common a reaction in the cat compared to other species.

Corneal edema can be seen in cases with glaucoma, because the increased intra-ocular pressure disrupts the endothelium, allowing aqueous to enter the stroma. The epithelium is usually intact.

WHERE?

Corneal epithelium stroma (keratocytes and matrix) and endothelium.

WHAT?

Most superficial corneal epithelial problems are caused by **trauma or infections, specifically herpesvirus-1**.

Corneal stromal problems are caused by trauma, herpesvirus or degeneration associated with corneal sequestrum. Cloudiness of the cornea is caused by edema or scarring.

Proliferative corneal lesions are usually caused by an immune-mediated reaction known as **eosinophilic keratoconjunctivitis**.

Corneal endothelial problems are caused by **trauma, uveitis, glaucoma,** and very rarely, endothelial dystrophy.

Non-specific reactions that cause edema and chronic keratitis can be seen with glaucoma.

Congenital diseases of the cornea are rare in cats.

DISEASES CAUSING ABNORMALITIES CONFINED TO THE CORNEA

FELINE HERPESVIRUS-1 (FHV-1) KERATITIS***

Classical signs

- Kittens may have swollen red eyes with a serous discharge. In very severe cases this may be followed by a cloudy appearance of the cornea. The cornea is covered by a conjunctival membrane and has a dull gray appearance, sometimes with superficial vascularization.
- Young cats may present with signs of ocular pain (blepharospasm and photophobia) and serous discharge. Microscopic examination of the cornea may show dendritic lesions seen as a faint branching within the epithelium. They may stain positive with rose bengal stain.
- Older cats develop chronic painful eyes that may have a slightly cloudy cornea with some faint blood vessels present. This is caused by shallow irregular ulceration (geographic ulcer) often with faint superficial vascularization.
- Older cats frequently have a history of acute episodes followed by quiescent periods, but close examination will reveal a slightly cloudy, scarred cornea.
- The condition is frequently unilateral but may be bilateral.

See main reference on page 1212 for details (The Cat With Ocular Discharge or Changed Conjunctival Appearance) and The Cat With Acute Sneezing or Nasal Discharge (page 7).

Pathogenesis

Herpesvirus infection is one of the most common causes of acute and chronic corneal disease in older cats

The condition is caused by infection with feline herpes virus-1 (FHV-1), a subfamily of Herpesvirinae. FHV-1 has poor tropism for corneal tissue. Corneal disease is usually the consequence of conjunctival infection in young cats.

FHV-1 affects the cornea through two different mechanisms.

Firstly, the virus has a **direct cytopathic effect on corneal epithelium** and produces the typical linear or branching (dendritic) lesions. The lesions rarely reach the depth of the epithelial basement membrane, and can therefore be difficult to detect. Staining the epithelium with rose bengal may reveal these pink branching lesions.

Secondly, **an immune response to viral antigen** causes a prolonged absence of epithelium. This is seen clinically as a **"geographic ulcer"**, that is, a large ulcer with an irregular shape that appears to look like a continent or land mass. There may be some fine superficial blood vessels within the anterior stroma in the area that is affected.

The virus is able to replicate and become latent in nerve tissue, most likely in trigeminal nerve sensory ganglia. Virus reactivation occurs after stress and after the administration of corticosteroids. Vaccination with live virus vaccines may exacerbate the condition in affected cases.

Clinical signs

The **earliest sign of classical** herpesvirus infection is paroxysms of sneezing or salivation. This is usually seen in kittens and cats that have not been immunized.

Systemic signs of upper respiratory disease are common and include anorexia, pyrexia and depression.

Acute conjunctivitis manifested by hyperemia and chemosis is seen at the same time as the respiratory signs. Prolapse of the third eyelid may occur as part of the inflammatory process in the eye.

Serous ocular discharge is seen in the acute phase and this progresses to a **mucopurulent discharge.**

In young cats, ulceration may occur in the buccal mucosa and on the tongue.

The ocular changes are **usually bilateral**, but may be unilateral in older cats.

The cornea may be affected in acute infections by formation of **symblepharon.** Necrosis of the epithelium, probably with stem cell damage, allows the conjunctiva to permanently adhere to the corneal stroma. The cornea then heals with a dull gray appearance, covered by a thin membrane of conjunctiva.

In older cats with a carrier status, **mild signs of herpesvirus** infection may be seen **after some form of stress.** In these cases, the inflammation is less intense and only a serous discharge is present. These cats may have a history of respiratory infection as a kitten.

The classical corneal lesions in **early infections** appear as **dendritic (branching) epithelial lesions** that can be very subtle in appearance and may require magnification to visualize. They usually occur after the primary conjunctival inflammation has decreased in intensity. The epithelium may be swollen in affected areas, and these branching lesions may stain pink with rose bengal stain. There may be a mild conjunctivitis with a serous ocular discharge

In chronic cases, a **stromal keratitis** develops. The condition is frequently unilateral. The epithelium is eroded and there may be mild edema with some superficial vascularization. The cornea develops an **irregular surface with scarring** that is obvious on clinical examination and this is known as a geographic ulcer. This is the calssical form of FHV-1 keratitis seen in older cats. It is **frequently only unilateral,** and may appear years after initial infection in cats with no previous history of eye disease.

Chronic stromal FHV-1 keratitis has a history of quiescent periods followed by signs of ocular pain with blepharitis, photophobia and corneal erosions. There is rarely conjunctivitis or ocular discharge.

A black staining color may develop in the center of the cornea known as a **corneal sequestrum** (keratitis nigrum). This is caused by a stromal coagulative necrosis, and it has been suggested that FHV-1 infection may be the cause of 80% of these lesions.

Diagnosis

Diagnosis is based on a **history of repeat ocular problems with subtle corneal changes**. It is difficult to establish a definitive diagnosis.

Cytology: intranuclear inclusions in epithelial cells can be demonstrated with immunoperoxidase stains in some acute primary infections. This is not very reliable.

Immunofluorescence: direct or indirect fluorescent antibody techniques on corneal/conjunctival smears or tissue sections. This has poor sensitivity.

Virus isolation by demonstration of cytopathic effects in cell culture. This is the gold standard for detection of herpesvirus, but is not often used because of logistical difficulties in getting rapid results.

Serology: antibody titers tend to be of low magnitude after primary infection, sometimes reaching only 1:64 at 60 days after infection. High titers are rarely seen after recrudescent infection.

Polymerase chain reaction (PCR) testing: DNA amplification of an amino acid sequence of the thymidine kinase gene is perhaps the most sensitive test available. Theoretically the test could pick up one strand of viral DNA. High sensitivity in nested PCR tests may reduce specificity by the detection of non-viral DNA contaminants. Although this test was initially heralded as an excellent diagnostic tool, in practice the results have been very disappointing. It would appear that sample collection and individual laboratories have a great influence on specificity.

- Conjunctival swabs and/or biopsies are used for PCR or virus isolation. Not all laboratories are equipped to do this work. Check with your laboratory, as you may have to send samples interstate or overseas for results.

Differential diagnosis

Ulcerative keratitis.
- Not common as a primary ocular disease, but is seen secondary to viral infection.
- It usually follows ocular trauma.

- The inflammation is more intense than herpesvirus keratitis with greater destruction of stromal tissue and more intense edema. Keratomalacia (melting cornea) can develop in cases with pseudomonas infections.
- Bacterial keratitis causes a mucopurulent discharge.
- Cytology from clean scrapings taken from the edge of the ulcer may demonstrate bacteria. Culture and sensitivity can be done from scrapings taken from the edge of the ulcerated cornea.
- Ulcers heal without recurrence.

Eosinophilic keratoconjunctivitis.
- This is a proliferative lesion that is usually accompanied by inflammation and a mucopurulent discharge.
- The presence of eosinophils on cytology is regarded as diagnostic.

Neoplasia.
- Squamous cell carcinoma of the cornea is reported, but it is a very rare condition in cats. The lesion is proliferative but there is little ocular discharge.
- Cytology or fine-needle biopsy will confirm this condition.

Treatment

Not all treatments useful for ocular herpesvirus infection are commercially available throughout the world.

Topical and probably systemic **corticosteroids are contraindicated** in all cases of ocular herpesvirus infections. The effect of topical NSAIDs has produced equivocal results experimentally. However, some cases of herpesvirus keratitis may only respond if corticosteroids are used in conjunction with antiviral agents.

Topical ocular antiviral agents include:
- **Idoxuridine** inhibits DNA synthesis by competing with thymidine for incorporation into viral DNA. It is no longer in production, but has been the most commonly used topical agent for treating FHV-1 infection. Topical drops are frequently made to order by a **compounding pharmacist** and produce excellent results. **Idoxuridine 0.1% drops are**

most commonly used. Drops need to be used at least three to four times daily.

- **Vidarabine** (adenine arabinoside. Vira-A, Parke-Davis) interferes with DNA polymerase and may be effective in cases that are resistant to idoxuridine. Use q 6–8 h.
- **Trifluorothymidine** (Viroptic, Glaxo Wellcome) has the best in vitro effect of all available topical agents. Use q 6–8 h.
- **Acyclovir** (Zovirax ophthalmic ointment, GlaxoSmithKline) may be the only commercially available drug in some countries. The efficacy against FHV-1 has been reported as poor. Use q 6–8 h.
- **Dilute povidine iodine** (diluted 50% in saline) has been used, but there is only anecdotal evidence of its efficacy in clinical situations, and at this strength can be very irritating to eyes.

Oral antiviral agents include:

- **Acyclovir** (Zovirax) seems very effective, even at doses far below the in vitro ED_{50}. The usual dose is 50 mg/kg, q 6–12 h, but watch for toxic signs of bone marrow suppression even at this dose. Often used in conjunction with oral α interferon and synergism significantly reduces ED_{50} of acyclovir.
- **Valaciclovir** (Valtrex, GlaxoSmithKline) is an acyclovir prodrug, but rapid absorption of this drug in cats appears to make it more readily able to cause toxicity, especially in sick acutely infected cats.
- **Interferon α**: α interferon is a cytokine produced naturally by leukocytes. It may prevent viral spread if given in the very early stages of infection in acutely infected cats. Most common regimen is a 7-day on/7-day off oral course, which is believed to work by absorption through the oral mucosa and tonsils. Treatment with this drug is controversial and dosages vary widely. Systemic courses are also used by giving 10 000 IU SC twice weekly in conjunction with topical idoxuridine or acyclovir.

Other therapies that are used:

- **Oral lysine**: Lysine has been used in human medicine to suppress clinical signs of herpes simplex infections. Lysine competes with arginine for incorporation in the viral genome. Arginine is necessary for the replication of the FHV-1 virus and incorporation of lysine produces a non-infective virus particle. It may be more effective in cats with corneal disease

than conjunctivitis alone. The recommended dose is 250 mg daily.

- **Topical and/or systemic tetracycline** antibacterials are commonly used because of their specific effect on chlamydial and mycoplasmal organisms which may be present together with herpesvirus infections.
  - Tetracyclines have a mild anti-inflammatory effect on ocular tissue. They suppress antibody production and chemotaxis of neutrophils, and inhibit lipases, collagenases and prostaglandin synthesis. Research also shows that tetracyclines exert other pleotrophic properties independent of their antimicrobial activity which include inhibition of metalloproteases, blockade of nitrous oxide synthetase (a potent mediator of inflammatory activity), suppression of tumor progression, bone resorption and angiogenesis.

Ocular hygiene is important. Regular cleaning of infected eyes with poly-ionic eye wash solutions will make the cat feel more comfortable and suppress secondary bacterial infection.

Prognosis

The prognosis for a full and uneventful recovery of herpetic keratitis is **very guarded.**

In young cats with very severe corneal symblepharon formation it is nearly impossible to create a normal cornea. These cases will have permanent scarring and opacity of the cornea with virtually no vision.

In adult cats, a chronic recurrent state may develop, and in these cases the prognosis for permanent recovery is guarded.

Virus replication occurs in the cornea, and although not clinically obvious at the time of infection, this will manifest in older cats as a chronic geographic keratitis, sometimes years after the initial infection.

Transmission

FHV-1 is a ubiquitous viral organism found all over the world and is highly infectious.

Infection of kittens may occur through direct contact from a carrier state present in queens. Virus is shed 4–6 weeks after queening.

Infection is via contamination of mucous membranes (ocular, oral or inhalation of virus).

Prevention

Vaccination with live modified or killed vaccines (see page 10).

Elimination of carrier states in catteries.

Only use killed vaccines on clinically affected animals.

CORNEAL SEQUESTRUM (FELINE KERATITIS NIGRUM)**

Classical signs

- Area of pigmented cornea varying from a very light coffee-colored stain to an intense thick black plaque.
- +/– Blepharospasm and photophobia.
- Predominantly in brachycephalic breeds such as Persians and Himalayans.
- Usually unilateral.

Pathogenesis

This disease is unique to cats and has an unknown cause.

Recent research suggests that **FHV-1 keratitis may play a role** in about 80% of cases.

Other causes include corneal ulceration, chronic corneal trauma from medial entropion, and disruption of the tear film on exposed globes.

It is a corneal stromal disease characterized by **degeneration of collagen and fibro-blasts**. The surrounding stroma is usually infiltrated with a mixed population of white blood cells including neutrophils, lymphocytes, plasma cells, and less commonly macrophages and giant cells. The degree of pigmentation varies with the degree of stromal degeneration.

Lesions vary in depth from superficial stromal degeneration to full-thickness degeneration as deep as Descemet's membrane.

The source of pigmentation has not been established, but is probably absorbed by the damaged stroma from the tear film pigments, particularly porphyrins.

Clinical signs

Clinical signs vary from a faint **coffee-colored staining** of the axial (central) super-ficial cornea to a **dense black plaque**.

There may be a history of previous infection with FHV-1 as a kitten, or later in life, herpetic keratitis.

The disease is **initially seen unilaterally**, but eventually both eyes may become involved.

Initially the cat may not show any signs of discomfort, but as the lesion progresses **blepharospasm and photophobia** develop.

Early, light-staining lesions have an intact epithelium and do not stain with fluorescein. Lesions that have developed a dense plaque may have a **fine ring of ulceration surrounding the lesion** which may stain positive with fluorescein.

The surrounding cornea will not show signs of edema or vascularization in mild cases, but as the degree of degeneration progresses, corneal edema with marked deep stromal vascularization may be prominent.

Eyes that have a faint stain usually do not have any ocular discharge. Eyes that have a dark plaque with surrounding ulceration and intense corneal vascularization often have a mucopurulent ocular discharge.

The disease is seen predominantly in **Persians and Himalayans**, but any breed can be affected.

There is no sex or age predilection, but it is more common in adults.

Diagnosis

Diagnosis is based on the clinical signs of a mild brown-staining cornea to a dense black plaque with keratitis.

Histopathology of resected cornea will show a typical pattern of degenerated stroma surrounded by a ring of inflammatory cells.

PCR tests on resected cornea may confirm the presence of FHV-1 infection but results are usually unequivocal.

Differential diagnosis

There are no other ocular presentations that present with a brown discoloration.

Herpetic keratitis.

- Very chronic cases may have a dense white superficial scar with degrees of corneal vascularization. This scarred area may slowly develop a faint stain and progress to a dense black plaque, typical of corneal sequestrum. The initial changes in corneal sequestration are subtle and may be missed.
- PCR tests may help to associate this disease with corneal sequestrum.

Eosinophilic keratitis.

- The lesion is proliferative with an intense corneal edema and vascularization. There is no brown staining.
- Cytology shows the presence of eosinophils.

Ulcerative keratitis.

- There is a positive stain to fluorescein in the initial stages.
- Chronic healing ulcers may be vascularized and have edema (white). There is no brown pigment, but occasionally ulcers may progress to form a corneal sequestrum.

Treatment

Try to identify the cause and eliminate this. **Medial entropion and FHV-1 keratitis** are the two most common causes that need to be addressed. Surgically correct medial entropion and treat FHV-1 keratitis with an anti-viral agent (see Herpes keratitis, page 1239).

Conservative management is encouraged by some ophthalmologists, as some lesions may spontaneously slough and the cornea heals with a scar. **Broad-spectrum antibiotic ointments** such as neomycin and polymixin, chloramphenicol or fucidic acid are used to lubricate the eye and guard against bacterial infection. **Antiviral agents** are often used to suppress the effects of herpetic keratitis. **Artificial tear solutions** may provide some relief from irritation and corneal drying.

Surgical management is the preferred option by the majority of ophthalmologists. The diseased stroma is resected by lamellar keratectomy, and the stromal defect closed with either a pedicle conjunctival graft or a sliding corneo-scleral graft. Partial- or full-thickness keratoplasty (corneal graft) has been used in an attempt to minimize corneal scarring, but results have not been very encouraging as the cornea vascularizes and scars. For surgical techniques readers should refer to an

ophthalmology text which describes the surgery in detail (see references).

Prognosis

The prognosis in cases that slough after medical management is reasonable. Some of these lesions may recur, and scarring will be intense causing vision impairment. However, cats with axial scarring seem to be able to lead a reasonably normal lifestyle.

Healing after pedicle grafts or cornea–scleral grafts is good, but scarring is present. Scarring is less intense after a sliding corneo–scleral graft as the opaque grafted scleral tissue is confined to the outer cornea.

Keratoplasty has not been widely embraced by veterinary ophthalmologists because rejection, vascularization and scarring of grafts occurs in other animal species. However, the cat cornea reacts more like human cornea to grafting than other animals, and therefore, is supposed to be amenable to full-thickness keratoplasty.

Transmission

Apart from FHV-1 infection, there is no known transmission of this disease from one cat to another. Cases with herpetic keratitis have the same etiopathogenesis as is described under this heading.

Prevention

There is no known prevention, apart from palliative treatment of corneal ulcers and herpetic keratitis. Cases associated with medial entropion should have surgical correction of the eyelid problem.

ULCERATIVE KERATITIS CAUSED BY CORNEAL PERFORATION (CAT FIGHT WOUNDS)**

Classical signs

- Acute very painful eye guarded with blepharospasm. Serous discharge, often containing blood.
- Very cloudy cornea usually with a linear wound or triangular tear that is plugged with fibrin.

Classical signs—Cont'd

- Collapsed anterior chamber with varying degrees of hyphema (blood) and protein.
- Iris prolapse may be seen as black bulge in the wound.
- If the wound has not sealed and is leaking aqueous humor, there will appear to be excessive amounts of tearing and the face will be wet.

Pathogenesis

Cat claw wounds are the most common cause of corneal perforation.

When the cornea is perforated the **anterior chamber collapses**. If the wound is large enough, the iris comes forward to plug the defect causing an **iris prolapse.**

An immediate prostaglandin reaction is set up within the eye, **causing leakage of protein** from the iris and ciliary body blood vessels.

The sudden decompression of the globe causes **hemorrhage in the anterior chamber**. The hemorrhage may also be caused by an injury to the iris by the penetrating claw.

The anterior lens capsule may be torn, causing **lens rupture**. This causes a severe antigenic reaction to the released lens proteins within the globe.

The wound is plugged by fibrin in cases where there is no iris prolpase. This forms a platform for fibroblasts to develop and the healing process in the wound is begun.

Secondary complications are common with anterior synechia (adhesion of iris to cornea) and posterior synechia (adhesion of iris to anterior lens capsule). This causes distortion of the pupil (dyscoria).

Secondary glaucoma may develop if the iridocorneal angle becomes obstructed.

Cats with ruptured lenses are at risk for developing an **intra-ocular sarcoma** (see The Cat With a Cloudy Eye, page 1276).

Clinical signs

Corneal perforations are severe corneal injuries that present as **ocular emergencies.** Cat claw injuries are the most common cause of corneal perforation, and there may be other evidence of skin wounds from the fight.

The perforated corneal lesion is usually with a **linear wound or triangular tear that is plugged with fibrin** surrounded by a **dense area of edema.** The injured cornea may be covered with a layer of fibrin.

The **eye is held tightly closed,** and cats with this injury will resist any handling of the eye.

There will be a **serous discharge** often tinged with fresh blood.

The **anterior chamber may be very shallow and the globe very soft.**

If the wound has not sealed and is leaking aqueous humor, the face will be wet and there will appear to be excessive amounts of tearing.

A black, bulging area in the wound is a sign of an **iris prolapse**. In lightly pigmented irises, the bulge may be brown in color.

Another sign of iris prolapse is a distorted pupil with the affected iris leaflet presenting towards the wound. This can only be visualized if the anterior chamber is not filled with blood.

Cats that have a penetrating corneal lesion should be **examined carefully for signs of lens rupture.** This can be very difficult to ascertain. An obvious tear in the anterior capsule may be seen in the pupil space if the pupil is not miotic, and the anterior chamber is not very cloudy or full of blood. Sometimes leakage of lens protein seen as **thick transparent jelly-like material** can be seen in the anterior chamber. However, if the tear in the lens capsule is under a small wound in the peripheral iris, it may be impossible to see. In such cases, watch for **intense uveitis that will not respond to therapy**. A cataract will form in the injured lens.

These cases need to be referred to a veterinary ophthalmologist whenever possible.

Iris prolapse may be difficult to differentiate from a descemetocele in cases that have a very painful eye.

Differential diagnosis

Keratomalacia (melting ulcer).
- A very cloudy cornea with soft gelatinous stroma covering a large area.

- Usually with history of previous ulcer, and is therefore not an acute injury.
- May be some hypopyon (protein and cells in the anterior chamber) present.

Descemetocele.
- Usually history of ulceration.
- The lesion is mostly axial (central) and there is rarely blood or protein in the anterior chamber.
- The globe is not soft and maintains normal to slightly lower IOP.
- The surrounding cornea is frequently quite healthy.

Treatment

If the corneal tear is small, near the limbus, and is well sealed with a fibrin plug, **conservative treatment** can be used.
- **Protect the cornea** with a third eyelid flap or temporary tarsorrhaphy.
- **Dilate the pupil with topical 1% atropine.**
- Use a **topical broad-spectrum antibiotic** drop and protect the eye from infection with **systemic broad-spectrum antibiotics. NEVER use an ointment** when there has been a penetrating corneal injury, as ointment bases that enter the anterior chamber will cause an intense and chronic foreign body uveitis.
- Cats with acute eye injuries should be given **systemic NSAIDs** to minimize the effects of an intra-ocular prostaglandin reaction.

Do not use topical corticosteroids when the cornea is ulcerated as this will predispose keratomalacia.

When there is a large tear or there is an iris prolapse, microsurgery is required to suture the cornea. The iris needs to be gently teased back into the anterior chamber, which should be flushed to remove blood and fibrin. Viscoelastic solutions are then used to space the anterior chamber, and the corneal deficit is sutured with interrupted 8/0 to 10/0 nylon or absorbable suture material. This is very specialized surgery that requires specialist training, magnification and specialized instrumentation.
- The pupil is then dilated with atropine, infection prevented with broad-spectrum topical and systemic antibiotics, and NSAIDs given to minimize inflammation.

If the lens has been ruptured, a **lensectomy** has to be performed. Remember that these cases may develop intra-ocular sarcoma at a later date, so owners must be warned of the danger.

Prognosis

Cases with no damage to the iris or lens have a good prognosis.

Cases with iris tears, prolapsed iris and ruptured lenses have a favorable to poor prognosis.

Glaucoma may be a sequela in cases with complications.

KERATITIS SECONDARY TO UVEITIS**

Classical signs
- Cloudy blue cornea and a red sclera/conjunctiva.
- +/− Keratic precipitates (mutton fat deposits) on cornea.
- A hypopyon (cloudiness) in the anterior chamber.

See the main reference on page 1259 for details (The Cat With a Cloudy Eye).

Clinical signs

The cat presents with a **cloudy blue cornea and injected red sclera and conjunctiva**.

The corneal cloudiness is caused by edema from compromised endothelial function.

Keratic precipitates (mutton fat deposits) may be present on the inferior endothelium of the cornea.

A **hypopyon (protein and white blood cells)** may be present in the anterior chamber, and evident as a cloudiness of the aqueous fluid.

The pupil will usually be **miotic** (constricted).

The cat will usually have a systemic disease such as **toxoplasmosis, cryptococcosis, FeLV, FIV or FIP or systemic mycoses**.

Diagnosis

A **tentative diagnosis is based on signs** of a red, cloudy eye and other classic signs of uveitis such as hypopyon and keratic precipitates.

Cats with acute uveitis need to be worked up for systemic diseases. The most common rule outs are toxoplasmosis, cryptococcosis, FeLV, FIV, FIP (in young cats) and systemic mycoses in North America.

EOSINOPHILIC KERATITIS*

Classical signs

- Irregular white to pinkish plaque on the cornea.
- Corneal edema and vascularization.
- +/− Similar conjunctival lesion.
- Unilateral or bilateral.
- Poor response to a variety of antibacterial agents.

Pathogenesis

The disease is thought to be **immune-mediated or an allergic response** peculiar to cats.

There is no age, sex or breed predisposition.

Eosinophilic keratitis is a **proliferative lesion** with an intense infiltration of inflammatory cells including plasma cells, lymphocytes, eosinophils and occasional histiocytes and mast cells. The corneal stroma shows edema and intense vascularization, both superficial and deep.

Insect bites from (insects) and food allergies have been documented as causes of this condition. It has also been suggested that this response may be an ocular form of the "Eosinophylic granuloma disease complex", particulary the linear granuloma response. See The Cat With Salivation (page 586).

Clinical signs

Signs **begin unilaterally**, but may become bilateral.

Seen as a cloudy, red cornea. This is a proliferative lesion producing **whitish to pink, plaque-like tissue** that may be covered by a thick white discharge.

The corneal epithelium is usually intact, but may show **patchy staining with fluorescein.** There is usually an **intense neovascularization** (superficial and deep) in chronic cases. There is varying degrees of edema, usually involving the entire cornea.

The conjunctiva is usually involved secondary to the cornea, and may present with a **similar white, proliferative plaque** and mucopurulent ocular discharge.

The third eyelid may also show proliferative lesions.

There is often a history of a **poor response to a variety of antibacterial agents.**

Diagnosis

There is usually a history of an **edematous, vascularized** cornea that will **not respond to antibiotic therapy**.

Clean the eye with saline or eye wash, and take a scraping of the lesion using a scalpel blade, spatula or cytology brush. Gently spread the tissue onto a glass microscope slide and stain with a Wright or Romanofski stain. The presence of **eosinophils is diagnostic**. If conjunctival lesions are present, preferably take a sample from the conjunctiva.

The use of cytology brushes on the cornea and conjunctiva will give the best results for examination of cell structure.

Small conjunctival biopsies can be submitted in formalin for histopathology. The presence of eosinophils is diagnostic. These may be easily taken by applying local anesthetic (preferably proxymetacaine) in the eye, and removing a small snip of conjunctiva from under the upper or lower eyelid with a fine pair of forceps and scissors.

Hematology may reveal a peripheral eosinophilia.

Differential diagnosis

Chronic ulcerative conjunctivitis.
- Ulcers that heal with proliferative granulation tissue are rare in the cat. However, chronic ulcers may present with intense vascularization and granulation of the stroma.
- Eosinophils will not be present in cytology of such lesions.

Keratomalacia (melting cornea).
- This is usually an acute corneal problem with severe edema and loss of stromal tissue forming a deep extensive ulcer. There is rarely vascularization. These lesions may be infected with

Pseudomonas aeruginosa, which can be cultured from the edge of the ulcer with a swab moistened in sterile saline.

Chronic herpetic keratitis.
- Chronic herpetic keratitis may present with a large irregular area of corneal scarring and mild superficial corneal vascularization, but the lesion usually has superficial ulceration and is not proliferative. The cornea rarely shows the same intense vascularization and edema seen in eosinophilic keratitis.
- There will be a history of poor response to antibiotic therapy.
- Cytology will not reveal eosinophils.
- PCR tests on conjunctival and corneal tissue may help to differentiate.

Neoplasia.
- Squamous cell carcinoma of the cornea has been seen, but it is a very rare condition in cats. The lesion is proliferative but there will not be much ocular discharge.
- Cytology or fine-needle biopsy will confirm this condition.

Treatment

The condition will rapidly respond to systemic corticosteroids dosed at 1 mg/kg q 12 h PO.

Topical prenisolone acetate 0.5 or 1% drops applied q 8–12 h are excellent providing there is no ulceration of the cornea.

If tips of the ears show alopecia, pruritis and crusting the condition may be caused by biting insects. Such cases have been documented in Queensland, Australia. These cats should be housed in conditions that are insect free to prevent reoccurrence.

Allergic states caused by diet have been implicated. **Dietary exclusion tests** may be useful to eliminate this as a cause. See "The Cat With Signs of Chronic Small Bowel Diarrhea" (page 739).

Prognosis

The prognosis is very favorable in cases that respond to corticosteroids. Corneal scarring may be a sequela after chronic keratitis.

The prognosis is improved if the cause of the allergic state can be found and controlled.

ULCERATIVE KERATITIS (NOT ASSOCIATED WITH SPECIFIC CORNEAL DISEASE OR CORNEAL PERFORATION)*

Classical signs

- Ocular pain with serous discharge, blepharospasm and photophobia.
- Varying degrees of corneal cloudiness.
- Very cloudy cornea with a soft gelatinous appearance (melting ulcers or keratomalacia).
- Black area within a cloudy cornea, and a thin, bulging membrane at the center (Descemetocele).
- Positive staining of the stroma with fluorescein dye, except where a Descemetocele is present.

Pathogenesis

Most ulcers that are not associated with a specific corneal disease state are caused by **corneal trauma**. Foreign bodies such as **grass seeds and thorns**, or **blunt trauma from motor vehicle** accidents are the most common causes of corneal trauma. Trauma may cause a superficial ulcer, a deep ulcer or penetrating wound.

Ulcers may **vary from a superficial loss of epithelium to a deep stromal defect.**

Corneal edema develops when there is loss of epithelium, because the stroma absorbs fluid causing the stromal matrix to swell.

A **Descemetocele** forms when there is **no stromal tissue present**, but Descemet's membrane is intact. In cats, Descemet's membrane is very elastic and can bulge considerably within the corneal defect.

Melting ulcers (keratomalacia) develop when the stromal tissue undergoes some form of **autolysis**. This may occur from **proteolytic enzymes** present in **damaged epithelial cells**, from enzymes produced by **neutrophils and macrophages** in the tear film, and **from**

bacteria especially *Pseudomonas* spp., which produce proteolytic enzymes.

Clinical signs

Eyes with ulceration are **invariably very painful**. Cats show serous ocular discharge, blepharospasm, photophobia and ocular guarding in severe injuries.

Ulcers stain **positive with fluorescein dye**. A very deep ulcer that has formed a **Descemetocele may not show any staining** because Descemet's membrane will not hold dye.

Examination of the cornea with magnification will show a deficit in the corneal surface due to loss of epithelium and stroma.

Corneal edema will be present in cases that have loss of epithelium, because fluid will be absorbed by the stromal matrix. This will show as a **cloudy cornea.** Edema may be focal, around the ulcer or diffuse when large ulcers are present.

A **Desemetocele** usually looks like a **thin, bulging membrane** in an area where there is a very deep ulcer. It may have a **black appearance** caused by a reflection from the pupil behind. It is usually a more **chronic condition** in the cat where there has been an ulcer for some time.

Cats with chronic ulcers often **do not show much inflammatory reaction** in the cornea. It is common to see chronic ulceration in cats with **no sign of neovascularization.**

Ulcers that develop into a **melting cornea** are devastating conditions that appear with a **rapidly developing cloudy edematous cornea that has a gelatinous soft appearance**. The eye is extremely painful and the threat of rupture is very high. They are often infected with *Pseudomonas* spp.

Diagnosis

There may be a **history of trauma or a cat fight**. The **diagnosis is made on clinical examination** by finding a painful eye showing a stromal deficit.

The ulcer will stain with fluorescein except in the case of a Descemetocele.

If the center of the ulcer is dark, and the area bulges, there may be a Descemetocele. Descemet's membrane is very elastic in cats and can bulge forward quite noticeably.

Where the cornea is soft and gelatinous, a **swab should be taken from the lesion** and sent to the laboratory for culture and sensitivity.

Perforating injuries are very painful, and show changes in the anterior chamber such as hyphema and protein leakage with fibrin, whereas non-perforating ulcers such as descemetocele rarely show changes in the anterior chamber.

Differential diagnosis

Herpetic keratitis.
- Usually appears as a superficial ulcer with an irregular appearance.
- PCR tests may be helpful to differentiate from chronic superficial ulceration.

Eosinophilic keratitis.
- This is a proliferative lesion, but the epithelium may be eroded with a positive fluorescein stain.
- Cytology should show the presence of eosinophils.

Iris prolapse (differential for descemetocele).
- An acute, very painful eye with cloudy cornea and usually hemorrhage in the anterior chamber. The eye will be soft and the anterior chamber shallow. The prolapsed iris tissue may be black or brownish in color depending on the degree of pigmentation in the iris. There may be a fibrin clot present over the iris, plugging the wound. The wound is usually linear in shape rather than oval to round as seen in ulcers.

Treatment

As a general rule, **eliminate the cause of the ulcer** and provide **protection for the cornea** using lubrication, appropriate antibiotics where necessary and surgical techniques to close and protect the eye.

Superficial epithelial erosions heal rapidly with minimal treatment. The use of antibiotics is not encouraged as they are rarely infected. **Support with artificial tear solutions** will make the eye more comfortable.

Corneas with deep ulcers that have stromal loss **need to be protected with surgical techniques** such as third eyelid flaps or temporary tarsorrhaphies (see references for texts that show details of these surgical techniques).

- **Antibiotics** are often used topically to prevent secondary infection. If the ulcer is infected, then appropriate antibiotics should be used after culture of a swab taken from the edge of the ulcer.
- **Artificial tear solutions** will lubricate the eye and make the cat feel more comfortable.
- **Atropine ophthalmic drops** (most commonly 1%) are used to dilate the pupil and to prevent ciliary muscle spasm. They should be used two to three times daily until the pupil is dilated, and daily thereafter (NOTE: atropine drops are very bitter and often make cats salivate profusely). For this reason 1% atropine ointment is often used, as the drug does not run down the tear duct as fast.

NEVER use topical corticosteroids when a corneal ulcer is present, as this will predispose to keratomalacia (melting ulcer).

BACTERIAL ULCERATIVE KERATITIS*

> ### Classical signs
>
> - Painful, edematous eye.
> - Mucopurulent discharge.
> - Cornea may have a soft gelatinous appearance (melting ulcer/keratomalacia).
> - Ulcers are not as well defined.
> - Anterior chamber, where visible may be cloudy.
> - Positive staining of the stroma with fluorescein dye, except where a descemetocele is present.

Pathogenesis

There are no specific primary bacterial conditions that affect the cornea in cats. **Infections are secondary to injury.**

Ulcers become infected secondarily, usually with *Streptococcus* spp. or *Staphylococcus* spp., which are the common pathogens associated with eye infections.

Pseudomonas infection may cause a "**melting ulcer**" (keratomalacia). The cornea loses definition and becomes quite soft and jelly-like. This is caused by **protease enzymes** secreted by the bacteria, and by self-digestion of stroma by enzymes secreted from dying epithelial cells and neutrophils and macrophages present in the ocular discharges.

Clinical signs

Signs are the same as for **ulcerative keratitis**

Eyes with bacterial ulceration may be much **more painful** than an eye with an uninfected ulcer. The **discharge** is likely to be **mucopurulent** rather than serous, and can be quite copious as there may be concurrent conjunctivitis.

Eyes are **photophobic** and there is guarding of the affected eye. Cats will resist handling of the eye.

Ulcers stain **positive with fluorescein dye**, except where a descemetocele is present.

Corneal edema will be much more obvious and intense when there is infection. The entire cornea may be quite cloudy and look very soft and jelly-like when there is a melting ulcer or keratomalacia. Ulcers are not as well defined.

When visible, **the anterior chamber may be cloudy**. Often there is **secondary uveitis** causing cloudiness of the anterior chamber, because protein and cells are excreted from the iris and ciliary body.

Ulcers that develop into a **melting cornea** are devastating conditions. They appear as a **rapidly developing cloudy edematous cornea that has a gelatinous soft appearance**. The eye is extremely painful, and the threat of rupture is very high. They are often infected with *Pseudomonas* spp.

Diagnosis

There may be a **history of trauma or a cat fight**. The **diagnosis is made on clinical examination** by finding a painful eye showing a stromal deficit.

The ulcer will stain with **fluorescein,** except in the case of a descemetocele.

Where the cornea is soft and gelatinous, a **swab should be taken from the lesion,** and sent to the laboratory for culture and sensitivity.

Cytology is useful to help choose immediate treatment. Using a Wrights stain, *Streptococcus* spp. and *Staphylococcus* spp. appear as single **cocci** or bunches of round, purple-staining cocci, free or in cells. One slide should also be stained with a Gram stain. *Pseudomonas* bacteria are seen as **rods**, and stain positively with a Gram stain.

Treatment

Infected ulcers need aggressive treatment.

As a general rule, **frequent use of appropriate antibiotic drops** is required every 15 min to hourly for at least 24 hours, followed by drops every 4 hours. Ointments can be used where there is no keratomalacia, and do not need to be used as frequently. **Superficial ulcers** heal rapidly and need less-frequent treatment.

- When an ulcer is infected, appropriate **antibiotics should be used based on culture** of a swab taken from the edge of the ulcer. If in doubt, use a broad-spectrum antibiotic that will control both Gram-positive and Gram-negative bacteria.
- Where a *Pseudomonas* **infection** is suspected or confirmed by laboratory analysis, the cat must be treated vigorously with **aminoglycoside** (commonly gentomycin or tobramycin in gentomycin-resistant cases) or **fluoroquinalone** (some generations such as flucloxacillin are effective) antibiotics **topically every 15 minutes to 1 hour** until the infection is controlled. They may also be used systemically but particular care should be used with aminoglycosides in cats, as they are ototoxic and nephrotoxic. Toxicity may occur from frequent topical use, so monitor cases carefully.

Corneas with deep ulcers that have stromal loss **need to be protected with surgical techniques** such as **third eyelid flaps or temporary tarsorrhaphies** (see references for texts that show details of these surgical techniques).

Artificial tear solutions will lubricate the eye and make the cat feel more comfortable.

Atropine ophthalmic drops (most commonly 1%) are used to dilate the pupil and to prevent ciliary muscle spasm. They should be used two to three times daily until the pupil is dilated, and daily thereafter (NOTE: atropine drops are very bitter and often make cats salivate profusely). For this reason 1% atropine ointment is often used, as the drug does not run down the tear duct as fast.

In cases where secondary uveitis is present, systemic treatment with NSAIDs at appropriate doses and systemic antibiotics are recommended.

NEVER use topical corticosteroids when a corneal ulcer is present, as this will predispose to keratomalacia (melting ulcer).

Prognosis

Prognosis is good in cases with simple superficial ulcers.

Prognosis is guarded if the entire cornea has keratomalacia, or if there is hypopyon and secondary uveitis.

BLUNT TRAUMA

Classical signs

- Painful, cloudy and red eye.
- Cornea may have superficial ulcer or be ruptured (usually around the limbus).
- Conjunctiva may be red from subconjunctival hemorrhage.
- The anterior chamber may be filled with blood (hyphema).
- Eye may be bulging (exophthalmos) from edema and hemorrhage in the orbit.

Pathogenesis

Blunt trauma causing corneal damage is usually the result of a **motor vehicle accident**.

Clinical signs

The blunt trauma may cause an **abrasion on the surface of the cornea,** usually with loss of epithelium. This is evident as positive staining with **fluorescein dye.**

Rupture of the cornea may be evident, and is **usually at the limbus** because this appears to be the area that is weakest and absorbs most of the force when the cornea is flattened inwards. The **iris may protrude from the wound** and is seen as **brownish pigmented tissue**.

Hemorrhage from iris root tears and ciliary body trauma is common with this type of injury, and is seen as **hyphema.**

Subcutaneous and scleral hemorrhage may also be present.

In cats with **orbital hemorrhage**, the eye will bulge forward (**exophthalmos**) and the cat may have difficulty closing the eye. **Rapid drying of the cornea** then occurs causing further loss of epithelium, which results in **severe ulceration**.

Diagnosis

Diagnosis is based on a **history of trauma**, and the **clinical appearance.** Typically there is a corneal ulcer or rupture, and hyphema with subcutaneous hemorrhage, with or without exophthalmos.

Ocular ultrasound is a useful tool when the anterior chamber cannot be visualized because of hyphema. Look for lens displacement and check if there is a normal scleral contour at the back of the eye. Vitreous hemorrhage is seen as a dark hyperechoic area between the lens and scleral contour.

Treatment

Superficial ulcers can be treated with lubrication using artificial tear solutions. If infection is present, a topical antibiotic drop or ointment may be used.

In cats with **limbal rupture,** treatment depends on whether there is iris prolapse or not. If there is a **simple tear without complication,** then the condition may be treated conservatively with **antibiotic drops, systemic NSAIDs and systemic broad-spectrum antibiotics. Do not use ointment** in cats with **corneal rupture,** as the ointment base may enter the eye and cause **severe uveitis.**

In cats with **limbal rupture complicated with iris prolapse, microsurgery** needs to be done to correct the iris prolapse and suture the corneo–scleral wound. If possible, referral to an ophthalmologist is encouraged. **Topical and systemic antibiotics** should be used in conjunction with a **systemic NSAID**.

Where **exophthalmos** is present, the eye must be closed with a **third eyelid flap** or preferably a **tarsorrhaphy**. Use nylon sutures in a mattress (preferably) or interrupted pattern through the middle of the eyelids.

Prognosis

For eyes with **superficial ulceration** and mild hyphema, the prognosis is very good.

Eyes with a **limbal rupture** have a good prognosis if the lesion is not very large and is not complicated with iris prolapse.

Eyes with **severe trauma** and hyphema, complicated by lens luxation or rupture and vitreous hemorrhage, have a poor prognosis.

Eyes with exophthalmos from orbital swelling and corneal desiccation, can develop **very deep and complicated ulcers** if not treated correctly.

NEUROTROPIC KERATITIS

Classical signs

- Chronic mild keratitis with superficial ulceration and superficial vascularization.
- Cornea looks dry and lusterless.
- Poor blink reflex or poor corneal reflex or both.

Pathogenesis

Cats that have **facial nerve damage** may have a **poor to absent blink reflex**. This results in drying of the cornea, as the tear film is not distributed over the cornea. The consequence is poor **epithelial health and superficial ulceration**.

Some cats cope well with paralyzed lids, as the third eyelid acts as a sweep to distribute tears over the cornea.

Cats with injury or infection affecting the **trigeminal nerve** may show complete **lack of corneal sensation** (reflex). When the cornea has no innervation, chronic keratitis may develop producing **superficial ulceration and neovascularization**.

Clinical signs

Neurotropic keratitis appears as a **chronically sore eye with poor blink reflex**. To test for this condition, gently touch the eyelids and they should automatically close if normal.

A **dry and lusterless cornea** with **superficial ulceration** and superficial neovascularization is typically seen.

Lack of eyelid closure or corneal sensation is evident. To test corneal sensation, use a thin piece of rolled cotton wool or a thread of cotton, and touch the cornea from the side of the eye. Try not to allow easy visualization of the test material, otherwise the animal will respond to the visual stimulus and not the touch stimulus. In a normal cornea, the eyelids should close immediately the cornea is touched.

Cases with corneal denervation have the same signs as those with lack of blink reflex. Even when the blink reflex is normal, and the tear film is normal, **if the cornea has no innervation** it will develop a **neurotropic keratitis**.

Diagnosis

A diagnosis is based on history and signs of **trauma or ear infection affecting the facial or trigeminal nerve**. Lack of corneal reflex or blink reflex is definitive.

Chronic keratitis which is usually mild, and accompanied by varying degrees of **superficial ulceration and vascularization**.

Differential diagnosis

Herpetic keratitis.
- These cases have superficial ulcers with neovascularization of varying degrees, but the blink and corneal reflex remains intact.

Treatment

Topical treatment with artificial tear solutions is of great benefit. The eyes need to be treated frequently for best results.

Temporary closure of the eyelids with a tarsorrhaphy is useful short term.

In chronic cases, the **eyelids may be permanently closed centrally to protect the cornea.** Refer to ophthalmology texts for surgical techniques.

Prognosis

Signs often **improve after a period of 3–6 months** when nerve function is improved or restored. Other cases need to be managed for life.

FLORIDA KERATOPATHY ("FLORIDA SPOTS")/MYCOBACTERIAL KERATITIS

Classical signs

- Focal gray-white opacities in the anterior stroma of the cornea.
- Usually affects both eyes.
- Only recognized in the southeastern USA.

Clinical signs

One, or more commonly both, **corneas have focal white to gray opacities** in the anterior stroma, varying in diameter from 1–8 mm in size.

The **condition is asymptomatic** as cats show no signs of ocular pain or irritation, and there is no associated inflammation in the cornea.

The condition has **only been described in the USA**, and is suspected to be **associated with infection.**
- **Rhinosporidium** was initially diagnosed from histological samples. However, ultrastructural examination of affected cornea showed vacuoles with amorphous material and **rod-like organisms characteristic of mycobacteria** that stain positively with Ziehl–Neelsen carbolfuchsin stain.

Diagnosis

A tentative diagnosis is based on geographical location and signs of a cornea with multiple focal opacities in the anterior stroma and the cat shows no irritation or inflammation.

A definitive diagnosis is based on histological findings.

Differential diagnosis

A focal lesion with **acid-fast bacilli** that progresses to form a fleshy white lesion has been described in the **northwest USA.**

Histology shows an inflammatory response with infiltration of neutrophils and mononuclear cells.

This lesion is said to resemble the skin lesion in **cat leprosy,** and is thought to be a different disease to "Florida spots".

Treatment

Treatment with antibiotics and corticosteroids does not alter the appearance of the lesions.

STROMAL DYSTROPHY OF MANX CATS

Classical signs

- Young Manx cats.
- Begins with stromal edema that progresses to a cornea filled with large bullae.

Clinical signs

Rare disease of young Manx cats. Cats present with an axial (central) **stromal edema** which progresses to diffuse corneal edema and a **thickened corneal stroma filled with bullae** (fluid-filled vesicles).

Affected cats become blind.

Histology demonstrates progressive disintegration of stromal collagen fibers which are replaced with fluid-filled vesicles. Eventually the epithelium separates from its basement membrane and ulceration occurs.

Diagnosis

A tentative diagnosis is based on the presentation of a young Manx cat with corneal edema.

A **definitive diagnosis** is based on **histopathology**.

Differential diagnosis

There is no similar condition seen in Manx cats.

Treatment

There is **no definitive treatment**, and cats will become blind.

If ulceration occurs, methods used to **protect the cornea** such as third eyelid flaps and tarsorrhaphies may keep the cat comfortable. Resolution of ulceration will be difficult, and conjunctival grafts may have to be used to seal the corneal defects.

ENDOTHELIAL DYSTROPHY

Classical signs

- Progressive corneal edema that eventually leads to blindness.

Clinical signs

Rare condition in **young (4-month-old) Domestic Shorthair cats**.

Endotheial dystrophy results in **progressive corneal edema seen as a cloudy blue cornea, which leads to blindness**.

The corneal **epithelium is intact**, and there is no staining with fluorescein dye.

If the anterior chamber can be examined, there is no sign of inflammation such as flare or hypopyon indicating the presence of protein and white blood cells.

The cause of the condition is not known, and no treatment is possible.

Diagnosis

A tentative diagnosis is based on the signs in a young cat of progressive corneal edema, no staining with fluorescein dye, and no history of trauma to the eye or inflammation.

There is **no definitive diagnosis.**

CALCIFIC DEGENERATION

Classical signs

- Linear deposit of calcium in the anterior stroma with a shiny, gritty appearance that may be vascularized.
- Rare condition associated with chronic herpetic keratitis.

Clinical signs

Calcific degeneration is seen as a **linear deposit of calcium in the anterior stroma,** known as a **band keratopathy.** The affected area has a shiny, gritty appearance and may be vascularized.

There will be a **history of herpes keratitis** with chronic ulceration and scarring of the cornea.

This is a rare condition in the cat.

Diagnosis

A **tentative diagnosis is based on signs** of a focal shiny, gritty lesion on the cornea associated with a chronic herpetic keratitis.

LYSOSOMAL STORAGE DISEASES WITH OPHTHALMIC MANIFESTATIONS

Classical signs

- A very rare condition in the cat.
- Young cats that develop progressive corneal opacity with a "ground glass" appearance.
- Usually neurological signs such as ataxia, muscular tremor and paralysis.

See the main reference on page 935 for details (The Cat With Ataxia Without Weakness).

Clinical signs

Signs begin in **young cats** around 3–6 months of age.

The **cornea develops a ground-glass appearance** that is seen as a corneal opacity. This is caused by vacuole formation in keratocytes and endothelial cells.

Affected cats usually have **neurological signs**, which include ataxia, muscular and head tremors, paralysis and hypermetria.

The retinal ganglion cells and cells in the inner nuclear layer can be affected with vacuole formation.

Diagnosis

A **tentative diagnosis is based** on the **clinical presentation** in a young cat with neurological signs and ocular signs such as corneal opacity.

A **definitive diagnosis** is made based on **histopathological examination** of neural tissue using specific staining techniques usually from tissues obtained at post mortem. A specialist pathologist will be needed to make the diagnosis.

Lysosomal storage diseases with ophthalmic manifestations include:
- GM 1 gangliosidosis.
- GM 2 gangliosidosis.
- Alpha mannosidosis.
- Mucopolysaccharidosis 1 (MPS1).
- Mucopolysaccharidosis 2 (MPS2).

RECOMMENDED READING

Barnett KC. A Color Atlas of Veterinary Ophthalmology. Wolfe Publishing Ltd, London, 1990.

Gelatt Kirk N (ed). Veterinary Ophthalmology, 2nd edn. Lea & Febiger, Philadelphia, 1991.

Gelatt Kirk N. Veterinary Ophthalmology, 3rd edn. Lippincott, Williams and Wilkins, Philadelphia, 1998.

Gelatt Kirk N. Essentials of Veterinary Ophthalmology. Lippincott Williams and Wilkins, Philadelphia, 2000.

Gelatt Kirk N. Color Atlas of Veterinary Ophthalmology. Lippincott Williams and Wilkins, Philadelphia, 2001.

Gelatt Kirk N, Gelatt J P. Handbook of Small Animal Ophthalmic Surgery, Vol. 1. Extraocular Procedures. Permagon Veterinary Handbook Series, Florida, 1994.

Gelatt Kirk N, Gelatt JP. Handbook of Small Animal Ophthalmic Surgery, Vol. 2. Intra-ocular Procedures. Permagon Veterinary Handbook Series, Florida, 1995.

Ketring KL, Glaze MB. Atlas of Feline Ophthalmology. Trenton, NJ, Veterinary Learning Systems, 1994.

Peiffer RL, Petersen-Jones S. Small Animal Ophthalmology, A Problem Oriented Approach, 3rd edn. Saunders, Philadelphia, 2001.

61. The cat with a cloudy eye

Richard IE Smith

KEY SIGNS

- Cloudiness of the cornea, anterior chamber, lens or vitreous.

MECHANISM

- A cloudy eye is usually caused by a change in the transparency of the clear structures of the eye.

WHERE?

- Cornea.
- Anterior chamber.
- Lens.
- Vitreous.

WHAT?

- The most common causes of a cloudy eye are diseases that cause edema or scarring of the cornea, and uveitis, which causes cloudiness in the aqueous humor and/or vitreous as a result of protein and cells leaking through inflamed uveal blood vessels. Hereditary cataract (opacity of the lens) is rare in cats, but cataracts may develop secondary to uveitis. Nuclear sclerosis is a common cause of lens cloudiness in old cats.

QUICK REFERENCE SUMMARY

Diseases causing a cloudy eye

WHERE?

CORNEA

DEGENERATIVE

- **Corneal sequestrum (feline keratitis nigrum)** (p 1260)**
Presents with an axial (central) area of staining (light brown to black) in the cornea, and is usually unilateral. Most common in brachycephalic breeds such as Persians and Himalayans. Approximately 80% are associated with herpetic keratitis. In the early stages there is no ulceration, but chronic lesions may have ulcerated borders surrounded by an inflammatory zone with intense vascularization.

ANOMALY

- Corneal (stromal) dystrophy of Manx cats (p 1264)

A rare condition in young Manx cats that starts with axial stromal edema and progresses to a diffuse corneal edema with a thickened stroma full of bullae (fluid-filled vesicles). It is a blinding corneal disease with no treatment possible.

INFLAMMATION/INFECTIOUS

- **Feline herpesvirus-1 keratitis*** (p 1259)**

Cats may have a history of FHV-1 infection as kittens. Often appears as a unilateral disease in older cats. The epithelium may show dendritic lesions (finger-like projections of thickened epithelium that stain with rose bengal stain) in early cases. Chronic cases show irregular (geographic) ulceration to the level of the superficial stroma. Scarring and vascularization of the cornea follows after repeated inflammatory episodes.

- Mycobacterial keratitis ("Florida spots") (p 1264)

Focal grayish opacities seen in the stroma caused by a mycobacterium. Only seen in the southeast USA.

INFLAMMATORY/NON-INFECTIOUS

- **Ulcerative keratitis* (p 1262)**

A very painful, cloudy eye with serous discharge, blepharospasm and photophobia. Usually occurs secondary to corneal trauma. Superficial ulcers have loss of epithelium, which is seen as an erosion of the surface, and stains green with fluorescein dye. Deeper ulcers have a hollow caused by loss of stroma.

Immune-mediated:

- **Eosinophilic keratitis* (p 1261)**

Seen as a cloudy, red cornea, sometimes with a muco-purulent discharge. A proliferative white to pinkish plaque develops on the cornea, with superficial and in chronic cases, deep vascularization. Usually a history of poor response to antibiotic therapy. Eosinophils demonstrated on cytology from corneal scrapings are diagnostic.

Trauma:

- **Cornea scarring from injury* (p 1263)**

Opaque areas on cornea, which vary in size and intensity. There is no pain or discharge associated with these opacities, and usually there is a history of previous severe ocular inflammation or trauma.

WHERE?

ANTERIOR CHAMBER

METABOLIC

- Lipemic aqueous (p 1270)

The anterior chamber looks milky, but intra-ocular architecture can be visualized. Signs may be unilateral or bilateral, and may have a sudden onset. Occurs secondary to anterior uveitis in cats on a high-fat diet, or is associated with hyperlipidemia. Idiopathic in Burmese cats.

continued

continued

NEOPLASTIC

● Ocular neoplasia* (p 1267)

Most cases present as anterior uveitis with corneal edema and a cloudy aqueous, and have some form of swelling seen in the iris, which may cause distortion of the pupil (dyscoria). The retina may be distorted and have a color change. Lymphosarcoma is the most common tumor and often presents as bilateral iris swelling with a "creamy" color change, and anterior chamber hypopyon and/or hemorrhage in a young cat, with or without other signs suggesting multicentric neoplasia. The pupil may be distorted (dyscoria).

INFLAMMATION/INFECTIOUS

● Feline leukemia virus* (p 1266)

FeLV may present as a cloudy aqueous associated with white cells and fibrin in the eye caused by a uveitis. Changes to iris appearance and abnormal pupil size and shape occur. It may or may not be associated with lymphosarcoma.

● Feline infectious peritonitis (p 1266)

Ocular form usually occurs in cats 6–12 months old. Ocular signs may be unilateral or bilateral. Typically there is fibrinous anterior uveitis and hypopyon, and initially no systemic signs. Advanced cases show serous retinal detachment and may have neurological signs.

● *Toxoplasma gondii* (toxoplasmosis)** (p 1265)

Most common sign is a cloudy anterior chamber from anterior uveitis and hypopyon. Older cats may develop small translucent nodules in the iris from lymphocytic–plasmocytic uveitis. Advanced cases may develop serous retinal detachment. Occasionally systemic signs are present including fever, weight loss, and respiratory, neurological and hepatic signs.

● *Cryptococcus neoformans* (cryptococcosis) (p 1268)

Usually presents as anterior uveitis with a cloudy aqueous secondary to leakage of white cells and protein. Examination of the retina shows focal granulomas with a cloudy vitreous. Blindness occurs in advanced cases.

● Other systemic fungal infections (*Blastomyces dermatitidis, Candida albicans, Coccidioides immitis, Histoplasma capsulatum*) (p 1268)

Typically there is a cloudy aqueous secondary to white cells and protein leaking into eye from anterior uveitis. Pre-iridal fibrovascular membranes are seen in chronic cases. Hemorrhage is associated with the PFIMs. Retinal hemorrhage is seen occasionally in areas of granuloma formation and appears as focal cloudy swelling in the retina.

WHERE?

LENS

DEGENERATIVE

● Nuclear sclerosis and senile cataract** (p 1271)

In nuclear sclerosis, the central part of the lens (nucleus) becomes slightly cloudy but the cat is still visual. Sclerosis is a normal aging process that starts from 8 years and becomes progressively cloudier with age. Senile cataract is seen in much older cats from 12–20 years of age. Nuclear cells finally break down so the nucleus becomes very cloudy and vision deteriorates. The lens cortex may also start to degenerate resulting in cortical changes in addition to nuclear changes.

METABOLIC

- Diabetic cataract (p 1273)

Rare finding in aged diabetic cats. Lens is cloudy with an immature to mature cataract and impaired vision.

INFLAMMATION/INFECTIOUS

• Cataract secondary to infectious uveitis** (p 1271)

The lens becomes very cloudy because of a cortical cataract developing from poor nutrition and toxic states within the eye. Signs of uveitis are present such as a cloudy eye due to aqueous flare and fibrovascular membranes on the iris (PFIMs).

INFLAMMATION/NON-INFECTIOUS

- Cataract secondary to non-infectious uveitis (p 1273)

Nuclear cataract in a young healthy cat with no evidence of ocular inflammation. Rare.

Trauma:

• Cataract secondary to lens trauma* (p 1272)

Penetrating injuries that rupture the lens capsule will disrupt normal lens physiology and cause cataract development. This causes an acute uveitis from the released lens proteins within the eye (lens-induced uveitis). Blunt trauma to the eye may also rupture the lens. A tentative diagnosis is based on a history or signs of eye trauma and the presence of a mature or immature cataract.

WHERE?

VITREOUS

METABOLIC

• Cloudy vitreous associated with systemic hypertension*** (p 1274)

Vitreous may appear cloudy due to detached retina bulging into vitreous. Hemorrhage occurs into the vitreous from ruptured retinal blood vessels. Seen in older cats with a history of sudden blindness. Common secondary to chronic renal disease or hyperthyroidism.

NEOPLASTIC

- Feline intra-ocular sarcoma (p 1276)

Affected cats range from 7–15 years of age and have a history of prior ocular trauma. Cats present with signs of anterior uveitis and may show glaucoma and white to pink masses in the vitreous, if it can be visualized.

INFLAMMATION/INFECTIOUS

• Feline immune deficiency virus* (p 1275)

FIV infection causes pars planitis which is a "Snowbank" inflammation of the pars plana and thought to be almost pathognomonic for FIV infection. It results in a cloudy vitreous.

INTRODUCTION

MECHANISM?

The eye is an organ with various media that normally maintain **clarity for transmission of light** by very specialized means.

- The **corneal stoma** maintains optical clarity by the highly organized structure of the collagen fibrils, lack of blood vessels and lack of pigment.
- The **lens fibers** (cells) are also laid down in a very orderly fashion and contain soluble lens proteins known as crystallins.
- The **aqueous humor** is a clear fluid secreted by the ciliary body to maintain the anterior chamber.
- The **vitreous is a complex, transparent living tissue** made mainly from complex carbohydrates.

Cloudiness of the eye results from changes in structure and composition of the cornea, aqueous (anterior chamber), lens or vitreous (posterior chamber).

Cloudy cornea

For details on the structure and function of the cornea see "The Cat With Abnormalities Confined to the Cornea" (page 1236).

The **cornea becomes cloudy from edema** when the surface develops an **ulcer** (**ulcerative keratitis**). Loss of epithelial cells allows the stroma to absorb fluid. This causes the intercellular matrix to swell, which in turn, disrupts the normal pattern of the keratocytes and the cornea becomes cloudy.

Corneal edema is also seen in cases of glaucoma and uveitis where the endothelial pump mechanism is disturbed, so that aqueous enters the stroma from the anterior chamber.

Inflammatory conditions in the cornea cause cloudiness by disrupting the normal cellular matrix, either with cellular infiltrates or by changing the normal cellular structure, such as scar tissue formation.

Cloudy anterior chamber

The anterior chamber is a **fluid-filled compartment bounded by the cornea anteriorly and the lens and ciliary body posteriorly**.

The fluid is called aqueous humor and is produced by a process of ultrafiltration and active secretion in the ciliary body. Aqueous exits the anterior chamber through the trabecular meshwork in the iridocorneal angle to reach the vascular system via the scleral vessels. The dynamics of aqueous humor production and drainage is very complex, but simply, it keeps the eye inflated at a predetermined pressure known as the intra-ocular pressure (IOP). **Interference of aqueous drainage causes glaucoma**. The increased intra-ocular pressure disturbs the corneal physiology resulting in corneal edema and a cloudy eye. See "The Cat with Abnormal Globe Position or Size" (page 1312).

Aqueous is a clear fluid that also supplies nutrients to the inner structures of the eye. When the anterior uveal tract (ciliary body and iris) becomes inflamed this is called **anterior uveitis**. Inflammation of the vascular-rich uveal tract causes the blood vessels to leak protein and white blood cells into the aqueous causing "**aqueous flare**". Accumulations of protein and white blood cells may form opaque clots known as "**hypopyon**". This causes a cloudy anterior chamber. See "The Cat With Abnormal Iris Appearance" (page 1294).

At the same time, anterior uveitis disturbs the endothelial pump mechanism, allowing aqueous to enter the stroma. This causes edema of the cornea seen as a cloudy eye.

Cloudy lens

A **cloudy lens** is seen when the lens develops a **cataract**.

A cataract is defined as an opacity of the lens. Lens fibers become opaque when they are no longer viable. A cataract is classified according to the position in the lens, and according to whether it is immature or mature.

The lens consists of an anterior and posterior capsule on the outer surface of the cortex. The central part of the lens is known as the nucleus. The lens is suspended by fibers known as zonules, which extend from the equator (outer circumference) of the lens to the ciliary processes. Lens cells are known as lens fibers and are continually produced from the lens epithelium, which is most active at the equator.

The lens has no blood supply, and therefore relies on the nutrients in the aqueous humor and the vitreous for its nutritional requirements. Disturbance to the nutrition of the lens will result in death of lens fibers and development of a cataract.

Genetic cataract is rare in the cat.

Most cataracts in cats are secondary to disease processes within the eye such as uveitis or neoplasia.

Lens fibers in the nucleus become slightly opaque with age. This is known as **nuclear sclerosis** and may be seen from about 8 years of age. This is not a true cataract as the fibers are viable and the eye is usually visual. With age, the nuclear fibers may die, so nuclear sclerosis may develop into a nuclear cataract.

Cloudy vitreous

The vitreous is a living tissue (mainly mucopolysaccharide; also called glycosaminoglycans) that fills the space between the retina, ciliary body and lens.

Inflammation or hypertension of the inner retinal blood vessels will allow protein and white/red blood cells to leak into the vitreous causing "**vitreous flare**". This may present as a cloudy eye behind the pupil.

Inflammation of the choroid (posterior uvea) leads to leakage of protein and blood cells into the outer retinal space leading to a serous retinal detachment. **Retinal detachment** can present as a cloudy eye behind the pupil.

Vitreous degeneration is rare in the cat.

WHERE?

Disease affecting the **cornea, anterior chamber, lens or vitreous** may result in a cloudy eye.

Decide which of the media have become cloudy and go to that part of the text for greater detail.

WHAT?

Cloudiness of cornea, anterior chamber, lens or vitreous may be caused by:
- **Infiltrates of inflammatory cells** or infusion of **tissue fluid** (edema), which produces swelling of the corneal stroma, will result in a cloudy cornea.
- **Alteration of the cellular matrix in** the **cornea and lens** causes a change in the refractive index, because of changed chemical properties of these

structures. For example, the change in the structure of the crystallins in the lens results in cataract formation.
- **Accumulation of protein and cells** in the aqueous humor causes a cloudy aqueous called hypopyon.
- On rare occasions **lipid** may be seen in the **aqueous (aqueous lipid)** forming a very cloudy eye.
- **Leakage of cells and protein** into the vitreous from inflammation of the ciliary body and/or choroid causes a cloudy vitreous.

The most common causes of corneal cloudiness are from **inflammation** associated with herpesvirus keratitis or eosinophilic keratitis, or from **trauma** resulting in edema, cellular infiltrates, ulcerative keratitis, and/or scarring or corneal sequestrum.

The most common causes of anterior chamber cloudiness are **inflammation** from **infectious agents** such as *Toxoplamsa gondii, Cryptococcus*, other systemic fungi, feline infectious peritonitis virus, feline leukemia virus or from **neoplasia**.

The most common causes of lens cloudiness are from **nuclear sclerosis** or **cataract** secondary to **infectious uveitis or trauma**.

The most common cause of posterior chamber cloudiness is from systemic hypertension.

DISEASES CAUSING A CLOUDY CORNEA

FELINE HERPESVIRUS-1 KERATITIS***

Classical signs
- FHV-1 keratitis is primarily a disease of older cats.
- Frequently unilateral but may be bilateral.
- Shallow irregular ulceration (geographic ulcer) often with superficial vascularization and edema.
- History of acute episodes followed by quiescent periods.

See main references on pages 1212, 1237 for details (The Cat With Ocular Discharge or Changed Conjunctival Appearance, The Cat With Abnormalities Confined to the Cornea) and page 7 (The Cat With Acute Sneezing or Nasal Discharge).

Clinical signs

Herpesvirus is one of the most common causes of acute and chronic corneal disease in older cats.

Acute primary infection with herpesvirus may result in the following signs:
- **Conjunctival hyperemia** and serous ocular discharge that becomes purulent by days 5–7 of infection.
- Mild to moderate **chemosis and blepharospasm**.
- Non-specific **upper respiratory signs** such as sneezing and serous nasal discharge.
- Fine-branching (microdendritic) **corneal lesions** may be seen, especially if the cornea is stained with rose bengal. They result from the direct cytopathic effect of the virus, and are finger-like projections of epithelium.

Symblepharon formation with adhesion of conjunctiva to conjunctiva and conjunctiva to cornea may follow severe inflammation especially in young kittens.

Recrudescent infections may show any of the following signs:
- Dendritic ulcers.
- Corneal sequestrum.
- Superficial indolent epithelial ulcers.
- Serous ocular discharge.
- Stromal edema and scarring.

FHV-1 keratitis is primarily a disease of older cats.

Frequently unilateral but may be bilateral.

A large shallow ulcer with an irregular shape that appears to look like a continent or land mass (**geographic ulcer**) may be evident, and is often associated with superficial vascularization. It is the result of an immune response to viral antigen. There may be edema and in chronic cases scarring with calcific degeneration (calcium deposition in the anterior stroma).

Typically there is a history of **acute episodes followed by quiescent periods**, but close examination will reveal a slightly cloudy, scarred cornea.

Diagnosis

A **tentative diagnosis** is usually based on the **clinical signs.**

A **definitive diagnosis** requires specific techniques, which are available from some la oratories. These are used infrequently and vary in their sensitivity. PCR is the most useful of these.
- **Cytological examination** of corneal/conjunctival smears stained with immunoperoxidase may demonstrate intranuclear inclusions in epithelial cells in some acute primary infections, but is not very reliable.
- **Immunofluorescence** using direct or indirect fluorescent antibody techniques on corneal/conjunctival smears or tissue sections may demonstrate the virus, but has poor sensitivity.
- **Virus isolation** is the gold standard for detection, but is not often used because of logistical difficulties in getting rapid results. It depends on demonstration of cytopathic effects of the virus in cell culture.
- **Serological techniques** are not very useful because antibody titers tend to be of low magnitude after primary infection sometimes reaching only 1:64 at 60 days after infection. High titers are rarely seen after recrudescent infection.
- **Polymerase chain reaction (PCR)** testing depends on DNA amplification of an amino acid sequence of the thymidine kinase gene, and is perhaps the most sensitive test available. Theoretically the test could pick up one strand of viral DNA. High sensitivity in nested PCR tests may reduce specificity by the detection of non-viral DNA contaminants.

CORNEAL SEQUESTRUM (FELINE KERATITIS NIGRUM)**

> ### Classical signs
>
> - Area of pigmented cornea varying from a very light coffee-colored stain to an intense thick black plaque.
> - +/– Blepharospasm and photophobia.
> - Predominantly in brachycephalic breeds such as Persians and Himalayans.
> - Usually unilateral.

See the main reference on page 1234 (The Cat With Abnormalities Confined to the Cornea).

Clinical signs

The classic presentation is an **area of pigmented cornea**. The degree of pigmentation varies from a very light **coffee-colored stain to an intense thick black plaque**.

Approximately 80% are associated with herpetic keratitis. There may be a **history of previous infection with FHV-1** as a kitten, or later in life, with herpetic keratitis. However, cases may develop after corneal ulceration or from medial entropion.

The disease is initially seen **unilaterally**, but eventually both eyes may become involved.

Initially the cat may not show any signs of discomfort, but as the lesion progresses **blepharospasm and photophobia develop**.

Early, light-staining lesions have an intact epithelium and do not stain with fluorescein. Lesions that have developed a dense plaque may have a **fine ring of ulceration** surrounding the lesion, which may stain positive with fluorescein.

In mild cases, the surrounding cornea will not show signs of edema or vascularization, but as the degree of degeneration progresses, **corneal edema with marked deep stromal vascularization** may be prominent.

Eyes that have a faint stain usually do not have any ocular discharge. Eyes that have a dark plaque with surrounding ulceration and intense corneal vascularization often have a **mucopurulent ocular discharge**.

The condition is seen in any breed of cat, but it occurs predominantly in **brachycephalic breeds such as Persians and Himalayans**. There is no sex or age predilection.

Diagnosis

A tentative diagnosis is based on the **signalment and clinical signs**. Typically there is a mild brown-staining cornea to a dense black plaque with keratitis.

A definitive diagnosis is based on **histopathological examination of resected cornea**. There is a typical pattern of degenerated stroma surrounded by a ring of inflammatory cells.

PCR tests on resected cornea may confirm the presence of FHV-1 infection.

EOSINOPHILIC KERATITIS*

Classical signs

- Irregular white to pinkish plaque on the cornea.
- Corneal edema and vascularization.
- +/– Similar conjunctival lesion.
- Unilateral or bilateral.
- Poor response to a variety of antibacterial agents.

See the main reference on page 1245 (The Cat With Abnormalities Confined to the Cornea).

Clinical signs

Signs **begin unilaterally**, but may become **bilateral**.

Seen as a **cloudy, red cornea**. This is a **proliferative lesion** producing **whitish to pink, plaque-like tissue** that may be covered by a thick white discharge.

The corneal epithelium is usually intact, but may show **patchy staining with fluorescein**. There is usually an **intense neovascularization** (superficial and deep) in chronic cases. There are varying degrees of edema, usually involving the entire cornea.

The **conjunctiva** is usually involved secondary to the cornea, and may present with a **similar white, proliferative plaque** and mucopurulent ocular discharge.

The third eyelid may also show proliferative lesions.

There is often a history of a **poor response to a variety of antibacterial agents**.

Diagnosis

A tentative diagnosis is based on the history of an **edematous, vascularized cornea** that will not respond to antibiotic therapy.

Clean the eye with saline or eye wash and take a scraping of the lesion using a scalpel blade, spatula or cytology brush. Gently spread the tissue onto a glass microscope slide and stain with a Wright or Romanofski stain. **The presence of eosinophils is diagnostic**. If conjunctival lesions are present, preferably take a sample from the conjunctiva.

Small conjunctival biopsies can be submitted in formalin for histopatholgy. The presence of eosinophils is diagnostic.

Hematology may reveal a peripheral eosinophilia.

Treatment

The condition will **rapidly respond to systemic corticosteroids** dosed at 1 mg/kg daily.

If the tips of the ears show alopecia, pruritis and crusting, the condition may be caused by biting insects. Such cases have been documented in Queensland, Australia. In such cases the cats must be housed in conditions that are insect free.

Allergic states caused by diet have been implicated. Dietary elimination tests may be useful to exclude this as a cause (see The Cat With Signs of Large Bowel Disease (page 766), The Cat With Abnormalities Confined to the Cornea (page 1246), The Cat With Miliary Dermatitis (page 1030), The Pruritic Cat Without Miliary Dermatitis (page 1046).

Try to minimize known causes of allergy such as insect bites by fleas and mosquitoes. Where there is a dietary component involved maintain cat on a **low-antigen diet**.

ULCERATIVE KERATITIS*

Classical signs

- Severe pain with serous discharge, blepharospasm and photobia.
- Variable severity from a superficial epithelial erosion to a deep stromal ulcer followed by a Descemetocele.
- Positive staining of the stroma with fluorescein dye, except where a Descemetocele is present.
- Varying degrees of corneal edema seen as a cloudy cornea. Corneal perforation is surrounded by a dense area of edema with a dark brown or black center if the iris has prolapsed into the corneal wound. A layer of fibrin may cover the injured cornea.

See the main reference on page 1242 (The Cat With Abnormalities Confined to the Cornea).

Clinical signs

There may be **evidence of the underlying cause**. Most ulcers that are not associated with a specific corneal disease are caused by **corneal trauma. Foreign bodies such as grass seeds and thorns**, or blunt trauma from **motor vehicle accidents** are the most common causes of corneal trauma. Trauma may cause a superficial ulcer, a deep ulcer or penetrating wound.

Eyes with ulceration are invariably **very painful**. Cats show serous **ocular discharge, blepharospasm**, photophobia and ocular guarding in severe injuries.

Ulcers stain positive with fluorescein dye. A very deep ulcer that has formed a Descemetocele may not show any staining because **Descemet's membrane will not stain with fluorescein**.

Examination of the cornea with magnification will show a deficit in the corneal surface because of loss of epithelium and stroma.

Corneal edema will be present in cases that have loss of epithelium, because fluid will be absorbed by the stromal matrix. This will show as a cloudy cornea. Edema may be focal around the ulcer, or diffuse when large ulcers are present.

Penetrating injuries are common after **cat fights**. They present with a perforation of the cornea surrounded by a dense area of edema and swelling. A **fibrin plug** may be present in the corneal wound. If the iris has prolapsed into the wound, the center of the perforation will be dark brown or black in color. The anterior chamber may be collapsed and contain blood (hyphema) and fibrin.

Perforating injuries that are not sealed by fibrin and/or iris, will **leak aqueous** so the cat will have a very wet eye and face.

Diagnosis

There may be a **history of trauma** or a **cat fight**. The diagnosis of ulcerative keratitis is based on clinical signs of a painful eye showing a stromal deficit.

The ulcer will **stain with fluorescein** except in the case of a Descemetocele. If the center of the ulcer is dark, and the area bulges, there may be a Descemetocele. Descemet's membrane is very elastic in cats and can bulge forward quite noticeably.

Perforating injuries are very painful and show **changes in the anterior chamber** such as hyphema and protein leakage with fibrin.

Treatment

As a general rule, **eliminate the cause of the ulcer** and provide **protection for the cornea** using lubrication, appropriate antibiotics where necessary and surgical techniques to close and protect the eye.

Superficial epithelial erosions heal rapidly with minimal treatment. The use of antibiotics is not encouraged as they are rarely infected. **Support with artificial tear solutions** will make the eye more comfortable.

Corneas with deep ulcers that have stromal loss **need to be protected with surgical techniques** such as third eyelid flaps or temporary tarsorrhaphies (see references for texts that show details of these surgical techniques).

- **Antibiotics** are often used topically to prevent secondary infection. If the ulcer is infected, then appropriate antibiotics should be used after culture of a swab taken from the edge of the ulcer.
- **Artificial tear solutions** will lubricate the eye and make the cat feel more comfortable.
- **Atropine ophthalmic drops** (most commonly 1%) are used to dilate the pupil and to prevent ciliary muscle spasm. They should be used two to three times daily until the pupil is dilated, and daily thereafter (NOTE: atropine drops are very bitter and often make cats salivate profusely). For this reason 1% atropine ointment is often used, as the drug does not run down the tear duct as fast.

Where a *Pseudomonas* infection is suspected or confirmed by laboratory analysis, the cat must be treated vigorously with **aminoglycoside** (commonly gentomycin or tobramycin in gentomycin-resistant cases) or fluoroquinalone (some generations such as flucloxacillin are effective) antibiotics **topically every 15 minutes to 1 hour** until the infection is controlled. They may also be used systemically but particular care should be used with aminoglycosides in cats as they are ototoxic and nephrotoxic. Toxicity may occur from frequent topical use, so monitor cases carefully.

NEVER use topical corticosteroids when a corneal ulcer is present, as this will predispose to keratomalacia (melting ulcer).

If there is a **penetrating corneal lesion**, examine the eye carefully for signs of **iris prolapse and lens rupture**. These cases need to be referred to a veterinary ophthalmologist whenever possible.

- If there is a **corneal tear that is well sealed with a fibrin plug**, protect the cornea with a third eyelid flap or **temporary tarsorrhaphy**. Dilate the pupil with atropine and use a **topical broad-spectrum antibiotic** drop. **NEVER use an ointment** when there has been a penetrating corneal injury, because ointment bases that enter the anterior chamber will cause an intense and chronic foreign body uveitis. Animals with acute eye injuries should be given **systemic NSAIDs** to minimize the effects of an intra-ocular prostaglandin reaction. The eye should also be protected from infection with **systemic broad-spectrum antibiotics**.

When there is an **iris prolapse, microsurgery is required** to suture the cornea. The iris needs to be gently teased back into the anterior chamber, and the chamber flushed to remove blood and fibrin. **Viscoelastic solutions** are then used to space the anterior chamber, and the corneal deficit is sutured with interrupted 8/0 to 10/0 nylon or absorbable suture material. This is very specialized surgery that requires specialist training, magnification and specialized instrumentation. The pupil is then dilated with atropine, infection prevented with broad-spectrum topical and systemic antibiotics and NSAIDs given to minimize inflammation.

CORNEAL SCARRING FROM INJURY*

Classical signs

- Range from faint cloudiness of the superficial stroma to dense opacity.
- Variable position, size, shape and density of scar.
- History of previous severe inflammation or trauma.

Pathogenesis

Scarring may be secondary to **disease processes or trauma**.

Scars form secondary to stromal damage. When stroma is infected or lost from ulceration, **keratocytes metaplase into fibrocytes**.

Corneal healing is achieved by **epithelial regeneration and stromal repair**.

Epithelial regeneration occurs by:
- Sliding of cells to cover the surface.
- Mitosis to reconstruct the layers.

Stromal repair occurs via avascular and vascular healing.
- **A vascular healing** occurs in small uncomplicated wounds and involves:
  - Infiltration of neutrophils from the tear film and limbal blood vessels.
  - Macrophages invade, and digest the cellular debris.
  - Keratocytes transform to fibrocytes that migrate into the damaged area.
  - Collagen fibrils are laid down in an irregular pattern that disrupts the corneal transparency.
- **Vascular healing** occurs when there is extensive stromal loss.
  - Cellular infiltration is more extensive.
  - Blood vessels invade from the limbus.
  - **Granulation tissue forms** and this heals in a dense scar.

Clinical signs

Scars present as **cloudy areas on the cornea**. Superficial scarring of the cornea is seen as a faint cloudiness of the superficial stroma. Dense opacity is seen with deep scars that involve the deep layers of the cornea.

Scars **vary considerably in position, size, shape and density** depending on the depth and area of corneal stroma that has been damaged.

Usually there is **no inflammation in the affected eye**.

Vision is always affected by corneal scarring.

Diagnosis

A diagnosis is based on **clinical findings and history**. Typically the cornea has cloudy areas of varying density, there is no positive staining with fluorescein, and the eye has no sign of inflammation, pain or discharge.

Usually, there is **a history of previous severe inflammation or trauma**, with healing of the cornea.

MYCOBACTERIAL KERATITIS (FLORIDA SPOTS)

Classical signs

- An asymptomatic keratitis recognized in the southeastern USA.
- The cornea has focal gray-white opacities in the anterior stroma, varying in diameter from 1–8 mm in size.
- The lesions usually affect both eyes.

See the main reference on page 1251 (The Cat With Abnormalities Confined to the Cornea).

Clinical signs

One, or more commonly, both **corneas have focal white to gray opacities** in the anterior stroma.

The **condition is asymptomatic**, as cats show no signs of ocular pain or irritation, and there is no associated inflammation in the cornea.

The condition has only been described in the USA.

Diagnosis

A **tentative diagnosis** is based on **clinical signs** – multiple focal opacities in the anterior stroma of the cornea, not associated with irritation or inflammation.

Rhinosporidium was initially diagnosed from histological samples. However, ultrastructural examination of affected cornea showed vacuoles with amorphous material and **rod-like organisms** characteristic of **mycobacteria** that stain positively with Ziehl–Neelsen carbolfuchsin stain.

CORNEAL (STROMAL) DYSTROPHY OF MANX CATS

Classical signs

- Young Manx cats.
- Begins with stromal edema that progresses to a cornea filled with large bullae.
- Eventually causes blindness.

See the main reference on page 1252 (The Cat With Abnormalities Confined to the Cornea).

Clinical signs

Rare disease of young Manx cats. Cats present with an axial (central) **stromal edema** which progresses to diffuse corneal edema and a thickened corneal stroma filled with **bullae (fluid-filled vesicles)**.

Affected cats become **blind**.

Diagnosis

A tentative diagnosis is based on the presentation of a **young Manx cat with corneal edema**.

A **definitive diagnosis** is based on histopathology.
- **Histology** demonstrates **progressive disintegration of stromal collagen fibers,** which are replaced with fluid-filled vesicles. Eventually the epithelium separates from its basement membrane and ulceration occurs.

DISEASES CAUSING A CLOUDY ANTERIOR CHAMBER

TOXOPLASMA GONDII (TOXOPLASMOSIS)**

Classical signs

- Cloudy anterior chamber from anterior uveitis is the most common sign.
- +/– Gray to tan-colored nodules on the iris surface (lymphocytic-plasmacytic uveitis).
- Cloudy vitreous (chorioretinitis and optic neuritis).
- Rarely, systemic signs may be seen concurrently with ocular signs.
- These include fever, weight loss, +/– muscular pain, +/– signs of respiratory or neurological disease.

See the main reference on pages 1296, 1169 (The Cat With Abnormal Iris Appearance and The Blind Cat or Cat With Retinal Disease).

Clinical signs

Systemic signs are rare but may include:
- **Fever, weight loss and muscle pain**.
- **Respiratory** signs associated with pneumonia.

- Signs of **multifocal neurologic** disease.
- Liver disease.

Ocular signs are more common, and may include one or all of the following signs:
- **Anterior uveitis** is the **most common sign** and is seen as a **cloudy anterior chamber**. This is caused by leakage of protein and white blood cells from inflamed iris and ciliary body blood vessels into the aqueous humor. It is also known as hypopyon.
- In severe cases of uveitis, the **cornea may be cloudy due to edema** caused by aqueous leakage through a compromised endothelium.
- **Keratic precipitates** may be seen on the surface of the endothelium. These are the so-called "mutton fat" deposits that consist of white cells and protein attached to the endothelium. They are more common in the inferior cornea.
- **Cloudy vitreous** caused by chorioretinitis; white cells and protein leak into the vitreous through inflamed retinal and choroidal blood vessels.
- **Lymphocytic plasmocytic uveitis** is seen as pale nodules on the iris surface.
- **Secondary cataract formation** is common in chronic cases, and will be seen as a cloudy eye within the pupil space.
- Glaucoma is a sequel to chronic uveitis.
- Signs may be **unilateral or bilateral**.

Diagnosis

A tentative diagnosis may be based on the **clinical signs**.

A **definitive diagnosis** requires supportive laboratory data which may include:
- **Serology**.
  - Demonstration of a **rise in IgM titers** indicates a recent active infection.
  - **Comparison of** levels of **aqueous humor** *T. gondii* antibody levels with **serum levels** (Goldman–Witmer coefficient or C-value) has been advocated, with higher aqueous levels suggesting the anterior uveitis was caused by *T. gondii*. The use of C-values is still controversial.
- **Polymerase chain reaction (PCR)** testing for parasite DNA in tissue or fluid samples.

FELINE INFECTIOUS PERITONITIS

Classical signs

- Young cats 6–12 months of age.
- Anterior uveitis with large fibrin clots (hypopyon).
- Large brownish to pink keratic precipitates on the inferior endothelial surface of the cornea.
- Chorioretinitis causing variable vision loss and/or abnormal pupil reflexes.
- Neurological signs, including behavioral changes, cranial nerve abnormalities, seizures and head tremor.

See the main reference on page 1179 (The Blind Cat or Cat With Retinal Disease).

Clinical signs

The ocular form of the disease is usually seen in young cats from **6 months to 1 year of age**.

Ocular signs may be **unilateral or bilateral**.

The **main presenting sign is uveitis. Large fibrin clots** mixed with exudated white and red blood cells form a **hypopyon. Keratic precipitates** are common and appear as large pinkish, brown spots on the inferior endothelial surface of the cornea ("mutton fat deposits").

The vitreous may be hazy due to a similar exudation of cells from the ciliary body.

The retina may show a **focal or total exudative retinal detachment**. It is common to see an inflammatory exudate sheathing the major retinal blood vessels, which form a **cloudy sheath around the vessels**.

Blindness may be seen with **abnormal pupil reflexes** (miotic in early stages with uveitis, followed by dilation in blind cases) and abnormal pupil size (anisocoria).

Cats with ocular signs frequently develop **neurological signs**, and die or are euthanized as a result of meningioencephalitis and its associated signs, which include behavioral changes, cranial nerve abnormalities, seizures and head tremor (seizures most common).

Cats with ocular signs of FIP **rarely show systemic signs** of illness such as fever, inappetence and weight loss **at the initial presentation**. As the disease becomes chronic, weight loss and neurological signs develop.

Diagnosis

There is no definitive diagnosis for FIP.

A tentative diagnosis is initially based on clinical signs; **a young cat with uveitis showing hypopyon and keratic precipitates**.

Serology is usually regarded as being of dubious benefit in the diagnosis, as the FIP organism cross-reacts with enteric forms of coronavirus.

Diagnosis can only be confirmed on **characteristic histopathology** of affected tissues on biopsy or necropsy examination. The typical change is described as a **pyogranulomatous vasculitis**. Necrosis and a fibrinoid response are seen in some cases. The ocular cellular response includes neutrophils, lymphocytes, plasma cells, macrophages and large, spindle-shaped histiocytes.

Cats often have a **large increase in plasma total protein, globulin** and **IgG** concentration, because of the chronic nature of the inflammatory disease process. The polyclonal increase in gammaglobulins is caused by virus antigen and cell destruction from the intense inflammation associated with the infection.

FELINE LEUKEMIA VIRUS*

Classical signs

- Discrete iris or ciliary body masses (FeLV-associated lymphosarcoma).
- Anterior uveitis.
- Intermittent asymmetric changes in pupil size, shape or response.
- Other FeLV-associated signs, e.g. anemia.
- Retinal detachment.

See the main reference on page 1300 (The Cat With Abnormal Iris Appearance).

Clinical signs

FeLV may cause **ocular lymphosarcoma**, which appears as **discrete iris or ciliary body masses**, usually bilateral, which may cause gross distortion of the iris structure.

FeLV more commonly presents as a uveitis, with changes to iris appearance, and abnormal pupil size and shape. The **anterior chamber** may contain **fibrin and/or blood**. Anterior uveitis may occur in the absence of discernible intra-ocular neoplasia.

Some cats develop **spastic pupil syndrome**, which presents as otherwise unexplainable intermittent asymmetric **changes in pupil size, shape or response**. For more detail see page 1300 (The Cat With Abnormal Iris Appearance).

It is possible to see **retinal detachment** when the neoplastic process involves the choroid.

There may be other signs of FeLV-associated disease, e.g. anemia or multicentric lymphosarcoma.

Diagnosis

Diagnosis is based on the clinical signs observed in the eye, in association with other signs suggestive of FeLV, e.g. multicentric lymphoma, FeLV-associated anemia.

Diagnosis is confirmed on **clinical pathology**, for example on cytology of lymph nodes or aqueous centesis samples, or occasionally on hematology.

A positive serological test using an **antigen-based test for FeLV** is supportive evidence of the disease. For more detail see page 543 (The Anemic Cat).

OCULAR NEOPLASIA*

Classical signs

- Diffuse pigmentary change across the anterior iris surface, most often a pale fleshy change.
- Mass lesions bulging forward from the anterior iris stroma or distorting normal pupil shape, or causing generalized iris thickening.

Classical signs—Cont'd

- Cloudy anterior chamber filled with white blood cells and protein.
- Varying degrees of hyphema.

See the main reference on pages 1184, 1297 for details (The Blind Cat or Cat With Retinal Disease, The Cat With Abnormal Iris Appearance).

Clinical signs

Most cases present as **anterior uveitis with corneal edema and a cloudy aqueous**, and have some form of **swelling seen in the iris**, which may cause distortion of the pupil (dyscoria).

Various tumors occur in the eye. They may **arise from the iris** such as melanoma, lymphosarcoma, sarcoma and ciliary body tumors or **arise from the retina** including **lymphosarcoma and adenocarcinoma from lung, uterus and undetermined origin**.

Lymphosarcoma is the most common ocular neoplasm, and may be FeLV-associated, although more commonly does not appear to be associated with FeLV.

Lymphosarcoma often presents as bilateral iris swelling, and anterior chamber hypopyon and/or hemorrhage in a young cat, with or without other signs suggesting multicentric neoplasia.

Signs of lymphosarcoma typically include:

- The **anterior chamber is cloudy** from white blood cells and proteins that have leaked from diseased iris blood vessels.
- **The iris may have red cells on the surface** mixed with protein and white blood cells caused by disruption of the endothelial cells on the blood vessel walls. Lymphosarcoma does not usually cause frank hemorrhage. Varying degrees of hyphema are present.
- The **iris appears thickened** with a pale fleshy color change, and may be tinged with blood.
- The pupil is distorted (dyscoria) if the iris is grossly distorted with infiltrated cells.
- Glaucoma is often an associated complication.
- Corneal edema may be present.
- Regional lymph nodes may be increased in size.

Diffuse iris melanoma typically appears as an enlarging area over months to years of light tan to dark brown pigmentation on the iris surface. Usually the neoplasm does not form an obvious discrete mass, but the iris may become diffusely thickened. The disease is usually unilateral and typically occurs in older cats.

- Presentation may more resemble uveal inflammation than neoplasia.
- Sometimes the disease may present in an advanced state with secondary glaucoma.
- Amelanotic diffuse iris melanomas have also been reported. These are difficult to diagnose unless the effects of the tumor on angle obstruction and resultant glaucoma are observed.

Post-traumatic sarcoma more commonly forms **discrete masses** within the eye.

Ciliary body adenoma is a rare slow-growing neoplasm, which appears as a whitish to cream mass behind the pupil margin.

Metastatic neoplasia from an extra-ocular primary tumor appears as an intra-ocular neoplasm involving the iris, and is associated with a similar neoplasm remote from the eye, e.g. mammary or uterine adenocarcinoma.

Diagnosis

A tentative diagnosis is based initially on the **appearance of the eye (uveitis, iris swelling and/or distortion of the retina)** and consideration of the history.

Examination of the buffy coat is useful for diagnosis of lymphosarcoma. The presence of abnormal plump lymphocytes with large prominent nucleoli is highly suggestive.

Biopsy of **regional lymph nodes** is useful if there is lymphomegaly.

Definitive diagnosis may be obtained by **fine-needle aspirate biopsies** or anterior chamber centesis and cytology.

Serology for FeLV may support the diagnosis of lymphosarcoma.

Chest and abdominal radiology and/or ultrasound may be indicated.

CRYPTOCOCCUS NEOFORMANS

Classical signs

- Sudden blindness with retinal detachment.
- Vitreous flare may be present making the retina difficult to examine.
- Anterior uveitis (anterior chamber flare, miosis, inflamed discolored iris).
- Exophthalmos (eye bulging forward).
- +/− Mucopurulent discharge with sneezing and a swollen nose.
- Neurological signs.
- Chronic skin granulomas.

See the main reference on pages 1174, 16, and 1089 (The Blind Cat or Cat With Retinal Disease, The Cat With Signs of Chronic Nasal Disease and The Cat With Non-healing Wounds).

Clinical signs

Cryptococcosis is the most common fungal infection affecting cats, and **occurs throughout the world**.

The initial ocular site for establishment of infection is usually the **choroid**, and the **anterior uveal tract** is often involved later in the course of the infection.

Cats may present with **sudden blindness** caused by **multifocal granulomatous chorioretinitis** with varying degrees of **retinal detachment**.

- **Vitreous flare (cloudy vitreous)** is present, and makes the retina difficult to examine in cases with severe inflammation.
- If the retina can be visualized, the granulomas appear as small swollen brownish discolored areas in the tapetal and non-tapetal retina.

There is usually **anterior uveitis with corneal edema, anterior chamber flare** (with or without hypopyon and keratic precipitates), **swollen iris with varying degrees of posterior synechia** causing a **distorted pupil**, and in chronic cases, new vascular growth on the anterior surface of the iris (pre-iridal fibrovascular membrane formation).

Complications include **secondary cataract and glaucoma**.

Some cats present with **exophthalmos** (eye bulging forward), where there has been an extension of the disease from the sinuses and nasal cavity into the orbital tissues.

In cases with nasal infection, there may be a **mucopurulent discharge with sneezing. Distortion and swelling** over the **bridge of nose**, or a **polyp-like mass** projecting from the nasal cavity are present in 70% of cats with the respiratory form.

Chronic skin granulomas may be present. Skin lesions consist of **papules or nodules** varying from 0.1–1 cm in diameter. Lesions may **ulcerate and exude serous fluid, or remain as intact nodules**.

Cats with disseminated disease may show neurological signs.

Cats may **present** with **chronic nasal or skin disease**, and the ocular involvement is identified secondarily on physical examination. Cats may also be presented **primarily for the ocular signs**, where the owner has seen the development of a cloudy eye and the cat has gone blind.

Diagnosis

A tentative diagnosis is based on typical clinical signs of nasal or skin disease and concurrent ocular signs. The presence of small swollen brownish discolored areas in the retina suggests fungal disease. The frequency of occurrence of individual fungal diseases in the geographical area helps establish a tentative diagnosis.

Cytology can be very useful in the diagnosis of *C. neoformans*. Demonstration of the organism can be made via **anterior chamber centesis** or by fine-needle biopsy (using a 25-gauge needle) taken from the subretinal space. The sample is best stained with **new methylene blue, Indian ink or Diff-Quick**.

Serology to detect **capsule antigen** is sensitive using serum, CSF fluid or urine.

Histopathology from tissue biopsies demonstrates the organism.

Radiology of the nasal cavity, sinuses and chest may be useful in cases that do not demonstrate nasal or skin signs.

Ocular ultrasound can be used to **detect retinal detachment** when anterior chamber flare, cataract or vitreal flare prevents ophthalmoscopic examination of the fundus. It is also used in cases of exophthalmos to examine, and do ultrasound-guided biopsies of the orbital tissue.

OTHER SYSTEMIC FUNGAL INFECTIONS (BLASTOMYCES DERMATITIDIS, CANDIDA ALBICANS, COCCIDIOIDES IMMITIS, HISTOPLASMA CAPSULATUM)

Classical signs

- Chorioretinitis progressing to anterior uveitis (cloudy eye) and endophthalmitis, in a geographical area where fungal infections occur.
- Vision loss and reduced pupil light reflexes.
- Other organ system disease, e.g. renal, CNS, nasal cavity.

See the main references on pages 1176, 1300 and 1283 for details (The Blind Cat or Cat With Retinal Disease, The Cat With Abnormal Iris Appearance and The Cat With Abnormal Pupil Size, Shape or Response).

Clinical signs

Most intra-ocular fungal infections cause similar ocular signs.

- **Choroidal granulomas** are the most characteristic sign on fundoscopy, and appear as a raised area of tapetal hyporeflectivity, or small swollen brownish discolored areas in the retina.
- A **generalized chorioretinitis and secondary retinal detachments**, with ballooning of the retina into the vitreous.
- **Optic neuritis** may be present, seen as a red, swollen optic nerve that is hyperemic.
- **Anterior uveitis** seen as cloudy, red eye with corneal edema, hypopyon and inflamed conjunctiva.

Affected cats show **varying degrees of blindness**, depending on the severity of the ocular infection.

Systemic signs can involve many other organs, especially the lungs, brain, nasal cavity, as well as the periorbital tissues, lymph nodes, bones, toenails and skin.

Diagnosis

A tentative diagnosis is based on the presenting signs of a cat with rapidly progressive, usually bilateral **chorioretinitis, progressing to anterior uveitis**, with signs of other systemic disease, and occurring in a geographic area where such fungal disease is known to occur.

Imaging techniques can be used to obtain more supportive evidence of a deep fungal infection:
- Thoracic radiography to demonstrate pulmonary granulomas.
- Nasal cavity radiography.
- Ocular ultrasound; signs of retinal detachment.

Confirmation of the diagnosis is based on the **demonstration of the respective organism** in:
- Cerebrospinal fluid.
- Samples taken by centesis of vitreous or subretinal exudate.
- Histopathology of enucleated globes.
- Bone marrow biopsy samples (histoplasmosis).

Serological tests can be performed, looking for elevated antibodies (blastomycosis, histoplasmosis, coccidiodomycosis).

LIPEMIC AQUEOUS

Classical signs

- Eye may suddenly become very cloudy with a "milky appearance".
- Unilateral or bilateral.
- Idiopathic in Burmese cats associated with hyperlipidemia.
- May occur in cats with uveitis that are on a high-fat diet.

Pathogenesis

High concentrations of lipid can enter the anterior chamber **from the uveal vessels** if there is either:

- Breakdown of the blood–aqueous barrier in **anterior uveitis**.
- Abnormally high concentrations of serum lipids, which can be secondary or primary **hyperlipidemia**.

Lipemic aqueous is **idiopathic in Burmese cats** associated with hyperlipidemia.

Clinical signs

Typically there is a **diffusely and uniformly cloudy anterior chamber**. The aqueous appears as if it is full of milk.

Usually the iris, pupil and tapetal reflex can still be visualized.

Lipemic aqueous is **often unilateral** and may be **sudden in onset**.

Occasionally it is associated with cats that have **uveitis** caused by systemic diseases such as **toxoplasmosis, FIP, fungal infections**, when they have hyperlipidemia caused by a **high-fat content in the diet**.

Diagnosis

A tentative diagnosis is based on **clinical signs**.

A definitive diagnosis is based on **biochemical analysis of aqueous centesis** samples and demonstration of high serum lipid concentrations. Lipid electrophoretograms may be performed on the sample.

Diagnosis of the underlying cause should be pursued, if lipemic acqueous is not in a predisposed breed such as the Burmese. If it is the result of a systemic disease combined with a high-fat diet, the underlying disease should be identified (see The Cat With Abnormal Iris Appearance, page 1294 and With Retinal Disease, page 1186).

Treatment

Reduce plasma lipid concentrations using a **low-fat diet.**

Treat other underlying medical problems, which are associated with hyperlipidemia such as diabetes mellitus, and systemic diseases causing uveitis (see The Cat With Abnormal Iris Appearance, page 1294).

DISEASES CAUSING A CLOUDY LENS

CATARACT SECONDARY TO INFECTIOUS UVEITIS**

Classical signs

- Cloudy lens, unilateral or bilateral.
- Frequently only unilateral.
- Poor vision if bilateral. Iris may be distorted from posterior synechia.
- Iris may show fibrovascular membranes on surface.
- History of chronic uveitis caused by infectious agent such as toxoplasmosis or fungal disease.

Pathogenesis

Inflammation in the eye results in changes to the lens nutrition and accumulation of toxic products in the eye which results in death of cells. This will cause a cloudy lens (cataract).

Cataract is often associated with chronic uveitis caused by infectious agent such as toxoplasmosis or fungal disease.

Clinical signs

The lens appears cloudy due to the formation of a cortical cataract.

The cataract may be **unilateral or bilateral**, but is more often unilateral. Vision is poor if bilateral.

Other **signs of uveitis** will be present such as aqueous flare and fibrovascular membrane growth on the iris. The iris may have a darker color than the opposite eye, or have changes in contour due to adhesions of the iris to the anterior lens capsule (posterior synechia).

There may be **changes in the cornea such as edema or scarring**, with or without superficial vascularization.

Hypopyon or keratic precipitates may be evident.

Some cats develop **secondary glaucoma**.

Diagnosis

A **tentative diagnosis** is based on the signs of a cloudy lens or cataract.

Signs of uveitis or history of past uveitis indicate the origin of the cataract. See page 1303 (The Cat With Abnormal Iris Appearance).

The eye should be checked for glaucoma by measuring the intra-ocular pressure.

Treatment

Cataract surgery can be done if the inflammation has been controlled.

- It is prudent to do a diagnostic work-up for systemic diseases that cause uveitis prior to doing surgery. See page 1199 (The Blind Cat or Cat With Retinal Disease) and page 1304 (The Cat With Abnormal Iris Appearance).
- Check the eye for retinal detachment with ultrasound prior to surgery.
- An **electroretinogram** is indicated to ensure that the eye has normal retinal function prior to surgery.

NUCLEAR SCLEROSIS AND SENILE CATARACT**

Classical signs

- Milky appearance of lens in cats older than 10 years of age.
- Cats are usually visual and leading a normal lifestyle.
- The fundus can be seen clearly with an ophthalmoscope.

Pathogenesis

Nuclear sclerosis is a **normal aging process** in the lens which starts in animals from about 8 years of age and is evident by 10 years.

Lens fibers are produced throughout life, but the lens does not increase in size. Therefore, the fibers in the center become **thinner and pack closer together** causing a slight opacity, termed **sclerosis**. As the lens ages further some of these fibers may **break-down** and then a **nuclear cataract** develops. In very old cats, the nuclear cataract may become quite dense with secondary changes in the surrounding cortex leading to a **mature cataract**.

Clinical signs

The **center of the lens** becomes **slightly cloudy**, but the cat will be able to see quite well until the changes are advanced and become a cataract.

Nuclear sclerosis is seen from **10 years of age** and **cataracts** typically occur in cats **12–20 years of age**.

On ophthalmoscopic examination, the fundus will be clearly visible until a true cataract forms.

Diagnosis

Diagnosis of nuclear sclerosis is **based on clinical signs** of a slightly cloudy lens in an older cat, with vision intact. The fundus can be clearly seen with an ophthalmoscope.

Diagnosis of senile cataract is **based on clinical signs** of a cloudy lens in an older cat, with no history or signs of preceding ocular trauma or inflammation.

Treatment

There is **no definitive treatment** for this aging change.

If a cataract develops and the cat is healthy, **cataract surgery** can be performed. Because senile cataract occurs in aged cats, it is important to check renal function and blood pressure before proceeding with surgery.

CATARACT SECONDARY TO LENS TRAUMA*

> ### Classical signs
>
> - History of previous eye injury, frequently caused by a cat claw.
> - Cornea has scar from old wound.
> - ± Anterior or posterior synechia (iris adhesions to cornea or lens).
> - Lens may be partially or completely cloudy.
> - ± Chronic inflammation (uveitis) caused by lens protein outside the capsule.

Pathogenesis

Any injury to the lens fibers will **disrupt the normal lens metabolism**, and cause death of lens fibers leading to cataract formation.

The **most common cause of lens injury** in cats is from **cat fights** when a cat claw penetrates the globe and tears the anterior lens capsule. This may be obvious when the tear is visible through the pupil, but some injuries occur under the iris root in the equator of the lens and are not possible to visualize.

Other causes of injury are **blunt trauma**, which is frequently associated with motor vehicle accidents. With blunt trauma, the sudden compression of the eye followed by rapid decompression causes rupture of the lens capsule.

Once the nutrition of the lens fibers is disturbed, the **cells will start to die and become opaque**, resulting in typical cloudy lens and cataract formation.

An injured lens in a cat can lead to **sarcoma formation** due to metaplasia of the lens epithelial cells. See pages 1276 (Feline intra-ocular sarcoma).

Clinical signs

Typically, there is a **history or signs of eye trauma**, usually a cat-fight claw injury or blunt trauma. The cornea may have a scar from an old wound.

Lens may be partially or completely cloudy because of an **immature or mature cataract**.

In anterior capsule tears, **lens material** can be seen in the anterior chamber as a **cloudy flocculent material**. There is intense inflammation associated with leakage of lens material, and it may be difficult to see through a very cloudy cornea.

Tears in the equatorial region of the lens may often be sealed by the ciliary body and iris root, and only develop a **local cataract**. Generally, an injury to the lens fibers will lead to a mature cataract.

Where the eye has hyphema (red eye), the lens will not be able to be seen ophthalmoscopically.

Often the tear in the lens capsule has **iris pigment adhered** to it, visible as a black area. Anterior or posterior synechia (iris adhesions to cornea or lens) may be evident.

Be aware that cats with **chronic inflammation after trauma** often have a ruptured lens causing chronic lens-induced uveitis.

Diagnosis

A tentative diagnosis is based on a **history or signs of eye trauma** and the presence of a **mature or immature cataract**.

In acute cases, lens material is visible in the anterior chamber.

In chronic cases, chronic uveitis is evident after an eye injury.

Ocular ultrasound is a very useful tool for detecting lens rupture. Look for the normal position of the lens as seen by the anterior and posterior hyperechoic line defining the anterior and posterior lens capsule. In high-quality machines with a 10-MHz probe, the lens shape and position can be visualized quite easily. Any change to the appearance or lack of hyperechoic lines is suspicious for lens rupture.

Treatment

If there is corneal edema and the anterior chamber is filled with blood and protein, treat the eye with **broad-spectrum antibiotics** topically and systemically. Inflammation should be controlled initially with **NSAIDs**. If the lens is ruptured, **corticosteroids systemically** will be needed to control the lens-induced uveitis, which is an immune reaction in the eye against the exposed lens fibers.

If the injury has recently occurred, and the cornea and anterior chamber allows visualization of the lens, a **lentectomy** should be performed immediately. This treatment is controversial because of the danger of sarcoma formation later in life.

Cataract surgery can be performed later if a mature cataract develops.

Cats with an injured lens have a high risk of developing ocular sarcoma, and enucleation should be considered.

CATARACT SECONDARY TO NON-INFECTIOUS UVEITIS

Classical signs

- Nuclear cataract in a young healthy cat that with no evidence of ocular inflammation.

Pathogenesis

In contrast to dogs, genetic cataract is rare in cats, but has been reported.

Congenital cataract is seen when the lens development is disrupted or altered in the early embryonic development of the eye.

As the nucleus is the first part of the lens to develop, this is the usual area of cataract development seen in young cats (**nuclear cataract**). As the cat ages, the lens cortex may become cataractous and the eye develops a mature cataract.

Clinical signs

Cloudy lens in a young cat with no history of illness and no sign of inflammation in the eye.

Vision is reduced or absent if both eyes are affected.

Diagnosis

Diagnosis is based on the classical appearance of a cloudy lens in a young healthy cat, which has no evidence of ocular inflammation.

Treatment

Cataract surgery can be done by a trained ophthalmologist if the globe and retina is normal.
- **Ocular ultrasound** should be done to determine whether the retina is detached. A 10-MHz probe should be used. Detached retinas are seen as faint lines bulging into the vitreous between the optic disc and ora serrata.
- **Electroretinography** can be done to determine whether the retina has normal rod and cone function.

DIABETIC CATARACT

Classical signs

- Rare finding in older cat with diabetes mellitus.
- Cloudy lens with immature to mature cataract.

Pathogenesis

Diabetic cataract forms because the lens is bathed in a solution that is very high in glucose. The lens cells cannot metabolize the excess glucose by normal anaerobic glycolysis, and therefore uses aerobic glycolysis using the **sorbitol pathway** and the enzyme **aldose reductase** as the catalyst. The by-product of this process is **sugar alcohol (sorbitol), which kills the cell**. The sugar alcohol is a large molecule that cannot escape through the cell wall, and results in a more concentrated intracellular fluid than the surrounding fluid. Water is therefore imbibed into the cell, which causes it to swell and rupture. This in turn causes an immune reaction within the eye called **lens-induced uveitis**.

Diabetic cataracts are **rare in cats**. This is thought to be due to **low levels of the enzyme aldose reductase** in old cats, which prevents the lens cells from using the sorbitol pathway to the same degree as other animals.

Clinical signs

Cloudy lens and poor vision in a cat with diabetes mellitus.

Diagnosis

A tentative diagnosis is based on the signs of a cloudy lens consistent with an immature to mature cataract in a cat with diabetes mellitus.

Treatment

Cataract surgery can be done successfully by a trained ophthalmologist.

DISEASES CAUSING A CLOUDY VITREOUS

CLOUDY VITREOUS ASSOCIATED WITH SYSTEMIC HYPERTENSION***

Classical signs

- Acute onset of vision loss in an old cat, usually bilateral.
- Dilated pupils, non-responsive or poorly responsive to light.

Classical signs—Cont'd

- Cloudy vitreous with red areas of hemorrhage.

See the main reference on page 1171 (The Blind Cat or Cat With Retinal Disease).

Pathogenesis

Hypertension causes **vasoconstriction of pre-capillary retinal arterioles. Hypoxia** of the arteriole causes smooth muscle necrosis, which leads to **vascular dilatation**, and leakage of serum and blood.

Leakage from vessels causes **serous retinal detachment**, and subretinal, intraretinal or preretinal **hemorrhage**.

Retinal blood vessels may rupture, causing hemorrhage into the vitreous.

Hypertensive retinopathy occurs most commonly secondary to **chronic renal disease** and **hyperthyroidism**.

Clinical signs

Classical signs are **acute onset of vision loss** in an **old cat**, which is usually **bilateral**. The cat suddenly starts to bump into things, appears to be lost, and has very cautious movements.

The **pupils** are usually **dilated**, and non-responsive or **poorly responsive light**.

Affected **eyes appear slightly cloudy**, and there may be focal red areas visible through the pupil, as a result of retinal hemorrhage. The vitreous may appear red. Early cases may show hemorrhage along the larger retinal blood vessels.

It is difficult to visualize the **retina** on fundoscopic examination, as it **appears out of focus**. This is caused by retinal detachment, with the retina ballooning into the vitreous, **and appears as a thin veil of pale tissue**.

These cats may have **cardiomegaly**, and left ventricular hypertrophy.

There may be other signs suggestive of hypertension, for example, a **bounding cardiac apex beat**.

Systolic arterial blood pressure is usually **greater than 160 mmHg**.

Other signs suggestive of renal and/or thyroid disease, such as progressive weight loss, polydipsia, polyuria and azotemia may be present.

Diagnosis

Clinicians should suspect this problem in **any old cat that has suddenly gone blind**.

Ophthalmoscopy will demonstrate **vitreal hemorrhage**. The retina will appear out of focus, and hemorrhage adjacent to the major retinal blood vessels is visible.

Blood pressure is most commonly measured in the cat using Doppler technology. Arterial blood pressure greater than 160 mmHg confirms a diagnosis of hypertensive retinopathy. Most cats with clinical signs have a blood pressure of **greater than 200 mmHg**.

BUN, creatinine and urine protein:creatinine ratios are useful clinical pathology parameters to check renal function.

Thyroid function should be checked by measuring **plasma thyroxine (T4) concentration**.

Further useful procedures include **cardiac ultrasound**, and in some cases, imaging of the thyroid with radioisotopes.

Treatment

Amlodipine (Norvasc, Pfizer) is a **calcium channel blocker**, which has a greater effect on vascular smooth muscle cells than on cardiac muscle cells. The dose is approximately 0.625 mg/cat/day, i.e. 1/4 of a 2.5 mg tablet (USA) or 1/8 of a 5 mg tablet (Australia).

The use of corticosteroids is controversial.

If hypertension is associated with **hypertrophic cardiomyopathy**, then calcium channel blockers such as **diltiazem** may be used. For more detail see main reference on page 162 for details (The Cat With Tachycardia, Bradycardia or an Irregular Rhythm).

β-blockers such as propranolol (Inderal) can also be used in the management of the cardiac disease at 1/4 of a 10 mg tablet q 8 h.

Hyperthyroidism when present, should be treated using surgery, radioactive iodine (131-I) or anti-thyroid drugs such as carbimazole or methimazole. For more detail see main reference on page 305 (The Cat With Weight Loss and a Good Appetite).

Cats with renal disease should be placed on appropriate medical and dietary management. For more details see the main reference on page 337 (The Thin, Inappetent Cat).

FELINE IMMUNODEFICIENCY VIRUS*

Classical signs

- Show signs of mild uveitis.
- "Snowbank" inflammation of the pars plana seen through dilated pupil. Appears as cloudy outer vitreous in this area.
- May be other systemic signs such as loss of weight, inappetence and fever.

Pathogenesis

Infection with the virus usually occurs as a result of a bite from another FIV-positive cat. Transmission in saliva by grooming is thought possible, but rare.

After infection a viremic phase occurs, which may be associated with a transient fever, generalized lymphadenopathy and neutropenia. An asymptomatic carrier state or chronic disease then follows.

Clinical signs

Cats that develop signs of FIV may have evidence of generalized systemic disease such as weight loss, and poor body and coat condition. Pyrexia, lymphadenopathy and infections of the oral cavity, respiratory tract, skin and other sites may occur.

In the eye**, pars planitis** or **"snow bank" inflammation of the pars plana** resulting in **vitreous cloudiness** is thought to be almost pathognomonic for FIV infection. Other signs of uveitis can also be seen, such as cloudy aqueous and iris inflammation.

Diagnosis

A tentative diagnosis is based on the **clinical signs of vitreous cloudiness** described as "snow bank" inflammation, in a FIV-positive cat.

Treatment

Supportive treatment is indicated, and depends on the organ system affected.

The use of steroid anti-inflammatory drugs for the ocular lesion has to be weighed against the potential immunosuppressive effects.

FELINE INTRA-OCULAR SARCOMA

Classical signs

- Rare, primary neoplasia that occurs in older cats (7–15 years).
- History of previous severe trauma to eye.
- Anterior uveitis, keratitis (corneal edema and pigmentation) and glaucoma.
- White to pinkish masses may be visible in the vitreous.

Clinical signs

Intra-ocular sarcoma is a **rare primary neoplasia** reported only in cats.

It is occurs in **older cats 7–15 years of age**, that have had a **history of ocular trauma 3–10 years** previously.

There may be signs of **anterior uveitis** with **keratitis**, with edema and pigmentation of the cornea. These changes may prevent visualization of the intra-ocular structures.

Secondary glaucoma is common at this stage of the disease. The eye will show **buphthalmos (enlarged globe)** with engorged scleral vessels.

If the posterior segment of the eye can be visualized, **white to pink masses** may be seen in the vitreous.

The condition is thought to occur after lens trauma, which triggers the lens **epithelial cells to undergo metaplasia**.

The neoplasia rapidly extends through the choroid and **infiltrates the optic nerve**. Metastasis has been reported.

Survival rate is very low.

Diagnosis

A tentative diagnosis is based on the **signalment, history and signs** of an old cat with a prior history of trauma and signs of glaucoma, uveitis and keratitis.

A definitive diagnosis is based on **histological examination** of tissue.
- **Fine-needle biopsy** can be attempted, but may not yield a diagnostic sample if the tumor contains fibrous and cartilagenous tissue.
- **Histopathology of enucleated globes** shows changes that may include **granulation tissue, fibrosarcoma, osteosarcoma and anaplastic spindle cell sarcoma**.

All blind globes with chronic uveitis should be watched for the development of this condition.

Treatment

Early enucleation with histopathology should be done on all globes with a prior history of trauma whenever there are changes in the size and shape of the globe, or changes in the anterior chamber and cornea indicative of intra-ocular disease.

Severely traumatized blind eyes in cats should be enucleated to prevent the occurrence of this condition, particularly if there has been lens rupture.

Check for metastases to regional lymph nodes and other organs such as lungs and liver prior to surgery.

RECOMMENDED READING

Barnett KC. A Colour Atlas of Veterinary Ophthalmology. Wolfe Publishing Ltd, London, 1990.
Gelatt Kirk N (ed). Veterinary Ophthalmology, 2nd edn. Lea & Febiger, Philadelphia, 1991.
Gelatt Kirk N. Veterinary Ophthalmology, 3rd edn. Lippincott, Williams and Wilkins, Philadelphia, 1998.
Gelatt Kirk N. Essentials of Veterinary Ophthalmology. Lippincott Williams and Wilkins, Philadelphia, 2000.
Gelatt Kirk N. Colour Atlas of Veterinary Ophthalmology. Lippincott Williams and Wilkins, Philadelphia, 2001.

Gelatt Kirk N, Gelatt JP. Handbook of Small Animal Ophthalmic Surgery, Vol. 1. Extraocular Procedures. Permagon Veterinary Handbook Series, Florida, 1994.

Gelatt Kirk N, Gelatt JP. Handbook of Small Animal Ophthalmic Surgery, Vol. 2. Intraocular Procedures. Permagon Veterinary Handbook Series, Florida, 1995.

Ketring KL, Glaze MB. Atlas of Feline Ophthalmology. Trenton, NJ, Veterinary Learning Systems, 1994.

Peiffer RL, Petersen-Jones S. Small Animal Ophthalmology, A Problem Oriented Approach, 3rd edn. Saunders, Philadelphia, 2001.

62. The cat with abnormal pupil size, shape or response

Michael E. Bernays

KEY SIGNS

- Slow or absent pupillary light reflex.
- Unequal pupil size or abnormal pupil shape.

MECHANISM

Abnormal pupil sizes or responses are usually due to processes which affect either the:

- Retina: inflammatory, degenerative or hypertensive retinopathies.
- Afferent or efferent nervous pathways involved in the pupillary light reflex or dilation of the pupil, particularly cranial nerve II and autonomic nerves, i.e. neuropathies.
- Iris: inflammatory or occasionally degenerative diseases.

WHERE?

Pathways involved in the pupillary light reflex.

- Retina, optic nerve, optic chiasm, optic tracts, midbrain, oculomotor nucleus parasympathetic preganglionic fibers, ciliary ganglion, parasympathetic fibers in long ciliary nerve, iris pupillary sphincter muscle.

Pathways involved in sympathetic dilation of the pupil.

- Thalamus, cervical spinal cord long tracts, T1–T3 spinal nerves, sympathetic preganglionic fibers, cranial cervical ganglion, sympathetic postganglionic fibers (middle ear**, orbit), iris dilator muscle.

WHAT?

- The most common diseases causing abnormalities of pupil response include hypertensive retinopathy and infectious diseases of the retina and central nervous system.

QUICK REFERENCE SUMMARY

Diseases causing abnormal pupil size, shape or response

RETINA AND OPTIC NERVE

DEGENERATIVE

- Hereditary progressive retinal photoreceptor dysplasia or degeneration (p 1290)

Young to middle-aged cat with a history of gradual onset vision loss, especially in Abyssinian cats, but also described in Persians and Siamese. Rare.

- Feline central retinal degeneration (FRCD) (p 1285)

Slow onset of vision loss and loss of normal papillary light reflex. Possible history of a diet poor in taurine.

METABOLIC

- **Hypertensive retinopathy*** (p 1282)**

Old cat with sudden onset of vision loss, dilated and poorly or non-responsive pupils. Fundoscopic signs ranging from retinal hemorrhage and localized subretinal exudate to extensive bullous retinal detachment.

- Anemic retinopathy (p 1288)

Blind, weak cat with profound anemia and retinal hemorrhages and partial to complete loss of papillary light reflexes.

- Hyperviscosity retinopathy (p 1288)

Rare condition causing blindness and loss of pupil reflexes due to retinal damage. Extremely dilated tortuous retinal vessels with monoclonal globulin spike on protein electrophoresis.

NUTRITIONAL

- **Taurine deficiency retinopathy* (p 1285)**

Slow onset of vision loss and loss of normal papillary light reflex. History of a diet poor in taurine, e.g. dry dog food diet, or a diet high in plant fiber.

INFECTION

- **Infectious chorioretinitis** (p 1283)**

Caused by protozoa (*Toxoplasma gondii*), fungi (*Cryptococcus neoformans,* blastomycosis, histoplasmosis, coccidoidomycosis), parasites (ophthalmomyiasis (fly larval migration)). Abnormal pupil responses result from retinopathy or central nervous system involvement. Variable signs occur including retinal detachments, retinal hemorrhages, subretinal exudates, subretinal granulomas, pre-retinal hemorrhages, together with systemic signs of infection such as fever, depression, inappetence and weight loss.

- **Feline infectious peritonitis (FIP) virus** (p 1284)**

Fibrinous peritonitis, CNS disease or fibrinous uveitis in a young cat with variable vision loss and/or abnormal pupil reflexes. Anorexia and/or pyrexia.

TOXIC

- **Drug toxicity to fluoroquinolones*-** (p 1284)**

Sudden-onset blindness and absent papillary light reflexes associated with recent administration of a fluoroquinolone, e.g. enrofloxacin.

continued

continued

IRIS

DEGENERATIVE

● **Iris atrophy* (p 1287)**

Dilated pupil with sluggish pupillary light reflex in an old cat with normal vision. Visible defects around the pupil margin may occur with atrophy.

● Feline dysautonomia (p 1289)

Variable ocular signs, including reduced lacrimation, dilated non-responsive pupils, anisocoria, prolapsed third eyelids, photophobia in conjunction with other systemic signs such as constipation, vomiting and regurgitation, dry mouth or dry nostrils.

ANOMALY

● Iris coloboma (p 1290)

Wedge-like or radial sectorial defect in appearance of the iris.

● Persistent pupillary membranes (PPM) (p 1289)

Small strand-like structures going from one part of the iris collarette to another, to the anterior lens capsule or to the posterior corneal surface.

● **Anisocoria associated with blue irides and deafness in white cats* (p 1287)**

Uneven-sized pupils in a white cat, with the larger pupil on the same side as a unilateral blue iris.

INFECTION

● **Infectious anterior uveitis – protozoal, fungal or parastic (*Toxoplasma, Cryptococcus neoformans*, blastomycosis, coccidioidomycosis, histoplasma capsulatum, ophthalmomyiasis)** (p 1283)**

These infectious organisms may cause chorioretinitis with variable pupil responses, vision loss and retinal changes, which typically include retinal detachment, subretinal exudates or granulomas. Signs of anterior uveitis may also be present such as flare, hyperemia of the iris surface, keratic precipitates and fibrin. Systemic illness is present, typically with pyrexia, inappetence, weight loss and malaise, and often with dyspnea.

● **Feline leukemia virus infection/feline spastic pupil syndrome* (p 1286)**

History of variable pupil behavior with pupils alternating between miotic or dilated, in one or both eyes, over weeks to months. Intervening periods of normality with equal pupils and/or neoplastic disease affecting the iris, iris thickening and inflammation.

● **Feline infectious peritonitis (FIP) virus* (p 1284)**

Fibrinous peritonitis, CNS disease or fibrinous uveitis in a young cat with variable vision loss and/or abnormal pupil reflexes. Anorexia, malaise and/or pyrexia are typically present.

IATROGENIC

● **Use of parasympatholytic drugs** (p 1284)**

Dilated non-responsive pupil associated with a history of recent use of a drug such as atropine or tropicamide in the same eye.

TRAUMA

- **Dyscoria associated with iris synechia or prolapse into a corneal wound* (p 1286)**
  Pear- or tear-shaped pupil, with adhesion of the acute angle of the tear to the lens capsule or to a traumatic defect in the cornea.

- **Feline hemidilated pupil syndrome* (p 1287)**
  D shape (left eye) or reverse D (right eye) shaped pupil, which becomes accentuated on stimulation of the pupil with bright light.

INTRODUCTION

This chapter refers only to diseases within the globe causing an abnormal pupil size, shape or response.

For other disease processes occurring remotely from the eye see main reference on page 1282 for details (The Cat With Anisocoria or Abnormally Dilated or Constricted Pupils).

For infectious conditions affecting the iris and therefore pupil size or response see main reference on page 1295 for details (The Cat With Abnormal Iris Appearance).

MECHANISM?

Disease processes affecting pupil size or response can generally be divided into:

- Those which affect **afferent** pathways, i.e. going towards the central nervous system (CNS) from the retina.
- Those which affect **efferent** pathways, i.e. going away from the CNS towards the effector organ, in this case the dilator and constrictor muscles of the iris.
- Those which affect the **effector organ**, the **iris** (these diseases are largely covered in The Cat With Changed Iris Appearance).

The term **anisocoria** refers to a difference in pupil size between the two eyes of the same animal.

The term **dyscoria** refers to an abnormality in shape.

The terms **mydriasis** and **miosis** refers to the states of pupil dilation and pupil constriction, respectively.

To demonstrate complete normality of pupil function, the pupil must be shown to dilate in a dark environment and to constrict after stimulation by bright light.

Dynamic contraction anisocoria, where the direct response of an eye to light stimulation is greater than the indirect response in the opposite eye is regarded as normal in cats. Only static anisocoria (i.e. where one eye is not being stimulated by a light source) is regarded as abnormal.

Disease processes therefore either involve the retina, afferent and efferent nerve pathways or iris and are most often **degenerative, hypertensive, infectious or toxic** in nature.

WHERE?

Abnormalities in pupil size or response can originate from lesions or dysfunction in any of the following regions:

- **Retina, optic nerve, optic chiasm, optic tracts or midbrain** which form the **afferent arm for reflexes** which regulate pupillary responses, i.e. they detect the amount of light getting into the system and transmit information about the light levels to the midbrain.
- **Parasympathetic nervous system**. The efferent arm for pupillary constriction consists of the parasympathetic nucleus of the oculomotor nerve, parasympathetic fibers in cranial nerve III (oculomotor nerve), ciliary ganglion and long ciliary nerves.
- **Sympathetic nervous system**. The efferent arm for pupillary dilation consists of the thalamus, cervical spinal cord long tracts, T1–T3 spinal nerves, preganglionic fibers in the cervical region, cranial cervical ganglion and postganglionic fibers especially as they course through the middle ear.
- **Iris**. Diseases which affect pupil size or response can affect either the dilator or constrictor muscles.

WHAT?

The most common causes of abnormalities of pupil size or response are:

- Diseases of the retina.
- Diseases of the central nervous system.

Less frequent causes of abnormal size or response are:

- **Neuropathy** of the **parasympathetic fibers** within cranial nerve III, which supply the pupillary constrictor muscle, or disease confined to the iris involving the **constrictor muscle**.
- **Injury** to the **sympathetic fibers** supplying the iris dilator, most commonly trauma in the cranial thoracic or cervical region, disease of the middle ear or disease confined to the iris affecting the dilator muscle.
- **Hypertensive retinopathy, fungal or** *Toxoplasma* **infection causing chorioretinitis or anterior uveitis, feline infectious peritonitis (FIP) and retinal degeneration from inherited or nutritional (taurine deficiency)** causes are the most **common intra-ocular causes** of abnormal pupil size, shape or response.

DISEASES CAUSING SIGNS OF ABNORMAL PUPIL SIZE, SHAPE OR RESPONSE

HYPERTENSIVE RETINOPATHY***

Classical signs

- Acute-onset vision loss in an old cat.
- Acute onset, usually bilateral, dilated pupils non-responsive or poorly responsive to light.

Pathogenesis

Hypertension causes vasoconstriction of pre-capillary retinal arterioles. Hypoxia of the arteriole causes **smooth muscle necrosis**, eventually leading to **vascular dilatation and leakage of serum and blood**.

Leakage from vessels causes **serous retinal detachment**, subretinal, intraretinal or preretinal **hemorrhage**.

Hypertension is most commonly the result of **hyperthyroidism, renal disease or is idiopathic**.

Clinical signs

Typical history is of **acute onset of vision loss in an old cat, or acute onset of bilaterally (usually) dilated pupils that are non-responsive or poorly responsive to light**.

Fundoscopic findings range from **retinal hemorrhage and localized subretinal exudates**, to extensive bullous retinal detachment.

Other signs suggestive of hypertension such as a **bounding cardiac apex beat** may be evident.

Other signs suggestive of **renal and/or thyroid disease** such as progressive weight loss, polydypsia, polyuria or azotemic breath may be detected from the history or physical examination.

Diagnosis

Diagnosis is initially based on the **characteristic clinical signs**.

Confirmation of the diagnosis is based on a workup involving:

- Blood pressure measurement.
- Clinical pathology suggestive of renal and/or thyroid disease.
- Other procedures such as imaging of the thyroid with radio-isotopes or cardiac ultrasound.

Treatment

Amlodipine (Norvasc, Pfizer) is a **calcium channel blocker** which has a greater effect on vascular smooth muscle cells than on cardiac muscle cells. Dose is approx 0.625 mg/cat/day, i.e. $\frac{1}{4}$ of a 2.5 mg tablet (USA) or $\frac{1}{8}$ of a 5 mg tablet (Australia) q 24 h.

If hypertension is associated with hypertrophic cardiomyopathy then calcium channel blockers such as **Diltiazem** may be used. For more detail see main reference on page 162 for details (The Cat With Tachycardia, Bradycardia or An Irregular Rhythm).

β-blockers such as propranolol (Inderal) can also be used in the management of the cardiac disease at $\frac{1}{4}$ of a 10 mg tablet q 8 h.

Hyperthyroidism, when present, should be treated by surgery, radioactive iodine (131-I) or anti-thyroid drugs such as carbimazole or methimazole. For more details see main reference on page 305 (The Cat With Weight Loss and a Good Appetite).

INFECTIOUS CHORIORETINITIS**

ANTERIOR UVEITIS** (PROTOZOAL, FUNGAL OR PARASITIC) (*TOXOPLASMA, CRYPTOCOCCUS NEOFORMANS,* BLASTOMYCOSIS, COCCIDIOIDOMYCOSIS, *HISTOPLASMA CAPSULATUM,* OPHTHALMOMYIASIS)

> **Classical signs**
>
> ● Abnormal pupil light reflexes.
> ● Variable degrees of vision loss.
> ● Variable signs on fundoscopy including retinal detachments, retinal hemorrhages, subretinal exudates, subretinal granulomas, pre-retinal hemorrhages.
> ● Signs of anterior uveitis.

For more details see main reference on page 1300 (The Cat With Abnormal Iris Appearance) or page 1172 (The Blind Cat or Cat With Retinal Disease).

Clinical signs

Organisms that may produce signs of chorioretinitis or uveitis include protozoa (*Toxoplasma gondii*), fungi (*Cryptococcus neoformans,* blastomycosis, histoplasmosis, coccidioidomycosis), parasites (ophthalmomyiasis (fly larval migration)).

Systemic clinical signs of fever, dyspnea, gastrointestinal disease, upper respiratory disease or other organ involvement suggest infection with *Toxoplasma* or any of the systemic fungal diseases.

Abnormal pupil responses occur due to retinopathy or to central nervous system involvement.

Variable degrees of vision loss result, depending on degree of retinal or central nervous tissue injury.

Variable signs on fundoscopy including retinal detachments, retinal hemorrhages, subretinal exudates, subretinal granulomas, and pre-retinal hemorrhages consistent with chorioretinitis.

Signs of **anterior uveitis** such as flare, hyperemia of the iris surface, keratic precipitates, and/or fibrin.

Diagnosis

Diagnosis is based initially on the identification of suspicious signs on careful examination of the fundus and the anterior segment.

Diagnosis is confirmed by serology, or **identification** of the characteristic morphology of a pathogen from the subretinal exudate or anterior chamber fluid, or from another site such as lymph node, bone marrow, liver or lung aspirate.

● **Technique of anterior chamber aqueous centesis**: Prepare the eye using a 1:20 Povidine solution. Under sedation using topical anesthesia and using illumination and magnification, pass a 30-G needle obliquely into the anterior chamber. It is important to visualize the needle passing into the anterior chamber anterior to the iris. Drain approximately $1/2$ a needle hub, then withdraw the needle.

● **Technique of subretinal fluid centesis**: Under general anesthesia, prepare the conjunctival surfaces with 1:20 Povidone iodine and with the pupil dilated (if possible), rotate the globe ventrally and immobilize with Colibri forceps. Insert a 27-G needle perpendicularly, and if possible, visualize the needle passing through the sclera and choroid into the subretinal space, and aspirate 0.1–0.2 ml of fluid.

Many infectious agents may not actually be present within the eye to cause ocular disease, but cause pathology by the presence of immunocompetent cells within the uveal tissue, which have been stimulated by antigens in sites remote from the eye. *Toxoplasma gondii* is thought to cause uveitis in this way.

An important differential diagnosis is hypertensive retinopathy. This is usually a very acute disease occurring mainly in old cats, which have other signs such as weight loss, and renal or cardiac disease. It is not associated with anterior uveitis, and is not usually associated with other CNS signs, although seizures may occur.

FELINE INFECTIOUS PERITONITIS (FIP) VIRUS**

Classical signs

- Fibrinous peritonitis, central nervous system disease or fibrinous uveitis in a young cat.
- Variable vision loss and/or abnormal pupil reflexes.
- Systemic signs including anorexia, lethargy and fever.

For more detail see main reference on page 1295 for details (The Cat With Abnormal Iris Appearance) and page 352 (The Thin, Inappetent Cat).

Clinical signs

FIP typically causes fibrinous peritonitis and/or signs of central nervous system disease and/or fibrinous uveitis in a young cat.

Anorexia, pyrexia, weight loss and malaise are usually present. Other signs including icterus, abdominal distention, dyspnea and multifocal neurological signs are variably present.

In the eye, the most common presenting sign is a fibrinous uveitis. Fibrinous exudation results in cream to red-colored solid opacities in the anterior chamber, or over the surface of the iris.

Other signs of anterior uveitis such as blood or cloudiness in the anterior chamber, miosis, general reddening or thickening of the iris, and injection of deep episcleral vessels may be evident.

Variable vision loss and/or abnormal pupil reflexes may be present.

Usually occurs in a cat less than 3 years of age, which has been housed with other cats in the previous 18 months, for example, in a cattery or multi-cat household.

Diagnosis

Diagnosis is based initially on the suspicious clinical signs. The "wet" forms (fibrinous peritonitis) and "dry" forms of the disease usually occur separately.

Serology is usually regarded as being of dubious benefit in the diagnosis, as the FIP organism cross-reacts with enteric forms of coronavirus.

Diagnosis can only be confirmed on characteristic histopathology of affected tissues on biopsy or necropsy examination. Typical change is described as a pyogranulomatous vasculitis. Necrosis and a fibrinoid response are seen in some cases.

USE OF PARASYMPATHOLYTIC DRUGS**

Classical signs

- Dilated non-responsive pupil associated with normal vision.
- History of recent use of one of these drugs in the same eye.

Clinical signs

Dilated non-responsive pupil(s) associated with normal vision.

History of use of eye drops containing a parasympatholytic drug such as atropine or tropicamide in the previous 1–2 weeks.

Diagnosis

Diagnosis is based purely on the clinical signs, and the history of recent use of one of these drugs in the same eye.

Diagnosis is usually confirmed by the return of normal pupil reflexes within 1–2 weeks of cessation of use of the drug in the eye.

DRUG TOXICITY TO FLUOROQUINOLONES*-**

Classical signs

- Acute onset of bilaterally dilated pupils, non-responsive to light.
- Acute onset vision loss.
- History of recent use of a fluoroquinolone, especially at higher than recommended dose.

Clinical signs

Acute onset of **bilaterally dilated pupils** that are non-responsive to light.

Acute onset of **vision loss**.

There is a history of **recent use of a fluoroquinolone**, especially at higher than recommended dose rate. Blindness may also occur at the recommended dose, and appears to be an idiosyncratic reaction to the drug.
- Anecdotal personal communication suggests that the problem is seen frequently when Enrofloxacin is given at a daily dose rate of 20 mg/kg (the standard recommended dose rate is 5 mg/kg q 24 h).

The retina has a normal appearance on fundoscopy.

Diagnosis

Diagnosis is based on the **acute onset of the clinical signs** and the history of recent use of a **fluoroquinolone**, especially at a higher than recommended dose.

Prognosis

Prognosis for vision is **usually guarded**, but may be improved if the toxicity is recognized in the early stages and the drug withdrawn immediately.

TAURINE DEFICIENCY RETINOPATHY*

FELINE CENTRAL RETINAL DEGENERATION (FCRD)

Classical signs

- Vision loss in advanced cases.
- Typical ophthalmoscopic signs starting in the area centralis progressing to involve the whole of the retina.
- History of inadequate diet.

Pathogenesis

The disease occurs in **cats fed an inadequate diet**, especially cats fed commercial dog foods, or a diet high in plant fiber.

Taurine deficiency is regarded as being the primary factor leading to **photoreceptor degeneration**.

The syndromes feline central retinal degeneration (FCRD) and taurine deficiency retinopathy are regarded by many authors as being the same disease. The disease is still **occasionally seen in cats which appear to have adequate levels of dietary taurine**, but the overall incidence of the disease throughout the world appears to have declined as the taurine content of commercial diets has been increased.

Taurine deficiency also causes **dilated cardiomyopathy**. See main references on page 151 for details (The Cat With Abnormal Heart Sounds and/or an Enlarged Heart).

Clinical signs

Vision loss occurs in **the later stages** of the disease, and is associated with a poor pupil light reflex.

Characteristic retinal lesions are evident on fundoscopy.
- **Focal degeneration** occurs in the **area centralis at first**. The area centralis at first develops a granular appearance, then becomes hyper-reflective.
- A second hyper-reflective lesion then develops nasal to the optic disc, which eventually coalesces with the area centralis lesion to form a broad hyper-reflective band dorsal to the optic disc.
- Finally, **generalized retinal degeneration develops**, with generalized tapetal hyper-reflectivity and retinal vessel attenuation.

Diagnosis

Diagnosis is based on clinical signs, in particular observation of the typical retinal lesions.

Electroretinography (ERG) can be performed to identify altered photoreceptor function. **Cones appear to be affected more than rods**, so these cats will have reduced b waves in photopic (light) conditions and better responses in scotopic (dark-adapted) conditions.

Treatment

Administer taurine supplementation. A minimum intake of **110 mg/kg body weight per day** is needed for maintenance of normal retinal function.

Prognosis

Effects of prolonged deficiency are **only partially reversible**, and supplementation is of no value where there is advanced retinal degeneration with blindness. The appearance of the lesions evident at time of diagnosis will remain the same, even though the ERG signs associated with rod degeneration may reverse.

DYSCORIA ASSOCIATED WITH IRIS SYNECHIA OR PROLAPSE INTO A CORNEAL WOUND*

Classical signs

- Pear- or tear-shaped pupil, with adhesion of the acute angle of the tear to the lens capsule or to a traumatic defect in the cornea.

Clinical signs

Pear- or tear-shaped pupil, with the acute angle of the tear **sticking to either the lens capsule**, or to a traumatic defect in the **cornea**.

The abnormal shape is often accentuated by stimulating the papillary light reflex with a bright light.

Diagnosis

Diagnosis is based purely on **careful examination of the eye** by focal light examination or slit lamp biomicroscopy.

Treatment

Treatment is usually either medical or surgical.
- **Medical treatment with mydriatics** such as atropine, mydriacyl or 10% phenylephrine will sometimes pull the iris away from the lens or cornea, if used in the very early stages.
- **Surgical repair** by a veterinary ophthalmic surgeon is recommended. Repair the corneal laceration and replace the iris and tamponade away from the corneal wound, using viscoelastics.

FELINE LEUKEMIA VIRUS INFECTION/FELINE SPASTIC PUPIL SYNDROME*

Classical signs

- History of variable pupil behavior with pupils at different times alternating between miotic or dilated, in one or both eyes, over weeks to months. Intervening periods of normality with equal pupils.
- Normal vision.
- Pupils may fail to dilate or incompletely dilate in semi-darkness.

Pathogenesis

Viral neuritis is caused by feline leukemia virus (FeLV) and affects the parasympathetic and/or sympathetic efferent fibers to the iris.

Clinical signs

Cats retain vision, but the **pupils fail to dilate**, or incompletely dilate in semi-darkness.

The history often reveals **paradoxically varying pupil behavior**, with pupils alternating between miotic or dilated, in one or both eyes in the weeks to months prior to presentation. There may have been intervening periods of normality with equal pupils.

Other ocular signs may be seen, for example, FeLV-associated **lymphoma** involving the iris, may cause swelling and hemorrhage of the iris surface. See main reference on page 1300 for more details (The Cat With Abnormal Iris Appearance).

Diagnosis

Diagnosis is based on the history of an intermittent, **bizarre, inexplicable variation in pupil response**.

Supportive evidence is based on positive testing for FeLV.

Treatment

There is no treatment for this condition. This syndrome is thought to have a very poor prognosis with most cats dying within 2 years from other manifestations of the feline leukemia complex.

FELINE HEMIDILATED PUPIL SYNDROME*

Classical signs

- D-shaped pupil in the left eye or reverse D-shaped pupil in the right eye.

Pathogenesis

Cats have two short ciliary nerves carrying only parasympathetic fibers from the ciliary ganglion, referred to as the malar (lateral) and nasal (medial) nerves. The **malar nerve innervates the lateral half of the iris sphincter**, while the **nasal nerve innervates the medial half**. The dog in contrast has 5–8 short ciliary nerves which contain both sympathetic and parasympathetic fibers.

Damage to the malar nerve results in constriction of only the medial half of the pupillary constrictor muscle, while **damage to the nasal nerve** will cause constriction of only the lateral half of the muscle during miosis.

Clinical signs

Pupil appears as **D shaped in the left eye or reverse D shaped in the right eye**. The D shape is accentuated by stimulating the pupillary light reflex with a bright light.

Diagnosis

Based entirely on the observation of a D- or reverse D-shaped pupil.

Treatment

No specific treatment is indicated. Some will reverse over time, provided the nerve has not been completely transected.

ANISOCORIA ASSOCIATED WITH BLUE IRIDES AND DEAFNESS IN WHITE CATS*

Classical signs

- White cat with behavioral signs suggesting deafness.
- With a unilateral blue iris, pupils are uneven sized (anisocoria) with a larger pupil on side of blue iris.

Clinical signs

Reduced pigmentation of the iris causes blue iris coloration in a white cat. These cats also have **reduced pigment in the retinal pigment epithelium and choroid, and have no tapetum**. Where the lack of pigment is unilateral, there will always be an anisocoria, with the **non-pigmented side having a larger pupil**. This is thought to be the result of an **abnormality of the pupillary light reflex**, caused by the effect of lack of pigment on the development of the afferent pathways to the lateral geniculate nucleus and pretectal nucleus.

White cat with behavioral signs suggesting **deafness**.

Diagnosis

Diagnosis is based purely on the clinical signs occurring in a white cat.

IRIS ATROPHY*

Classical signs

- Loss of normal iris color associated with increased transparency of the iris in an old cat.
- Dilated pupil with sluggish pupillary light reflex (PLR).

Pathogenesis

Age-related atrophy and thinning of iris structures occur, especially involving the anterior stroma, pupil margin and associated pupillary constrictor muscle.

Clinical signs

Cat is **older than 10 years of age**.

There is **loss of normal coloration** because of **loss of pigment** in the anterior iris stroma. This may be especially obvious in old Siamese or other color-dilute cats with blue irides (e.g. Himalayan). The iris can become so thin, that it may take on a transparent appearance. Vision is normal.

Loss of normal pupillary light reflex is associated with atrophy of the pupillary sphincter. This sign is less commonly seen in the cat than in the dog, as the pupillary sphincter shape is more often conserved in feline iris atrophy, resulting in a **sluggish pupillary light reflex** rather than a dilated non-responsive pupil. Visible defects may occur around the pupil margin with atrophy.

Diagnosis

Diagnosis is based purely on consideration of the **age and breed of the cat**, that is, an old color-dilute cat greater than 10 years of age, and on the **clinical signs** of a sluggish pupillary light reflex, and loss of iris pigmentation.

Treatment

No treatment is possible for iris atrophy.

ANEMIC RETINOPATHY

Classical signs

- Blind, weak cat with profound anemia.
- Retinal hemorrhages and attenuated, pale retinal vessels.
- Partial to complete loss of pupil light reflex.

See main reference on page 1186 (The Blind Cat or The Cat With Retinal Disease).

Clinical signs

Blind cat with partial to complete loss of pupil light reflex.

Retinal hemorrhages and attenuated, pale retinal vessels.

Other **signs of severe anemia**, e.g. pale mucous membranes, increased respiratory rate and lethargy. Anemia must be **profound** for this syndrome to occur, i.e. **usually the PCV is less than 10%** or hemoglobin less than 5 g/dl.

Diagnosis

Diagnosis is based initially on the clinical signs of a severely anemic cat with poor papillary light reflexes and multiple small retinal hemorrhages.

Diagnosis is confirmed on hematology. The cause of the anemia should be identified. Common causes of profound anemia include FeLV-associated anemia or *Mycoplasma haemofelis* infection. FeLV-associated anemia may also be accompanied by thrombocytopenia which may contribute to the retinal hemorrhages.

HYPERVISCOSITY RETINOPATHY

Classical signs

- Blindness and loss of pupil reflexes.
- Extremely dilated tortuous retinal vessels, retinal hemorrhages, retinal detachment, perivascular effusion, optic disc edema.
- Monoclonal globulin spike on protein electrophoresis.

Clinical signs

Blindness and loss of pupil reflexes occur due to retinal damage.

Extremely dilated, tortuous retinal vessels, retinal hemorrhages, retinal detachment, perivascular effusion and optic disc edema are evident on fundoscopy.

A variety of **other clinical signs** including lethargy, weight loss, inappetence, pale mucous membranes, neurological signs and lameness may be exhibited.

Rare condition in cats.

Diagnosis

Diagnosis is initially based on the suspicious signs seen on fundoscopy, especially the presence of **bizarre, dilated, tortuous retinal vessels**.

Diagnosis is confirmed by demonstration of a **monoclonal globulin spike** on protein electrophoresis.

FELINE DYSAUTONOMIA

Classical signs

- Variable ocular signs, including reduced lacrimation, dilated non-responsive pupils, anisocoria, prolapsed third eyelids, photophobia.
- Other systemic signs such as constipation, vomiting and regurgitation, dry mouth or dry nostrils.

For more details see main reference on page 792 (The Constipated or Straining Cat) or page 203 (The Incontinent Cat).

Clinical signs

Ocular signs are due to abnormalities of autonomic innervation to eye structures and can include reduced lacrimation, **dilated non-responsive pupils, anisocoria, prolapsed third eyelids** and photophobia in a cat with vision.

Other systemic signs such as **constipation, vomiting and regurgitation, dry mouth or dry nostrils** are related to effects of the disease on autonomic nerves supplying secretory glands or the gastrointestinal system.

Typically, the onset of signs is **acute over 48 h and associated with depression and anorexia**.

Rare disease, and most common in the United Kingdom.

Diagnosis

The disease can be suspected in any cat showing combinations of the clinical signs.

Definitive diagnosis is based on histopathology of autonomic ganglia at necropsy.

PERSISTENT PUPILLARY MEMBRANE (PPM)

Classical signs

- Strands of iris-like tissue arising from the iris collarette and crossing the pupil space, or attaching to the cornea or lens.

Classical signs—Cont'd

- Dot-like opacities on the endothelial surface of the cornea or the anterior capsule of the lens.
- Thin strands of iris tissue crossing the pupil space.

Pathogenesis

The pupillary membrane is a mesodermal embryonic structure, which, until regression, forms a solid sheet of tissue bridging the pupil space and the anterior chamber.

The **pupillary membrane arises from the iris collarette**. In adult cats, the collarette appears as a slightly raised region halfway between the pupil margin and the iris root.

The pupillary membrane remains as **persistent strands of tissue** in the anterior segment of the eye, **if it fails to rarify in late fetal life**.

Clinical signs

Fibrous strands of iris-like tissue extend **from the iris collarette** (raised area approximately half way between the iris root and the pupillary margin) to either another region of the collarette, the anterior capsule of the lens, or the **posterior corneal surface** (most commonly). The strands can be very thin, and magnification may be required to visualize them.

Dot-like gray to black opacities may be visible on the endothelial surface of the cornea or the anterior capsule of the lens, and are associated with strands attaching the opacity to the iris. The opacities are unassociated with a history of previous inflammation within the eye.

The condition is **rare in cats** compared to the frequency with which it is seen in dogs, and rarely seems to affect the pupillary light reflex or pupil shape.

Diagnosis

Diagnosis is based on the **characteristic appearance** of the persistent pupillary membranes on careful ocular examination.

Differential diagnosis

The gray opacities formed by persistent pupillary membranes, which attach to the corneal endothelium should be differentiated from **keratic precipitates (KPs)**, formed as a result of anterior uveitis. A strand of tissue attaching the opacity to the iris, and the absence of other signs of anterior uveitis is diagnostic of a persistent pupillary membrane.

Treatment

No treatment is indicated.

IRIS COLOBOMA

> **Classical signs**
> - Wedge-like or radial sectorial defect in the iris.

Clinical signs

Wedge-like or radial sectorial defect in the iris.

Occurs as a **congenital anomaly**, but can be first noticed in a cat of any age.

The defect may enable structures behind the iris, for example the lens equator or lens zonules, to be visualized more readily in the affected sector.

Diagnosis

The condition is quite rare in cats, and should be differentiated from **iris atrophy** seen in old color-dilute (Himalayan or Siamese) type cats.

HEREDITARY PROGRESSIVE RETINAL PHOTORECEPTOR DYSPLASIA OR DEGENERATION

> **Classical signs**
> - Progressive vision loss especially in a young Abyssinian cat.
> - Slow loss of pupillary light reflexes.
> - Fundoscopic signs of tapetal hyper-reflectivity and retinal vessel attenuation.

Pathogenesis

Although rare, genetically determined **progressive retinal rod–cone degeneration** has been described in Abyssinian, Siamese and Persian cats.

The best-described degeneration occurs in the **Abyssinian cat**. In this breed, both autosomal dominant rod–cone dysplasia (onset 2–3 months of age), and autosomal recessive rod–cone degeneration (onset 1–2 years of age) modes of inheritance have been described. The disease in Abyssinians is now seen rarely.

Clinical signs

Typically there is a history of **progressive vision loss**.

Slow loss of pupillary light reflexes progresses to dilated pupils non-responsive to light.

Occasionally other signs, such as variable or intermittent **nystagmus**, are seen, especially in the rod–cone dysplasia in Abyssinian kittens.

In the adult-onset form, the fundoscopic signs start as a **subtle grayish discoloration in the central retina** on each side of the optic nerve head. The lesion progresses to a more diffuse gray tapetal discoloration with early retinal vessel attenuation. Later, hyper-reflective areas start to appear within the discolored tapetum. Finally, there is extensive tapetal hyper-reflectivity with severe attenuation of retinal vessels.

In the early-onset form there is tapetal fundus dullness and loss of detail evident at 8–12 weeks of age. Progression of the disease is fairly rapid, with development of tapetal hyper-reflectivity, loss of pigmentation in the non-tapetum and vessel attenuation. There is end-stage degeneration by 12 months of age.

Diagnosis

Diagnosis is based on the history of a **slow onset of vision loss**, with slow deterioration of the pupillary light reflex and characteristic fundoscopic changes in an Abyssinian cat.

Diagnosis can be confirmed by demonstration of progressive reductions in b-wave amplitude on electroretinography.

Differential diagnosis

Other retinal diseases can usually be differentiated by age and breed of the cat, other systemic signs and the fundoscopic changes.

- **Taurine deficiency retinopathy** may also produce the signs associated with dilated cardiomyopathy.
- **Hypertensive retinopathy** is usually sudden in onset in an old cat, and typically there is retinal detachment and associated renal and/or thyroid disease.

- **Feline infectious peritonitis** usually causes signs in young cats. Typically systemic signs of anorexia, lethargy and fever are also seen.

Treatment

There is no treatment for progressive retinal degeneration.

RECOMMENDED READING

Aguirre GD. Retinal degeneration associated with the feeding of dog foods to cats. J Am Vet Med Assoc 1978; 172: 791–796.

Bellhorn RW, Aguirre GD, Bellhorn M. Feline central retinal degeneration. Invest Ophthalmol 1974; 608–616.

Bercovitch M, Krohne S, Lindley D. A diagnostic approach to anisocoria. Compend Contin Educ Pract Vet 1995; 17: 661–672.

Glaze MB, Gelatt KN. Diseases of the anterior uvea. In: Stiles J (ed) Ocular Manifestations of Systemic Disease, Part 2. The Cat. In: Gelatt KN (series ed) Veterinary Ophthalmology, 3rd edn. Baltimore, Maryland, Lippincott, Williams & Wilkins, 1999, pages 1018–1028, 1448–1467.

Miller W, Johnson B. How ocular signs reveal systemic disease in cats. Vet Med 1989; 780–788.

Sansom J, Barnett KC, et al. Ocular disease associated with hypertension in 16 cats. J Small Anim Pract 1994; 35: 604–611.

Stiles J, Polzin DJ, Bistner SI The prevalence of retinopathy in cats with systemic hypertension and chronic renal failure or hyperthyroidism. J Am Anim Hosp Assoc 1994; 30: 564–571.

63. The cat with abnormal iris appearance

Michael E. Bernays

KEY SIGNS

- Abnormal iris shape.
- Abnormal iris coloration.

MECHANISM?

- Inflammatory processes, either idiopathic or associated with infectious agents, are the most common cause of changed iris appearance. Neoplasia, immune-mediated inflammation and degeneration are less frequent mechanisms for change.

WHERE?

- Iris.
- Other organ systems.

WHAT?

- Most diseases which alter iris appearance are inflammatory associated with infectious agents such as FIP, FIV, FeLV and *Toxoplasma*, or are idiopathic. Iris neoplasia from melanoma or lymphosarcoma are less common. Iris atrophy associated with age-related degeneration is common in old cats.

QUICK REFERENCE SUMMARY

Diseases causing abnormal iris appearance

DEGENERATIVE

● **Iris atrophy* (p 1299)**
Thinning of the iris with loss of normal iris color. Loss of normal pupillary constrictor function resulting in sluggish pupil light reflex in an old cat.

ANOMALY

● **Iris coloboma (p 1304)**
Notch-like or sectorial defect in structure of the iris. Unusual.

● **Persistent pupillary membranes (p 1304)**
Small strand-like structures going from one part of the iris collarette to another, to the anterior lens capsule or to the posterior corneal surface. Rare.

- Iris cyst (p 1305)

Small brown to black cyst-like structures commonly found at the pupil margin which may become more obvious with pupil dilation. May be semi-transparent.

METABOLIC

● Pre-iridal fibrovascular membranes* (p 1303)

New vessels growing across the anterior surface of the iris giving the iris a pink injected appearance. An intra-ocular neoplasm, a retinal detachment or signs of chronic inflammation may be evident. There may be secondary hyphema or glaucoma.

NEOPLASTIC

● Iris neoplasia*** (p 1297)

Diffuse iris melanoma appears as a brown to light tan discoloration, which is rapidly progressive over the iris surface over weeks to months. It usually occurs in older cats, and is usually unilateral. Lymphosarcoma appears as bilateral iris swelling, and anterior chamber hemorrhage, in a young cat with or without other signs suggesting a multicentric location. Ciliary body adenoma is rare, and appears as a slow-growing whitish to cream mass behind the pupil margin. Metastatic neoplasia from an extra-ocular primary tumor is an intra-ocular neoplasm involving the iris, and is associated with a similar neoplasm remote from the eye, e.g. mammary or uterine adenocarcinoma.

INFECTIOUS

Viral:

● Feline leukemia virus (FeLV)** (p 1300)

Signs of anterior uveitis such as blood, fibrin or cloudiness in the anterior chamber, miosis, or general reddening or thickening of the iris in a FeLV-positive cat. Bilateral iris swelling from lymphosarcoma may be present.

● Feline immunodeficiency virus (FIV)** (p 1302)

Signs of anterior uveitis such as blood, fibrin or cloudiness in the anterior chamber, miosis, or general reddening or thickening of the iris and/or swelling associated with lymphosarcoma in a FIV-positive cat.

● Feline infectious peritonitis (FIP) virus*** (p 1295)

Severe anterior fibrinous uveitis, usually bilateral, in a young cat. Other signs of FIP such as anorexia, weight loss, depression, pyrexia, abdominal or chest effusions and/or multifocal neurological disease.

Bacterial:

● *Bartonella henselae* (cat-scratch fever) (p 1305)

Typically, naturally infected cats only develop subclinical disease, although anterior uveitis has been reported.

Protozoal:

● *Toxoplasma gondii*** (p 1296)

Signs may be acute, or chronic and intermittent. Fever, lethargy and anorexia with various combinations of respiratory, hepatic, ocular and neurological signs.

continued

continued

Fungal:

- **Fungal infections (*Cryptococcus neoformans*, blastomycosis, coccidioidomycosis, *Histoplasma capsulatum*)** (p 1302)**

  Fever, depression, anorexia and weight loss combined with signs of other organ disease such as involvement of lung, liver, bone marrow, lymph nodes, CNS and/or eyes. Typically there is chorioretinitis progressing to anterior uveitis and endophthalmitis associated with positive serological evidence of an infectious cause, or identification of an organism in anterior chamber fluid. Fungal uveitis has a geographic distribution.

Parasitic:

- Cuterebra larval migration (ophthalmomyiasis) (p 1305)

  Vision loss, poor PLR and characteristic track-like lesions in the tapetal fundus, with or without anterior uveitis.

- Ocular dirofilariasis (p 1305)

  Uveitis occurs associated with presence of adult filaria in the eye. Rare.

Immune:

- **Lymphocytic-plasmacytic uveitis* (p 1302)**

  Chronic gray to slightly tan nodules in the anterior stromal surface of the iris.

Idiopathic:

- **Idiopathic uveitis* (p 1302)**

  Uveitis in a cat where extensive investigation does not reveal a possible etiology.

Trauma:

- **Penetrating injuries to the iris** (p 1299)**

  Changes may occur in the iris appearance associated with trauma, including fibrinous adhesions to adjacent structures, tears in the iris proper or iris prolapse through the outer ocular coats, i.e. the cornea and sclera. Penetrating foreign bodies may or may not be obvious.

INTRODUCTION

MECHANISM?

The most common cause of changed iris appearance is inflammation, most commonly associated with infectious agents, although inflammation secondary to neoplasia and immune-mediated disease may also occur.

Important pathophysiologic processes involved in iris inflammation (anterior uveitis) include breakdown of the blood–aqueous barrier associated with increased vessel permeability, release of chemical mediators following tissue damage, and chemotaxis of polymorphonuclear and mononuclear leukocytes.

The most important chemical mediators are probably the **arachidonic acid derivatives** released from damaged cell membranes, which then participate in the cyclo-oxygenase and the lipoxygenase pathways. Prostaglandins produced by the cyclo-oxygenase pathway are regarded as the most important chemical mediators. Oxygen free radicals may also be important.

While most types of immunologic responses are thought to occur in the eye, types II (antibody-mediated cytotoxic responses), III (immune-complex deposition and complement activation) and IV (cell-mediated cytotoxic responses) are thought to be the most important. Monocytes and macrophages are important in phagocytosis, antigen processing and presentation to T cells.

Immune-mediated responses to retinal or lens antigens may be important in immune-mediated uveitis where no infectious cause is identified.

Some neoplastic diseases, e.g. intra-ocular lymphosarcoma can look very inflammatory, whereas others (e.g. diffuse iris melanoma) tend to cause gross pigment changes without necessarily causing an inflammatory response until the disease becomes very advanced.

Changes which can be seen in association with inflammation of the iris (anterior uveitis) include:

- **Generalized reddening** (hyperemia) and thickening of the iris.
- **Frank hemorrhage** from the iris surface.
- Fibrinous exudation resulting in **cream to red-colored solid opacities** in the anterior chamber, or over the surface of the iris.
- **Miosis**.
- **Grayish nodules** on the iris surface which represent localized aggregations of lymphoid cells.
- Gray to tan, dot-like, or sometimes coalescing opacities on the endothelial surface of the cornea (called **keratic precipitates**).
- **Cloudiness** of the aqueous fluid (called aqueous flare).
- Deposits of pigment or inflammatory cell debris on the anterior lens capsule. Adhesions of the pupil margin to the lens may occur (called **posterior synechiae**). If synechia are extensive, there may be anterior bowing of the iris (called iris bombé) and a shallow anterior chamber.
- Anterior cortical **cataract**.
- **Iris cysts**, either attached to the pupillary margin or free floating in the anterior chamber.
- **Anterior vitreous opacity** due to inflammation of the pars plana of the ciliary body ("pars planitis"). This change is especially associated with feline immunodeficiency virus (FIV) infection.
- **Corneal vascularization**.
- Engorgement of the deep episcleral vessels.
- **Lens subluxation or luxation**. This is usually due to inflammatory destruction of ciliary zonules, but may result from secondary glaucoma, which causes globe enlargement and zonule stretching.

WHERE?

Diseases which alter iris appearance can arise in and be confined to the iris, they can result from disease processes involving other parts of the eye, or they can be a localized manifestation of systemic disease.

WHAT?

Most diseases which alter iris appearance are inflammatory. Investigation of many cases of anterior uveitis for a possible infectious cause may not identify an etiologic agent, and so **many cases of uveitis in the cat are regarded as "idiopathic"**. Most cases of idiopathic uveitis probably involve an autoimmune response to an unidentified endogenous antigen.

Severe inflammation in a young cat is more likely to have an infectious etiology and **feline infectious peritonitis (FIP)** should be considered as one of the more likely possibilities.

A change in pigmentation in an older cat is more likely to be due to **neoplasia**.

Iris atrophy secondary to degenerative changes is a common incidental finding in may old cats.

Congenital abnormalities such as persistent pupillary membranes or iris colobomas are seen far less commonly.

DISEASES CAUSING ABNORMAL IRIS APPEARANCE

FELINE INFECTIOUS PERITONITIS VIRUS***

Classical signs

- Severe anterior fibrinous uveitis, usually bilateral, in a young cat.
- Other signs of FIP such as anorexia, weight loss, pyrexia, abdominal or chest effusions, multifocal neurological disease.

See main references on page 372 for details (The Pyrexic Cat).

Pathogenesis

Infection is thought to be acquired by inhalation or ingestion.

The virus replicates in the tonsils, epithelial cells of pharynx, respiratory mucosa and small intestine then infects monocytes, which disseminate the virus throughout the body.

The effusive form of the disease is thought to occur in cats with poor cell-mediated immune (CMI) responses, and the non-effusive form in cats with partial cell-mediated immunity.

The effusive form is associated with **immune complex-mediated vasculitis**.

The non-effusive form is characterized by **pyogranulomatous and granulomatous lesions in many organs** in particular eyes, brain, liver and kidney.

Clinical signs

Initially mild upper respiratory tract signs may occur, but usually go unnoticed.

Generally the disease is seen in young cats less than 1–2 years of age.

Anorexia, pyrexia, weight loss and malaise are typical. Other signs including icterus, abdominal distention, dyspnea and multifocal neurological signs are variably present.

In the eye, the most common presenting sign is a fibrinous uveitis. Fibrinous exudation results in **cream to red-colored solid opacities** in the anterior chamber, or over the surface of the iris.

Other signs of anterior uveitis such as blood or cloudiness in the anterior chamber, miosis, general reddening or thickening of the iris, and injection of deep episcleral vessels may be evident.

Diagnosis

A presumptive diagnosis is initially based on a combination of the clinical signs and laboratory findings. FIP should be **suspected especially when a bilateral fibrinous uveitis occurs in a young cat**.

Hematology and biochemistry may be helpful but are not definitive. Changes typical of FIP include a mild normocytic, normochromic anemia, neutrophilic leukocytosis and lymphopaenia, elevated total serum proteins, and a **polyclonal gammopathy** due to elevated alpha-2 globulins and gamma globulins.

Serology is usually regarded as being of dubious benefit in the diagnosis, as the FIP coronavirus cross-reacts with enteric forms of coronavirus.

Diagnosis can only be confirmed on characteristic histopathology of affected tissues on biopsy or necropsy examination. Typical change is described as a pyogranulomatous vasculitis. Necrosis and a fibrinoid response are seen in some cases.

Treatment

No treatment will cure the disease, which is invariably fatal. There is no prognosis for long-term survival, especially for cases with the effusive form. Cases with uveitis only may have a slightly better long-term prognosis.

Recent interest has been shown in the use of recombinant **alpha interferon** at doses ranging between 10 000–30 000 IU/kg given SQ daily for **short-term remission of signs**.

Palliative therapy traditionally has included the use of corticosteroids, including **topical 0.5% prednisolone** acetate applied to the eyes q 6–8 h for cases with uveitis.

Cats which are anorexic and depressed, and do not respond to supportive therapy, should be euthanized.

TOXOPLASMA GONDII INFECTION***

> ### Classical signs
>
> - Fever, weight loss, inappetence, malaise.
> - +/– Muscle or joint pain.
> - +/– Signs of respiratory, hepatic and/or neurological disease.
> - Typical signs of anterior uveitis.

See main references on page 375 for details (The Pyrexic Cat) and page 958 (The Cat With Generalized Weakness).

Pathogenesis

Infection occurs by:

- Ingestion of tissue cysts (bradyzoites) from an intermediate host (most common) or
- Ingestion of sporulated oocysts from soil or water (far less common) or
- Transplacental transmission (rare).

After ingestion a **gut replication cycle occurs**. The cat is the definitive host and is the only species in which this occurs. This results in the production of unsporulated (non-infective) oocysts which are passed in feces. The oocysts **sporulate in the environment after 1–5 days** and become **infective**. Intestinal replication will also result in the formation of **tachyzoites (active acute infection)** or **bradyzoites (inactive latent infection)**.

Activation of bradyzoites, typically found in muscle, brain and liver, may occur because of other disease states such as FIV, which act as stressors or immunosuppressors. High-dose corticosteroid use has been known to activate dormant *T. gondii* infections.

When bradyzoites are activated, they undergo rapid replication causing destruction of tissue and inciting an inflammatory response in various tissues, notably the **central nervous system, uveal tract of the eye, liver and lungs**.

Clinical signs

Signs may be acute, or chronic and intermittent. The acute fatal form occurs mostly in kittens.

Fever, anorexia, depression, weight loss.

Muscle or joint pain may be evident.

Dyspnea is common in kittens and cats with the acute form, and is associated with pneumonia.

Multifocal neurologic signs.

Signs of liver disease such as jaundice, enlarged liver, ascites or elevated liver enzymes.

Ocular signs, especially anterior uveitis, chorioretinitis and optic neuritis. The organism may cause a lymphocytic-plasmacytic uveitis evidenced by gray to tan-colored nodules on the iris surface.

Diagnosis

Diagnosis may be based initially on the clinical signs, but obtaining supportive laboratory data is essential in making a definitive diagnosis.

Serology.

- Demonstration of a **rise in IgM titers** indicates a recent active infection.
- **Comparison of levels of aqueous humor *T. gondii* antibody levels with serum levels** (Goldman–Witmer coefficient or C-value) has been advocated to determine that anterior uveitis has been caused by *T. gondii*, although the use of C-values is still controversial.

Definitive diagnosis requires demonstration of the organism **in inflamed tissues or fluid samples by histology, immunohistochemistry, or polymerase chain reaction (PCR) techniques**.

Treatment

Clindamycin (Antirobe, Upjohn) at a dose rate of 12.5 mg/kg twice daily for 3–4 weeks is usually effective against the organism. If no response is evident after 3 weeks of antibiotic therapy, reconsider the diagnosis.

Concurrent anti-inflammatory therapy decreases the anterior uveitis, e.g. topical 0.5% **prednisolone** acetate drops applied bid–qid.

IRIS NEOPLASIA***

Classical signs

- Diffuse pigmentary change across the anterior iris surface.
- Mass lesions bulging forward from the anterior iris stroma or distorting normal pupil shape.

Pathogenesis

Various tumors occur in the iris such as melanoma, lymphosarcoma, sarcoma and ciliary body tumors.

Diffuse iris melanoma arises as a primary neoplasia of the iris stroma, and is the most common primary intra-ocular neoplasm seen in cats.

Lymphosarcoma results from invasion of neoplastic lymphocytes from the peripheral circulation.

Intra-ocular sarcoma usually occurs as a sequel after (usually years) trauma causing penetrating injury to the lens. It is believed that the sarcoma arises from trans-formed lens epithelium. This neoplasm forms solid masses within the eye, which metastasize rapidly, usually via the optic nerve.

Ciliary body tumors may represent primary neoplasia or metastatic neoplasia from an extra-ocular site.

Clinical signs

Diffuse iris melanoma typically appears as an enlarging area over months to years of light tan to dark brown pigmentation on the iris surface. Usually the neoplasm does not form an obvious discrete mass, but the iris may become diffusely thickened. The disease is usually unilateral and typically occurs in older cats.

- Presentation may more resemble uveal inflammation than neoplasia.
- Sometimes the disease may present in an advanced state with secondary glaucoma.
- Amelanotic diffuse iris melanomas have also been reported.

Lymphosarcoma and post-traumatic sarcoma more commonly form **discrete masses** within the eye. Lymphosarcoma often presents as bilateral iris swelling, and anterior chamber hemorrhage in a young cat, with or without other signs suggesting multicentric neoplasia.

Ciliary body adenoma is a rare, slow-growing neo-plasm, which appears as a whitish to cream mass behind the pupil margin.

Metastatic neoplasia from an extra-ocular primary tumor appears as an intra-ocular neoplasm involving the iris, and is associated with a similar neoplasm remote from the eye, e.g. mammary or uterine adeno-carcinoma.

Diagnosis

Diagnosis is based initially on the appearance of the iris and consideration of the history.

Amelanotic diffuse iris melanomas are difficult to diag-nose unless the effects of the tumor on angle obstruc-tion and resultant glaucoma are observed.

Definitive diagnosis may be obtained by **fine-needle aspirate biopsies** or anterior chamber centesis and cytology.

Differential diagnosis

Diffuse iris melanoma needs to be differentiated from other causes of pigmentation of the iris and can look similar to:

- **A benign pigmented nevus,** which appears as a flat pigment spot in the iris. A nevus will be observed not to have changed in size with serial examination.
- **Post-inflammatory pigmentation**. A detailed history may reveal previous bouts of anterior uveitis within the eye. This pigmentation will not be progressive.

Treatment

Enucleation of an eye with diffuse iris melanoma is recommended if:

- There is evidence of rapid spread of a diffuse iris melanoma. The eye should be reassessed frequently to determine if the pigmentary change is progressive.
- Pigmentary change is seen near or in the irido-corneal angle on gonioscopy.
- A change in pupil shape or mobility occurs.
- Secondary glaucoma develops.

Evidence of metastasis may still occur as late as 2–3 years after enucleation.

If there is a high suspicion or confirmation of an **intra-ocular sarcoma** it requires **immediate enucleation** with exenteration of orbital tissue. Prognosis is still guarded and most cats will eventually die from metastatic disease within months.

Systemic chemotherapy for **lymphosarcoma** can be attempted unless the eye is already affected by secondary glaucoma. For more detail see main reference on page 432 (The Yellow Cat or Cat With Elevated Liver Enzymes).

PENETRATING INJURIES TO THE IRIS**

> **Classical signs**
>
> - Corneal lacerations.
> - Mis-shapen pupil margin and bulging of iris tissue into the corneal defect.
> - Visible iris tear.
> - Blood and fibrin in the anterior chamber.

Pathogenesis

Injuries to the iris usually occur in conjunction with injuries to the adjacent cornea or sclera.

If the corneal injury is large, the iris may prolapse through the cornea and plug the defect.

Clinical signs

Trauma to the eye may result in a variety of changes to the iris including:

- **Visible iris tears**.
- **Iris prolapse through the corneal wound**. A black, bulging membrane will be seen with associated fibrin. The pupil margin is mis-shapen associated with the iris moving forward into the corneal defect.
- **Fibrinous adhesions** to adjacent structures.

Fibrin and blood in the anterior chamber (hyphema) are often present with trauma.

Associated **lens injury may occur**, which may be difficult to appreciate without removing fibrin from the anterior chamber and dilating the pupil.

A penetrating foreign body may or may not be evident.

Diagnosis

Diagnosis is based purely on the appearance of the iris on careful examination.

Treatment

Surgical repair is recommended. This might include replacement of iris tissue into the anterior chamber with suturing of the corneal defect. Viscoelastic substances and mydriatics can be used to push the iris away from the cornea.

Partial iridectomy may be necessary if a prolapsed section of iris is badly damaged or atonic.

Intra-ocular surgery may be required to **remove a damaged lens** to prevent destruction of the eye by severe lens-induced intra-ocular inflammation. If the lens is severely traumatized then eye ablation would be recommended to reduce the possibility of later post-traumatic intra-ocular sarcoma development.

IRIS ATROPHY**

> **Classical signs**
>
> - Loss of normal iris color and increased transparency of the iris in an old cat.
> - Sluggish pupillary light reflex (PLR).

Pathogenesis

Iris atrophy is an **age-related atrophy and thinning of iris structures**, especially the anterior stroma, pupil margin and associated pupillary constrictor muscle.

Clinical signs

Iris atrophy occurs in old cats, and appears as **loss of normal coloration and increased transparency of the iris because of loss of pigment** in the anterior iris stroma. This may be **especially obvious in old Siamese cats or other color-dilute cats** with blue irides. The iris can become so thin that it may take on a transparent appearance.

There may be **some loss of normal pupillary light reflex** (PLR) associated with atrophy of the pupillary sphincter. In old cats with iris atrophy, pupil shape is often retained, but the PLR is not as brisk as in a younger cat. It is unusual to see atrophy to the degree sometimes seen in old dogs, where notch-like defects occur, with thin connecting strands across the defect.

If the pupil becomes very dilated, the equator of the lens may become visible.

Diagnosis

Diagnosis is based principally on a consideration of age and clinical signs.

Treatment

There is no treatment for iris atrophy.

FELINE LEUKEMIA VIRUS (FELV)**

Classical signs

- Discrete iris or ciliary body masses (FeLV-associated lymphosarcoma).
- Anterior uveitis, fibrin and blood in the anterior chamber.
- Otherwise unexplainable intermittent asymmetric changes in pupil size, shape or response.
- Other FeLV-associated signs, e.g. anemia.

See main references on page 540 for details (The Anemic Cat) and page 350 (The Thin, Inappetent Cat).

Pathogenesis

Following oral or nasal exposure to the virus, there is viral **replication in oropharyngeal lymphoid tissue**. If the immune response to the virus is ineffective in eliminating it, there is **replication of virus in bone marrow**, which leads to viremia, FeLV-related diseases or latent infection.

Infection with the virus is known to **cause a number of neoplasms**, including alimentary, mediastinal, renal, spinal, retrobulbar or lymph node forms as well as a number of hematologic lymphoid malignancies involving different bone marrow precursors.

Malignant lymphoid cells can invade intra-ocular uveal structures, generally as part of a wider syndrome of multicentric lymphosarcoma.

A **viral neuritis** can also be caused by FeLV, and affect parasympathetic or sympathetic efferent fibers to the iris in feline spastic pupil syndrome.

FeLV is also associated with uveitis.

Clinical signs

Discrete iris or ciliary body masses, which cause gross distortion of iris structure, and are usually bilateral.

Fibrin and/or blood may be evident in the anterior chamber indicating the presence of anterior uveitis.

Spastic pupil syndrome is associated with FeLV neuritis. Vision is retained, but one or both pupils are intermittently miotic or dilated over weeks or months, and they do not dilate appropriately with darkness. For more detail see main reference on page 878 (The Cat With Anisocoria or Abnormally Dilated or Constricted Pupils).

Diagnosis

Diagnosis is based on the clinical signs observed in the eye, in association with other signs suggestive of FeLV, e.g. multicentric lymphoma, FeLV-associated anemia.

Diagnosis is confirmed on **clinical pathology** including hematology and cytology of lymph nodes or aqueous centesis samples which demonstrate neoplasia.

A positive serological test for FeLV antigen suggests association of the neoplasm or spastic pupil syndrome with FeLV infection. For more details of testing see main reference on page 543 (The Anemic Cat).

Treatment

For more detail see main reference on page 544 (The Anemic Cat)

Treatment of the ocular condition in conjunction with systemic chemotherapy might include topical corticosteroids such as **0.5% prednisolone acetate drops** given q 6–12 h. Prognosis for the eye will be poor to guarded if secondary glaucoma has occurred.

FUNGAL INFECTIONS** (*CRYPTOCOCCUS NEOFORMANS*, BLASTOMYCOSIS, COCCIDIOIDOMYCOSIS, *HISTOPLASMA CAPSULATUM*)

Classical signs

- Chorioretinitis progressing to anterior uveitis and endophthalmitis, occurring in a geographical area where fungal infections are known to occur.
- Vision loss and reduced pupil light reflexes in affected eyes.
- Signs of other organ system disease, e.g. renal, CNS, nasal cavity.

See main references on page 16 for details (The Cat With Signs of Chronic Nasal Disease) for cryptococcosis and pages 371, 379, 387 (The Pyrexic Cat) for other fungi.

Pathogenesis

In general, all deep fungal infections enter the body by the **inhalation of aerosolized spores** leading to either **fungal rhinitis** (e.g. *Cryptococcus*) or **pneumonia** (e.g. blastomycosis, histoplasmosis) with subsequent dissemination to other parts of the body, including the eye, by hematogenous or lymphatic spread.

The initial ocular site for establishment of infection is usually the choroid, while the anterior uveal tract is often involved later in the course of the infection.

The different intra-ocular fungi vary in their geographical distribution.

- **Blastomycosis** is caused by a dimorphic fungus, which grows as a yeast in mammalian tissue and as a mycelial form in the environment. Found in the USA (in the midwestern and southeastern states along the Mississipi, Ohio and Missouri Rivers and occasionally mid Atlantic states), Central America, parts of Asia, Africa, Europe and Israel. Close proximity to water may be a factor in its geographical distribution.
- **Cryptococcosis** is caused by a budding capsulated yeast-like fungus with more worldwide distribution. *C. neoformans* is shed in pigeon feces and can be found in soil or in avian excreta. *C. neoformans* var. *gatti* is found in the developing flower of some Australian Eucalypt trees (red river gums and forest red gums). High concentrations of organisms are found in the bark and the accumulated debris surrounding the base of the tree. These trees have been widely exported around the world from Australia.
- **Histoplasmosis** is caused by a dimorphic fungus which forms a free-living mycelial form and yeast-like organisms in mammalian tissues. Found in central USA especially in Ohio, Mississippi and Missouri River basins and in Central and South America. There is association with moist humid conditions, nitrogen-rich soils, and bat and bird excrement.
- **Coccidioidomycosis** is caused by a soil mycelial organism with a natural resevoir in desert soils and around animal burrows. Found in Southwestern USA, Mexico, Central and South America. Animal infection occurs by inhalation of arthrospores, which can transform into spherules and then endospores in lung tissue.

Clinical signs

Typically, there is **anorexia, depression, fever and weight loss** combined with other systemic signs which can involve many other organs, especially the **lungs, brain, nasal cavity but also the orbital tissues, lymph nodes, bones, toenails and skin**.

Most **intra-ocular fungal infections** cause either:

- **Choroidal granulomas** which are typically evident on fundoscopy as a raised area of tapetal hyporeflectivity, or **small swollen brownish discolored areas** in the tapetal and non-tapetal retina.
- **Generalized chorioretinitis** and secondary retinal detachments. This may progress to anterior uveitis and endophthalmitis.
- **Optic neuritis,** which is seen as a red, swollen optic nerve that is hyperemic.
- **Anterior uveitis,** which appears as anterior chamber flare, miosis and an inflamed discolored iris.
- Vision loss and **reduced pupil light reflexes** in affected eyes.

Diagnosis

Initial diagnosis is based on the clinical presentation of a cat with a rapidly progressive, usually bilateral chorioretinitis progressing to anterior uveitis, with signs of other systemic disease, and occurring in a geographic area where such fungal disease is known to occur.

Imaging techniques can be used to obtain more supportive evidence of a deep fungal infection:

- Thoracic radiography for pulmonary granulomas.
- Nasal cavity radiography.
- Ocular ultrasound for signs of retinal detachment.

Confirmation of the diagnosis is based on the demonstration of the organism in:

- Cerebrospinal fluid.
- Samples taken by centesis of vitreous or subretinal exudate.
- Histopathology of enucleated globes.
- Bone marrow biopsy samples (histoplasmosis).
- Lung or lymph node aspirates or draining tracts.

Serological tests can be performed, looking for elevated:

- Antibodies (blastomycosis, histoplasmosis, coccidiodomycosis).
- Antigen – Cryptococcal capsular antigen in blood, CSF, or urine is sensitive and specific.

Treatment

Antifungal medications. Drug chosen should be based on results of fungal culture and sensitivity where possible. Treatment may need to be prolonged, depending on response.

- Itraconazole 100 mg PO daily with food.
- Fluconazole 50 mg PO q 8 hours.
- Amphotericin B. See page 26 (The Cat With Signs of Chronic Nasal Disease) for description of administration in a subcutaneous infusion of glucose and sodium chloride to reduce the renal toxicity.

Avoid use of systemic corticosteroids in systemic fungal disease.

Topical steroids or non-steroidals may be used to control the anterior uveitis.

Supportive therapy is important until anti-fungal medication is effective.

Enucleation of the eye is recommended if endophthalmitis and/or secondary glaucoma develop.

Prognosis

Guarded to grave in most cases where there is systemic involvement.

FELINE IMMUNODEFICIENCY VIRUS (FIV) INFECTION**

Classical signs

- Signs of uveitis.
- Bilateral iris swelling associated with neoplasia.

See main references on page 330 for details (The Thin, Inappetent Cat) and page 399 (The Cat With Enlarged Lymph Nodes).

Pathogenesis

Ocular disease including uveitis, glaucoma, infiltration of inflammatory cells in the posterior chamber (pars planitis), focal retinal chorioretinitis and retinal hemorrhages have been reported associated with FIV infection.

Neoplasia including lymphoma (often extra-nodal) have been associated with the terminal stage of the disease, although the exact role of FIV in the neoplastic process is unclear.

Clinical signs

Signs of anterior uveitis, e.g. miosis, injected iris surface, anterior chamber flare, fibrin.

Discrete iris or ciliary body masses causing iris swelling, which is associated with lymphosarcoma.

Diagnosis

Diagnosis is based on the clinical signs of uveitis or lymphosarcoma in a FIV-positive cat, and failure to identify any other possible cause.

LYMPHOCYTIC-PLASMACYTIC UVEITIS*

Classical signs

- Gray to tan nodules on the anterior surface of the iris.
- Keratic precipitates.

PATHOGENESIS

Lymphocytic-plasmacytic uveitis stems from an **immune-mediated process**, which results in the formation of **numerous lymphoid nodules within the anterior uveal tract**. It is probably a response to endogenous antigens, and in some cats, *Toxoplasma* is regarded as a possible cause.

Clinical signs

Typically there are **gray to tan nodules on the anterior surface of the iris**.

Opacities occur on the **endothelial surface of the cornea** (keratic precipitates)

Aqueous flare (cloudiness of the anterior chamber due to suspended proteins and cells)

Pre-iridal fibrovascular membranes occur in the chronic stages.

Secondary glaucoma, lens luxation and globe enlargement occur in the chronic stages.

Diagnosis

Diagnosis is based principally on the appearance of the iris.

Cytology of aqueous humor usually reveals lymphocytes and occasional plasma cells.

Treatment

There is no cure for this disease. Once the nodules have been formed they will never go away completely with therapy, however treatment will control the inflammation and reduce the incidence of the secondary sequelae.

Topical corticosteroids.
- **Prednisolone** acetate
  Prednefrin Forte (Allergan - 1%) applied q 8–12 h.
  Sterofrin (Alcon - 0.5%) q 6–8 h reducing to effect.

Topical NSAIDs.
- **Flurbiprofen** (Ocufen 0.03%) applied q 8–12 h.

Mydriatics such as atropine are rarely indicated because of the side effects of salivation seen in cats and the chronic nature of the disease.

Treat glaucoma with:
- Continuing steroid or NSAID therapy.
- Topical carbonic anhydrase inhibitors (Dorzolamide 2% topically tid).
- Topical beta-blockers, e.g. timolol maleate 0.5% applied bid–tid.

Laser cyclo-photo-coagulation in chronic cases non-responsive to medical treatment.

Glaucoma will often be refractory to treatment.

PRE-IRIDAL FIBROVASCULAR MEMBRANES*

Classical signs

- New vessels growing across the anterior surface of the iris giving the iris a pink injected appearance.
- ± Intra-ocular neoplasm, detached retina and/or uveitis.

Pathogenesis

Pre-iridal fibrovascular membrane (PIFM) formation is associated with angiogenic factors released by proliferating intra-ocular neoplasms, retinal hypoxia or chronic inflammation.

Clinical signs

PIFMs appear as **new vessels growing across the anterior surface of the iris**, giving the iris a pink discoloration.

Because PIFM formation is associated with **intra-ocular neoplasms, retinal detachment or chronic inflammation**, these abnormalities may be evident on careful examination of the eye.

PIFMs may be associated with secondary **hyphema or glaucoma**.

Occasionally the vessels in PIFMs may be visible leaving the pupil margin and migrating across the anterior lens capsule.

Diagnosis

Diagnosis is based on the characteristic appearance of the fibrovascular membranes on the anterior stromal surface of the iris.

Occasionally an underlying cause may be apparent, e.g. a ciliary body epithelial tumor at the pupil space or a total retinal detachment.

Differential diagnosis

Iris neoplasia, especially secondary neoplasms of the iris arising in some other part of the body, e.g. lymphosarcoma resulting in hyphema.

Acute inflammation resulting in pinkish injection of the anterior iris surface.

Treatment

There is no treatment for PIFMs except for treatment of the underlying chronic diseases, which may be associated with the condition. Once formed the PIFMs will remain permanently on the iris surface.

IDIOPATHIC UVEITIS*

Classical signs

- Signs of uveitis.
- Extensive laboratory investigations fail to identify possible etiology.

Clinical signs

Idiopathic uveitis is characterized by any signs of anterior uveitis such as miosis, injected iris surface, anterior chamber flare, and fibrin, where **extensive laboratory investigations fails to identify a possible etiology**.

One study showed there may be a significant positive association of idiopathic anterior uveitis with **high aqueous titers to herpesvirus**.

Diagnosis

Diagnosis is based on the clinical signs of uveitis with failure to identify a possible cause.

PERSISTENT PUPILLARY MEMBRANES

Classical signs

- Strands of iris-like tissue arising from the iris collarette and crossing the pupil space, or attaching to the cornea or lens.
- Dot-like gray to black opacities on the endothelial surface of the cornea or the anterior capsule of the lens unassociated with history of previous inflammation within the eye.
- Rare in cats.

Pathogenesis

Persistent papillary membrane is an embryonic structure, and results from **failure of the pupillary membrane to rarify in late fetal life**.

The pupillary membrane is formed from mesoderm, which, until regression, forms a solid sheet of tissue bridging the pupil space from the iris collarette. In normal adult cats, the collarette appears as a slightly raised region halfway between the pupil margin and the iris root.

The condition is seen rarely in cats compared to the frequency with which it is seen in dogs, and rarely seems to affect the pupil light response or pupil shape.

Clinical signs

Persistent papillary membrane appears as **fibrous strands of iris-like tissue** running from the:

- Iris collarette to another region of the iris collarette. The iris collarette is a raised area approximately half way between the iris root and the pupillary margin.
- Iris to anterior capsule.
- Iris to posterior corneal surface (most common).

The strands can be very thin and magnification may be required to visualize them.

Persistent papillary membrane may also appear as **dot-like gray to black opacities on the endothelial surface of the cornea** or the anterior capsule of the lens, unassociated with history of previous inflammation within the eye.

Diagnosis

Diagnosis is based on the characteristic appearance of the PPMs on careful ocular examination.

Differential diagnosis

The gray opacities formed by PPMs which attach to the corneal endothelium should be differentiated from **keratic precipitates**, formed as a result of anterior uveitis. A strand of tissue attaching the opacity to the iris and the absence of other signs of anterior uveitis is diagnostic of a PPM.

Treatment

No treatment is indicated for PPMs.

IRIS COLOBOMA

Classical signs

- Segmental full-thickness defect of the iris with lens visible behind the defect.
- Remaining iris is normal.
- May also cause an abnormal pupil shape.
- Rare in cats.

Clinical signs

The defect is a **rare anomaly** that may be detected in a young cat, and results in a **notch-like or sectorial defect in the iris**.

Iris coloboma appears as **thinned to absent iris stroma in a radial sector of the iris**. The remaining iris appears normal.

Small strands, which are remnants of the iris dilator muscle, may be seen **bridging the space** formed by the defect.

Abnormal pupil shape (dyscoria) may be present.

Diagnosis

Diagnosis is based on the **characteristic appearance** of iris coloboma on ocular examination.

IRIS CYST

> **Classical signs**
> - Pigmented cyst-like structures, translucent on illumination, in the anterior chamber or attached to the pupil margin.
> - Rare in cats.

Clinical signs

Iris cysts appear as **brown- or black-pigmented cyst-like structures** freely floating in the anterior chamber, or attached to the posterior pigmented epithelium of the iris at the pupil margin. They may be more obvious with pupil dilation.

Iris cysts occur as a congenital abnormality, or occur as a result of inflammation, and are uncommon in cats.

Iris cysts are usually **partly translucent** on focal light illumination.

Diagnosis

Diagnosis is based purely on the characteristic appearance of iris cysts on ocular examination.

CUTEREBRA LARVAL MIGRATION (OPHTHALMOMYIASIS)

> **Classical signs**
> - Vision loss.
> - Cloudy posterior segment with linear track-like lesions on fundoscopy.

> **Classical signs—Cont'd**
> - Typical signs of anterior uveitis associated with larva in the anterior chamber.

Clinical signs

Migration of cuterebra larva through the eye causes vision loss and poor pupillary light reflexs.

Characteristic signs on fundoscopy include **linear hyper-reflective "tracks" in the tapetal fundus**, linear light gray areas of **reduced pigmentation in the non-tapetum** and cloudy posterior segment. The white body of a fly larva is sometimes seen associated with one of the tracks.

Sometimes the larva is seen in the anterior chamber with associated signs of anterior uveitis.

Diagnosis

Diagnosis is based on **appearance of the suspicious fundoscopic lesions**, or on the observation of the parasite in the anterior chamber with the associated uveitis.

OCULAR DIROFILARIASIS

> **Classical signs**
> - White filarial worm in the anterior chamber associated with typical signs of anterior uveitis.

Clinical signs

Immature adult dirofilaria are rarely found in the anterior chamber, and are associated with signs of **corneal edema and/or anterior uveitis**.

Diagnosis

Diagnosis is on observation of a filarial-like parasite within the anterior chamber on ocular examination.

BARTONELLA HENSELA (CAT-SCRATCH FEVER)

Classical signs

- Subclinical or mild fever.
- Occasionally ocular signs associated with anterior uveitis.

See main reference on page 366 (The Pyrexic Cat) for more details.

Clinical signs

Naturally infected cats **usually only develop subclinical infection**.

Mild, self-limiting fever **lasting 48–72 hours has been documented in some experimentally infected cats**.

Anterior uveitis was documented in one naturally exposed cat.

Diagnosis

Diagnosis is based on a positive blood culture, however, intermittent bacteremia may occur for longer than 1 year following infection.

The organism is present within erythrocytes, therefore, hemolyzing red blood cells **increases the sensitivity of the culture**.

RECOMMENDED READING

Davidson MG. English RV Feline ocular toxoplasmosis. Vet Ophthalmol 1998; 1: 70–80.

Maggs DJ, Lappin MR, Nasisse MP. Detection of feline herpesvirus – specific antibodies and DNA in aqueous humour from cats with or without uveitis, Am J Vet Res 1999; 60: 932–936.

Malik R, Martin P, Wigney DI, et al Nasopharyngeal cryptococcosis. Aust Vet J 1997; 75: 483–488.

64.   The cat with abnormal globe position or size

Michael E. Bernays

KEY SIGNS

- Increased globe prominence.
- Increased globe size.
- Reduced globe prominence.
- Reduced globe size.

MECHANISM?

- A globe which is more prominent may be either enlarged (buphthalmic) or a normal-sized globe which is abnormally positioned, usually displaced cranially (exophthalmic).
- A globe which is less prominent may be shrunken (pthisis), or it may be a normal-sized globe which is positioned more caudally or deeper in the orbit (enophthalmic).

WHERE?

- Globe.
- Orbit.

WHAT?

- The most common causes of abnormal globe positioning or size in the cat are:
- Increased prominence: orbital cellulitis or orbital neoplasia.
- Increased size: chronic glaucoma causing enlargement.
- Reduced prominence: shrinkage of orbital tissue related to loss of orbital fat.
- Reduced size: pthisis (shrinkage) due to intractable inflammation causing low intra-ocular pressure or globe leakage due to a persistent corneal or scleral defect.

QUICK REFERENCE SUMMARY

Diseases causing abnormal globe position or size

INCREASED GLOBE SIZE OR PROMINENCE

WHERE?

GLOBE

INFLAMMATION

- **Buphthalmos associated with glaucoma** (p 1312)**

Enlarged globe results from glaucoma, which occurs as a sequel to chronic anterior uveitis. Usually unilateral.

TRAUMA

- Traumatic globe proptosis** (p 1313)

Globe is located external to eyelids and is usually associated with evidence of severe trauma.

WHERE?

ORBIT

NEOPLASTIC

- **Orbital neoplasia*** (p 1310)**

Lymphosarcoma usually results in bilateral globe prominence and peri-ocular tissue swelling. Sometimes it is associated with anterior uveitis evidenced by intra-ocular fibrin, hemorrhage and/or iris masses. It may occur in conjunction with other signs of multicentric lymphoma. Squamous cell carcinoma more often causes unilateral globe prominence, and there is evidence of co-existent neoplasia involving oral or nasal mucous membranes or pre-existent eyelid or conjunctival neoplasia in a cat with non-pigmented eyelid margins. Fibrosarcoma or osteosarcoma typically produce a unilateral, slow-onset increase in globe prominence or globe displacement, and peri-ocular swelling.

INFECTION

- **Bacterial orbital cellulitis*** (p 1310)**

Exophthalmos, peri-ocular swelling, conjunctival chemosis, and pain on palpation, retropulsion or opening of the mouth occurs secondary to periodontal disease of the caudal maxillary teeth, penetrating injury caudal to the upper M1 tooth, or blood-borne infection.

IATROGENIC

- Non-septic orbital cellulitis or hemorrhage (p 1310)

Exophthalmos and peri-ocular swelling which becomes more pronounced following blind surgical orbital exploration procedures.

TRAUMA

- **Fractures of bones around the orbit or orbital emphysema* (p 1314)**

Severe peri-ocular swelling, abnormalities in outline of the skull and/or proptosis of varying degrees may occur as a sequel to trauma. Palpable zygomatic arch, vertical ramus of the mandible and/or frontal bone fractures are often evident. Orbital emphysema may occur with trauma, and appears as peri-orbital swelling which has a crepitant or "puffy" sensation on palpation.

DECREASED GLOBE SIZE OR PROMINENCE

WHERE?

GLOBE

DEGENERATIVE

- Pthisis (p 1315)

Reduced globe size occurs secondary to a known history of severe trauma, chronic intra-ocular inflammation or hemorrhage. Unusual in cats.

ANOMALY

- Microphthalmos (p 1316)

Rare in cats. Appears as small eye with small corneal dimensions sometimes and associated with other ocular defects, e.g. cataract.

TRAUMA

- **Collapse of the globe* (p 1315)**

Small globe and signs of aqueous leakage (wetting of the skin and haircoat around the eye), which occurs in association with rupture of the cornea or sclera.

WHERE:

ORBIT

DEGENERATIVE

- **Enophthalmos secondary to orbital fat loss or muscle wastage** (p 1314)**

Bilateral, non-painful, caudal displacement of the globe occurs associated with generalized muscle wastage and weight loss. The third eyelid is prominent.

INTRODUCTION

MECHANISM?

A globe which appears to be more prominent may be either enlarged (buphthalmic) or a normal-sized globe which is abnormally positioned, usually displaced cranially (exophthalmic). Likewise a globe which is less prominent may be so because it is shrunken (pthisis) or it may be a normal-sized globe which is positioned more caudally or deeper in the orbit (enophthalmic).

WHERE?

Globe.

Orbit.

WHAT?

The **most common causes of abnormal globe positioning or size in the cat** are:

- **Cranial displacement (exophthalmos)** from orbital cellulitis or orbital neoplasia.
- **Increased size (buphthalmos)** from chronic glaucoma.
- **Caudal displacement (enophthalmos)** as a result of shrinkage of orbital tissue related to loss of orbital fat.
- **Reduced size (pthisis)** from shrinkage of the globe due to intractable inflammation causing low intra-ocular pressure or leakage due to a persistent corneal or scleral defect.

Unilateral prominence or enlargement can best be appreciated by comparing with the opposite eye especially from the dorsal aspect.

Bilateral abnormalities are more likely to be **associated with systemic disease**, whereas unilateral problems are more likely to reflect local phenomena, for example, lymphoma involving the orbit will usually cause bilateral exophthalmos.

The final decision as to whether there is a change in size or a change in position might lie with a consideration of the associated ocular signs, for example:

- If **buphthalmos rather than an exophthalmos** is suspected, then look for associated signs which one might expect to see with glaucoma and buphthalmos, that is, dilated to mid-dilated non-responsive pupil, deep episcleral vessel injection, high intra-ocular pressure measured with a tonometer, vision loss, and fundoscopic suggestion of retinal degeneration.
- If **exophthalmos is suspected rather than buphthalmos,** then look for pain on opening the mouth, poor retropulsion, signs of ventral orbital swelling behind the last upper molar teeth, and swelling of peri-ocular tissue.
- If **enophthalmos is suspected rather than pthisis**, look for a prominent but not swollen third eyelid.
- If **reduced size** is suspected, look for signs of chronic intra-ocular inflammation, low intra-ocular pressure on tonometry and/or possible signs of globe rupture and aqueous leakage.

DISEASES CAUSING INCREASED GLOBE SIZE OR PROMINENCE

BACTERIAL ORBITAL CELLULITIS*** OR NON-SEPTIC CELLULITIS OR HEMORRHAGE

Classical signs

- Acute in onset over a few days.
- Exophthalmos.
- Pain on opening mouth.
- Prominent nictitating membrane.
- ± Fever.
- Occasionally bulging of oral mucosa caudal to upper M1 tooth.
- Chemosis.

Pathogenesis

Cellulitis is induced by bacterial infection of the orbital soft tissue. Bacteria are introduced into the tissue by several routes:

- Blood-borne via vessels within the orbit.
- Traumatic inoculation through the oral mucous membranes caudal to the upper molar tooth from sharp foreign bodies such as a bone, or by iatrogenic introduction during orbital exploration.
- Spread of infection associated with periodontal disease of caudal maxillary teeth.
- Spread from an area of osteomyelitis involving bone around the orbit.

Iatrogenic non-septic cellulitis can occur by trauma of orbital tissues during surgical exploration behind the upper M1 tooth with serrated cutting devices such as hemostats.

Clinical signs

Typically there is a very acute onset of signs over a few days.

Pain is evident, especially on opening the mouth.

A normal-sized globe is pushed cranially (exophthalmos).

Prominent nictitating membrane.

Fever is variably present.

Peri-orbital swelling causes swelling of conjunctival tissue around the globe (chemosis), and conjunctiva become exposed and dry.

Occasionally bulging of oral mucosa caudal to upper M1 may be evident.

If the cellulitis, hemorrhage and/or edema are associated with blind surgical orbital exploration, signs of exophthalmos and peri-ocular swelling become more pronounced following the procedure.

Diagnosis

History is usually of a rapid onset of signs over a few days.

Classical signs are exophthalmos, chemosis, third eyelid prominence, and peri-ocular swelling, which are usually associated with pain on palpation, retropulsion or opening of the mouth.

Imaging techniques which are useful include:

- **Ultrasound**: anechoic or hypo-echoic regions are suggestive of a fluid-filled cavity while complex echogenicity is more suggestive of cellulitis.
- **Plain radiographs** of the maxilla and zygomatic arch may demonstrate signs suggestive of osteomyelitis such as proliferation or lysis of bone. A frontal sinus view may be helpful.
- **Dental radiography** might demonstrate a rarified area of alveolar bone around the tooth root apical region.
- **CT or MRI** in special circumstances might be helpful for demonstrating soft tissue detail.

Laboratory examination of aspirates or swabs of orbital contents are valuable. Look for neutrophils, macrophages, signs of bacterial lysis.

Differential diagnosis

Orbital neoplasia usually causes more slowly progressive onset of signs with less acute pain.

Treatment

Treatment involves careful surgical drainage via a small incision caudal to upper molar tooth. Blunt probes are preferable to hemostats, which cause more trauma to orbital tissue.

Use oral antibiotics based on culture and sensitivity of aspirates, or treat empirically with antibiotics directed particularly at anaerobes, such as clindamycin (5.5 mg/kg q 12 h). Administer for 7–10 days, but for severe infections use for up to 28 days.

Anti-inflammatory drugs help to reduce inflammation and achieve more rapid reduction of peri-orbital swelling.

- Oral prednisolone 1 mg/kg q 24 h for the first 7 days or
- NSAIDs.
  - Ketoprofen: Ketofen 2 mg/kg SC continuing 1 mg/kg orally q 24 hourly for up to 5 days.
  - Carprofen: Rimadyl 4 mg/kg SC or IV. Oral dose not approved for use in cats.
  - Meloxicam: Metacam 0.1 mg/kg (one drop/kg) PO as an initial loading dose then 1–2 drops q 24 hourly for up to 3 days.

ORBITAL NEOPLASIA***

> ### Classical signs
>
> - Usually slow in onset over weeks to months. Lymphosarcoma of the orbit can however progress more rapidly.
> - Not usually associated with pain on opening the mouth except in advanced stages.
> - Exophthalmos with a prominent nictitating membrane.

Pathogenesis

Lymphosarcoma can localize in the orbit in multicentric disease, and is often bilateral when it involves the orbit.

Squamous cell carcinoma invades from the oral mucous membrane, the nasal cavity or from the frontal sinus into the medial orbit.

Fibrosarcoma is a primary neoplastic disease originating from the periosteum of the bone surrounding orbit.

Clinical signs

Clinical signs are usually slow in onset over weeks to months. Lymphosarcoma of the orbit can however progress more rapidly.

Exophthalmos is present and the severity is dependent on the degree of proliferation of the neoplasm.

A **prominent nictitating membrane** might be seen especially in the later stages.

Chemosis of the conjunctiva occurs with subsequent exposure and drying.

Bulging of oral mucosa caudal to the upper M1 tooth is occasionally seen, especially in the later stages of the disease.

Pain on opening mouth is variable, and the majority of cases do not show signs of pain. Neoplastic disease may become more painful if the affected tissue becomes inflamed. If pain does occur, it is more likely to occur in the later stages of the disease, when there is more gross disruption of normal tissue architecture.

Blindness or abnormality of the pupillary light reflex occurs if the optic nerve or CN III is affected by the neoplastic process but this is uncommon.

Lymphosarcoma usually results in bilateral globe prominence and peri-ocular tissue swelling. Sometimes it is associated with anterior uveitis evidenced by intra-ocular fibrin, hemorrhage and/or iris masses. It may occur in conjunction with other signs of multicentric lymphoma.

Squamous cell carcinoma more often causes unilateral globe prominence, and there is evidence of co-existent neoplasia involving oral or nasal mucous membranes or pre-existent eyelid or conjunctival neoplasia in a cat with non-pigmented eyelid margins.

Fibrosarcoma or osteosarcoma typically produce a unilateral, slow-onset increase in globe prominence or globe displacement and peri-ocular swelling.

Diagnosis

Orbital neoplasia should be suspected in any case of non-painful or mildly painful exophthalmos with a slow onset and progression of signs.

Ultrasound is a particularly useful imaging technique. Plain radiographs of the maxilla, frontal bone and zygomatic arch may be useful, and CT or MRI may be needed in special circumstances.

Differential diagnosis

Orbital cellulitis usually causes a more painful exophthalmos of more rapid onset.

Treatment

Chemotherapy is used for treatment of **lymphosarcoma**. See main reference on page 432 for details (The Cat With Enlarged Lymph Nodes).

Squamous cell carcinoma and fibrosarcoma can be treated by surgery with or without irradiation.
- Radical surgical excision is required, and aim to remove 1–2 planes of normal tissue with the affected tissue.
- Megavoltage or orthovoltage irradiation of the orbit can be used to attempt prevention of regrowth of invasive neoplasms where surgical excision does not achieve clean margins.

Prognosis

Prognosis is poor for invasive orbital fibrosarcoma or squamous cell carcinoma.

Orbital lymphosarcoma has a guarded prognosis.

BUPHTHALMOS ASSOCIATED WITH GLAUCOMA**

> ### Classical signs
> - Enlarged globe.
> - Deep episcleral vessel injection.
> - Associated with signs of chronic anterior uveitis, uveal neoplasia and secondary glaucoma.

Pathogenesis

Buphthalmos occurs from stretching of the fibrous outer tunic of the eye associated with elevated intra-ocular pressure. In the cat, most cases of glaucoma are secondary to chronic anterior uveitis or iris neoplasia.

Primary glaucoma has been described in **Burmese** cats in Australia, which appears to be familial. In this condition there appears to be a genetically determined narrowing of the irido-corneal angle resulting eventually in reduced aqueous outflow and increased intra-ocular pressure.

Clinical signs

The globe is more prominent because it is enlarged (buphthalmos).

Deep episcleral vessels are injected secondary to increased intra-ocular pressure. Deep vessels are usually straighter and larger, do not move when the overlying bulbar conjunctiva is moved, and do not blanch with the topical application of 1:1000 epinephrine.

The **pupil is dilated or semi-dilated**, and the pupillary light response is either absent or poor.

Signs of chronic anterior uveitis are often present, especially abnormalities in the appearance of the iris surface. The iris may have a pinkish discoloration associated with fibrovascular membranes or grayish nodules.

The **anterior chamber** may appear to be very **shallow** in **aqueous misdirection glaucoma**, which is a poorly understood syndrome where the lens is positioned more anteriorly along the axis of the eye as a result of aqueous being diverted into the vitreous.

Signs of lens instability are typically present and include:
- Aphakic crescent (crescent shape produced by the clear space between the edge of the displaced lens and the adjacent pupillary margin).
- Anterior or posterior luxation (dislocation).
- Iridonesis (wobbling of the iris).

Signs of intra-ocular neoplasia such as mass lesions or discoloration of the iris may be present.

Diagnosis

Diagnosis is based on the appearance of buphthalmos with any or all of the other related signs of glaucoma, chronic anterior uveitis, intraocular neoplasia or lens instability.

Measurement of intra-ocular pressure by tonometry confirms the diagnosis. Normal range for intra-ocular pressure in the cat is 15–25 mmHg. Readings over 30 mmHg are supportive of a diagnosis of glaucoma.

Treatment

There are **no consistently reliable therapeutic protocols** which will lower intra-ocular pressure in all cats. Monitoring is necessary to confirm that chosen treatment is working. Type of therapy chosen and its predicted success will depend on several factors. These include:
- **Whether the angle is opened or closed**. When the angle is closed or obstructed, treatment regimes involving cyclo-destruction to reduce production of aqueous within the eye may not work as well as aqueous shunting procedures.
- **Whether the glaucoma is primary or secondary to other pathology**. If glaucoma occurs secondary to chronic anterior uveitis it is often more responsive to simple treatment with anti-inflammatories alone, without the use of other ocular hypotensive treatments.

Medical therapy includes:
- **Carbonic anhydrase inhibitors**.
  - Dorzolamide 2% (Trusopt): one drop q 8 h topically.

- **Anti-inflammatories** can be used, especially where the glaucoma has been secondary to chronic anterior uveitis.
  - Topical prednisolone acetate 1% (Prednefrin Forte, Allergan) 1 drop q 12–24 h.
  - Oral prednisolone up to 1 mg/kg q 12 h.

Surgical therapy.
- **Cyclo-destructive procedures** are used to selectively destroy parts of the ciliary body to reduce aqueous production to match reduced outflow.
- Transcleral diode laser cyclo-photo-coagulation only works well where the ciliary body is well pigmented, and so tends not to work well for color dilute cats, e.g. Burmese, Siamese, Himalayans.
  - Transcleral cyclo-cryo-ablation. This is the original technique described for cyclo-destruction, and is a suitable alternative for use in cats where laser surgery does not work well, i.e. Color Point cats with minimal pigmentation of the uveal tract.
- **Lens removal** is suggested wherever the lens is unstable because of chronic anterior uveitis. Inflammation is sometimes easier to control by removing the lens.

TRAUMATIC GLOBE PROPTOSIS**

Classical signs
- Globe located cranially to eyelid margins.
- Subconjunctival hemorrhage.
- Extra-ocular muscle tearing.

Pathogenesis

Proptosis occurs through **excessive blunt trauma to the globe or lateral orbit**. The condition is uncommon in cats because of skull shape. The globe is located deeper in the orbit with more protection laterally than in dogs, except in brachycephalic cats. Occasionally however, cats can be seen with this condition following motor vehicle trauma. Prognosis for the eye is usually poor because the forces required to proptose a feline globe are often so severe that severe globe trauma occurs with resultant permanent loss of normal globe structure and function.

Clinical signs

Proptosis of the eye, with eyelid margins located behind the globe.

Subconjunctival **hemorrhage**.

Extra-ocular muscle tearing.

Intra-ocular signs are variable. The pupil can be dilated or constricted, but is more commonly dilated after severe trauma, because of damage to the optic nerve and or the long ciliary nerves. Hyphema may be present.

Diagnosis

Diagnosis is obvious based on clinical signs.

Treatment

Irrigate the globe with a balanced electrolyte solution to remove debris.

Lubricate the cornea and bulbar conjunctiva with solutions containing hypromellose, polyvinyl alcohol or carboxymethyl cellulose.

Surgically attempt to replace the globe by manipulation of the eyelid margins. Often orbital soft tissue swelling makes this difficult. A technique using pre-placed tarsorrhaphy sutures has been described:

- 4/0 or 5/0 polypropylene or nylon sutures are inserted by passing through the dorsal and ventral eyelid.
- A flat object (e.g. scalpel handle) is placed on the corneal surface under the row of pre-placed sutures with sufficient lubricant to protect the cornea.
- The sutures are tightened over the scalpel handle to force the globe back into the orbit, at the same time, the eyelids are brought together and the sutures are tied to effect a temporary tarsorrhaphy, which can be left in place for 1–2 weeks, until peri-ocular and orbital swelling is resolved.

FRACTURES OF THE BONES AROUND THE ORBIT OR ORBITAL EMPHYSEMA*

Classical signs

- Orbital swelling.
- Fluctuant, puffy or crepitant feel on palpation.

Clinical signs

Peri-orbital edema, hemorrhage and/or emphysema associated with blunt trauma or surgery may result in exophthalmos and increased globe prominence.

Severe peri-ocular swelling, abnormalities in outline of the skull and/or proptosis of varying degrees may occur as a sequel to trauma. Palpable zygomatic arch, vertical ramus of the mandible and/or frontal bone fractures often evident.

Orbital emphysema may be present associated with trauma from a fall or motor car accident or following surgery. Emphysema is most commonly caused by a fracture of a bone lining one of the paranasal sinuses, in particular the frontal sinus. **Swelling** is evident and there is a **fluctuant, "puffy" or crepitant feel on palpation** of peri-ocular tissues.

Diagnosis

Diagnosis is usually based on the **characteristic clinical signs**, and a history of possible frontal bone fracture.

Plain skull radiography may show soft tissues dissected by air-containing compartments.

THE CAT WITH REDUCED GLOBE SIZE OR PROMINENCE

ENOPHTHALMOS SECONDARY TO ORBITAL FAT LOSS OR MUSCLE WASTAGE**

Classical signs

- Globe is caudally displaced into the orbit.
- ± Entropion especially of the lower lid.
- Generalized atrophy of facial muscles and prominence of zygomatic arch.
- Associated generalized poor body condition.

Pathogenesis

Loss of orbital fat caudal to the globe secondary to **weight loss**, or **generalized muscle wastage** causes caudal movement of a normal-sized globe.

Clinical signs

Globe is caudally displaced into the orbit (**enophthalmos**).

Generalized atrophy of the muscles of mastication and/or facial expression is evident, and the zygomatic arch is prominent.

Lower lid entropion is sometimes seen.

Ocular signs are usually **always bilateral** because they relate to systemic illness.

Generalized poor body condition is evident, and atrophy of other muscle groups and bony prominences are more obvious. There may also be associated loss of hydration of connective tissue, if the weight loss is secondary to chronic renal disease.

Diagnosis

Diagnosis is based on the appearance of a **normal-sized globe, which is sunken into the orbit, and a thin emaciated cat**.

Laboratory investigation is required to determine the cause of the weight loss. Common causes include hyperthyroidism and chronic renal disease.
- Hyperthyroidism is associated with increased thyroxine concentrations, and often increased alanine-amino-transferase (ALT) activity.
- Chronic renal disease is associated with variable increases in BUN, creatinine and serum phosphate and poorly concentrated urine (<1.030). Serum potassium may be low in the early stages, and high in the late stages of the disease.

Treatment

Treatment involves correcting or controlling the medical condition causing weight loss.

COLLAPSE OF THE GLOBE*

Classical signs
• Small globe size compared to the opposite side. • Painful closed eye. • Serous discharge from leaking aqueous.

See the main reference for details in "The Cat With Abnormalities Confined to the Cornea" on page 1243,

"Ulcerative keratitis caused by corneal perforation (cat fight wounds)" and on page 1246 "Blunt trauma".

Clinical signs

Painful, closed eye with serous discharge and sometimes bleeding.

Cornea is cloudy and anterior chamber may be full of blood and protein.

Globe appears small compared with the ipsilateral eye, and there are **signs of aqueous leakage** with wetting of the skin and haircoat around the eye, which occurs in association with rupture of the cornea or sclera.

Diagnosis

A presumptive diagnosis is based on clinical signs and history.

PTHSIS

Classical signs
• Small globe size compared to the opposite side. • Globe is covered by the third eyelid. • Signs of previous inflammation within the eye. • Intra-ocular pressure is usually low. • Rare in cats.

Clinical signs

The **globe size is small** compared with the ipsilateral eye.

There is unusual coverage of the globe by the nictitating membrane because of small size.

Pthisis occurs secondary to chronic uveal inflammation or severe penetrating trauma. **Signs of chronic uveal inflammation** are evident, for example:
- Abnormal pupil shape.
- Changes in iris color due to fibrovascular membranes on the anterior surface of the iris.
- Keratic precipitates, which are gray to tan-colored opacities on the posterior surface of the cornea, and are usually located ventrally.
- Synechia, which are visible as adhesions of the iris to the anterior lens capsule, and may cause irregularity

in pupil shape. Pigment deposition on the anterior capsule may be seen.
- Pupillary membranes, which are membranous structures spanning the pupil space. Immobility of the pupil often results.

Diagnosis

Diagnosis is **based on the appearance of a small globe with low intra-ocular pressure** and signs of previous inflammation.

Tonometry will usually reveal unusually low intraocular pressure (usually < 10 mmHg).

MICROPHTHALMOS

> **Classical signs**
>
> - Small globe unassociated with signs of previous inflammation.
> - ± Other ocular abnormalities such as congenital cataract or persistent pupillary membranes.
> - Rare in cats.

Clinical signs

Rare in cats.

The **globe is small, and there is no history or signs of previous inflammation**. The corneal diameter is usu-

ally obviously smaller than the opposite side, but the cornea does not have a significantly smaller radius of curvature than the scleral coat. In contrast, a pthisical globe will usually have an obviously smaller corneal radius of curvature than the scleral coat, causing the appearance of a bulging cornea.

There is unusual coverage of the globe by the nictitating membrane because of the small globe size.

Other ocular abnormalities are sometimes present, for example:
- Persistent pupillary membranes (PPM), which are small strands of tissue arising from the iris surface. They connect either to other points on the iris surface, the posterior surface of the cornea where they form gray focal opacities, or the anterior lens capsule. Persistent pupillary membranes are unassociated with other signs of intra-ocular inflammation.
- Congenital cataract resulting in opacity of the lens. Congenital cataracts are more likely to be nuclear in location, with the surrounding cortex clear.

Diagnosis

Diagnosis is **based on the clinical signs** of a small, but relatively normal looking eye.

If intra-ocular pressure can be measured, is usually normal (15–25 mmHg). In contrast, pressure is usually low in a pthisical globe.

RECOMMENDED READING

Gilger BC, McLaughlin SA, Whitley RD, et al. Orbital neoplasms in cats: 21 cases (1974–1990). J Am Vet Med Assoc 1992; 201: 1083.

Gilger BC, Hamilton HL, Wilkie DA, et al. Traumatic ocular proptoses in dogs and cats: 84 cases (1980–1993). J Am Anim Hosp Assoc 1995; 206: 1186.

Glaze MB, Gelatt KN. Feline ophthalmology. In: Gelatt KN (ed) Veterinary Ophthalmology, 3rd edn. Baltimore, Maryland, Lippincott, Williams & Wilkins, 1999, pages 998–999.

Hampson ECGM, Smith RIE Bernays ME. Primary glaucoma in Burmese cats. Aust Vet J Nov 2002; 80(11): 672–680.

Ramsay DT, Marretta SM, Hamor RE, et al. Ophthalmic manifestations and complications of dental disease in dogs and cats. J Am Anim Hosp Assoc 1996; 32: 215.

65. The cat with abnormal eyelid appearance

Michael E. Bernays

KEY SIGNS

- Misshapen or abnormal alignment of eyelid(s).
- Eyelid swelling or mass.
- Alopecia, erythema, crusting, discharge.
- Eyelid lacerations.

MECHANISM?

- Abnormal eyelid appearance can result from congenital abnormalities, inflammation, neoplasia, trauma or neurological disease.

WHERE?

- Eyelid skin.
- Eyelid margin.
- Conjunctiva.

WHAT?

- The most common causes of altered eyelid appearance include neoplasia, inflammation and trauma.

QUICK REFERENCE SUMMARY

Diseases causing abnormal eyelid appearance

ANOMALY

- **Eyelid agenesis/eyelid coloboma** (p 1323)**
Absence of an identifiable eyelid margin, usually bilateral and involving the upper lateral lid. Gradual transition from haired skin to conjunctiva, and often causing keratitis, corneal vascularization, ulceration and increased lacrimation with wetting of the irritating hairs. Usually first noticed in a young cat.

- Distichiasis (p 1329)
Cilia extending from meibomian gland openings at the eyelid margin. Rare.

continued

continued

MECHANICAL

● **Entropion* (p 1320)**

Lower eyelid margin rolled inwards, causing corneal irritation and serous to mucopurulent ocular discharge. Seen occasionally.

● Ectropion (p 1328)

Eyelid rolled outwards due to former injury associated with cicatricial scarring.

● **Upper lid ptosis* (p 1324)**

Upper eyelid droops or fails to be elevated. Usually from sympathetic neuropathy (Horner's syndrome) and associated with ipsilateral miosis, enophthalmos and third eyelid prominence. Less often from cranial nerve III paresis, and occasionally in associated with a dilated pupil unresponsive to light (internal ophthalmoplegia), or inability to elevate the eyeball during outward turning.

NEOPLASTIC

● **Squamous cell carcinoma*** (p 1321)**

Ulceration and crusting affecting the lid margins and non-haired skin or conjunctiva. Localized or diffuse eyelid swelling may be present. Only occurs on non-pigmented skin.

● **Basal cell carcinoma** (p 1321)**

Flat to slightly raised areas of red to dark brown discoloration with irregular edges.

● **Mast cell tumor* (p 1321)**

Rapidly growing nodular tumor often with poorly defined borders, with variable surface ulceration.

● **Fibrosarcoma* (p 1321)**

Usually rapidly growing diffuse swelling with involvement of adjacent facial or orbital tissues.

● Sebaceous gland adenoma or adenocarcinoma (p 1321)

Nodular or diffuse mass causing localized thickening of the eyelid. Tumor may have an ulcerated surface.

INFLAMMATION/INFECTIOUS

Bacterial:

● **Bacterial blepharitis, meibomitis, chalazion or hordoleum* (p 1324)**

Bacterial blepharitis causes eyelid swelling, erythema and ulceration. Lesions seen more commonly at the medial canthus. Meibomitis, chalazion and hordoleum are associated with acute or chronic swelling of single or multiple meibomian glands, causing erythema of lid conjunctiva, and eyelid swelling. In acute cases (hordoleum) the lids are painful and inflamed with inflammation around the glands. In chronic cases, inflammation may organize into large mass of caseous material with a tendency to be walled off in fibrous capsules within eyelid (chalazion). Only individual glands may be swollen (meibomitis). Mucoid to mucopurulent ocular discharge occurs.

Fungal:

● **Dermatophytosis** (p 1322)**

Alopecia and crusting or scaling of peri-ocular eyelid skin. Other similar lesions on the face or ears.

● Malasezzia (p 1327)

Alopecia and crusting of peri-ocular skin.

Parasitic:

● Demodecosis (p 1327)

Peri-ocular alopecia, erythema, scaling with variable pruritis.

● **Notoedres cati* (p 1327)**

Alopecia with pronounced pruritis, crusting and excoriation of the ears, eyelids face and neck.

● Parasitic myiasis (p @)

Fistulous opening with larvae visible in wound.

Inflammation/non-infectious:

● **Solar dermatitis** (p 1329)**

Erythema and crusting, with or without hemorrhage usually involving non-pigmented eyelid skin.

● **Allergic blepharitis** (p 1325)**

Associated with food allergy, atopy, insect bite hypersensitivity, staphylococcal allergy, or contact allergy to topical drugs. Variable erythema, swelling, pruritis, excoriation, exudation and crusting of eyelid skin.

Immune-mediated:

● Pemphigus foliaceous, pemphigus erythematosus, systemic lupus erythematosus (p 1328)

Alopecia, erythema, scaling and crusting of the eyelids additionally affecting nailbeds, nipples (foliaceous) and ears, muzzle and nose (erythematosus). Uncommon. Other immune-mediated disease (e.g. immune-mediated polyarthritis, glomerulo-nephritis) is present in SLE.

Trauma:

● **Eyelid trauma/wounds* (p 1326)**

Visible tears in the eyelid skin or discontinuities at the eyelid margin with loss of normal function. Discharge ranges from hemorrhagic, serous or purulent, depending on duration.

INTRODUCTION

MECHANISM?

Basic pathological mechanisms underlying an abnormal eyelid appearance include failure of embryonic tissues to differentiate or rarify, inflammation, neoplasia, trauma and neurological disease.

WHERE?

The location of disease processes within the eyelid can often be simply described according to whether the process affects the eyelid skin, the eyelid margin or the palpebral conjunctiva. Sometimes multiple tissues may be affected within the eyelid. Occasionally an eyelid may appear abnormal because of a neurological process occurring distant to the eye.

Altered eyelid function or structure may affect adjacent or remote structures, for example:

● Entropion or eyelid agenesis may cause corneal disease due to lack of a normal anatomical relationship between the eyelid and the cornea.

● Immune-mediated, allergic or parasitic skin disease may affect skin remote from the eyelid.

WHAT?

The most common causes of altered eyelid appearance include:

- **Failure of embryonic tissues to differentiate or rarify** resulting in eyelid agenesis or abnormal cilia. These conditions will commonly be first recognized in a young cat.
- **Inflammation of infectious or non-infectious etiology**.
  - Infectious causes include bacteria, dermatophyte fungi or external parasites.
  - Non-infectious causes include **allergic** causes such as food allergy, inhalant allergy, bacterial hypersensitivity, insect bite hypersensitivity or contact allergy to topical drugs; **immune-mediated responses to components of the skin around the eyelids** occur in pemphigus erythematosus or pemphigus foliaceous.
- **Neoplasia**.
  - **Squamous cell carcinoma** occurring in non-pigmented skin is the most common neoplastic disease seen in the eyelid.
  - Basal cell carcinomas, mast cell tumors or fibrosarcomas are less common, while sebaceous gland tumors occur rarely.
- **Neurological disease**.
  - **Sympathetic ptosis** or **ptosis due to injury to the dorsal branch of the oculomotor nerve** may occur with trauma, inflammation or neoplasia involving the nervous system.
- **Trauma**.
  - Cats are renowned for injuries caused by claws inflicted during fighting with other cats.

DISEASES CAUSING AN ABNORMAL EYELID APPEARANCE

ENTROPION**

Classical signs

- Lower eyelid is curled inwards.
- Chronic ulcerative keratitis caused by eyelid hair rubbing on the cornea.
- Mucoid to mucopurulent discharge.

Pathogenesis

The condition **appears to occur secondary to enophthalmos in cats**. Enophthalmos can be caused by loss of fat or reduction in masseter muscle mass within the orbit.

The defect can also occur **secondary to chronic blepharospasm** caused by painful corneal diseases.

Clinical signs

Usually the **central portion of the lower eyelid margin rolls inwards towards the globe**. Lid hair adjacent to the margin may appear moist or be coated in conjunctival mucus.

Corneal surface disease is present from the eyelid hair rubbing on the cornea. This can include superficial ulceration, sequestrum formation, and a vascular response from the limbus adjacent to the area of lid irritation.

Chronic discharge occurs ranging from mucoid to mucopurulent.

Diagnosis

Diagnosis is based on the characteristic sign of an inward rolling eyelid margin with secondary corneal changes and chronic ocular discharge.

Treatment

Surgical procedures such as the modified Hotz–Celsus procedure involving **removal of a strip of skin and orbicularis muscle adjacent to the area of entropion** seem to work adequately for cats. Some cats seem to have an oversized palpebral fissure, resulting in inadequate tension of the lower eyelid. Occasionally a permanent lateral canthal closure in addition to the Hotz–Celsus procedure is recommended to reduce palpebral fissure size.

The **condition will recur if the inciting cause is not corrected**.

EYELID NEOPLASIA (SQUAMOUS CELL CARCINOMA, BASAL CELL CARCINOMA, MAST CELL TUMOR, FIBROSARCOMA, AND SEBACEOUS GLAND ADENOMA OR CARCINOMA)****

Classical signs

- Localized or diffuse eyelid swelling.
- Ulceration, excoriation or discharging sinuses.
- Altered tissue color.

Pathogenesis

Squamous cell carcinoma is thought to be induced by prolonged exposure to solar radiation. This causes dysplastic changes in the surface squamous cells of lid epithelium, with eventual progression of the dysplasia to invasive carcinoma. **This neoplasm almost exclusively affects non-pigmented skin**, so is more common in white cats. It is the most common feline eyelid neoplasm.

Basal cell carcinoma arises from the basal cells of the epithelium. Solar radiation is a possible etiology. The tumor is less common.

Mast cell tumor is a neoplastic proliferation of mast cells in tissue. Inciting factors are unknown. Less common.

Fibrosarcomas arise from connective tissue fibroblasts of the dermis or subcutis. Feline sarcoma virus (FeSV) is implicated as a cause of multicentric fibrosarcoma in young cats. Less common.

Sebaceous gland adenomas or carcinomas are rare.

Clinical signs

Any of the following typical signs might be seen including **localized or diffuse areas of eyelid swelling, erosion, crusting, discharging sinuses (+/− necrotic material forming a core), or alterations in tissue color**.

Squamous cell carcinoma can have a flattened verrucous (cauliflower-like) appearance or can look erosive without swelling. Often there is ulceration and crusting affecting the lid margins and non-haired skin or conjunctiva. Localized or diffuse eyelid swelling

may be present. The lesion may invade into adjacent palpebral conjunctiva. These neoplasms generally only occur in **non-pigmented skin**.

Basal cell carcinomas are usually round and well circumscribed, but can become ulcerated. Appear as flat to slightly raised areas of red to dark brown discoloration with irregular edges.

Mast cell tumors can form either well or poorly circumscribed areas of swelling in the eyelid. They appear as rapidly growing nodular tumor, often with poorly defined borders, and variable surface ulceration.

Fibrosarcomas are generally focal nodular neoplasms in the subcutis, but can become ulcerated. Usually appear as a rapidly growing diffuse swelling, and involve adjacent facial or orbital tissues.

Sebaceous gland adenomas or carcinomas are seen as a nodular or diffuse mass causing localized thickening of the eyelid. The tumor may have an ulcerated surface.

Diagnosis

Tentative diagnosis is based on the appearance of the eyelid lesion.

Exfoliative cytology is useful in some cases that show ulceration.
- **Squamous cell carcinomas** typically appear as undifferentiated, single or grouped, round to square cells with large amounts of light basophilic cytoplasm and pleomorphic nucleolated nuclei. Sometimes more squamous, partly or fully keratinized cells can be seen.
- **Basal cell carcinomas** are usually more basophilic staining than SCC. Cells are more round to square than SCC, and have small amounts of basophilic cytoplasm, and relatively uniform round to oval, non-nucleolated nuclei.
- **Mast cell tumors** can be poor- to well-differentiated with intensely basophilic staining cytoplasmic granules, and small, round, centrally located nuclei. Accompanying eosinophils are usually seen.

Fine-needle biopsy can be useful in cases where there is discreet swelling.

Definitive diagnosis is based on histopathological examination of affected tissue.

Differential diagnosis

Autoimmune skin disease causes peri-ocular inflammation, alopecia and crusting with sites remote from the eyelid affected as well, for example, ear pinna, muzzle, nasal planum, nailbeds.

Allergic skin disease causes swollen inflamed lids, sometimes with conjunctival chemosis and ocular discharge. May respond rapidly to topical anti-inflammatory treatment or identification and removal of an offending antigen from the environment, e.g. stopping feeding of an allergenic food or reduce exposure to insects by enclosure in a gauzed cat house.

Infectious eyelid skin diseases respond to treatment with antibiotics, antifungals or antiparasitics.

Any lesion appearing in pigmented eyelid skin is very unlikely to be squamous cell carcinoma.

Treatment

Wide surgical excision is the treatment of choice for most neoplastic lesions. Wide excision is especially important in the treatment of mast cell tumor and squamous cell carcinomas as the borders between the neoplasm and normal tissue can be ill-defined. Large excisions may require plastic surgery procedures to replace removed sections of eyelid. As the lower lid is more frequently involved, lip-to-lid subdermal plexus flaps can be used. Lid-splitting techniques can be used for smaller defects.

Adjunctive modalities can include:
- **Squamous cell carcinoma: cryosurgery, β irradiation**.
- Basal cell carcinoma: cryosurgery.
- Mast cell tumor: chemotherapy with oral and intralesional steroids. Intralesional injections with hypotonic solutions (sterile distilled water) have also been used as an adjunctive therapy. See reference on page 1075 for more details (The Cat With Skin Lumps and Bumps).

Prognosis

Varies depending on the type and stage of the neoplasia, degree of local tissue and/or systemic involvement.

The prognosis is grave for cats affected by FeSV-induced fibrosarcoma.

SOLAR DERMATITIS**

Classical signs

- Erythema and crusting, with or without hemorrhage.
- Almost always involves non-pigmented eyelid skin only.

Clinical signs

Erythema and crusting is usually seen, occasionally associated with hemorrhage under the crusts. The lesion is regarded as a **precursor to the development of squamous cell carcinoma**.

Non-pigmented areas only are affected almost **without exception**.

The lesions are more **commonly seen on the lower lid** rather than the upper lid because of the more direct exposure to UV light.

Associated lesions may be seen on the nasal planum or the tips of the ears.

Diagnosis

Tentative diagnosis is based on the appearance of the lesions and location in non-pigmented areas of eyelid skin.

Definitive diagnosis is made on the histopathological examination of affected eyelid skin.

DERMATOPHYTOSIS**

Classical signs

- Alopecia and crusting or scaling of peri-ocular eyelid skin.
- Other similar lesions on the face or ears.

Clinical signs

Typical lesions include alopecia and crusting or scaling of peri-ocular eyelid skin.

Other similar lesions might be seen on the face or ears.

Diagnosis

Tentative diagnosis is based on appearance of the skin lesions, and the clinical history of exposure to other cats with similar lesions or a suspected carrier cat.

Some organisms (*Microsporum canis*) demonstrate **fluorescence under UV light**. Negative findings under UV light examination should not be used to rule out dermatophyte infection. "False" fluorescence of epidermal scales can sometimes be interpreted as a positive result.

Definitive diagnosis is made by **microscopic examination of hair shafts and by culture of the organism**. Microscopic examination may reveal the presence of small ectothrix, or endothrix spores on or in the keratin at the base of the hair shaft. *Microsporum canis* is the most common cause. *Microsporum gypseum* is identified less commonly, while *Trichophyton* species are rarely implicated in feline dermatophyte infections.

Differential diagnosis

Autoimmune skin disease can be ruled out by histopathological examination of affected skin.

Treatment

Many different treatments are recommended in the literature but more common ones include:

- **Griseofulvin** 12.5 mg/kg PO q 12 h for 4–6 weeks. Drug should be given with a fatty meal to enhance absorption. The drug is teratogenic if given to pregnant queens.
- **Ketoconazole** 10 mg/kg PO q 24 h.
- Topical treatments containing compounds such as miconazole or povidine iodine are also effective. Some other compounds such as chlorine may be irritant when used around the eye.

EYELID AGENESIS/EYELID COLOBOMA*

Classical signs

- Absence of normal eyelid margin, with transition from haired skin to conjunctiva.
- Often bilateral, usually involving lateral upper lids in a young cat.

Classical signs—Cont'd

- Trichiasis with secondary keratitis and corneal vascularization.

Pathogenesis

There is an abnormality in development and differentiation of surface ectoderm and possibly neural crest mesenchyme.

Breed predisposition may occur, as the disease appears to be seen more commonly in Persian kittens.

Clinical signs

Often seen as a bilateral abnormality, usually of the **upper lateral eyelid. There is gradual transition from haired skin to conjunctiva, with absence of a normal lid margin**.

Corneal disease occurs because of trichiasis (hair rubbing on the cornea) associated with the absence of a normal margin, which results in corneal ulceration and vascularization.

Diagnosis

Diagnosis is based on the characteristic appearance of the deficient eyelid margin in a young cat, with secondary keratitis caused by irritation of the trichiasis.

Treatment

Surgical techniques are aimed at removing the abnormal area of eyelid and joining normal lid margins together. The method depends on the size and position of the defect.

If the eyelid defect is small, a V-shaped wedge of the abnormal eyelid may be resected and the normal lid sutured together using a figure-of-eight suture to appose the margins.

If there are **larger, lateral upper lid defects**, the lower lid margin at the lateral canthus may be joined to the medial aspect of the upper lid defect, making a new lateral canthus.

Larger defects involve surgical correction by transposition of a strip of skin and associated orbicularis muscle from the lower eyelid to the upper defect. The conjunctiva is dissected from the upper defect and sutured to the edge of the transposition flap. Cryosurgery of hairs near the new conjunctiva–skin margin may be needed later to correct the remaining upper lid trichiasis.

More recently a new technique has been described involving injection of subdermal collagen into the colobomatous region, and use of a modified Stades technique to create a hairless scar in the region of the reconstructed margin. This technique overcomes the traditional problem of trichiasis and continuing irritation of the cornea by eyelid hairs in the reconstructed region.

UPPER LID PTOSIS*

Classical signs

- Upper lid droops over the globe and ocular fissure appears smaller.
- Poor performance of blink response in tests for palpebral or corneal blink.

See main reference on page 1335 for details (The Cat With an Abnormal Third Eyelid: sympathetic neuropathy of the third eyelid).

Pathogenesis

Sympathetic neuropathy causing denervation of Müller's muscle results in upper lid ptosis. Sympathetic neuropathies can be associated with pathology involving pre- or post-ganglionic fibers.

- **Pre-ganglionic fibers** can be damaged at a number of locations including the descending sympathetic fibers in the spinal cord (rare), thoracic spinal cord segments or nerve roots of T1–T3 (nerve root avulsion, brachial plexus injuries or anterior mediastinal disease) or the ascending fibers in the cervical region (e.g. abscess or cellulitis).
- **Post-ganglionic fibers** are most commonly damaged by middle ear disease.

Cranial nerve III (oculomotor nerve) dysfunction affecting the superior palpebral levator.

Clinical signs

The upper lid does not elevate properly compared to the opposite side, and the upper lid droops over the globe. The ocular fissure appears smaller than the other eye.

There is poor performance of the blink response in tests for palpebral or corneal blink.

Diagnosis

Diagnosis is usually based on the observation of clinical signs in association with other manifestations of either:
- **Sympathetic dysfunction – miosis, prominent nictitating membrane, enophthalmos.**
- **CN III dysfunction: internal ophthalmoplegia** occurs due to effects on parasympathetic fibers to the pupillary constrictor. Dysfunction will result in a **dilated pupil non-responsive to direct or indirect light**, but the **opposite eye will show a normal indirect response to light in the affected eye**. External ophthalmoplegia can result in lateral strabismus or inability to elevate the eyeball during outward turning, along with the upper lid ptosis.

Use of topical 10% epinephrine will help to differentiate between oculomotor and sympathetic ptosis. Oculomotor ptosis would not be expected to be reversed by application of this drug whereas sympathetic ptosis will disappear transiently.

Treatment

Identify and correct (if possible) the problem causing the neuropathy.

BACTERIAL BLEPHARITIS, MEIBOMITIS, CHALAZION OR HORDOLEUM*

Classical signs

- Eyelid swelling, erythema and ulceration.
- Mucoid to mucopurulent ocular discharge.
- ± Chronic meibomian gland swelling with caseous material or acute abscessation.

Pathogenesis

Bacterial infection is mostly by pathogenic staphylococci. The most common region of the eyelid involved is the **meibomian gland**.

Pyodermas involving the sebaceous glands of the skin and associated staphylococcal hypersensitivity are also seen.

Clinical signs

Eyelid swelling, erythema and ulceration occur with **bacterial blepharitis**. Lesions are seen more commonly at the medial canthus with staphylococcal hypersensitivity.

Meibomitis, chalazion or hordoleum involve acute or chronic swelling of single or multiple meibomian glands.

In acute cases (hordoleum), the lids are painful and inflamed with inflammation around the glands. The infection in the meibomian gland may organize into discrete abscesses containing purulent material. Occasionally sinuses form which discharge onto the skin. Chronic cases may organize into large masses of caseous material with a tendency to be walled off in a fibrous capsule within the eyelid (chalazion). In meibomitis, only individual glands are swollen.

Mucoid to mucopurulent ocular discharge occurs.

Diagnosis

Diagnosis is usually based on the appearance of the eyelid and response to treatment.

Samples of material drained from abscessed meibomian glands can be cultured to determine etiology and sensitivity to antibiotics.

Histopathology might be performed on eyelid skin where allergy or autoimmune disease is suspected in the differential diagnosis.

Differential diagnosis

Allergic skin disease must be ruled out by appropriate consideration of possible antigens, e.g. food proteins, insect bites, inhalant or contact allergens.

Immune-mediated skin disease can be ruled out by demonstration of characteristic histopathology.

Neoplasia can be differentiated from chronic meibomian gland swelling with caseous material or acute abscessation by cytology or histopathology.

Treatment

Use systemic antibiotics based on results of culture and sensitivity or empirically:

- Amoxil–clavulanic acid combinations at 12.5 mg/kg q 12 hourly.
- Doxycycline at 5 mg/kg q 12 hourly. There is now some suggestion in the literature that doxycycline may act as an immune-modulator by altering immune responses to meibomian or sebaceous lipid.
- Cephalexin 15 mg/kg q 12 hourly.

Topical antibiotics.
- Fusidic acid is not available in North America but is used in Australia and Europe. Apply topically q 12 hourly.
- Terramycin ophthalmic ointment q 12 hourly.

Surgical drainage and/or curettage of lesions may sometimes be necessary to control chalazia. This is best done via a caudal approach through bulbar conjunctiva. A chalazion clamp will help to immobilize the lid during drainage.

ALLERGIC BLEPHARITIS*

Classical signs

- Variable eyelid erythema, swelling and pruritis.
- Excoriation and exudation, with crusting of eyelid skin.
- ± Skin lesions involving other parts of the body.

See main reference on page 1025 for details (The Cat With Miliary Dermatitis).

Pathogenesis

Allergic skin disease affecting eyelid skin can be due to any of the following:
- Food allergy.
- Staphylococcal allergy.
- Insect bite hypersensitivity.
- Atopy.
- Contact allergy (to topical drugs).

Clinical signs

Clinical signs are variable and can include combinations of erythema, swelling, pruritis, excoriation, exudation and crusting of eyelid skin.

Lesions may be seen at other sites on the skin, e.g. neck and face, ears, ventral abdomen.

Diagnosis

A tentative diagnosis is based on the appearance of the erythematous, crusting and/or pruritic lesions around the eyelids, and the appearance of lesions on other parts of the body, e.g. ears, for insect bite hypersensitivity.

Confirmation of the diagnosis is based on the use of appropriate tests or trials.

- **Food allergy** diagnosis requires careful **questioning about dietary history, followed by an appropriate food elimination trial** using a single novel protein (1/3 cup) with potato or rice (2/3 cup), and demonstration of an improvement in the appearance of the skin. Dietary trials should be performed for at least one month.
- **Staphylococcal allergy** is indicated by **demonstration of an improvement after a trial course of antibiotics**, e.g. amoxicillin–clavulanic acid combination at a dose rate of 12.5 mg/kg q 12 hourly for at least 2 weeks.
- **Insect bite hypersensitivity** is diagnosed by **demonstration of an improvement after enclosing the cat in an insect-proof enclosure** for at least 2–3 weeks.
- **Atopy requires intradermal skin testing** to help identify the allergen.
- **Contact allergy** should be suspected when **withdrawal of the suspected offending drug from topical use** for 2–3 weeks results in resolution of signs.

Differential diagnosis

Immune-mediated skin disease can be ruled out on the basis of histopathology of skin biopsies by a competent dermatohistopathologist.

Treatment

Treatment is variable depending on the type of allergy:

- Food allergy: withdraw offending food protein from the diet.
- Staphylococcal allergy: continue antibiotic treatment for at least 4 weeks.
- Insect bite hypersensitivity: use insect repellants on or around the cat, or attempt to reduce insects by environmental control, e.g. use of mosquito coils,

electrical insect destruction appliances, reducing local mosquito or midge breeding grounds.

- Inhalant allergy: hyposensitization by a competent dermatologist. Judicious use of oral corticosteroids to control pruritis.
- Contact allergy (to topical drugs): Withdraw offending drug from use on the eye.

EYELID TRAUMA/WOUNDS*

Classical signs

- Linear defects or discontinuities.
- Puncture wounds with secondary cellulitis and abscessation.
- Abrasions, excoriations, hemorrhage and crusting.
- Swelling with purple to red discoloration (bruising).

Pathogenesis

Trauma can be variable in its effect on eyelid structure.

- **Sharp lacerating trauma** tends to create linear defects or discontinuities.
- **Puncturing trauma** may not be readily obvious unless infectious organisms introduced by the puncture wound later cause cellulites.
- **Abrading trauma** causes surface excoriation, hemorrhage and crusting.
- **Traumatic contusion** (bruising trauma) will cause significant swelling and purple to red discoloration of the eyelid tissue.

Clinical signs

Trauma to the eyelids should be suspected whenever any of the following are observed:

- Linear defects or discontinuities of the eyelid margin or skin surface.
- Swelling.
- Surface ulceration or excoriation.
- Surface hemorrhage or bruising.
- Serous ocular discharge and/or crusting.
- Associated trauma to the conjunctiva and/or globe.

Diagnosis

Diagnosis is based on the history of a known traumatic episode, and on the appearance of the eyelids suggesting trauma.

Treatment

Initial debridement is recommended to remove excessively traumatized tissue.

Accurate surgical apposition of wounds using 5/0 or 6/0 polypropylene or nylon sutures should be performed whenever there are sharp discontinuities of tissue. Debridement without suturing, followed by secondary intention healing (granulation) may be used whenever accurate apposition is not possible, however primary healing of eyelid structures is always preferable.

Antimicrobial therapy with antibiotics should be specifically directed against known common skin flora. Antibiotics should be considered whenever there is severe devitalization of tissue, loss of normal tissue perfusion due to disruption of arterial supply, or venous or lymphatic drainage. Appropriate empirical antibiotics selections include:
- Amoxicillin–clavulanic acid combinations at 12.5 mg/kg q 12 hourly.
- Cephalexin 15 mg/kg q 12 hourly.

Anti-inflammatory therapy with NSAIDs to reduce inflammation and swelling: Ketoprofen 1 mg/kg orally q 24 hours.

NOTOEDRES CATI INFECTION*

> **Classical signs**
> - Alopecia of the ears, eyelids, face and neck.
> - Crusting and excoriation.
> - Usually pronounced pruritis.

Clinical signs

Alopecia, crusting and excoriation of the ears, eyelids, face and neck.

Usually pronounced pruritis.

Diagnosis

If *Notoedres* infection is suspected, a tentative diagnosis is often made on the basis of the appearance of the lesions and the pruritis.

Other diseases which cause scaling and crusting such as **dermatophytosis** and **autoimmune skin diseases are usually not pruritic**.

Definitive diagnosis is based on the identification of the parasite in skin scrapings.

DEMODECOSIS

> **Classical signs**
> - Peri-ocular alopecia, erythema and scaling.
> - Variably pruritic.
> - Rare in cats.

Clinical signs

Typically there is alopecia, sometimes associated with scaling, erythema, crusting or alterations in pigmentation of the peri-ocular skin.

Often demodecosis is associated with other systemic disease such as FIV, FeLV, diabetes mellitus.

Diagnosis

Tentative diagnosis is based on suspicious skin lesions.

Definitive diagnosis is made on identification of mites in scrapings and/or histopathologic examination of affected eyelid skin.

MALASEZZIA

> **Classical signs**
> - Peri-ocular alopecia, and crusting.
> - Variably pruritic.
> - Rare in cats.

Pathogenesis

Rare in cats, and appears to be associated with **genetic factors in young cats**, for example Rex cats.

Adult-onset disease may be **allergy-associated**, and in aged cats *Malasezzia* has been associated with **thymomas and carcinomas** of the pancreas and liver.

Clinical signs

Typically there is **alopecia**, sometimes associated with **crusting** or pruritis, erythema and scaling.

Diagnosis

Diagnosis is made on **identification of yeast** organisms on cytological examination of a Diff-Quik-stained specimen obtained by adhesive tape or touching a cotton bud or slide to the affected area.

Because the organism is a normal commensal of the skin, diagnosis is based on identifying the organism associated with a typical skin lesion, and resolution of the lesion in response to treatment.

Treatment

Malasezzia is responsive to topical therapy such as **creams or lotions containing imidazoles**, but application is difficult because of the location.

Systemic antifungal therapy using **ketaconazole** or other **imidazole** may be better tolerated.

IMMUNE-MEDIATED BLEPHARITIS (PEMPHIGUS FOLIACEOUS, PEMPHIGUS ERYTHEMATOSUS, SYSTEMIC LUPUS ERYTHEMATOSUS)

Classical signs

- Alopecia, erythema, scaling and crusting of eyelids.
- Lesions on ears, muzzle, temporal skin and nose (pemphigus erythematosus), or nailbeds, nipples and other mucocutaneous junctions (pemphigus foliaceous).
- Other immune-mediated disease (e.g. immune-mediated polyarthritis, glomerulonephritis) in SLE.
- Uncommon.

Clinical signs

Uncommon disease in cats.

Alopecia, erythema, scaling and crusting of eyelids. Blisters are rarely seen as these are usually transient.

Additional areas affected are the **nailbeds, nipples and other mucocutaneous junctions** (foliaceous) and **ears, muzzle, temporal skin and nose** (erythematosus).

Systemic lupus erythematosus (SLE) is a very rare disease. It is more commonly seen in young cats with a reported higher incidence in Persian and Siamese breeds. Immune-mediated disease of other tissues is usually present by definition in SLE, for example:
- Immune-mediated polyarthritis: painful arthritic joints, lameness.
- Glomerulo-nephritis: chronic progressive signs of polydypsia/polyuria and azotemia.
- Cats usually have other systemic signs such as fever, lymphadenopathy.

Diagnosis

A provisional diagnosis is made on the appearance and location of the skin lesions.

Definitive diagnosis is made on histopathology of skin biopsies.

High ANA titers are usually seen in SLE.

Differential diagnosis

Similar eyelid lesions can be seen in allergic blepharitis, and in both conditions other lesions may also be seen on the face, but these cases can usually be differentiated from pemphigus and SLE on biopsy.

Dermatophyte infections can be identified by microscopic examination of hair shafts and culture.

Squamous cell carcinoma in the pre-cancerous stage ("solar dermatitis") can look similar to immune-mediated skin disease, but can be ruled out by biopsy of affected skin.

Treatment

Immunosuppressive doses of corticosteroids, e.g. prednisolone up to 2.5 mg/kg PO q 12 h, reducing as signs of disease abate.

In more aggressive immune-mediated skin disorders such as pemphigus foliaceous, other immune-modulating drugs may have to be used to achieve control, e.g. chlorambucil 0.1 mg/kg q 24 h.

ECTROPION

Classical signs

- Eyelid rolled outwards, making bulbar conjunctiva more visible.

Classical signs—Cont'd

- Cicatricial scarring from previous injury.
- Rare.

Clinical signs

Rare in cats.

Eyelid margin is rolled outwards, making bulbar conjunctiva more visible.

Usually it is caused by former injury. If the eyelid is examined carefully, signs of previous injury will be identified by cicatricial scarring causing the roll-out. This will make manual correction of the ectropion by lid tensioning at the time of examination difficult.

Diagnosis

Diagnosis is based on the characteristic appearance of a fixed ectropion with scarring.

DISTICHIASIS

Classical signs

- Cilia extending from meibomian gland openings at the eyelid margin.
- ± Ocular irritation with lacrimation.
- Rare in cats.

Clinical signs

Cilia are present extending from meibomian gland openings at the eyelid margin.

Irritation from the cilia may cause increased lacrimation and occasionally signs of corneal irritation, such as ulcerative or non-ulcerative keratitis, vascularization of the cornea or even corneal sequestration.

Rare in cats.

Diagnosis

Diagnosis is based on the detection of the fine cilia extending from the meibomian gland openings. Magnification and bright illumination will facilitate detection against a white scleral background.

PARASITIC MYIASIS

Classical signs

- Discharging fistulous opening onto the face.
- Fly larvae visible in wound.

Clinical signs

Discharging wound which may involve the eyelid. Usually fly larvae are visible inside a discharging fistulous opening.

Diagnosis

Diagnosis is based on the appearance of the fly larvae (maggots) in a discharging wound.

RECOMMENDED READING

Doherty M. A bridge flap blepharorrhaphy method of lower eyelid reconstruction in the cat. J Am Anim Hosp Assoc 1973; 9: 238.

Pavletic MM. Mucocutaneous subdermal plexus flap from the lip for lower eyelid restoration in the dog. J Am Vet Med Assoc 1982; 180: 921.

Scagliotti R. Comparative neuro-ophthalmology. In: Gelatt KN (ed) Veterinary Ophthalmology, 3rd edn. Baltimore, Maryland, Lippincott, Williams & Wilkins, 1999, pages 1362–1366.

Wolfer JC. Correction of eyelid coloboma in four cats using subdermal collagen and a modified Stades technique. Vet Ophth 2002; 5: 269–272.

66. The cat with an abnormal third eyelid

Michael E. Bernays

KEY SIGNS

- Abnormal prominence of third eyelid.
- Focal or generalized swelling of third eyelid.
- Erythemia, chemosis.
- Eyelid lacerations.
- Ocular discharge.

MECHANISM?

- Abnormalities of third eyelid appearance usually result from abnormalities in eyelid innervation, especially of the autonomic sympathetic nerves, or inflammation or neoplasia involving the conjunctiva of the third eyelid.

WHERE?

- Third eyelid cartilage.
  Conjunctiva covering the third eyelid.
  Gland of the third eyelid.

WHAT?

- The most common cause of altered third eyelid appearance is autonomic nervous system disease especially sympathetic neuropathy. Neoplasia and inflammatory disease is occasionally seen.

QUICK REFERENCE SUMMARY

Diseases causing an abnormal third eyelid

WHERE?

THIRD EYELID

METABOLIC

- **Third eyelid prominence related to severe weight loss* (p 1137)**
  Occurs secondary to loss of orbital fat and enophthalmos (caudal globe retraction).

NEOPLASTIC

- **Squamous cell carcinoma*** (p 1134)**

Proliferative pink mass growing from the third eyelid with verrucous or ulcerated surface.

- **Other neoplastic disease of the third eyelid (adenoma, adenocarcinoma, mast cell tumor, lymphoma, hemangioma)* (p 1138)**

Tumors result in generalized swelling, a localized mass lesion, or erosion on the third eyelid. Hemangioma may form a discrete mass on the third eyelid, usually red to purple in color, which may hemorrhage.

PHYSICAL

- Prolapsed gland of the third eyelid (p 1340)

Pink to red mass protruding from behind the leading edge of the third eyelid (rare).

- Everted nictitans cartilage (p 1331)

Folded edge of third eyelid margin, without fleshy mass suggestive of gland prolapse (rare).

- **Third eyelid prominence related to ocular pain* (p @)**

Occurs secondary to enophthalmos (globe retraction) due to the pain.

INFECTIOUS

- **Infectious disease involving the conjunctiva of third eyelid (feline herpesvirus-1**, *Chlamydophila felis*** *Mycoplasma**) (p 1337)**

Signs include acute onset of hyperemia and chemosis of conjunctival surfaces and serous or mucopurulent ocular discharge, often together with concurrent upper respiratory tract signs. Chlamydial and mycoplasmal conjunctivitis may involve one or both eyes initially, and herpesvirus causes bilateral involvement.

- Tetanus (p 1339)

Bilateral third eyelid prominence in association with contraction of facial muscles, and increased tone in muscles of mastication ("lockjaw"). Rare in cats.

IMMUNE

- **Eosinophilic keratoconjunctivitis** (p 1335)**

Pink to whitish plaque-like thickening of the third eyelid, sometimes associated with similar lesions on the cornea.

IDIOPATHIC

- **Third eyelid dysautonomia ("Haws")*** (p 1338)**

Acute onset of bilateral third eyelid prominence, which is non-painful, and resolves over days to weeks without treatment.

- Feline dysautonomia (p 1338)

Third eyelid prominence, in association with any of a range of other systemic signs, e.g. keratoconjunctivitis sicca, dilated non-responsive pupils, anisocoria, dry nose and/or mouth, bradycardia, constipation megaesophagus and urinary or fecal incontinence. Onset of signs is over 48 h, and is associated with depression and anorexia.

continued

continued

TRAUMA

● **Trauma to the third eyelid* (p 1330)**
Asymmetric notch-like defects in the third eyelid margin due to claw injury from fighting with other cat(s).

● **Sympathetic neuropathy of the third eyelid (Horner's syndrome)** (p 1335)**
Prominent third eyelid, usually unilateral, in association with any combination of enophthalmos, upper lid ptosis or miosis, in association with or without other localizing signs such as ipsilateral forelimb lameness, cervical lesions (e.g. abscess, cellulitis) or middle ear disease.

INTRODUCTION

MECHANISM?

The most common cause of change in third eyelid appearance is an abnormality in innervation, especially involving the autonomic sympathetic nerves.

The abnormal third eyelid is most often noticed because it is prominent.

Prominence or **protrusion of the third eyelid is a passive phenomenon** in most animal species. Protrusion is usually facilitated by active contraction of muscle in adjacent orbital structures, and occurs because either:

● The globe is retracted caudally into the orbit by the action of the rectus and retractor bulbi muscles (the normal position of the globe tends to push the third eyelid into its retracted position at the medial aspect of the globe) or

● Sympathetically innervated smooth muscle at the base of the third eyelid (arising from deep in the orbit around facial coverings of the medial and ventral rectus muscles) is not contracting, causing a failure of retraction of the third eyelid.

In the cat, the third eyelid may become actively protruded, independent of globe movement, by the action of skeletal muscle fibers, which are extensions of the levator palpebrae superioris and the lateral rectus muscles, innervated by the oculomotor (CN III) and abducens (CN VI), respectively.

Because the third eyelid is covered by conjunctiva on both its posterior and anterior surface, any disease which affects the conjunctiva (see The Cat With Ocular Discharge or Changed Conjunctival Appearance, page 1212) can also involve the surface of the third eyelid. Such conjunctival diseases are either:

● Inflammatory disease due to:
  – Infectious agents such as FHV1, *Chlamydophila felis*, *Mycoplasma*.
  – Non-infectious, allergic or other immune-mediated etiologies, e.g. eosinophilic keratoconjunctivitis or follicular conjunctivitis.
● Neoplastic disease, especially squamous cell carcinoma.

WHERE?

Disease anywhere along the **sympathetic neural pathways** (i.e. thalamus, cervical spinal cord long tracts, T1–T3 spinal nerves, ascending pre-ganglionic fibers, cranial cervical ganglion, sympathetic postganglionic fibers in middle ear or orbit), and the smooth muscle fibers innervated by them, may cause protrusion of the third eyelid.

Conjunctival surface diseases cause abnormal appearance of the third eyelid.

Cartilage of the third eyelid may fold causing an everted appearance.

WHAT?

The most common cause of altered third eyelid appearance is autonomic nervous system disease especially **primary third eyelid dysautonomia ("haws")**. Horner's syndrome is associated **with other clinical signs** such as enophthalmos, miosis and upper lid ptosis. Primary third eyelid dysautonomia is associated with **prominence of the third eyelid with lack of other signs** of sympathetic denervation.

Inflammatory disease is occasionally seen, and can be of infectious or non-infectious, immune-mediated or allergic etiology.

Neoplasia involving the conjunctiva of the third eyelid occurs infrequently.

DISEASES CAUSING ABNORMAL THIRD EYELID APPEARANCE

INFECTIOUS DISEASE INVOLVING CONJUNCTIVA OF THE THIRD EYELID*** (FELINE HERPESVIRUS-1**, *CHLAMYDOPHILA FELIS** AND MYCOPLASMA* INFECTION)

Classical signs

- Inflammation and chemosis (swelling) specifically involving the conjunctiva of the third eyelid.
- Discharge varies from serous or mucoid to mucopurulent.

See main references on feline herpesvirus, chlamydial and mycoplasmal infection on pages 1212, 1218 for details (The Cat With Ocular Discharge or Changed Conjunctival Appearance).

Clinical signs

Typically there is **inflammation and chemosis (swelling)** specifically involving the conjunctiva of the third eyelid. Usually the associated bulbar and palpebral conjunctivae are also affected.

There may be **signs of upper respiratory tract disease** in the early stages, although all these organisms may also cause conjunctivitis unassociated with typical upper respiratory tract signs. Conjunctivitis alone may occur in cats with previous exposure that have developed immunity, or it may represent recrudescence of signs in carrier cats.

Discharge varies from serous or mucoid to mucopurulent. The type of discharge seen is dependent on the stage of the infection, for example, FHV-1 herpesvirus infections usually cause a serous discharge in the early stages, which progresses to a mucopurulent discharge secondary to bacterial infection.

Although herpesvirus, *Chlamydophila felis* and *Mycoplasma* infection may be difficult to distinguish clinically in some cats, in other cats signs may be suggestive of the causative agent.

- **Herpesvirsus** typically causes bilateral serous conjunctivitis in conjunction with other upper respiratory signs (sneezing, nasal discharge). Discharge rapidly becomes mucopurulent and the cat is depressed, anorexic and febrile. In some cats, dendritic ulcerative keratitis may occur initially. Non-ulcerative stromal keratitis and/or corneal sequestration may occur several weeks to a few months after the initial infection, which may have been unnoticed. Symblepharon may be seen as a sequel in young cats.
- **Chlamydial conjunctivitis** typically appears as severe hyperemia and chemosis of conjunctival surfaces. It is associated with mucopurulent discharge, usually starting in one eye and later progressing to involve the contralateral eye.
- **Mycoplasmal conjunctivitis** appears as unilateral or bilateral conjunctivitis, associated with epiphora, papillary hypertrophy of conjunctiva, conjunctival follicles, chemosis, and occasionally thick white pseudomambrane.

Diagnosis

A tentative diagnosis is often made on the signs of inflammation, chemosis and discharge associated with upper respiratory tract signs.

A **definitive diagnosis** requires identification of the organism on conjunctival cytologic preparations stained with **Wright–Giemsa,** e.g.

- Membrane-bound basophilic intracytoplasmic inclusions indicate chlamydial infection.
- Small basophilic-staining pleomorphic organisms closely associated with the cell membrane surface indicate mycoplasmal infection.

Specific tests are available for the diagnosis of infectious disease especially in the early stages, e.g.

- Herpesvirus: immunofluorescent antibody (IFA), virus isolation (VI) and polymerase chain reaction (PCR).
- *Chlamydophila felis*: IFA and PCR.

Differential diagnosis

Infectious conjunctivitis is usually distinctive and differentiation between the infectious agents needs to be made. The chronic forms of infection may appear similar to **eosinophilic keratoconjunctivitis,** which can be differentiated based on cytological examination of deep scrapings or on histopathology.

Treatment

See The Cat With Ocular Discharge or Changed Conjunctival Appearance (page 1207) for more details.

Herpesvirus: topical trifluorothymidine, Idoxuridine, Vidarabine, topical or oral Acyclovir, topical or oral alpha interferon, oral lysine.

Chlamydophila felis: topical tetracycline, oral doxycycline, oral azithromycin.

Mycoplasma: topical tetracycline or chloramphenicol.

THIRD EYELID DYSAUTONOMIA ("HAWS")***

> ### Classical signs
>
> - Bilateral non-painful third eyelid prominence.
> - Usually acute onset, and often resolves rapidly without treatment within days to weeks.
> - Unassociated with other signs of sympathetic denervation.

Clinical signs

Bilateral, non-painful third eyelid prominence, usually acute in onset and resolves rapidly within days to weeks. Not associated with other signs of sympathetic denervation such as ptosis and a miotic pupil.

Sometimes seen in association with acute gastrointestinal signs, e.g. diarrhea. One report in the literature found an association with torovirus infection.

Diagnosis

Diagnosis is usually based solely on the clinical signs.

Differential diagnosis

Horner's syndrome results in acute onset of unilateral prominence of the third eyelid whereas Haws is bilateral. Horner's syndrome is associated with other signs such as ptosis and a miotic pupil.

Treatment

No treatment is necessary. All cases will resolve with time.

SQUAMOUS CELL CARCINOMA***

> ### Classical signs
>
> - Verrucous, raised mass usually arising from non-pigmented conjunctival surface.
> - Erosion and mucopurulent discharge.

Clinical signs

Pink, proliferative mass with a cauliflower-like (verrucous) or ulcerated surface usually arising from the non-pigmented conjunctival surface of the third eyelid. Typically the lesion is associated with erosion, loss of normal tissue architecture and mucopurulent discharge.

Diagnosis

Initial diagnosis is based on the appearance of the lesion.

Cytology and/or histopathology are required for a definitive diagnosis. Typical cytological appearance includes large clumps of eosinophilic keratinized epithelial cells, and sometimes loss of normal architecture is visible in the form of whorls or keratin "pearls".

Differential diagnosis

Eosinophilic keratitis is an uncommon proliferative disease of the third eyelid. It may also be associated with corneal disease and cytology is characteristically in the form of eosinophilic infiltrates.

Other neoplastic disease. Hemangiomas are not as common, have a smoother surface, and appear as a darker red to purple-colored mass.

Treatment

Surgical excision with good margins is required to ensure complete removal. The lesions can sometimes invade deep into the extra-ocular tissues by the time the lesion is recognized.

Cryosurgery using liquid nitrogen or nitrous oxide with double freeze thaws and slow controlled thawing can be effective for small tumors less than 0.5 cm diameter. Maximal destruction of tumor cells occurs when temperatures of between −20°C to −40°C are achieved at the center of the tumor.

β-irradiation with strontium 90 can be effective if available.

EOSINOPHILIC KERATOCONJUNCTIVITIS**

Classical signs

- Pink to whitish plaque-like thickening of the third eyelid.
- ± Similar lesions on the cornea.

Clinical signs

Appears as **pink to whitish plaque-like thickening of the third eyelid**. Similar lesions may appear on the cornea in some cats.

The pathogenesis is unknown, but is postulated to involve insect bite hypersensitivity or herpesvirus infection in some cats. Generally there is not a strong association with the presence of other feline eosinophilic disease.

Diagnosis

Tentative diagnosis is based on the presence of typical lesions on the third eyelid and cornea.

Cytological examination of deep scrapings of the lesion or histopathology of a biopsy specimen demonstrate an **infiltrate of plasma cells and lymphocytes** with variable numbers of eosinophils. Eosinophils may not always be the most numerous cell type.

Tests for herpesvirus infection, e.g. in situ PCR and (see The Cat With Ocular Discharge or Changed Conjunctival Appearance, page 1213, for more details).

Differential diagnosis

Squamous cell carcinoma usually causes more disfigurement of the third eyelid due to proliferation and ulceration.

Other neoplasms such as hemangioma have a characteristic appearance.

Chronic *Mycoplasma* and *Chlamydophila felis* infection may appear similar in some cats, but can be differentiated on cytological examination of Wright–Giemsa-stained slides, immunofluorescent antibody and PCR.

Treatment

Oral corticosteroids: Prednisolone 5 mg orally q 12–24 h, with dose reducing as effect is achieved.

Oral progestagens at a low dose (e.g. megestrol acetate 5 mg twice weekly) should be used only in cases refractory to oral prednisolone. Beware of possible side effects such as insulin resistance, diabetes and obesity.

Topical corticosteroids are usually contraindicated because of an underlying association with ocular herpesvirus infection. These drugs may potentiate the herpesvirus infection by local immunosuppression.

Treat the underlying cause if identified, e.g. treat the ocular herpesvirus infection.

SYMPATHETIC NEUROPATHY OF THE THIRD EYELID (HORNER'S SYNDROME)**

Classical signs

- Usually unilateral.
- Non-painful prominence of the third eyelid.
- Miosis of the ipsilateral pupil.
- Upper lid ptosis.
- Enophthalmos.

Pathogenesis

Protrusion of the third eyelid occurs where there is disruption of the sympathetic neural pathways innervating the smooth muscle of the third eyelid (Horner's syndrome). Disruption may occur anywhere along the pathway including in the thalamus, cervical spinal cord long tracts, T1–T3 spinal nerves or nerve roots, ascending pre-ganglionic fibers, cranial cervical ganglion and sympathetic post-ganglionic fibers in middle ear or orbit. Less commonly protrusion is the result of dysfunction of the smooth muscle fibers innervated by the sympathetic nerve.

More common causes in the cat include:
- **Middle ear disease** especially nasopharyngeal polyps. Nasopharyngeal polyps arise in the middle ear and emerge into the external ear canal or nasopharynx. Typically they occur in young cats (< 5 years), but any age can be affected.
- **Disruption of ascending sympathetic pathways** in the neck due to **injury or inflammation** associated with fight wounds.
- **Injury to nerve roots of T1–T3** associated with forelimb trauma, usually from motor vehicle accidents.
- **Anterior thoracic cavity disease,** e.g. mediastinal lymphoma.

Rarely, is third eyelid protrusion the result of nerve damage within the brain or spinal cord, or smooth muscle disease.

Clinical signs

Usually there is a **unilateral, non-painful prominence of the third eyelid**, together with other signs of sympathetic denervation, i.e. miosis, upper lid ptosis ("drooping"), enophthalmos.

Other signs may be present in some cases, which may enable further localization of the lesion, e.g.
- An **abscess or cellulitis of cervical soft tissue** structures suggests disruption of ascending preganglionic fibers.
- **Signs** of **middle or inner ear disease** such as a head tilt or circling. Nasopharyngeal polyp may be seen as a fibrous mass emerging into the external ear canal, or cause noisy breathing, dyspnea with or without nasal discharge, sneezing or coughing and gagging.
- **Ipsilateral forelimb lameness** may occur from damage to nerve roots or nerves innervating the leg. **Radial nerve paresis or paralysis** may occur concurrently with avulsion of T1–T3 nerve roots if C8 or T1 nerve roots are injured. If the **musculocutaneous nerve** roots (C5–7) are also injured, the

elbow cannot be flexed or the paw picked up, resulting in excoriation of the dorsum of the paw. Muscle atrophy is apparent within 5–7 days of injury to the motor nerve roots. Damage to C7–T1 may also result in loss of the **ipsilateral cutaneous trunci (panniculus)** reflex.

Diagnosis

Any cat with an apparently non-painful, non-inflamed prominent third eyelid, which also has miosis, upper lid ptosis and enophthalmos should be suspected as having Horner's syndrome.

Pharmacological testing with sympathomimetics is controversial, and the indirect-acting sympathomimetic hydroxyamfetamine is no longer available in some countries. Reliable diagnostic protocols are not available, however a rapid (within 5–8 minutes) reversal of signs following the administration of one drop of 10% phenylephrine is suggestive of post-ganglionic denervation hypersensitivity, indicating that the lesion is somewhere rostral to the cranial cervical ganglion. Anatomically this corresponds to localization of the lesion in the middle ear or orbital structures rostral to the middle ear. The response should always be compared with that in the contralateral normal eye.

Lesion localization will not be possible in many cases, and many cases seem to be idiopathic.

Differential diagnosis

Third eyelid dysautonomia (Haw's) is always bilateral, and is not associated with other signs of sympathetic denervation. Horner's syndrome is almost always unilateral.

Treatment

Where possible, treatment should be directed at the associated problems which may be causing interruption of sympathetic pathways.

The disfigurement created by Horner's syndrome can be reversed by frequent (at least 2–3 times daily) application of one drop of 10% phenylephrine in the affected eye. This treatment only alters the appearance of the eye and does nothing else for the cat's well-being, except that vision might be improved where the third eyelid prominence and enophthalmos is extreme, causing most of the globe to be covered by nictitans.

Prognosis

Depending on the cause many cases may resolve over time as denervated smooth muscle re-innervates, provided that oculosympathetic fibers are not totally destroyed.

TRAUMA TO THE THIRD EYELID MARGIN*

Classical signs

- Notch-like or linear tears arising from the third eyelid margin.
- Usually unilateral, with the contralateral eye unaffected.

Clinical signs

Trauma to the third eyelid may result in notch-like or linear tears starting at the margin of the third eyelid. These occur most commonly from cat fights.

Third eyelid trauma may be associated with other ocular signs, when seen in the acute stages, e.g. conjunctival chemosis and ocular discharge (see The Cat With Ocular Discharge or Changed Conjunctival Appearance, page 1211).

Diagnosis

Diagnosis is based on the clinical signs, and the history of unilateral third eyelid notch or tear occurring after a possible fight with another cat.

THIRD EYELID PROMINENCE RELATED TO OCULAR PAIN*

Classical signs

- Third eyelid prominence.
- Associated with other ipsilateral signs of ocular pain, e.g. enophthalmos, blepharospasm, corneal disease, pupil miosis.

Clinical signs

The third eyelid is prominent because of **retraction of the globe, associated with ocular pain**.

It is associated with **ipsilateral signs of ocular pain**, for example, enophthalmos, blepharospasm, corneal disease, pupil miosis or anterior uveitis.

Diagnosis

Diagnosis is based on signs of ocular pain together with prominence of a normal-appearing third eyelid.

Differential diagnosis

Horner's syndrome and **Haws** are usually non-painful.

Horner's syndrome, tetanus and feline dysautonomia each have their own specific associated clinical signs, which are more suggestive of that particular condition.

Treatment

Treat the cause of the ocular pain as indicated.

THIRD EYELID PROMINENCE RELATED TO SEVERE WEIGHT LOSS*

Classical signs

- Signs of generalized muscle wasting associated with chronic disease.
- Thin face with signs of muscle wastage around the lateral aspects of the orbit.
- Bilaterally symmetrical third eyelid prominence without miosis or upper lid ptosis.

Clinical signs

Typically these cats have a bilaterally symmetrical third eyelid prominence due to marked enophthalmos, and there are no other signs normally associated with other causes of third eyelid prominence such as miosis or upper lid ptosis.

Generalized whole-body muscle wasting is present in association with signs of other organ system disease, e.g. chronic renal failure, inflammatory bowel disease or hyperthyroidism.

Third eyelid prominence occurs secondary to loss of orbital fat and enophthalmos.

Diagnosis

Diagnosis is based on the generalized body muscle and fat loss, in association with the pronounced enophthalmos and third eyelid prominence.

OTHER NEOPLASTIC DISEASE OF THE THIRD EYELID* (ADENOMA, ADENOCARCINOMA, MAST CELL TUMOR, LYMPHOMA, HEMANGIOMA)

Classical signs

- Mass or erosive lesion involving the third eyelid.
- Ocular discharge.

Clinical signs

Tumors of the third eyelid **appear as a mass or erosive lesion** involving the third eyelid. Appearance depends on the type of tumor, which includes lymphoma, hemangioma, mast cell tumor, adenoma and adenocarcinoma.

- **Hemangiomas** are rare, are usually dark red to purple in color, and are fragile with a tendency to hemorrhage.
- **Lymphoma** will usually cause more generalized swelling of the third eyelid and the peri-orbital tissues, and may be associated with other systemic signs of multicentric lymphoma.
- **Mast cell tumors** can form either well- or poorly circumscribed areas of swelling in the eyelid. They appear as rapidly growing nodular tumor, often with poorly defined borders, and variable surface ulceration.
- **Adenomas or carcinomas** are seen as a nodular or diffuse mass causing localized thickening of the eyelid. The tumor may have an ulcerated surface.

The neoplastic mass may cause increased **ocular discharge** because of third eyelid dysfunction. The normal distribution of the precorneal tear film across the cornea is impaired because of an uneven eyelid margin.

Diagnosis

Diagnosis is initially based on the **appearance of the lesion**, which varies according to the type of tumor.

Definitive diagnosis is by cytological and histological examination.

FELINE DYSAUTONOMIA

Classical signs

- Unilateral or bilateral third eyelid prominence.
- Acute onset of anorexia and depression.
- Other signs of autonomic dysfunction such as keratoconjunctivitis sicca, mydriasis, anisocoria, dry nose or mouth, bradycardia, constipation, megaesophagus, urinary or fecal incontinence.

See main references on page 792 for details (The Constipated or Straining Cat).

Clinical signs

Third eyelid prominence, in association with any of a range of **other systemic signs suggestive of autonomic dysfunction** including keratoconjunctivitis sicca, dilated non-responsive pupils, anisocoria, dry nose and/or mouth, bradycardia, constipation, megaesophagus and urinary or fecal incontinence.

Typically, the onset of signs is **acute over 48 h and associated with depression and anorexia**.

Diagnosis

Diagnosis is based on signs of generalized autonomic dysfunction.

Condition is rare or at least uncommon, and most frequent in UK.

Definitive diagnosis is based on the demonstration of **characteristic ultrastructural lesions within cell bodies** in autonomic ganglia at post mortem.

Differential diagnosis

Abnormality of the third eyelid without the presence of other signs of autonomic dysfunction would suggest localized sympathetic dysfunction such as **Horner's or Haws syndrome**.

Treatment

No definitive treatment is available. Prognosis is generally guarded to poor, however supportive treatment is reported to be variably effective.

TETANUS

> ### Classical signs
>
> - Bilateral third eyelid prominence.
> - Contraction of facial muscles, increased tone in muscles of mastication ("lockjaw").
> - Stiffness of one or more limbs which worsens with stimulation.

Pathogenesis

Signs of tetanus result from the toxin produced by *Clostridium tetani*, a spore-forming, Gram-positive rod. *C. tetani* is found in the soil, and also occurs as part of the normal gastrointestinal tract flora of some animals.

Spores of the *Clostridium tetani* bacillus enter the body commonly via surface wounds. The toxin, **tetanospasmin**, is produced during cell growth, sporulation and lysis, if there is a suitable anaerobic environment for the bacteria. The toxin migrates along nerve axons from a local wound, to sites of action in the central nervous system, where it initially binds to presynaptic inhibitory motor nerve endings. The effect of the toxin is to block the release of inhibitory neurotransmitters (glycine and gamma-amino butyric acid) across the synaptic cleft. This results in uninhibited muscle contraction.

The **incubation period** for signs to develop varies from **3–21 days after an injury**, depending on the proximity of the injury to the CNS, the ability of the local tissue environment to support toxin production, and the number of organisms present.

Tetanus is **rare in cats**, because they are more **resistant to the toxin** than humans and horses. This innate resistance is related to the **inability of the toxin to penetrate and bind to nervous tissue**, and likely accounts for the frequency of localized signs in cats.

Tetanus has occurred after routine surgery (such as ovariohysterectomy), fetal death during pregnancy, and trauma.

Tetanus may occur in young cats associated with a gum wound secondary to losing a deciduous tooth.

Clinical signs

Signs of tetanus may be localized or generalized, or may begin with localized signs and progressively involve more muscle groups over a week or more, and become generalized. Generalization is more likely if there is inadequate wound management, or inadequate antibiotic therapy.

Diagnosis may be difficult in the early stages of the disease when characteristic signs of generalized tetanus are absent.

Classical signs of generalized tetanus include bilateral third eyelid prominence in association with **contraction of the facial muscles** giving the appearance of a "**sardonic smile**", and increased tone in the muscles of mastication ("lockjaw"). The cat may have a "startled" appearance.

Focal tetanus results in **stiffness of the muscles in closest proximity to the wound**, and is often evident as stiffness of one or two limbs.

In many cats, **a neglected wound with necrotic tissue** is found, suggesting a site for toxin production.

Tetanus may be associated with infection of the female reproductive tract, and may produce local signs in the pelvic limbs.

The history of a penetrating or neglected wound, and the **presence of persistent involuntary muscle rigidity in a mentally alert cat** is highly suggestive of tetanus.

If there is generalized muscle stiffness, the cat may have an **increased temperature** associated with the muscle contraction.

Diagnosis

Diagnosis is based on the characteristic clinical signs.

EMG testing of affected muscles is strongly suggestive of tetanus if it demonstrates **persistent spontaneous motor unit potentials**.

Differential diagnosis

Any condition which causes **bilateral third eyelid prominence** such as **haws or dysautonomia** should be considered. However, facial muscle or limb rigidity is not seen with these conditions.

Mild hypocalcemia in late pregnancy or following whelping could be confused with tetanus, especially as the reproductive tract may be a site of infection and toxin production. Rapid response to intravenous calcium in pregnancy-associated hypocalcemia will rule out tetanus.

Meningoencephalitis or encephalopathy including thiamine deficiency may occasionally have tetanic spasms worsened with touch or sound. In these animals mentation is usually depressed and other neurological signs are evident.

Treatment

Treatment involves appropriate **antibiotic therapy, wound care, supportive treatment**, and use of **tetanus antitoxin**.

It is important to **debride necrotic tissue**, so the tissue environment is less attractive for persistence of the organism and toxin production.

Antibiotics with anaerobic activity especially **metronidazole (10 mg/kg, q 8 h)**, and those belonging to the penicillin group, e.g. amoxicillin or **amoxycillin/clavulanate** are indicated to prevent further proliferation of bacteria in the wound.

- Metronidazole has been shown to be superior to penicillin G and tetracycline. It is bactericidal against most anaerobes and achieves effective therapeutic concentrations even in anaerobic tissues.

Tetanus antitoxin binds to circulating toxin, and cannot dislodge toxin within peripheral nerves. Its main purpose is to neutralize circulating toxin outside the nervous system. If the signs are localized and non-progressive, administering tetanus antitoxin systemically is not likely to be beneficial, and is associated with a risk of anaphylaxis.

- The dose of antitoxin is usually about 1000 U/kg IV administered slowly over 5–10 minutes, with some (1000 U) injected locally in the wound. As most tetanus antiserums are generally prepared in equines, consideration should be given to the pre-emptive use of corticosteroids and antihistamine to prevent possible anaphylaxis. Give a test dose (0.1–0.2 ml) intradermally or subcutaneously 15–20 minutes before IV administration and check for a wheal.

Muscle relaxants such as **diazepam** can be used to control the muscle rigidity and make the cat more comfortable. Efficacy of the drug varies between individual cats. Alternatively, small doses of **acepromazine** (1.25–2.5 mg/cat PO q 6 hours as required), **chlorpromazine** (IV) or **phenobarbital** may be effective in reducing muscle stiffness.

Other **supportive treatment** should be given as indicated, e.g. **alimentation, intravenous fluids**.

Keep the cat in a **quiet, dark area** to reduce the muscle spasms, which are stimulated by touch or sound

Difficulty urinating or defecating may occur, and needs to be managed.

Prognosis

The **prognosis is generally good** with appropriate treatment, and full resolution of signs usually occurs within 2–3 months.

Prognosis is poorer if signs develop very rapidly.

PROLAPSED GLAND OF THE THIRD EYELID

> **Classical signs**
>
> - Pink to red mass protruding from behind the third eyelid.
> - Variable inflammation and discharge.
> - Rare and only reported in Burmese cats.

Clinical signs

Pink to reddish mass with a smooth conjunctival surface protrudes from behind the leading edge of the third eyelid margin.

Prolapse may be accompanied by **variable degrees of inflammation and discharge**, ranging from mucoid to mucopurulent.

Rare in cats compared with dogs, and reported only in Burmese cats.

Diagnosis

Diagnosis is based on the appearance of the mass. Differential diagnosis would be a tumor or a folded (everted or inverted) third eyelid cartilage, also rarely reported, and only in Burmese cats.

EVERTED NICTITANS CARTILAGE

Classical signs

- Folded everted third eyelid margin.
- Rare and only reported in Burmese cats.

Clinical signs

Everted third eyelid margin occurs because **of folding of the cartilage** of the third eyelid. This condition should be distinguished from a prolapsed gland of the nictitans.

Rare in cats. Reported only in Burmese cats.

Diagnosis

Diagnosis is based on the appearance of the third eyelid margin. Usually there is no sign of a fleshy mass protruding from behind the third eyelid.

Treatment

Resection of the folded section of cartilage will enable straightening of the third eyelid.

RECOMMENDED READING

Glaze MB, Gelatt KN. Feline ophthalmology. In: Scagliotti R (ed) Comparative Neuro-ophthalmology. In: Gelatt KN (series ed) Veterinary Ophthalmology, 3rd edn. Baltimore, Maryland, Lippincott, Williams & Wilkins, 1999, pp. 1004–1010, 1366–1370.

Ketring KL, Glaze MB. Atlas of Feline Ophthalmology. Trenton, New Jersey, Veterinary Learning Systems, 1994, pp. 69–76.

Sharp NJH, Nash AS, Griffiths IR. Feline dysautonomia (the Key-Gaskell syndrome): a clinical and pathologic study of forty cases. J Small Anim Pract 1984; 25: 599–615.

PART 16

Drugs

67. Special considerations related to drug use in cats

Jill Elizabeth Maddison

KEY SIGNS

- Differences in dosing recommendations between dogs and cats are usually because of differences in drug metabolism.
- Cats are deficient in some glucuronyl transferases resulting in very prolonged half lives for some drugs such as aspirin.
- Feline hemoglobin is more susceptible to oxidation forming methemoglobin; oxidation occurs with drugs such as benzocaine.
- Some receptor sites for drug binding are more sensitive, for example with morphine.

Drugs not recommended for use in cats

Acetaminophen (paracetamol)	Methemoglobinemia and Heinz body anemia.
Apomorphine	Significant CNS depression.
Azathioprine	Bone marrow suppression.
Benzocaine	Methemoglobinemia. Laryngeal edema.
Cisplatin	Fatal, acute pulmonary edema.

continued

continued

Phenytoin	Sedation. Ataxia. Anorexia. Dermal atrophy.
Propylthiouracil	Lethargy. Weakness. Anorexia. Bleeding diathesis.
Scopolamine	Tendency to cause behavioral changes.
Sodium phosphate	Depression.
enemas	Ataxia. Vomiting. Bloody diarrhea.

Drugs which are therapeutically useful in cats but which may have different toxicity/activity profiles than in dogs

Aspirin	Hypernea. Hypersensitivity. Hyperthermia.
Chloramphenicol	Anemia.
Digoxin	Vomiting. Anorexia. Bradycardia. Arrhythmias.
Doxorubicin	Renal failure.
Enrofloxacin	Blindness.
Furosemide	Dehydration. Hypokalemia.
Griseofulvin	Leukopenia and thrombocytopenia. Non-reversible ataxia.
Ketoconazole	Dry hair coat. Weight loss.
Lignocaine	Myocardial and CNS depression.
Megestrol acetate	Mammary hypertrophy and neoplasia. Cystic endometritis. Diabetes mellitus.
Methimazole,	Anorexia.
carbimazole	Vomiting. Self-induced facial excoriation. Bleeding diathesis. Hepatopathy. Serious hematological side effects.

continued

continued

Metronidazole	Disorientation. Ataxia. Seizures. Blindness.
Opioids: morphine derivatives (excluding meperidine [pethidine], butorphanol and buprenorphine)	Inconsistent sedation. Increased risk of excitation.
Organophosphates	Acute toxicity – hypersalivation, vomiting, diarrhea, muscle tremors. Chronic or delayed toxicity – paresis or paralysis which may or may not be reversible.
Potassium bromide	Depression. Severe coughing.
Tetracyclines	Hepatic lipidosis. Increased ALT activity. Ptyalism. Anorexia.
Thiacetarsamide	Drug fever. Respiratory distress. Fulminant pulmonary edema.

INTRODUCTION

SPECIAL CONSIDERATIONS RELATED TO DRUG USE IN CATS

Why are cats different?

There are some important differences in drug disposition between dogs and cats that can have a profound influence on dosing recommendations for cats.

The majority of the difference in drug disposition between cats and dogs **relates to differences in drug metabolism.**

DRUG METABOLISM – GENERAL

Water-soluble drugs can be **excreted in urine** without being metabolized.

Drugs that are **lipid soluble** must be **converted to water-soluble metabolites** that can be excreted, usually by the kidney.

Drug metabolism occurs in the liver in two phases (I and II).

Most differences between dogs and cats in drug disposition relate to **differences in Phase II metabolism**, although deficiencies in Phase I metabolism may be involved in some drug toxicities in cats including chloramphenicol toxicity.

During Phase II metabolism, parent drugs or Phase I metabolites are bound (conjugated) to large molecules such as **glucuronide, glutathione, sulfate and acetyl groups, and amino acids** (e.g. glycine and taurine) resulting in a water-soluble, inactive compound.

FELINE DRUG METABOLISM

Cats are **deficient in some glucuronyl transferases** which are important for glucuronidation.

- Drugs that are excreted as glucuronide conjugates in other species such as aspirin, benzoic acid, acetaminophen (paracetamol) and hexachlorophene may have a **prolonged half-life in cats**.
- Increased half-life **increases the risk of toxicity** due to drug accumulation.

Not all drugs that are glucuronidated are a problem in cats. **Cats are only deficient in certain families of glucuronyl transferases.**

- The drug may have a wide safety margin and drugs may be metabolized by a different route in cats (although this can result in toxicity for some drugs).
- For example, **sulfation is well developed in cats** compared to dogs and **acetylation**, which is deficient in dogs, appears to be **well developed in cats**.

FELINE HEMOGLOBIN AND DRUGS

Feline hemoglobin is more susceptible to oxidation, and therefore methemoglobinemia formation, than in dogs. This increases the risk of adverse drug reactions.

There are a number of possible mechanisms including the different structure of feline hemoglobin, lower concentrations or activities of intracellular repair enzyme and differences in intracellular concentrations of glutathione-conjugating enzymes.

OTHER PHYSIOLOGIC FACTORS THAT INFLUENCE DRUG DISPOSITION

Other physiologic factors that may influence drug disposition are similar in dogs and cats.

Age-related differences should always be considered. **Pediatric and geriatric animals** are potentially more susceptible to adverse drug effects due to:
- **Alterations in drug distribution**.
  - Greater volume of distribution in pediatric animals.
  - Reduced lean body mass and total body water in geriatric animals.
  - Lower plasma protein in young and old animals.
- **Drug metabolism**.
  - Reduced hepatic metabolism in neonates.
  - Reduced hepatic blood flow and reduced hepatocyte mass and function in geriatric animals.
- **Drug elimination**.
  - Glomerular and tubular function are reduced in neonates and old animals.

Drug interactions and disease factors that influence drug disposition such as **hepatic, cardiac and renal pathology** have a similar importance in cats and dogs.

The effect of **inappetence in diseased cats is important** as dietary protein is an important source of sulfate and other compounds used in Phase II drug metabolism in cats. Taurine may also be important. Anorexic cats therefore may be more susceptible to adverse drug reactions because of reduced drug metabolism.

DRUGS NOT RECOMMENDED FOR USE IN CATS

ACETAMINOPHEN (PARACETAMOL)

Clinical action
Non-steroidal analgesic.

Why shouldn't it be used in cats?
Glucuronidation is the major pathway for metabolism of acetominophen in most species, but **cats have a low concentration of glucuronyl transferase**.

Sulfation is the major metabolic pathway in the cat, but its capacity is limited.

As the dose is increased, a greater percentage of the drug is oxidized, which results in toxic metabolites.

The metabolites are normally conjugated with glutathione, but **when hepatic glutathione is depleted**, the metabolite binds covalently to amino acid residues of protein in the liver **resulting in centrilobular hepatic necrosis**.

Glutathione is easily depleted in cats as the reserves are limited.

APOMORPHINE

Clinical action
Anti-emetic.

Why shouldn't it be used in cats?
Higher doses are required for anti-emetic action than in dogs.

Significant CNS depression is associated with its use.

AZATHIOPRINE

Clinical action
Cytotoxic.

Why shouldn't it be used in cats?
Although azathoprine has been used successfully to treat immune-mediated disease in cats, serious **bone marrow suppression** has been reported in cats treated

with doses used in dogs (2.2 mg/kg and 1.1 mg/kg on alternate days).

In addition to dose-related marrow toxicity, idiosyncratic severe, irreversible, fatal leukopenia and thrombocytopenia has also been reported in cats.

They may lack thiopurine methyl transferase (TPMT), the enzyme necessary to degrade the 6-mercaptopurine active metabolite of azathioprine although this is not proven.

The recommended dose in cats (0.3 mg/kg) and the single size tablet of 25 mg means that reformulation is necessary as clients must not split the coating of cytotoxic drugs.

Chlorambucil is a better alternative in cats.

BENZOCAINE

Clinical action

Topical local anesthetic.

Why shouldn't it be used in cats?

Topical application can cause **methemoglobinemia**, laryngeal application can cause **laryngeal edema.**

CISPLATIN

Clinical action

Cytotoxic.

Why shouldn't it be used in cats?

Cisplatin causes **fatal, acute pulmonary edema** in cats and should not be used in this species.

PHENYTOIN

Clinical action

Anti-convulsant.

Why shouldn't it be used in cats?

Prolonged half life (>40 hours) compared to dogs resulting in rapid accumulation and development of adverse signs such as sedation, ataxia and anorexia.

Dermal atrophy has also been reported in a cat treated with phenytoin.

PROPYLTHIOURACIL

Clinical action

Anti-thyroid.

Why shouldn't it be used in cats?

Adverse effects from PTU include lethargy, weakness, anorexia and bleeding diathesis due to induction of immune-mediated disease.

Nine of 105 cats developed serious side effects in a study of cats with hyperthyroidism.

Methimazole or carbimazole are the preferred drugs of choice for treating feline hyperthyroidism.

SCOPOLAMINE

Clinical action

Anti-emetic.

Why shouldn't it be used in cats?

Short half life.

Tendency to cause **behavioral changes.**

SODIUM PHOSPHATE

Clinical action

Retention enemas.

Why shouldn't it be used in cats?

Active ingredients can be rapidly absorbed through the rectal mucosa resulting in potentially **fatal hyperphosphatemia**, hypocalcemia, hypernatremia, hyperosmolality and metabolic acidosis.

Clinical signs observed include **depression, ataxia, vomiting and bloody diarrhea**.

Dehydrated or debilitated cats are particularly susceptible.

DRUGS WHICH ARE THERAPEUTICALLY USEFUL IN CATS BUT WHICH MAY HAVE DIFFERENT TOXICITY/ACTIVITY PROFILES THAN IN DOGS

ASPIRIN

Clinical action

Non-steroidal anti-inflammatory.

Adverse effects

The **half life of aspirin** in the cat is approximately four times longer (**38 hours** vs 9 hours) than in dogs because clearance depends on glucuronidation.

The dose should be reduced and the dosing interval extended when using aspirin in cats.

Clinical signs of toxicity include **hypernea, hypersensitivity and hyperthermia**.

Recommended dose

10–20 mg/kg q 48–72 h.

CHLORAMPHENICOL

Clinical action

Anti-microbial.

Adverse effects

Reversible non-regenerative anemia can occur in both dogs and cats.

Cats may be more susceptible, but the increased incidence is probably related to overdosing of cats by using the dog-dosing schedule, which is approximately five times higher per kg than what is recommended here. Note, many texts still recommend higher doses than 50 mg/cat bid.

Recommended dose

50 mg/cat bid.

DIGOXIN

Clinical action

Positive ionotropic, negative chronotropic.

Adverse effects

Cats are **more sensitive to digitalis-induced toxicosis** than dogs and the dosage should be reduced compared to dogs and further reduced if given concurrently with aspirin and furosemide.

The elixir form is not as well tolerated as the tablet form.

Dose

Cat 2–3 kg	0.0312 mg q 48 h.
Cat 4–5 kg	0.0312 mg q 24–48 h.
Cat > 6 kg	0.0312 mg q 12 h.

DOXORUBICIN

Clinical action

Cytotoxic.

Adverse effects

Doxorubicin when used at the "dog dose" of 30 mg/m^2 has been associated with induction of **renal failure in cats**. Therefore, it is used at a lower dose in cats.

Recommended dose

25 mg/m^2.

ENROFLOXACIN

Clinical action

Fluoroquinolone anti-microbial agent.

Adverse effects

An apparent species-specific toxicity is acute retinal degeneration recently reported in cats.

Blindness often results, but some cats may regain vision.

In a recent study of affected cats, the daily and total doses of enrofloxacin administered and the duration of treatment were highly variable.

Recommended dose
5 mg/kg sid.

FUROSEMIDE

Clinical action
Diuretic.

Adverse effects
Cats appear to be **more sensitive** to the effects of furosemide than dogs.

Dose
1–2 mg/kg bid.

GRISPEOFULVIN

Clinical action
Anti-fungal.

Adverse effects
Bone marrow hypoplasia manifested as leukopenia and thrombocytopenia. This is believed to be an idiosyncratic reaction. Cats with FIV infection appear to be at an increased risk.

Non-reversible ataxia has also been reported in a kitten treated with the drug.

Recommended dose
50 mg/kg/day PO (may be given in divided doses and should be administered with a fatty meal to enhance absorption).

KETOCONAZOLE

Clinical action
Anti-fungal.

Adverse effects
In contrast to dogs, ketoconazole does not alter production of steroid hormones such as cortisol, testosterone and progesterone. Adverse effects appear to be minimal, and limited to **dry hair coat and weight loss**.

Recommended dose
5–10 mg/kg q 8–12 h PO.

LIGNOCAINE

Clinical action
Anti-arrhythmic.

Adverse effects
Toxicosis results in **myocardial depression** and **CNS signs** including drowsiness, depression, ataxia and muscle tremors, and occurs more commonly in cats.

Dose
0.25–0.75 mg/kg IV slowly.

MEGESTROL ACETATE

Clinical action
Synthetic progestagen used for reproductive, behavioral and dermatologic disorders.

Adverse effects
The most serious side effects associated with megestrol acetate include **mammary hypertrophy and neoplasia, cystic endometritis and diabetes mellitus**.

The mechanism for diabetes mellitus appears to be different than in the dog (where it relates to increased growth hormone production).

Megestrol-induced diabetes in the cat may be transient or permanent. Megestrol acetate also causes adrenal suppression in the cat.

Recommended dose
Megestrol acetate is not recommended for the treatment of behavioral or dermatologic disorders due to the risk of serious side effects.

Control of estrus can be achieved by using 5 mg/cat for 3 days then 2.5–5 mg once/week for 10 weeks.

METHIMAZOLE, CARBIMAZOLE

Clinical action
Anti-thyroid.

Adverse effects
Side effects observed in about 18% of cats treated with methimazole (or its metabolite, carbimazole) include **anorexia, vomiting, self-induced facial excoriation, bleeding diathesis and hepatopathy.**

About 4% will develop serious hematological side effects.

Although about 20% develop autoantibodies, this does not appear to be associated with clinical immune-mediated disease.

Recommended dose
5 mg/cat q 8–12 h induction then 2.5–5 mg/cat q 8–12 h for maintenance.

METRONIDAZOLE

Clinical action
Antibiotic.

Adverse effects
Reversible CNS toxicity has been reported in cats resulting in disorientation, ataxia, seizures and blindness.

Dose
10–25 mg/kg q 24 h or 10–25 mg/kg q 12 h (for Giardia).

OPIOIDS

Some morphine derivatives (excluding meperidine [pethidine], butorphanol and buprenorphine).

Clinical action
Analgesia.

Adverse effects
Inconsistent sedation.

Increased risk of excitation.

This may reflect differences in the type or concentration of opioid receptors in cats or a relative overdosage.

Dose

Meperidine	3–5 mg/kg IM, IV.
Morphine	0.1 mg/kg SC, IM.
Butorphanol	0.4 mg/kg q 6 h SC or 0.2 mg/kg q 6 h IV.
Buprenorphine	0.01 mg/kg SC, IM q 8–12 h.

ORGANOPHOSPHATES

Clinical action
Insecticide.

Adverse effects
Cats are more sensitive to the effects of organophosphates than dogs although the mechanism for this is unknown.

It is not related to different hepatic metabolizing capacity as organophosphates are metabolized by cholinesterases located at nerve endings.

Toxicity may be acute (similar signs to dogs) or chronic or delayed.

Chronic or delayed toxicity manifests as **paresis or paralysis** which may or may not be reversible.

Toxic epidermal necrolysis has been reported in cats treated topically with organophosphate based flea rinses.

A survey of the effects of flea collars in cats revealed a high number of adverse reactions ranging from **dermatitis to death**.

POTASSIUM BROMIDE

Clinical action
Anti-convulsant.

Adverse effects

There appears to be a greater prevalence of adverse effects in cats compared to dogs (50%) in one study.

Coughing of sufficient severity to lead to euthanasia or discontinuation of medication has been reported.

Dose

30 mg/kg/day.

TETRACYCLINES

Clinical action

Antibiotic.

Adverse effects

Hepatic lipidosis, increased ALT activity, ptyalism and anorexia have been reported in a cat treated with tetracycline.

It has been speculated that cats may be more susceptible to tetracycline-induced **hepatotoxicosis** than other species due to their unique protein metabolism and requirements.

THIACETARSAMIDE

Clinical action

Adulticide (dirofilariasis).

Adverse effects

Cats appear to be relatively susceptible to the acute toxic effects of thiacetarsamide.

Drug fever and respiratory distress may develop.

In one study 25% of cats treated died from fulminant pulmonary edema.

Recommended dose

2.2 mg/kg q 12 h for 2 days.

RECOMMENDED READING

Boothe DM. Drug therapy in cats: mechanisms and avoidance of adverse drug reactions. J Am Vet Med Assoc 1990; 196: 1297–1305.
Boothe DM. Drug therapy in cats: a systems approach. J Am Vet Med Assoc 1990; 196: 1502–1511.
Boothe DM. Drug therapy in cats: a therapeutic category approach. J Am Vet Med Assoc 1990; 196: 1659–1669.
Boothe DM. Drug therapy in cats: recommended dosing regimens. J Am Vet Med Assoc 1990; 196: 1845–1850.
Boothe DM, George KL, Couch P. Disposition and clinical use of bromide in cats. J Am Vet Med Assoc 2002; 221: 1131–1135.
Plumb DC. Veterinary Drug Handbook, 3rd edn. Iowa State University Press, 1999.

68. Drug therapy in cats

A comprehensive list of recommended dosing regimens

Dawn Merton Boothe

The following index represents a compilation of doses recommended for the treatment or prevention of diseases in the cat. The information has been retrieved from multiple sources, including but not limited to: *Boothe's Formulary*, published by the American Animal Hospital Association (2nd printing 1997); *Kirk's Current Veterinary Therapy XIII* (John D. Bonagura (ed), published by WB Saunders Company, Philadelphia, USA), and the *Veterinary Drug Handbook* (Donald C Plumb, published by PharmaVet Publishing, White Bear Lake, MN).

Inclusion of a drug in the index should not be interpreted as an indication of safety of the drug. Most drugs are likely to be associated with adverse effects if used in excess. It is assumed that the reader is familiar with significant adverse effects, which may occur with drugs that are commonly used, regardless of the species. Many of the drugs tend to be uniquely associated with adverse effects in cats and the reader should refer to the text regarding the use of these drugs. Several drugs which have been effectively and safely used in the cat no doubt are missing from the table. Exclusion of a particular drug from the table may reflect a contraindication for the use of the drug in cats (e.g., acetaminophen). Also not addressed in the accompanying dosing index are drug interactions. Again, the reader is strongly encouraged to review the risks associated with drugs when administered simultaneously in a patient.

Of the drugs listed, 5% are approved for use in the cat in the United States. More specific information regarding the use of these drugs, or drugs approved for use in the dog but not the cat, may be obtained through *Veterinary Pharmaceuticals and Biologicals*, the Veterinarian's PDR, published by Veterinary Medicine Publishing Group, a subsidiary of Medical Economics Company, Inc, Oradell, New Jersey, USA. The remaining drugs are approved for use in humans; further information regarding these drugs can be obtained from the *Physician's Desk Reference* (PDR), published by Medical Economics. Comparable European resources are available for use.

The source of the dosing regimen recommended in the index varies with the drug. If an original source which referenced use of the drug in cats could not be found in the literature, the dose was obtained from either personal communication (noted as such), the manufacturer's drug packaging or from the above identified sources. In instances when recommended dosing regimens for a drug varied with the source, either a range or several doses were listed for the drug in the index. Doses which varied with the therapeutic intent of a drug were also listed as either a range or as separate subheadings for each intent. Dosing regimens for anticancer drugs have not been well established in the cat and vary with each author. Although a dosing regimen is offered for most anticancer drugs in the index, the reader is encouraged to refer to alternative and recent literature sources for more detailed discussion. For all drugs, an attempt should be made to titrate the drug to the individual animal's response. This approach is critical for avoiding adverse reactions to some drugs (e.g., insulin, dihydrotachysterol and others). Again, the reader is encouraged to review literature which addresses the use of these drugs more in depth.

Drug index

Drug	Indications	Dose	Route[a]	Frequency (h)[b]
Acarbose	Hyperglycemia (diabetes mellitus)	12.5–20 mg	PO	with each meal
Acemannan	Immunomodulation	2 mg, 1–2 mg/kg	intralesional, IP, or SC	weekly
Acepromazine	Restraint, sedation Arterial thromboembolism Amphetamine toxicosis	0.05–0.1 mg/kg, max 1 mg 0.05–2.25 mg/kg 0.15–0.3 mg/kg 0.05–1.00 mg/kg	IV IM, SC, IV, PO SC IV, IM, SC	8–12
Acetazolamide	Glaucoma	5–10 mg/kg	PO	8–12
Acetylcysteine	Acetaminophen toxicosis	140 mg/kg 70 mg/kg	IV PO	loading dose 4–6×5–7 treatments
Acetylsalicylic acid	Antipyretic Antithrombotic Anti-inflammatory Hypertrophic cardiomyopathy Analgesia	6–10 mg/kg 80 mg/cat or 25 mg/kg 10–20 mg/kg 162 mg/cat 10 mg/kg	PO PO PO PO PO	48–72 2 times/wk 48 2 times/wk 48
Activated charcoal	Gastrointestinal adsorbent	1 g/5 ml water: give 10 ml of slurry/kg 1–4 gm/kg (granules) 6–10 ml/kg (suspension)	PO	
Actinomycin–D	Anticancer	0.5–0.9 mg/m²	IV	
Acyclovir	Feline herpes	200 mg	PO	6
Albendazole	Lung worms	50 mg/kg	PO	24×21 days
Albuterol	Bronchodilation	20–50 (up to 100):μ/kg	PO	6–8
Allopurinol	Urate urolithiasis	10 mg/kg	PO	8–12 for 30 days then every 24 h
Aloe vera cream	Burns	thickness of 1/8–1/4 inch	topically	6× several days then 12–24
Alpha-Keri		1 capful to 1–2 quarts of water for final rinse or spray aerosol onto wet coat and rub well		

Drug	Indication	Dose	Route	Frequency
Alprazolam	Elimination behavioral problems	0.125–0.25 mg/cat	PO	12
Aluminum carbonate gel	Phosphate binder	10–30 mg/kg	PO w/meals	8
Aluminum hydroxide	Antacid / Phosphate binder	21–30 ml / 30–90 mg/kg	PO / PO w/meals	2–4 / 8–24
Aluminum magnesium hydroxide		2–10 ml	PO	2–4
Amantadine	Analgesia for chronic pain, e.g. DJD, used as combination therapy	3–5 mg/kg	PO	24 for 7–14 days
Amikacin	Susceptible infections	15–22 mg/kg	IM, SC, IV	24
Aminopentamide	Antidiarrheal	0.1 mg/cat	SC, IM, PO	8–12
Aminophylline	Bronchodilator	4–6.6 mg/kg / 2–5 mg/kg	PO / IV infusion	8–12 / 12
Aminopromazine	Smooth muscle relaxant	2.0–4.5 mg/kg	PO	12
6-aminosalicylic acid	Chronic inflammatory bowel disease see mesalamine, olsalazine			
Amitraz	Ear mites	Mix 1 ml amitraz in 10–20 ml mineral oil	apply topically	48 h for 3 wk
Amitryptyline	Behavior, urine spraying	2 mg/kg or 5–10 mg/cat	PO	24
Amlodipine besylate	Systemic hypertension	0.625 mg up to 1.25mg/cat	PO	24
Ammonium chloride	(Struvite dissolution)	800 mg/cat (approx 1/4tsp) or 1.5% of diet / 20 mg/kg	PO	24, mixed with food / 12
Amoxicillin	Susceptible infections	10 mg/kg	PO, SC, IV	8–12
	Cholangiohepatitis	20 mg/kg	PO, SC, IV, IM	6–12
	Cellulitis	22 mg/kg / 11.1 mg/kg	PO, SC / IM, SC	12 / 12
Amoxicillin/clavulinic acid	Resistant, serious infection	10–20 mg/kg / 62.5 mg/cat	PO / PO	8–12 / 12
Amfetamine SO₄	CNS stimulation during certain toxicoses, chlorpromazine toxicosis	5 mg/cat	PO	12
		5 mg	PO	24 × 4 days

Continued

Continued

Drug	Indications	Dose	Route[a]	Frequency (h)[b]
Amphotericin B	Systemic mycoses	0.25 mg/kg test dose 0.15–1 mg/kg in 5% dextrose	IV over 6–8 h	48 to a total cumulative dose of 10 mg/kg
	Leishmaniasis	0.5–0.8 mg/kg	IV	48 to cumulative dose of 8–16 mg/kg
		1–2.5 mg/kg	IV	48 × 4 weeks
liposomal	Leishmaniasis	3.0–3.3 mg/kg	IV	72–96 to cumulative dose of 15 mg/kg
	Mycoses	1–2.5 mg/kg	IV	48 for 4 weeks
lipid complex solution	Mycoses	0.5 mg/kg test dose then 1–2.5 mg/kg	IV	48 for 4 weeks to a cumulative dose of 12 mg
	Resistant filamentous fungi	2–2.5 mg/kg	IV	48 for a total cumulative dose
Ampicillin	Susceptible bacteria	20–60 mg/kg	PO	8–12
Ampicillin trihydrate	Susceptible bacteria	5.5–50 mg/kg	IM, SC	6–8
Ampicillin sodium salt		5.5–22 mg/kg	IV	6–8
Ampicillin–sulbactam	Susceptible bacteria	10–50 mg/kg	IV, IM	6–8
Amprolium	Coccidiosis	60–100 mg/kg	PO	24 × 5
		300–400 mg/kg on food	PO	24 × 5
		1.5 tsp/gallon or 3.8 liter water	PO	24 × 14
	with sulfadimethoxine (25 mg/kg)	150 mg/kg	PO	24 × 14
Antazoline 0.5%	Allergic conjunctivitis		Topically	24
Aprotinin	Protease inhibitor (pancreatitis)	5000 KUI (kallikrein inhibitor units)/kg	IV, IP (preferred)	6–8
Ascorbic acid	Feline infectious peritonitis	25–125 mg/kg/day	PO	24
	Acetaminophin toxicosis	30 mg/kg	PO, SC	6 × 7 treatments
		100 mg/cat	PO	24–8
Asparaginase	Lymphosarcoma	10,000 U/m²	IV	weekly as part of a protocol

Drug	Indication	Dose	Route	Interval/Notes
Aspirin	see acetylsalylic acid			
Atenolol	Hypertension	2 mg/kg or 6.25–12.5 mg/cat	PO	24
Atipamezole	Metadomidine reversal	volume equivalent to medetomidine volume	IV	As needed
Atovaquone	Antiprotozoal (pneumocystosis)	13.3 mg/kg with fatty meal	PO	8 × 21 days
Atracurium besylate	Paralytic agent	0.1–0.25 mg/kg	IV	initially, then
		0.15 mg/kg	IV	30 min later
Atropine	Sinus bradycardia	0.022–0.044 mg/kg	IM, SC, IV	PRN or
		0.04 mg/kg	PO	6–8
	Atropine response test	0.044 mg/kg	IV	Preanesthetic
	Hypersialism	0.02–0.045 mg/kg	SC, IM, IV	
		0.02 mg/kg	SC	PRN
	Cholinergic toxins	0.2–2 mg/kg	1/4 dose IV, the rest SC, IM	
Aurothioglucose	Pemphigus complex, plasmacytic stomatitis and podomatitis	2 mg	IM	then,
		1 mg/kg	IM	once weekly decreasing to once monthly
Azathioprine	Enteritis	0.2–0.3 mg/kg	PO	24–48
	Immune hemolytic anemia	1.0 mg/kg	PO	24–48
	Immune thrombocytopenia			
	Immunosuppression	1.1 mg/kg	PO	48
Azithromycin	Susceptible infection	5 mg/kg	PO	24–48
Aztreonam	Susceptible bacteria	12–25 mg/kg	IV, IM	8–12
BAL	Chelator	see dimercaprol		
Baquiloprim–sulfa methoxine or sulfadimidine	Coccidiosis	30 mg/kg	PO	48 × 2
	Susceptible infections	30 mg/kg	PO	24 × 2 then 48 × 10 to 21 days
Beclomethasone dipropionate	Anti-inflammatory	200 mg	Inhalant	PRN
Benazepril	Afterload reduction	0.25–0.5 mg/kg	PO	24

Continued

Continued

Drug	Indications	Dose	Route[a]	Frequency (h)[b]
Benzimidazole	Trypanosomiasis	5 mg/kg	PO	24 for 2 months
Benzocaine	Local anesthetic		Topical	
Benzoyl peroxide	Seborrheic, antibacterial	leave on skin for 10 min and rinse		every 3–4 days to once every 1–2 wk
Betamethasone	Antiinflammatory	0.1–0.2 mg/kg	PO	12–24
Bethanechol	Bladder atony, dysautonia	1.25–5.0 mg	PO	12–8
Bisacodyl	Stool softener	2–5 mg/cat 1–3 suppositories 1–2 ml enema	PO rectal rectal	24, PRN PRN PRN
Bismuth subcarbonate	GI tract protectant	0.3–3.0 gm	PO	4
Bismuth subsalicylate	Antidiarrheal, antiemetic	1–3 ml/kg	PO	divided every 4–6
Bleomycin	Chemotherapy	10 μ/m²	IV, SC	24 for 4 days, then weekly; max dose 200 mg/m²
Bran	Stool softener	1–2 TBS/400 g food	PO	PRN
Brewer's yeast	Source of B vitamins	0.2 μ/kg	PO	24–96
Bromide; Potassium or sodium	Anticonvulsant	30–60 mg/kg	PO	divided every 12 h; monitor to adjust dose
Bromocriptine mesylate	Hyperadrenocorticism, pseudo-pregnancy	10–30 μ/kg	PO	24 for 10–16 days
Bunamidine	Taenia, dipylidium	20–50 mg/kg	PO	
Bupivacaine hydrochloride		0.22–0.3 ml 5–10 μ/kg 2.5–15.0 mg	Epidural IM PO	after 3 h fast 12 12–8
Buprenorphine	Analgesia	0.005–0.01 mg/kg	IV, IM	4–8
Buspirone	Behavioral therapy	2.5–5 mg/cat	PO	12–24
Busulfan	Chronic myelocytic leukemia	3–4 mg/m² or 0.1 mg/kg	PO	24

Drug	Indication	Dose	Route	Interval
Butamisole	Hookworm, whipworms	2.2 mg/kg (0.22 ml/kg)	SC	repeat in 21 days
Butorphanol	Preanesthetic	0.05–0.4 mg/kg w/ acepromazine	IV, IM, SC	
	Antiemetic prior to cancer chemo.	0.2–0.6 mg/kg	SC, IM, IV	
	Analgesia	0.1–0.8 mg/kg	IM, SC, IV	6–12
		0.55–1.1 mg/kg	PO	6–12
Calcitriol	Hypoparathyroidism	2.5–3 mg/kg (0.0025–0.003(g/kg)	PO	24
Calcium carbonate	Nutritional supplement	1/2 tsp	with each meal	
	Phosphate binder	60–100 mg/kg		24
Calcium chloride 10%	Ventricular asystole	1 ml/9 kg or 0.1–0.3 ml/kg	IV (slowly)	
	Hypocalcemia	0.1–0.3 ml/kg	IV (slowly)	
Calcium citrate	Calcium replacement Urothiliasis	10–30 mg/kg	PO	8 (with meals)
Calcium EDTA	Lead poisoning	100 mg/kg/day = total dose make soution of 1 g Versenate/ 100 ml D₅W divide total quantity mls into 20 aliquots, 1 dose		5 days
			SC	6 for 5 days
Calcium gluconate 10%	Ventricular asystole	0.5–1.5 ml/kg	IV (slowly)	PRN
	Hypocalcemia, hyperkalemia	0.5–1.5 ml/kg	IV in 5% D/W over 20–30 min	6–8 intervals
		10–15 ml	IV infusion	24
		50–150 mg/kg		
		150–250 mg/kg	PO (tab)	8–12
		0.2–0.5 g	PO	
Calcium lactate	Calcium replacement	0.2–0.5 g/cat	PO	24
Captan powder 50%	Dermatomycoses	2 tbsp/gal water	topically, do not rinse	2–3 times/wk
Captopril	Vasodilator	2–3 mg/cat	PO	8–12
		3–6.25 mg/cat	PO	12
Carbenicillin	Susceptible bacterial infection	15–30mg/kg	IV	8

Continued

Continued

Drug	Indications	Dose	Route[a]	Frequency (h)[b]
Carbenicillin indanyl sodium	Urinary tract infection	15–110 mg/kg	IV, IM, SC	6–8
		10–55 mg/kg	PO	8
Carbimazole	Hyperthyroidism	5 mg/cat	PO	8–12
Carboplatin	Anticancer	200 mg/m²	IV	4 weeks
Carmustine	Anticancer chemotherapy	50 mg/m²	IV	6 weeks
Carprofen	Analgesic, perioperative	1–4 mg/kg	SC	once
		0.5–1 mg/kg	PO	24
Cascara sagrada	Laxative	0.5–1.5 ml/cat	PO	24
Cefaclor	Susceptible bacterial infection	4–20 mg/kg	PO	8 in fasted animal
Cefadroxil	Susceptible bacterial infection	22 mg/kg	PO	24
Cefamandole	Susceptible bacterial infection	6–40 mg/kg	IM, IV	6–8
Cefazolin sodium	Susceptible infections	20–35 mg/kg	IV, IM, SC	6–8
	Surgical prophylaxis	22 mg/kg	IV	1 to 2 during sugery
Cefepime	Susceptible infections	50 mg/kg	IV, IM	8
Cefixime	Susceptible infections	5–12.5 mg/kg	PO	12–24
Cefmetazole	Susceptible infections,	20 mg/kg	IV	6–12
	Surgical prophylaxis	20 mg/kg	IV	Single treatment
Cefoperazone	Susceptible infections	22 mg/kg	IV, IM	6–12
Cefotoaxime	Susceptible infections	20–80 mg/kg	IM, IV	8
Cefotetan	Susceptible bacterial infections	30 mg/kg	IV,SC	8
Cefoxicin	Susceptible bacterial infections	11–30 mg/kg	IM, IV	8
Cefpodoxime	Susceptible bacterial infections	5–10 mg/kg	PO	12–24
Ceftazidime	Suscpetible bacterial infections	15–30 mg/kg	IV, IM, SC	6–12
Ceftiofur	Susceptible urinary tractinfections	2.2–4.4 mg/kg	SC	12–24

Drug	Indication	Dose	Route	Interval
Ceftizoxime	Susceptible bacterial Infections	25–50 mg/kg	IV, IM	8–12
Ceftriaxone	Susceptible bacterial infections	15–50 mg/kg	IM, IV	12
	Surgical prophylaxis	25 mg/kg	IM, IV	Single treatment
Cefuroxime	Susceptible bacterial infections	10–30 mg/kg	PO, IV	8–12 with food
Cephalexin	Susceptible bacterial infections	10–35 mg/kg	PO	8–12
Cephaloridine	Susceptible infection	10 mg/kg	IM, SC	8–12
Cephalothin	Susceptible bacterial infection	10–44 mg/kg	IV, IM, SC	4–8
Cephamandole	Susceptible bacterial infection	6–40 mg/kg	IM, IV	6–8
Cephapirin	Susceptible bacterial infection	10–30 mg/kg	IM, IV, SC	4–8
Cephradine	Susceptible bacterial infection	10–40 mg/kg	PO, IV, IM	6–8
Cetacaine	Topical anesthetic	Use cautiously	Topical	May cause methemoglobinemia
Charcoal, activated	Adsorbent during poisonings	1–8 g/kg as slurry (1 gm: 5 ml water) 6–12 ml/kg (suspension)	PO	PRN
Chlorambucil	Anticancer	0.1–0.5 mg/kg	PO	48–72
		2–6 mg m^2	PO	14–21 days
		0.1 mg/kg	PO	24 w/prednisone once every 48 h w/prednisone
	Immune-mediated skin disease	0.1–0.2 mg/kg	PO	
Chloramphenicol	Susceptible bacterial infections	50 mg/cat	PO	12
Chloramphenicol succinate	Susceptible bacterial infections	12.5–20 mg/cat	IV, IM	12
Chlordiazepoxide–clidinium	Irritable colon syndrome	1–2 tab	PO	12
Chlorhexidine 0.5%	Burns	dilute 1:40 with saline and apply after cleansing area saturate wet dressing		PRN 12–24
Chlorothiazide	Diuretic	10–40 mg/kg	PO	12
	Partial ADH deficiency	20–40 mg/kg	PO	12
Chlorpheniramine	Antihistamine	1–2 mg/cat	PO	8–12
	Excessive grooming, self-trauma	2–4 mg/cat	PO	12–24
	Antiemetic	0.5 mg/kg	IM, IV	6–8
		0.5 mg/kg	IV, IM	6–8

Continued

Continued

Drug	Indications	Dose	Route[a]	Frequency (h)[b]
Chlortetracycline hydrochloride	Prior to cancer chemotherapy	2 mg/kg	SC	1 prior to therapy
	Susceptible infection	25 mg/kg	PO	6–8
Cholecalciferol (vitamin D)	Hypocalcemia	500–2,000 U/kg	PO	24
Cimetidine	Esophagitis, gastric ulceration, antiemetic, chronic gastritis, GI tract ulceration	5–15 mg/kg	PO, IV, IM	8–12
	Gastrinemia	5–15 mg/kg	PO, IV, SC	6
	Immunomodulator	10–25 mg/kg	IV, PO, IM	12
Ciprofloxacin	Not bioavailable in cats			
Clarithromycin	Atypical mycobacterial	62.5 mg/cat	PO	12
Clindamycin	Anaerobic infections	5–11 mg/kg	PO	12
		22 mg/kg	PO	24
	Stomatitis, acute pancreatitis	5–10 mg/kg	IV, IM	8
	Pancreatic exocrine insufficiency	5–10 mg/kg	PO	6–8 30 min before meals
	Enteroepithelial cycle	12.5–50 mg/kg	PO, IM	12
	Extraintestinal cycle toxoplasmosis	12.5–25 mg/kg	PO, IM	12 for 2 wk
Clofazimine	Feline leprosy	1 (up to 4–8) mg/kg	PO	24 for 6wks
		25–50 mg/cat	PO	24
		50 mg/cat	PO	48
Clomipramine	Behavior modification	1–5 mg/cat	PO	12–24
Clonazepam	Anticonvulsant, behavior therapy	0.5 mg/kg	PO	8–12
Clorazepate dipotassium	Anxiolytic drug	1–2 mg/kg	PO	8–12
Clotrimazole	Dermatophytosis	apply to lesions	topical	2×12 h $\times$ wk
	Antifungal	60 ml of 1 g/dl of polyethylene glycol intranasal		over 1 h (under general anesthesia) repeat in 3–4 wks as needed

Drug	Indication	Dose	Route	Interval (h)
Cloxacillin	Susceptible infections	20–40 mg/kg	PO, IM, IV	4–8
Coal tar shampoos	Seborrhea	keep in contact w/skin for 10 min		24
Cobalamin	see Vitamin B$_{12}$			
Cod liver oil		1tsp/10kg	PO	24
Codeine	Pain	0.5–4 mg/kg	PO	6–12
		60 mg with 300 mg acetaminophen	PO	8–12
	Antitussive, analgesia	0.1–0.3 mg/kg	PO	4–6
Colchicine	Antifibrotic	0.01–0.3 mg/kg	PO	4–6
Colony-stimulating factor	Neutropenia	2.5–5 mg/kg	SC	24
Corticotropin gel (ACTH)	Response test	preACTH sample 0.5–2.2 IU/kg	IM	
Cortisone acetate	Hypoadrenocorticism	1 mg/kg	PO, IM	24
Cosequin®	Osteoarthritis, joint damage	1 capsule RS	PO	24
Cosyntropin	preACTH sample	0.125 mg/cat	IV	12 for 2 treatments
		1–2 mg/kg	PO(w/caution)	
Cromolyn sodium 4%	Allergic conjunctivitis		topically	4–6
Cyanocobalamine	Vitamin B$_{12}$ deficiency	50–100 μ	PO, IM, SC	24
Cyclizine	Antiemetic	4 mg/kg	IM	8
Cyclophosphamide	Anticancer	100 mg/m2	IV	
	Feline mammary cancer	100 mg/m2	PO	every 3 wks w/ doxorubicin
	Immune hemolytic anemia	2 mg/kg, 50 mg/m^2	PO	24 for 4 days/wk
	Lymphosarcoma, myeloproliferative disorders	50 mg/m^2	PO	48
	Autoimmune skin diseases, SLE	50 mg/m^2	PO	24 h 4 days/wk or every 48 h
	Multiple myeloma	7 mg/kg	PO	once
	Feline infectious peritonitis	2–4 mg/kg	PO	24 h 4 days/wk
	Eosinophilic enteritis	6.6 mg/kg	PO	3 days,then
		2.2 mg/kg	PO	24
	Immunosuppressive therapy	2.2 mg/kg	PO	48, or 24 h 4 days/wk

Continued

Continued

Drug	Indications	Dose	Route[a]	Frequency (h)[b]
	Anticancer and immunosuppressive therapy	6.25–12.5 mg/cat	PO	24 h 4 days/wk
Cyclosporine	Immune thrombocytopenia, SLE, sebaceous adenitis	4–6 mg/kg	4 hour IV infusion	24 (avoid extravasation)
		3–7 mg/kg	PO	12 (adjust dose based on monitoring)
		10 mg/kg	PO	12
Cyclosporine ophthalmic	Keratoconjunctivitis sicca, pigmentary keratitis plasmoma of third eyelid	1–2% solution	drop in eye	12
Cyclothiazide	Diuretic	0.5–1 mg/kg	PO	24
Cyproheptidine	Appetite stimulant	2–4 mg/cat	PO	12–24
Cytarabine	Anticancer	30–50 mg/kg	IV, IM, SC	once a wk
		100 mg/m²	IV, IM, SC	24h for 4 days then
		20 mg/m²	Intrathecal	24 for 1–5 days
Cythioate	Tick prevention	1.5–3.3 mg/kg	PO	72 or 2x wk
		0.22 ml/kg	liquid (15 mg/ml)	72 or 2 wk
Dacarbazine	Lymphoreticular neoplasms	200–250 mg/m²	IV	24 for 5 days, every 21 days
	Soft tissue sarcomas	1000 mg/m²	IV drip	over 6–8 h, every 21 days
Dactinomycin	Anticancer	0.015 mg/kg	IV	24 for 3–5 days: wait 3 wks
		0.7–1.5 mg/m²	IV	weekly
Dalteparin (LMW heparin)	DIC, thrombosis	70 IU/kg	SC	24
Danazolol	Immune-mediated disorders	5–10 mg/kg	PO	12
Dapsone	Mycobacteriosis	1.1 mg/kg	PO	12 for 4–6 wks
	Brown recluse spider bite	0.7–1 mg/kg	PO	8
Deferoxamine mesylate	Iron chelator	10 mg/kg	IV, IM, SC	2 h for 2 doses then, 8 h for day

Drug	Indication	Dose	Route	Frequency/Notes
	Repertusion injuries	10 mg/kg; 50 mg/kg	IV, IM; IV	over 5 min
Demeclocycline	Innappropriate ADH secretion	3–12 mg/kg	PO	6–12
Deprenyl	Hyperadrenocorticism, Cognitive dysfunction	see selegiline		
Derm caps	Skin disorders	1 capsule per 9 kg	PO	24
Derm caps (liquid)	Skin disorders	to 4.5 kg give 0.35 ml		
Desmopressin acetate	Central diabetes insipidus	0.3 : µ/kg (diluted in 50 ml saline)	IN, conjunctival	infused over 15–30 min; repeat as needed
		2–4 drops	conjunctivally	12–24
		0.1 mg	PO	12–24
		1–2 drops	IN, conjunctival	12–24
Desoxycorticosterone acetate	Hypoadrenocorticism	0.2–0.4 mg/kg	conjunctivally	24, max 5 mg
Desoxycorticosterone pivalate	Hypoadrenocorticism	25 mg	IM = 1mg/day	DOCA released for 25 days
Dexamethasone	Cerebral edema, spinal cord trauma, fibrocartilaginous disk disease, other CNS trauma	2 mg/kg	IV	then,
	Hydrocephalus	1 mg/kg	IV, SC	8–12, then
		0.1 mg/kg	IV, SC, PO	8–12
		0.25 mg/kg	IV, PO, IM	6–8
	Shock, anaphylaxis	4–6 mg/kg	IV(slowly)	
	Immune-mediated disease	0.25–1.25 mg/kg	PO	12–24
		0.10–0.15 mg/kg	SC, PO	12 for 5–7 days, then taper dose with mineralocorticoids
	Adrenocortico collapse	0.1–0.5 mg/kg	SC, IV	then
		1 mg/kg	IV	8–24
	Feline bronchial asthma	0.25–1.0 mg/cat	PO	
Dexrazoxane	Iron chelation for doxorubicin Induced cardiotoxicity	25 mg/kg (ratio of 10–20:1 Dexrazoxane: doxorubicin)	IV	15 minutes before doxirubicin

Continued

Continued

Drug	Indications	Dose	Route[a]	Frequency (h)[b]
Dextran 40	Shock	10–20 ml/kg	IV	24
Dextran-70	Frostbite	20–40 ml/kg	IV	24 in 5% D/W
	Volume expander	10–20 ml/kg	IV	24 to effect
Dextroamfetamine	Narcolepsy	5–10 mg	PO	8 w/imipramine
	Hyperkinesis	0.2–1.3 mg/kg	PO	as needed
Dextromethorphan	Cough	0.5–2 mg/kg	PO, SC, IV	6–8
Dextrose, 50%	Hypoglycemia, insulin overdosage	2 ml/kg	PO	
		0.25–1.00 ml/kg	IV	
Dextrose, 5%	Hypoglycemia, insulin overdosage	40–50 ml/kg	IV, SC, IP	as needed
Diazepam	Sedation	0.5–2.2 mg/kg	PO	as needed
	Seizures	0.15–0.70 mg/kg or	PO	8
		2–5 mg/cat	PO, IV	8
		1–2 mg/kg	Rectal	as needed
	Status epilepticus, certain toxicoses	0.5–1.0 mg/kg	IV	in increments of 5–20 mg
	Strychnine induced seizures	2–5 mg/kg	IV	as needed
		0.5 mg/kg	IV	
	Reflex dyssynergia (urethral obstruction)	2.5–5.0 mg/cat	PO	6–8
		0.5 mg/kg	IV	
	Urinary disorder in cat	1.25–2.5 mg/cat	PO	8–12
	Appetite stimulant	0.05–0.4 mg/kg	IV, PO, IM	24 or 48
		1 mg/cat	PO	24
	Psychogenic alopecia	1–2 mg	PO	12
		1 mg/kg	PO	8–12
Dichlorphenamide	Glaucoma	3–5 mg/kg	PO	8–12
Dichlorvos	Hook-, whip-, roundworms	11–22 mg/kg	PO	repeat in 3wks
Dicloxacillin	Susceptible infections	10–50 mg/kg	PO	6–8
		50 mg/kg	PO	6–8

Drug	Indication	Dose	Route	Interval
Dicoumarol	Anticoagulant	5 mg/kg	PO	load, then
		1.3–2.6 mg/kg	PO	sid (monitor response)
Dicyclomine	Detrusor hyperspasticity or urge incontinence	10 mg/cat	PO	6–8
Diethylcarbamazine	Heartworm prophylaxis	6.6 mg/kg	PO	24
Diethylstilbestrol	Feline symmetrical alopecia	0.05–0.1 mg/cat	PO	24
Difloxacin	Susceptible bacterial infection	5–10 mg/kg	PO	24
Digoxin	Congestive heart failure	0.005–0.008 mg/kg/day	PO(tablet)	div 12
		0.18 mg/m²	PO(elixir)	12
		0.003–0.004 mg/kg	PO (Cardoxin)	48
		2–3 kg cat: 0.0312 mg	PO (Cardoxin)	24–48
		4–5 kg cat: 0.0312 mg	PO (Cardoxin)	12
		>6 kg cat: 0.0312 mg		
Dihydrostreptomycin	Susceptible infection	10–30 mg/kg	IM, SC	12–24
Dihydrotachysterol	Hypocalcemia	0.03–0.06 mg/kg	PO	24 for 3 then
		0.02–0.03 mg/kg	PO	24 for 3 then
		0.01–0.02 mg/kg	PO	24 (monitor calcium)
Diltiazem	Hypertension, hypertrophic cardiomyopathy, supraventricular tachyarrhythmias	0.125–0.35 mg/kg	IV	
		0.5–1.5 mg/kg	PO	8
		1.75–2.5 mg/kg	PO	8
Diltiazem XR, cardiazem CD	babesiosis, trypanosomiasis	½ of 60 mg or 10 mg/kg (C)	PO	24
Dimenhydrinate	Antihistamine	12.5 mg/cat	PO, IM, IV	
Dimercaprol (BAL)	Arsenic toxicosis	2.5–5.0 mg/kg	IM	4 for 2 days Rx then 8 for 3 then 12 for 10 days
Dimethylsulfoxide	Spinal cord trauma	0.5–1 g/kg	IV (10%)	6–8 over 45 min
Diminazine aceturate	Babesiosis, trypanosomiasis	2.0–3.5 mg/kg	IM	Once

Continued

Continued

Drug	Indications	Dose	Route[a]	Frequency (h)[b]
Diminazene aceturate	Babesiosis trypanosomiasis cytauxzoonosis	3.5 mg/kg	SC, IM	24×2 days
Dinoprost	see prostaglandin F2a			
Diphenhydramine	Antihistamine	2–4 mg/kg	PO	6–8
	Mast cell disease, anti-emetic	2 mg/kg	IM, IV	slowly 12 prn
	Anaphylaxis, urticaria angioneurotic edema	2 mg/kg	IM, IV	slowly 12 prn
		1 mg/kg	IM, IV	8
Diphenoxylate HCL	Acute colitis,	0.05–0.1 mg/kg 0.6–1.2 mg/cat	PO PO	12 8–12
Diphenylthiocarbazone	Thallium toxicosis	50–70 mg/kg	PO	8
Diphemanil methylsulfate	Anticholinergic (bronchodilator)	1.8 mg/kg	IM	12
Dipyridamole	Antithrombotic	4–10 mg/kg 25 mg/kg	PO	24 8 (low dose); 12–24 (high dose)
Disodium EDTA	Calcium keratopathy	0.37% soln.		lavage cornea for 15–20 min
Dithiazanine iodide	Microfilaricide	1% soln. 1–2 drops	topically	12 for several wk
DL Methionine	See methionine	6.6–11 mg/kg	PO	24 for 7–10 days
Dobutamine	Positive inotrope	0.5–2 μ/kg/min	IV infusion (caution)	1 min
Docusate calcium or sodium	Stool softener Disposable enema	50 mg/cat 250 mg/12 ml glycerin	PO Rectal	12–24 1 (repeat)
Dolansetron	Antiemetic	0.6 mg/kg	PO, IV, SC	24
Dopamine HCl	Inotropic agent	2–25 μ/kg (up to 50 μ/kg if severe hypotension or shock)	IV infusion	1 min
	Renal vasodilator: Acute renal failure Acute heart failure	2–5 μ/kg (low dose) 2–10 μ/kg	IV infusion in 5% D/W IV infusion 40 mg in 500 ml	1 min 1 min

Drug	Indication	Dose	Route	Interval (hours)
Doxapram	Respiratory stimulant	1–5 mg/kg	IV	as needed
	Neonate	1–2 drops (1–5 mg)	Sublingual	
		0.1 ml or 10 mg/m²	IV (umblilical vein)	
Doxorubicin	Antineoplastic	30 mg/m² or 10 mg/m²	IV	21 days or 7 days
		20–30 mg/m²	IV	21–28 days
Doxycyline HCL	Susceptible bacterial infection	5–10 mg/kg	PO, IV	12–24
Doxylamine succinate	Antihistamine	1.1–2.2 mg/kg	PO, SC, IM	8–12
Edetate calcium disodium	Lead poisoning	25 mg/kg of 1% solution (2 g max)	SC	6 for 5 days
Edrophonium	myasthenia gravis diagnosis	2.5 mg/cat	IV	
Emetine	vomiting	3.3 ml/kg, dilute 50:50 w/water	IV	
Enalapril	Hypertension, heart failure, valvular insufficiency	0.25–0.50 mg/kg	PO	12–24
Endotoxin antisera	endotoxemia	4–8 mg/kg	IV	once
Enflurane	Anesthesia	Induction: 2–3%		
		Maintenance: 1.5–3.0%		
Enilconazole 10%	Nasal aspergillosis	5% soln (1:1 in water)	topically	
		10–20 mg/kg (10% soln; 50:50 water) instill into nasal sinus dilute to 0.2% soln		
Enrofloxacin	Dermatophytes		wash	72–96 for 4
	Susceptible bacterial infection	5.0–20.0 mg/kg	PO, SC, IM, IV	12–24
Ephedrine	Bronchodilator	2–5 mg/kg	PO	8–12
	Urininary incontinence	2–4 mg/kg	PO	8–12
Epinephrine	Cardiac arrest	Use 1:10000 (0.1 mg/ml)	Intratracheal, IV	PRN every 5–15 min
		Dilute 1:1000 in 10 ml saline		
		0.2 ml/kg (0.5–5.0 ml)	IV	
		10–20 μ/kg	IT	
	Anaphylaxis	200 μ/kg	SC, IM, IV	PRN every 5–15 min
		0.1 ml/kg	IV	
		2.5–5 μ/kg	IT	
	Feline asthma	50 μ/kg	IM, SC, IV	PRN every 5–15 min
		0.1 ml/kg	IM, IV, SC	PRN every 5–15 min
		0.1 mg (1 ml)/cat		
Epsiprantel	Diylidium, Taenia	2.5–2.75 mg/kg	PO	once
Ergocalciferol	Vitamin D	500–2000 U/kg/day	PO	

Continued

Continued

Drug	Indications	Dose	Route[a]	Frequency (h)[b]
Erythromycin	Susceptible infections	10–22 mg/kg	PO, IV	8
Erythropoietin	Anemia from renal failure	50–100 U/kg	SC	3x/wk for 12 wks then 2x/wk as needed to maintain HCT >35% week (adjust to hematocrit of 30–34%)
		400 U/kg	IV, SC	
Esmolol	Selective B₁ blockade,	0.05 mg/kg	slow IV bolus	loading dose then
		50–200 µ/kg	IV infusion	per min
Estradiol cypionate after mating	replacement	125–250 µ/cat	IM	b/w 40 h and 5 days
Ethacrynic acid	Diuretic: pulmonary edema	0.2–0.4 mg/kg	IV, IM	4–12
Ethanol (20%)	ethylene glycol toxicosis	5 ml/kg	IV	6 h for 5, then q 8 h for 4
Ethosuximide	Seizures	40 mg/kg	PO	load, then
		20 mg/kg	PO	
Etidronate disodium	Hypercalcemia	10 mg/kg	PO	2
Etomidate	Anesthetic induction	0.5–3 mg/kg	IV	as needed
	With opioids	0.5–1 mg/kg	IV	
Etretinate	Dermatopathy	1–2 mg/kg/day	PO	24
Euthanasia solution	Pentobarbitol	120 mg/kg for first 4.5 kg 60 mg/kg thereafter	IV	
	with phenytoin	1 ml/4.5 kg	IV	
Famotidine	gastric antisecretory	0.5 mg/kg	IM, SC, PO	12–24
Fatty acids (essential)	Atopy, fatty acid deficiency	Derm cap–1 cap/10–20 kg or 1 ml/10 kg EFA-2 plus–2.5 ml/5 kg Pet tabs/FA granules–1 tsp/5 kg <6.7 kg: 3.7 ml/day	PO PO PO PO	24 24 24 24

Drug	Indication	Dose	Route	Interval
Febantel	Antiparasiticide	10 mg/kg of febantel/1 mg/kg praziquantel	PO	24 for 3 days
Fenbendazole	Capillaria Sp	25–50 mg/kg	PO	12 for 3–14 days depending on organism
	Hook-, whip-, roundworms; *Taenia, Giardia*	50 mg/kg	PO	24 for 3–5 days; repeat in 3 wk
	Mesocestoides	50–100 mg/kg	PO	12–24 × 28 days, repeat in one week
Fentanyl citrate	Analgesia	0.02–0.04 mg/kg	IV, IM, SC	
		0.01 mg/kg	IV, IM, SC	
	Transdermal patch	25 µ/h	transdermal	
Fenthion (20%:Spotton) (Pro Spot 10:5.6%)	Fleas	0.35 ml/5 kg	Top (head)	every 72–96 h
Ferric cyanoferrate	Thallium toxicosis	4–8 mg/kg	PO	8
Ferrous sulfate	anemia	50–100 mg/cat	PO	24
Flavoxate	Detrusor hyperspasticity, urge incontinence	100–200 mg/cat	PO	6–8
Florfenicol	Susceptible bacterial infection	22–50 mg/kg	PO, IM, SC	12
Fluconazole	Antifungal	2.5–10 mg/kg	PO w/food	12–24
	Cryptococcosis	50–100 mg/cat	PO w/food	12–24
Flucytosine	Cryptococcus	30–50 mg/kg	PO	6–8
		50–75 mg/kg (up to 100 mg/kg)	PO	8
	Urinary candidiasis	67 mg/kg	PO	8
Fludricortisone	Hypoadrenocorticism	0.1–0.2 mg/cat	PO	24
Flumazenil	Hepatic encephalopathy	0.2 mg/cat	IV	as needed
		0.1 mg/kg	IV	
Flumethasone	Anti-inflammatory	0.15–0.3 mg/kg	IV, IU, SC Intralesional	24
		0.125–1 mg		
Flunixin meglumine	Anti inflammatory	0.5–2.2 mg/kg	IV, IM, SC	once
Fluoxetine	Behavioral therapy	0.5–4 mg/cat	PO	24
Flurazepam	Appetite stimulant	0.2–0.4 mg/kg	PO	q 4–7 days
Flurbiprofen (0.03% solution)	Allergic conjunctivitis	0.2–0.4 mg/kg	topically	8–12
Folic acid	Dietary supplement	2.5 mg/cat	PO	24

Continued

Continued

Drug	Indications	Dose	Route[a]	Frequency (h)[b]
Folinic acid	Supplement to pyrimethamine	1 mg	PO	24
	"Rescue" for sulfonamides	1 mg/kg	PO	24
Follicle stimulating hormone	Induction of estrus	500 IU HCG 5–15 mg FSH–P–2 mg	IV, IM, SC IM	24 for 2 days 24 for 5 days
Fomepizole	see 4-methylpyrazole			
Foscarnet sodium (phosphonoformate)	Susceptible viral infections	13.3 mg/kg	IV, PO	8
Furazolidone	Giardia Amebic colitis Coccidiosis	4 mg/kg 2.2 mg/kg 8–20 mg/kg	PO PO PO	12 for 7–10 days 8 for 7–10 days 24 for 5 days
Furosemide	Diuresis	2–4 mg/kg (up to 8 mg/kg for acute renal failure)	IV, IM, PO	8–12 or as needed, adjust to lowest dose possible
	Hypertension Hydrocephalus, brain edema Ascites from hepatic failure Hypercalcemia	0.5–2.0 mg/kg 1–2 mg/kg 1–2 mg/kg 5 mg/kg	PO PO PO, SC IV, IM, SC, PO	12 12 12–24 8–12 or each h IV infusion
		2–5 mg/kg	IV	PRN
Gabapentin	Seizures (add-on)	10 mg/kg	PO	8–12
Gamma globulin	Immune mediated disease	1 g/cat	IV	6–12
Gentamacin	Susceptible injections	6–8 mg/kg	IM, SC, IV	24
Gentamicin SO₄ 0.1%	Topical	Apply light coating		12–24
Glimipiride	Non-insulin-dependent diabetes mellitus	1–2 mg/cat	PO	24
Glipizide	Non-insulin-dependent diabetes mellitus	0.25–0.5 mg/kg 2.5–7.5mg/cat	PO PO	8–12 8–12 (gradual increase to maximum dose as needed based on serum glucose)
Glucose 40%	Corneal edema, non-healing erosions	Apply 1/8 inch or 0.32 cm	topically to affected eye	2–6 times daily

Drug	Indication	Dose	Route	Frequency
Glyburide	Hyperglycemia (Non-insulin dependent diabetes mellitus)	0.2 mg/kg	PO	daily
Glycerin	Acute glaucoma	0.625 mg/cat	PO	daily
Glyceryl guaiacolate	Muscle relaxation during certain toxicoses	1–2 ml/kg of 50% solution	PO	repeat once at 8 h
Glyceryl monoacetate	Sodium fluoroacetate toxicosis	110 mg/kg	IV	PRN
Glycopyrrolate	Sinus bradycardia, SA block, AV block	0.55 mg/kg hourly to 2–4 mg/kg	IM	
		0.005–0.010 mg/kg	IV, IM	PRN or
		0.01–0.02 mg/kg	SC	8–12
	Hypersialism	0.01 mg/kg	SC	PRN
	Preanesthetic	0.01–0.02 mg/kg	SC, IM	
Gold sodium thiomalate	Immune-mediated disease	1–5 mg/cat	IM	1st wk X 1
		2–10 mg/cat	IM	2nd wk X 1
		1 mg/kg	IM	once/wk; maint.
	Challenge test	125–250 mg/kg		
Gonadotropin-releasing hormone	Ovarian follicular cyst	50–100 μ/cat	IM	for 1–3 Rx
		25 μ/cat	IM	after mating, or on day 2 of estrus
Graunlocyte colony stimulating factor (hematopoietic growth factor, filgrastim, granisetron)	Neutropenia	3–10 μ/kg	SC	12
		3–10 μ/kg	SC	24
Griseofulvin	Microsize (with fat meal)	10–30 mg/kg	PO	24 (or div 8–12)
		50 mg/kg	PO	24 (or div 8–12)
	Ultramicrosize	25 mg/kg	PO	24 (or div 8–12)
		5–10 mg/kg	PO	24
Guaifenesin	Alone	20–50 mg/kg	PO	24
		44–88 mg/kg	IV	or
	With thiamylal (2.2–6.6 mg/kg)	33–88 mg/kg	IV	

Continued

Continued

Drug	Indications	Dose	Route[a]	Frequency (h)[b]
	With ketamine (1.1 mg/kg) Muscle relaxation w/strychnine or tetanus	33–88 mg/kg	IV	
Haloperidol	Psychogenic alopecia	2 mg/cat	PO	12
Halothane	Anesthesia	Induction: 3%		
		Maintenance: 0.5–1.5%		
Hemoglobin (polymerized bovine)	Blood replacement	10–30 ml/kg	IV	once
Heparin	Arterial thromboembolism, thrombophlebitis	Initial dose: 100–200 IU/kg	IV	then
		375 IU/kg Maintenance dose: 50–100 IU/kg	SC	6–8
		Low dose: 10–50 IU/kg	SC	6–8
	Feline thromboembolism associated with cardiomyopathy	Induction: 1000 IU/kg	IV	then
		Maintenance: 50 IU/kg	SC	8
	During acute pancreatitis	50–100 IU/kg	SC	8–12
	DIC	75–100 IU/kg	IV, SC	6
		5000 IU/500 ml blood		
	Low dose	5–10 IU/kg	IV infusion	Hr
	Burns	100–200 IU/kg	IV, SC	8 for 1–4 Rx
	Closed chest lavage	1000 IU/L fluid, 20 ml/kg		12
	Lipoprotein lipase provocative test	100 U/kg	IV	test lipids before and 15 min after heparin
Heparin, LMW	see Dalteparin			
Hetacillin	Susceptible infections	10–20 mg/kg	PO	8–12 not associated with feeding

Drug	Indication	Dose	Route	Interval
		20–40 mg/kg	PO	8
		50 mg/cat	PO	12
Hetastarch (Hydroxyethyl starch)	Plasma volume expander	10–20 ml/kg	IV	to effect
Human gamma globulin	Immune-mediated diseases	0.5–1.5 g/kg	IV	12 hr infusion
Hycodan (hydrocodone)	Antitussive	0.22 mg/kg	PO	12
Hyaluronate Na	Synovitis	3–5 mg/cat	IA	7 days
Hydralazine	Vasodilator: heart failure	0.5 mg/kg titrate up to 0.5–0.8 mg/kg	PO	12
		2.5 mg; up to 10 mg/cat	PO	12
Hydrochlorothiazide	Antihypertensive agent	0.5–2.0 mg/kg	PO	12–24
	Nephrogenic diabetes insipidus	0.5–5.0 mg/kg	PO	12
	Hypoglycemia	2–4 mg/kg	PO	12
	Calcium oxalate uroliths	2 mg/kg	PO	12
Hydrocortisone	Replacement therapy	0.5–1.0 mg/kg	PO	24
	Anti-inflammatory	2.5–5.0 mg/kg	PO	12
Hydrocortisone aurate	Hypoadrenocorticism	0.1–0.2 mg/kg	IM	8–12
	Immune mediated hemolytic anemia	2–4 mg/kg	IM	12–24
Hydrocortisone sodium succinate	Shock	8–20 mg/kg	IV	or
		50–150 mg/kg	IV	
Hydrogen peroxide 3%	Emetic	5–10 ml/cat	PO	for 1–2 Rx
Hydroxyurea	Primary polycythemia	25–30 mg/kg	PO	3 days/wk
		0.5 g/m^2	PO	12 for 5–7 days, then
		15 mg/kg	PO	24 until remission, then taper to min. effective dose
	Chronic granulocytic leukemia	0.5 g/m^2	PO	12 for 4–6 wk, then halve dosage

Continued

Continued

Drug	Indications	Dose	Route[a]	Frequency (h)[b]
Hydroxyzine	Antihistamine	5–10 mg/cat	PO	12
		6.6 mg/kg	PO	8
Hypertonic saline	Shock	2–6 ml/kg	rapid IV infusion	
Idarubicin hydrochloride	Viral infection	2 mg/kg/day		1 day for 2 days; repeat every 21 days
Idoxuridine	Ocular herpes virus infection	0.1 % soln: 1 drop	apply topically	3–6 times daily
		0.5 % ointment:	topically	1
Imipenem-cilastin	Susceptible bacterial infection	2–10 mg/kg	IM or slow IV infusion	6–8
Imipramine	Behavior modification	2.5–5.0 mg/cat	PO	12
Insulin, glargine	Diabetes mellitus	0.25–0.5 U/kg	SC	12, adjust as needed
Insulin, lente	Diabetes mellitus	Intial dose: Blood glucose < 20 mmol/L 0.25 U/kg Blood glucose > 20 mmol/ L 0.5 U//kg	SC	12–24; adjust as needed
Insulin, NHP	Diabetes mellitus	0.25–0.5 U/kg/day	SC	12–24
		1–3 U/cat	SC	12–24
		3–5 U/cat	SC	24 to effect
Insulin, PZI	Diabetes mellitus	0.3–1 U/kg	SC	12–24
		1–3 U/cat	SC	12–24
Insulin, regular	Diabetic ketoacidosis	1 unit/100 ml IV fluid, 0.025–0.05 U/kg/h	IM	1
		<3 kg: 1 U/cat initially then 1 U/cat	IM	1
		3–10 kg: 2 U/cat initially, then 1 U/cat 0.2 U/kg, then 0.1 U/kg	IM	hourly until glucose <250 mg/dl to effect, 6 h
		2–5 U	SC	3–8
		0.25 U/kg	SC	
Insulin, ultralente	Diabetes mellitus	0.25–0.5 U/kg	SC	24
		1–3 U/cat	SC	12–24

Drug	Indication	Dose	Route	Interval (h)
Interferon-α_2 (human recombinant)	Non-neoplastic FeLV-associated disease	15–30 U/cat	IM, SC, PO	24 on alternate weeks
	FeLV appetite stimulation	0.5–5.0 U/kg	PO	24
	FIP (nonexudative)	1 U/cat	PO	24
	FIP (exudative)	30 U/cat	PO	24 on alternate weeks
	Ocular herpes	20000 U/cat	IM	24
		10 U/cat	PO	24
Interferon, feline recombinant	omega Immunostimulation (FIP)	1 million U/kg	SC	48; reduce to 1/wk if response
Interferon, human recombinant α 2b	Immunostimulation	15–30 units/cat	PO, SC, IM	24 × 7 D
Iodine	Hyperthyroidism	50–100 mg/cat	PO	24
Iodide sodium, potassium 20% solution	Hyperthroidism, Sporotrichosis	20 mg/kg	PO	12–24
Iopamidol	Myelography	0.25 ml/kg		
Ipecac syrup	Emetic	2–6 ml/cat	PO	
Ipodate	Hyperthyroidism (short term)	15 mg/kg	PO	12
Iron dextran	Anemia	50 mg/cat	IM	at 18 days of age
Isoflurane	Anesthesia	Induction: 5% Maintenance: 1.5–2.5%		
Isometheptene	Urethical antispasmodic	0.25–0.50 ml/cat	IM	12
		0.5 tablet/cat	PO	12
Isoniazid	Tuberculosis	10–20 mg/kg	PO	24
Isopropamide iodide	Sinus bradycardia, SA or AV block	0.2–0.4 mg/kg	PO	8–12
	Antidiarrheal	0.2–1.0 mg/kg	PO	12
Isopropamide/prochlor perazine		0.5–0.8 mg/kg	IM, SC	12

Continued

Continued

Drug	Indications	Dose	Route[a]	Frequency (h)[b]
Isoproterenol	Bradycardia, AV block, cardiac arrest	0.04–0.08 μ/kg 0.4 mg in 250 ml 5% dextrose 0.2 mg in 100 ml 5% dextrose	IV infusion IV slowly	minute
	Feline asthma	0.004–0.006 mg	IV	to effect at 8 hrs
		0.44 mg/kg	IM	30 min PRN
		10 μ/kg	PO	6–12
		1–2 μ/min	IM, SC	6
		0.5 ml of 1:200 dilution	Inhalant	4 for 3
Isosorbide dinitrate	Vasodilator	2.5–5.0 mg/cat	PO	12
Isotretinoin	Feline acne	5 mg/kg	PO	24
Itraconazole	Systemic mycoses or generalized dermatomycosis	5–10 mg/kg	PO	12–24
Ivermectin	Heartworm prophylaxis	24 μ/kg	PO	once monthly
	Microfilaricide	50 μ/kg	PO	
	Endoparasites	200–400 μ/kg	IM, SC, PO	
	Cheyletiellosis, notoedric mange	200–400 mg/kg	SC	weekly
Jenotone	Urinary tract obstruction	2 mg/kg	IM, SC	12
Kanamycin	Susceptible infections	10–15 mg/kg	IV, IM, SC	12
		5–7.5 mg/kg	IV, IM, SC	24
	GI tract bacterial overgrowth	10–20 mg/kg 10–12 mg/kg	PO	8–12
Kaolin/pectin	GI tract protectant	1–2 ml/kg	PO	2–6
Ketamine HCl	Sedation	Xylazine (1.1–2.2 mg/kg IM) 7–11 mg/kg	IV	
		Xylazine (1.1 mg IM) 22 mg/kg	IM	
		Diazepam (0.3–0.5 mg/kg IV) 5.5–10.0 mg/kg	IV	
		Midazolam (0.066–0.22 mg/kg IM or IV) 6.6–11.0 mg/kg	IM	
		Acepromazine mg/kg (0.22 mg/kg) 33 mg.kg	IM	
	Anesthesia	Acepromazine (0.66 mg/kg) 16	IV	
		22–33 mg/kg 2.2–4.4 mg/kg	IM	
Ketoconazole	Systemic and cutaneous mycoses,	10 mg/kg	PO	12–24
	sporotrichosis	5–10 mg/kg	PO	12–24
	CNS mycoses	15–20 mg/kg	PO	12

Drug	Indication	Dose	Route	Interval
Ketoprofen	Hyperadrenocorticism	10 mg/kg	PO	12
	Anti-inflammatory	0.5–1 mg/kg	PO	24 once
		2 mg/kg	IV	once
		2 mg/kg	SC, IM	24, up to 3 days
		1 mg/kg	PO	24, up to 5 days
L-asparaginase	See Asparaginase			
Lactated Ringer's solution		40–50 ml/kg/day	IV for maintenance or septic shock	
		60 ml/kg	IV	
Lactilol	Stool softener, hepatic encephalopathy	250 mg/cat	PO	12
Lactoferrin	FIV stomatitis	40 mg/kg	Topical	24
Lactulose	Hepatic encephalopathy	2.5–5 ml/cat	PO	8
		5–10 ml diluted 1:3 with water	Rectal	
	Stool softener	1 ml/cat	PO	8 (to effect)
Lenperone	Opioid preanesthetic	0.22–0.88 mg/kg	IM, IV	
Leucovorin	Counteract methotrexate toxicity	3 mg/m^2	IM	w/in 3 h of methotrexate
	Pyrimethamine antidote	1 mg/kg	PO	
Levallorphan	Narcotic antagonist	0.02–0.20 mg/kg	IV	as needed
Levamisole	Microfilaroide	10 mg/kg	PO	24 for 7 days
	Filaroides, aleurostrongylus	25 mg/kg	PO	48 for 10–14 days
		25 mg/cat	PO	48 for 3 treatments for 2 days
	Hookworms	up to 10 mg/kg	PO	48 for 5–6 days
		20–40 mg/kg	PO	
	Immune stimulant	4.4 mg/kg	PO	once
Levarterenol	(see norepinephrine)			
Levetiracetam	Seizures (add-on)	15 to 20 mg/kg	PO	8–12 h
Levodopa	Hepatic encephalopathy	6.8 mg/kg initially, then 1.4 mg/kg	PO	6
Levothyroxine (T4)	Hypothyroidism	10–30 μ/kg	PO	12
		50–100 μ/kg)	PO	div 12
Lidocaine	Ventricular arrhythmias	0.25–1.00 mg/kg	IV bolus, then	minute
		10–40 μ/kg	IV infusion	once
	epidural	4.4 mg/kg of 2% solution	epidural	

Continued

Continued

Drug	Indications	Dose	Route[a]	Frequency (h)[b]
Lime sulfur	Sarcoptic mange	1:40 dilution	Dip, air–dry;	repeat weekly for 6 wk
Lime water	Alkaline gastric lavage	5 ml/kg	PO	
Lincomycin	Susceptible infections	11–33 mg/kg	PO, IV, IM	12–24
Liothryonine (T3)	Hypothyroidism	4.4 µ/kg	PO	8–12
Lisinopril	Afterload reduction (vasodilator)	0.25–0.50 mg/kg	PO	24
Lobaplatin	Anticancer chemotherapy	35 mg/m²	IV	3
Loperimide	Antidiarrheal	0.1–0.3 mg/kg	PO	12–24
Lufeneron	Immunomodulator	15–30 mg/kg	PO	24 with meal × 30 days
	Flea control	10 mg/kg	SC	
	Antifungal (ringworm)	80 mg/kg	PO	Repeat in 2 wks
		100 mg/kg (cattery)	PO	Repeat in 2 wks
Lufeneron/milbemycin	Heartworm preventative	1 tablet per appropriate-sized cat	PO	
Luteinizing hormone (LH)	Stimulate ovulation	50 IU/cat	IM	after mating
L-lysine	Herpes keratitis–rhinitis	250–500 mg	PO in food	12
Lysine-8-vasopressin	Central diabetes insipidus	1–2 sprays	conjunctival	8–24
Magnesium citrate	Laxative	2–4 ml/kg	PO	
Magnesium hydroxide	Antacid	5–10 ml/cat	PO	8–24
	Cathartic	2–6 ml/cat	PO	24
Magnesium salts	Laxative	2–5 g/cat	PO	24
Magnesium sulfate (25%)	Hypomagnesemia	5–15 mmol/cat	IM, IV	over 1–2 h
Mannitol 5–20%	Oliguric renal failure	0.25–1 g/kg of 15–25% solution	IV over 15–60 min	repeat every 4–6 h to maintain urine flow
	Glaucoma	1–3 mg/kg	IV over 15–20 min	
	CNS edema	1.5 mg/kg	IV	once
Marbofloxacin	Susceptible infections	2.75–5.5 mg/kg	PO	24

Drug	Indication	Dose	Route	Schedule
Mebendazole	Hook-, whip-, and roundworms	22 mg/kg with food	PO	24 for 3 days
Meclizine	Motion sickness	12.5 mg/cat	IM	24, 1 h before driving
Medetomidine HCl	Chemical restraint, sedation analgesia, muscle relaxant	750 μ/m² IV or 1000 μ/m²	IM	
Medium-chain triglycerides	Chylothorax, Primary lymphangiectasis, pancreatic exocrine insufficiency	1 oz or 28 ml/10 kg with each meal; 0.5–1.0 oz or 28 ml/10 kg (max 1 tbsp per meal)	PO	divided daily every 6–8 hrs
Medroxyprogesterone acetate	Prevent abortion	1–2 mg/kg	IM	once weekly: stop 7–10 days before parturition
	Urine marking, anxiety, intraspecies aggression	10–20 mg/kg	SC	PRN up to 3 injections per year
	Skin conditions	50–100 mg/cat	SC, IM	repeat in 3–6 months if needed
	Behavioral disorders	100 mg/cat; 30–50 mg/cat	IM	then, 30 days
Megestrol acetate	Feline plasma cell gingivitis	2.5–5.0 mg/cat	PO	24 for 10 d, then 48 for 5 treatments, then PRN
	Urethritis, FUS	2.5–5.0 mg/cat	PO	24–48 for 14–21 until remission, then 1–2 wk
	Endocrine alopecia	2.5–5.0 mg/cat	PO	24 for 10 days, then 48
	Eosinophilic granulomas	0.5 mg/kg/day	PO	for 7–14 days
	Eosinophilic ulcers	5–10 mg/cat	PO	48 for 10–14 treatments then every 2nd wk
	To prevent estrus	5 mg/cat for 3 days, then 2.5–5.0 mg/cat wk for 10 wk	PO	
		2.5–5.0 mg	PO	7 days
		5 mg	PO	24 for 5 days
		25 mg	IM	6 months
	Unaceptable masculine behavior, urine marking, anxiety, intraspecies aggression	2–4 mg/kg reduce to 1/2 dose at 8 days	PO	1 daily
	Skin conditions	2.5–5.0 mg/cat	PO	24 for 5–10 days, then once weekly
		5 mg	PO	24 for 5ᵉ, then twice weekly
	Asthma	5 mg/cat	PO	24 for 4 m then wkly for 4
	Chemical contraception	5.0 mg/cat	PO	24 for 3, then wk for 10
		2.5 mg/cat		24 for 8 wk

Continued

Continued

Drug	Indications	Dose	Route[a]	Frequency (h)[b]
	Chemical contraception (continued)	2.5 mg/cat	PO	wk for 18 mnths
Meglumine antimonate	Leishmaniasis	5–30 ml/cat	IV, IM, IP	48–72 h
Meloxicam	Anti-inflammatory	0.1 mg/kg 0.1 mg/cat	PO PO	24 × 4 days 24
Melphan	Multiple myeloma	0.05 mg/kg 0.05 mg/kg	PO PO	24 for 2 wk. then 48
	Ovarian carcinoma, multiple myeloma, lymphoreticular neoplasms, osteosarcoma, mammary or pulmonary neoplasms FIP, chronic lymphocytic leukemia	2 mg/m^2	PO	48
Mepiridine	Sedation	1–5 mg/kg 2.2–4.4 mg/kg	IM IM	2–4 h
Mepivacaine	Local analgesic	local infiltration as needed 0.5 ml (1–5 ml) of 2%	local epidural	every 30 seconds until
6-Mercaptopurine	Chronic myelocytic leukemia, lymphoma	50 mg/m^2 or 2 mg/kg	PO PO	24 24, in a protocol
Meropenem	Susceptible bacterial infections, meningitis	20 mg/kg 40 mg/kg	IV IV	8 8
Mesna	Hemorrhagic cystitis associated With cyclophosphamide	40% of cyclophosphamide dose	PO, IV, SC, IM	3 × 6 at time of cylcophosphamide treatment follow with repeat dose(24 hour infusion)
Metamucil	Laxative	2–4 g/cat	in moistened food	12–24
Metaproterenol sulfate	Bronchodilation	0.325–0.65 mg/kg	PO	4–6
Metaraminol	Vascular support during shock	0.01–0.10 mg/kg or 10 mg in 250 ml 5% dextrose	IV slowly IV to effect	
Metformin	Hyperglycemia (non-insulin-dependent diabetes mellitus)	2 mg/kg	PO	12

Drug	Indication	Dose	Route	Frequency
Methazolamide	Glaucoma	1–2 mg/kg	PO	12
Methenamine hippurate	Urinary antiseptic	250 mg/cat	PO	12 (extreme caution)
Methicillin	Susceptible bacterial infections	20 mg/kg	IM, IV	6
Methimazole	Hyperthyroidism	5 mg/cat (induction)	PO	8–12, followed by
		2.5–5.0 mg/cat	PO	8–12
(DL) Methionine	Urinary acidifier	0.2–1.5 g/cat (Adult cats only)	PO, added to food	24
Methocarbamol	Muscle relaxation	20–66 mg/kg	PO	8–12
	Relief of moderate conditions	44 mg/kg	IV	
	Controling effects of strychnine and tetanus	55–220 mg/kg; give 1/2 dose rapidly until relaxation occurs and continue (not to exceed 330 mg/kg/day)		
		20–66 mg/kg	IV	8–12
		If no response in 5 days, discontinue	PO	
Methohexital	Anesthesia induction	2.5% solution: 11 mg/kg	IV	
Methotrexate Na	Chemotherapy	2.5 mg/m² or	PO	24 or 2–3x wkly
		0.3–0.5 mg/m²	IV	weekly, in a protocol
		0.3–0.8 mg/kg	IV	on day 14 w/5 mg prednisone PO 12 h
	Carcinomas, sarcomas	2.5–5.0 mg/m²	PO	24
		10–15 mg/m²		1–3 wks
Methoxamine	Vasopressor: cardiac arrest, shock	200–250 μ/kg or	IM	
		40–80 μ/kg	IV	
Methoxyflurane	Anesthesia	Induction: 3%		
		Maintenance: 0.5–1.5%		
Methscopolamine bromide	Anti-emetic	0.3–1.0 mg/kg	PO	8 (use cautiously)
Methylcellulose	Laxative	1.0–1.5 g/cat	PO	
Methylene blue 0.1%	Indicator dye	3 mg/250 ml 0.9% NaCl	IV over 30–40 min	staining maximal at 25 min daily
Antidote		1–1.5 mg/kg	IV, slowly	
Methylprednisolone	Anti-inflammatory	0.5–1.0 mg/kg	PO	12
		0.22–0.44 mg/kg	PO	12–24

Continued

Continued

Drug	Indications	Dose	Route[a]	Frequency (h)[b]
Methylprednisolone acetate	Eosinophilic ulcers			
	Linear granulomas	10–40 mg	SC, IM, intralesional	2 wk for 2–6 Rx
	Asthma	1–2 mg/kg	IM	7 days
	Others	5.5 mg/kg	SC, IM	1–24 wk
Methylprednisolone sodium succinate	Spinal trauma	15 – 30 mg/kg	IV	2 h later, then
		10 mg/kg	IV, SC	6 for 2 days, then taper dose over 5–7 days
4-Methylpyrazole	Antifreeze toxicity	20 mg/kg	IV	followed by
		15 mg/kg	IV	12 × 2 then
		5 mg/kg	IV	at 36 h
Methyltestosterone	Anabolic drug	1–2 mg/kg	PO	24
	Testosterone-responsive dermatosis	1–2.5 mg/cat	PO	48
Metoclopramide	Gastric motility disorders, anti-emetic	0.2–0.5 mg/kg	PO, SC, IM	8
		1.0–2.0 mg/kg	IV infusion	24 h
	Gastric reflux	0.2–0.4 mg/kg	PO	8, 30 min before meals and at bedtime
	Dysautonomia	0.3 mg/kg	PO	8
Metoprolol	Atrial fibrillation, hypertrophic cardiomyopathy	2–15 mg/cat	PO	8
		12.5–25.0 mg/cat	PO	12
Metronidazole	GI tract bacterial overgrowth, acute colitis *Entamoeba, Trichomonas,*	10 mg/kg/day	PO	12–24 for 5 days
		10–25 mg/kg	PO	24 for 5 days
	Anaerobic infections	10–25 mg/kg	PO	8–12 for 2–3 wks
	Hepatic lipidosis	25–30 mg/kg	PO	24
	Plasmacytic/lymphocytic enteritis	10 mg/kg	PO	24
	Gingivits	50 mg/kg		
	Other	10–25 mg/kg; max dose:		
		50 mg/kg	PO	24
	Giardia	17 mg/kg	PO	24 for 8 days

Drug	Indication	Dose	Route	Frequency
Miconazole	Dermatophytosis Ocular fungal infections	apply topically as directed apply topically		4–12 times daily
Midazolam	Preanesthetic, sedation	0.066–0.22 mg/kg	IM, IV	
Milbemycin oxime	Heart-, hook-, round-, whipworm prophylaxis	0.5–2 mg/kg	PO	once monthly
Mineral oil	Laxative	5–10 ml/cat	PO, per rectum	
Minocycline	Susceptible infections	5–15 mg/kg	PO	12
Mithramycin	Hypercalcemia	0.25–0.50 μ/kg	IV	12
Mitotane (o,p-DDD)	Pituitary – dependent hyperadrenocorticism	25 mg/kg 75–100 mg/kg/wk (adjust dose based on cortisol measurements)	PO PO	24 for 2 Rx 7 days (maintenance)
Mitoxantrone	Chemotherapy (part of protocol)	6.0–6.5 mg/m²	IV	3–4 wks for 4–6 treatments
Morphine sulfate	Antitussive, analgesic	0.05–0.10 mg/kg	SC, IM	4–6
Mycobacterial cell wall extract	Immunostimulation	1.5 ml	IV, deep IM	24 × 1
Nadolol	Beta blockade	0.25–0.50 mg/kg	PO	12
Nafcillin	Resistant staphylococcal infections	10 mg/kg	PO, IM	6
Nalbuphine hydrochloride	Analgesic	0.75–1.50 mg/kg 0.2–0.3 mg/kg	IV SC	6–8 6–8
Nalorphine	Narcotic antagonist	0.1 mg/kg (max 1 mg) 0.44 mg/kg 1 mg for every 10 mg of morphine	IV IV, IM, SC	
Naloxone HCl	Stereotypic behavior Shock Opoid reversal	20 mg 2 mg/kg 0.01–0.04 mg/kg 0.02–0.1 mg/kg	SC IV infusion IV IV	1 to effect, repeat PRN
Naltrexone (Trexan)	Test dose Behavior problem, lick granulomas	0.01 mg/kg 2.2 mg/kg	SC PO	12–24
Nandrolone decanoate	Anemia	10–50 mg/cat 1 mg/kg	IM IM	wkly wkly
Natamycin	Ocular fungal infections		topically	3–8

Continued

Continued

Drug	Indications	Dose	Route[a]	Frequency (h)[b]
N-acetylcysteine	see Acetylcysteine			
Neo-Darbazine	Antiemetic	4.5–9.0 kg:one #1 capsule	PO	12
Neomycin	Susceptible infections Hepatic encephalopathy	7 mg/kg 10–20 mg/kg	IM, IV, SC rectal (dilute in water)	24 (nephrotoxic) 6
Neostigmine	Diagnostic aid for myasthenia gravis	20 µ/kg with 0.04 mg/kg of atropine 2 mg/kg/day	IV IV PO	divided to effect
Niacin (Niacinamide)	Hypertriglyceridemia Vacor toxicosis	50–100mg/day 500–1000 mg 200–300 mg 200 mg	PO IM IM PO	24 then 4 24 for 2 wk
Nikethamide	Combat CNS depression from central depressant drugs	7.8–31.2 mg/kg	IV, IM, SC	
Nitrofurantoin	Urinary tract infections Prophylactic dose	2.5–4 mg/kg 4 mg/kg	PO PO	6–8 24
Nitroglycerin 2% ointment	Pre-load reduction	1/8–1/4 inch (0.3–0.6 cm)	cutaneously	6–8
Nitroprusside	Vasodilator for acute congestive heart failure	0.5–10 µ/kg (3 µ/kg)	IV infusion	1 min (use 50 µ/ml dilution)
Norepinephrine bitartrate	Positive intotrope	0.05–0.30 µ/kg 5 mg/kg	IV PO	1 min
Nortriptyline	Behavior disorders	0.5–2.0 mg/kg	PO	12–24
Novobiocin	Susceptible infections	10 mg/kg	PO	8
Nystatin	Susceptible infections	100 000 U	PO	8
Ofloxacin	Susceptible bacterial infections	2.5–10 mg/kg	PO	12
Olsalazine sodium	Inflammatory bowel disease	10–20 mg/kg (human dosage is 500 mg twice daily)	PO	12–24
Omega fatty acids	See derm caps			

Drug	Indication	Dose	Route	Interval/Notes
Omeprazole	Gastric antisecretory drugs	<5 kg 1/4 capsule (5 mg)	PO	24
		0.5–1.0 mg/kg	PO	24
Ondansetron	Antiemetic	0.5–1 mg/kg	PO	followed by
		0.5 mg/kg (loading dose)	IV	1 h infusion for 6 h
		0.5 mg/kg		
Orbifloxacin	Susceptible bacterial infections	2.5–7.5 mg/kg	PO	24
				48 for 8 days
Ormetoprim/sulfa	See sulfadimethoxine/ormetoprim			
Ormetoprim	See sulfadimethoxine/ormetoprim			
Oxacillin	Susceptible infections	22–40 mg/kg	PO	8
Oxazepam	Appetite stimulant	2.0–2.5 mg/cat	PO	12
Oxtriphylline	Bronchodilator	6 mg/kg	PO	8–12
		10–15 mg/kg	PO	6–8
Oxybutinin	Detrusor hyperspasticity	0.5 mg/cat	PO	8–12
Oxymetholone	Anabolic agent	1 mg/kg	PO	12–24
		0.1–1.1 mg/kg	PO	24
		1–5 mg/kg	PO	24
Oxymorphone	Preanesthetic	0.1–0.2 mg/kg	IM, IV	w/acepromazine,gly copyrrolate or atropine
		0.05–0.15 mg/kg	IM, IV	w/acepromazine
		Acepromazine: 0.05–0.10 mg/kg	IM, IV	
	Analgesia	0.1–0.4 mg/kg	IV	
	Restraint/sedation	0.02–0.03 mg/kg	IV, IM	w/acepromazine
Oxytetracycline	Susceptible infections	55–82.5 mg/kg	PO	8
		15–30 mg/kg	PO	8
		20–40 mg/kg	PO	8 for 3 wks
	Hemobartonellosis	7–12 mg/kg	IM, IV	12
Oxytocin	Acute metritis	0.5–1.0 U/kg	IV, IM	repeat in 1–2 h
		0.5 U/kg	IM, IV	max dose:3 U/cat
	Stimulate milk letdown	spray	Intranasal	5–10 min before nursing
		10 U in 5% D/W	IV	over 30 min

Continued

Continued

Drug	Indications	Dose	Route[a]	Frequency (h)[b]
Paclitaxel	dystocia	2.5–5.0 U/cat	IM, IV infusion, SC	may repeat in 45 min
	Anticancer chemotherapy	5 mg/kg	IV	pretreat for anaphylactoid reaction
Pancreatic enzymes	Pancreatic exocrine insufficiency	1 tablet, 1–2 tsp	PO (crush tablets)	in food 20 min prior to feeding
Pancreatin	Pancreatic exocrine insufficiency	0.5–1.0 tsp	PO	in food
Pancuronium bromide	Paralytic agent for controlled anesthesia	1–2 tablets	PO	in food
		0.044–0.11 mg/kg	IV	
Paregoric	Antidiarrheal	0.05–0.06 mg/kg (5 ml of paregoric corresponds to approx 2 mg of morphine)	PO	8–12
Paromomycin (aminosidine)	Cryptosporidiosis	125–165 mg/kg	PO	12 × 5 days
Paroxetine	Behavior modification	1/8–1/4 of 10 mg tablet	PO	24
Parvaquone	Antiprotozoal	10–30 mg/kg	IM	24
D-Penicillamine	Progressive hepatitis	10–15 mg/kg	PO	12
Penicillin G, aqueous (K or Na)	Meningitis,bacterial endocarditis	20 000–55 000 U/kg	IV	4–6
Potassium	Actinomycosis, tetanus	22 000 U/kg	IM, IV, SC	6
Sodium	Leptospirosis	20 000–55 000 U/kg	PO	4
		40 000 U/kg	IM, IV, SC	6 on empty stomach
		20 000–55 000 U/kg		4
Penicillin G, benzathine	Susceptible bacterial infections	50 000 U/kg	IM	5 days
Penicillin G, phenoxymethyl Potassium	Susceptible bacterial infections Susceptible bacterial infections	20–30 mg/kg	PO	6–8
Penicillin G, procaine[1]	Leptospirosis, actinomycosis	20 000–100 000 U/kg	IM, SC	12
Penicillin V, potassium	Susceptible bacterial infections	10 mg/kg	PO	8
Pentazocine	analgesic	2.2–3.3 mg/kg	IV, IM, SC	4 h
Pentobarbital	General anesthesia	25–30 mg/kg	IV	to effect

Drug	Indication	Dose	Route	Interval (h)
Pentobarbital	Status epilepticus, sedation	5–15 mg/kg	IV	to effect
	Sedation	2–4 mg/kg	IV, PO	6
		25 mg/kg	IV	
Pentosan polysulfate	Disease modifying agent: arthritis	3 mg/kg	IM, SC	7 days
Pentoxifylline	Dermatomyositis	100 mg/cat	PO	8–12
	Immune-mediated dermatologic diseases	10–15 mg/kg	PO	sid
Pepto bismol	See bismuth subsalicylate			
Petrolatum, white	Laxative	1–5 ml/cat	PO	24
Phenamidine isethionate	Babesiosis	7.5 mg/kg	IM, SC	24 × 2
		15 mg/kg	IM, SC	24 × 1
Phenobarbital	Status epilepticus	2–30 mg/kg	PO, IM, IV	loading dose (in 3 mg/kg increments)
	Maintenance	1–2 mg/kg	IV, PO	12: monitor to adjust dose
	Sedation	1 mg/kg	PO	12
	Psychogenic alopecia	4–8 mg	PO	12
Phenoxybenzamine HCl	Acute hypertension from pheochromocytoma	0.5 mg/kg	PO	12
	Detrusor areflexia	2.5–10 mg/cat	PO	8–12
	Relaxation of urinary sphincter	0.5 mg/kg	IV	
	Endotoxemia	2.5–10.0 mg/cat	PO	24
		0.5 mg/cat	PO	12
Phentolamine	Hypertension from pheochromocytoma	0.02–0.1 mg/kg	IV	
Phenylephrine	Vasopressor	0.15 mg/kg	IV slowly	PRN
Phenylpropanolamine HCl	Urethral sphincter incompetence	1.5–2.0 mg/kg	PO	8
		12.5 mg/cat	PO	8
		75 mg (sustained release)	PO	24
Phenytoin	Seizures, ventricular arrhythmia	2–3 mg/kg	PO	24
Phosphate (K or Na)	Hypophosphatria	4.5 mg/dl serum phosphate	IV	over 6 h
		0.06–1.80 mM/kg	IV	per h (discontinue when phosphorus > 2 mg/dl)
		0.01–0.03 mM/kg	IV	per h (discontinue when phosphorus > 2 mg/dl)

Continued

Continued

Drug	Indications	Dose	Route[a]	Frequency (h)[b]
Physostigmine	Muscarinic mushroom intoxication	0.25–0.50 mg/cat 0.02 mg/kg	IM IV	12, over 5 min period
Physostigmine 0.5% o.o	Dysautonomia	apply 1/8 inch or 0.3 cm	topically	8
Phytomenadione (phytonadione)	See Vitamin K1			
Pilocarpine 1% ophthalmic soln	Dysauronomia	1 drop	topically	6
Piperacillin sodium	Susceptible bacterial infections	25–50 mg/kg	IV, IM	8–12
Piperacillin-tazobactam	Susceptible bacterial infections	25–50 mg/kg (based on piperacillin)	IV	6–8
Piperazine	Roundworms	44–66 mg/kg	PO	repeat in 3 wks
Piroxicam	Anagesic, anticancer	0.3 mg/kg	PO	24–72
Plicamycin	see Mithramycin			
Polyethylene glycol	Cathartic	25 ml/kg	PO, stomach tube	then repeat in 2–4 before lower GI exam
Polyethylene glycol electrolyte solution	Electrolyte replacement	25 ml/kg	PO	repeat in 2–4 hours
Polysulfated glycosam-inoglycans	Degenerative joint disease	2–5 mg/kg	IM	3–5 days
Potassium chloride	Potassium supplementation Hypokalemia	0.10–0.25 ml/kg 0.5 mEq/kg	PO IV	8:dilute 1:1 w/water not to exceed 0.5 mEq/kg/h
		1–3 mEq	PO, IV	24
		10–40 mEq/500 ml of fluid, depending on serum potassium	IV, SC	
Potassium citrate	Calcium oxalate urolithiasis	50–75 mg/kg	PO	12
Potassium gluconate	Hypokalemic polymyopathy	5–8 mEq/cat	PO	12–24
Kaon elixer		2.2 mEq/100 kal of energy	PO	24
Tumil-K		1/4 tsp/4.5 kg	PO	12–24

Drug	Indication	Dose	Route	Interval (h)
Potassium iodide	Sporotrichosis, pythiosis	30–100 mg/cat		daily (in single or divided doses) for 10–14 days
Potassium permanganate (1:2000)	Strychnine toxicosis	5 ml/kg in gastric lavage		
Potassium phosphate	See phosphate			
Povidone-iodine	Burns	Apply light coating		
Pralidoxime Cl (2-PAM)	Organophosphate toxicosis	20 mg/kg	IV, IM, SC	12–24
Praziquantel	Antiparasiticide	<1.8 kg: 6.3 mg/kg	PO	12, initial dose IV slow
		>1.8 kg: 5 mg/kg	PO	once
		5 mg/kg	IM, SC	once
	Paragonimiasis	25 mg/kg	PO	8–12 for 2 days
Prazosin	After load reductions	0.5 and 2 mg/cat	PO	8–12
	Urethral obstruction	0.5–2 mg/cat; 0.07 mg/kg	PO	8–12
Prednisolone/prednisone	Eosinophilic ulcers, plasma cell gingivitis	1–2 mg/kg	PO	24
		0.5–1.5 mg/kg	PO	24 divided daily, taper over 3 months
	Plasmacytic/lymphocytic enteritis	1–2 mg/kg	PO	12, then taper dose weekly
	Urethritis, persistent hematuria	2.5–5.0 mg	PO	24–48
	Anti-inflammatory	2.2 mg/kg	IV, IM, PO	12–24, then taper to every 2 days
	Hypoadrenocorticism	1 mg/kg	PO, IM	12
	Hypoglycemia	0.25–3.00 mg/kg	PO	12
	Chronic therapy	2–4 mg/kg	PO	48
	Hypercalcemia			
	Immune skin diseases, systemic lupus erythematosus	1.1–2.2 mg/kg	PO	12 until remission, then taper
	SLE, rheumatoid arthritis	1.5–2.0 mg/kg	PO	12–24, then taper to
	Immune polymyositis, masticatory myositis	<1 mg/kg	PO	48
		2 mg/kg	PO, IM	24
	Blepharitis, episcleritis uveitis,	0.5–2.0 mg/kg	PO	12

Continued

Continued
Continued

Drug	Indications	Dose	Route[a]	Frequency (h)[b]
	Feline infectious peritonitis	4 mg/kg	PO	24 w/cyclophosphamide
	Allergy	1 mg/kg	PO, IM	12
	Immunosuppression	3 mg/kg	PO, IM	12
		2–5 mg/kg	PO, IM, SC	12–24
		2.2–6.6 mg/kg	IM, PO, IV	24 initially, then taper to 48
	Shock	2–4 mg/kg		
	Lymphosarcoma, myelo-	15–30 mg/kg	IV	repeat in 1, 3, 6 or 10 h
	proliferative disorders, eosinophilic	1 mg/kg	PO	24, then every other 48 h
	leukemia, in a protocol	30–40 mg/m²	PO	24, then every other 48 h
	Mast cell tumors, mastocytosis	30–40 mg/m²	PO	24 for 4wk, then every other 48 h
	Multiple myeloma, macroglobulinemia	0.5 mg/kg	PO	24 in a protocol
Prednisolone acetate	Hypoadrenocorticism	0.1–0.2 mg/kg	IM	12
Prednisolone sodium phosphate	Shock	15 mg/kg	IV	repeat in 4–6 h
Prednisolone sodium succinate	Allergic bronchitis, asthma	15–30 mg/kg	IV, IM	to effective dose
	Shock	15–30 mg/kg	IV	repeat in 4–6 h
	Hypoglycemia	1–2 mg/kg	IV	
	CNS trauma	15–30 mg/kg	IV	then taper to effective dose
		1–2 mg/kg		
Primaquine PO₄ (not available in US)	Babesiosis	0.5 mg/kg	PO, IM	once
Procainamide	Ventricular arrhythmias	62.5 mg/cat	PO	6
		3–8 mg/kg	IM, PO	6–8
Prochlorperazine	Antiemetic	0.1 mg/kg	IM	6
		0.13 mg/kg	IM	12
		0.5 mg/kg	PO	6–8
Prochlorperzine/ isopropamide	See isopropamide			
Promazine hydrochloride	Preanesthetic	2.2–6.6 mg/kg	IV	

Drug	Use	Route	Dose	Interval (h)
Promethazine HCl	Sedative	IM	2.2–4.4 mg/kg	4–6
	Anti-emetic	IM, IV	1–2 mg/kg	4–6
	Other	IM, IV	2–4 mg/kg	4–6
Propantheline bromide	Antihistamine, anti-emetic	IV, IM, PO	0.2–0.4 mg/kg (max dose: 1 mg/kg)	6–8
	Acute colitis, irritable colon syndrome, anti-emetic	PO	0.22–0.25 mg/kg	8 up to 3 days
	Detrusor hyperspasticity, urge incontinence	PO	0.2 mg/kg	6–8
		PO	5–7.5 mg/cat	24–72; up to every 8 h
Propiomazine	Sedation	IV, IM	1.1–4.4 mg/kg	12–24
Propionibacterium acnes	Immunostimulation IFA and ELISA (FeLV-associated disease)	IV	0.5 ml 2 inj	biweekly for 2–3
		IV	15 µ/kg	
	Feline retrovirus infection	IV	0.25–2.00 ml	
Propiopromazine	Tranquilization	IM	1.1–4.4 mg/kg	12–24
Propofol	Anesthesia	IV	Induction: 6–8 mg/kg	
		IV	Induction: 2.5–4.0 mg/kg	w/ premedication
		IV infusion	Maintenance: 0.51 mg/kg	min
Propranolol	Ventricular hypertrophy aortic stenosis	PO	0.4–1.2 mg/kg	8–12
	Ventricular arrhythmias	IV	0.02–0.06 mg/kg	over 2–3 min; every 8 h followed by
		IV slowly	0.25–0.50 mg	8
		PO	2.5–5.0 mg	8–12
	Hypertrophic cardiomyopathy valvular insufficiency	PO	2.5 mg/cat	
	Hypertension	PO	≥5.0 kg 5.0 mg	8–12
	Tachyarrhythmias from endocrinopathies	PO	2.5–5.0 mg	8–12
		PO	2.5–5.0 mg	8–12
Propylthiouracil (PTU)	Hyperthyroidism	PO	10 mg/kg	8
		PO	50 mg/cat	8–12
		PO	11 mg/kg	12
Prostaglandin F2 alpha	Pyometritis, open cystic endometrial hyperplasia	SC	0.10–0.25 mg/kg	24 for 3–5 days
	Abortion	SC	0.5–1.0 mg/kg; 40 days post conception	for 2 injections; 24 h apart
Protamine sulfate	Heparin antagonist		1.0–1.5 mg for every 100 IU heparin	

Continued

Continued

Drug	Indications	Dose	Route[a]	Frequency (h)[b]
		to be antagonized	IV	over 10 min, then reduce dose by 50% decrease dose by 50% for each hour since heparin administration
Pseudoephedrine	Nasal decongestant	15–30 mg/cat	PO	8–12
	Urinary incontinence	0.2–0.4 mg/kg	PO	8–12
Psyllium	Bulk laxative	1–3 tsp	PO	8–12 in food w/food
		3–10 g	PO	
Pyrantel pamoate	Round-, hookworms	10 mg/kg	PO	once, repeat in 2 wks
Pyridostigmine bromide	Myasthenia gravis/acquired	1–5 mg	PO	
		0.25 mg/kg	PO	
	Antidote (curariform)	0.15–0.30 mg/kg	IM, IV	24
Pyrilamine maleate	Antihistamine	12.5–25.0 mg	PO	6
Pyrimethamine	Neosporosis	0.25–1 mg/kg	PO	24
	With trimethoprim/sulfonamide	15 mg/kg	PO	12
	Toxoplasmosis	0.5–2.0 mg/kg	PO	12 for 14–28 days
	Enteroepithelial cycle	2 mg/kg	PO	24 for 14–28 days
Quinacrine	Giardia, coccidiosis	11 mg/kg	PO	24 for 5 days
Racemethionine	Urinary acidifier	see DL Methionine		
Ranitidine	Chronic gastritis, GI tract ulceration, gastrinoma Hypergastrinemia from chronic renal failure	0.5 mg/kg	IV, PO, SC	12
		3.5 mg/kg	PO	12
		2.5 mg/kg	IV	12
Retinol (Vitamin A)	Dermatologic lesions	625–800 IU/kg	PO	24
Ribavirin	Susceptible viral infections	11 mg/kg	PO, IM, IV	24 × 7 days
Riboflavin (Vitamin B$_{12}$)	Bartonellosis (with doxycycline)	5–10 mg/kg	PO	24 × 14 days
Rifampin	Susceptible infections	10–20 mg/kg	PO	24
Ringer's solution		40–50 ml/kg/day	IV, SC, IP	for maintenance
Roxithromycin	Susceptible infections	15 mg/kg	PO	24

Rutin	Chylothorax, limb lymphedema	50 mg/kg		PO	8
Selegiline	Cognitive disorders	0.5 mg/kg		PO	24
	Hyperadrenocorticism	1–2 mg/kg		PO	24
Selamectin	Parasiticide	6 mg/kg		topical	30 days (fleas, ticks [*Dermacentor variabilis*], Heartworm preventative) 1–2 × 30 days apart (*Ootodectes, Sarcoptic scabie*). Once (*Ancyclostoma tubaeforme, Tanei cati*).
Selenious acid, sodium selenite	Supplementation	0.3 mg/kg		PO	
Selenium	Pancreatitis	0.1 mg/kg	IV infusion		
Senna	Constipation	5 ml/cat (syrup) 1/2 tsp/cat w/food (granules)			24 24
Silver nitrate solution 0.5%	Burns	Saturate wet dressings			12–24
Silver sulfadiazine	Burns	Apply light coating			12 for several days, then 2
	Otitis externa	Dilute 1:1 with water	Pack cleaned ears		12
Sodium bicarbonate	Renal failure	10–15 mg/kg		PO	8
	Certain toxicoses	50 mg/kg (1 tsp is approx 2 g)		PO	8–12
	Acidosis	0.3 × wt (kg) × (target bicarb-patient bicarb)		IV, dose for acidosis	
		0.5–1.0 mEq/kg (8.5% soln=1 mEq/ml of NaHCO₃)		IV, dose for acidosis	
	Hyperkalemic crisis	2–3 mEq		IV	over 30 min
	Urine alkalization	0.65–5.85 g		PO	maint. pH 7.0 up to 7.5
Sodium chloride	Hypoadrenocorticism	1–5 g/day		PO	
	Hyponatremia: acute renal failure	1–4 g/day		PO	divided every 8
	(0.9% soln)	40–50 ml/kg/day		IV, SC, IP	

Continued

Continued

Drug	Indications	Dose	Route[a]	Frequency (h)[b]
Sodium chloride 5% 0.0 (Muro 128)	Corneal edema, non-healing erosions	1/8 inch /0.3cm	topically	2–6 times daily
Sodium chloride 7.5%	Shock therapy	2–8 ml/kg	IV	to be followed w/ balanced crystalloids
Sodium iodide, 20% soln	Sporotrichosis	0.5 ml/5 kg/day	PO	for 4–6 wk
	Susceptible infections	20 mg/kg/day	PO	
Sodium phosphate	Hypercalcemia	Dilute 1–3 g with water (1:1); give 10–20 ml	PO	8–24 until stools are soft
Sodium polystyrene sulfonate	Hypercalcemia	2 g/kg in 3–4 ml H$_2$O	PO	8
		15 gm in 100 ml of 1% methylcellulose or glucose	Rectal	div. every 8 h
		2–5 g/cat	IV	
			PO	4 for 6
Sodium thiopental	Anesthesia	3–15 mg/kg	IV	to effect
Sorbitol	Stool softener	3 ml/kg of 70% solution	PO	
Sotalol	Ventricular arrhythmias	1–2 mg/kg	PO	12
Spectinomycin	Susceptible infections	5–12 mg/kg	IM	12
Spiramycin	Toxoplasmosis	12.5–23 mg/cat	PO	24
Spironolactone	Diuretic: heart failure	2–4 mg/kg/day	PO	
	Primary hyperaldosteronism, hepatic insufficiency	1 mg/kg	PO	12
		12.5 mg/cat	PO	24
Spironolactone/ hydrochlorothiazide	Diuretic, antihypertensive agent	2 mg/kg	PO	12–24

Drug	Indication	Dose	Route	Interval/Notes
Stanozolol	Anabolic agent; anemia	1–2 mg/cat	PO	12
		0.5–2.0 mg/cat	PO	24
		10–25 mg/kg	PO	7 days
		1 mg/cat	PO	12
		25 mg/cat	IM	7 days with caution
		1–4 mg	PO	12
Staphage lysate	Immune stimulant	0.1–0.2 ml/cat incremental doses to 1.0 ml	SC	then 1–2 for a wk
		0.5 ml 0.5–1.0 ml	SC	wkly for 10–12 wk, then every 1–2 wk increasing the dosing interval to the longest that maintains clinical control.
Staphylococcal A	Immune stimulant twice weekly	20 μ/2.75 kg	IP	3.5 days
Streptomycin, dihydro	Leptospirosis, endocarditis, tuberculosis *Yersinia pestis*	10 mg/kg	IM	6
		10–20 mg/kg	IM	12
Styrid caricide (styryl-pyridinium chloride plus diethylcarbamazine)	Antiparasiticide	6.7 mg/kg diethylcarbamazine and 5.5 mg/kg styrylpyridinium chloride	PO	24
Succinyl choline	Paralysis	0.06–0.11 mg/kg	IV	
Sucralfate	Gastrointestinal ulceration	250–500 mg/cat	PO	8–12
		40 mg/kg	PO	8
Sufentanil	Premedicant, with acepromazine	2 μ/kg (max dose 5 μ/kg)	IV	
Sulfadiazine	Nocardiosis	220 mg/kg	PO	for 1 Rx, then
		50–110 mg/kg	PO	12
	Toxoplasmosis	15–50 mg/kg/day, with pyrimethamine	PO	div. 12 for 14 days

Continued

Continued

Drug	Indications	Dose	Route[a]	Frequency (h)[b]
		50 mg/kg (loading)	PO	12
		25 mg/kg		
		100 mg/kg (loading)	IV, PO	12
		50 mg/kg		
Sulfadiazine/trimethoprim	Susceptible infection	30 mg/kg	PO, SC	24
	Meningitis	15 mg/kg	PO, IV	8–12
	Nocardiosis	30–60 mg/kg	PO, SQ	12
Sulfadimethoxine	Susceptible infections	25–50 mg/kg	PO, IM, IV	12–24 followed by 24 once daily for a max. of 21 days
	Coccidiosis	55 mg/kg (loading)	PO	24
		27.5 mg/kg		
Sulfaguanidine	Coccidiosis	100–200 mg/kg	PO	8 for 5 days
Sulfamethazine, sulfamerazine	Coccidiosis	100 mg/kg (loading)	PO	12
		50 mg/kg	PO	
Sulfamethoxazole	Susceptible infections	100 mg/kg (loading)	PO	12
		50 mg/kg	PO	
Sulfamethoxazole/ trimethoprim	Susceptible infections	15 mg/kg	PO	12
Sulfasalazine	Lymphocytic–plasmacytic enteritis	250 mg/cat	PO	8 for 3, then 24 h
	Inflammatory bowel disease	20–25mg/kg	PO	12–24
	Susceptible bacterial infections	20 mg/kg	PO	12
Sulfisoxazole	U.T. infection	50 mg/kg	PO	8
Sulfobromophthalein sodium	Hepatic function testing	5 mg/kg	IV	collect serum 30 min after BSP injection
Suprofen 1% ophthalmic soln	Allergic conjuntivitis	Apply topically		8–12
Tamiflu	Viral disease	2–4 mg/kg	PO	12 within 48 hr of infection
Taurine	Taurine deficiency dilated cardiomyopathy	250–500 mg/cat	PO	12
	Central retinal degeneration	250 mg/cat	PO	12–24

Drug	Indication	Dose	Route	Interval
Telazol	Restraint	6.6 mg/kg	IM	
	Anesthesia	11–15 mg/kg	IM	
Temaril-P (trimeprazine plus prednisolone)	Allergy	0.7–1.1 mg/kg (of trimeprazine)	PO	12–24
Terbinafine	Dermatophytosis	3–10 mg/kg	PO	24
Terbutaline	Bronchodilator	0.01 mg/kg	SC, IM	4
		1.25–2.50 mg/cat	PO	8
Testosterone cypionate	Hormone replacement	2.2 mg/kg	IM	2–3 days
Testosterone, methyl	Anabolic effects	1–2 mg/kg; max 30 mg/day	PO	once daily
Testosterone propionate	Feline symmetrical alopecia	12.5 mg with estrogen	IM	
	Urinary incontinence	5–10 mg	IM	
		0.5–1 mg/kg	IM	2–3/week
Tetanus toxoid	Tetanus treatment	0.2 ml (test dose) then give 100–500 units/kg	SC	watch for anaphylaxis for 30 min
Tetracycline HCl	Acute bronchitis	10–25 mg/kg	PO	8–12
	GI bacterial overgrowth, acute colitis			
	Rickettsial and Lyme disease	15 mg/kg	PO	8 for 21 days
	Mycobacterial infections	22 mg/kg	PO	8
	Susceptible infections	10–25 mg/kg	IV, IM	8–12
Theophylline	Bronchodilator	4 mg/kg	PO, IM	8–12
Sustained release Theo-Dur, Slo Bid		20–25 mg/kg	PO	24 at night
Thiabendazole	Heartworm adulticide	35 mg/kg	PO	12 for 20 days
	Strongyloides	125 mg/kg		q 24 for 3 days
Thiacetarsamide	Heartworm adulticide	2.2 mg/kg	IV	12 for 2 days; entire dose should be given (36 h; use cautiously)
Thiamine (Vitamin B$_{12}$)	Thiamine deficiency	1–2 mg/cat	IM	12 until regression of symptoms
		5–30 mg/cat	PO	12 until regression of symptoms
		100–250 mg/kg	SQ	
		10–20 mg/kg	IM, SC	8–12 until signs abate,

Continued

Continued

Drug	Indications	Dose	Route[a]	Frequency (h)[b]
		10 mg/kg	PO	then 24 for 21 days
Thiamylal sodium	Induction of anesthesia	4% soln: 8-10 mg/kg up to 20 mg/kg 8.8-13.3 mg/kg 4.4-6.6 mg/kg	IV IV IV	in incremental doses after tranquilization after narcotic premedication
Thioguanine	Lymphocytic and granulocytic leukemia	25 mg/m²	PO	24 for 1-5, then 30
Thyroid	Hypothyroidism	15-20 mg/kg/day	PO	24
Thyrotropin (TSH)	Provocative testing	1 IU/kg	IM	Collect baseline sample and post-TSH sample
	Acantosis nigrans, hypothyroidism	at 8-12 h 1-2 IU	SQ	24 for 5
L-thyroxine (levothyroxine)	Hypothyroidism	0.5 mg/m² 20-30 µ/kg/day	PO PO	12 24 or dd 12
Ticarcillin	Susceptible infections	33-50 mg/kg 55-110 mg/kg	IM, IV IM, IV	6-8 4-8
Ticarcillian/clavulanate	As above			
Tiletamine/zolazepam	minor procedure	9.7-11.9 mg/kg	IM	
	Castration, lacerations	10.6-12.5 mg/kg	IM	Do not exceed 72 mg/kg with repeat doses
	Spay, declaw	14.3-15.8 mg/kg	IM	
Tinidazole	Stomatitis	15 mg/kg	PO	24
Tiopronin	Cystine urinary calculi	15-20 mg/kg	PO	12
Tolazoline	Reversal for xylazine and other sedatives	2 mg/kg	IV	
Tolfenamic acid	Analgesic	4 mg/kg	PO	24, up to 5; 3 out of 7 days for chronic
Toluene	Anthelmintic	267 mg/kg	PO	repeat in 2-4 wks
Tramadol	analgesia	1-2 mg/kg 12.5 mg/cat	PO PO	8-12 h 12

Drug	Indication	Dose	Route	Interval
Tretinoin	Canine and feline acne, nasal hyperkeratosis	0.25–0.50 mg	topically	24
Triamcinolone	Feline plamacytic pharyngitis, pododermatitis	0.11–0.22 mg/kg	PO	24 for 7 d
	Feline polymyopathy	2–4 mg	PO, IM, SC	24–48
	Anti inflammatory	0.5–1.0 mg/kg	PO	24–48
Triamcinolone acetonide	Esophageal stricture	1–2 mg/cat	submucosal infiltration	at time of dilation
	Glucocorticoid effects	0.11–0.22 mg/kg	PO	24
		0.1–0.2 mg/kg	IM, SC	24
		Intralesional: 1.2–1.8 mg or 1 mg for every 1 cm diameter of tumor	IM, SC	q 2 wk
Triamcinolone	Pannus, eosinophilic keratitism episcleritis	4 mg	subconjunctivally	
Triamterene	Diuretic	1–2 mg/kg	PO	12
Trientine hydrochloride	Chelating agent	10–15 mg/kg	PO	12
Triethylene thio-phosphoramide	Bladder neoplasia	30 mg/m^2	intravesicularly	q 3–4 wk
Triethylperazine	Antipsychotic	0.13–0.2 mg/kg	IM	8–12
Trifluoperazine	Antipsychotic	0.03 mg/kg	IM	12
Triflupromazine	Behavior modification	0.1–0.3 mg/kg	IM, PO	8–12
Trifluridine ophthalmic soln	Ocular herpesvirus infection	0.1% soln: 1–2 drops	Apply topically	3–8 times daily
Triiodothyronine (T3)	Hypothyroidism	4.4 µg/kg	PO	8–12
Trimethoprim/sulfadiazine	Routine infections	15 mg/kg	PO, SC	12
	Meningitis	15 mg/kg	PO, IV	8–12
Tripelennamine	Antihistamine	1 mg/kg	PO, IM	12
Trypan blue	Babesiosis	4 mg/kg	IV	
Tylosin	GI bacterial overgrowth, chronic colitis	6.6–11 mg/kg	IM	12–24
		25 mg	PO	8
Urea	Osmotic	300 mg	IV	1
Urofollitropin	Hypogonadotropic anovulation	2 mg/cat	IM	24

Continued

Continued

Drug	Indications	Dose	Route[a]	Frequency (h)[b]
Ursodeoxycholic acid (Ursodiol)	Chronic hepatitis	5–15 mg/kg	PO	24
Valproic acid	Seizures	25–65 mg/kg 10–105 mg/kg	PO PO	8, w/phenobarbital
Vanadium	Hyperglycemia (early non-insulin-dependent diabetes mellitus)	0.2 mg/kg	PO	24
Vasopressin, aqueous	Central diabetes insipidus	10 mU/cat	IV,IM	PRN
Vasopressin, tannate in oil	Central diabetes insipidus	2.5–5.0 U/cat	IM	q 1–7 days
Vecuronium bromide	Paralytic agent for controlled anesthesia	40 μ/kg 20–40 μ/kg	IV IV	over 30 minutes
Verapamil	Supraventricular arrhythmias	10–15 mg/kg/day 1.1–2.9 mg/kg	PO PO	div. 8–12 8
	Conversion of rapid supraventricular tachycardia	1.1–4.4 mg/kg 0.11–0.33 mg/kg	PO slow IV	8–12
Vidarabine	Ocular herpesvirus infection	1/8 inch or 0.3 cm	topically	3–6 times daily
Vinblastine	Mast cell tumors, lymphosarcoma	0.1–0.4 mg/kg 2 mg/m^2	IV	q 7–14 days
Vincristine	Immune mediated thrombocytopenia	0.010–0.025 mg/kg	IV	q 7–10 days
	Lymphosarcoma Neoplasia	0.50–1.0 mg/m^2 0.5–0.75 mg/m^2	IV IV	once wkly, in a protocol q 7–14 days
Viokase	Pancreatic exocrine insuffiency	1 (325 mg tabs) or 1.1–2.2 g (0.5–1.0 tsp) of powder w/ each meal		
Vitamin A	Dietary supplement	400 U/kg 625–800 U	PO PO	24 for 10 days 24
Vitamin B$_1$		see Thiamine		
Vitamin B$_2$		5–10 mg/cat 50–100 μ/day	PO PO, SC	24
Vitamin B complex	Vitamin B deficiency	0.5–1.0 ml	IV, IM, SC	24

Drug	Indication	Dosage	Route	Interval (h)
Vitamin C (ascorbic acid)		See Ascorbic acid		
Vitamin D (dihydrotachysterol)	Hypocalcemia	0.02 mg/kg	PO	Initially, then
		0.01–0.02 mg/kg	PO	24–48
Vitamin D$_2$, ergocalciferol	Hypocalcemia	4000–6000 U/kg/day (initial)	PO	
		500–2000 U/kg/day (maintenance)	PO	@T body:
Vitamin D$_3$, calcitriol (1-25, dihydroxy vitamin D$_3$)	Hypocalcemia	0.03–0.06 μ/kg/day	PO	
	Chronic renal failure	0.025 μ/kg/day	PO	
Vitamin E	Vitamin E-deficient myositis, Steatitis	10–20 IU/kg	PO	12
	Immune-mediated skin disease	400–600 IU/cat	PO	12
		100–400 IU/cat	PO	12
		100 mg/cat	PO	
Vitamin K$_1$ (phytonadione)	Deficiency	1–3 mg/kg	SC, PO	12, recheck coagulation at 2 days and 3 weeks for 4–6 wk
		1 mg/kg/day	PO	12–24
		5 mg/kg	IM	divided 8–12 h
		0.25–2.5 mg/kg	PO	divided 8–12 h
		5 mg/kg	PO	24 for 7 days
		15–25 mg/cat	IV	24 for 3–4 weeks until coagulation normal, check 1–2 days after therapy discontinued
		15–25 mg/cat	IV	
	Short-acting rodenticides	1 mg/kg/day	SC, PO	for 5–7 days
	Long-acting rodenticides	3–5 mg/kg/day	SC, PO	for 4–6 wk
Warfarin	Thromboembolism	0.06–0.20 mg/kg	PO	24, Maintain PT 2.0–2.5 times normal
Xylazine	Muscle relaxation	1.1–2.2 mg/kg	IM, SC	
	Emetic	0.44 mg/kg	IM	
Zafirlukast	Leukotriene receptor antagonist	0.15–0.2 up to 2 mg/kg	PO	12–24
Zidovudine	Antiviral	5–20 mg/kg	SQ, PO	8–12

aPO = oral, IV = intravenous, SC = subcutaneous, IM = intramuscular, IP = intraperitoneal; DJD = degenerative joint disease

bh = hours (default time unit unless otherwise noted); PRN = as needed; TBS = tablespoon; tsp = teaspoon.

Subject Index

Page numbers in *italics* denote figures and tables. Page numbers in **bold** denote main discussions (where necessary).

Propiomazine, 1393
Propionbacterium acnes, 1393
Propionibacterium acnes, 545
Propofol, 1393
Proprandol, 973
Propranolol, **1393**
    atrial fibrillation, 163
    cardiomyopathy, restrictive and
        unclassified, 137
    hypertensive retinopathy, 1172, 1282
    hyperthyroid heart disease, 132
    sinus tachycardia, 161
    supraventricular/atrial tachycardia,
        162
    supraventricular premature beats,
        166
    tetralogy of Fallot, 150
    ventricular premature beats, 167
    ventricular tachycardia, 165
Propylthiouracil, 1343, **1346, 1393**
Prostaglandin PGF$_{2a}$, 1163, **1393**
Prostaglandin therapy, 1162
Protamine sulfate, 1393–1394
Protamine zinc insulin (PZI), 238, 313
Protein, dietary
    glomerulonephritis, 328
    restriction, renal failure, 337
Protein:creatinine ratio, protein-losing
    nephropathy, 359
Protein hydrosylates, food allergy diet,
    709
Protein levels, feline infectious
    peritonitis, 457
Protein-losing enteropathy, 72, 89, **760**
    diarrhea, chronic small bowel, 737,
        760
    inflammatory bowel disease and,
        349
Protein-losing nephropathy, 72, 89,
    358–359
    clinical signs, 332, **358–359**
    diagnosis, 359
    pathogenesis, 358
    prognosis, 359
    pulmonary thromboembolism, 59
    thin, inappetent, 358–359
    see also Glomerulonephritis
Proteins induced by vitamin K
    antagonism or absence (PIVKA),
    491–492
    liver disease, 492
    vitamin K antagonist
        rodenticides/drugs, 508–509

Proteinuria
    glomerulonephritis, 327
    protein-losing nephropathy, 359
    renal failure, chronic, 236, 336, 339
Proteus, 187
Prothrombin time, 490–491
    vitamin K antagonist
        rodenticides/drugs, 508
Proton pump inhibitors
    esophagitis, 616
    gastritis/gastric ulcers, 638, 680
Protopam chloride (2-PAM),
    organophosphate toxicity, 595,
    862, 948
Prototheocosis, 418
Protozoal infections, 396
Protozoans, 314
Pruritus, 1045–1051
    causes/diseases causing, 1045–1046,
        1046–1050
    flea dermatitis, 1028
    food hypersensitivity, 1029, 1030
    location, 1045, 1046
    mechanisms, 1045, 1046
    miliary dermatitis and, 1025
    paw/pad problems, 1116
    peri-ocular, 1211
Prussian blue, thallium poisoning, 1125
Pseudoanorexia, 266
Pseudochylous effusions, chylothorax,
    79
Pseudoephedrine, 1394
Pseudomembranous colitis, 763,
    777–778
Pseudomonas infection, ulcerative
    keratitis, 1248, 1263
Pseudomycetoma, 1084, 1094–1095
Pseudonaja (Brown snake)
    envenomation, 950–953
Pseudorabies (Aujesky's disease, mad
    itch), 297, 752
Psychogenic alopecia, 1013,
    1015–1017, 1053, **1056–1058**
Psychological problems, infertility,
    1150
Psychotropic medication, pica, 1020
Psyllium, 1394
Pthisis, 1309, 1310, 1315–1316
Ptosis, upper lid, 1318, 1324
Ptyalism
    causes, 581–601
    mechanism of, 581
    see also Salivation

Puberty, age variations, 1148
Pudendal nerve damage, 200
Puffer fish, 973
Pulmonary arterial angiography, 59
Pulmonary arterial obstruction, 59
Pulmonary arteriovenous fistula, 143
Pulmonary artery
    banding, 142
    dilation
        pulmonary stenosis, 148
        tetralogy of Fallot, 150
    heartworm disease, 140
Pulmonary disease, chronic, 562–563
    causes, 562–563
    clinical signs, 554, 562, 563
    diagnosis, 563
    differential diagnosis, 563
    pathogenesis, 562–563
    polycythemia, 562–563
    prognosis, 563
    treatment, 563
    see also specific diseases/disorders
Pulmonary edema, 54, 105, 144
Pulmonary fibrosis, 50, 69–70
Pulmonary function testing, asthma, 94
Pulmonary infiltrates, heartworm
    disease, 140
Pulmonary infiltrates with eosinophils
    (PIE), 91, 96–97
Pulmonary inflammation, 105
Pulmonary neoplasia, **66–67,** 87, 91,
    100–101
    clinical signs, 97
    coughing, 100–101
    dyspnea/tachypnea, 49, 66–67
    hydrothorax, 72
Pulmonary stenosis, **148–149**
    abnormal heart sounds/enlarged
        heart, 148–149
    atrial septal defect, 145
    clinical signs, 125, 142, **148,** 150
    diagnosis, 148
    differential diagnosis, 148–149
    pathogenesis, 148
    prognosis, 149
    tetralogy of Fallot, 150
    treatment, 149
Pulmonary thromboembolism, 58–60
    cyanosis, 110, 116
    dyspnea/tachypnea, 49, 58–60
    heart worm disease associated, 116
Pulmonary venous congestion, 146
Pulmonary venous distention, 147

Septic exudate, 447
Septic focus, 331, 344–345
Septic peritonitis, 446, 450, **467–468**
Septic shock, 722
 definition, 269
 treatment, 119
Seroconversion delay, feline leukemia
  virus, 1142
Serology
 atopic dermatitis, 1031
 bacterial infection in non-healing
   wounds, 1087
 cryptococcosis, 16, 26, 37, 812
 Cryptococcus neoformans, 1175
 feline herpes virus-1 keratitis, 1239,
   1260
 feline infectious peritonitis, 431, 811
 flea allergic dermatitis, 1026
 heartworm disease, 140
 herpes conjunctivitis, 1213
 histoplasmosis, 438
 inflammatory retinal disease, 1205
 intra-ocular fungal infections, 1270
 iris abnormality in fungal infections,
   1301
 ocular toxoplasmosis, 1173
 toxoplasmosis, 432, 815, 1265, 1297
Serosa membrane, abdominal
  distention/ fluid, 447–449
Serotonin
 anxiety-related behavior problems,
   1011
 feline asthma, 93
 obsessive compulsive disorders,
   1015
Serotonin antagonists, feline asthma,
  95
Serum amylase, pancreatitis, 274
Serum antibody tests, feline infectious
  peritonitis, 457
Serum bile acids
 hepatic diseases and, 675
 portosystemic shunts, 362, 589
Serum biochemistry
 alimentary lymphosarcoma, 317
 cholangiohepatitis, 348, 747
 diabetes mellitus, 681
 encephalitis, 930
 ethylene glycol poisoning, 288
 gastrointestinal lymphosarcoma, 676
 hypernatremic myopathy, 904
 hyperthyroidism, 671
 lymphocytic cholangiohepatitis, 321

pancreatitis, 274, 319
 see also specific assays
Serum cholinesterase, organophosphate
  poisoning, 645
Serum cobalamin assay, exocrine
  pancreatic insufficiency, 731
Serum folate
 exocrine pancreatic insufficiency,
   731
 folic acid deficiency, 549
Serum fructosamine, diabetes mellitus,
  312
Serum insulin concentration, metabolic
  encephalopathy, 831
Serum lipase, pancreatitis, 274
Serum potassium level
 hypokalemia, acute, 272
 hypokalemic myopathy, 946
Serum sodium, hypernatremia, 298
Sewing needle as foreign body, 40
Sex hormone-secreting adrenal tumor,
  232, 258–259
Sexual development disorders, 1147
Sexual maturity, aggression, 998
Shaker cat syndrome, 803
Shampoo, *Notoedres cati* (notoedric
  mange), 1040
Shelters, disease control, 11
Shock, 722
 clinical signs, 722
 diagnosis, 722
 diarrhea, acute small bowel, 698,
   722
 endotoxic, 722
 hypovolemic, 722
 motor vehicle injuries, 493
 septic *see* Septic shock
 treatment, 119, 818
"Shock triad," 969, 970
Short bowel syndrome, 730, 760–761
 clinical signs, 730, 761
 diagnosis, 730, 761
 diarrhea, acute small bowel, 698,
   730
 diarrhea, chronic small bowel, 735,
   760–761
 differential diagnosis, 730, 761
 pathogenesis, 730, 760–761
 prognosis, 730, 761
 treatment, 730, 761
Short colon syndrome, 763, 779
Siamese cats
 anemia, 536

antral pyloric hypertrophy/stenosis,
  694
cholesterol ester storage disease, 576
colonic adenocarcinoma, 774
feline mucopolysaccharidosis, 988
hydrocephalus, 826
hypercalcemia, 247
hypotrichosis, 1056
intestinal adenocarcinoma, 677, 750
intussusception, 643
megaesophagus, 621
myasthenia gravis, 622, 955
nervous system, degenerative
  diseases, 867
Niemann–Pick type A disease, 925,
  936
pancreatitis, 273
pica, 1019
vestibular disease, congenital, 925,
  933
"Sick euthyroid syndrome," 561
Silicone elastomer catheters, 182
Silver nitrate, 1395
Silver sulfadiazine, 1395
Sinoatrial node, 159, 165
Sinus arrhythmia, 166, 167
Sinus bradycardia, 159, 168
Sinusitis, 356–357
 clinical signs, 331, 356
 diagnosis, 356–357
 feline rhinotracheitis virus, 9, 22
Sinus tachycardia, **160–161**
 clinical signs, 158, **160–161,** 162
 diagnosis, 161, *161*
 differential diagnosis, 161
 high cardiac output heart disease,
   138
 hyperthyroid heart disease, 132
 mitral valve dysplasia/stenosis, 146
 pathogenesis, 160
 prognosis, 161
 treatment, 161
Situation anxiety, 263, 270–271
Skin biopsy
 cutaneous asthenia (Ehlers–Danlos
   syndrome), 519
 flea allergic dermatitis, 1026
 telogen defluxion, 1063
Skin disorders, 1022–1080
 aggression when patted, 1001
 alopecia, 1052–1066
 lymph nodes, enlarged, 394
 miliary dermatitis, 1022–1044

Vitamin A, 454–455, **1394, 1402**
deficiency, 1146, 1158–1159
excessive intake *see*
Hypervitaminosis A
supplementation, 1159
Vitamin B supplements, **1402–1403**
cholangitis, 711
ethylene glycol poisoning treatment,
289
feline panleukopenia virus, 724
pancreatitis, 278
Vitamin C *see* Ascorbic acid
Vitamin D, **1403**
deficiency, rickets, 991
hypocalcemia, 962–963
parathyroid hormone elevation in
chronic renal failure, 338
toxicosis, 246, 249
see also Cholecalciferol (vitamin
D₃)
Vitamin E, **1403**
cholangiohepatitis, 349
deficiency, 1082, 1104
lymphocytic cholangiohepatitis, 322
pancreatitis, 320
traumatic panniculitis, 1103
Vitamin K
antagonists, 485
see also Rodenticide poisoning
deficiency
diet, 484, 523
exocrine pancreatic insufficiency,
752
inflammatory bowel disease, 517
hepatic lipidosis, 427
Vitamin K₁, **1403**
cholangiohepatitis, 349
lymphocytic, 322
inflammatory bowel disease, 310,
517
pancreatitis, 320
supplementation
exocrine pancreatic insufficiency,
732
factor abnormalities, 539
vitamin K antagonist
rodenticides/drugs, 509–510
vitamin K responsive coagulopathy,
516
Vitamin K₂ (menaquinone)
hemorrhage, 523
inflammatory bowel disease,
517–518

Vitamin K₃, inflammatory bowel
disease, 518
Vitamin K responsive coagulopathy,
473, 484
Devon Rex, 515–516
Vitamins, cirrhosis, 435
Vitiligo, 1122
Vitreal hemorrhage, 1206
hypertensive retinopathy, 1171
systemic hypertension, 1275
Vitreous flare, 1175, 1259, 1268
Vitreous humor, 1258, 1259
cloudy, 1195, 1257, 1259,
1274–1276
red coloration, 1193–1194,
1202–1204
Vocalization
inappropriate, 1017–1018
normal response, 1017
Voice changes
laryngeal paralysis, 44
laryngeal stenosis, 43
Vomiting
acute, 630–661
causes/diseases causing, 630–634,
634–661
mechanism, 630, 634
chronic, 662–696
causes/diseases causing, 663–666,
667–696
diagnosis, 667
mechanism, 662, 666
hepatic lipidosis, 427
induction
acetaminophen toxicity, 122
ciguatoxin, 972
ethylene glycol poisoning, 289
intoxications, 814
lead poisoning, 693
poisoning, 286
vitamin D toxicosis, 249
vitamin K antagonist
rodenticides/drugs, 509
inflammatory bowel disease, 307,
349
renal failure, chronic, 334
weight loss and, 303
*see also specific diseases/
disorders*
Vomiting center stimulation, 666
Vomitus
components of, 634, 666
pH, 634, 666

worms in, 654, 690, 717
Von Willebrand's disease, 482, 521

W

Walking dandruff, 1037
Wallerian degeneration,
encephalopathy, 939
Warfarin, **1403**
aortic thromboembolism, 917
cardiomyopathy, 137, 153
factor abnormalities, 539
rodenticides containing, 507
Wasp stings, 285
Water administration
hypernatremic myopathy, 904
metabolic encephalopathy, 832
Water deprivation test, diabetes
insipidus, 244
Water intake, diabetes mellitus, 239,
313
Water retention, 450
Weakness
ataxia and *see* Ataxia, with
weakness
generalized, 941–975
causes/diseases causing, 941–945,
945–975
location, 945
mechanism, 945
Weaning
pica, 1019
stress, 1127, 1140
Weight loss, 301–362
diabetes mellitus and, 312
good appetite and, 301–329
causes/diseases causing, 302, 303,
304–328
*see also specific
diseases/disorders*
diagnosis, 303–304
mechanisms of, 303
physical examination, 304
hypertensive heart disease, 133
inappetent and, 330–363
causes/diseases causing, 333–362
*see also specific
diseases/disorders*
mechanism, 330–332, 332
inflammatory bowel disease, 307
obesity, 454
Wheezing, 92, 99
Whipworm eggs, 775
Whistling *see* Stridor

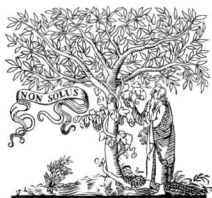